W9-BSM-678

Clinical Practice
of the
DENTAL HYGIENIST

EIGHTH EDITION

CLINICAL PRACTICE
OF THE
DENTAL HYGIENIST

Esther M. Wilkins, BS, RDH, DMD
Department of Periodontology
Tufts University, School of Dental Medicine
Boston, Massachusetts

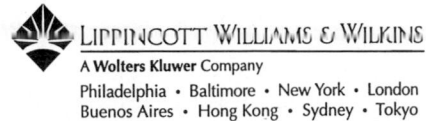
LIPPINCOTT WILLIAMS & WILKINS
A **Wolters Kluwer** Company
Philadelphia • Baltimore • New York • London
Buenos Aires • Hong Kong • Sydney • Tokyo

Acquisitions Editor: Lawrence McGrew
Editorial Assistant: Holly Chapman
Associate Managing Editor: Barbara Ryalls
Senior Production Manager: Helen Ewan
Senior Production Coordinator: Nannette Winski
Design Coordinator: Doug Smock
Indexer: Katherine Pitcoff

Eighth Edition

Copyright © 1999 by Lippincott Williams & Wilkins.
Copyright © 1994, 1989, 1982, 1976, 1971, 1964, 1959 by
Williams & Wilkins / All rights reserved. This book is protected by copyright. No part of it may be reproduced, stored in a retrieval system, or
transmitted, in any form or by any means—electronic, mechanical,
photocopy, recording, or otherwise—without the prior written permission of the publisher, except for brief quotations embodied in critical articles and reviews and testing and evaluation materials provided by
publisher to instructors whose schools have adopted its accompanying
textbook. Printed in the United States of America. For information
write Lippincott Williams & Wilkins, 530 Walnut Street, Philadelphia,
PA 19106-3621 USA.

Materials appearing in this book prepared by individuals as part of their
official duties as U.S. Government employees are not covered by the
above-mentioned copyright.

9   8   7   6   5   4   3

Library of Congress Cataloging-in-Publication Data

Wilkins, Esther M.
    Clinical pratice of the dental hygienist / Esther M. Wilkins. —
8th ed.
      p. cm.
    Includes bibliographical references and index.
    ISBN 0-683-30362-7 (alk. paper)
    1. Dental hygiene. I. Title.
    [DNLM: 1. Dental Prophylaxis outlines. 2. Dental Hygienists
outlines. WU 18.2 W684c 1999]
    RK60.5.W5 1999
    617.6'01—dc21
DNLM/DLC
for Library of Congress   98-51355
                                       CIP

    Care has been taken to confirm the accuracy of the informa-
tion presented and to describe generally accepted practices.
However, the authors, editors, and publisher are not responsible
for errors or omissions or for any consequences from application
of the information in this book and make no warranty, express
or implied, with respect to the contents of the publication.

    The authors, editors and publisher have exerted every effort
to ensure that drug selection and dosage set forth in this text are
in accordance with current recommendations and practice at the
time of publication. However, in view of ongoing research,
changes in government regulations, and the constant flow of information relating to drug therapy and drug reactions, the
reader is urged to check the package insert for each drug for any
change in indications and dosage and for added warnings and
precautions. This is particularly important when the recommended agent is a new or infrequently employed drug.

    Some drugs and medical devices presented in this publication
have Food and Drug Administration (FDA) clearance for limited
use in restricted research settings. It is the responsibility of the
health care provider to ascertain the FDA status of each drug or
device planned for use in their clinical practice.

DEDICATION

The Contributors to the 8th Edition of Clinical Practice of the Dental Hygienist lovingly dedicate this book to Dr. Esther Wilkins in honor of her lifetime of devotion and service to the dental hygiene profession

CONTRIBUTORS

Susan Anderson, RDH, BS, MEd
Dental Hygiene Department
Allegany College of Maryland
Cumberland, MD

Lois Rigmont Barber, RDH, BSEd
Professional Education
Oral-B Laboratories
Melbourne, FL

Caren Barnes, RDH, BS, MS
Department of Surgical Specialties
College of Dentistry
University of Nebraska Medical Center
Lincoln, NE

Kathy B. Bassett, BSDH, RDH, MEd
Dental Hygiene Department
Pierce College
Tacoma, WA

Cynthia R. Biron, RDH, EMT, MA
The Dental Hygiene Programs
Tallahassee Community College
Tallahassee, FL

Patricia A. Cohen, RDH, BS, MS
Private Practice
Post Office Square Dental Practice
Boston, MA

Marilyn B. Cortell, RDH, MS
Cortell Presentation Resources
Lexington, MA

Christina B. DeBiase, BSDH, MA, EdD
Department of Dental Hygiene
West Virginia University School of Dentistry
Morgantown, WV

Loraine DiPietro, BA, MA
National Information Center on Deafness
Gallaudet University
Washington, DC

Peggy Ellingson, RDH, BA, MA
Department of Dental Hygiene
Eastern Washington University
Spokane, WA

Kathryn Jean Falcone, RDH, AS
Philadelphia, PA

Dorathea Foote, RDH, MEd
Department of Dental Hygiene
Springfield Technical Community College
Springfield, MA

Carol A. Jahn, RDH, MS
Teledyne Water Pik
Warrenville, IL

Nancy Sisty LePeau, RDH, MS, MA
Child Health Clinic
Johnson County Department of Public Health
Iowa City, IA

Deborah Mancinelli Lyle, RDH, MS
Teledyne Water Pik
Morris Plains, NJ

Arthur S. Miller, DMD, MSD
Department of Pathology
Temple University School of Medicine
Philadelphia, PA

Laura Mueller-Joseph, RDH, EdD
Department of Dental Hygiene
State University of New York at Farmingdale
Farmingdale, NY

Anna Matsuishi Pattison, RDH, MS
Department of Dental Hygiene
School of Dentistry
University of Southern California
Los Angeles, CA

Frieda Atherton Pickett, RDH, MS
Department of Dental Hygiene
East Tennessee State University
Johnson City, TN

Kathryn Ragalis, RDH, MS, DMD
Tufts University School of Dental Medicine
Boston, MA

Judith E. Romano, RDH, MA
Department of Dental Hygiene
Hudson Valley Community College
Troy, NY

Dale Scanlan, DipDH
Children's Hospital of Eastern Ontario Dental Clinic
Ottawa, ON, Canada

Donna J. Stach, BS, RDH, MEd
Department of Dental Hygiene
School of Dentistry
University of Colorado, Health Sciences Center
Denver, CO

Cynthia A. Stegeman, RDH, MEd, RD, CDE
Dental Hygiene Department
Raymond Walters College, University of Cincinnati
Cincinnati, OH
and
Cardiac Rehabilitation and Diabetes Center
The St. Luke Hospitals
Ft. Thomas, KY

Kathleen Sweeney, RDH, BS, MS
Department of Dental Hygiene
Middlesex Community College
Lowell, MA

Janet H. Towle, RN, RDH, MEd
Forsyth School for Dental Hygienists
Forsyth Dental Center
Boston, MA

Margaret Waring, RDH, BS, MS, EdD
Department of Dental Hygiene
College of Allied Health Sciences
University of Tennessee
Memphis, TN

Nancy L.J. Williams, RDH, MS, EdD
Department of Dental Hygiene
College of Allied Health Sciences
and
University of Tennessee Cancer Center
Memphis, TN

Charlotte J. Wyche, RDH, MS
Department of Dental Hygiene
School of Dentistry
University of Detroit Mercy
Detroit, MI

Dental hygienists are preventive oral healthcare specialists. As clinicians, health educators, and counselors, their professional goals center on the prevention and control of disease, with emphasis on the maintenance of health, both for general as well as oral health. Over the past 50 years, research advancements and application of preventive measures have brought a decline in the debilitating dental, periodontal, and other oral conditions that were widespread in the past. Dental hygienists have played a major role in the preventive, clinical, and educational interventions that have brought oral health to large segments of the population.

OBJECTIVES AND ORGANIZATION

The basic objective of the new eighth edition of **Clinical Practice of the Dental Hygienist** has not changed from previous editions, namely, to make available in a concise format integrated comprehensive information essential to the professional practice of dental hygiene. As expected with a new edition, all chapters have been thoroughly reviewed and updated to ensure that the material reflects current information and developments.

Selected contributors have been invited to provide review and revision in the areas of their expertise. New topics have been added in keeping with the improved opportunities for dental hygienists to recognize individual patient problem areas that can be managed by dental hygiene care. Many new illustrations and tables have been introduced. As in the previous edition, the book is divided into six parts.

Part 1 introduces the features of the professional dental hygienist and factors influencing the practice of dental hygiene, with emphasis placed on ethical responsibilities. New to Chapter 1 is the detailed introduction to the dental hygiene process of care. Each of the five categories of the process are described; namely, patient assessment, formulation of the dental hygiene diagnosis and care plan, implementation of the treatment aspects selected to meet the specific needs of a patient, and evaluation with follow-up.

Part 2 details the preparation for dental hygiene appointments. Emphasis is on the orally transmitted diseases and exposure control for the individual pa-

tient and clinician. Positioning of patient and clinician with principles of ergonomics is essential to the continued participation of the clinician in the clinical aspects of the dental hygiene profession.

Part 3 addresses the many details of patient assessment. In the completely revised Chapter 21, essential recordings and chartings are brought together for preparation of the dental hygiene diagnosis and care plan.

Part 4 introduces the first essential for implementation of care—the teaching and motivation for the patient's own oral care. For positive continuing results, the patient must take responsibility for self-care by carrying out selected preventive measures for dental caries and periodontal disease.

Prevention is introduced in a new Chapter 22 that brings together the individual prevention care plan, principles of learning, and a suggested teaching sequence for helping a patient learn bacterial plaque control. The chapter also includes sections on xerostomia and halitosis, two conditions closely related to the problems of disease prevention.

The new Chapter 27, *The Patient Who Uses Tobacco,* has been included to promote anti-tobacco education as a part of the total oral health program. Research concerning the specific relationships of tobacco use to oral health has mandated the dental hygienist to inform all tobacco-using patients of the detrimental effects and to encourage elimination of tobacco-related habits. Many dental hygienists are learning how to introduce personalized programs for smoking cessation for patients.

Part 5 leads into the professional treatment areas of nonsurgical periodontal therapy. Essential to complete care of the patient with a moderate to severe periodontal infection that requires deep pocket scaling is the use of pain control. The new Chapter 31, *Anxiety and Pain Control,* outlines the basic products, procedures and indications for use of nitrous oxide–oxygen sedation, local anesthesia, and topical anesthesia. Anesthesia is used extensively in the practice of dental hygiene around the world, and more dental hygienists become legally allowed to administer local anesthetics each year.

Supplemental care may include a variety of needs exemplified by the chapters in Part 5. In completely revised Chapter 34, supplemental antimicrobial therapy includes not only irrigation as a selective treatment option but also techniques using the tetracycline fiber, the chlorhexidine chip, and the doxycycline gel.

All dental hygiene care culminates in a plan for maintenance over the lifetime of each patient. Revised Chapter 42 includes recommendations for a comprehensive continuing care plan to prevent recurrence of disease.

Part 6, as in previous editions, is devoted to patients with special needs. Dental hygienists are involved in many aspects of dental and oral care. Patients turn to their dental hygienist for clarification of questions about total treatment. The research that relates periodontal infections as risk factors for cardiovascular diseases, diabetes, preterm low-birth-weight newborns, and many systemic conditions has definite impact on the practice of dental hygiene. The dental hygienist applies anticipatory guidance for disease prevention and health promotion at all ages.

In all chapters, References and Suggested Readings from the literature have been updated. They are included to enhance the text content, to substantiate the research background for the scientific foundation for evidence-based patient care, and to encourage self-education through reading. Self-education is essential for continuing competence after entering professional practice. The habit and appreciation of reading of the current dental and dental hygiene literature is one method for self-education that can be acquired during college days and continued through life.

THE CHALLENGE

Personal integrity and competence in patient care are foremost factors in assuring quality control within the dental hygiene profession. It is hoped that this book will facilitate learning, and, by preparing knowledgeable ethical dental hygiene practitioners/clinicians, the dental hygiene care and instruction for each patient will be the best possible, and the image of dental hygiene will continue to be elevated.

ACKNOWLEDGMENTS

Many dental hygiene students, faculty, and practitioners around the world have influenced the preparation of this eighth edition. Individual ideas, requests, and recommendations range from a single word change or brief comment to requests about a whole chapter or the color of the cover. Each is acknowledged with humble gratitude and sincere thanks.

Appreciation goes to the contributors of the various chapters, as listed in the Contents. As the first official contributors of this book, they deserve particular commendation for their patience.

A special note of gratitude goes to Tanya Lazar who started when the revision was first underway as the Managing Editor and later carried the book through as Development Editor until Williams & Wilkins merged with Lippincott-Raven. Since the changeover, my thanks go to Lawrence McGrew, Editor, and Holly Chapman, Editorial Assistant, for their expertise and careful attention to the necessary details.

The illustrations for this and the previous edition have been the work of a talented artist, Marcia Williams of Newton Highlands, Massachusetts. Her personal interest and patience in preparing the new artwork is sincerely appreciated. Thanks to Laurie Brown, who has been our computer specialist, and a personal thank-you to my friend Patricia Cohen, who, besides editing a chapter, has made numerous contributions to the progress and mechanisms of this major undertaking.

Boston, Massachusetts   *Esther M. Wilkins*

CONTENTS

3 Exposure Control: Barriers for Patient and Clinician 42

Esther M. Wilkins, BS, RDH, DMD
Kathryn Jean Falcone, RDH, AS

4 Infection Control: Clinical Procedures 55

5 Patient Reception and Positioning   73

PART III
ASSESSMENT   81

6 Personal, Dental, and Medical Histories   87
Esther M. Wilkins, BS, RDH, DMD
Lois Rigmont Barber, RDH, BSEd
Carol Jahn, RDH, MS
Frieda Atherton Pickett, RDH, MS

7 Vital Signs   106

8   Extraoral and Intraoral Examination   116

Esther M. Wilkins, BS, RDH, DMD
Arthur S. Miller, DMD, MSD

9   Dental Radiographs   134

Dorathea Foote, RDH, MEd

10 Study Casts   171

16 Bacterial Plaque and Other Soft Deposits   264

17 Dental Calculus   277

18 Dental Stains and Discolorations   285

19 Indices and Scoring Methods   293

20 Records and Charting   314

21 Planning Dental Hygiene Care   320

Charlotte J. Wyche, RDH, MS

24   Interdental Care and Chemotherapy   370

Esther M. Wilkins, BS, RDH, DMD
Deborah Mancinelli Lyle, RDH, MS

25 Care of Dental Prostheses   394

26 The Patient With Oral Rehabilitation and Implants   411

27 The Patient Who Uses Tobacco   425

Nancy L.J. Williams, RDH, EdD

28 Diet and Dietary Assessment 441

Cynthia A. Stegeman, RDH, MEd, RD, CDE
Esther M. Wilkins, BS, RDH, DMD

29 Fluorides 455

30 Sealants 480

Kathleen Sweeney, RDH, BS, MS
Esther M. Wilkins, BS, RDH, DMD

PART V

TREATMENT 489

33   Nonsurgical Periodontal Instrumentation   544

Caren Barnes, RDH, MS
Margaret Waring, RDH, BS, MS, EdD
Esther M. Wilkins, BS, RDH, DMD

34 Nonsurgical Periodontal Therapy: Supplemental Care Procedures 566

35 Acute Periodontal Conditions 576

36   Sutures and Dressings   585

Esther M. Wilkins, BS, RDH, DMD
Marilyn B. Cortell, RDH, MS

37   Dentin Sensitivity   595

Kathy B. Bassett, BSDH, RDH, MEd
Peggy Ellingson, RDH, BA, MA

38   Extrinsic Stain Removal   603

Esther M. Wilkins, BS, RDH, DMD
Caren Barnes, RDH, MS

39 The Porte Polisher 619

40 Care of Dental Restorations 623

Susan Anderson, RDH, BS, MEd
Esther M. Wilkins, RDH, BS, DMD

41 Debonding 636

49 The Patient With Cancer   721
Christina B. DeBiase, BSDH, MA, EdD

50 Care of Patients With Disabilities   736
Esther M. Wilkins, BS, RDH, DMD
Charlotte J. Wyche, RDH, MS

51 The Patient Who Is Homebound, Bedridden, or Helpless 761

Esther M. Wilkins, BS, RDH, DMD
Charlotte J. Wyche, RDH, MS

52 The Patient With a Physical Impairment 768

59   The Patient With a Blood Disorder   865

Christina B. DeBiase, BSDH, MA, EdD
Esther M. Wilkins, BS, RDH, DMD

60   The Patient With Diabetes Mellitus   880

Kathryn Ragalis, RDH, MS, DMD

61   Emergency Care   892

Cynthia R. Biron, RDH, EMT, MA

ORIENTATION TO CLINICAL DENTAL HYGIENE PRACTICE

The Professional Dental Hygienist

The dental hygienist is a licensed primary health-care professional, oral health educator, and clinician who provides preventive, educational, and therapeutic services supporting total health for the control of oral diseases and the promotion of oral health. Dental hygiene services are available for general and specialty dental practices, programs for research, professional education, community health, and hospital and institutional care of disabled persons, as well as federal programs, the armed services, and dental product promotion. Key words relating to dental hygienists and their practice are defined in Box 1-1.

I. TYPES OF SERVICES

The clinical and educational responsibilities of the dental hygienist are divided into preventive and therapeutic services. Clinical and educational activities are inseparable and overlap as patient care is planned and accomplished.

A. Preventive
Preventive services are the methods employed by the clinician and/or patient to promote and maintain oral health.

Preventive services fall into three groups: primary, secondary, and tertiary. *Primary prevention* refers to measures carried out so that disease does not occur and is truly prevented. *Secondary prevention* involves the treatment of early disease to prevent further progress of potentially irreversible conditions that, if not arrested, may lead eventually to extensive rehabilitative treatment or loss of teeth. *Tertiary prevention* uses methods to replace lost tissues and to rehabilitate the patient to a level where function is as near normal as possible after secondary prevention has not been successful.

An example of a primary preventive measure is the application of a topical fluoride preparation for dental caries prevention. Removal of subgingival calculus and debriding the root surface in a relatively shallow pocket is an example of a secondary prevention procedure in that the treatment contributes to the prevention of a deep pocket and further clinical attachment loss. For tertiary prevention, an example is the placement of a fixed partial denture to replace a missing tooth and therefore restore function.

B. Educational
Educational services are the strategies developed for an individual or for groups to elicit behaviors directed toward health.

BOX 1-1 KEY WORDS AND ABBREVIATIONS: Professional Dental Hygienist

CEU: continuing education unit; 1 unit commonly refers to 1 clock hour of instruction.

Competency: the skills, understanding, and professional values of an individual ready for beginning dental hygiene practice.

Continuing education: postlicensure short-term educational experiences for refresher, updating, and renewal; continuing education units may be required for relicensure.

Cotherapist: term used to describe the relationships between patient, dentist, and dental hygienist when coordinating the efforts to attain and maintain the oral health of the patient.

Deductive reasoning: interpretation of information from generalizations to specific facts.

Dental hygiene care: the science and practice of the prevention of oral diseases; the profession of the dental hygienist.

Dental hygiene diagnosis: the actual or potential oral health problems that are amenable to resolution by a dental hygienist's clinical and educational performance; a dental hygiene diagnosis identifies an existing or potential oral health problem that the dental hygienist is qualified and licensed to treat.

Dental hygiene process of care: an organized systematic group of activities that provides the framework for delivering quality dental hygiene care.

Dental hygiene care plan: after assessment, the pertinent interventions are selected and a care plan outlined; the plan consists of those services to be performed by the dental hygienist within the total care plan for dental care.

Dental hygienist (hī-jĕ′nĭst): dental health specialist whose primary concern is the maintenance of oral health and the prevention of oral disease (see also opening paragraph, page 3).

Dentistry: the evaluation, diagnosis, prevention, and/or treatment (nonsurgical, surgical, or related procedures) of diseases, disorders, and/or conditions of the oral cavity, maxillofacial area, and/or the adjacent and associated structures and their impact on the human body, provided by a dentist, within the scope of his/her education, training, and experience, in accordance with the ethics of the profession and applicable law (ADA, October, 1997).

Ethics (ĕth′ĭks): a sense of moral obligation and a system of moral principles governing the conduct of a professional group, planned by them for the common good of people; principles of morality.

Health: state of physical, mental, and social well-being, not only the absence of disease.

Health promotion: the process of enabling people to increase control and improve their health through self-care, mutual aid, and the creation of healthy environments.

Hygiene (hī-jēn): the science of health and its preservation; a condition or practice, such as cleanliness, that is conducive to the preservation of health.

Oral hygiene: procedures for preservation of health of the oral cavity; personal maintenance of cleanliness and other measures recommended by dental professionals.

Inductive reasoning: interpretation of information whereby specific facts form general inferences.

Interdependent interventions: functions of the dental hygienist that are carried out in conjunction with other health-care team members.

Intervention: an action taken by the dental hygienist to maintain or restore the patient's optimal oral health.

License by credential: acceptance for licensure by a regulatory body (state, province) on the evidence from a license obtained in another state where equivalent standards and requirements are required; also called reciprocity, a mutual or cooperative exchange.

Primary health care: employs the techniques and agents to abort the onset of disease, to reverse the progress of the initial stages of disease, or to arrest the disease process before treatment becomes necessary.

Profession: occupation or calling that requires specialized knowledge, methods, and skills, as well as preparation, from an institution of higher learning, in the scholarly, scientific, and historic principles underlying such methods and skills; a profession continuously enlarges its body of knowledge, functions autonomously in formulation of policy, and maintains high standards of achievement and conduct; members of a profession are committed to continuing study, place service above personal gain, and are committed to providing practical services vital to human and social welfare.

Prognosis (prŏg-nō′-sĭs): a forecast of the probable course and outcome of the treatment of a condition or disease.

Supervision: term applied to the legal relationship between dentist and dental hygienist in practice. Each practice act defines the type of supervision required.

General supervision: means that the dentist has authorized the procedure for a patient of record, but need not be present when the authorized procedure is carried out. The procedure is carried out in accordance with the dentist's diagnosis and treatment plan.

(continued)

BOX I-I KEY WORDS AND ABBREVIATIONS: (Continued)

Direct supervision: means that the dentist has diagnosed and authorized the condition to be treated, remains on the premises while the procedure is performed, and approves the work performed before dismissal of the patient.

Personal supervision: means that while the dentist is personally treating a patient, the dental hygienist is authorized to aid in the treatment by concurrently performing a supportive procedure.

Collaborative Practice of Dental Hygiene: the science of the prevention and treatment of oral disease through the provision of educational, assessment, preventive, clinical and other therapeutic services in a collaborative working relationship with a consulting dentist, but without general supervision.

Educational aspects of dental hygiene service permeate the entire patient care system. The preparation for specific treatment, the success of treatment, and the long-term success of both preventive and therapeutic services depend on the patient's understanding of each procedure and daily care of the oral cavity.

C. Therapeutic

Therapeutic services are clinical treatments designed to arrest or control disease and maintain oral tissues in health.

Dental hygiene treatment services are an integral part of the total treatment procedures. All scaling and root debridement, along with the steps in postoperative care, are parts of the therapeutic phases in the treatment of periodontal infections. Placement of a pit and fissure sealant is both a preventive and a therapeutic service.

II. DENTAL HYGIENE CARE

The term *dental hygiene care* is used to denote all integrated preventive and treatment services administered to a patient by a dental hygienist. This term is parallel to the commonly used term *dental care,* which refers to the services performed by the dentist.

Clinical services, both dental and dental hygiene, have limited long-range probability of success if the patient does not understand the need for cooperation in daily procedures of personal care and diet, and for regular appointments for professional care. Educational and clinical services, therefore, are mutually dependent and inseparable in the total dental hygiene care of the patient.

Dr. Alfred C. Fones, the "father of dental hygiene," emphasized the important role of education. In the first textbook for dental hygienists, he wrote:

"It is primarily to this important work of public education that the dental hygienist is called. She must regard herself as the channel through which dentistry's knowledge of mouth hygiene is to be disseminated. The greatest service she can perform is the persistent education of the public in mouth hygiene and the allied branches of general hygiene."[1]

Dental hygiene has been studied and the scope of practice has developed from Dr. Fones' original concept. Scientific information about the prevention of oral diseases has been advancing steadily. The public has become increasingly aware of the need for dental hygiene care and the importance of oral health instruction. The clinical practice of the dental hygienist integrates specific care with instructional services required by the individual patient.

DENTAL HYGIENE PROCESS OF CARE

Quality dental hygiene care is more than the rote performance of clinical procedures. It requires dental hygienists to think critically about treatment options and develop individualized care plans that meet the needs of their patients. The practice of dental hygiene has moved from an intuitive process that focused on treatment of current conditions to an evidence-based process that includes a complex grouping of assessment indices, treatments, education, and evaluation of therapies.

The current practice of dental hygiene comprises five categories: assessment, dental hygiene diagnosis (with prognosis), planning, implementation, and evaluation.[2] Since the five categories are part of an integrated whole and the procedures performed overlap or occur simultaneously, the structure has been termed a *process.*

The dental hygiene process of care is a sequence of actions that are continual in nature (Figure 1-1). Data gathered on a patient in the assessment phase are used to make judgments concerning diagnoses, which in turn direct the plan of care. Evidence gathered during implementation and evaluation coupled with the clinician's knowledge base completes and continues the process.

The purpose of the dental hygiene process of care is to provide a framework within which the individualized needs of a patient can be met. The dental hygiene process is a deliberate, logical, and rational activity performed systematically. Inherent in the process is a series of actions that identifies the causative or influencing factors of a condition that can be reduced, eliminated, or prevented by the den-

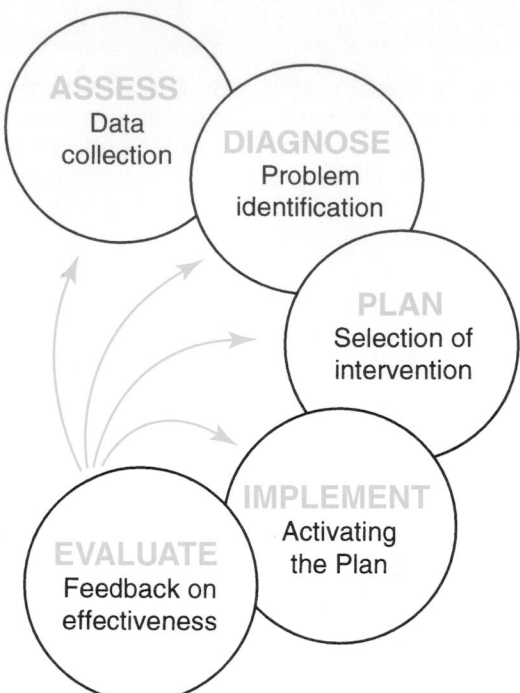

FIGURE 1-1 The Five Components of the Dental Hygiene Process of Care. All components are interrelated and depend upon evaluation to determine the need for change in the care plan.

tal hygienist. The process is designed to provide dental hygiene care that will maintain or restore the patient's optimal oral health.

I. ASSESSMENT

The assessment component represents the first phase of the dental hygiene process.[3] It is an organized, systematic process of collecting data from multiple sources to evaluate the health status of a patient. An accurate, complete assessment provides the foundation for patient care. During this phase, data are collected and documented in the patient's record. The data collected should be comprehensive and multifocal, representing a variety of sources.

A. Subjective
Subjective data are obtained by observation and interaction with the patient. The patient's chief complaint, feelings, perception of health care, and value of oral health are included.

B. Objective
Objective data are measurable and include both a comprehensive physical and oral assessment. Such a database requires the dental hygienist to be consistent in the use of descriptive statements to describe clinical findings and technical procedures such as periodontal probing.

II. DENTAL HYGIENE DIAGNOSIS[4]

The dental hygiene diagnosis identifies the patient's problems for which the dental hygienist would be responsible and provides the basis on which the dental hygiene treatment plan is designed, implemented, and evaluated. During this phase the data collected from assessment are critically analyzed and interpreted.

Many models have been developed for diagnostic decision-making. All models analyze and synthesize data collected during assessment through deductive and inductive reasoning. The dental hygiene diagnostic model is based on the nursing model and broadens the already established dental model to include the health behaviors of individuals. The actual or potential health problem that dental hygienists are licensed to treat is described. Specifically, the two steps involved in the development of a diagnosis include data processing and diagnosis formulation.

A. Data Processing
Dental hygienists and other health-care professionals use critical thinking skills to assist in the processing of data, to collect and interpret information, and to make sound judgments that lead to appropriate decisions. Although data processing is a component of diagnosis, it is not isolated. The phases are active and occur continuously throughout the process of care. Data processing includes the classification, interpretation, and validation of information collected during the assessment phase.
1. *Classification.* Classification of data involves the sorting of information into specific categories such as general systemic, oral soft tissue, periodontal, or oral hygiene. As information is organized, data interpretation that focuses on data pertinent to the patient's needs begins.
2. *Interpretation.* Data interpretation relies upon critical thinking skills to identify significance, compare with standards or norms, recognize deviations or abnormalities, and analyze the abnormalities with respect to significance. The cognitive processes of analysis, synthesis, inductive reasoning, and deductive reasoning are included.
3. *Validation.* Validation is an attempt to verify the accuracy of data interpretation. Validation can assist in recognizing errors, isolating discrepancies, and identifying the need for additional information. The validation procedure may be accomplished by direct interaction with the patient or significant other, consultation with other health-care professionals, or comparison of data with an authoritative reference.

B. Diagnosis Formulation
The diagnostic statement focuses on a patient's individual needs. The potential or actual problems that can be prevented, minimized, or re-

solved by independent or interdependent interventions are determined. Dental hygiene diagnostic statements:

1. Focus on the patient's individual needs.
2. Determine potential or actual problems that can be prevented, minimized, or resolved by independent or interdependent interventions.
3. Identify the patient's condition or potential for risk.
4. Specify the cause and contributing factors. Contributing factors reflect the environmental, psychological, sociocultural, and physiological factors believed to be related or contributing to the patient's health condition.

Sample diagnostic statements are suggested:

1. *Halitosis* related to plaque accumulation on the tongue.
2. *Dental abrasion* related to incorrect toothbrushing.
3. *Potential for dental caries* related to deep occlusal pits and fissures.
4. *Bleeding on probing* related to marginal plaque accumulation.
5. *Anxiety* related to dental phobia.

III. DENTAL HYGIENE CARE PLANNING[5]

The planning phase develops strategies to meet the individual needs of the patient as identified by the dental hygiene diagnosis. Several steps are involved that include establishing priorities for the identified needs, setting goals, determining interventions, and developing expected outcomes.

A. Establishing Priorities
1. Priorities are determined by the immediacy of the condition, severity of the problem, and available resources.
2. Patients are active participants in the identification of priorities.

B. Setting Goals
1. Each problem is accompanied by a goal.
2. Goals are directly related to the problem and represent the anticipated level of achievement.

C. Determining Interventions
1. Interventions are dental hygiene therapies or patient educational activities that reduce, eliminate, or prevent the cause of the problem.
2. For the prevention of halitosis, dental hygiene interventions may include tongue brushing, tongue scraping, and patient education about the papilla found on the tongue that trap plaque microorganisms.

D. Identifying Expected Outcomes
1. Expected outcomes represent measurable criteria for each intervention.

2. They are selected according to the anticipated effectiveness of the interventions.
3. They provide a way to evaluate the results of the intervention.
4. An expected outcome following a patient education intervention about tongue anatomy, for example, would be that the patient could perform a self-evaluation of tongue cleanliness.

IV. IMPLEMENTATION

Implementation is the phase in which the care plan is put into action. The activities identified in the care plan that are to be performed by the patient, dental hygienist, or others are carried out at this time. Before any specific procedures are performed, the patient is informed and consent is obtained for the planned course of treatment. Informed consent is described on page 328.

V. EVALUATION

During the evaluation phase, the patient's current status is compared with the baseline data, and progress or lack thereof toward the stated goal is assessed. The evaluation phase is the component of the dental hygiene process that provides the opportunity to change or modify the care plan. The evaluation phase uses the expected outcomes identified during planning as tools to assist in determining if particular interventions were appropriate and successful.

At this point the process comes full circle. The evaluation phase is used to determine if the patient should be retreated, referred, or placed on a supportive therapy program that maintains the patient's current health status.

FACTORS INFLUENCING CLINICAL PRACTICE

I. LEGAL

The law must be studied and respected by each dental hygienist practicing within the state, province, or country. Although the various practice acts have certain basic similarities, differences in scope and definition exist. Terminology varies, but each practice act regulates the patient services that may be practiced by the licensed dental hygienist. Changes may be made from time to time. Frequent review of the practice acts and/or regulations is recommended to keep dental health professionals up to date.

II. ETHICAL

The ethics of a profession provide the general standards of right and wrong that guide the behavior of the members of that profession. Each profession has its own code of ethics. The *Code of Ethics for Dental Hygienists* of the American Dental Hygienist Association is found in Appendix 1 (page 934). The purpose of the code is to define a standard of conduct that will give the individual a strong sense of ethical consciousness not only in professional practice but in all phases of life. Each dental hygienist must study the code of ethics of the particular association in which membership is held.

Dental hygienists are ethically and morally responsible to provide dental hygiene care for all patients without discrimination. Ethical decision-making and professional behavior must be reflected in all aspects of dental hygiene practice. Foremost is the responsibility to put the best interests of the patient first. Commitment to life-long learning is an ethical duty to society in order to ensure the best care for each patient, to maintain competency, and to learn from new research the scientific advances.

Professional people in the health services are set apart from others by virtue of the dignity and responsibility of their work. Others look to the health-care professional person for leadership and expect more than ordinary demonstration of good human relationships. Being professional requires interpersonal, interprofessional, and community relationships of a high standard.

III. PERSONAL

Each dental hygienist may represent the entire profession to the patient being served. The dental hygienist's expressed or demonstrated attitudes toward dentistry, dental hygiene, and other health professions, as well as toward health services and preventive measures, are apt to be reflected in the subsequent attitude of the patient toward other dental hygienists and dental hygiene care in general.

Members of health professions must exemplify the traits they hold as objectives for others if response and cooperation are to be expected. Many personal factors of general physical health, oral health, cleanliness, appearance, and mental health are to be considered. A few of these are mentioned as follows:

1. *General Physical Health.* Optimum physical health depends primarily on a well-planned diet, a sufficient amount of sleep, and an adequate amount of exercise.

   Because of the occupational hazards of dental personnel, routine examinations at least annually should include tests for hearing, sight, urinary mercury, and certain communicable diseases. Immunizations are described on pages 43 to 44.
2. *Oral Health.* The maintenance of a clean, healthy mouth demonstrates by example that the dental hygienist follows the teachings of the dental and dental hygiene professions relative to prevention and control of disease.
3. *Mental Health.* The mental health of the dental hygienist is reflected in interpersonal re-

lationships and the ability to inspire confidence through a display of professional and emotional maturity. Adequate physical health, recreation, and participation in professional and community activities contribute to optimum mental health.

SPECIAL PRACTICE AREAS

A wide range of settings is available for the practice of a dental hygienist. Likewise, a wide range of patient problems brings out the need for specialized knowledge and skills.

A. Dental Specialties

There are eight areas of dentistry in which a dentist may conduct an ethical limited practice. They are the following: dental public health, endodontics, oral and maxillofacial pathology, oral and maxillofacial surgery, orthodontics and dentofacial orthopedics, pediatric dentistry, periodontics, and prosthodontics.[6] Education and training for certification in the dental specialties require a minimum of 2 or 3 years of graduate or postdoctoral study and the successful completion of written and practical examinations. Masters and postdoctoral specialty degrees require 3 or more years beyond basic dental education.

B. Dental Hygiene Specialties

Although dental hygienists have not been required to complete examinations for practice within a specialty, educational curricula exist for certain areas. For example, advanced degree programs to prepare for dental hygiene education and public health have been available for many years.

In other special areas, short-term courses have been developed, such as for instruction in the care of patients with disabilities. In-service training may be available in long-term care institutions, hospitals, and skilled nursing facilities. Some dental hygienists have learned how to practice in a specialty through private study, special conferences, and personal experience.

Dental hygienists are needed to practice with dentists in specialty areas, particularly orthodontics, pediatric dentistry, and periodontics. Others are involved in special clinics with a variety of health specialists, where patients with dental deformities, such as cleft lip and/or palate or patients with oral cancer, are under care. In other facilities, dental hygienists serve with a combined medical and dental team in the treatment of patients with severe systemic diseases; patients with physical, mental, or emotional handicapping conditions; or patients with combinations of any of the problems mentioned.

OBJECTIVES FOR PROFESSIONAL PRACTICE

The dental hygienist's self-assessment is essential in attaining goals of perfection in service to the patient and in collaboration with the dentist in a total dental and dental hygiene care program. Personal objectives should be outlined and reviewed frequently in a plan for continued self-improvement.

The goal with respect to patient care is *to aid individuals and groups in attaining and maintaining optimum oral health*. Other objectives are related to this primary one.

The professional dental hygienist will:

A. Strive toward the highest degree of professional ethics and conduct.
B. Plan and carry out effectively the dental hygiene services essential to the total care program for each individual patient.
C. Apply knowledge and understanding of the basic and clinical sciences in the recognition of oral conditions and prevention of oral diseases.
D. Apply scientific knowledge and skill to all clinical techniques and instructional procedures.
E. Recognize each patient as an individual and adapt techniques and procedures accordingly.
F. Identify and care for the needs of patients who have unusual general health problems that affect dental hygiene procedures.
G. Demonstrate interpersonal relationships that permit attending the patient with assurance and presenting dental health information effectively.
H. Provide a complete and personalized instructional service to help each patient to become motivated toward changes in oral health behavioral practices.
I. Practice safe and efficient clinical routines for the application of universal precautions for infection control.
J. Apply a continuing process of self-development and self-evaluation in clinical practice throughout professional life.
　1. Be objective and critical of procedures used in order to perform the best possible service.
　2. Appreciate the need for acquiring new knowledge and skills by regular enrollment in continuing education courses.
K. Maintain membership and participate actively in the local, national, and international dental hygiene professional associations.

FACTORS TO TEACH THE PATIENT

A. The role of the dental hygienist as a cotherapist with each patient and with members of the dental profession.
B. The scope of service of the dental hygienist as defined by various practice acts.
C. The interrelationship of instructional and clinical services in dental hygiene patient care.
D. The patient's potential state of oral health and how it can be developed and maintained.

REFERENCES

1. **Fones**, A.C., ed.: *Mouth Hygiene*, 4th ed. Philadelphia, Lea & Febiger, 1934, p. 248.
2. **Mueller-Joseph**, L. and Petersen, M.: *Dental Hygiene Process: Diagnosis and Care Planning*. Albany, Delmar, 1995, pp. 9–14.
3. Ibid., pp. 20–25.
4. Ibid., pp. 46–55.
5. Ibid., pp. 89–104.
6. **American Dental Association**: *Principles of Ethics and Code of Professional Conduct*. Revised January, 1998.

SUGGESTED READINGS

Boyer, E.M. and Gupta, G.C.: Clinical Dental Hygienists' Perceptions of Quality Dental Hygiene Care, *J. Dent. Hyg.*, *66*, 216, June, 1992.

Brutvan, E.L.: Current Trends in Dental Hygiene Education and Practice, *J. Dent. Hyg.*, *72*, 44, Fall, 1998.

Gaston, M.A.: Managing Change, (Editorial), *J. Dent. Hyg.*, *71*, 179, Fall, 1997.

King, C.C. and Craig, B.J.: The Role of the Dental Hygienist as Change Agent, *Canad. Dent. Hyg. Assoc./Probe, 31*, 81, May/June, 1997.

Luxmore, J.S., Mattana, D., Wyche, C., Zager, S., and Zarkowski, P.: Learning the Process of Collaborative Clinical Research, *J. Dent. Hyg.*, *71*, 207, Fall, 1997.

McFall, D.B.: The Future of Allied Health Education, *Educ. Update, 12*, 1, December, 1992.

McIntyre, L.: The Evolution of Health Promotion, *Canad. Dent. Hyg. Assoc./Probe, 26*, 15, Spring, 1992.

Mickelson, L.M.: Back to the Future: Appropriating Our Traditions, *Canad. Dent. Hyg. Assoc./Probe, 27*, 55, March/April, 1993.

Pack, A.R.C.: Hygienists and Their Role in Dental Practice, *N. Zeal. Dent. J., 91*, 57, June, 1995.

Sisty-LePeau, N.: A Credible Image, (Editorial), *J. Dent. Hyg.*, *65*, 403, November–December, 1991.

Sisty-LePeau, N.: Life-long Learning, (Editorial), *J. Dent. Hyg.*, *66*, 331, October, 1992.

Sisty-LePeau, N.: What's in a Name? (Editorial), *J. Dent. Hyg.*, *71*, 3, January–February, 1997.

Slavkin, H.C.: Preparing for Change in the 21st Century, *J. Dent. Hyg.*, *70*, 220, November–December, 1996.

Uldricks, J.M., Hicks, M.J., Whitacre, H.L., Anderson, J., and Moeschberger, M.L.: Dental Hygienists' Utilization of Periodontal Assessment Skills and Perceived Collaboration with Dentist-Employer, *J. Dent. Hyg.*, *67*, 22, January, 1993.

Professionalism and Ethics

Devore, C.H.: Legal Risk Management for the Dental Hygienist, *J. Pract. Hyg., 6*, 59, July/August, 1997.

Fleming, W.C.: The Attributes of a Profession and Its Members, *J. Am. Dent. Assoc., 69*, 390, September, 1964.

Frankel, M.S.: Taking Ethics Seriously. Building a Professional Community, *J. Dent. Hyg., 66*, 386, November–December, 1992.

Gaston, M.A., Brown, D.M., and Waring, M.B.: Survey of Ethical Issues in Dental Hygiene, *J. Dent. Hyg., 64*, 217, June, 1990.

Giangrego, E.: The Ethics of Everyday Practice, *J. Dent. Hyg., 64*, 208, June, 1990.

Hine, M.K.: The Professional Concept—Its History and Meaning to Health Service, *J. Am. Coll. Dent., 37*, 19, January, 1970.

Lautar, C.: Is Dental Hygiene a Profession? A Literature Review, *Canad. Dent. Hyg. Assoc./Probe, 29*, 127, July/August, 1995.

MacQuarrie, E.E.: Factors in the Development of Professional Attitude, *J. Am. Dent. Hyg. Assoc., 45*, 86, March–April, 1971.

Motley, W.E.: *Ethics, Jurisprudence and History for the Dental Hygienist*, 3rd ed. Philadelphia, Lea & Febiger, 1983, 217 pp.

Walker, B., Juchli, J., and Pimlott, J.: Self-regulation in Alberta, Canada: The Achievement of a Goal, *Canad. Dent. Hyg. Assoc./Probe, 27*, 59, March/April, 1993.

II

PREPARATION FOR DENTAL HYGIENE APPOINTMENTS

2

Infection Control: Transmissible Diseases

For dental health-care workers infection and communicable disease can lead to illness, disability, and loss of work time. In addition, patients, family members, and community contacts can become exposed and may become ill and lose productive time or suffer permanent after-effects.

In oral health-care practice, the objective is to protect patients, dental personnel, and others that may become exposed by acquiring infection in the environment of the office or clinic. Health services facilities, including dental facilities, must be places for cure and prevention, not for dissemination of disease due to inadequate precautionary measures and habits of the professional personnel.

The first responsibility of the entire dental team is to organize and maintain a system for the sterilization, disinfection, and care of instruments and equipment. The second step is to develop and maintain work practices for all appointments that will prevent direct or indirect cross-infections between dental personnel and patients, and from one patient to another. Box 2-1 lists and defines terms that apply to the transmission of infectious agents.

BOX 2-1 KEY WORDS AND ABBREVIATIONS: Disease Transmission

Aerosol (ār'o-sol): an artificially generated collection of particles suspended in air.

> **Microbial aerosol:** suspension of particles in the air that consists partially or wholly of microorganisms; it may be capable of causing an infection.

Anergy (ăn'er-jē): diminished reactivity to specific antigen(s); inability to react to skin-test antigen (even if person is infected with the organism tested) because of immunosuppression.

Antibody (ăn'tĭ-bod"ē): a soluble protein molecule produced and secreted by body cells in response to an antigen; it is capable of binding to that specific antigen.

Antigen (ăn'tĭ-jen): a substance that is capable, under appropriate conditions, of inducing a specific immune response and of reacting with the products of that response, that is, with the specific antibody.

Carrier: a person who harbors a specific infectious agent in the absence of discernible clinical disease and serves as a potential source of infection. The carrier state may be temporary, transient, or chronic.

> **Asymptomatic carrier:** an individual who harbors pathogenic organisms without clinically recognizable symptoms; a carrier may infect those he/she contacts.

CDCP: United States Centers for Disease Control and Prevention, Department of Health and Human Services, Public Health Service, Atlanta, GA 30333.

Communicable period of a disease: the time during which an infectious agent may be transferred directly or indirectly from an infected person to another person; the communicable period may include or overlap the incubation period.

Droplet (drop'let): diminutive drop, such as the particles of moisture expelled while coughing, sneezing, or speaking, that may carry infectious agents.

ELISA or EIA: an enzyme-linked immunosorbent assay; a laboratory test to detect antibody in the blood serum.

> **Western blot (WB):** a laboratory test for antibody that is more specific than EIA and is used to validate seropositive reactions to the EIA.

Endemic (ĕn-dĕm'ik): the constant presence of a disease or infectious agent within a geographic area.

Epidemic (ĕp"ĭ-dĕm'ik): widespread occurrence of cases of an illness in a community or region; greater than the expected number of cases for the particular population.

Fomite (fō'mīt) or **fomes** (fō'mēz): an inanimate object or material on which disease-producing agents (microorganisms) may be conveyed.

HCW: health-care worker; **DHCW:** dental health-care worker.

Immunity (ĭ-mū'nĭ-tē): the resistance that a person has against disease; it may be natural or acquired.

> **Passive immunity:** short-duration immunity either naturally attained by transplacental transfer from the mother or artificially acquired by inoculation of specific protective antibodies.

> **Active immunity:** immunity either naturally attained by infection, with or without clinical manifestations, or artificially acquired by inoculation of the agent in a killed, modified, or variant form; in response, the body produces its own antibodies; usually lasts for years.

Incubation period (ĭn"kū-bā'shun): the time interval between the initial contact with an infectious agent and the appearance of the first clinical sign or symptom of the disease.

Infection: a state caused by the invasion, development, or multiplication of an infectious agent into the body.

> **Primary infection:** first time; no pre-existing antibodies.

> **Latent infection:** persistent infection following a primary infection in which the causative agent remains inactive within certain cells.

> **Recurrent infection:** symptomatic reactivation of a latent infection.

(continued)

BOX 2-1 KEY WORDS AND ABBREVIATIONS: Disease Transmission (Continued)

Infectious agent: organism capable of producing an infection.

Jaundice (jawn'dĭs): yellowness of skin, sclerae, mucous membranes, and excretions due to hyperbilirubinemia and deposition of bile pigments. Also called *icterus.*

Microbiota (mī"krō-bī-ō'tah): the microscopic living organisms of a region.

Pandemic (pan-dem'ik): widespread epidemic usually affecting the population of an extensive region, several countries, or sometimes the entire globe.

Parenteral (pah-rĕn'ter-al): injection by a route other than the alimentary tract, such as subcutaneous, intramuscular, or intravenous.

Parotitis (păr"ŏ tī'tis): inflammation of the parotid gland.

Pathogen (păth'ō-jen): a virus, microorganism, or other substance that causes disease.

   Opportunistic pathogen: capable of causing disease only when the host's resistance is lowered.

Percutaneous (pĕr"kū-tā'nē-us): by way of, or through, the skin.

Permucosal (pĕr"mū-kō'sal): by way of, or through, a mucous membrane.

Prodrome (prō'drōm): early or premonitory symptom (adj: prodromal).

Replication: process by which viruses reproduce and multiply.

Retrovirus (rĕt'rō-vī"rus): virus with RNA as its core genetic material; requires the enzyme reverse transcriptase to convert its RNA into proviral DNA.

Serologic diagnosis: the identification of a disease by serum markers of that specific condition.

Seroconversion (sē"rō-kon-ver'zhun): after exposure to the etiologic agent of a disease, the blood changes from negative ("seronegative") to positive ("seropositive") for the serum marker for that disease; the time interval for conversion is specific for each disease.

Serum marker: a specific finding (such as an antibody or antigen) by laboratory blood analysis that identifies an existing disease state.

Shedding (viral): presence of virus in body secretions, in ex-

cretions, or in body surface lesions with potential for transmission.

STD: Sexually transmitted disease.

Surveillance (sŭr-vāl'ans) (of disease): continuing scrutiny of all aspects of occurrence and spread of a disease that are pertinent to effective control.

Susceptible host: host not possessing resistance against an infectious agent.

Transmission (horizontal): passage of an infectious agent from one individual to another.

   Vertical transmission: passage of an infectious agent from one generation to another by breast milk or across the placenta.

Universal precautions: an approach to infection control in which all human blood and certain human body fluids are treated as if known to be infectious for HIV, HBV, and other blood-borne pathogens.

Vector (vĕk'tor): a carrier that transfers an infectious microorganism from one host to another.

   Biologic vector: an arthropod, insect, or other living carrier in whose body the infecting organism multiplies before becoming infective to the recipient.

Vehicle (vē'ĭ-kĭl): a substance or object that serves as an intermediate means by which an infectious agent is transported and introduced into a susceptible host through a suitable portal of entry.

Virion (vī'rē-ŏn): complete virus particle made up of the **nucleoid** (the genetic material) and **capsid** (the shell of protein that protects the nucleoid).

Virulence (vĭr'ū-lens): the degree of pathogenicity or disease-evoking power of an infectious agent.

Virus (vī'rus): a subcellular genetic entity capable of gaining entrance into a limited range of living cells and capable of replication only within such cells; a virus contains either DNA or RNA but not both. (DNA and RNA are defined in Box 2-2.)

Window period: the time between exposure resulting in infection and the presence of detectable serum antibody; antibody test is negative but infectious agent is transmissible during the window period.

MICROORGANISMS OF THE ORAL CAVITY

In utero the oral cavity is sterile, but after birth within a few hours to 1 day a simple oral flora develops.[1] As the infant grows there is continuing introduction of microorganisms normal for an adult oral cavity. The microbiota of the adult is very complex.

Most of the salivary bacteria come from the dorsum of the tongue, but some are from other mucous membranes. Much higher counts of total microorganisms are found in bacterial plaque, periodontal pockets, and carious lesions than in saliva.

The intact mucous membrane of the oral cavity protects against infection to a degree. However, when the gingival tissues are inflamed and are manipulated during instrumentation, microorganisms can be introduced into the underlying tissues by way of the gingival sulcus or periodontal pocket.

Pathogenic (disease producing), potentially pathogenic, or nonpathogenic microorganisms may be present in the oral cavity of each patient. Pathogenic organisms may be transient. Patients may be carriers of certain diseases. Inadvertent transmission to subsequent susceptible patients or to dental personnel may occur as a result of inappropriate work practices, such as careless handwashing, unhygienic personal habits, or inadequate sterilization and handling of sterile instruments and materials.

Cross-contamination refers to the spread of microorganisms from one source to another: person to person, or person to an inanimate object and then to another person. Recognition of the many possibilities for the transfer of infection in a dental office or clinic provides a basis for planning the system of sterilization, disinfection, and handling of instruments and equipment.

THE INFECTIOUS PROCESS

A chain of events is required for the spread of an infectious agent. The six essential links are shown in Figure 2-1.

I. ESSENTIAL FEATURES FOR DISEASE TRANSMISSION

  A. An *infectious agent,* the *invading organism* (bacterium, virus, fungus, rickettsia, or protozoa). Each organism has its own specific reaction in an infected host.
  B. A *reservoir* where the invading organisms live and multiply. The infectious agent has its own essential environment, which may be inanimate matter, an insect, or human cells or blood. For example, soil is the reservoir for tetanus,

and humans are reservoirs for herpetic infections.
  C. A *mode of escape,* the port of exit from the reservoir. Organisms exit through various body systems, such as the respiratory tract, or through skin lesions. Escape from the blood stream may be through skin abrasions, hypodermic needles, or dental instruments.
  D. A *mode of transmission,* which may be direct, person to person, or indirect by way of an intermediate vehicle, such as contaminated hands or hypodermic needle. Transmission by a droplet may be direct from the respiratory tract of one person to the oral cavity of the receiving host. Droplets also may pass indirectly to hands or inanimate objects to be transferred indirectly to the susceptible host.
  E. A *mode of entry,* the port of entry of the infectious agent into the new host. Modes of entry may be similar to modes of escape, such as the respiratory tract, mucous membranes, or a break in the skin.
  F. A *susceptible host* that does not have immunity to the invading infectious agent.

II. FACTORS THAT INFLUENCE THE DEVELOPMENT OF INFECTION

The presence of an infectious agent does not lead inevitably to infection or disease. Factors involved include, but are not limited to, the following:
  A. Number of organisms and duration of exposure.
  B. Virulence of the organisms: their ability to survive interim exposure.
  C. Immune status of the host; antibody response; defense cell reaction.
  D. General physical health and nutritional status of the host. In health, disease is resisted, whereas in a deprived state, the body can be susceptible to infection.

III. FACTORS THAT ALTER NORMAL DEFENSES

The patient's complete medical and dental history must be reviewed to identify specific problems and take necessary precautions. Examples of situations that alter the normal defenses are included under the following topics.

  A. Abnormal Physical Conditions
    A heart valve may be defective as a result of a congenital or acquired condition. Such a valve may be susceptible to infective endocarditis resulting from a bacteremia created during dental or dental hygiene instrumentation. Prevention of infective endocarditis is described on page 851 and the antibiotic regimen is in Table 6-4 and Figure 6-2 (pages 102 to 103).

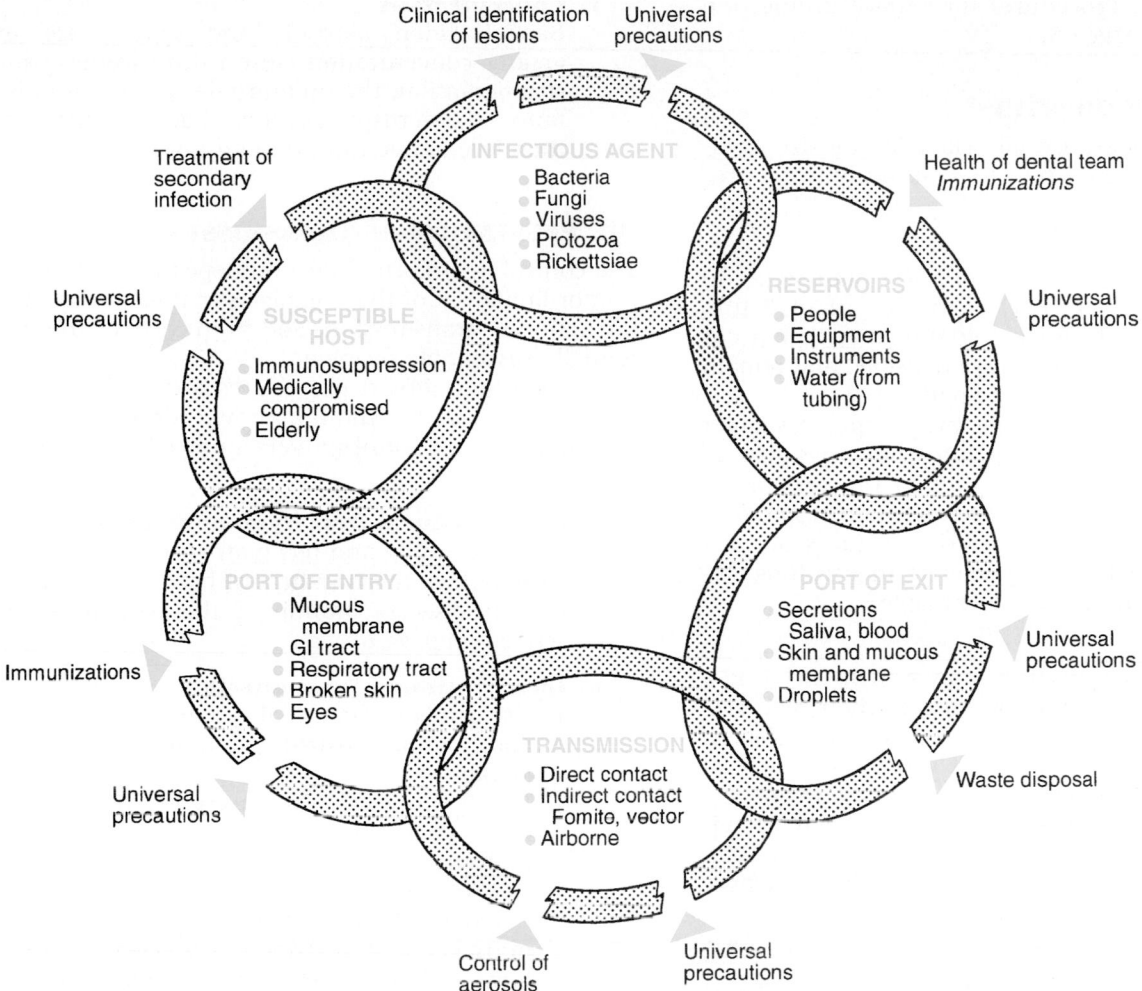

FIGURE 2-1 Interventions to Break the Chain of Disease Transmission. A break in the chain of six major links is required for the spread of an infectious agent. Universal precautions are applied to interrupt the chain.

B. Systemic Diseases

Examples of systemic conditions in which susceptibility to infection is increased are diabetes mellitus, alcoholism, leukemia, glomerulonephritis, acquired immunodeficiency syndrome, and all causes of immunosuppression.

C. Drug Therapy

Certain drugs used in the treatment of systemic disease alter the body's defenses. Examples are steroids and chemotherapeutic agents that are immunosuppressive. Special precautions, such as prophylactic antibiotics, may be indicated to prevent infection.

D. Prostheses and Transplants

A patient with, for example, a joint replacement, cardiac prosthesis, ventriculoatrial shunt for hydrocephalus, or an organ transplant may require antibiotic premedication.

AIRBORNE INFECTION

I. DUST-BORNE ORGANISMS

Clostridium tetani (tetanus bacillus), *Staphylococcus aureus,* and enteric bacteria are among the organisms that may travel in the dust brought in from outside and that moves in and about dental treatment areas. When doors are opened and closed and people pass in and out, dust is set into motion that can settle on instruments, other objects, or people.

Infectious microorganisms also reach dust from the oral cavities of patients by way of large airborne particles. Dust-borne organisms can be sources of contamination for dental instruments and the hands of dental personnel.

Surface disinfection of all equipment contacted during an appointment contributes to control of dust-borne pathogens. Procedures for surface disinfection are described on page 68.

II. AEROSOL PRODUCTION[2]

Airborne particles are usually classified by size as either *aerosols* or *spatter.* They are constantly being produced.

A. Aerosols

A particle of a true aerosol is less than 50 µm in diameter, and nearly all are less than 5 µm. Aerosols are biologic contaminants that occur in solid or liquid form, are invisible, and remain suspended in air for long periods.

Aerosol particles that are 5 µm or smaller may be breathed deep into the lungs. Larger particles get trapped higher in the respiratory tree. The tiny particles may contain respiratory disease–producing organisms or traces of mercury or amalgam that collect in the lung because they are not biodegradable.

B. Spatter

Heavier, larger particles may remain airborne a relatively short time because of their own size and weight. They drop or spatter on objects, people, and the floor. The spatter is composed of particles greater than 50 µm in diameter.

In contrast to aerosols, spatter may be visible, particularly after it has landed on skin, hair, clothing, or environmental surfaces where gross contamination can result.

C. Origin

Aerosols and spatter are created during breathing, speaking, coughing, or sneezing. They are produced during all intraoral procedures, including examination and manual scaling. When produced by air spray, air–water spray, handpiece activity, or ultrasonic scaling, the number of aerosols increases to tremendous proportions.[2–5]

D. Contents

1. *Microorganisms.* An aerosol may contain a single organism or a clump of microorganisms adhered to a dust or debris particle. The organisms may be contained within a liquid droplet.
2. *Particles from Cavity Preparation.* Tooth fragments; microorganisms from saliva, plaque, and/or oropharynx/nasopharynx; oil from a handpiece; and water from the cooling equipment may be in aerosols following cavity preparation.
3. *Ultrasonic Scaling.* The many microorganisms found in the aerosols from ultrasonic scalers include *Staphylococcus aureus, albus,* and *pyogenes, Streptococcus viridans,* lactobacilli, actinomyces, pneumococci, and diphtheroids.[4,5] Viruses also may be spread by ultrasonic instruments.

E. Concentration

Bacteria-laden aerosols and spatter are in greater concentration close to the scene of instrumentation; the quantity decreases with distance. The aerosols travel with air currents and, therefore, move from room to room.

III. PREVENTION OF TRANSMISSION

The control of airborne infection depends on elimination or limitation of the organisms at their source, interruption of transmission, and protection of the potentially susceptible recipient.

Carefully monitored procedures are necessary for all patients with or without a known serious communicable disease. A list of universal procedures appears on page 69.

A. Preprocedural Oral Hygiene Measures

Tooth brushing and using an antiseptic mouthrinse reduce the numbers of bacteria contained in aerosols. Preparation of the patient is described on page 68.

B. Interruption of Transmission

1. Use rubber dam, high-volume evacuation, and manual instrumentation as much as possible.
2. Install air-control methods to supply adequate ventilation, filtration, and relative humidity.
3. Employ vacuum cleaning to remove dirt and microorganisms rather than dust-arousing housekeeping methods. The cleaner must have a filter to prevent the escape of organisms after they are suctioned.[6]

C. Clean Water

Run water through all tubings to handpieces, ultrasonic scalers, and air–water spray for at least 2 minutes at the start of the day and at least 30 seconds after each appointment during the day. Contamination by spatter and aerosols is reduced by this method.[7]

D. Protection of the Clinician

The use of masks and protective eyewear can prevent direct contact of spatter and aerosols with the faces of the dental team.

PATHOGENS TRANSMISSIBLE BY THE ORAL CAVITY

Selected pathogens that may be transmitted by way of the oral cavity, and their disease manifestations, mode of transfer, incubation, and communicability periods are listed in Table 2-1.

Tuberculosis, viral hepatitis, acquired immunodeficiency syndrome, and herpetic infections are described in detail in this chapter because of the special problems they create in personal and patient care.

TABLE 2-1 Infectious Diseases

Infectious Agent	Disease or Condition	Route or Mode of Transmission	Incubation Period	Communicable Period	Vaccine
Human immuno-deficiency virus (HIV)	Acquired immuno-deficiency syndrome (AIDS) HIV infection	Blood and blood products (infected IV needles) Sexual contact Transplacental and perinatal	3 months to 12 years or more	From asymptomatic through life	*
Hepatitis A virus (HAV)	Type A hepatitis "infectious" hepatitis	Fecal–oral Food, water, shellfish	15 to 50 days (average 28 to 30 days)	2 to 3 weeks before onset (jaundice) through 8 days after	Yes
Hepatitis B virus (HBV)	Type B hepatitis "Serum" hepatitis	Blood Saliva and all body fluids Sexual contact Perinatal	2 to 6 months (average 60 to 90 days)	Before, during, and after clinical signs Carrier state: indefinite	Yes
Hepatitis C virus (HCV) PT-NANB	Type C hepatitis Parenterally transmitted non-A, non-B	Percutaneous Blood Needles	2 weeks to 6 months (6 to 9 weeks)	1 week before onset of symptoms Carrier state: indefinite	No
Delta hepatitis virus (HDV) Delta agent	Delta hepatitis	Coinfection with HBV Blood Sexual contacts Perinatal	2 to 8 weeks	All phases	HBV vaccine
Hepatitis E virus (HEV) ET-NANB	Type E hepatitis Enterically transmitted non-A, non-B	Fecal–oral Contaminated water	15 to 64 days	Not known	No
Herpes simplex virus Type 1 (HSV-1) Type 2 (HSV-2)	Acute herpetic gingivostomatitis Herpes labialis Ocular herpetic infections Herpetic whitlow	Saliva Direct contact (lip, hand) Indirect contact (on objects, limited survival) Sexual contact	2 to 12 days	Labialis: 1 day before onset until lesions are crusted Acute stomatitis: 7 weeks after recovery Asymptomatic infection: with viral shedding Reactivation period: with viral shedding	No
Varicella-zoster virus (VZV)	Chickenpox Herpes zoster (shingles)	Direct contact Indirect contact Airborne droplet	2 to 3 weeks	5 days prior to onset of rash until crusting of vesicles	Yes

*Vaccine progress.

(continued)

TABLE 2-1 Infectious Diseases (Continued)

Infectious Agent	Disease or Condition	Route or Mode of Transmission	Incubation Period	Communicable Period	Vaccine
Epstein-Barr virus (EBV)	Infectious mononucleosis	Direct contact Saliva	4 to 6 weeks	Prolonged Pharyngeal excretion 1 year after infection	No
Cytomegalovirus (CMV)	Neonatal cytomegalovirus infection Cytomegaloviral disease	Perinatal Direct contact (most body secretions) Blood transfusion Saliva	3 to 12 weeks after delivery 3 to 8 weeks after transfusion	Months to years	No
Mycobacterium tuberculosis	Tuberculosis	Droplet nuclei Sputum Saliva	4 to 12 weeks	As long as viable bacilli are discharged in sputum	B.C.G. (Bacille Calmette-Guérin)
Treponema pallidum	Syphilis Congenital syphilis	Direct contact Transplacental	10 days to 3 months	Variable and indefinite May be 2 to 4 years	No
Neisseria gonorrhoeae	Gonorrhea Gonococcal pharyngitis	Direct contact Indirect (short survival of organisms)	2 to 7 days	During incubation Continued for months and years if untreated	No
Bordetella pertussis	Whooping cough Pertussis	Direct contact with discharges	6 to 20 days	Not treated: from early catarrhal stage to 3 weeks after paroxysmal cough	Yes
Mumps virus (paramyxo-virus)	Infectious parotitis (mumps)	Direct contact (saliva) Airborne droplet	12 to 25 days (average 18 days)	12 to 25 days after exposure From 6 to 7 days before symptoms until 9 days after swelling	Yes
Poliovirus types 1, 2, 3	Poliomyelitis	Direct contact (saliva) Droplet Fecal–oral	7 to 14 days	Probably most infectious 7 to 10 days before and after onset of symptoms	Yes
Influenza viruses (A, B, C)	Influenza	Nasal discharge Respiratory droplets	1 to 5 days	3 days from clinical onset	Yes
Measles virus (Morbillivirus)	Rubeola (measles)	Direct contact Saliva Airborne droplet	7 to 18 days to fever, 14 days to rash	Few days before fever to 4 days after rash appears	Yes
Rubella virus (togavirus)	Rubella (German measles)	Nasopharyngeal secretions Direct contact Airborne droplets	16 to 23 days	From 1 week before to at least 4 days after rash appears Highly communicable	Yes
	Congenital rubella syndrome	Maternal infection first trimester		Infants shed virus for months after birth	

(continued)

TABLE 2-1 Infectious Diseases (Continued)

Infectious Agent	Disease or Condition	Route or Mode of Transmission	Incubation Period	Communicable Period	Vaccine
Group A streptococci (beta-hemolytic) *Streptococcus pyogenes*	Stretococcal sore throat Scarlet fever Impetigo Erysipelas	Respiratory droplets Direct contact	1 to 3 days	10 to 21 days, untreated Many nasal oropharyngeal carriers	No
Staphylococcus aureus *Staphylococcus epidermidis*	Abscesses Boils (furuncle) Impetigo Bacterial pneumonia	Saliva Exudates Nasal discharge	4 to 10 days Variable and indefinite	While lesions drain and carrier state persists	No
Candida albicans	Candidiasis	Secretions Excretions (oral, skin, vagina)	Variable 2 to 5 days for "thrush" in children	While lesions are present	No
Streptococcus pneumoniae	Pneumonia Pneumococcal pneumonia	Droplet Direct contact Indirect	1 to 3 days Not well determined	While virulent organisms are discharged	Yes

The general preventive measures described for these diseases should be applied during all appointments.

The etiologic agents of many communicable diseases enter the body by way of the oral cavity. Many infectious diseases have specific oral manifestations from which the disease can be identified. Pathogens are often present within the oral cavity without producing oral signs or symptoms, a fact of particular importance to the total consideration of prevention of disease transmission.

TUBERCULOSIS[8]

Mycobacterium tuberculosis, the etiologic agent in tuberculosis, is a resistant organism that requires special consideration when sterilization and disinfection methods are selected and administered. Tuberculosis is a serious disease that can involve many months and years of lost time during the active stages of illness and the following convalescence. Clinical procedures must be planned to prevent exposure and infection from this debilitating disease.

Tuberculosis is a common communicable disease throughout the world and a major public health problem. The incidence has increased in population groups with a high prevalence of HIV infection. Tuberculosis is an AIDS-defining illness.[9]

I. TRANSMISSION

A. Inhalation

Tuberculosis is contracted by the inhalation of fresh droplets containing tubercle bacilli. The organisms are disseminated from sputum and saliva of the infected individual by coughing, breathing heavily, or sneezing (Figure 2-2). During the use of ultrasonic and other handpieces, and of air–water spray, aerosols are created that can carry the bacilli.

When the organisms are in tiny aerosols, they can pass readily into the lungs and the respiratory bronchioles. There, they can invade the tissue and establish an infection.

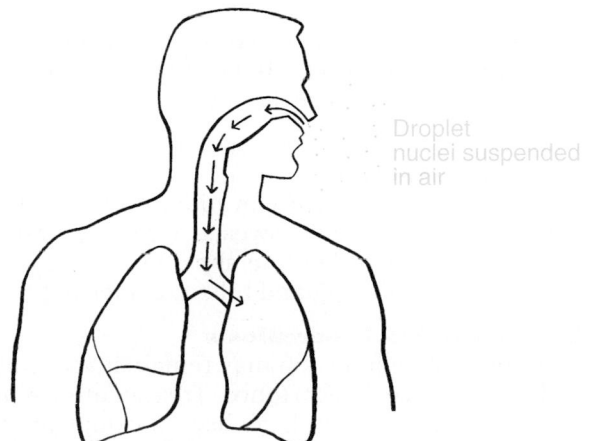

Droplet nuclei suspended in air

FIGURE 2-2 Droplet Nuclei. Many potentially pathogenic microorganisms are disseminated by aerosols and spatter. The primary mode of transmission of tubercle bacilli is by droplet nuclei breathed directly into the lung. (Adapted from McInnes, M.E.: *Essentials of Communicable Disease,* 2nd ed. St. Louis, The C.V. Mosby Co., 1975.)

B. Factors Affecting Transmission

Transmission of tuberculosis is dependent on the following: (1) the degree to which the infected person produces infectious droplets, (2) the amount and duration of exposure, and (3) the susceptibility of the recipient. Some patients are more contagious than are others. Maximum communicability is usually just before the disease is diagnosed, when the person may have a severe cough and other respiratory symptoms.

C. Other Modes of Transmission

The tubercle bacillus may enter the body by ingestion or direct inoculation, as well as by inhalation. Infection of the lungs is most common, but the tubercle bacillus also infects lymph nodes, meninges (tuberculous meningitis), kidneys, bone, skin, and the oral cavity.[8]

II. DISEASE PROCESS

A. Predisposing Factors

Any debilitating or immunosuppressive condition can predispose a person to invasion by the tubercle bacillus. Systemic conditions that may be related to lowered resistance to infection include diabetes, congenital heart disease, chronic lung disease, alcoholism, and the acquired immunodeficiency syndrome (page 35 and Table 2-5).

B. Incubation Period

As shown in Table 2-1, the incubation period may be as long as 12 weeks. After such an extended period, the origin of the disease can be difficult or impossible to trace.

C. Early Symptoms

In the early stages before marked symptoms appear, the patient may have a low-grade fever, loss of appetite, and weight loss and may tire easily. There may be a slight cough, and eventually sputum, indicating the possible presence of tubercle bacilli in the throat and saliva.

D. Later Symptoms

Definite temperature elevation, particularly in the afternoon, night sweats, weakness, and a persistent cough become apparent. Diagnosis is by chest radiograph and tuberculin testing.

E. Reactivation Tuberculosis

A focus of an infection may remain inactive and later produce a recurrence. Treatment of a primary infection may have been incomplete. Reactivity may be related to a debilitating condition or immunosuppression.

Reactivation of latent tuberculous infection may occur after many years. Usually a patient with a healthy immune system is asymptomatic and cannot spread the disease to others. The infection can be eliminated with antituberculosis drugs. ■

F. Multidrug-Resistant Tuberculosis

Multiple antituberculosis drugs are taken daily or several times a week for 6 months to treat active tuberculosis (TB). Three of the principal drugs used are isoniazid, pyrazinamide, and rifampin.

If medications are not prescribed properly or are not taken by the patient regularly, the tubercle bacilli can become resistant. The drug-resistant organisms can be transmitted and can cause disease in the recipient. Multidrug-resistant TB is difficult and expensive to treat.

The first line of prevention for multidrug-resistant TB is supervision of treatment so the medication is used properly. The second approach is to locate and treat persons with latent TB, particularly those at a high risk for reactivation. Direct supervision to assure completion of the full course of treatment is required.

III. CLINICAL MANAGEMENT

A. Official Recommendations (CDC)[10]

1. *Periodic Risk Assessment.*
2. *Medical History.* Routine questioning of patients about a history of tuberculosis and symptoms suggestive of disease; updating history regularly.
3. *Referral.* Prompt referral of patients with symptoms or history suggestive of tuberculosis for medical evaluation.
4. *Deferral of Elective Dental Treatment.* Obtain a physician's confirmation of the state of the patient's health. If the patient is diagnosed with active tuberculosis, elective treatment should be deferred until the patient is no longer infectious.
5. *Urgent Dental Care.* For a patient suspected of having infectious tuberculosis, use of a facility that can offer isolation and optimal ventilation and wearing respiratory protection (highest filtration level mask) are needed.
6. *Dental Health-Care Workers.* Prompt medical evaluation for a dental worker with a persistent cough (3 weeks) especially if with weight loss, fever, and other symptoms.
7. *Separation of Suspected or Confirmed Tuberculosis Patients.* A separate reception area where the patient can wait may be indicated. Appointments arranged to prevent a waiting period are preferred.

B. Extraoral and Intraoral Examination

Tuberculosis is primarily a lesion of the lungs, but any organ or tissue may be involved.

1. *Lymphadenopathy.* Regional lymph nodes may be enlarged.
2. *Oral Lesions.*[11] Oral lesions are relatively rare, but when they occur, they are usually ulcers. They may be located on the soft or hard palate and, occasionally, on the tongue.

C. Patient Under Treatment

Chemotherapy can control the patient's contagious condition. Isoniazid, rifampin, and pyrazinamide are used, sometimes in combinations. After a few weeks from the beginning of therapy, bacilli in the sputum, the cough, and the infectivity are decreased.

VIRAL HEPATITIS

Hepatitis means inflammation of the liver. Viruses cause a variety of types of hepatitis. Some of the viruses have been specifically identified, and hepatitis A, hepatitis B, hepatitis C, hepatitis D (delta), and hepatitis E are described in this section. New viruses designated non-ABCDE and HGV have emerged from viral hepatitis in posttransfusion patients or injection-drug users.[12–14]

The incidence of hepatitis B has increased significantly over the past 20 years. It has been a serious occupational hazard for health-care workers. Among professional personnel, both medical and dental, the use of strict sterilization of equipment and materials, aseptic techniques, and self-protection measures is mandatory.

Table 2-2 lists the hepatitis terminology with abbreviations and significance.

HEPATITIS A[15]

Hepatitis A occurs much more frequently in children and young adults than in older adults. It is more severe in adults. Early immunization is indicated.

I. TRANSMISSION

A. Fecal–Oral Route

The most common transmission is through close contact in unsanitary conditions. Unwashed hands of an infected person can contaminate anything touched.

B. Waterborne and Food-borne

Epidemics may occur when sanitation is inadequate. Contaminated water may carry hepatitis A virus directly to those using the water, or it may contaminate shellfish grown in the water.

Infected food handlers can contaminate uncooked food or food handled after cooking.

C. Blood

In the earliest days of active disease, the blood contains transient hepatitis A viruses; however, transmission by blood transfusion is rare.

II. DISEASE PROCESS

A. Incubation and Communicability

The incubation period is from 15 to 50 days, with an average of 28 to 30 days. During the 2- to 3-week period before the onset of jaundice, the infection is communicable. Shortly after jaundice appears, the communicability begins to diminish. A carrier state has not been demonstrated.

B. Signs and Symptoms

The stages are defined by the incidence of jaundice as preicteric (before jaundice appears) and icteric (while jaundice is present). Hepatitis A without jaundice (anicteric) is two to three times more prevalent than the icteric form. A diagnosis of hepatitis is not always made, because without jaundice, symptoms may resemble influenza or other diseases.

1. *Preicteric Phase.* Typically, there is an abrupt onset of an influenza-like illness, with fever, headache, fatigue, nausea, vomiting, and abdominal pain. The liver may be enlarged and tender to palpation.
2. *Icteric Phase.* Jaundice may appear in adults, but rarely in children. Other symptoms become prolonged, and the patient may be ill for a few days to a month. Occasionally, chronic hepatitis follows, but 85% to 90% of patients recover completely.

III. IMMUNITY

Anti-HAV is usually detectable in the serum within 2 weeks of onset. Immunity to reinfection follows with recovery.

In addition to those who are known to have had the disease, many more people acquire immunity from undetected disease.

Vaccines for active immunization are available.

IV. PREVENTION

A. Sanitation and Personal Hygiene

Because the principal means of transmission is by way of the feces, prevention on that level is indicated.

1. Public health control of food handlers and of water contamination.
2. Personal hygiene control through scrupulous handwashing by a patient and all contacts, as well as by all health-care workers involved in patient care.

B. Application in Dental Setting

Instrument sterilization, use of disposable materials, and all related precautions for persons and objects contacted by the patient.

HEPATITIS B[15]

Hepatitis B differs in many respects from hepatitis A, particularly in mode of transmission, the length of the incubation period, the onset, and the existence of a chronic carrier state. Hepatitis B occurs at any age. Figure 2-3 shows a diagram of the hepatitis B virus.

TABLE 2-2 Viral Hepatitis: Abbreviations

Abbreviation	Term	Significance
Hepatitis A		
HAV	Hepatitis A virus	Etiologic agent for hepatitis A
anti-HAV	Antibody to hepatitis A virus	Acute or resolved infection
		Protective immune response to infection
		Passively acquired antibody
		Response to vaccination
IgM anti-HAV	IgM antibody to hepatitis A virus	Recent HAV infection
HAV-RNA	RNA of HAV	Detected by nucleic acid amplification and/or hybridization
Hepatitis B		
HBV	Hepatitis B virus (Dane particle)	Etiologic agent for hepatitis B
		Current HBV infection
HBsAg	Hepatitis B surface antigen	Surface marker in acute disease and carrier state
		Antigen used in hepatitis B vaccine
anti-HBs	Antibody to hepatitis B surface antigen	Indicates
		(1) Active immunity to HBV (past infection)
		(2) Passive immunity from HBIG
		(3) Immune response from HB vaccine
HBeAg	Hepatitis B e antigen	High titer HBV in serum indicates high infectivity
		Persists into carrier state
anti-HBe	Antibody to hepatitis B e antigen	Low titer HBV
		Low degree infectivity
HBcAg	Hepatitis B core antigen	Indicates acute, chronic, or resolved HBV infection
		Not elicited by vaccination
anti-HBc	Antibody to hepatitis B core antigen	Indicates prior HBV infection
IgM anti-HBc	IgM class antibody to hepatitis B core antigen	Indicates recent HBc infection
HBV-DNA	DNA of HBV	Detected by nucleic acid amplification and/or hybridization
Hepatitis C		
HCV	Hepatitis C virus (formerly parentally transmitted non-A, non-B)	Etiologic agent for hepatitis C
anti-HCV	Antibody to hepatitis C virus	Indicates acute disease and chronic state
		Resembles hepatitis B
HCV-RNA	RNA of HCV	Defines viremia; detected by nucleic acid amplification
Hepatitis D		
HDV	Hepatitis delta virus	Etiologic agent for hepatitis D
		Only infectious in presence of acute or chronic HBV infection
HDV-Ag	Delta antigen	Detectable during early acute HDV infection
anti-HDV	Antibody to hepatitis D virus	Indicates acute, resolved, or chronic infection
IgM anti-HDV	IgM-class antibody to HDV	Indicates either acute or chronic infection with active viral replication
HDV-RNA	RNA of HDV	Detected by nucleic acid amplification or hybridization
Hepatitis E		
HEV	Hepatitis E virus (formerly enterically transmitted non-A, non-B)	Etiologic agent for hepatitis E
anti-HEV	Antibody to hepatitis E virus	Indicates acute or resolved infection
IgM anti-HEV	IgM-class antibody to hepaptitis E virus	Indicates acute infection
Non-ABCDE		
Parenterally transmitted	Diagnosis of exclusion	Epidemiologic evidence of parenteral or sexual transmission
Enterically transmitted	Diagnosis of exclusion	Epidemiologic evidence of fecal–oral transmission
Immune globulins		
IG	Immune globulin	Contains antibodies to HAV and low-titer HBV antibodies
HBIG	Hepatitis B immune globulin	Contains high-titer antibodies to HBV

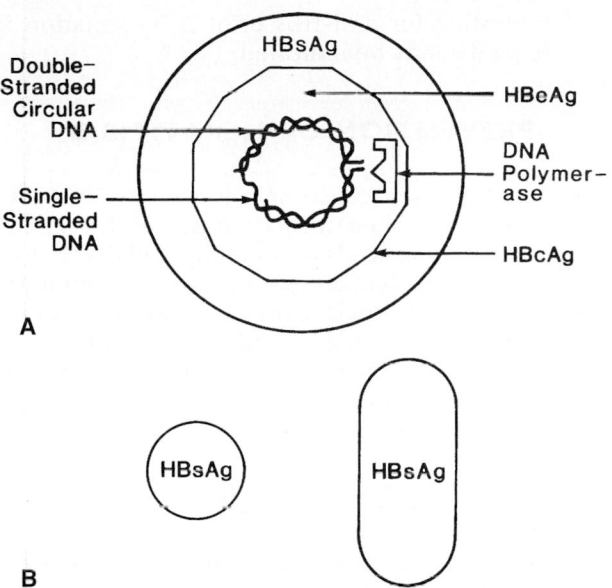

FIGURE 2-3 Diagram of the Hepatitis B Virus. (A) The virus is composed of an outer component of HBsAg and an inner component of HBcAg. Inside the core particle is a single molecule of circular, partially double-stranded DNA, an endogenous DNA polymerase, and HBeAg. **(B)** Spherical and tubular particles of HBsAg circulate in infected blood in great numbers. (Redrawn from Hoofnagle, J.H. & Schafer, D.F.: Serologic Markers of Hepatitis B Virus Infection, *Semin. Liver Dis.*, 6, 1, No. 1, 1986.)

I. TRANSMISSION

A. Blood and Other Body Fluids

Nearly all body fluids carry the virus, but only blood, saliva, semen, and vaginal fluids have been shown infectious. Hepatitis B viruses also have been found in gingival sulcus fluid, menstrual blood, tears, urine, perspiration, and nasopharyngeal secretions.

B. Modes of Transmission

Hepatitis B is transmitted by percutaneous and permucosal exposure.

1. Percutaneous (intravenous, intramuscular, subcutaneous).
2. Accidents with needle stick or other sharp instruments.
3. Perinatal exposure.
4. Exchanging of contaminated needles, syringes, and other paraphernalia by users of intravenous drugs.
5. Sexual exposure.
6. Infection from blood transfusion and blood products (extremely rare because all donors are screened and all blood has been tested since 1985).

C. Perinatal Transmission

During pregnancy, transmission of the hepatitis virus to the fetus can occur, and the newborn may be exposed during birth. An infant in-fected perinatally is at a high risk for chronic infection, which can lead to chronic liver disease or cancer of the liver later in life. Preventive measures are possible when pregnant women are tested for HBsAg and HBeAg.

II. INDIVIDUALS AT RISK OR WITH RISK BEHAVIORS FOR HEPATITIS B[15]

Risk populations are those that have an increased prevalence of infection, increased chances or likelihood of infection, and increased prevalence of disease carriers. High risk in HBV infection can be related to a variety of factors, including occupation, place of residence, lifestyle, confinement to an institution, other diseases and their treatments, and parenteral drug abuse. A person may belong to more than one of the risk groups listed here.

Health-care workers are included in the list; however, when they adhere to universal precautions with the use of protective barriers (gloves, masks, eyewear) and follow essential precautions for blood and other body fluid infection control, as well as have immunity following vaccination or acquired antibody to hepatitis B, they are really at a low risk.

A. Infants born to HIV-infected mothers.
B. Users of parenteral drugs (swapping contaminated needles).
C. Homosexually active men not practicing safe sex.*
D. Heterosexually active persons with multiple partners, including prostitutes, not practicing safe sex.*
E. Persons who have repeatedly contracted sexually transmitted diseases.
F. Clients and staff in institutions for the mentally retarded and current or former residents, particularly individuals with Down's syndrome.
G. Patients and staff in hemodialysis units.
H. Recipients of blood products used for treating clotting disorders, particularly before all blood was screened (prior to 1985).
I. Patients with active or chronic liver diseases.
J. Health-care workers with frequent blood contact are at a higher risk than are other health-care workers who have no or infrequent blood contact. Included are emergency room staff, hospital surgical staff, dental hygienists, dentists, and blood bank and plasma fractionation workers.
K. Household contacts of HBV carriers.
L. Male prisoners.
M. Military populations stationed in countries with high endemic HBV.
N. Returned travelers from areas of endemic HBV who stayed longer than 3 months or who were treated medically by transfusion while there.

---

*"Practice safe sex" is meant to include barrier protection and no exchange of body fluids (saliva, semen, vaginal secretions), in accord with recommended guidelines.

O. Morticians and embalmers.

P. Immigrants and refugees from areas of high endemic HBV.

III. DISEASE PROCESS

A. Incubation and Communicability

The incubation period is longer than that for hepatitis A and ranges from 2 to 6 months, with an average of 60 to 90 days. The period of communicability varies, but HBsAg may be detected in the blood as early as 30 days after exposure to the disease.

The presence of serum HBsAg indicates communicability. HBsAg may no longer be detected in the blood from a few days to 3 months after the icteric or jaundice stage of illness.

B. Transient Subclinical Infection

The majority of patients do not have an icteric stage but have subclinical disease. Many remain undiagnosed for hepatitis but develop antibodies and permanent immunity.

The infection is transient because the individual has a rapid, strong immune response to the hepatitis virus, and the HBV is cleared before it can become established.

C. Acute Type B Hepatitis

Hepatitis B cannot be distinguished from other viral hepatitis infections on the basis of the clinical signs and symptoms. The onset or preicteric stage with fever, malaise, and influenza-like symptoms is typical of all types of acute viral hepatitis. The onset may be slower and more insidious for hepatitis B and may include skin rash, itching, and joint pains.

The period of illness extends from 4 to 6 weeks for hepatitis A and usually longer for hepatitis B.

Convalescence begins with the disappearance of jaundice. During this period, serum antibody (anti-HBs) rises except in those who become permanent carriers.

D. Carrier State

A chronic carrier of HBV is defined as an individual with the HBsAg marker in the blood serum for more than 6 months. From 5% to 10% of infected persons develop a chronic carrier state.

A carrier state may also result following a subclinical undiagnosed exposure and, therefore, may be unknown to the individual. Many carriers eventually develop cirrhosis or cancer of the liver.

E. Immunity

The presence of anti-HBs in the serum shows that the person had a previous exposure to hepatitis B and is, therefore, immune to reinfection. The anti-HBs may be present, although unknown, because immunity may have been acquired following a subclinical, anicteric, or otherwise unrecognized case of hepatitis B.

Pretesting for anti-HBs prior to vaccination for hepatitis may be indicated.

PREVENTION OF HEPATITIS B

Hepatitis B viruses cause serious illness, including acute and chronic hepatitis, cirrhosis, and liver cancer, that sometimes leads to disability and death. Hepatitis is a critical occupational hazard for dental personnel because of their close association with the potentially infected body fluids of patients. Every health-care individual should be immunized so that the possibilities of disease acquisition and transmission can be minimized.

I. COMPREHENSIVE PREVENTIVE PROGRAM[15,16]

A. Eliminate Transmission During Infancy and Childhood

1. Prenatal testing of all pregnant women for HBsAg
   a. To locate newborns who require immunoprophylaxis to prevent perinatal infection.
   b. To identify household contacts who should be vaccinated.
2. Universal immunization of infants and children to be accomplished during routine health-care visits when vaccinations are usually administered. Hepatitis vaccine can be combined with diphtheria-tetanus-pertussis (DTP) or with influenza vaccine to reduce the number of injections.
3. Immunization of uninfected children in special education classes.
4. Immunization of adolescents and adults, particularly those at high risk. Eventually, as the universal vaccination of children continues, adult requirements will be lessened.

B. Enforce Blood Bank Control Measures[16]

1. Screening of donors; rejection of individuals who have a history of viral hepatitis, who show evidence of drug addiction, or who have received a blood transfusion or tattoo within the preceding 6 months.
2. Strict testing for all donated blood.

C. Enforce Sterilization or Use of Disposable Syringes and Needles

1. For acupuncture, skin testing, parenteral inoculations, body piercing, and all types of clinic treatments available to the public.
2. Education of public to expect certain standards.

II. ACTIVE IMMUNIZATION: THE VACCINES[15]

Hepatitis B vaccines are available for pre- and postexposure prophylaxis. They are administered intramuscularly in three doses, the first at the outset, then at 1 and 6 months.

The vaccine should be given only in the deltoid

muscle for adults and children and in the anterolateral thigh muscle for infants and neonates.

A. Plasma-derived HB Vaccine[†]

The original vaccine was prepared using purified and formalin-treated HBsAg from the plasma of chronic HBsAg carriers. In its preparation, the treatment steps inactivated all classes of viruses so that transmission of any other disease became impossible.

B. Recombinant DNA HB Vaccine[‡]

Recombinant DNA technology has been used to synthesize HBsAg in a culture of *Saccharomyces cerevisiae,* a yeast. The HBsAg is purified and sterilized.

C. Effectiveness

1. Both vaccines act in a comparable manner to stimulate antibody, and both convey the same degree of immunity.
2. In healthy 20- to 39-year-old adults, immunity is conferred in more than 95%. In children, protective antibodies are shown in 99%.
3. Postvaccination testing for anti-HBs within 1 to 6 months is recommended for a hemodialysis patient or other at-risk person having frequent exposure, including dental personnel.
4. Lower responses have been noted in older people, in hemodialysis patients, and in people receiving the injection in the buttock rather than in the deltoid muscle.[17]
5. The vaccines have no effect on a person who is already a carrier and no effect on a person who already has antibodies.
6. Immunization is not contraindicated during pregnancy. An HBV infection during pregnancy can be severe, and the newborn can become a permanent carrier.

D. Booster

1. The higher initial peak of response usually means longer persistence of antibody. Even when the antibody level drops there can still be protection.
2. A 7-year booster is suggested; however, the antibody level can be tested to determine individual needs.
3. For certain at-risk patients, particularly hemodialysis patients, annual antibody testing has been recommended.

III. POSTEXPOSURE PROPHYLAXIS

A. Indications for Prophylaxis

1. Newborn of HBsAg-positive mother.
2. Significant hepatitis B exposure to HBsAg-positive blood (page 70).

[†]Heptavax, Merck Sharp & Dohme.
[‡]Recombivax HB, Merck Sharp & Dohme; (Engerix B, Smith Kline Biologicals).

B. Hepatitis B Immune Globulin (HBIG)

High-titer anti-HBs immune globulin (HBIG) is available. Its primary use is for postexposure prophylaxis.

IG contains low-titer anti-HBs of varying amounts. It is effective against HBV to a lesser degree than is HBIG, but it should be used when HBIG is not available. IG is recommended when protection for exposure to hepatitis C and E is needed.

C. Procedure for Newborn of HBsAg-Positive Mother

1. *Immediate Treatment.* HBIG and HBV vaccine intramuscularly within 12 hours of birth and subsequently as recommended for a specific vaccine.
2. *Effect.* The combined treatment prevents up to 94% of infants from developing a carrier state.
3. *Risk.* Breast-feeding poses no risk of infection when prophylaxis has been started.

D. Procedure for Percutaneous Exposure or Wound From a Contaminated Instrument
(pages 69 to 70 and Table 4-6)

HEPATITIS C[15,18]

Hepatitis that developed as a result of transfusion but could not be classified with hepatitis A or B was originally called hepatitis non-A, non-B. When studied over time, two patterns of non-A, non-B hepatitis were recognized. The first, associated with blood transfusion and the use of contaminated needles, became hepatitis C. The second type was associated with waterborne epidemics and is now called hepatitis E.

Hepatitis C, caused by the hepatitis C virus (HCV), has been recognized as the former chief cause of transfusion-associated non-A, non-B hepatitis. HCV also has a role in many cases of chronic liver disease. Now, a serologic test for antibody to HCV has been developed and is an established test for blood donors. This advance in making blood transfusion safe is highly significant.

I. TRANSMISSION

Hepatitis C can be acquired by percutaneous exposure to contaminated blood and plasma derivatives, contaminated needles and syringes, transfusion, or accidental needle stick. HCV has been demonstrated in saliva. Nonpercutaneous routes include sexual transmission and perinatal exposure.

II. DISEASE PROCESS

The onset of viral hepatitis C can be insidious, with no clinical symptoms, or the patient can have abdominal discomfort, nausea, and vomiting and can progress to jaundice. Chronic liver disease is more common than with hepatitis B.

III. PREVENTION AND CONTROL

Measures recommended for hepatitis B can be applied to hepatitis C. Testing of all donated blood is basic to control.

HEPATITIS D[15,18]

The delta hepatitis virus, also called the delta agent, cannot cause infection except in the presence of HBV infection. The diagram in Figure 2-4 shows the delta antigen surrounded by HBsAg.

I. TRANSMISSION

Most frequently, the delta infection is superimposed on HBsAg carriers. It occurs primarily in persons who have multiple exposures to HBV, particularly patients with hemophilia and intravenous drug users.

Transmission is similar to that of HBV, that is, by direct exposure to contaminated blood and serous body fluids, contaminated needles and syringes, sexual contacts, and perinatal transfer.

II. DISEASE PROCESS

Delta hepatitis is more severe and the mortality rate is greater than with hepatitis B alone. The onset is abrupt and signs and symptoms resemble hepatitis B. Infection can occur in the following ways.

A. Coinfection

Acute delta hepatitis occurring with acute HBV infection may lead to resolution of both types. Clearance of HBV may lead to clearance of delta virus.

B. Superinfection

Acute delta hepatitis is superimposed on an existing carrier HBV state. The HBV carrier state remains unchanged, and a delta carrier state may develop in addition.

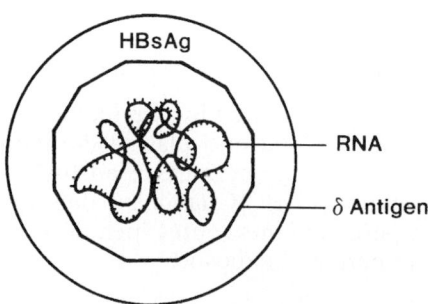

■ **FIGURE 2-4 Diagram of the Hepatitis Delta Virus.** The delta agent antigen is surrounded by the hepatitis B surface antigen. (Redrawn from Hoofnagle, J.H.: Type D Hepatitis and the Hepatitis Delta Virus, in Thomas, H.C. & Jones, E.A.: *Recent Advances in Hepatology.* Edinburgh, Churchill Livingstone, 1986.)

C. Superimposition

Chronic delta hepatitis superimposes on the chronic HBsAg carrier.

III. PREVENTION

All measures used to prevent hepatitis B prevent delta hepatitis because HDV is dependent on the presence of HBV. Immunization with hepatitis B vaccine also protects the recipient from delta hepatitis infection.

HEPATITIS E[15,18]

Hepatitis E (HEV) was formerly known as enterically transmitted non-A, non-B hepatitis. The clinical course and distribution are like those of hepatitis A.

I. TRANSMISSION

Hepatitis E is transmitted by contaminated water, as well as person-to-person by the fecal–oral route. Reported large outbreaks have been associated with fecally contaminated water sources after heavy rains where sewage disposal was inadequate. Adults have been affected more than have children. The mortality rate in pregnant women has been high.

II. PREVENTION AND CONTROL

A. Sanitary disposal of wastes.
B. Handwashing, especially before handling food.

HERPESVIRUS DISEASES[19]

The herpesvirus infections represent a wide variety of disease entities that are highly infectious. Each virus is antigenically distinct. Herpesviruses produce diseases with latent, recurrent, and sometimes malignant tendencies. For example, herpes simplex type 2 has been implicated in cervical cancer and herpes simplex type 1 in oral cancer.

Immunosuppressed patients have more frequent and severe herpes infections. Herpesviruses are among the opportunistic organisms in acquired immunodeficiency syndrome (AIDS) (page 34, and Table 2-5).

Table 2-3 lists herpesviruses, their abbreviations, and some of the infections they cause.

VIRAL LATENCY

I. GANGLIA

The herpesviruses have the ability to travel along sensory nerve pathways to specific ganglia. The specific ganglia are usually the following:

A. Herpes simplex type 1 (HSV-1) travels to the trigeminal nerve ganglion (Figure 2-5).
B. Herpes simplex type 2 (HSV-2) goes to the thoracic, lumbar, and sacral dorsal root ganglia.

TABLE 2-3 Herpesviruses

Abbreviation	Name of Virus	Infections
VZV	Varicella-zoster	Varicella (chickenpox) Herpes zoster (shingles)
EBV	Epstein-Barr	EBV mononucleosis
HCMV	Human cytomegalo-virus	Cytomegalovirus disease Fetal infection
HSV-1 HSV-2	Herpes simplex virus, types 1 and 2	Herpes labialis Herpetic gingivosto-matitis Herpetic kerato-conjunctivitis Herpetic whitlow Encephalitis Neonatal herpes
HHV-6	Human herpesvirus 6	Mononucleosis-like rash

C. Varicella-zoster virus (VZV) goes to the sensory ganglia of the vagal, spinal, or cranial nerves.

II. PRIMARY INFECTION: SEQUENCE OF EVENTS

A. Exposure of person to the virus at the mucosal surface or abraded skin.
B. Replication begins in the cells of the dermis and epidermis.
C. Infection of sensory or autonomic nerve endings.
D. Virus travels along the nerve to the ganglion.

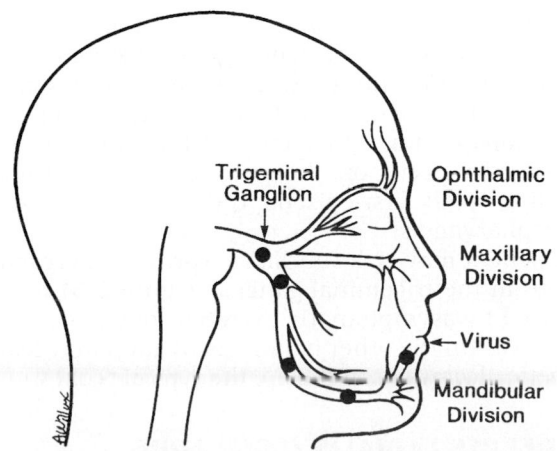

FIGURE 2-5 Latent Infection of Herpes Simplex Virus. Path of the virus traced from point of viral penetration on lip to establishment of latent infection in the trigeminal ganglion.

E. After primary disease resolves, the virus becomes latent in the ganglion.
F. Reactivation at a later date is precipitated by a stimulus, such as sunlight, immunosuppression, infection, or stress (physical or emotional).
G. Virus transports along the nerve to the body surface where replication takes place and a lesion forms, usually in the same spot as the previous activation.

VARICELLA-ZOSTER VIRUS (VZV)[20]

Chickenpox (varicella) and shingles (herpes zoster) are caused by the same virus, the varicella-zoster virus.

I. CHICKENPOX

A. Transmission

Chickenpox is a highly contagious disease transmitted by direct contact, droplet (possibly airborne), or by indirect contact with articles soiled by discharges from the vesicles and the respiratory tract.

B. Disease Process

Primarily a disease of children, chickenpox is occasionally found in adults not previously exposed. Chickenpox can be life threatening in children who are immunocompromised, such as children with HIV infection.

When primary maternal VZV occurs during pregnancy or during the peripartum period, fetal infection may result in congenital malformations.

The disease is characterized by a maculopapular rash that becomes vesicular in a few days and then scabs. The lesions appear anywhere on the body, more abundantly on the covered than on the exposed parts. When oral lesions occur, they may spread into the upper respiratory tract.

If the itchy, crusted lesions of the skin are scratched, a secondary bacterial infection can result. Other complications are rare, but neurologic and ocular disorders are possible.

II. SHINGLES

A. Recurrent Infection

Chickenpox leaves a lasting immunity, but the VZV remains latent in the dorsal root ganglia. Reactivation in adulthood may result from immunosuppression, such as from drug therapy or from HIV infection, and in people with advanced neoplastic disease.

B. Disease Process

Shingles consists of localized unilateral eruptions associated with the nerve endings of the area innervated by the infected sensory nerves. When the second division of the trigeminal nerve is involved, intraoral lesions may occur.

Pain, burning, and itching are characteristic. Eye infections and complications of the lungs, central nervous system, liver, and pancreas have been secondary developments.

EPSTEIN-BARR VIRUS (EBV)[21]

One type of infectious mononucleosis is caused by infection with the EBV. It has also been shown that the EBV replicates within the epithelial cells in hairy leukoplakia, the lesion associated with subsequent development of the acquired immunodeficiency syndrome (pages 34 and 36). EBV is also a factor in the development of certain lymphomas.

Infectious mononucleosis is generally a disease of adolescents and young adults. It is characterized by fever, lymphadenopathy, and sore throat, and is identified by specific atypical lymphocytes called mononucleosis cells.

The disease is transmitted orally by direct contact and by droplet. Viruses are excreted through the saliva even when the patient has no symptoms of disease, so there may be a long period of communicability or a lasting carrier state. EBV can remain latent and become reactivated, particularly when the immune system is compromised by disease or drug therapy.

CYTOMEGALOVIRUS (HCMV)[22]

Cytomegalovirus infections appear in various forms. The most affected age groups are from 1 to 2 years and from 16 to 50 years. The infections are sometimes latent or subclinical in adults. HCMV has been found in the tumor cells of Kaposi's sarcoma.

I. TRANSMISSION

A. Congenital and Neonatal
The virus from the mother's primary or recurrent infection may infect the infant *in utero*, in the birth canal, or through breast milk.

B. Direct Infections
The virus is excreted in urine, saliva, cervical secretions, and semen. Infection can result from the following:
1. Blood transfusion.
2. Graft transplant from a donor with latent infection.
3. Sexual transmission through semen, vaginal fluid, or saliva.
4. Respiratory droplet, especially among children. Children attending day-care centers have a high prevalence of HCMV infection.

II. DISEASE PROCESS

A. Infants
Cytomegalic inclusion disease in a fetus is the most severe form of the infection. Survivors may be premature, anemic, and have mental retardation, microcephaly, motor disabilities, deafness, and chronic liver disease.

B. Adult Infection
Symptomatic infection is relatively rare, but infectious mononucleosis, pneumonitis, and other infections may be caused by HCMV.

C. Immunosuppression and Debilitation
HCMV, an opportunistic agent, is a common cause of both primary and reactivated infections in immunodeficient or immunosuppressed patients. Infection with HCMV is a serious complication of the acquired immunodeficiency syndrome.

III. PREVENTION
A. Personal hygiene: handwashing.
B. Universal precautions by health-care workers.
C. Seropositivity of donor checked before organ transplant.

HERPES SIMPLEX VIRUS INFECTIONS[19,23]

Primary infection usually occurs in children but may occur at any age. Antibodies (anti-HSV) are produced but do not guarantee immunity to recurrent herpes or to other herpesvirus infections.

Sulcular epithelium serves as a reservoir for the viruses.[24] Anti-HSV is present in the gingival sulcus fluid. The possibility exists that trauma to the oral area during a dental or dental hygiene appointment may bring about herpetic recurrence.

Acyclovir, an antiviral drug, has been used in topical, oral, and intravenous forms. Acyclovir is a selective inhibitor of replication of HSV and VZV. It is established as the drug of choice for treatment of a wide range of infections caused by HSV and VZV.

I. PRIMARY HERPETIC GINGIVOSTOMATITIS
The primary infection may be asymptomatic. When clinical disease is evident, gingivostomatitis and pharyngitis are the most frequent manifestations, with fever, malaise, inability to eat, and lymphadenopathy for 2 to 7 days. Painful oral vesicular lesions may occur on the gingiva, mucosa, tongue, and lips. Both first-episode HSV-1 and HSV-2 can cause pharyngitis.

A patient may be a subclinical carrier, and reactivation from the trigeminal ganglia (Figure 2-5) may be followed by asymptomatic excretion of the viruses in the saliva. On the other hand, reactivation may lead to herpetic ulcerations of the lip, the typical "cold sore."

II. HERPES LABIALIS (COLD SORE, FEVER BLISTER)
Both HSV-1 and HSV-2 cause genital and oral–facial infections that cannot be distinguished clinically. Re-

activations of oral–facial HSV-1 infections are more frequent than of oral–facial HSV-2 infections. Reactivations of genital HSV-2 are more frequent than of genital HSV-1 infections.

Recurrent (HSV) lesions occur at or near the primary lesion at indefinite intervals. They are usually triggered by stress, sunlight, illness, or trauma. Not infrequently, they relate to the patient's dental appointment, when emotional stress and oral trauma may be involved.

A. Prodrome
Before the local lesion appears, there may be burning or slight stinging sensations with slight swelling as a forewarning or prodrome. Most frequently, the recurrent lesion is at the vermilion border of the lower lip, although less commonly, the lesions may occur intraorally on the gingiva or the hard palate.

B. Clinical Characteristics
A group of vesicles forms and eventually ruptures and coalesces. Crusting follows, and healing may take up to 10 days. The lesions are infectious, with viral shedding. Care must be taken by the patient because autoinfection (to the eye, nose, or genitals, for example) is possible, as is infection of others.

III. HERPETIC WHITLOW[19]

Herpetic whitlow is the herpes simplex infection of the fingers that results from the virus entering through minor skin abrasions. The most frequent location is around a fingernail, where cracks in the skin often occur.

A. Transmission
A whitlow may be a primary or recurrent infection of HSV-1 or HSV-2. Transmission results from direct contact with a vesicular lesion on a patient's lip or with saliva that contains the viruses.

Members of the dental team who do not wear protective gloves will have whitlow on the index fingers and thumbs that are in close contact with the patient's saliva where instrumentation and retraction are performed.

Autoinfection from a lip or intraoral herpetic lesion is possible while nail biting.

B. Disease Process
The whitlow usually starts suddenly as an area of irritation that becomes tender and painful. Groups of vesicles coalesce, and the whole healing process may last up to 2 weeks. The lesions are infectious and transmissible even before the whitlow appears and is diagnosed. Recurrences are not unusual.

IV. OCULAR HERPES[19]

Herpes simplex lesions in the eye can be a primary or recurrent infection of HSV-1 or HSV-2.

A. Transmission
1. Splashing saliva or fluid from a vesicular lesion directly into an unprotected eye.
2. Extension of infection from a facial lesion.
3. Infection of an infant's eye *in utero* or during birth.

B. Disease Process
Symptoms include fever, pain, blurring of vision, swelling, excess tears, and secondary bacterial infection. Herpes keratoconjunctivitis can cause deep inflammation and, when left untreated, is a leading cause of loss of sight.

CLINICAL MANAGEMENT

I. PATIENT HISTORY
All patient histories need questions to determine experiences with herpesviruses. Terminology may be a problem, so such terms as "fever blisters" or "cold sores" need to be used to assure patient understanding.

II. POSTPONE APPOINTMENT WITH PATIENT WITH ACTIVE LESION

A. Problems of Transmission
Explain the following to patient:
1. Contagiousness, with possible transmission to other patients.
2. Autoinoculation possible from instrumentation that can splash viruses to the patient's eye or extend lesion to nose.

B. Irritation to Lesions
Irritation to the lesions can prolong the course and increase the severity of the infection.

C. Prodromal State May Be the Most Contagious
The patient should be requested to call ahead to change an appointment when it is known that a lesion is developing.

HIV-1 INFECTION[25]

The acquired immunodeficiency syndrome (AIDS) is a severe condition caused by infection with the *human immunodeficiency virus* (HIV-1). A second virus, HIV-2, isolated in West Africa and later in Europe and North America, has been shown to have similar characteristics and transmission as the original HIV-1. Both are slow, progressive, often lethal diseases and have the ability to persist within cells such as macrophages for long periods of time.

HIV-1-infected patients may present with manifestations that range from mild abnormalities in immune response without apparent signs and symptoms to profound immunosuppression associated with a variety of life-threatening infections and rare malignant conditions. Box 2-2 provides abbreviations and terminology relating to HIV-1 infection and AIDS.

TRANSMISSION

The HIV-1 virus has been found in most body fluids. Transmission has been demonstrated by way of blood, semen, vaginal secretions, and breast milk.

I. ROUTES OF TRANSMISSION

A. Sexual Contact (Heterosexual or Homosexual)
The virus from an infected person's blood, semen, or vaginal secretions enters the blood circulation through tiny breaks in the rectum, vagina, or penis.

B. Blood and Blood Products
1. Injection drug users: contaminated, shared needles carry the infection.
2. Transfusion and use of blood products by patients with blood disorders. The serologic testing of all donor blood has nearly eliminated the threat of infection from transfusion or blood products.
3. Occupational accidental injuries: low risk of infection.

C. Perinatal
1. Placenta: viruses can be transmitted across the placenta.
2. During delivery: exposure during passage through infected genital tract.
3. Postnatally: through breast-feeding.

II. INDIVIDUALS AT HIGH RISK FOR INFECTION

A. Sexually active homosexual and bisexual men having multiple partners without practicing safe sex.§
B. Users or former users of intravenous drugs, particularly when contaminated needles are shared.
C. Recipients of blood transfusions or blood products prior to mandatory testing for HIV-1 antibodies in 1985. People with hemophilia or other coagulation disorders are included.
D. Male and female prostitutes who do not practice safe sex.§
E. Health-care workers who do not adhere to strict barrier procedures and do not follow essential blood and other body fluid precautions for infection control.

§"Practice safe sex" is meant to include barrier protection and no exchange of body fluids (saliva, semen, vaginal secretions) in accord with recommended guidelines.

BOX 2-2 KEY ABBREVIATIONS: HIV and AIDS

AIDS: acquired immunodeficiency sydrome.

AZT (ZDV): zidovudine, retrovir; drug used for the treatment of HIV infection and AIDS; first antiviral drug approved by the United States Food and Drug Administration (FDA).

CD4+: T-helper lymphocyte; primary target cell for HIV infection; CD4+ count decreases with the severity of HIV-related illness.

DNA: deoxyribonucleic acid; a nucleic acid found in a cell nucleus; a carrier of genetic information.

HIV: human immunodeficiency virus; causes AIDS.

HIV-1 antibody: antibody to human immunodeficiency virus type 1; antibody can be detected in the blood 6 to 8 weeks after infection.

HL: hairy leukoplakia.

IDU: injection-drug user.

KS: Kaposi's sarcoma; a malignant vascular tumor; an opportunistic neoplasm that may occur in people with HIV infection.

LAV: lymphadenopathy-associated virus; one of the former names for HIV.

MMWR: *Morbidity and Mortality Weekly Report;* publication of the United States Centers for Disease Control and Prevention **(CDCP)**, Atlanta, GA.

PCP: pneumocystis pneumonia; caused by *Pneumocystis carinii;* an opportunistic infection that occurs in people with HIV infection.

PGL: persistent generalized lymphadenopathy.

PWA: person with AIDS.

RNA: ribonucleic acid; a nucleic acid found in cytoplasm and in the nuclei of certain cells; RNA directs the synthesis of proteins and replaces DNA as a carrier of genetic codes in some viruses.

F. Females artificially inseminated with HIV-1-infected semen.

G. Recipients of HIV-1-infected organ transplants.

H. Steady sexual partners of all those previously listed who do not practice safe sex.[||]

I. Steady sexual partners of those infected with AIDS or at high risk for AIDS who do not practice safe sex.[||]

J. Infants born to HIV-1-infected mothers.

K. Infants fed breast milk from HIV-1-infected mothers.

LIFE CYCLE OF THE HIV-1[26]

HIV-1 is a retrovirus, and in a retrovirus, RNA is the core genetic material. The enzyme reverse transcriptase is essential for replication. a diagram of the HIV-1 virus is shown in Figure 2-6.

The complex life cycle of the HIV-1 can be divided into two general phases: the establishment of infection, and the production of new virus particles.

I. ESTABLISHMENT OF INFECTION

A. Binding to a Target/Host Cell

1. HIV-1 enters the body and passes by way of the blood to a target cell surface, where it binds to a specific cellular receptor, CD4+.

2. Target cells that have CD4+ receptors include T-helper lymphocytes, monocytes, macrophages, and certain neurons and glial cells of the brain tissue.

B. Entry Through Wall of the Target/Host Cell

Fusion occurs between the virion and the target cell membrane, and the virus becomes uncoated. Only the viral RNA and the enzymes enter the cell.

C. Reverse Transcription

1. Viral RNA is changed into single-stranded DNA by the enzyme *reverse transcriptase*. Another enzyme, *ribonuclease*, destroys the RNA, which is no longer needed. Single-stranded DNA is then translated to a double-stranded DNA, which is called the *provirus*.

2. The provirus migrates to the nucleus of the host cell, enters the nucleus, and becomes permanently integrated with host DNA.

D. Infection Is Established

Once the viral DNA enters the host nucleus, infection is established. Succeeding progeny of the host cell are HIV-1 infected.

E. Latent Period

The integrated proviral DNA stays latent indefinitely.

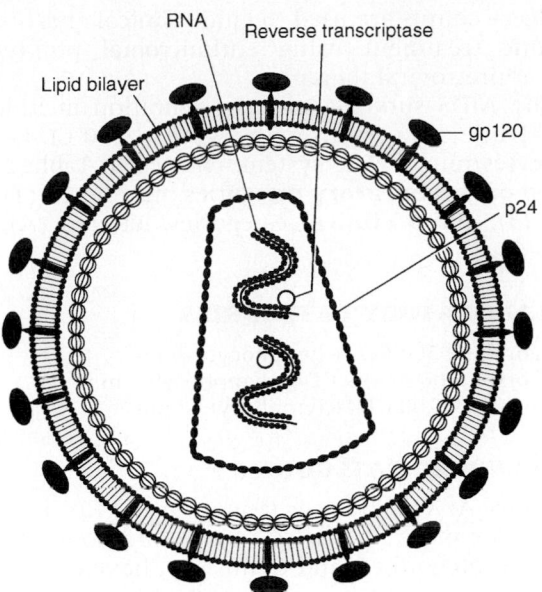

■ **FIGURE 2-6 Diagram of the Human Immunodeficiency Virus (HIV-1).** The envelope of the virion is composed of the lipid bilayer with glycoproteins (gp120). The core contains two strands of RNA, enzymes, and core proteins (p24).

II. PRODUCTION OF NEW VIRUS

A. Activation of the Host Cell

1. Stimulation causes activation. The DNA of the infected host cell can form new viral RNA and protein.

2. Viral proteins are broken down to form "building blocks" for progeny viral particles.

3. DNA is transcribed into RNA for the new virus.

B. Budding From Host Cell: Release

1. Host cell membrane is used to make a new viral envelope.

2. Free new virion is released into the blood stream; it proceeds to find another CD4+ for attachment.

D. Host Cell Outcome

1. Loss of normal function.

2. Destruction; reduced numbers of host CD4+ cells lead to immune suppression.

3. The CD4+, or T-helper lymphocyte, is the primary target cell for HIV-1 infection. A decrease in the number of the CD4+ cells correlates with the risk and severity of HIV-1-related illnesses.

HIV-1 CLASSIFICATION SYSTEM FOR ADOLESCENTS AND ADULTS[27]

The CDC classification system emphasizes the importance of the CD4+ lymphocyte count in the clinical management of HIV-1-infected individuals. Measures

---

[||]"Practice safe sex" is meant to include barrier protection and no exchange of body fluids (saliva, semen, vaginal secretions) in accord with recommended guidelines.

of CD4+ counts are used to guide clinical and/or therapeutic treatment using antimicrobial prophylaxis and antiretroviral therapies.

The AIDS surveillance case definition includes all HIV-1-infected persons with less than 200 CD4+ lymphocytes/mm^3.[27] The system, charted in Table 2-4, is based on **3 laboratory** categories, numbered (1), (2), and (3), and **3 clinical** categories, lettered (A), (B), and (C).

I. LABORATORY CATEGORIES

Category 1: ≥ 500 CD4+ lymphocytes/mm^3
Category 2: 200 to 499 CD4+ lymphocytes/mm^3
Category 3: < 200 CD4+ lymphocytes/mm^3

II. CLINICAL CATEGORIES

Category A: Asymptomatic (acute primary) HIV-1 or PGL
One or more of the following conditions. (Conditions in categories B and C must not have occurred.)

- Asymptomatic HIV-1 infection
- Persistent generalized lymphadenopathy (PGL)
- Acute (primary) HIV-1 infection or history of acute HIV-1 infection

Category B: Symptomatic (not A or C)

Examples of conditions in category B follow. They must be attributed to HIV-1 infection, indicative of a defect in cell-mediated immunity, and not listed under category C.

- Bacillary angiomatosis
- Candidiasis, oropharyngeal (thrush)
- Candidiasis, vulvovaginal: persistent, frequent, or poorly responsive to therapy
- Cervical dysplasia (moderate or severe)/cervical carcinoma in situ
- Constitutional symptoms, such as fever (38.5° C) or diarrhea lasting > 1 month
- Hairy leukoplakia, oral

- Herpes zoster (shingles), involving at least two distinct episodes or more than one dermatome
- Idiopathic thrombocytopenic purpura
- Listeriosis
- Pelvic inflammatory disease, particularly if complicated by tubo-ovarian abscess
- Peripheral neuropathy

Category C: AIDS-Indicator Conditions

Conditions that follow in category C are strongly associated with severe immunodeficiency, occur frequently in HIV-1-infected individuals, and cause serious morbidity or mortality.

- Candidiasis of bronchi, trachea, or lungs
- Candidiasis, esophageal
- Cervical cancer, invasive**
- Coccidioidomycosis, disseminated or extrapulmonary
- Cryptococcosis, extrapulmonary
- Cryptosporidiosis, chronic intestinal (> 1 month's duration)
- Cytomegalovirus disease (other than liver, spleen, or nodes)
- Cytomegalovirus retinitis (with loss of vision)
- Encephalopathy, HIV-1-related
- Herpes simplex: chronic ulcer(s) (> 1 month's duration); or bronchitis, pneumonitis, or esophagitis
- Histoplasmosis, disseminated or extrapulmonary
- Isosporiasis, chronic intestinal (> 1 month's duration)
- Kaposi's sarcoma
- Lymphoma, Burkitt's (or equivalent term)
- Lymphoma, immunoblastic (or equivalent term)
- Lymphoma, primary, of brain
- *Mycobacterium avium* complex of *M. kansasii*, disseminated or extrapulmonary
- *Mycobacterium tuberculosis*, any site (pulmonary** or extrapulmonary)

**Added in the 1993 expansion of the AIDS surveillance case definition.

TABLE 2-4 1992 Revised Classification System for HIV Infection and Expanded AIDS Surveillance Case Definition for Adolescents and Adults*

Laboratory CD4+ Cell Categories	Clinical Categories		
	[A] Asymptomatic, or PGL†	[B] Symptomatic, not (A) or (C) conditions	[C] AIDS-indicator conditions‡
(1) ≥ 500/mm^3	A1	B1	C1
(2) 200–499/mm^3	A2	B2	C2
(3) <200/mm^3 AIDS-indicator cell count	A3	B3	C3

*The shaded boxes illustrate the expansion of the AIDS surveillance case definition. Persons with AIDS-indicator conditions (category C) are currently reportable to the health department in every state and U.S. territory. In addition to persons with clinical category C conditions (categories C1, C2, and C3), persons with CD4+ lymphocyte counts of less than 200/mm^3 (categories A3 or B3) also have been reportable as AIDS cases in the United States and its territories since April 1, 1992.
†PGL = persistent generalized lymphadenopathy. Clinical category A includes acute (primary) HIV infection.
‡See text.

- *Mycobacterium,* other species or unidentified species, disseminated or extrapulmonary
- *Pneumocystis carinii* pneumonia
- Pneumonia, recurrent[††]
- Progressive multifocal leukoencephalopathy
- *Salmonella* septicemia, recurrent
- Toxoplasmosis of brain
- Wasting syndrome caused by HIV-1

CLINICAL COURSE OF HIV-I INFECTION[28]

A detectable antibody level usually can be detected within 1 to 3 months after exposure to the HIV-1 virus. Antibody presence indicates infection. Viral production is high throughout all stages of infection.

I. INCUBATION PERIOD

The incubation period ranges from the time of infection until the time when symptoms of AIDS are evident, which may be 15 years or longer.

II. THE ACUTE SEROCONVERSION SYNDROME

A. Initial Infection

After exposure, approximately one-half of those infected will have flulike or mononucleosis-like symptoms within 2 to 6 weeks. They are often unsuspected as associated with HIV-1 infection.

1. *Symptoms.* A wide variety of possible symptoms have been experienced, especially fever, lymphadenopathy, pharyngitis, fatigue, muscle pain, and a skin rash.
2. *Viremia.* Within 2 to 4 weeks after the initial infection, high levels of virus occur related to dissemination and development of antibody.

III. EARLY HIV-1 DISEASE

A. CD4+ Count: greater than 500 cells/mm^3.

B. Symptoms: with CD4+ count high, no symptoms usually, but if any, lymphadenopathy and dermatologic lesions.

C. Oral Lesions: more common in later stages.

1. Aphthous ulcers, herpes simplex labialis.
2. Hairy leukoplakia: pathognomonic for underlying HIV-1 infection; when occurring in early HIV-1 disease, it is considered an indicator of disease progression.

IV. INTERMEDIATE STAGE OF HIV-1 DISEASE

A. CD4+ Count: between 200 and 500 cells/ mm^3.

B. Symptoms: skin and oral lesions become more common; recurrent herpes simplex, varicella-zoster, fever, weight loss, candidiasis (oropharyngeal or vaginal), myalgias, headaches, fatigue.

C. Oral Lesions: more common; candidiasis is

considered a predictor for *Pneumocystis carinii* pneumonia.

V. LATE STAGE DISEASE: AIDS

A. CD4+ Count: 50 to 200 cells/mm^3.

B. Symptoms: AIDS-indicator conditions (Table 2-4).

1. *Opportunistic Infections.* An opportunistic infection is caused by a microorganism that is capable of taking advantage of a compromised immune system as an opportunity to develop in a person in whom the disease would not otherwise develop. When the immune reactions of the person with HIV-1 infection decrease, as monitored by the lowered CD4+ lymphocyte count, opportunistic infections can become more frequent, extensive, and severe.
2. *Constitutional Disease: HIV-1 Wasting Syndrome.* Long-term fever, severe weight loss, anemia, chronic diarrhea, and chronic weakness are all effects of loss of immune response and repeated opportunistic diseases. The wasting syndrome symptoms, along with organic mental disorders (HIV-1 dementia), contribute to the severe degeneration during the terminal AIDS illness.
3. *Encephalopathy: Organic Mental Disorders.* Disabling cognitive and/or motor dysfunction may develop with symptoms of apathy, inability to concentrate, poor memory, and depression.
4. *Neoplasms.* Several neoplasms, related to the underlying immunodeficiency, are common indicators of HIV-1 infection and AIDS. These include Kaposi's sarcoma, primary B-cell lymphoma of the brain, and non-Hodgkin's lymphoma.

ORAL MANIFESTATIONS OF HIV-I INFECTION

Many HIV-1-infected patients have head and/or neck manifestations. Certain oral findings have been identified as indicators of HIV-1 infection.

Oral symptoms can be integrated with information from the patient's medical history. From the complete assessment, an early recognition by dental clinicians, or at least a suspicion, of HIV-1 infection may result. Referral for medical evaluation and testing can be recommended.

Early recognition of an HIV-1-seropositive condition is important because drugs available for treatment can slow down the process of the disease. With early intervention, severe complications may be prevented, and the long-term quality of life can be improved.

Table 2-5 lists oral lesions according to whether the

[††]Added in the 1993 expansion of the AIDS surveillance case definition.

TABLE 2-5 Oral Lesions Associated with HIV Infection Classification

Group I. Lesions Strongly Associated with HIV Infections	Group III. Lesions seen with HIV Infection

Candidiasis
    Erythematous
    Pseudomembranous
Hairy Leukoplakia
Kaposi's sarcoma
Non-Hodgkin's lymphoma
Periodontal disease
    Linear gingival erythema
    Necrotizing (ulcerative)
        gingivitis
    Necrotizing (ulcerative)
        periodontitis
	Bacterial infections
	    Actinomyces israelii
	    Escherichia coli
	    Klebsiella pneumoniae
	Cat-scratch disease
	Drug reactions (ulcerative
	    erythema multiforme,
	    lichenoid, toxic
	    epidermolysis)
	Epithelioid (bacillary)
	    angiomatosis
	Fungal infection other than
	    candidiasis
	    *Cryptococcus
	        neoformans*
	    Geotrichum candidum
	    Histoplasma capsulatum
	    *Mucoraceae
	        (mucormycosis/
	        zygomycosis)*
	    Aspergillus flavus
	Neurologic disturbances
	    Facial palsy
	    Trigeminal neuralgia
	Recurrent aphthous
	    stomatitis
	Viral infections
	    Cytomegalovirus
	    Molluscum contagiosum

Group II. Lesions Less Commonly Associated with HIV Infection	

Bacterial infections
    *Mycobacterium avium-
        intracellulare*
    *Mycobacterium
        tuberculosis*
Melanotic
    hyperpigmentation
Necrotizing (ulcerative)
    stomatitis
Salivary gland disease
    Dry mouth due to
        decreased salivary flow
        rate
    Unilateral or bilateral
        swelling of major
        salivary glands
Thrombocytopenic purpura
Ulceration NOS (not
    otherwise specified)
Viral infections
    Herpes simplex virus
    Human papillomavirus
        (warty-like lesions)
    Condyloma
        acuminatum
    Focal epithelial
        hyperplasia
    Verruca vulgaris
    Varicella-zoster virus
    Herpes zoster
    Varicella	

(From European Commission Clearinghouse on Oral Problems Related to HIV Infection and World Health Organization Collaborating Centre on Oral Manifestations of the Human Immunodeficiency Virus, 1990, with revisions, 1992.)

condition is strongly associated, less commonly associated, or possibly associated with HIV-1 infection.

I. EXTRAORAL EXAMINATION

A careful extraoral assessment is essential and must be conducted at each appointment.

A. Lymphadenopathy

Palpation for enlarged lymph nodes is a routine part of every extraoral examination. In Chapter 8 (pages 118 to 120), procedures for palpation are described; the location of nodes is shown in Figure 8-4.

B. Skin Lesions

Several conditions listed in Table 2-5 develop in the skin. Examples are Kaposi's sarcoma, purpura, and herpetic lesions.

II. INTRAORAL EXAMINATION

Of the intraoral lesions listed as strongly associated with HIV-1 infection (group I in Table 2-5), candidiasis, Kaposi's sarcoma, and hairy leukoplakia have been highly correlated with the subsequent development of advanced HIV-1 infection. All three lesions are readily observable during an oral examination.

A. Fungal Infections[29]

Oral candidiasis, the most frequently occurring oral infection, appears in various forms. They are listed in Table 2-5.

Although usually recognized by clinical examination, the dentist may request the use of exfoliative cytology for differential distinction (Chapter 8, pages 126 to 127).

B. Viral Infections[29]

Herpes simplex, hairy leukoplakia, oral lesions of chickenpox, verruca vulgaris, condyloma acuminatum, and cytomegalovirus ulcer are all examples of lesions that may be seen.

C. Bacterial Infections: Gingival and Periodontal Infections

As with other oral manifestations, gingival changes may be an initial indicator of undiagnosed HIV-1 infection. On the other hand, there may not be any unusual gingival or periodontal changes that can be associated with HIV-1 infection, especially when the patient maintains a high level of personal and professional oral care.

The general clinical sequelae are that periodontal infections associated with HIV-1 infection tend to show more severe symptoms and to progress more rapidly than do periodontal conditions in people who are not immunosuppressed.

1. *Gingivitis: Linear Gingival Erythema.* Unusual degrees of severity of gingivitis may be observed. A 2- to 3-mm red band may appear along the gingival margin with petechia-like and/or diffuse red lesions of the attached

gingiva. Spontaneous bleeding and bleeding on gentle probing occur. Scaling, root planing, and an increased bacterial plaque control effort on a frequent maintenance plan are necessary but may not reach the degree of health usually expected.

2. *Necrotizing Ulcerative Gingivitis (NUG).* An increased incidence of NUG has been observed in HIV-1-positive patients. Ulceration and destruction of interdental papillae with spontaneous bleeding and pain may develop rapidly.

3. *Periodontal Infection.* A range of severity of periodontal involvement may be observed in HIV-1-infected patients. Severe soft tissue necrosis and rapid destruction of periodontal attachment characteristic of a rapidly progressive periodontitis can occur in a few months. In extreme cases, loss of crestal alveolar bone has led to bone exposure and sequestration.

Severe pain and difficulty in mastication contribute to patient discomfort and malnutrition.

D. Dental Assessment

Dental caries and dental erosion can be problems for patients medicated with zidovudine (AZT) or retrovir. Common side effects of AZT are nausea and vomiting. The patient who uses the medication several times each day and vomits each time could have dissolution of the enamel in the form of dental erosion. Personal daily and periodic professional fluoride applications must be included in the preventive oral hygiene program.

E. Xerostomia

Xerostomia, as a result of salivary gland diseases (Table 2-5, group II) or as a side effect of medications, can contribute to dental caries and discomfort from dry mucosa. In addition to fluoride therapy for dental caries control, the patient's diet should be reviewed and instruction given in the selection of noncariogenic foods and snack items. Other information on xerostomia can be reviewed on pages 345 to 346.

HIV-1 INFECTION IN CHILDREN[30]

An increasing number of patients with HIV-1 infection are children younger than 13 years of age. Children older than 13 years are diagnosed and treated as adults.

I. CHILDREN AT RISK

A. Perinatal Transmission

Infants born to mothers infected with HIV-1; approximately 25% to 40% of infants born to HIV-1-seropositive mothers become infected.

B. Breast-fed Infants

HIV-1 has been demonstrated in human milk, and postpartum transmission does occur. Human milk contains components, such as immunoglobulins and leukocytes, that could reduce the infectivity of the HIV-1. Many questions remain unanswered. The World Health Organization has recommended that women in developing countries whose water supplies are unsafe for preparation of infant formulas continue to breast-feed their infants.[31]

C. Infected Blood and Blood Products

Infants or children who received transfusions or treatments with infected blood or blood products are at risk. This mode of transfer is under control in countries where blood donors are screened and all donated blood is tested.

D. Sexual Abuse

Children who have been sexually abused by an infected perpetrator.[32]

II. CLASSIFICATION

The classification system for HIV-1 infection in children younger than 13 years of age has been developed by the United States Centers for Disease Control and Prevention. In the revised 1994 system infected children are classified by three parameters: the infection status, the clinical status, and the immunologic status.[33]

III. CLINICAL MANIFESTATIONS

A. Incubation or Latent Period

The progression of HIV-1 in infants is more severe and faster than in adults due to the immature immune system, which provides less resistance to infection. The time before clinical symptoms appear is variable and may range from months after birth to several years.

B. Diagnosis

Initial diagnosis is based on blood screening for the presence of virus or HIV-1 antibody. Diagnosis of HIV-1 infection in the neonate during the first year is complicated by the persistence of maternal antibody, which has been passively transferred across the placenta to the fetus.

When the mother is without symptoms and has never been tested for HIV-1, the child's diagnosis may be the index case in the family. Testing of family members and parental counseling are indicated.

C. Systemic Findings[30]

The wide range of symptoms includes disorders of nearly every body organ system. Oral lesions are common clinical signs of HIV-1 infection in children. Bacterial infections tend to be more frequent and more severe than those in adults. Following is a partial list of frequently found conditions:

1. Failure to thrive; developmental delay.
2. Hepatomegaly; splenomegaly.
3. Generalized lymphadenopathy.
4. Chronic pneumonitis.
5. Progressive encephalopathy.

D. Oral Findings[34]

Oral lesions are common clinical signs of HIV-1 infection in children. They are frequently among the earliest symptoms to appear and may be used to diagnose HIV-1.

1. Persistent oral candidiasis; *Candida* esophagitis.
2. Parotiditis; swelling of the parotid glands.
3. Herpetic gingivostomatitis; sore mouth and poor oral intake lead to malnutrition and dehydration.
4. Aphthous ulcers.
5. Hairy leukoplakia.
6. Linear gingival erythema.
7. Necrotizing ulcerative gingivitis and periodontitis (less frequently).

IV. TREATMENT/MANAGEMENT

A. Counseling

Family counseling can be essential to the patient's care. Family and caregivers of the child need to watch for symptoms that are significant to disease progression. They also need to understand the reasons for frequent follow-up for testing and to attend faithfully to the medications program.

Counseling for oral health becomes an important part of the child's care. The healthy mouth, free from pain, can allow comfort during eating and thereby contribute to the nutritional status and the overall welfare and quality of life.

B. Medications: Threat to Dental Caries[35,36]

Children with HIV-1 infection or AIDS take many types of medications. Many children's medications have a base with a high percentage of sucrose, some of which may be taken by the child several times each day. They may be prepared for the children as an elixir, in a sweet, sticky form to disguise an unpleasant flavor.

Other children's preparations with high sucrose are nutritional supplements. Multivitamins, given as drops for infants and toddlers, contain high quantities of sucrose. Mycostatin (for oral candidiasis) may be recommended for several applications a day and may have a sucrose content as great as 50%.[36]

All these preparations can contribute to the initiation of dental caries. Infants and toddlers with HIV-1 infection can be at great risk for early childhood caries (page 240). When a parent is counseled concerning oral care, recommendations must be given relative to the nursing bottle and pacifiers, as well as to cleaning the mouth immediately after giving the various medications (pages 660 and 663).

PREVENTION OF HIV-1 INFECTION

Until a vaccine is available, prevention depends to a large degree on community education for attitudinal and behavioral changes. People need to understand the modes of transmission of the HIV-1 and the preventive measures necessary to halt its transmission. Dental personnel must keep well informed with accurate, current information that can be applied in practice and give support to community health programs.

The goal of *primary prevention* (for those not infected) is to lower the rate at which new cases of HIV-1 infection appear. Programs for women, particularly of childbearing age; intravenous drug users who share needles; and teenagers are focused to reach the most vulnerable groups. HIV-1 testing should be offered for all pregnant women, and all newborns should be tested in the attempt to control the increasing numbers of children with HIV-1 infection.

The goals of *secondary prevention* (for seropositive individuals) are to reduce the rate of transmission and to introduce treatment early. Early intervention may postpone severe clinical manifestations of advanced illness. A leading part of the program is to counsel the HIV-1-infected individuals to practice safe sex[§§] and to cooperate with the program to screen and counsel their sexual contacts and families.

Ongoing programs include strict testing for blood donors and all tissue organ donors, as well as identification and counseling of recipients of blood transfusions before 1985 and their sexual partners. The incubation period has been shown to be much longer than was originally thought. With early diagnosis and medical intervention, people with HIV-1 infection can be symptom free and healthy and can live longer than was possible earlier in the epidemic.

TECHNICAL HINTS

I. BLOOD BANKS

Blood banks are required to test all blood received for hepatitis B and C, syphilis, and the HIV-1 antibody. Frequently used tests for HIV-1 antibody have been the EIA (ELISA) and the WB (Western blot). When the test result is positive, the blood is rejected and the person is notified and counseled.

[§§]"Practice safe sex" is meant to include barrier protection and no exchange of body fluids (saliva, semen, vaginal secretions) in accord with recommended guidelines.

II. RESOURCES

CDC National AIDS Clearinghouse
P.O. Box 6003
Rockville, MD 20849-6003
CDC National AIDS Hotline
1-800-342-2437 (English)
1-800-344-7432 (Spanish)
1-800-243-7889 (TDD service for the deaf)
AIDS Clinical Trials Information Service (ACTIS)
1-800-874-2572

FACTORS TO TEACH THE PATIENT

I. Reasons for postponing an appointment when a herpes lesion ("fever blister" or "cold sore") is present on the lip or in the oral cavity.
   A. Importance of not touching or scratching the lesion because of self-infection to fingers or eyes, for example.
   B. How the viruses can survive on objects and transfer infection to other people.
II. How to help by keeping the medical history up-to-date by informing of additional exposures and immunizations to communicable diseases for self and family members.
III. Preparation for a dental or dental hygiene appointment by thorough mouth cleaning with toothbrush and dental floss to lower the bacterial count and thus lessen acrosol contamination in the treatment room.

REFERENCES

1. **Socransky**, S.S. and Manganiello, S.D.: The Oral Microbiota of Man From Birth to Senility, *J. Periodontol., 42,* 485, August, 1971.
2. **Miller,** R.L. and Micik, R.E.: Air Pollution and Its Control in the Dental Office, *Dent. Clin. North Am., 22,* 453, July, 1978.
3. **Miller,** R.L.: Generation of Airborne Infection—by High Speed Dental Equipment, *J. Am. Soc. Prev. Dent., 6,* 14, May/June, 1976.
4. **Larato**, D.C., Ruskin, P.F., and Martin, A.: Effect of an Ultrasonic Scaler on Bacterial Counts in Air, *J. Periodontol., 38,* 550, November–December, 1967.
5. **Holbrook**, W.P., Muir, K.F., MacPhee, I.T., and Ross, P.W.: Bacteriological Investigation of the Aerosol from Ultrasonic Scalers, *Br. Dent. J., 144,* 245, April 18, 1978.
6. **Pokowitz,** W. and Hoffman, H.: Dental Aerobiology, *N.Y. State Dent. J., 37,* 337, June–July, 1971.
7. **Gross,** A., Devine, M.J., and Cutright, D.E.: Microbial Contamination of Dental Units and Ultrasonic Scalers, *J. Periodontol., 47,* 670, November, 1976.
8. **Benenson,** A.S., ed.: *Control of Communicable Diseases in Man,* 16th ed. Washington, D.C., American Public Health Association, 1995, pp. 488–499.
9. **United States Centers for Disease Control:** Revised Classification System for HIV Infection and Expanded Surveillance Case Definition for AIDS Among Adolescents and Adults, *MMWR, 41,* 1–19, RR-17, December 18, 1992.
10. **United States Centers for Disease Control and Prevention:** Guidelines for Preventing the Transmission of *Mycobacterium tuberculosis* in Health-care Facilities, 1994, *MMWR, 43,* 52, October 28, 1994.
11. **Robinson,** H.B.G. and Miller, A.S.: *Colby, Kerr, and Robinson's Color Atlas of Oral Pathology,* 5th ed. Philadelphia, J.B. Lippincott Co., 1990, p. 91.
12. **Miyakawa,** Y. and Mayumi, M.: Hepatitis G Virus—A True Hepatitis or an Accidental Tourist? (Editorial), *N. Engl. J. Med., 336,* 795, March 13, 1997.
13. **Alter**, H.J., Nakatsuji, Y., Melpolder, J., Wages, J., Wesley, R., Shih, J.W.-K., and Kim, J.P.: The Incidence of Transfusion-associated Hepatitis G Virus Infection and Its Relation to Liver Disease, *N. Engl. J. Med., 336,* 747, March 13, 1997.
14. **Alter**, M.J., Gallagher, M., Morris, T.T., Moyer, L.A., Meeks, E.L., Krawczynski, K., Kim, J.P., and Margolis, H.S.: Acute Non-A-E Hepatitis in the United States and the Role of Hepatitis G Virus Infection, *N. Engl. J. Med., 336,* 741, March 13, 1997.
15. **Benenson:** op. cit., pp. 217–233.
16. **United States Centers for Disease Control:** Hepatitis B Virus: a Comprehensive Strategy for Eliminating Transmission in the United States Through Universal Childhood Vaccination, *MMWR, 40,* 1–25, RR-13, November 22, 1991.
17. **United States Centers for Disease Control:** Suboptimal Response to Hepatitis B Vaccine Given by Injection into the Buttock, *MMWR, 34,* 105, March 1, 1985.
18. **Porter**, S., Scully, C., and Samaranayake, L.: Viral Hepatitis. Current Concepts for Dental Practice, *Oral Surg. Oral Med. Oral Pathol., 78,* 682, December, 1994.
19. **Merchant,** V.A.: Herpesviruses and Other Microorganisms of Concern in Dentistry, *Dent. Clin. North Am., 35,* 283, April, 1991.
20. **Benenson:** op. cit., pp. 87–91.
21. **Benenson:** op. cit., pp. 312–314.
22. **Cheeseman,** S.H.: Cytomegalovirus, in Gorbach, S.L., Bartlett, J.G., and Blacklow, N.R.: *Infectious Diseases.* Philadelphia, W.B. Saunders Co., 1992, pp. 1715–1720.
23. **Benenson:** op. cit., pp. 233–236.
24. **Amit,** R., Morag, A., Ravid, Z., Hochman, N., Ehrlich, J., and Zakay-Rones, Z.: Detection of Herpes Simplex Virus in Gingival Tissue, *J. Periodontol., 63,* 502, June, 1992.
25. **Benenson:** op. cit., p. 1–8.
26. **Folks,** T.M. and Hart, C.E.: The Life Cycle of Human Immunodeficiency Virus Type I, in DeVita, V.T., Hellman, S., and Rosenberg, S.A., eds.: *AIDS. Etiology, Diagnosis, Treatment and Prevention,* 4th ed., Philadelphia, Lippincott-Raven, 1997, pp. 29–39.
27. **United States Centers for Disease Control and Prevention:** 1993 Revised Classification System for HIV Infection and Expanded Surveillance Case Definition for AIDS Among Adolescents and Adults, *MMWR, 41,* 1–19, No. RR-17, December 18, 1992.
28. **Saag**, M.S.: Clinical Spectrum of Human Immunodeficiency Virus Diseases, in DeVita, V.T., Hellman, S., and Rosenberg, S.A., eds.: *AIDS. Etiology, Diagnosis, Treatment and Prevention,* 4th ed. Philadelphia, Lippincott-Raven, 1997, pp. 203–213.
29. **Greenspan**, D., Greenspan, J.S., Schiødt, M., and Pindborg, J.J.: *AIDS and the Mouth. Diagnosis and Management of Oral Lesions.* Copenhagen, Munksgaard, 1990, pp. 91–102, 113–134.
30. **Mueller**, B.U. and Pizzo, P.A.: Pediatric Human Immunodeficiency Virus Infections, in DeVita, V.T., Hellman, S., and Rosenberg, S.A., eds.: *AIDS. Etiology, Diagnosis, Treatment and Prevention,* 4th ed. Philadelphia, Lippincott-Raven, 1997, pp. 443–464.
31. **World Health Organization**: Global Program on AIDS. Consensus Statement from WHO/UNICEF Consultation on HIV Transmission and Breast-feeding, *Weekly Epidemiol. Rec., 67,* 177, 1992.
32. **Gutman,** L.T., St. Claire, K.K., Weedy, C., Herman-Giddens, M.E., Lane, B.A., Niemeyer, J.C., and McKinney, R.E.: Human Immunodeficiency Virus Transmission by Sexual Abuse, *Am. J. Diseases Child., 145,* 137, February, 1991.
33. **United States Centers for Disease Control and Prevention**: 1994 Revised Classification System for Human Immunodeficiency Virus Infection in Children Less Than 13 Years of Age, *MMWR, 43,* 1–19, No. RR-12, September 30, 1994.
34. **Chigurupati**, R., Raghavan, S.S., and Studen-Pavlovich, D.A.: Pediatric HIV Infection and Its Oral Manifestations: A Review, *Pediatr. Dent., 18,* 106, March/April, 1996.

35. **Gehrke,** F.S. and Johnsen, D.S.: Bottle Caries Associated with Anti-HIV Therapy (Letter), *Pediatr. Dent., 13,* 73, January/February, 1991.
36. **Howell,** R.B. and Houpt, M.: More Than One Factor Can Influence Caries Development in HIV-positive Children (Letter), *Pediatr. Dent., 13,* 247, July/August, 1991.

SUGGESTED READINGS

Bagg, J.: Common Infectious Diseases, *Dent. Clin. North Am., 40,* 385, April, 1996.

Bentley, C.D., Burkhart, N.W., and Crawford, J.J.: Evaluating Spatter and Aerosol Contamination During Dental Procedures, *J. Am. Dent. Assoc., 125,* 579, May, 1994.

Harfst, S.: Infection Control Update: Vaccinations, *J. Pract. Hyg., 5,* 43, July/August, 1996.

Laskaris, G.: Oral Manifestations of Infectious Diseases, *Dent. Clin. North Am., 40,* 395, April, 1996.

Slavkin, H.C.: First Encounters: Transmission of Infectious Oral Diseases from Mother to Child, *J. Am. Dent. Assoc., 128,* 773, June, 1997.

Tuberculosis

Abou-Shala, N. and Mauldin, G.: Tuberculosis: An Old Nemesis Returns, *Am. Acad. Phys. Assist., 6,* 639, October, 1993.

Bagg, J.: Tuberculosis: a Re-emerging Problem for Health Care Workers, *Br. Dent. J., 180,* 376, May 25, 1996.

Bednarsh, H.S. and Eklund, K.J.: TB Prevention Through Screening and Therapy, *Access, 10,* 4, July, 1995.

Brown, B.S.: Oral Manifestations of Tuberculosis, *Pros and Contra Angles, 20,* 5, April, 1998.

Harlow, R.F. and Rutkauskas, J.S.: Tuberculosis Risk in the Hospital Dental Practice, *Spec. Care Dent., 15,* 50, March/April, 1995.

Iseman, M.D.: Treatment of Multidrug-resistant Tuberculosis, *N. Engl. J. Med., 329,* 784, September 9, 1993.

Molinari, J.A.: Tuberculosis Infection Control: A Reasonable Approach for Dentistry, *Compend. Cont. Educ. Dent., 16,* 1080, November, 1995.

Phelan, J.A., Jimenez, V., and Tompkins, D.C.: Tuberculosis, *Dent. Clin. North Am., 40,* 327, April, 1996.

Shearer, B.G.: MDR-TB. Another Challenge from the Microbial World, *J. Am. Dent. Assoc., 125,* 43, January, 1994.

Villanueva, A.V. and Chandrasekar, P.H.: Emergence of Antimicrobial-resistant Pathogens: a Growing Concern, *J. Pract. Hyg., 6,* 37, September/October, 1997.

Woods, R.G., Amerena, V., David, P., Fan, P.L., Heydt, H., and Marianos, D.: Additional Precautions for Tuberculosis and a Self Assessment Checklist, *FDI World, 6,* 10, May/June, 1997.

Hepatitis

Hoofnagle, J.H. and Lau, D.: Chronic Viral Hepatitis: Benefits of Current Therapies, *N. Engl. J. Med., 334,* 1470, May 30, 1996.

Hoofnagle, J.H. and DiBisceglie, A.M.: The Treatment of Chronic Viral Hepatitis, *N. Engl. J. Med., 336,* 347, January 30, 1997.

Lee, W.M.: Hepatitis B Virus Infection, *N. Engl. J. Med., 337,* 1733, December 11, 1997.

Lemon, S.M. and Thomas, D.L.: Vaccines to Prevent Viral Hepatitis, *N. Engl. J. Med., 336,* 196, January 16, 1997.

Molinari, J.A.: Hepatitis. Vaccination Information, *DentalHygienistNews, 9,* 15, Number 3, 1996.

Najm, W.: Viral Hepatitis: How to Manage Type C and D Infections, *Geriatrics, 52,* 28, May, 1997.

Reddi, S. and Garg, A.K.: Patients with Chronic Hepatitis: Potential Risks When Undergoing Dental Surgery: Review and Case Report, *Spec. Care Dentist., 14,* 241, November/December, 1994.

Slavkin, H.G.: The A,B,C,D, and E of Viral Hepatitis, *J. Am. Dent. Assoc., 127,* 1667, November, 1996.

Szmuness, W., Stevens, C.E., Harley, E.J., Zang, E.A., Oleszko, W.R., William, D.C., Sadovsky, R., Morrison, J.M., and Kellner, A.: Hepatitis B Vaccine. Demonstration of Efficacy in a Controlled Clinical Trial in a High-risk Population in the United States, *N. Engl. J. Med., 303,* 833, October 9, 1980.

Hepatitis C

Alter, M.J., Margolis, H.S., Krawczynski, K., Judson, F.N., Mares, A., Alexander, W.J., Hu, P.Y., Miller, J.K., Gerber, M.A., Sampliner, R.E., Meeks, E.L., and Beach, M.J.: The Natural History of Community-acquired Hepatitis C in the United States, *N. Engl. J. Med., 327,* 1899, December 31, 1992.

Donahue, J.G., Muñoz, A., Ness, P.M., Brown, D.E., Yawn, D.H., McAllister, H.A., Reitz, B.A., and Nelson, K.E.: The Declining Risk of Post-transfusion Hepatitis C Virus Infection, *N. Engl. J. Med., 327,* 369, August 6, 1992.

Kelen, G.D., Green, G.B., Purcell, R.H., Chan, D.W., Qaquish, B.F., Sivertson, K.T., and Quinn, T.C.: Hepatitis B and Hepatitis C in Emergency Department Patients, *N. Engl. J. Med., 326,* 1399, May 21, 1992.

Pereira, B.J.G., Milford, E.L., Kirkman, R.L., Quan, S., Sayre, K.R., Johnson, P.J., Wilber, J.C., and Levey, A.S.: Prevalence of Hepatitis C Virus RNA in Organ Donors Positive for Hepatitis C Antibody and in the Recipients of Their Organs, *N. Engl. J. Med., 327,* 910, September 24, 1992.

Pereira, B.J.G., Milford, E.L., Kirkman, R.L., and Levey, A.S.: Transmission of Hepatitis C Virus by Organ Transplantation, *N. Engl. J. Med., 325,* 454, August 15, 1991.

Weintrub, P.S., Veereman-Wauters, G., Cowan, M.J., and Thaler, M.M.: Hepatitis C Virus Infection in Infants Whose Mothers Took Street Drugs Intravenously, *J. Pediatr., 119,* 869, December, 1991.

Herpesvirus

Fons, M.P., Flaitz, C.M., Moore, B., Prabhakar, B.S., Nichols, C.M., and Albrecht, T.: Multiple Herpesviruses in Saliva of HIV-infected Individuals, *J. Am. Dent. Assoc., 125,* 713, June, 1994.

Foreman, K.E., Friborg, J., Kong, W.-P., Woffendin, C., Polverini, P.J., Nickoloff, B.J., and Nabel, G.J.: Propagation of a Human Herpesvirus from AIDS-associated Kaposi's Sarcoma, *N. Engl. J. Med., 336,* 163, January 16, 1997.

Gibbs, R.S. and Mead, P.B.: Preventing Neonatal Herpes—Current Strategies (Editorial), *N. Engl. J. Med., 326,* 946, April 2, 1992.

Gilden, D.H.: Herpes Zoster With Postherpetic Neuralgia—Persisting Pain and Frustration, (Editorial), *N. Engl. J. Med., 330,* 932, March 31, 1994.

Greenberg, M.S.: Herpesvirus Infections, *Dent. Clin. North Am., 40,* 359, April, 1996.

Manzella, J.P., McConville, J.H., Valenti, W., Menegus, M.A., Swirkosz, E.M., and Arens, M.: An Outbreak of Herpes Simplex Virus Type I Gingivostomatitis in a Dental Hygiene Practice, *JAMA, 252,* 2019, October 19, 1984.

Martin, J.N., Ganem, D.E., Osmond, D.H., Page-Shafer, K.A., Macrae, D., and Kedes, D.H.: Sexual Transmission and the Natural History of Human Herpesvirus 8 Infection, *N. Engl. J. Med., 338,* 948, April 2, 1998.

Poland, J.M.: Current Therapeutic Management of Recurrent Herpes Labialis, *Gen. Dent., 42,* 46, January–February, 1994.

Pruksananonda, P., Hall, C.B., Insel, R.A., McIntyre, K., Pellett, P.E., Long, C.E., Schnabel, K.C., Pincus, P.H., Stamey, B.A., Dambaugh, T.R., and Stewart, J.A.: Primary Human Herpesvirus 6 Infection in Young Children, *N. Engl. J. Med., 326,* 1446, May 28, 1992.

Robbins, D.L.: Human Herpesviruses: Research and Threats to Health Professionals, *Gen. Dent., 42,* 418, September–October, 1994.

Scott, D.A., Coulter, W.A., and Lamey, P.J.: Oral Shedding of Herpes Simplex Virus Type I: A Review, *J. Oral Pathol. Med., 26,* 441, November, 1997.

HIV: General

American Dental Association, Health Foundation: Dental Management of the HIV-infected Patient, Chicago, *J. Am. Dent. Assoc., Supplement,* 1995.

Cao, Y., Qin, L., Zhang, L., Safrit, J., and Ho, D.D.: Virologic and

Immunologic Characterization of Long-term Survivors of Human Immunodeficiency Virus Type I Infection, *N. Engl. J. Med., 332,* 201, January 26, 1995.

Chaisson, R.E., Keruly, J.C., and Moore, R.D.: Race, Sex, Drug Use, and Progression of Human Immunodeficiency Virus Disease, *N. Engl. J. Med., 333,* 751, September 21, 1995.

de Vincenzi, I., for the European Study Group on Heterosexual Transmission of HIV: A Longitudinal Study of Human Immunodeficiency Virus Transmission by Heterosexual Partners, *N. Engl. J. Med., 331,* 341, August 11, 1994.

Johnson, A.M.: Condoms and HIV Transmission, *N. Engl. J. Med., 331,* 391, August 11, 1994.

Katz, M.H. and Gerberding, J.L.: Postexposure Treatment of People Exposed to the Human Immunodeficiency Virus Through Sexual Contact or Injection-drug Use, *N. Engl. J. Med., 336,* 1097, April 10, 1997.

Levy, J.A.: Infection by Human Immunodeficiency Virus—CD4 is Not Enough, *N. Engl. J. Med., 335,* 1528, November 14, 1996.

Lipton, S.A. and Gendelman, H.E.: Dementia Associated With the Acquired Immunodeficiency Syndrome, *N. Engl. J. Med., 332,* 934, April 6, 1995.

Pantaleo, G., Graziosi, C., and Fauci, A.S.: The Immunopathogenesis of Human Immunodeficiency Virus Infection, *N. Engl. J. Med., 328,* 327, February 4, 1993.

Phillips, K.A., Flatt, S.J., Morrison, K.R., and Coates, T.J.: Potential Use of Home HIV Testing, *N. Engl. J. Med., 332,* 1308, May 11, 1995.

Royce, R.A., Sena, A., Cates, W., and Cohen, M.S.: Sexual Transmission of HIV, *N. Engl. J. Med., 336,* 1072, April 10, 1997.

Waddell, C.: Perception of HIV Risk and Reported Compliance With Universal Precautions: A Comparison of Australian Dental Hygienists and Dentists, *J. Dent. Hyg., 71,* 17, January–February, 1997.

HIV: Oral Complications

Begg, M.D., Panageas, K.S., Mitchell-Lewis, D., Bucklan, R.S., Phelan, J.A., and Lamster, I.B.: Oral Lesions as Markers of Severe Immunosuppression in HIV-infected Homosexual Men and Injection Drug Users, *Oral Surg. Oral Med. Oral Pathol. Oral Radiol. Endod., 82,* 276, September, 1996.

Brady, L.J., Walker, C., Oxford, G.E., Stewart, C., Magnusson, I., and McArthur, W.: Oral Diseases, Mycology and Periodontal Microbiology of HIV-I-infected Women, *Oral Microbiol. Immunol., 11,* 371, December, 1996.

Glick, M., Abel, S.N., Muzyka, B.C., and Delorenzo, M.: Dental Complications After Treating Patients With AIDS, *J. Am. Dent. Assoc., 125,* 296, March, 1994.

Glick, M., Muzyka, B.C., Lurie, D., and Salkin, L.M.: Oral Manifestations Associated With HIV-related Disease as Markers for Immune Suppression and AIDS, *Oral Surg. Oral Med. Oral Pathol., 77,* 344, April, 1994.

Grbic, J.T., Lamster, I.B., and Mitchell-Lewis, D.: Inflammatory and Immune Mediators in Crevicular Fluid From HIV-infected Injecting Drug Users, *J. Periodontol., 68,* 249, March, 1997.

Tillis, T.S.I. and Vojir, C.P.: Identification of HIV/AIDS-Associated Oral Lesions, *J. Dent. Hyg., 67,* 30, January, 1993.

HIV Children

Asher, R.S., McDowell, J., Acs, G., and Belanger, G.: Pediatric Infection With the Human Immunodeficiency Virus (HIV): Head, Neck, and Oral Manifestations, *Spec. Care Dentist., 13,* 113, May/June, 1993.

Bryson, Y.J., Pang, S., Wei, L.S., Dickover, R., Diagne, A., and Chen, I.S.Y.: Clearance of HIV Infection in a Perinatally Infected Infant, *N. Engl. J. Med., 332,* 833, March 30, 1995.

Cohen, F.L. and Nehring, W.M.: Foster Care of HIV-positive Children in the United States, *Public Health Rep., 109,* 60, January–February, 1994.

Howell, R.B., Jandinski, J.J., Palumbo, P., Shey, Z., and Houpt, M.I.: Oral Soft Tissue Manifestations and CD4 Lymphocyte Counts in HIV-infected Children, *Pediatr. Dent., 18,* 117, March/April, 1996.

Laskaris, G., Laskaris, M., and Theodoridou, M.: Oral Hairy Leukoplakia in a Child With AIDS, *Oral Surg. Oral Med. Oral Pathol., 79,* 570, May, 1995.

Madigan, A., Murray, P.A., Houpt, M., Catalanotto, F., and Feuerman, M.: Caries Experience and Cariogenic Markers in HIV-positive Children and Their Siblings, *Pediatr. Dent., 18,* 129, March/April, 1996.

Moniaci, D., Cavallari, M., Greco, D., Bruatto, M., Raiteri, R., Palomba, E., Tovo, P.A., and Sinicco, A.: Oral Lesions in Children Born to HIV-1 Positive Women, *J. Oral Pathol. Med., 22,* 8, January, 1993.

Valdez, I.H., Pizzo, P.A., and Atkinson, J.C.: Oral Health of Pediatric AIDS Patients: A Hospital-based Study, *ASDC J. Dent. Child., 61,* 114, March–April, 1994.

Ethics

Bayer, R.: AIDS Prevention: Sexual Ethics and Responsibility, *N. Engl. J. Med., 334,* 1540, June 6, 1996.

Chiodo, G.T. and Tolle, S.W.: The Ethical Foundations of a Duty to Treat HIV-positive Patients, *Gen. Dent., 45,* 14, January–February, 1997.

Keyes, G.G. and Waithe, M.E.: HIV Infection in Dentistry: Ethical and Legal Issues, in Weinstein, B.D.: *Dental Ethics.* Philadelphia, Lea & Febiger, 1993, pp. 81–100.

Romano, J.E.: AIDS Social Policy Education for the Dental Hygienist, Thesis submitted in partial fulfillment for the Master of Arts, State University of New York, Empire State College, Saratoga, New York, 1997.

Exposure Control: Barriers for Patient and Clinician

Exposure control refers to all procedures during clinical care necessary to provide top-level protection from exposure to infectious agents for members of the dental team and their patients. Dental health-care workers (DHCW) have a professional obligation to serve *all* patients with comprehensive oral care, including patients with known or unknown communicable diseases. The practice of *universal precautions* means that the body fluids of all patients are treated as if they were infectious.

An organized system for exposure control is needed. First, a written exposure control plan is prepared to serve as a guide for the entire team.[1] Consistency between DHCWs is necessary to maintain standards of asepsis and to prevent cross-contamination. The written plan can be the basis for training new personnel. As new research and commercial products become available, the written protocol must be revised.

Using the protocol and transferring the objectives and overall aims to the clinical setting are the responsibilities of each member of the dental team. It should be realized that physical barriers and other requirements of the protocol provide safety for both the DHCW and the patient. Selected terms from the application of exposure control and immunizations are defined in Box 3-1.

PERSONAL PROTECTION OF THE DENTAL TEAM

The continuing health and productivity of dental health personnel depend to a large degree on the control of cross-contamination. Loss of work time, personal suffering, long-term systemic effects, and even exclusion from continued practice are possible results from communicable diseases. The only safe procedure is to practice defensively at all times, with specific precautions for personal protection.

In this section, topics include immunizations and periodic tests; clothing; barriers to infectious microor-

BOX 3-I KEY WORDS AND ABBREVIATIONS: Exposure Control

Allergen (ăl′er-jĕn): substance, protein or nonprotein, capable of inducing allergy or specific hypersensitivity; can enter the body by being inhaled, swallowed, touched, or injected.

> **Hypoallergenic:** property of a substance that indicates it does not create a hypersensitive reaction; may apply to various chemicals; not specified on manufacturer's labels.

Antimicrobial soap: a soap containing an active ingredient against skin microorganisms.

Atopy (at′o-pē): clinical hypersensitivity state or allergy with a hereditary predisposition; includes hay fever, eczema, and asthma.

Barrier protection: refers to placing a physical barrier between the patient's body fluids (such as blood and saliva) and the health-care worker (HCW) to prevent disease transmission.

> **Barriers for HCW:** include gloves, mask, protective eyewear, and protective clothing (gown).

> **Barriers for patient:** include protective eyewear, headcover during surgeries, and rubber dam during restorative and sealant procedures.

Booster dose: amount of immunogen (vaccine, toxoid, or other antigen preparation), usually smaller than the original amount, injected at an appropriate interval after the primary immunization to sustain the immune response to that immunogen.

Exposure incident: a specific eye, mouth, mucous membrane, nonintact skin, or parenteral contact with blood or other potentially infectious material that results from the performance of one's usual professional duties.

Immunization (ĭm″ū-nĭ-zā′shun): the process of rendering a subject immune to a particular disease by stimulation with a specific antigen to promote antibody formation in the body.

Inoculation (ĭ-nŏk″ū-lā′shun): introduction of antigenic material or vaccine; more frequently used to refer to introduction of material into a culture medium.

Latex allergy: an acquired hypersensitivity reaction to the proteins found in natural rubber latex (NRL).

Occupational exposure: reasonably anticipated skin, eye, mucous membrane, or parenteral contact with blood or other potentially infectious materials that may result from the performance of one's usual duties.

PPD: purified protein derivative for tuberculin intracutaneous skin test for tuberculosis; positive reaction means previous infection with *Mycobacterium tuberculosis* (mĭ″ko-băk-tēr′ē-′m too-ber″kū-lō′sĭs).

Rhinitis (rī-nī′tĭs): inflammation of the mucous membrane of the nose; may result from infection by bacteria or virus, or may be a seasonal (hay fever) or nonseasonal allergic reaction.

Toxoid (tok′soid): toxin treated by heat or chemical agent to destroy its deleterious properties without destroying its ability to combine with, or stimulate the formation of, antitoxin; examples of toxoids used for active immunization are tetanus and diphtheria.

Tuberculin test (Mantoux) (too-ber′ku-lĭn test [mann-too′]): a test for the presence of active or inactive tuberculosis; a positive test is denoted by redness and induration at the injection site by 48 to 72 hours after injection.

Vaccination (văk″sĭ-nā′sh′n): process of introducing a vaccine into the body to produce immunity to a specific disease.

Vaccine (văk-sēn′): a suspension of attenuated or killed microorganisms administered for the prevention or treatment of an infectious disease.

---

ganisms, such as face mask and protective eyewear; personal hygiene; handwashing; gloves; and habits.

IMMUNIZATIONS AND PERIODIC TESTS

Dental personnel in a hospital setting are subject to the rules and regulations for all hospital employees. Policies usually require certain immunizations for new employees if written proof of immunizations is not available and tests for antibodies prove to be negative.

In private dental practices, individual initiative is required to maintain standards of safety for all dental team members. All staff members should be well aware of the signs and symptoms of diseases that are occupational hazards. All must be encouraged to seek early diagnosis and treatment of a seemingly minor condition that could be the initial symptom of a more serious communicable disease.

At the time of employment, it is reasonable for a dentist-employer to request of employees a record of current immunizations and their most recent updating, as well as specific tests, such as for tuberculosis.

Immunization for rubella is particularly important for female employees of childbearing age.

I. IMMUNIZATIONS

A. Basic Schedule[2,3]

The immunization schedule for infants and children includes protection against poliomyelitis, diphtheria, tetanus, pertussis (whooping cough), measles, mumps, rubella (German measles), influenza, and hepatitis B.

Immunization is required for children either at school entry or at entry into middle or junior high school (at 5 to 6 years or 11 to 12 years of age) if not immunized previously.

For adolescents ages 11 to 21 years, which includes college students, planned immunizations aim to vaccinate those that had not been previously vaccinated, provide booster shots, as well as to promote preventive health services.[3]

B. Booster and Reimmunization

Each agent requires booster or reimmunization on a specific plan, which may range from 1 to 10 years, or reimmunization only upon intimate contact or exposure. The needs differ in different climates, countries, and locations. Persons moving or traveling need to become aware of specific precautions.

For tetanus boosters, intervals of 10 years are indicated. If an injury occurs, however, a booster should be given on the day of the injury.[4]

C. Adult Immunizations

Table 3-1 summarizes the vaccines and toxoids recommended for most adults by age groups.[5] Hepatitis B vaccine is also recommended, especially for members of risk groups (page 25) and all DHCWs.

II. MANAGEMENT PROGRAM

A. Recommended Tests

1. Annual tuberculin test (Mantoux); chest radiograph as indicated.

2. Periodic throat culture for possible hemolytic streptococcus carrier.

B. Obtaining Tests

Obtain tests promptly when exposed to certain infectious diseases and seek prophylactic immunization as indicated and available.

C. Written Records

Keep confidential written records of immunizations, boosters, and reimmunizations; plan for regular follow-up. When the status of current immunizations is known, time is saved by not needing a susceptibility test prior to initiating passive immunizations when accidental exposure occurs.

CLINICAL ATTIRE

The wearing apparel of clinicians and their assistants is vulnerable to contamination from splash, spatter, aerosols, and patient contact. The gown or uniform should be designed and cared for in a manner that minimizes cross-contamination.

I. GOWN, UNIFORM, OR SCRUB SUIT

Gowns, uniforms, or scrub suits are expected to be clean and maintained as free as possible from contamination. Wearing clinic coats over street clothes is not recommended because of the exposure of the street clothes to infectious material.

A. Solid, Closed Front

The garment should be closed at the neck and tie in back, preferably. The fabric should be disposable or able to be washed commercially and withstand washing with bleach.

B. No Pockets

Pockets are too readily available for placing contaminated objects, such as writing implements or keys. Gloved hands, prepared for patient treatment, must be kept from touching objects or being placed in pockets.

Age Groups (years)	Vaccine/toxoid					
	Id*	Measles	Mumps	Rubella	Influenza	Pneumococcal Polysaccharide
18–24	X	X	X	X		
25–64	X	X†	X	X		
≥65	X				X	X

TABLE 3-1 Vaccines and Toxoids Recommended for Adults, by Age Groups, United States

*Td = Tetanus and diphtheria toxoids, adsorbed (for adult use), which is a combined preparation containing < 2 flocculation units of diphtheria toxoid.

†Indicated for persons born after 1956.

(From United States Centers for Disease Control: Update on Adult Immunization Recommendations of the Immunization Practices Advisory Committee [ACIP], *MMWR*, *40*, 56, No. RR-12, November 15, 1991.)

C. Long garment to cover lap when seated for patient treatment.

Long sleeves with fitted cuffs permit protective gloves to extend over the cuffs.

II. HAIR AND HEAD COVERING

A. Hair must be worn off the shoulders and fastened back away from the face. When longer, it should be held within a head cover. Because the hair is exposed to much contamination, an appropriate head cover is advised when using handpieces, ultrasonic, or air-powder polishing instruments.

B. Facial hair should be covered with a face mask and/or face shield.

III. PROTECTION OF UNIFORM

A plastic washable or a disposable apron may be used when clinical services are performed that usually involve blood, spatter, or aerosols.

IV. OUTSIDE WEAR

Clinic uniforms and shoes should not be worn outside the clinic practice setting.[6] When clinical clothing is worn outside, contamination can be carried from, and brought into, the treatment area.

Commercial laundry services are preferred. When laundered at home, the items from a dental office or clinic should be kept separate and treated with household bleach for disinfection.

USE OF FACE MASK: RESPIRATORY PROTECTION

Basic personal barrier protection is composed of face mask, protective eyewear, and gloves. The use of the face mask is described first because it should be positioned first when preparing for clinical care procedures. The protective eyewear is placed second. After that, the hands can be washed prior to gloving.

Dispersion of particles of debris, polishing agents, calculus, and water, all of which are contaminated by the patient's oral flora, occurs regularly during instrumentation. The greatest aerosols are created following the use of a handpiece, prophylaxis angle, or power-driven scaler. Evidence of the spread of particles appears on the splashed face, protective eyewear, and uniform and on the coverall placed over the patient for protection from the spray. Aerosol production was described on page 18.

I. MASK EFFICIENCY

A. Criteria: Essential Characteristics (Table 3-2)
1. *Filtration* (measured in BFE = bacterial filtration effectiveness). Standard masks block filtration of particles as small as 3 μm with a filter efficiency greater than 95%. Particles

---

TABLE 3-2 Characteristics of an Ideal Mask

1. No contact with the wearer's nostrils or lips
2. Has high bacterial filtration efficiency rate
3. Fits snugly around the entire edges of the mask
4. No fogging of eyewear
5. Convenient to put on and remove
6. Made of material that does not irritate skin or induce allergic reaction
7. Does not collapse during wear or when wet

(Adapted from Molinari, J.A.: Face Masks: Effective Personal Protection, *Compend. Cont. Educ. Dent., 17,* 818, September, 1996.)

---

of 3 μm and smaller can penetrate to the alveoli of the lower respiratory tract, where their infectivity is increased. Droplet nuclei (*Mycobacterium tuberculosis*) range from 0.5 to 1 μm and are a risk in health-care settings.[7]
2. *Fit.* Proper fit over face is vital to protect against inhaling droplet nuclei from aerosols.
3. *Moisture Absorption.* Soak through is an important factor. Lining should be impervious. Mask must be changed for each patient and not worn longer than 1 hour.
4. *Comfort.* Degree of comfort should encourage compliance in wearing.

B. Materials
Various materials have been used for masks, including gauze and other cloth, plastic foam, fiberglass, synthetic fiber mat, and paper. In research studies, foam, paper, and cloth were found to be the least adequate filters of aerosols, whereas glass fiber and synthetic fiber mat were shown to be the most effective.[8,9]

II. USE OF A MASK

A. Adjust the mask and position eyewear before a scrub or handwash.
B. Use a fresh mask for each patient.
   1. Change mask each hour or more frequently when it becomes wet.
   2. Chin-cover face shield needs to be supplemented with fitted mask.
C. Keep the mask on after completing a procedure while still in the presence of aerosols. Particles smaller than 5 μm remain suspended longer (up to 24 hours) than do larger particles and can be inhaled directly into terminal lung alveoli. Removal of a mask in the treatment room immediately following the use of aerosol-producing procedures permits direct exposure to airborne organisms.
D. Mask Removal
   1. Grasp side elastic or tie strings to remove (Figure 3-1).
   2. Never handle the outside of a contami-

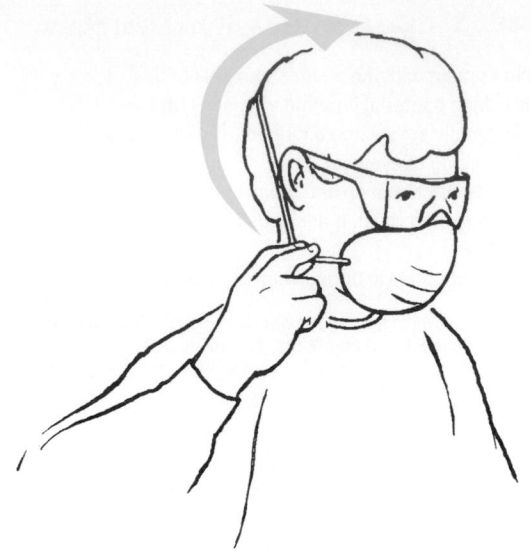

FIGURE 3-1 Removal of Mask. Handle only by the elastic or tie strings, carefully avoiding the contaminated mask.

nated mask with gloved or bare hands. Never place the mask under the chin.

USE OF PROTECTIVE EYEWEAR

Eye protection for the dental team members and patients is necessary to prevent physical injuries and infections of the eyes.

Severe and disabling eye accidents and infections have been reported.[10-12] Eye involvement may lead to pain, discomfort, loss of work time, and, in certain instances, permanent injury. Accidents can occur at any time, and as with most accidents, they occur when least prepared for or expected.

Eye infections can follow the accidental dropping of an instrument on the face or the splashing of various materials from a patient's oral cavity into the eye. Contamination can be introduced from saliva, plaque, carious material, pieces of old restorative materials during cavity preparation, bacteria-laden calculus during scaling, and any other microorganisms contained in aerosols or spatter as described on page 18. An aerosol created by a power-driven scaler can be heavily contaminated with oral microorganisms.

Careful, deliberate techniques and instrument management, with evacuation and other procedures for the control of oral fluids, contribute to the prevention of accidents and infections of the eyes. All measures described for prevention of airborne disease transmission by aerosols and spatter apply to eye protection. The most effective defense is the use of protective eyewear by all involved, dental team members and patients.

I. INDICATIONS FOR USE OF PROTECTIVE EYEWEAR

A. Dental Team Members
Protective eyewear should be worn for all procedures. For dental personnel who do not require a corrective lens for vision, protective eyewear with a clear lens should be a routine part of clinical dress.

B. Patients
Protective eyewear is essential for each patient at each appointment. The patient's medical history should reflect types of eye surgery, implants, or other special concerns.

Patients with their own prescription lenses may prefer to wear them, but for the safety of the patient's glasses, the use of the protective eyewear provided in the office or clinic may be advisable.

II. PROTECTIVE EYEWEAR

A. General Features of Acceptable Eyewear
1. Wide coverage, with side shields, to protect around the eye.
2. Shatterproof; made of strong, sturdy plastic.
3. Lightweight.
4. Flexible and with rounded smooth edges to prevent discomfort if pressed against the nose or ears.
5. Easily disinfected.
   a. Surface areas should be smooth to prevent accumulation of infectious material.
   b. Frames and lens should not be damaged or distorted by the disinfectant used.
6. A clear or lightly tinted lens, rather than a very dark lens, permits the dental team members to watch the patient's reactions and maintain contact and response.
7. Protection against glare. Certain patients may request tinted lenses or prefer to wear their own sunglasses when their eyes are especially sensitive to the dental light.

B. Types of Eyewear
Many styles, including regular eyeglass shapes and those described as follows, have been used.
1. *Goggles* (Figure 3-2A). Shielding on all sides of the glasses may give the best protection, provided they fit closely around the edges. Goggle-style coverage is especially necessary for protection during laboratory work.
2. *Eyewear With Side Shields.* (Figure 3-2B and C). A side shield can provide added protection. For the member of the dental team who depends on a prescription lens, separate side shields are available that can be connected to the bow on each side.
3. *Eyewear With Curved Frames.* When the sides of the eyewear are curved back, they may

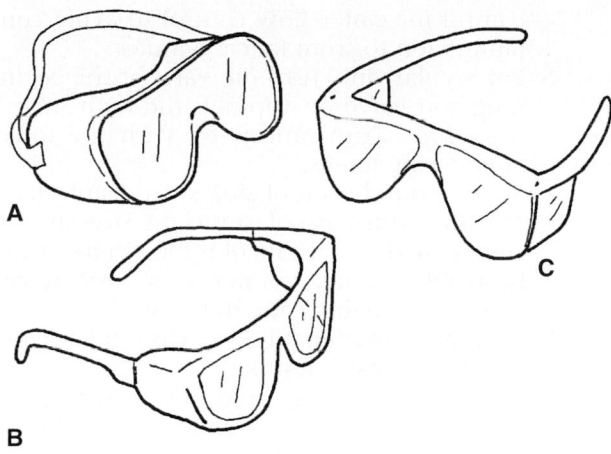

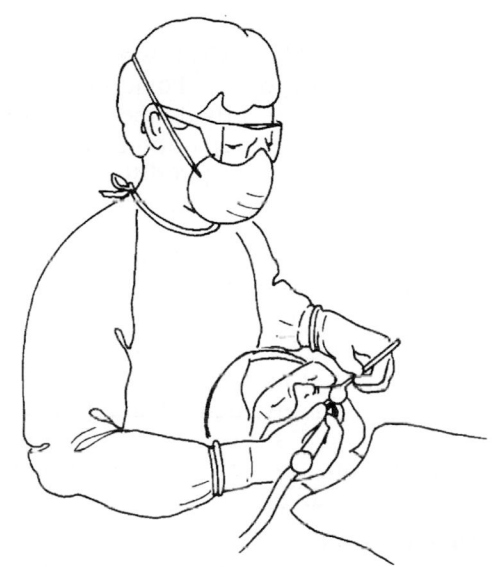

FIGURE 3-2 Protective Eyewear. Protective cover for both patient and clinician may be **(A)** goggles-style, or **(B)** and **(C)** glasses with side shields.

provide a protection somewhat similar to that offered by those with the side shield.
4. *Postmydriatic Spectacles Used by Ophthalmologist.* Disposable glasses are available that are made of flexible plastic.
5. *Child-Sized.* Child-sized sunglasses and children's play spectacles have been used.

C. Availability
Several pairs of goggles or protective eyewear are maintained to facilitate cleaning and disinfection after each use.

III. SUGGESTIONS FOR CLINICAL APPLICATION
A. Patient Instruction
A patient who has not been asked to wear pro-

tective eyewear at previous appointments will appreciate a simple explanation of the reasons for doing so.

B. Contact Lens
Dental team members and patients who wear contact lenses should always wear protective eyewear over them during dental and dental hygiene procedures.

C. Care of Protective Eyewear
1. Run eyewear under water stream to remove abrasive particles. Rubbing an abrasive agent over the plastic lens can create scratches.
2. Materials used for protective lens may be damaged by some disinfectants. Clean with detergent and rinse thoroughly.[13] Air dry.
3. Check periodically for scratches on the lens, and replace appropriately.

HAND CARE

In the infectious process of disease transmission (Figure 2-1, page 17), the hands may serve as a *means of transmission* of the blood, saliva, and bacterial plaque from a patient, and the hands, especially under the fingernails, may serve as a *reservoir* for microorganisms. Skin breaks in the hands may serve as a *port of entry* for potentially pathogenic microorganisms.

By caring properly for the hands, using effective washing procedures, and following the basic rules for gloving, primary cross-contamination can be controlled. A conscious effort must be made to keep the gloved hands from touching objects other than the instruments and disinfected parts of the equipment prepared for the immediate patient.

I. BACTERIOLOGY OF THE SKIN[14]
A. Resident Bacteria
Many relatively stable bacteria inhabit the surface epithelium or deeper areas in the ducts of skin glands or depths of hair follicles; they are ultimately shed with the exfoliated surface cells, or with excretions of the skin glands. The flora may be altered by newly introduced pathogens or reduced by washing. Resident bacteria tend to be less susceptible to destruction by disinfection procedures.

B. Transient Bacteria
Transient bacteria reflect continuous contamination by routine contacts; some bacteria are pathogens and may act temporarily as residents. They may be washed away or, in the event that a skin break exists, may cause an autogenous infection. Most transients can be removed with soap and water by washing thoroughly.

II. HAND CARE

A. Fingernails

1. Maintain clean, smoothly trimmed, short fingernails with well-cared-for cuticles to prevent breaks where microorganisms can enter.
2. Effects of short nails.[15]
   a. Make handwashing more effective because of fewer microorganisms harbored under the nails.[16]
   b. Prevent cuts from nail in disposable gloves.
   c. Permit selection of a closer fit of glove; longer glove fingers may be required to protect nails.
   d. Allow greater dexterity during instrumentation.
   e. Decrease chance of patient discomfort.

B. Wristwatch and Jewelry

Remove hand and wrist jewelry at the beginning of the day. Microorganisms can become lodged in crevices of rings, watchbands, and watches, where scrubbing is impossible.

C. Gloves

1. After handwashing, don gloves. Never expose open skin lesions or abrasions to a patient's oral tissues and fluids. Gloves and gloving are described on pages 50 to 51.
2. After glove removal, wash hands to remove microorganisms.

HANDWASHING PRINCIPLES

I. RATIONALE

Effective and frequent handwashing can reduce the overall bacterial flora of the skin and prevent the organisms acquired from a patient from becoming skin residents. It is impossible to sterilize the skin, but every attempt must be made to reduce the bacterial flora to a minimum.

II. PURPOSES

The objective of all scrub procedures is to reduce the bacterial flora of the hands to an absolute minimum. An effective scrub procedure can be expected to accomplish the following:
A. Remove surface dirt and transient bacteria.
B. Dissolve the normal greasy film on the skin.
C. Rinse and remove all loosened debris and microorganisms.
D. Provide disinfection with a long-acting antiseptic.

III. FACILITIES

A. Sink

1. Use a sink with a foot pedal or electronic control for water-flow control to avoid contamination to/from faucet handles.
2. For regular sink, turn on water at the beginning and leave on through the entire scrub procedure. Turn faucets off with the towel after drying hands.
3. Scrub around brim of sink with disinfectant. The sink must be of sufficient size so that contact with the inside of the wash basin can be avoided easily. A sink cannot be sterilized and can be highly contaminated.
4. Prevent contamination of clothing by not leaning against the sink.
5. Use a separate area and sink reserved for instrument washing. Contaminated instruments must be removed from the treatment room prior to preparation for the next patient.

B. Soap

1. Use a liquid surgical scrub containing an antimicrobial agent. Povidone-iodine (iodophore) has a broad spectrum of action. Chlorhexidine preparations are used extensively to provide rapid disinfection and a cumulative, persistent (residual) action.
2. Apply from a foot- or knee-activated or electronically controlled dispenser to avoid contamination to and from a hand-operated dispenser or cake soap.
3. Do not use foam hand preparations, alcohol wipes, or other substitutes for handwashing, because many pathogenic microorganisms cannot be destroyed by disinfecting preparations. Rinsing is a very important part of the handwashing procedure.

C. Scrub Brushes

1. Clean brushes with a detergent, and sterilize after each use.
2. Avoid overvigorous use of a brush to minimize skin abrasion. Skin irritation and abrasion can leave openings for additional cross-contamination.
3. Disposable sponges are available commercially and may be preferred when a scrub brush is traumatic to the skin.

D. Towels

1. Obtain disposable towel from a dispenser that requires no contact except with the towel itself, which hangs down from the container (Figure 3-3).
2. Cloth towels are not recommended.

METHODS OF HANDWASHING

The three methods described here are called the *short scrub, short standard handwash,* and *surgical scrub.* Handwashing methods more often are defined by numbers of latherings and rinsings. Scrub techniques,

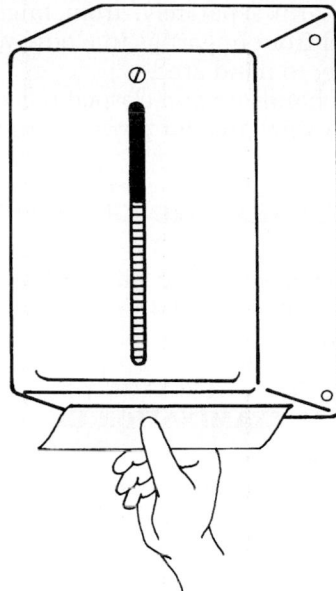

FIGURE 3-3 Towel Dispenser. Correct type of dispenser that requires no contact except with the towel itself, which hangs down from the container.

on the other hand, are best learned in time periods or specific numbers of scrub strokes applied to each area of each hand and arm. The aim of either method is to provide complete coverage and to develop a sequence of performance that can be completed efficiently.

I. SHORT SCRUB

The short scrub handwashing is recommended for the beginning of the day prior to the first gloving, and just prior to the first gloving of any series of appointments. The word "scrub" is used more from a traditional viewpoint, and it does not imply that a scrub brush must be used. A sterile soft brush or nail brush may be used, but hard brushing should be avoided if breaks in the skin could result.

The objectives are to remove surface transient bacteria, dirt, and oils from the hands and wrists and to clean under the fingernails.

The procedure outlined here may be expected to take 2 to 3 minutes. Hands are held higher than forearms to allow water to run away from the clean hands.

A. Preliminary Steps

1. Remove watch and all jewelry. Fasten hair back securely. Don protective eyewear and mask.
2. Wash hands and wrists briefly, using liquid antimicrobial surgical scrub soap. Leave water running at a moderate speed that does not allow splashing from base and sides of sink. Use cool water.
3. Clean under fingernails with orangewood stick from sterile package. Orangewood stick and soft scrub brush may be packaged to-

gether for sterilization when the use of a brush is preferred by the clinician.
4. Rinse from fingertips toward wrists. Keep hands higher than elbows through the entire procedure.

B. Lather Hands

C. First Hand

1. Brush back and forth across nails and fingertips five times.
2. Begin with the thumb, use small circular strokes (five strokes each area) on each side of thumb and each finger, then palm, and back of hand. Extend fingers to gain access to each crevice and line.
3. Scrub wrist on all sides and move to forearm.
4. When completed, rinse well, from fingertips on up over the wrist.

D. Second Hand

1. Rinse the brush and transfer to other hand.
2. Repeat entire procedure.
3. Rinse the hand and arm generously and thoroughly to wash away all transient microorganisms.
4. Dry hands thoroughly.
   a. Take care not to recontaminate hands while drying them.
   b. Use a separate paper towel for each hand.

E. Don Gloves

II. SHORT STANDARD HANDWASH

Handwashing is mandatory before each patient contact, whenever gloves are donned, after gloves are removed, and before leaving the treatment area. The short standard handwash is the general procedure for all times except those indicated under the short scrub technique.

Handwashing is considered the most important single procedure for the prevention of cross-contamination.

A. Remove watch and all jewelry. Fasten hair back securely. Don protective eyewear and mask.
B. Use cool water and liquid antimicrobial surgical scrub soap.
C. Lather hands, wrists, and forearms quickly, rubbing all surfaces vigorously. Interlace fingers and rub back and forth with pressure.
D. Rinse thoroughly, running the water from fingertips down the hands. Keep water running.
E. Repeat two more times. One lathering for 3 minutes is less effective than are three short latherings and three rinses in 30 seconds. The lathering serves to loosen the debris and microorganisms and the rinsings wash them away.
F. Use paper towels for drying, taking care not to recontaminate.

III. SURGICAL SCRUB

Each hospital or oral surgery clinic has rules and regulations for scrub procedures. These should be posted over the scrub sinks.

A surgical scrub performed as the initial scrub of a day should be 10 minutes and subsequent scrubs may be 3 to 5 minutes. Following treatment of a contagious or isolated patient, the scrub should take at least 5 minutes.

A. Preliminary Steps

1. Remove watch and jewelry. Place hair and beard coverings and make sure hair is completely covered. Don protective eyewear and mask.
2. Open sterile brush package to have ready.
3. Wash hands and arms, using surgical liquid antimicrobial soap to remove gross surface dirt before using the scrub brush. Lather vigorously with strong rubbing motions, 10 on each side of hands, wrists, and arms. Interlace the fingers and thumbs to clean the proximal surfaces.
4. Rinse thoroughly from fingertips across hands and wrists. Hold hands higher than elbows throughout the procedure. Leave water running.
5. Use orangewood stick from the sterile package to clean nails. Rinse.

B. First Hand

1. Lather the hands and arms and leave the lather on during the scrub to increase the exposure time to the antimicrobial ingredient.
2. Apply surgical liquid soap, and begin the brush procedure. Scrub in an orderly sequence without returning to areas previously scrubbed.
3. First hand and arm.
   a. Brush back and forth across nails and fingertips, passing the brush under the nails.
   b. Fingers and hand. Use small circular strokes on all sides of the thumb and each finger, overlapping strokes for complete coverage.
   c. Continue to wrist. Apply more soap to maintain a good lather.
   d. When arm is completed, leave lather on.

C. Second Hand

1. Repeat on other arm. Some systems require the use of a second sterile brush for the second hand. When this is so, discard the first brush into the proper container and obtain second brush.
2. At one-half of scrub time, rinse hands and arms thoroughly, first one and then the other, starting at the fingertips and letting water pass down over the arm.
3. Lather and repeat.
4. At end of time (or counts), rinse thoroughly, each arm separately, from fingertips. Apply towel from fingertips to elbow without reapplying to hand area.
5. Hold hands up and clasped together. Proceed to dressing area for gowning and gloving.

GLOVES AND GLOVING

Wearing gloves has become standard practice to protect both the patient and the clinician from cross-contamination.

I. CRITERIA FOR SELECTION OF TREATMENT/EXAMINATION GLOVES

A. Safety Factors

1. Effective barrier; evidence from manufacturer of quality control standards.
2. Impermeable to patient's saliva, blood, and bacteria.
3. Strength and durability to resist tears and punctures.
4. Impervious to materials routinely used during clinical procedures.
5. Nonirritating or harmful to skin; use nonlatex gloves when patient or clinician is allergic.

B. Comfort Factors

1. Fit hand well; no interference with motion; glove cuff extends to provide coverage over cuff of long sleeve.
2. Tactile sense minimally decreased.
3. Taste and odor not unpleasant for patient.

II. TYPES OF GLOVES

A. Material

1. Latex.
2. Nonlatex: neoprene, block copolymer, vinyl, N-nitrile.[17]

B. For Patient Care

1. *Nonsterile Single-Use Examination/Treatment.* Latex, nonlatex.
2. *Presterilized Single-Use Surgical.* Latex, nonlatex.

C. Utility Gloves

1. *Heavy duty.* Latex, nonlatex (puncture resistant for clinic cleanup).
2. *Plastic.* Food handler's glove to wear as overglove.

D. Dermal Underglove: to reduce irritation from latex or nonlatex.

III. PROCEDURES FOR USE OF GLOVES

A. Mask and Eyewear Placement

Place mask and protective eyewear prior to handwashing and gloving to prevent the need for manipulating the mask around the face and hair after washing the hands.

B. Pregloving Handwash
1. First wash of the day is performed with the short scrub; all other times require the short standard procedure.
2. Hands must be dried thoroughly to control moisture inside glove and thus discourage growth of bacteria.

C. Glove Placement
1. Always glove and deglove in front of the patient; a patient may need assurance that gloves are new and used only for that appointment.
2. Place gloves over the cuff of long-sleeved clinic wear to provide complete protection of arms from exposure to contamination.

D. Avoiding Contamination
Keep gloved hands away from face, hair, clothing (pockets), telephone, patient records, clinician's stool, and all parts of the dental equipment that have not been predisinfected and covered with a barrier material.

E. Torn, Cut, or Punctured Glove
Remove immediately, wash hands thoroughly, and don new gloves.

F. Removal of Gloves
1. Develop a procedure whereby gloves can be removed without contaminating the hands from the exposed external surfaces of the gloves. Figure 3-4 illustrates one system for glove removal.
2. Wash hands promptly after glove removal. Organisms on the hands multiply rapidly inside the warm, moist environment of the glove, even when no external contamination has occurred.

LATEX HYPERSENSITIVITY

Patients and clinicians may have or may develop a sensitivity to natural rubber latex. Symptoms of a hypersensitive reaction range from a dermatitis to a life-threatening anaphylactic shock. The only available treatment for latex allergy is avoiding all contact.

Latex sensitivity is due to the protein allergens and to additives used when the commercial latex is prepared. Latex allergens occur in any equipment or product used that contains natural rubber latex. Table 3-3 lists a few of the possible sources. Gloves are the most frequently used, and when powdered (cornstarch), the allergen can become airborne and be dispersed throughout the clinical area and on the personnel.

Equipment listed in Table 3-3 may contain NRL. However, many of the items also are made of alternative materials. When the label on a product does not list the contents, the manufacturer should be contacted to identify latex-free items.

I. CLINICAL MANIFESTATIONS
A. Methods of Exposure
1. Aeroallergen inhalation (from powdered gloves)
2. Donning gloves
3. Mucosal contact

B. Type I Hypersensitivity (immediate reaction)
1. Urticaria: hives
2. Dermatitis: rash, itching
3. Nasal problems: sneezing, itchy nose, runny nose

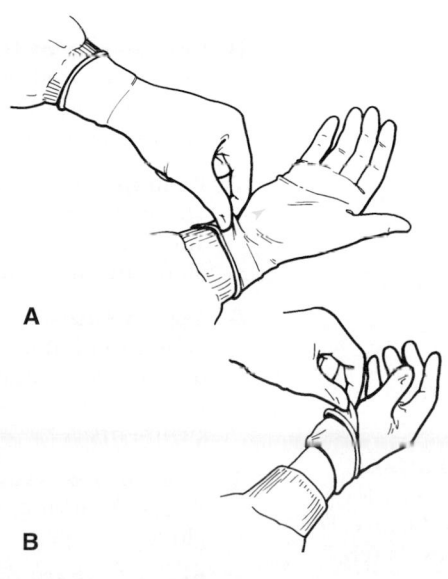
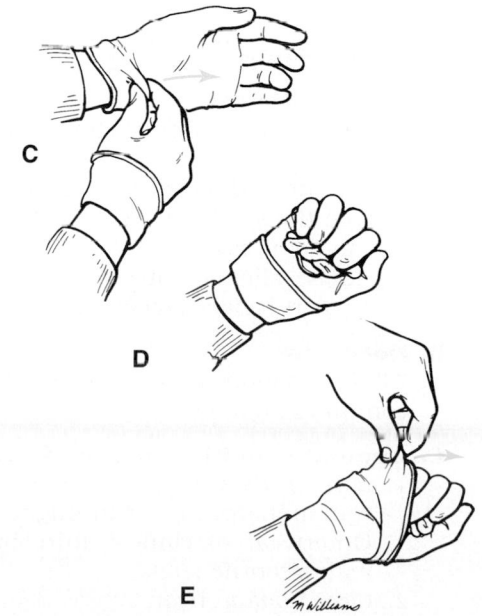

FIGURE 3-4 Removal of Gloves. (A) Use left fingers to pinch right glove near edge to fold back. **(B)** Fold edge back without contact with clean inside surface. **(C)** Use right fingers to contact outside of left glove at the wrist to invert and remove. **(D)** Bunch glove into the palm. **(E)** With ungloved left hand, grasp inner noncontaminated portion of the right glove to peel it off, enclosing other glove as it is inverted.

TABLE 3-3 Equipment That May Contain Latex

Gloves	Stopper in anesthesia
Masks (elastic head band)	Carpule
Goggles	Orthodontic elastics
Rubber dam	Bite blocks
Nitrous oxide nosepiece	Mixing bowl
and tubing	Suction adapter
O ring (on ultrasonic insert)	Blood pressure cuff
Lead apron cover	Stethoscope
Rubber polishing cup	

4. Respiratory reaction: breathing difficulty, asthmalike wheezing, coughing
5. Eyes: watery, itchy
6. Drop in blood pressure: shock
7. Anaphylaxis (Table 61-5, page 913)

C. Type IV Hypersensitivity (delayed reaction)
Contact dermatitis develops 6 to 72 hours after contact.

II. INDIVIDUALS AT HIGH RISK FOR LATEX SENSITIVITY

A. Have Had Frequent Exposure to Latex Products
1. Occupational exposure: health-care workers who wear latex gloves regularly for patient care.
2. Multiple medical surgeries or treatments requiring placement of rubber tubes or drains. Examples: genitourinary anomalies, spina bifida.

B. Have Other Documented Allergies
Examples: food allergies (avocado, banana, kiwi fruit, chestnuts, papaya).

C. Worker in a Rubber-Manufacturing Plant

III. MANAGEMENT

A. Medical History
1. Questions in history should reveal all allergies.
2. Questions directed to latex may not suffice. Questions about other specific products should be asked.
3. Advise allergic patients to obtain and wear an alert badge (bracelet).

B. Document
All information should be carefully recorded for continuing reference.

C. Appointment Planning for Allergic Patient
1. *Early in the Day.* Meet before glove powder contaminates the air throughout the facility. Outerwear of clinical attire becomes laden with airborne latex.
2. *Clean Clinical Areas*

a. Person preparing room must wear non-latex gloves.
b. Wipe all surfaces to remove allergen.
3. *No Latex in the Treatment Room.* Use nonlatex products for high-risk patients (whether or not specific latex sensitivity has been known and reported in the history).
4. *Prepare Latex-free Carts.*[18] Materials and gloves, for use when seeing high-risk patients, can be readied in advance.

E. Emergency Treatment Equipment and Drugs Ready
1. Inform the entire dental team of appointment.
2. Have a latex-free emergency cart available.[18]
3. Alert for emergency.

TECHNICAL HINTS

I. EYE WASH STATION

The eye wash station equipment should not be connected to a sink used by clinicians for patient preparation. It must not be connected to the regular faucets unless the hot water source is turned off permanently.

II. SKIN INTEGRITY

Small abrasions or cracks of the fingers should be covered with a clear liquid bandage for safety under gloves.

III. FACTORS AFFECTING GLOVE INTEGRITY

A. Length of Time Worn
New pair for each patient is the basic requirement; total time worn should be no longer than 1 hour; when gloves develop a sticky surface, remove, wash hands, and reglove with a fresh pair.

B. Complexity of the Procedure
Certain procedures are more likely to promote perforations, especially when sharp instruments must be changed frequently.

C. Packaging of the Gloves
Top gloves of a new package are tightly packed and can be torn when removed; must be handled carefully until pressure is relieved.

D. Size of Glove
When too long, the extra material at the fingertips can get caught, torn, or in the way; picking up small objects is difficult, especially sharp instruments.

E. Pressure of Time
Stress; working too fast increases the risk of glove damage.

F. Storage of Gloves
Keep in cool, dark place; exposure to heat, sun,

or fluorescent light increases potential for deterioration and perforations.

G. Agents Used
Certain chemicals react with the glove material; for example, petroleum jelly, alcohol, and products made with alcohol tend to break down the glove integrity.

H. Hazards From the Hands
Long fingernails, rings worn inside gloves.

FACTORS TO TEACH THE PATIENT

I. Importance of the patient's complete history for the protection of both the patient and the professional person.
II. Necessity for use of barriers (face mask, protective eyewear, and gloves) by the clinician for the benefit of the patient.
III. Importance of eye protection.

REFERENCES

1. **United States Department of Labor,** Occupational Safety and Health Administration: Controlling Occupational Exposure to Bloodborne Pathogens in Dentistry, OSHA 3129, 1992. United States Government Printing Office: 1992–312–410/64790.
2. **United States Centers for Disease Control and Prevention, Advisory Committee on Immunization Practices (ACIP):** Recommended Childhood Immunization Schedule—United States, 1998, *MMWR, 47,* 8, January 16, 1998.
3. **United States Centers for Disease Control and Prevention:** Immunization of Adolescents, *MMWR, 45,* 1–13, No. RR-13, November 22, 1996.
4. **Benenson,** A.S., ed.: *Control of Communicable Disease in Man,* 16th ed. Washington, D.C., American Public Health Association, 1995, p. 464.
5. **United States Centers for Disease Control:** Update on Adult Immunization. Recommendations of the Immunization Practices Advisory Committee (ACIP), *MMWR, 40,* 1–94, No. RR-12, November 15, 1991.
6. **Federation Dentaire Internationale,** Commission on Dental Practice: Technical Report: Recommendations for Hygiene in Dental Practice, *Int. Dent. J., 29,* 72, March, 1979.
7. **United States Centers for Disease Control:** Guidelines for Preventing the Transmission of *Mycobacterium tuberculosis* in Health-care Facilities, *MMWR, 43,* 1–132, No. RR-13, October 28, 1994.
8. **Micik,** R.E., Miller, R.L., and Leong, A.C.: Studies on Dental Aerobiology: III. Efficacy of Surgical Masks in Protecting Dental Personnel from Airborne Bacterial Particles, *J. Dent. Res., 50,* 626, May–June, 1971.
9. **Miller,** R.L. and Micik, R.E.: Air Pollution and Its Control in the Dental Office, *Dent. Clin. North Am., 22,* 453, July, 1978.
10. **Cooley,** R.L., Cottingham, A.J., Abrams, H., and Barkmeier, W.W.: Ocular Injuries Sustained in the Dental Office: Methods of Detection, Treatment, and Prevention, *J. Am. Dent. Assoc., 97,* 985, December, 1978.
11. **Wesson,** M.D. and Thornton, J.B.: Eye Protection and Ocular Complications in the Dental Office, *Gen. Dent., 37,* 19, January–February, 1989.
12. **Roberts-Harry,** T.J., Cass, A.E., and Jagger, J.D.: Ocular Injury and Infection in Dental Practice. A Survey and a Review of the Literature, *Br. Dent. J., 170,* 20, January 5, 1991.
13. **Office of Safety and Asepsis Procedures Research Foundation:** The Dental Infection Control Program, *OSAP Monthly Focus,* Focus no. 2, p.2, 1998.
14. **Gröschel,** D.H.M. and Pruett, T.L.: Surgical Antisepsis, in Block, S.S.: *Disinfection, Sterilization, and Preservation,* 4th ed. Philadelphia, Lea & Febiger, 1991, pp. 642–648.
15. **Harfst,** S.A.: Personal Barrier Protection, *Dent. Clin. North Am., 35,* 357, April, 1991.
16. **Allen,** A.L. and Organ, R.J.: Occult Blood Accumulation Under the Fingernails: A Mechanism for the Spread of Blood-borne Infection, *J. Am. Dent. Assoc., 105,* 455, September, 1982.
17. **Snyder,** H.A. and Settle, S.: The Rise in Latex Allergy: Implications for the Dentist, *J. Am. Dent. Assoc., 125,* 1089, August, 1994.
18. **Falcone,** K.J. and Powers, D.O.: Latex Allergy: Implications for Oral Health Care Professionals, *J. Dent. Hyg., 72,* 25, Summer, 1998.

SUGGESTED READINGS

Cottone, J.A., Terezhalmy, G.T., and Molinari, J.A.: *Practical Infection Control in Dentistry,* 2nd ed. Philadelphia, Williams & Wilkins, 1996, pp. 127–145.
Fedson, D.S.: Adult Immunization: Summary of the National Vaccine Advisory Committee Report, *JAMA, 272,* 1133, October 12, 1994.
Foley, E.S.: Update on Clinical Attire Requirements in Dental Hygiene Programs, *J. Dent. Hyg., 68,* 131, May–June, 1994.
Harfst, S.: Infection Control Update: Vaccinations, *J. Pract. Hyg., 5,* 43, July/August, 1996.
Hill, J.G., Grimwood, R.E., Hermesch, C.B., and Marks, J.G.: Prevalence of Occupationally Related Hand Dermatitis in Dental Workers, *J. Am. Dent. Assoc., 129,* 212, February, 1998.
McDonnell, W.M. and Askari, F.K.: Molecular Medicine: DNA Vaccines, *N. Engl. J. Med., 334,* 42, January 4, 1996.
Miller, C.H. and Palenik, C.J.: *Infection Control and Management of Hazardous Materials for the Dental Team.* St. Louis, Mosby, 1994, pp. 106–131.
Molinari, J.A.: Dermatitis in Dental Professionals: Causes, Treatment, and Prevention, *J. Pract. Hyg., 5,* 13, July/August, 1996.

Eye Protection

Christensen, R.P., Robison, R.A., Robinson, D.F., Ploeger, B.J., and Leavitt, R.W.: Efficiency of 42 Brands of Face Masks and Two Face Shields in Preventing Inhalation of Airborne Debris, *Gen. Dent., 39,* 414, November/December, 1991.
Ing, E., Ing, H.C., Ing, M., Fusco, D., and Ing, T.G.E.: Diagnosing Oral Diseases That Affect the Eyes, *J. Am. Dent. Assoc., 125,* 608, May, 1994.
Miller, C.: Make Eye Protection a Priority to Prevent Contamination and Injury, *RDH, 15,* 40, October, 1995.
Pacak-Carroll, D.: Remember Eye Protection is Necessary for Patients Too, *RDH, 12,* 14, June, 1992.
Shingleton, B.J.: Eye Injuries, *N. Engl. J. Med., 325,* 408, August 8, 1991.
Stokes, A.N., Burton, J.F., and Beale, R.P.: Eye Protection in Dental Practice, *N.Z. Dent. J., 86,* 14, January, 1990.

Gloves

Boyer, E.M.: The Effectiveness of a Low-chemical, Low-protein Medical Glove to Prevent or Reduce Dermatological Problems, *J. Dent. Hyg., 69,* 67, March–April, 1995.
Brownson, K.M. and Gobetti, J.P.: Fluorescein Dye Evaluation of Double-gloving, *Gen. Dent., 38,* 362, September–October, 1990.
Drunick, A.L., Burns, S., Gross, K., Tishk, M., and Feil, P.: A Comparative Study: The Effects of Latex and Vinyl Gloves on the Tactile Discrimination of First Year Dental Hygiene Students, *Clin. Prev. Dent., 12,* 21, June–July, 1990.
Burke, F.J.T. and Wilson, N.H.F.: The Incidence of Undiagnosed Punctures in Non-sterile Gloves, *Br. Dent. J., 168,* 67, January 20, 1990.
Chua, K.L., Taylor, G.S., and Bagg, J.: A Clinical and Labora-

tory Evaluation of Three Types of Operating Gloves for Use in Orthodontic Practice, *Br. J. Orthod., 23,* 115, May, 1996.

European Panel for Infection Control in Dentistry (EPICD): Hand Hygiene, Hand Care and Hand Protection for Clinical Dental Practice, *Br. Dent. J., 176,* 129, February 19, 1994.

Molinari, J.A.: Handwashing and Hand Care: Fundamental Asepsis Requirements, *Compend. Cont. Educ. Dent., 16,* 834, September, 1995.

Munksgaard, E.C.: Permeability of Protective Gloves to (di)Methacrylates in Resinous Dental Materials, *Scand. J. Dent. Res., 100,* 189, June, 1992.

Patton, L.L., Campbell, T.L., and Evers, S.P.: Prevalence of Glove Perforations During Double-Gloving for Dental Procedures, *Gen. Dent., 43,* 22, January–February, 1995.

Powell, B.J., Winkley, G.P., Brown, J.O., and Etersque, S.: Evaluating the Fit of Ambidextrous and Fitted Gloves: Implications for Hand Discomfort, *J. Am. Dent. Assoc., 125,* 1235, September, 1994.

Schwimmer, A., Massoumi, M., and Barr, C.E.: Efficacy of Double Gloving to Prevent Inner Glove Perforation During Outpatient Oral Surgical Procedures, *J. Am. Dent. Assoc., 125,* 196, February, 1994.

Shah, M., Lewis, F.M., and Gawkrodger, D.J.: Delayed and Immediate Orofacial Reactions Following Contact With Rubber Gloves During Treatment, *Br. Dent. J., 181,* 137, August 24, 1996.

Tinsley, D. and Chadwick, R.G.: The Permeability of Dental Gloves Following Exposure to Certain Dental Materials, *J. Dent., 25,* 65, January, 1997.

Latex Hypersensitivity

Brick, P. and Berthold, M.: Latex Allergies: The Hidden Occupational Hazard, *Access, 10,* 17, December, 1996.

Field, E.A. and Fay, M.F.: Issues of Latex Safety in Dentistry, *Br. Dent. J., 179,* 247, October 7, 1995.

Haman, C.P., Turjanmaa, K., Rietschel, R., Siew, C., Owensby, D., Gruninger, S.E., and Sullivan, K.M.: Natural Rubber Latex Hypersensitivity: Incidence and Prevalence of Type I Allergy in the Dental Professional, *J. Am. Dent. Assoc., 129,* 43, January, 1998.

Miller, C.: Offices Manage Allergies to Latex Material by Understanding Risks, Reducing Exposure, *RDH, 17,* 43, May, 1997.

Roy, A., Epstein, J., and Onno, E.: Latex Allergies in Dentistry: Recognition and Recommendations, *J. Can. Dent. Assoc., 63,* 297, April, 1997.

Safadi, G.S., Safadi, T.J., Terezhalmy, G.T., Taylor, J.S., Battisto, J.R., and Melton, A.L.: Latex Hypersensitivity: Its Prevalence Among Dental Professionals, *J. Am. Dent. Assoc., 127,* 83, January, 1996.

Spina Bifida

Engibous, P.J., Kittle, P.E., Jones, H.L., and Vance, B.J.: Latex Allergy in Patients With Spina Bifida, *Pediatr. Dent., 15,* 364, September/October, 1993.

Nelson, L.P., Soporowski, N.J., and Shusterman, S.: Latex Allergies in Children With Spina Bifida: Relevance for the Pediatric Dentist, *Pediatr. Dent., 16,* 18, January/February, 1994.

Peters, H.C.: Latex Allergy and Spina Bifida, (Letter), *J. Can. Dent. Assoc., 60,* 177, March, 1994.

Infection Control: Clinical Procedures

4

The success of a planned system for control of disease transmission depends on the cooperative effort of each member of the dental health team. The aim is to provide the highest level of infection control possible and practical that will ensure a safe environment for both patient and clinicians.

The presence of specific disease-producing organisms is rarely known; therefore, application of protective, preventive procedures is needed prior to, during, and following *all* patient appointments. Definitions and abbreviations related to infection control are provided in Box 4-1.

BOX 4-1 KEY WORDS AND ABBREVIATIONS: Infection Control

ADA: American Dental Association, 211 E. Chicago Ave., Chicago, IL 60611.

Antimicrobial agent (ăn″tĭ-mī-krō′bē-al): any agent that kills or suppresses the growth of microorganisms.

Antiseptic (ăn″tĭ-sĕp′tĭk): a substance that prevents or arrests the growth or action of microorganisms either by inhibiting their activity or by destroying them; term used especially for preparations applied topically to living tissue.

Asepsis (ā-sĕp′sĭs): free from contamination with microorganisms; includes sterile conditions in tissues and on materials, as obtained by exclusion, removing, or killing organisms.

   Chain of asepsis: a procedure that avoids transfer of infection. The "chain" implies that each step, related to the previous one, continues to be carried out without contamination.

Aseptic technique: procedures carried out in the absence of pathogenic microorganisms.

Bioburden: a microbiologic load, that is, the number of contaminating organisms present on a surface prior to sterilization or disinfection.

Biofilm: the surface film that contains microorganisms and other biologic substances.

Biohazard: a substance that poses a biologic risk because it is contaminated with biomaterial with a potential for transmitting infection.

Biologic indicator: a preparation of nonpathogenic microorganisms, usually bacterial spores, carried by an ampule or a specially impregnated paper enclosed within a package during sterilization and subsequently incubated to verify that sterilization has occurred.

Broad spectrum: indicates a range of activity of a drug or chemical substance against a wide variety of microorganisms.

Chemical indicator: a color change stripe or other mark, often on autoclave tape or bag, used to monitor the process of sterilization; color change indicates that the package has been brought to a specific temperature, but it is not an indicator of sterilization.

Contamination (kon-tam″ĭ-nā′shun): introduction of microorganisms, blood, or other potentially infectious material or agent onto a surface or into tissue.

Decontamination (dē″kon-tăm-ĭ-na′shun): disinfection; use of physical or chemical means to remove, inactivate, or destroy pathogenic microorganisms on a surface or item to the extent that they are no longer capable of transmitting infectious disease; the surface or item is rendered safe for handling, use, or disposal.

Disinfectant (dĭs″ĭn-fek′tant): an agent, usually a chemical, but may be a physical agent, such as x rays or ultraviolet light, that destroys microorganisms but may not kill bacterial spores; refers to substances applied to inanimate objects.

EPA: United States Environmental Protection Agency, Washington, DC.

   EPA registered: number on a label indicates that the product has the acceptance of EPA.

FDA: United States Food and Drug Administration, 5600 Fishers Lane, Rockville, MD 20857; regulates food, drugs, biologic products, medical devices, radiologic products.

Infection control: the selection and use of procedures and products to prevent the spread of infectious disease.

Infectious waste: contaminated with blood, saliva, or other substances; potentially or actually infected with pathogenic material; officially called "regulated" waste.

Invasive procedure: entry into tissues during which bleeding occurs or the potential for bleeding exists.

Nosocomial (nŏs″ō-kō′mē-al) **infection:** an infection occurring in a patient while in a health-care facility that was not present at the time of admission; includes infections acquired in the health-care facility but appearing after dismissal.

OSAP: Organization for Safety and Asepsis Procedures Research Foundation, P.O. Box 6297, Annapolis, MD 21401.

OSHA: United States Occupational Safety and Health Administration, Department of Labor, Washington, DC 20210.

(continued)

BOX 4-I KEY WORDS AND ABBREVIATIONS: Infection Control (Continued)

PPE: personal protective equipment.

Sanitation: the process by which the number of organisms on inanimate objects is reduced to a safe level. It does not imply freedom from microorganisms and generally refers to a cleaning process.

Shelf life: stability of an item after it has been prepared; length of time a substance or preparation can be kept without changes occurring in its chemical structure or other properties.

Sporicide (spo′rĭ-sīd): substance that kills spores.

Sterilization: process by which all forms of life, including bacterial spores, are destroyed by physical or chemical means.

Synergism (sĭn′er-jĭzm): the joint action of agents so that their combined effect is greater than the sum of their individual parts.

Waste:

Infectious waste: capable of causing an infectious disease.

Contaminated waste: items that have contacted blood or other body secretions.

Hazardous waste: poses a risk to humans or the environment.

Toxic waste: capable of having a poisonous effect.

Regulated waste: liquid blood or saliva, sharps contaminated with blood or saliva, and nonsharp solid waste saturated with or caked with liquid or semisolid blood or saliva or tissue including teeth (OSHA).

I. OBJECTIVES OF INFECTION CONTROL

The following are necessary to prevent the transmission of infectious agents and eliminate cross-contamination:

A. Reduction of available pathogenic microorganisms to a level at which the normal resistance mechanisms of the body may prevent infection.

B. Elimination of cross-contamination by breaking the chain of infection (Figure 2-1, page 17).

C. Application of universal precautions by treating each patient as if all human blood and body fluids are known to be infectious for HIV, HBV, and other blood-borne pathogens.

II. BASIC CONSIDERATIONS FOR SAFE PRACTICE

Basic factors involved in the conduct of safe practice include the material in Chapter 3 and the following, to be described in this chapter:

A. Treatment room features.
B. Instrument management.
1. Precleaning.
2. Sterilization and disinfection.
C. Preparation for appointment.
D. Unit water lines.
E. Environmental surfaces.
F. Care of sterile instruments.
G. Patient preparation.
H. Summary of procedures for the prevention of disease transmission.
I. Disposal of waste.

TREATMENT ROOM FEATURES

The design of many treatment rooms may not be conducive to ideal planning for infection control. Changes can be made in routines so that updated, preferred systems can be adapted. When renovations or a new dental office or clinic are anticipated, plans must reflect the most advanced knowledge available relative to safety and disease control.

A partial list of notable features is included here and illustrated in Figure 4-1. The objective is to have materials, shapes, and surface textures that facilitate the effective use of infection control measures.

1. UNIT
   —Designed for easy cleaning and disinfection, with smooth, uncluttered surfaces.
   —Removable hoses that can be cleaned and disinfected.
   —Hoses that are not mechanically retractable, but are straight, not coiled, with round smooth outer surfaces.
   —Syringes with autoclavable tips or fitted with disposable tips.
   —Handpieces with anti-retraction valves.
   —Handpieces that can be autoclaved.
2. DENTAL CHAIR
   —Controls all foot operated. If manually operated, need disposable barrier cover for buttons (switches).
   —Surface and seamless finish of easily cleaned plastic material that withstands chemical disinfection without damage or discoloring; cloth upholstery to be avoided.
3. LIGHT
   —Foot-activated switches.

OPTIMAL TREATMENT ROOM FEATURES

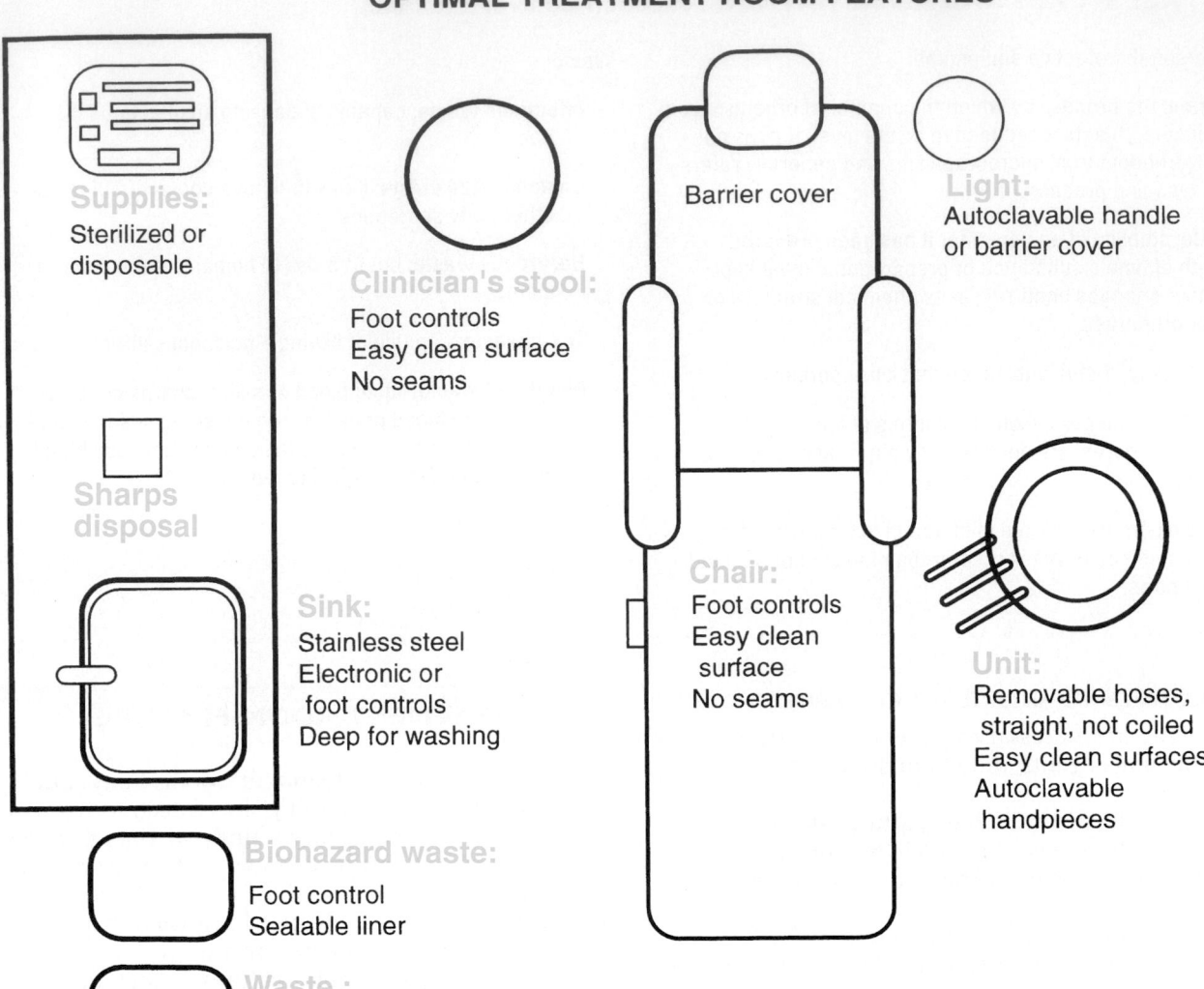

Supplies:
Sterilized or disposable

Sharps disposal

Sink:
Stainless steel
Electronic or foot controls
Deep for washing

Biohazard waste:
Foot control
Sealable liner

Waste :
Large opening
Heavy-duty liner

Clinician's stool:
Foot controls
Easy clean surface
No seams

Barrier cover

Chair:
Foot controls
Easy clean surface
No seams

Light:
Autoclavable handle or barrier cover

Unit:
Removable hoses, straight, not coiled
Easy clean surfaces
Autoclavable handpieces

Floor: Smooth, easy clean, nonabsorbent, no carpeting

FIGURE 4-1 Optimal Treatment Room Features.

—Removable handle for sterilization or disposable barrier cover.
4. CLINICIAN'S STOOL
 —Smooth, plastic material that is easily disinfected and has a minimum of seams and creases.
 —Foot-operated controls. If manually operated, must have a barrier cover for the control.
5. FLOOR
 —Carpeting should be avoided.
 —Floor covering should be smooth, easily cleaned, nonabsorbent.
6. SINK
 —Smooth material (stainless steel).
 —Wide and deep enough for effective handwashing without splashing.

—Water faucets and soap dispensers with electronic, "knee," or foot-operated controls.
 —Separate room or area for contaminated instrument care.
7. SUPPLIES
 —All sterilizable or disposable.
8. WASTE
 —Receptacle with opening large enough to prevent contact with sides when material is dropped in; heavy-duty plastic bag liner to be sealed tightly for disposal.
 —Sharps disposal.
 —Small biohazard receptacle near treatment area to receive contaminated sponges and other waste, for disposal in large waste container clearly marked for contaminated waste.

INSTRUMENT PROCESSING CENTER

The successful practice of universal precautions to prevent cross-contamination depends on the development of, and strict adherence to, a planned program for instrument management. A good rule is to learn the most effective, safe system and then to follow that method without exception. A specific routine is easier for the entire dental team to follow, and peer review is built-in.

The basic steps in the recirculation of instruments from the time an appointment procedure is completed until the instruments are sterilized and ready for use in the next clinical appointment are shown in the flowchart in Figure 4-2. Each of the steps is described in the following sections.

HOLDING STEP

Cleaning is more difficult when saliva and blood are left on instruments for a period of time after use. If the cleaning process cannot be accomplished immediately, a container with a holding solution of a mild disinfectant/detergent should be available in which to place the used instruments.

When a cassette is not used, the instruments can be placed directly into the basket for later submergence into the ultrasonic cleaner. The basket can be placed in the soaking solution. By doing so, less handling of the instruments is required. When a cassette is used, the instruments are arranged in the cassette, which then holds the instruments through the entire preclean and sterilization process.

The instrument holding step is intended for a short period of time. Nonstainless instruments can corrode and discolor unless removed for cleaning within a reasonable time period.

Contaminated instruments must be moved to a separate area set aside for the specific purpose of infection control. Cleaning and preparation for sterilization are accomplished away from treatment rooms.

CLEANING STEP[1]

Ideally the instruments are contained within a cassette so that little or no handling is required. When instruments are not in a cassette, transfer forceps are used for transferring contaminated instruments.

For all cleaning processes, heavy-duty, puncture-resistant gloves must be used, and a face mask and protective eyewear must be worn. The two methods for cleaning instruments are ultrasonic processing and manual cleaning.

I. ULTRASONIC PROCESSING

Ultrasonic cleaning prior to sterilization is safer than manual cleaning. Manual cleaning of instruments is

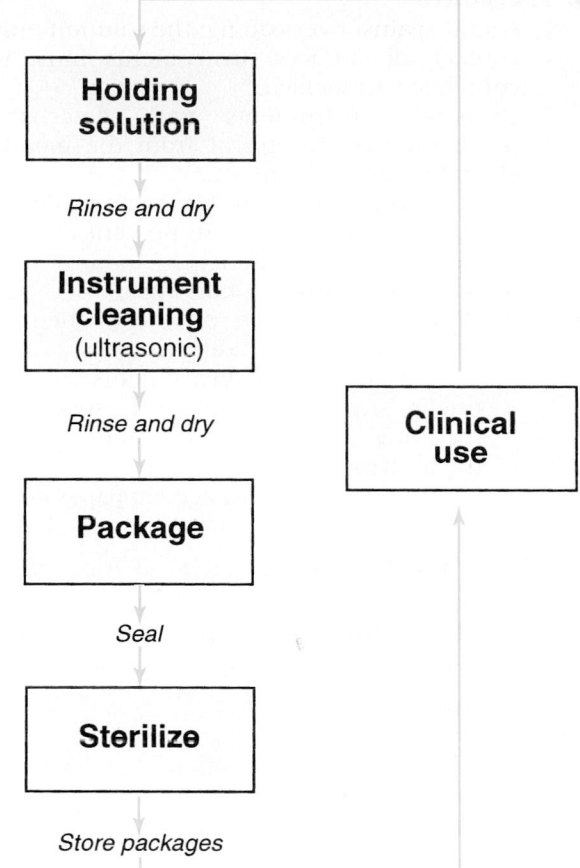

FIGURE 4-2 Recirculation of Instruments. Flowchart shows step-by-step process. At the completion of treatment, instruments are cleaned, packaged, sterilized, and stored. They are kept sealed until patient appointment begins.

a dangerous, difficult, and time-consuming procedure.

Ultrasonic equipment is maintained and used according to manufacturer's guidelines. *Ultrasonic processing is not a substitute for sterilization; it is only a cleaning process.*

A. Advantages

Benefits from the use of ultrasonic cleaning include the following:

1. Increased efficiency in obtaining a high degree of cleanliness.
2. Reduced danger to clinician from direct contact with potentially pathogenic microorganisms.
3. Improved effectiveness for disinfection.
4. Elimination of possible dissemination of microorganisms through release of aerosols and droplets, which can occur during the scrubbing process.
5. Penetration into areas of the instruments where the bristles of a brush may be unable to contact.
6. Removal of tarnish.

B. Procedure
1. Guard against overloading; the solution must contact all surfaces. Instruments must be completely immersed.
2. Dismantle instruments with detachable parts, such as the mirror from the handle. Open jointed instruments.
3. Time accurately by manufacturer's guide.
4. Drain, rinse, and air dry to prevent dilution of the ultrasonic solution.
5. Indications for thorough drying:
   a. When sterilizing by dry heat, chemical vapor, or ethylene oxide.
   b. Nonstainless steel instruments require predip in rust inhibitor before steam autoclaving; water on instruments dilutes the antirust solution.
   c. Instruments to be packaged in paper wrap.

II. MANUAL CLEANING

Ultrasonic processing is the method of choice, but when manual cleaning is the only alternative, precautions must be taken to prevent contamination.

A. Procedure
1. Wear heavy-duty gloves and mask.
2. Dismantle instruments with detachable parts. Open jointed instruments.
3. Use detergent and scrub with a long-handled brush under running water; hold the instruments low in the sink.
4. Brush with strokes away from the body; use care not to splash and contaminate the surrounding area.
5. Rinse thoroughly.
6. Dry on paper towels (same reasons as those listed for ultrasonic processing).

B. Care of Brushes
1. Color code brushes to distinguish from hand-wash brushes.
2. Soak and wash contaminated brushes in detergent; rinse thoroughly and sterilize.

PACKAGING STEP[1]

I. PURPOSES
A. To prevent contamination of newly sterilized instruments as soon as they are removed from the sterilizer.
B. To provide a means of storing instruments to keep them in sets for individual appointment use and sterilized and ready for immediate use on opening.

II. INSTRUMENT ARRANGEMENT
A. Preset cassettes, trays, or packages can be preplanned to contain all the items usually needed for a particular appointment.
B. Each tray or package should be dated and marked for identification of contents: for example, *Adult Scaling and Root Planing; Examination.*
C. Clear packages with self-seal permit instrument identification without special labeling. Figure 4-3 shows clear, "see-through" packages for easy identification of package contents.

III. PREPARATION

A. Materials
Each method of sterilization has specific requirements, and the manufacturer's recommendations can be reviewed. Sturdy wrapping is necessary to prevent punctures or tears that break the chain of asepsis and require a repeat of the process. The wrap must permit the steam or chemical vapor to pass through the contents.

B. Seal
Indicator tape is used. Pins, paper clips, or other types of metal fasteners are not used because they provide holes for the entry of microorganisms.

IV. CHEMICAL INDICATOR FOR CYCLE MONITORING

Chemical indicator tape is used to seal all packages, except when the wrap has built-in indicators. The chemical, usually in the form of a series of stripes, changes color during the sterilization process. The change of color means that the autoclave reached a designated temperature required for penetration and that the contact time was adequate (Figure 4-3). Distinct black stripes should appear. A lighter color change may be a warning signal that the autoclave function should be checked.

Indicator tape does not serve to test for true sterilization. A biologic indicator in the form of microbial spores must be used to test each sterilizer routinely.

The striped indicator tape is left on the sealed package and thereby serves to identify those packages ready for use. Packages are kept completely sealed until unwrapped in front of the patient.

STERILIZATION

I. APPROVED METHODS
Each of the methods listed here is described in detail in the sections following. Table 4-1 summarizes the operating requirements of each.
A. Moist heat: steam under pressure.
B. Dry heat.
C. Chemical vapor.
D. Ethylene oxide.

II. SELECTION OF METHOD
All materials and items cannot be treated by the same system of sterilization. It is necessary to supplement with disposable single-use products when sterilization is not possible.

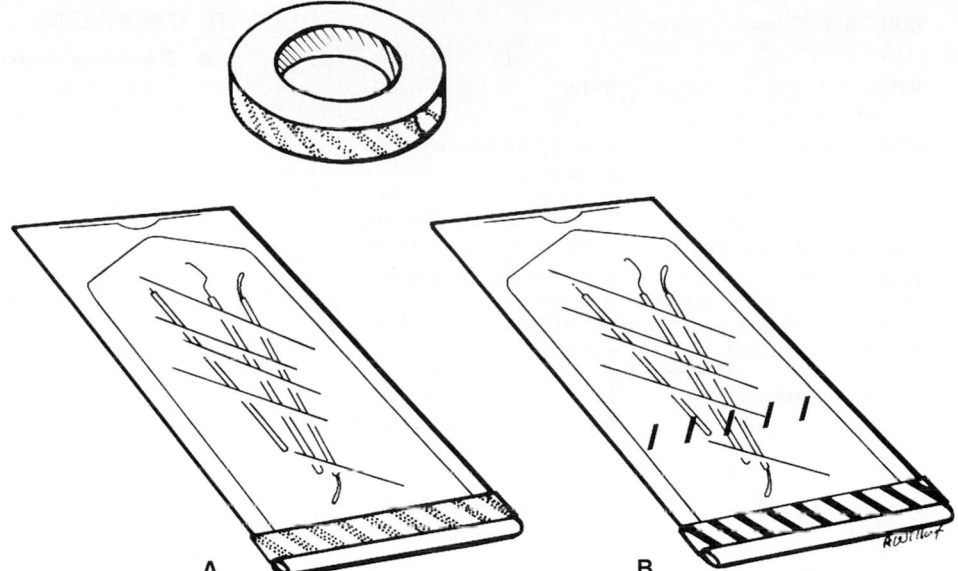

■FIGURE 4-3 Process Indicator Tape (A) Before autoclaving. **(B)** After autoclaving. The change of color in the stripes indicates that the package has been subjected to the proper temperature for sterilization, but does not show sterilization. A biologic indicator is also needed for periodic monitoring to determine that the autoclave is functioning properly and that sterilization is actually taking place.

The method for sterilization that is selected must provide complete destruction of all microorganisms, viruses, and spores and yet must not damage the instruments and other materials. In addition, the procedures must not be overly complex, or many errors in the processing can occur.

Careful, specific use of sterilizing equipment in accord with the manufacturer's specifications is necessary. Incomplete sterilization most frequently results from inadequate preparation of the materials to be sterilized (cleaning, packaging), misuse of the equipment (overloading, timing, temperature selection), or inadequate maintenance.

III. TESTS FOR STERILIZATION

Sterilization is the process by which all forms of life are destroyed. That definition provides the rationale for testing whether a sterilizer is working properly.

The testing system requires the use of selected test microorganisms that are put through a regular cycle of sterilization and then are cultured. When no growth occurs, the sterilizer has performed with maximum efficiency.

A. Microorganisms Used

1. *Steam Autoclave. Bacillus stearothermophilus* in vials, ampules, or on strips.
2. *Dry Heat Oven. Bacillus subtilis* strips.
3. *Chemical Vapor. Bacillus stearothermophilus* on strips.
4. *Ethylene Oxide. Bacillus subtilis* strips.

B. Procedures

The ampule, vial, or strip is placed in the center of a package, which in turn is placed in the middle of the load of packages to be sterilized. After the cycle has been completed at the customary time and temperature, the ampule or strip is incubated. Ampules and vials show the color change associated with no living microorganisms, whereas the strip organisms are cultured and show no growth if the sterilizer has performed properly.

Table 4-2 shows indications for performing spore tests in dental settings. Records that are kept should show dates and outcomes.

C. Frequency

At least weekly testing is recommended. Equipment can be obtained for performing the testing, or commercial mail-in services are available.

IV. THE CHEMICAL INDICATOR

In contrast to spore testing, the chemical indicator is related only to the temperature to which the autoclave was heated. As described on page 60, a chemical indicator is used routinely when packaging instruments (Figure 4-3).

	TABLE 4-1 Methods of Sterilization		

Method	Sterilizing Requirement		
	Time	Temperature	Pressure
Moist heat Steam under pressure (steam autoclave)	15–30 min	250°F 121°C	15 psi
Dry heat oven	120 min	320°F 160°C	
Unsaturated chemical vapor	20 min	270°F 132°C	20–40 psi
Ethylene oxide gas	10–16 hr	75°F 25°C	

TABLE 4-2 Spore Testing

When	Why
Once per week	To verify proper use and functioning
Whenever a new type of packaging material or tray is used	To ensure that the sterilizing agent is getting inside to the surface of the instruments
After training of new sterilization personnel	To verify proper use of the sterilizer
During initial uses of a new sterilizer	To make sure unfamiliar operating instructions are being followed
First run after repair of a sterilizer	To make sure that the sterilizer is functioning properly
With every implantable device and hold device until results of test are known	Extra precaution for sterilization of item to be implanted into tissues
After any other change in the sterilizing procedure	To make sure change does not prevent sterilization

Adapted from Miller, C.H. and Palenik, C.J.: Sterilization, Disinfection, and Asepsis in Dentistry, in Block, S.S.: *Disinfection, Sterilization, and Preservation,* 4th ed. Philadelphia, Lea & Febiger, 1991, p. 680.

MOIST HEAT: STEAM UNDER PRESSURE

Destruction of microorganisms by heat takes place as a result of inactivation of essential cellular proteins or enzymes. Moist heat causes coagulation of protein.

I. USE

Moist heat may be used for all materials except oils, waxes, and powders that are impervious to steam, or for materials that cannot be subjected to high temperatures.

II. PRINCIPLES OF ACTION

A. Sterilization is achieved by action of heat and moisture; pressure serves only to attain high temperature.
B. Sterilization depends on the penetrating ability of steam.
   1. Air must be excluded, otherwise steam penetration and heat transfer are prevented.
   2. Space between objects is essential to ensure access for the steam.
   3. Materials must be thoroughly cleaned and air dried; adherent material can provide a barrier to the steam.
   4. Air discharge occurs in a downward direction; load must be arranged for free passage of steam toward bottom of autoclave.

III. OPERATION

A. Packing Autoclave
Pack loosely to permit steam to reach all instruments in all packages; place jars and tall vessels on their sides to permit air to leave as steam enters.

B. Standard Procedure
The temperature must remain at 121°C (250°F) at 15 pounds pressure for 15 minutes after the meters show that proper pressure and temperature have been reached. Use 30 minutes for heavy loads to ensure penetration.

C. Cooling
1. *Dry Materials.* Release steam pressure, turn operating valve, and open the door; required time for drying is about 15 minutes.
2. *Liquids.* Reduce chamber pressure slowly at an even rate over 10 to 12 minutes to prevent boiling or escape of fluids into the chamber; it is preferable to turn off the autoclave and let the pressure fall before opening the door. Check heat sensitivity of each solution and avoid prolonged exposure, as indicated.

IV. CARE OF AUTOCLAVE

Manufacturer's instructions must be followed.

A. Daily
Maintain proper level of distilled water; wash trays and interior surfaces of chamber with water and a mild detergent; clean removable plug, screen, or strainer.

B. Weekly
Flush chamber discharge system with an appropriate cleaning solution, such as hot trisodium phosphate or a commercial cleaner.

V. EVALUATION OF STEAM UNDER PRESSURE

A. Advantages
1. All microorganisms, spores, and viruses are destroyed quickly and efficiently.
2. Wide variety of materials may be treated; most economical method of sterilization.

B. Disadvantages
1. May corrode carbon steel instruments if precautions are not taken.
2. Unsuitable for oils or powders that are impervious to heat.

DRY HEAT

The action of dry heat is oxidation.

I. USE

A. Primarily for materials that cannot safely be sterilized with steam under pressure.

B. For oils and powders when they are thermostabile at the required temperatures.

C. For small metal instruments enclosed in special containers or that might be corroded or rusted by moisture.

II. PRINCIPLES OF ACTION

A. Sterilization is achieved by heat that is conducted from the exterior surface to the interior of the object; the time required to penetrate varies among materials.

B. Sterilization can result when the whole material is treated for a sufficient length of time at the required temperature; therefore, timing for sterilization must start when the entire contents of the sterilizer have reached the peak temperature needed for that load.

C. Oil, grease, or organic debris on instruments insulates and protects microorganisms from the sterilizing effect.

III. OPERATION

A. Temperature
A temperature of 160°C (320°F) maintained for 2 hours; 170°C (340°F) for 1 hour. Timing must start after the desired temperature has been reached.

B. Penetration Time
Heat penetration varies with different materials, and the nature and properties of various materials must be considered.

C. Care
Care must be taken not to overheat because certain materials can be affected. Temperatures over 160°C (320°F) may destroy the sharp edges of cutting instruments.

IV. EVALUATION OF DRY HEAT

A. Advantages
1. Useful for materials that cannot be subjected to steam under pressure.
2. When maintained at correct temperature, it is well suited for sharp instruments.
3. No corrosion as compared with steam under pressure.

B. Disadvantages
1. Long exposure time required; penetration slow and uneven.
2. High temperature critical to certain materials.

CHEMICAL VAPOR STERILIZER

A combination of alcohols, formaldehyde, ketone, water, and acetone heated under pressure produces a gas that is effective as a sterilizing agent.

I. USE

Chemical vapor sterilization cannot be used for materials or objects that can be altered by the chemicals that make the vapor or that cannot withstand the high temperature. Examples are low-melting plastics, liquids, or heat-sensitive handpieces.

II. PRINCIPLES OF ACTION

Microbial and viral destruction results from the permeation of the heated formaldehyde and alcohol. Heavy, tightly wrapped, or sealed packages would not permit the penetration of the vapors.

III. OPERATION

A. Temperature
From 127° to 132°C (260° to 270°F) with 20 to 40 pounds pressure in accord with the manufacturer's directions.

B. Time
Minimum of 20 minutes after the correct temperature and pressure have been attained. Time should be extended for a large load or a heavy wrap.

C. Cooling at the Completion of the Cycle
Instruments are dry. Instruments need a short period for cooling.

IV. CARE OF STERILIZER

Depending on the amount of use, refilling is needed by at least every 30 cycles. In accord with manufacturer's instructions, the condensate tray is removed, the exhausted solution emptied, and the tray cleaned.

V. EVALUATION OF CHEMICAL VAPOR STERILIZER

A. Advantages
1. Corrosion- and rust-free operation for carbon steel instruments.
2. Ability to sterilize in a relatively short total cycle.
3. Ease of operation and care of the equipment.

B. Disadvantages
1. Adequate ventilation is needed; cannot use in a small room.
2. Slight odor, which is rarely objectionable.

ETHYLENE OXIDE[2]

Gaseous sterilization using ethylene oxide is not commonly found in a private dental office or clinic, but rather in hospitals and larger clinics.

I. USE

Nearly all materials, whether metal, plastic, rubber, or cloth, can be sterilized in ethylene oxide with little or no damage to the material.

II. PRINCIPLES OF ACTION

Ethylene oxide vapor is effective against all types and forms of microorganisms provided sufficient time is allowed.

III. OPERATION

Specific operation is related to the type of equipment. Operation in a well-ventilated room is necessary. Overnight processing is usually the most practical.

A. Time and Temperature

The time may vary from 10 to 16 hours, depending on both the temperature and the concentration of ethylene oxide used.

B. Aeration After Completion of the Cycle

Plastic and rubber products need to be aerated at least 24 hours. Metal instruments are ready for immediate use.

IV. EVALUATION OF ETHYLENE OXIDE

A. Advantages

1. Many types of materials (including plastic and rubber items) can be sterilized with minimum or no damage to the material itself.
2. Low temperature for operation.

B. Disadvantages

1. High cost of the equipment.
2. Problems of dispersement of gaseous exhaust. Need for planned and tested ventilation system.
3. Increased time of operation.
4. Gas absorption requires airing of plastic, rubber, and cloth goods for several hours.

CARE OF STERILE INSTRUMENTS

Instruments stored without sealed wrappers are only momentarily sterile because of airborne contamination.

Labeled, sterilized, and sealed packages are stored unopened in clean, dry cabinets or drawers. Paper-wrapped packages must be handled carefully to prevent tearing. All stored packages should be dated and used in rotation.

Packages wrapped and sealed in paper usually do not need resterilizing for several months to 1 year.[3] Plastic or nylon wrap with a tape or heat seal may be expected to remain sterile longer. However, the expected shelf life before resterilizing depends on the area surrounding the stored packages. A closed, protected area without exposure, such as a cabinet or drawer that can be disinfected routinely, is preferred.

CHEMICAL DISINFECTANTS

Chemical disinfectants are used in several forms, including the surface disinfectants, immersion disinfectants, immersion sterilants, and hand antimicrobials. Each variety has specific chemicals, dilutions, and directions for application.

I. CATEGORIES[4]

Disinfectants are categorized by their biocidal activity as high level, intermediate level, or low level. Biocidal activity refers to the ability of the chemical disinfectant to destroy or inactivate living organisms.

A. High Level

High-level disinfectants inactivate spores and all forms of bacteria, fungi, and viruses. Applied at different time schedules, the high-level chemical is either a disinfectant or a sterilant.

B. Intermediate Level

Intermediate-level disinfectants inactivate all forms of microorganisms but do not destroy spores.

C. Low Level

Low-level disinfectants inactivate vegetative bacteria and certain lipid-type viruses but do not destroy spores, tubercle bacilli, or nonlipid viruses.

II. USES

A. Environmental Surfaces Disinfection

Following each appointment, the treatment area is cleaned and disinfected (pages 66 to 68).

B. Precleaning: Holding Solution

After use, instruments are placed in a disinfecting solution until cleaning and preparation for sterilization can be accomplished (page 59).

C. Dental Laboratory Impressions and Prostheses

Impressions can be carriers of infectious material to a dental laboratory, and completed prostheses must be disinfected before delivery to a patient. References may be found with the Suggested Readings at the end of Chapter 10 (page 185).

III. PRINCIPLES OF ACTION

A. Disinfection is achieved by coagulation, precipitation, or oxidation of protein of microbial cells or denaturation of the enzymes of the cells.
B. Disinfection depends on the contact of the solution at the known effective concentration for the optimum period of time.
C. Items must be thoroughly cleaned and dried,

because action of the agent is altered by foreign matter and dilution.

D. A solution has a specific shelf life, use life, and reuse life. Some may be altered by changes in pH, or the active ingredient may decrease in potency. Check manufacturer's directions.

IV. CRITERIA FOR SELECTION OF A CHEMICAL AGENT

The objective is to select a product that is effective in the control of microorganisms and practical to use. Properties of an ideal disinfectant are shown in Table 4-3.

The manufacturer's informational literature and container labels must provide facts about the product that ensure its effectiveness. After the product has been selected, it is the responsibility of the dental personnel to use it as directed to obtain the best possible infection control. When the label has insufficient information, the manufacturer should be contacted and instructions obtained.

The criteria should include at least the following:

A. EPA approval.

B. Chemicals must be tuberculocidal, bacteriocidal, virucidal, and fungicidal.

C. Label must state
   1. Effectiveness and stability expressed by
      a. *Shelf life:* the expiration date indicating the termination of effectiveness of the unopened container.
      b. *Use life:* the life expectancy for the solution once it has been activated but not actually put to use with contaminated items.
      c. *Reuse life:* the amount of time a solution can be used and reused while being challenged with instruments that are wet or coated with bioburden.
   2. Directions for activation (mixing proportions).
   3. Type of container for storage and place (conditions such as heat and light).
   4. Directions for use
      a. Precleaning and drying of items to be submerged.
      b. Time/temperature ratio.
   5. Instructions for disposal of used solution.
   6. Warnings
      a. Toxic effects (on eyes, skin).
      b. Specific directions for emergency care in the event of an accident (for example, splash in eye).
      c. Keep manufacturer's *Materials Safety Data Sheets* for reference.

RECOMMENDED CHEMICAL DISINFECTANTS[5]

The agents that have been shown adequate for use in dentistry are glutaraldehydes, chlorine compounds, iodophores, and complex phenolics. These are listed in Table 4-4 and are described in sections that follow.

Alcohols are not approved for instrument or environmental surface disinfection. The alcohols, eth-

---

TABLE 4-3 Properties of an Ideal Disinfectant

1. Broad spectrum:
   Should always have the widest possible antimicrobial spectrum.
2. Fast acting:
   Should always have a rapidly lethal action on all vegetative forms and spores of bacteria and fungi, protozoa, and viruses.
3. Not affected by physical factors:
   Active in the presence of organic matter, such as blood, sputum, and feces.
   Should be compatible with soaps, detergents, and other chemicals encountered in use.
4. Nontoxic
5. Surface compatibility:
   Should not corrode instruments and other metallic surfaces.
   Should not cause the disintegration of cloth, rubber, plastics, or other materials.
6. Residual effect on treated surfaces
7. Easy to use
8. Odorless:
   An inoffensive odor would facilitate its routine use.
9. Economical.
   Cost should not be prohibitively high.

From Molinari, J.A., Gleason, M.J., Cottone, J.A., and Barrett, E.D.: Comparison of Dental Surface Disinfectants, *Gen. Dent., 35,* 171, May–June, 1987.

TABLE 4-4 Chemical Disinfecting Agents

GLUTARALDEHYDES

Glutaraldehyde, 2% neutral
Glutaraldehyde, 2% alkaline
Glutaraldehyde, 2% alkaline with phenolic buffer
Glutaraldehyde, 2% acidic

CHLORINES

Chlorine dioxide
Sodium hypochlorite, 5.25% household bleach

IODOPHORS

Iodophor (1% available iodine)

PHENOLICS

o-phenylphenyl 9% with *o*-benzyl-*p*-chlorophenol 1%

anol and isopropanol, have been widely accepted and used for the preparation of the skin prior to injections or blood-taking procedures. The use of alcohol for this purpose is as a cleansing agent; the length of time involved is not enough for antibacterial effect.

I. GLUTARALDEHYDES

As shown in Table 4-4, the three types of glutaraldehydes are the alkaline, acidic, and neutral preparations.

A. Action
At the designated time exposure, they are high-level disinfectants and act to kill microorganisms by damaging their proteins and nucleic acids.

B. Preparation
The solutions become activated when the components of the two containers are mixed. The manufacturers' labels must show shelf life and reuse life, because the various preparations differ.

C. Limitations
1. Caustic to skin; use forceps and wear gloves.
2. Irritating to eyes; need protective eyewear.
3. Corrosive to some metal instruments.
4. Items must be rinsed in sterile water after removal from immersion bath.
5. Not used as a surface disinfectant because of toxic effects of fumes; surfaces wiped with glutaraldehyde should have residual film wiped off with sterile water.

II. CHLORINE COMPOUNDS

A. Action
Chlorine compounds have been used in a variety of ways for disinfection. Their use in water purification is well known. Solutions of sodium hypochlorite are used in cleaning dentures (page 404). Microorganisms are destroyed primarily by oxidation of microbial enzymes and cell wall components.

B. Chlorine Dioxide
The use life of chlorine dioxide is only 1 day. The preparation is economical and generally nontoxic but is corrosive to nonstainless steel instruments.

C. Sodium Hypochlorite
Daily fresh solutions are needed because sodium hypochlorite tends to be unstable. Use distilled water for mixing to improve the stability. The solutions can harm the eyes, skin, and clothing, and can corrode certain instruments; the strong odor may be offensive. In spite of certain disadvantages, it is widely used and economical.

III. IODOPHORS

A. Action
Iodine is released slowly from the iodophor compound and creates a disinfecting action as a broad-spectrum antimicrobial.

Povidone-iodine preparations are widely used in the forms of surgical scrubs, liquid soaps, mouthrinses, and surface antiseptics prior to hypodermic injection.

B. Environmental Surface Disinfectant
Concentrated solutions of iodophor contain less free iodine; therefore, the correct dilution for hard-surface disinfection is 1 part iodophor concentrate to 213 parts soft or distilled water. Hard water inactivates iodophors. The solution changes from amber to clear as it loses its activity.

IV. COMBINATION PHENOLICS (SYNTHETIC)

Phenolics may be water-based or alcohol-based.[5]

A. Action
High-concentration phenols act as protoplasmic poisons that destroy the cell wall and precipitate the protein. The lower concentrations used as surface disinfectants inactivate enzyme systems.

B. Use
As with iodophores, the synthetic phenolic disinfectants are broad spectrum, with residual biocidal activity.

CHEMICAL STERILANTS (IMMERSION)

Immersion in a chemical sterilant is used only for items that cannot be sterilized by heat. Because the immersion chemicals cannot be verified by spore testing, their use is limited. When ethylene oxide sterilizers are available, many of the items may be treated by that method.

A chemical that may require only 10 to 30 minutes for disinfection requires as many as 10 hours for sterilization at the same or different concentrations. Temperature may also be a factor. Manufacturer's instructions must be followed explicitly.

Instruments cannot be packaged, so maintenance of strict asepsis is not possible after chemical sterilization. Also, because of toxic effects to skin and mucosa, the chemical must be rinsed away with sterile water and the instruments dried before clinical use.

PREPARATION OF THE TREATMENT ROOM

The cleanliness and neatness of the treatment room reflect the character and conscientiousness of the dental personnel. The patient, with limited knowledge of dental science, may judge the ability of the dental personnel by the appearance of the office or clinic. Other patients may inquire about sterilization and infection control.

The patient's attitude is important, but more important is the relationship of cleanliness to the presence of microorganisms. The need is to provide clinical services in an environment that minimizes cross-contamination.

The orderliness and immaculate cleanliness of the treatment rooms result from continuing care. An excellent test for the effects of care and any minor oversights is for each dental team member to sit in the dental chair occasionally and look around at what the patient sees from that vantage point.

I. OBJECTIVES

Effective care of instruments and equipment contributes to the following:
A. Control of disease transmitted by way of environmental surfaces.
B. An increase in the working efficiency of the office personnel.
C. An atmosphere of cleanliness and orderliness that contribute to the patient's and the clinician's well-being.
D. An increase in the patient's confidence in the ability of the dental personnel.
E. The maintenance of the working efficiency of office equipment and instruments
   1. To prolong their span of usefulness.
   2. To contribute to patient safety.
F. A decrease in the occurrence of unpleasant odors in the office.

II. PRELIMINARY PLANNING

Preparation of the treatment room when time between appointments is limited requires an efficient procedural system. The classification of inanimate objects (Table 4-5) provides a guide for analysis.[4]

First, all surfaces and items that will be used or contacted during the appointment can be categorized and listed as critical, semicritical, or noncritical. The most logical and scientific sequence for preparation for the appointment can then be outlined.

A. Hand Contacts
Only contacts essential to the service to be performed should be made. Planning ahead to have materials ready so that cabinet knobs or drawer handles do not have to be contacted is an example.

B. Sterilizable Items
Critical and semicritical items are sterilized or are disposable.

C. Disposable Items
Disposable items should be used wherever possible.

D. Items That May Be Covered
Barrier coverings prevent contamination from reaching surfaces. Covers for light handles, counter tops, x-ray machine parts, and water faucets are examples. Care must be taken when removing the covers not to contaminate the object beneath.

E. Items That Require Chemical Disinfection
Objects and surfaces that cannot be included in one of the preceding categories must be treated with a chemical disinfectant. If the material is not compatible with the chemical action of the disinfectant, a substitute item, which is either disposable or coverable, will be needed.

TABLE 4-5 Classification of Inanimate Objects[4]

Surface Category	Definition	Sterilization/Disinfection	Examples
Critical	Penetrate soft tissue or bone	Sterilize or disposable	Needles Curets Explorers Probes
Semicritical	Touch intact mucous membrane, oral fluids Does not penetrate	Sterilize after each use High level disinfection when sterilization cannot be used	Radiographic biteblock Ultrasonic handpiece Amalgam condenser Mirror
Noncritical	Do not touch mucous membranes (only contact unbroken epithelium)	Cleaning and tuberculocidal intermediate level disinfection	Light handles Certain x-ray machine parts Safety eyewear
Environmental surfaces	No contact with patient (or only intact skin)	Cleaning and intermediate to low disinfection	Counter tops Equipment surfaces Housekeeping surface

III. CLEAN AND DISINFECT ENVIRONMENTAL SURFACES

A. Agent

1. Approved effective agents are iodophors, sodium hypochlorite, or complex phenols (Table 4-4).
2. The effectiveness of the disinfection procedure is the result of two actions:
   a. The physical rubbing and removal of contaminated material.
   b. The chemical inactivation of the living microorganisms.
3. Do not store gauze sponges in the solution. Use a spray bottle to dispense the disinfectant.

B. Procedure

1. Wear heavy-duty household gloves and mask.
2. Use several large gauze sponges or paper towels. The use of small sponges wastes time. A disinfectant-soaked sponge in each hand can decrease the time of cleaning certain objects, and contaminated objects, such as tubings, can be held with one sponge while scrubbing with the other sponge.

   Spraying of a disinfectant must be followed by vigorous scrubbing for cleaning. When applied only by spray without scrubbing, the agent does not penetrate or remove the film of microorganisms.
3. Scrub the disinfectant over the entire surface, with attention to irregularities where contaminated material can aggregate.
4. Spray and leave the surfaces wet.

UNIT WATER LINES

A biofilm of microorganisms forms on the inside of the water line tubings after overnight standing. Tests have been made on tubings to handpieces, water syringes, and ultrasonic scalers. When the lines were flushed for 2 minutes, the microbial counts were reduced.[6]

Contaminated water should not be used for surgical purposes or during the irrigation of pocket areas, because infective microorganisms can be introduced. If contaminated water is directed forcefully into a pocket, microorganisms can enter the tissue and infection or bacteremia can result.

I. PROCEDURES FOR CLINICAL USE

A. Flush all water lines at least 2 minutes at the beginning of each day.
B. Run water through water syringes for 30 seconds before and 30 seconds after each patient appointment.

II. WATER RETRACTION SYSTEM

To correct saliva and debris suck-back in the water line of a handpiece, the water retraction valve should be removed and a check valve or antiretractor valve installed.[7] Originally, handpieces were made with a retraction valve to prevent dripping when the instrument was turned off. Material sucked into the line, possibly filled with microorganisms including hepatitis viruses, tubercle bacilli, and other pathogens, then was discharged when the handpiece was used for the next patient.

PATIENT PREPARATION

The use of preprocedural rinsing and toothbrushing has been shown to lower the numbers of oral bacteria and, therefore, to lower the numbers of infected aerosols created during instrumentation.

Oral procedures that require penetration of tissues, such as giving anesthesia by injection or scaling subgingival pocket surfaces, can introduce bacteria into the tissues and hence into the blood stream. Organisms injected into the tissue could multiply and create an abscess. Because of natural resistance, the body can handle and destroy invading microorganisms, provided the numbers can be kept to a minimum.

Practical procedures for the preparation of a patient include preprocedural oral hygiene measures and rinsing with an antimicrobial mouthrinse. These contribute to the prevention of disease transmission.

I. PREPROCEDURAL ORAL HYGIENE MEASURES

A. Toothbrushing

Toothbrushing disturbs and removes microorganisms. When a patient is being trained in bacterial plaque control measures and needs supervision at each appointment, a double purpose can be accomplished. Demonstration of plaque removal from the teeth, tongue, and gingiva contributes to lowering the microbial count prior to treatment procedures.

B. Rinsing

The numbers of bacteria on the gingival or mucosal surfaces can be reduced by the use of a preprocedural antiseptic mouthrinse.[8]

The substantivity of 0.12% chlorhexidine provides a lowered bacterial count for more than 60 minutes. Preprocedural rinsing before injections is advised.

II. APPLICATION OF A SURFACE ANTISEPTIC

A. Prior to Injection of Anesthetic[9,10]

As a needle is introduced into the mucosa for penetration to deeper tissues, microorganisms on the surface can be carried into the tissue. During positioning of the instrument for injection, the needle might accidentally contact a tooth surface and pick up some plaque, which could be carried to and into the injection site.

An antiseptic applied prior to the injection can decrease the risk of introducing septic material into the soft tissue.

1. Dry the surface (gauze square).
2. Apply antiseptic (swab).
3. Apply topical anesthetic (swab).

B. Prior to Scaling and Other Dental Hygiene Instrumentation[11]

1. *Instrumentation* in a sulcus or pocket and around the gingival margin can create breaks in the tissue where bacteria can enter. Subgingival instrumentation in a pocket with broken down sulcular epithelium contributes to the entrance of bacteria into the underlying tissues and bacteremia.
2. *Procedure.* Dry the surface and swab the area prior to instrumentation. Use an antiseptic solution to irrigate the sulci and pockets carefully.

SUMMARY OF UNIVERSAL PROCEDURES FOR THE PREVENTION OF DISEASE TRANSMISSION

Basic procedures for clinical management are listed here. For many items, a detailed description has been provided in Chapter 3 or elsewhere in this chapter.

I. PATIENT FACTORS

A. Prepare a comprehensive patient history. Refer patients suspected of carrying infectious disease for medical evaluation.
B. Avoid elective procedures for a patient who is suffering from a communicable condition, such as a respiratory infection, or who has an open lesion on or about the lips or oral tissues, for the benefit of all who would be subjected to exposure.
C. Ask the patient to rinse with germicidal mouthrinse to reduce the numbers of oral microorganisms.
D. Provide protective eyewear.

II. CLINIC PREPARATION

A. Run water through all water lines, including the air–water syringe, handpieces, and ultrasonic unit, for 2 minutes at the start of the day and for at least 30 seconds before and after each use during the day.
B. Disinfect all environmental surfaces that may be touched during the appointment. Make an orderly sequence for surface disinfection. Apply barrier covers as indicated.
C. Sterilize instruments and all other equipment that can be sterilized by one of the methods for complete sterilization.

III. FACTORS FOR THE DENTAL TEAM

A. Have medical examinations; keep immunizations up to date; have appropriate testing on a periodic basis.
B. Always use mask, protective eyewear, gloves, and a clean closed-front gown with fitted wrist cuffs.
C. Wash hands and dry thoroughly using a short scrub at the start of the day and handwashes with three latherings and thorough rinsings before donning and after removal of gloves. Use antimicrobial soap.
D. Develop habits that minimize contacts with switches and other parts of the dental unit, dental chair, light, and clinician's stool, and avoid all environmental contacts unrelated to the procedure at hand.

IV. TREATMENT FACTORS

A. Hypodermic Needles

1. Use a safe recapping method to prevent accidental penetration or self-inoculation (Figure 31-5, page 508).
2. Place used needles into a puncture-resistant sharps container.
3. Dispose of all partially emptied Carpules of anesthetics.

B. Removable Oral Prostheses

Routinely, gloves should be worn to receive a septic prosthesis from a patient. Place the prosthesis in a disposable cup and cover with a disinfectant. Use a fresh solution of 0.05% iodophor in water, or a 1:5 dilution of 5% sodium hypochlorite. Clean by ultrasonics.

When a lathe is used for cleaning the denture, wear goggles and a mask and use a sterile ragwheel and fresh pumice. Pumice is used only once and caught on a disposable paper liner in the dustbin and discarded.

V. POST-TREATMENT

A. Transport holding solution container to the sterilization area. Use heavy household gloves to handle used instruments.
B. Follow routines on pages 59 to 60 to disinfect, clean in ultrasonic cleaner, and prepare the instruments for sterilization.
C. Contaminated waste is secured in plastic disposal bags. See Disposal of Waste, page 70.
D. Disinfect safety eyewear for patient and dental team members.

OCCUPATIONAL ACCIDENTAL EXPOSURE MANAGEMENT

Accidents happen even to the most skillful clinician. Accidental percutaneous (laceration, needle stick) or permucosal (splash to eye or mucosa) exposure to blood or other body fluids requires prompt action.

A. Significant Exposures

1. Percutaneous or permucosal stick or wound with needle or sharp instrument contaminated with blood or saliva.
2. Contamination of any obviously open wound, nonintact skin, or mucous membrane with blood, saliva, or a combination.
3. Exposure of patient's body fluids to unbroken skin is not considered a significant exposure.

B. Procedure Following Exposure

1. Immediately wash the wound with soap and water; rinse well.
2. Obtain permission for blood testing and arrange for counseling.
3. On the same day
   a. Patient (source person) should be tested for HBsAg and anti-HIV.
   b. Exposed person should be tested for anti-HBs and anti-HIV (anti-HBs would not be needed if recent postvaccine confirmation showed positive immunization).
4. Table 4-6 outlines the necessary procedures.

C. Follow-up

1. Report signs and symptoms associated with HIV seroconversion.
2. Obtain medical evaluation of any illness involving fever, rash, lymphadenopathy.
3. Pursue counseling and further testing.

DISPOSAL OF WASTE[12]

Types of waste are defined in Box 4-1. Each type of waste requires special handling.

I. REGULATIONS

Investigate the regulations of each town or city sanitation division for rules concerning disposal of contaminated waste.

Figure 4-4 illustrates the universal label required by OSHA. The labels must be attached to containers used to store or transport hazardous waste materials.

II. GUIDELINES

A. Disposable materials, such as gloves, masks, wipes, paper drapes, or surface covers, that are contaminated with blood or body fluids should be carefully handled and discarded in sturdy, impervious plastic bags to minimize human contact.
B. Blood, suctioned fluids, or other liquid waste may be carefully poured into a drain that is connected to a sanitary sewer system in compliance with applicable local regulations.
C. Sharp items, such as needles and scalpel blades, should be placed intact into a puncture-resistant, leak-proof container.

TABLE 4-6 HIV and HBV Postexposure Management

Patient (Source)	Exposed DHCW	Treatment
HBsAg positive or Refuses testing or Cannot be identified	Not HBV immunized	Start vaccine series Give HBIG (single dose)
	HBV vaccine received	Test for anti-HB 1. Adequate titer level: no treatment 2. Inadequate titer level: Give vaccine booster HBIG (single dose)
HBsAg negative	Not HBV immunized	Start vaccine series
	HBV vaccine received	No treatment necessary
Has AIDS or is HIV seropositive or Refused testing or Cannot be identified	Counsel concerning the risk Test for anti-HIV	Negative for anti-HIV: Test again in 6 weeks 12 weeks 6 months 1 year Counsel: 1. Do not donate blood 2. Use appropriate protection during sexual intercourse

Key: DHCW = dental health-care worker
HBsAg = hepatitis B surface antigen
HBIG = hepatitis B immune globulin
Anti-HBs = antibody to hepatitis B surface antigen
Anti-HIV = antibody to human immunodeficiency virus

D. Human tissue and contaminated solid wastes can be disposed of according to the requirements established by local or state environmental regulatory agencies and published recommendations.
E. Infectious medical waste, including tissues and culture media, should be handled in a manner consistent with local regulations before disposal.
F. Liquid chemicals should be carefully poured into a drain connected to a sewer while flushing with copious amounts of water unless labeling or local regulations prohibit such a practice. Disposal methods for solid chemicals vary with the type of chemical and local regulations governing waste-management practices.

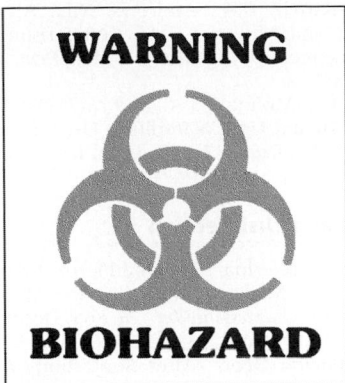

WARNING

BIOHAZARD

■ **FIGURE 4-4 Universal Label for Hazardous Material.** A hazard-warning label should be fluorescent orange or orange-red with lettering or a symbol in a contrasting color. The label must be attached to containers used to store or transport waste. A label is not required for regulated waste that has been decontaminated (such as dental waste that has been autoclaved).

TECHNICAL HINTS

I. CLEANING THE FACE

Check and clean the exposed parts of the face not covered by mask or protective eyewear, where spatter collects, as an aid to disease control as well as for general sanitation. The face should be cleaned several times each day and washed before eating. When washing the face, an effort should be made not to spread spatter material into the eyes or the mouth.

II. SMOKING AND EATING

Neither smoking nor eating should be permitted in treatment areas.

III. TOYS

Select toys and other reception area items that can be cleaned and disinfected.

IV. HANDPIECE MAINTENANCE

Keep records of handpiece purchase, maintenance, and other information pertinent to longevity and effectiveness. Maintain a sufficient number of handpieces to permit rotation and routine sterilization.

V. STERILIZATION MONITORING

Keep a written record of dates when processing tests and biologic monitor tests were performed for each sterilizer. Indicate advance dates for the next testing clearly on a calendar or other reference point. Tests made weekly should be performed on the same day to simplify remembering.

VI. OFFICE POLICY MANUAL

Include in the clinic or office policy manual outlines of procedures to follow for universal precautions. Addresses for sources of various materials can be kept in a special reference section of the manual. Emergency procedures to follow when accidentally exposed should also be defined clearly.

FACTORS TO TEACH THE PATIENT

I. The meaning of "universal precautions" and what is included under the term; how these precautions protect the patient and the dental team members.

II. The contribution of the accurately completed medical and dental personal history to the provision of the best, safest treatment possible.

III. Methods for sterilization of instruments, including handpieces; how the autoclave or other sterilizer is tested daily or weekly.

IV. Facts about the normal oral flora and the factors that influence an increased number of bacteria on the tongue, mucosa, and in the bacterial plaque on the teeth.

V. Methods for personal daily control of the oral bacteria through plaque control and tongue brushing.

VI. Reasons for preprocedural rinsing.

VII. Method for thorough rinsing (page 384).

REFERENCES

1. **Office Safety and Asepsis Procedures Research Foundation:** The Sterilization Process, *OSAP Monthly Focus*, 1–3, Number 5, 1997.

2. **Parisi,** A.N. and Young, W.E.: Sterilization with Ethylene Oxide and Other Gases, in Block, S.S.: *Disinfection, Sterilization, and Preservation,* 4th ed. Philadelphia, Lea & Febiger, 1991, pp. 580–595.

3. **Butt,** W.E., Bradley, D.V., Mayhew, R.B., and Schwartz, R.S.: Evaluation of the Shelf Life of Sterile Instrument Packs, *Oral Surg. Oral Med. Oral Pathol., 72,* 650, December, 1991.

4. **United States Centers for Disease Control and Prevention:** Recommended Infection-Control Practices for Dentistry, 1993, *MMWR, 42,* 1–10, RR-8, May 28, 1993.

5. **Miller,** C.H.: Infection Control Strategies for the Dental Office, in American Dental Association: *ADA Guide to Dental Therapeutics.* Chicago, ADA Publishing Co., 1998, pp. 489–504.

6. **Gross,** A., Devine, M.J., and Cutright, D.E.: Microbial Contamination of Dental Units and Ultrasonic Scalers, *J. Periodontol., 47,* 670, November, 1976.

7. **Bagga,** B.S.R., Murphy, R.A., Anderson, A.W., and Punwani, I.: Contamination of Dental Unit Cooling Water With Oral Microorganisms and Its Prevention, *J. Am. Dent. Assoc., 109,* 712, November, 1984.

8. **Veksler,** A.E., Kayrouz, G.A., and Newman, M.G.: Reduction of Salivary Bacteria by Pre-procedural Rinses With Chlorhexidine 0.12%, *J. Periodontol., 62,* 649, November, 1991.

9. **Malamed,** S.F.: *Handbook of Local Anesthesia,* 4th ed. St. Louis, Mosby, 1996, p. 134.

10. **Connor,** J.P. and Edelson, J.G.: Needle Tract Infection, *Oral Surg. Oral Med. Oral Pathol., 65,* 401, April, 1988.

11. **Fine,** D.H., Korik, I., Furgang, D., Myers, R., Olshan, A., Barnett, M.L., and Vincent, J.: Assessing Preprocedural Subgingi-

val Irrigation and Rinsing With an Antiseptic Mouthrinse to Reduce Bacteremia, *J. Am. Dent. Assoc., 127,* 641, May, 1996.

12. **Miller**, C.H. and Palenik, C.J.: *Infection Control and Management of Hazardous Materials for the Dental Team.* St. Louis, Mosby, 1994, pp. 210–219.

SUGGESTED READINGS

American Dental Association Council on Scientific Affairs and Council on Dental Practice: Infection Control Recommendations for the Dental Office and the Dental Laboratory, *J. Am. Dent. Assoc., 127,* 672, May, 1996.

Harte, J., Davis, R., Plamondon, T., and Richardson, B.: The Influence of Dental Unit Design on Percutaneous Injury, *J. Am. Dent. Assoc., 129,* 1725, December, 1998.

Legnani, P., Cheechi, L., Pelliccioni, G.A., and D'Achille, C.: Atmospheric Contamination During Dental Procedures, *Quintessence, Int., 25,* 435, June, 1994.

Miller C.H.: Infection Control, *Dent. Clin. North Am., 40,* 437, April, 1996.

Wooten, R.K. and Barata, M.-C.: Procedure-specific Infection Control Recommendations for Dentistry, *Compend. Cont. Educ. Dent., 14,* 332, March, 1993.

Occupational Exposure

Beekman, S.E. and Henderson, D.K.: Managing Occupational Risks in the Dental Office: HIV and the Dental Professional, *J. Am. Dent. Assoc., 125,* 847, July, 1994.

Chenoweth, C.E. and Gobetti, J.P.: Postexposure Chemoprophylaxis for Occupational Exposure to HIV in the Dental Office, *J. Am. Dent. Assoc., 128,* 1135, August, 1997.

Ramos-Gomez, F., Ellison, J., Greenspan, D., Bird, W., Lowe, S., and Gerberding, J.L.: Accidental Exposures to Blood and Body Fluids Among Health Care Workers in Dental Teaching Clinics: A Prospective Study, *J. Am. Dent. Assoc., 128,* 1253, September, 1997.

Dental Unit Water

Andrews, N.: Management of Biofilm and Water Quality in Dental Devices, *J. Pract. Hyg., 5,* 33, July/August, 1996.

Bednarsh, H.S., Eklund, K.J., and Mills, S.: Check Your Dental Unit Water IQ, *Access, 10,* 37, November, 1996.

Challacombe, S.J. and Fernandes, L.L.: Detecting *Legionella Pneumophila* in Water Systems: A Comparison of Various Dental Units, *J. Am. Dent. Assoc., 126,* 603, May, 1995.

Karpay, R.I., Plamondon, T.J., Mills, S.E., and Dove, S.B.: Validation of an In-office Dental Unit Water Monitoring Technique, *J. Am. Dent. Assoc., 129,* 207, February, 1998.

Murdoch-Kinch, C.A., Andrews, N.L., Atwan, S., Jude, R., Gleason, M.J., and Molinari, J.A.: Comparison of Dental Water Quality Management Procedures, *J. Am. Dent. Assoc., 128,* 1235, September, 1997.

Williams, J.F., Molinari, J.A., and Andrews, N.: Microbial Contamination of Dental Unit Waterlines: Origins and Characteristics, *Compend. Cont. Educ. Dent., 17,* 538, June, 1996.

Sterilization and Disinfection

Andrés, M.T., Tejerina, J.M., and Fierro, J.F.: Reliability of Biologic Indicators in a Mail-return Sterilization-Monitoring Service: A Review of 3 Years, *Quintessence Int., 26,* 865, December, 1995.

Burkhart, N.W. and Crawford, J.: Critical Steps in Instrument Cleaning: Removing Debris After Sonication, *J. Am. Dent. Assoc., 128,* 456, April, 1997.

Chau, V.B., Saunders, T.R., Pimsler, M., and Elfring, D.R.: Indepth Disinfection of Acrylic Resins, *J. Prosthet. Dent., 74,* 309, September, 1995.

Larsen, T., Andersen, H.-K., and Fiehn, N.-E.: Evaluation of a New Device for Sterilizing Dental High-speed Handpieces, *Oral Surg. Oral Med. Oral Pathol. Oral Radiol. Endod., 84,* 513, November, 1997.

McGivern, T.: The Use of Glutaraldehyde for Disinfection and Sterilization, *J. Pract. Hyg., 6,* 1, Supplement, September/October, 1997.

Miller, C.H.: Update on Heat Sterilization and Sterilization Monitoring, *Compend. Cont. Educ. Dent., 14,* 304, March, 1993.

Molinari, J.A., Gleason, M.J., and Merchant, V.A.: The Evolution of Sterilization Monitoring Services, *Compend. Cont. Educ. Dent., 15,* 1422–1487 (8 articles), Special Issue, 1994.

Sheldrake, M.A., Majors, C.D., Gaines, D.J., and Palenik, C.J.: Effectiveness of Three Types of Sterilization on the Contents of Sharps Containers, *Quintessence Int., 26,* 771, November, 1995.

Young, J.M.: Dental Air-powered Handpieces: Selection, Use, and Sterilization, *Compend. Cont. Educ. Dent., 14,* 358, March, 1993.

Preprocedural Rinse

Buckner, R.Y., Kayrour, G.A., and Briner, W.: Reduction of Oral Microbes by a Single Chlorhexidine Rinse, *Compend. Cont. Educ. Dent., 15,* 512, April, 1994.

Logothetis, D.D. and Martinez-Welles, J.M.: Reducing Bacterial Aerosol Contamination with a Chlorhexidine Gluconate Prerinse, *J. Am. Dent. Assoc., 126,* 1634, December, 1995.

Rahn, R., Schneider, S., Diehl, O., Schafer, V., and Shah, P.M.: Preventing Post-treatment Bacteremia: Comparing Topical Povidone-Iodine and Chlorhexidine, *J. Am. Dent. Assoc., 126,* 1145, August, 1995.

5

Patient Reception and Positioning

The patient's well-being is the all-important consideration throughout the appointment. At the same time, the clinician must function effectively and efficiently in a manner that minimizes stress and fatigue.

The physical arrangement and interpersonal relationships provide the setting for specific services to be performed. Key words related to the positioning of patient and clinician are defined in Box 5-1.

The patient's presence in the office or clinic is an expression of confidence in the dentist and the dental hygienist. The confidence is inspired by the reputation for professional knowledge and skill, the appearance of the office, and the action of the workers in it.

I. PREPARATION FOR THE PATIENT

A. Treatment Area

The procedures for the prevention of disease transmission were described in Chapters 3 and 4. The requirements are universal precautions for all patients whether or not the presence of a communicable disease is known.

1. *Environmental Surfaces.* All contact areas must be thoroughly disinfected or covered to control cross-contamination.

2. *Instruments.* Sterile packaged instruments remain sealed until the start of the appointment.

3. *Equipment.* Prepare and make ready other materials that will be used, such as for the determination of blood pressure and patient instruction. Anticipate specific needs for assessment procedures.

B. Records

By leaving the record open for reference, the need for handling the record after handwashing and gloving may be avoided. Radiographs can be placed on the viewbox and the light left on.

1. Review the patient's medical and dental history for pertinent appointment information and need for updating.

2. Read previous appointment case records to focus the current treatment needs.

3. Anticipate examination procedures and new record making for a new patient.

C. Position Chair

1. Upright, in low position.
2. Chair arm adjusted for access.

BOX 5-1 KEY WORDS: Chair Positioning

Body language: a set of nonverbal signals, including body movements, postures, gestures, and facial expressions, that gives expression to various physical, mental, and emotional states.

Body mechanics: the field of physiology that studies muscular actions and functions in the maintenance of the posture of the body.

Cumulative trauma: disorders of the musculoskeletal, autonomic, and peripheral nervous system caused by repeated, forceful, and awkward movements of the human body, as well as by exposure to mechanical stress, vibration, and cold temperatures.

Ergonomics (er"gō-nŏm'ĭks): a branch of ecology dealing with human factors in the design and operation of machines and the physical environment; in dentistry, the science encompassing all factors that relate to quality and quantity of dental care delivered in comparison to the physical and mental fatigue generated.

Postural hypotension (pos'chu-ral hī"pō-ten'shun): also called orthostatic (ōr"thō-stăt'ĭk) hypotension; a fall in blood pressure associated with dizziness, syncope, and blurred vision that occurs upon standing or when standing motionless in a fixed position.

Supine (soo'pīn): flat position with head and feet on the same level.

Trendelenburg (trĕn-dĕl'ĕn-berg): the modified supine position when the head is lower than the heart.

Work simplification: application to clinical procedure of time and motion studies, analysis of instruments and equipment, and body mechanics to provide the patient with a smooth, systematic, simplified approach for comprehensive dental hygiene therapy.

---

3. Clear pathway to chair of obstacles: rheostat, clinician's stool.

II. PATIENT RECEPTION

A. Introductions
1. The dental assistant or the dentist may introduce the new patient to the dental hygienist, but more frequently, a self-introduction is in order. The patient is greeted by name and the hygienist's name is clearly stated, for example, "Good morning, Mrs. Smith; I am Miss Jones, the dental hygienist." Wearing a name-tag for the patient's convenient observation is helpful.
2. Procedure for introducing the patient to others:
   a. A lady's name always precedes a gentleman's.
   b. An older person's name precedes the younger person's (when of the same sex and when the difference in age is obvious).
   c. In general, the patient's name precedes that of a member of the dental personnel.
3. An older patient is not called by the first name except at the patient's request.

B. Escort Patient to Dental Chair
1. Invite patient to be seated.
   a. For the average patient, stand ready to adjust the chair.
   b. Assist the elderly, the infirm, or very small children; guide into the chair by supporting the patient's arm. Procedure for assisting a patient who is blind is described on pages 792 to 793.

2. Assist with wheelchair. Bring wheelchair adjacent to the dental chair and provide assistance when indicated. Wheelchair transfers and assistance for a patient with a walker or crutches are described on pages 743 to 745.
3. Place handbag in a safe place, if possible within the patient's view.
4. Apply drape and napkin. Stabilization aids for patients with disabilities are described on pages 745 to 746.
5. Receive removable prostheses and cover with water in a protective container.
6. Provide protective eyewear. For information about the types and care of protective eyewear, see pages 46 to 47. When a patient removes personal corrective eyeglasses to substitute those provided by the office or clinic, make sure the personal glasses are placed in their case in a safe place.

III. THE TREATMENT AREA

The treatment area centers around the patient's oral cavity. The entire "work area" refers to the dental chair with patient, the unit, and the instrument tray as they are positioned for the convenience and accessibility of the clinician on the clinician's stool.

Patient and clinician positioning is described in detail in this chapter. In summary, the general features of an appropriate work area include the following:
   A. Unit and instruments positioned for visibility and convenient selection by the clinician, and for ready access without stretching or reaching over the patient.

B. Clinician's shoulders, elbows, and wrists are comfortably in neutral position.

C. The patient is in supine position adjusted so that the oral cavity is at the elbow height of the clinician.

D. The dental light is directed from a height that illuminates as large an area as possible, yet allows the clinician to adjust conveniently.

POSITION OF THE CLINICIAN

The position of the patient is contingent upon the position of the clinician. Attention to the patient's comfort must always be foremost, but when the working arrangement is considered, it is realistic to remember that the patient's position will be assumed for a relatively short time compared with that of the clinician, who may conduct a major portion of a full day's professional activity in close proximity to the chairside. The patient, therefore, is positioned so that a thorough, biologically oriented service may be performed conveniently and efficiently within a reasonable length of time.

I. OBJECTIVES

Objectives concern the health of the clinician, the service to be performed, and the effect on the patient. The *preferred* position attempts to accomplish the following:

A. Contribute to, rather than detract from, the health of the clinician.

B. Provide physical comfort and mental tranquility that reduce stress.

C. Apply principles of body mechanics that reduce fatigue and maintain stamina for prolonged periods of peak efficiency.

D. Contribute to ease and efficiency of performance.

E. Transmit to the patient a sense of well-being, security, and confidence, as well as a need for cooperation with dental personnel.

F. Develop better patient–clinician relationships because of greater comfort, lessened physical stress, and reduced appointment time.

G. Be flexible in relation to individual needs of physically challenged patients with special health problems, where limitations of physiologic or pathologic conditions require variations in chair positions.

II. CHARACTERISTICS OF AN ACCEPTABLE CLINICIAN'S STOOL[1,2]

A. Base
Broad and heavy for stability, with no fewer than four casters. A stool with five casters has greater stability.

B. Mobility
Completely mobile; not connected to other dental equipment; built with free-rolling cast-ers; allows free movement around the patient's head for instrumentation from either side.

C. Seat
Relatively large to provide complete body support; padded firmly, yet not too hard; without a welt on the leaning edge that could dig into the upper part of the thigh.

D. Height
Adjustable to provide exactly the correct level for the individual so that feet can be flat on the floor and thighs parallel with the floor.

E. Adjustment
In accord with universal precautions, the stool is adjusted by a foot control mechanism.

F. Assistant's Stool
Needs additional support at the base, with at least five casters recommended for maximum stability; should be freely adjustable for height. A footrest is needed at the base of the chair, because the assistant is positioned 4 to 6 inches higher than the clinician, and generally, the feet cannot reach the floor.

III. USE OF THE CLINICIAN'S STOOL

Once the stool is adjusted for the individual, it does not need changing, unless other personnel also use it. Once adjusted, the height remains constant, and other dental equipment is arranged to accommodate for optimum usage. Positioning that incorporates principles of good body mechanics benefits both the clinician and the patient. Basic positioning includes the following features related to posture and the treatment area.

A. Feet are flat on the floor; thighs parallel with the floor (Figure 5-1*A*).

B. Back is straight; head is relatively erect; shoulders are relaxed and parallel with floor.

C. Body weight is completely supported by the chair; balancing on the edge of the stool should be avoided (Figure 5-1*B*).

D. Eyes are directed downward in a manner that prevents neck strain and eye strain; it is not necessary to bend the head.

E. Distance from the patient's mouth to the eyes of the clinician should be 14 to 16 inches (Figure 5-2).

F. With elbows close to the sides, the treatment area (patient's mouth) is adjusted to elbow height.

G. Forearm and wrist are kept in a straight line.

POSITION OF THE PATIENT

I. GENERAL POSITIONS

Four commonly used body positions are shown in Figure 5-3. Body positions are of extreme importance during emergency care; they are identified in Tables

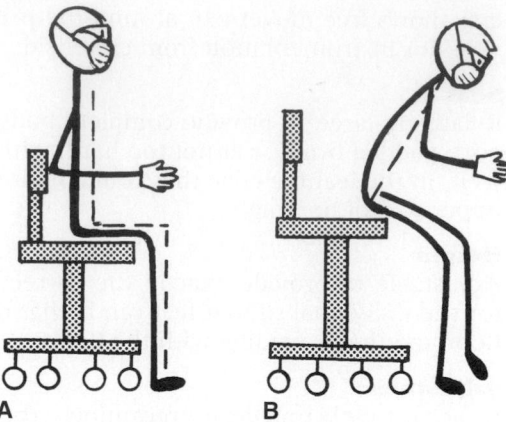

■ FIGURE 5-1 **Clinician's Use of Stool.** **(A)** Correct position, with feet flat on the floor, thighs parallel with floor, and body weight supported by the stool. **(B)** Incorrect position, with seat high, body balanced on the edge of the stool, and back bent forward.

61-5 and 61-6, with outlines for emergency procedures.

A. Upright

This is the initial position from which chair adjustments are made.

B. Semi-upright

A patient with certain types of cardiovascular or respiratory problems may need to be in a semi-upright position during treatment.

C. Supine

The patient is flat, with the head and feet on the same level.

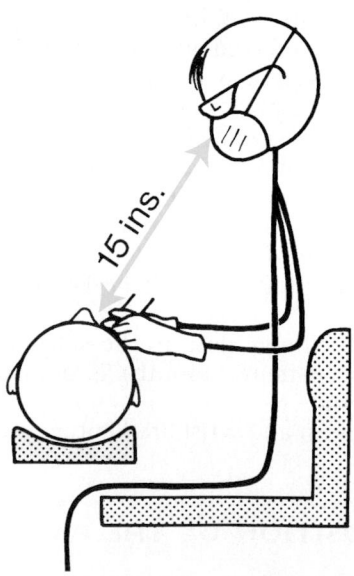

■ FIGURE 5-2 **Distance from Clinician to Patient.** Acceptable positioning shows the patient at the clinician's elbow level and the oral cavity of the patient approximately 15 inches from the clinician's eyes.

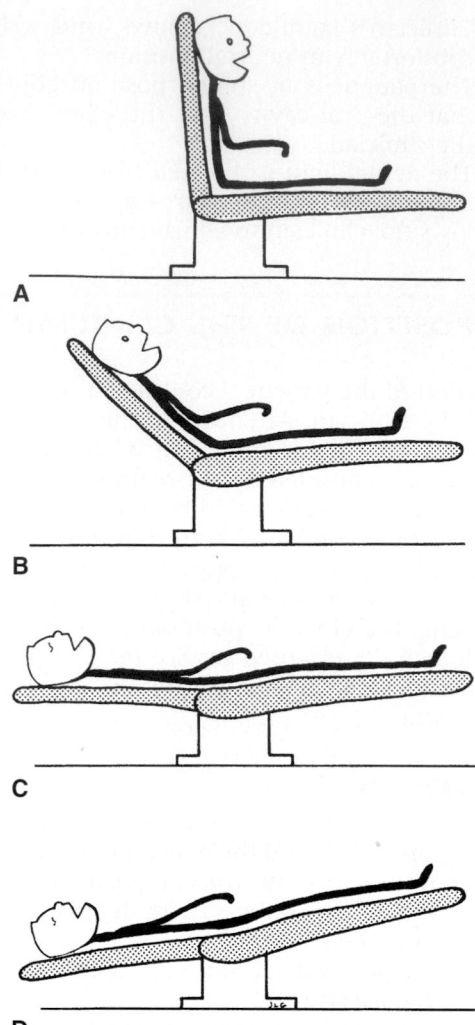

■ FIGURE 5-3 **Basic Patient Positions.** **(A)** Upright. **(B)** Semi-upright. **(C)** Supine or horizontal, with the brain on the same level as the heart. **(D)** Trendelenburg, with the brain lower than the heart and the feet slightly elevated.

D. Trendelenburg

The patient is in the supine position and tipped back and down 35° to 45° so that the heart is higher than the head (Figure 5-3D).

II. CHARACTERISTICS OF A DENTAL CHAIR FOR EFFICIENT UTILIZATION

A dental chair provides complete body support for the patient, which increases patient relaxation. The clinician can be in a comfortable working position with good access, light, and visibility, which in turn contribute to an efficient performance.

In a supine position, a patient is ideally situated for support of the circulation. Rarely could a patient faint while lying in a supine position.

A. Provides complete body support.

B. Seat and leg support move as a unit; back and headrest move as a unit; both are power controlled.

C. Has a thin back without protruding adjustment devices so that the chair may be lowered close to the clinician's elbow height.

D. Has supports that hold the patient's arms as the chair is lowered into the supine position; otherwise the hands hang down or the patient must hold them up forcibly.

E. Chair base should be shallow to permit the chair to be lowered as close to the floor as needed for correct treatment position.

F. Foot controls for the back and seat should be readily available to both the assistant and clinician.

III. USE OF DENTAL CHAIR

A. Prepositioning for Patient Reception
1. Chair at low level; back upright.
2. Chair arm raised on side of approach.

B. Adjustment Steps
1. Patient is seated first with back upright.
2. Chair seat and foot portion are raised first to help the patient settle back.
3. Backrest is lowered until the patient reaches the supine position for maxillary instrumentation. For mandibular teeth, chair back is adjusted to a 20° angle with the floor (Figure 5-4).
4. Patient is requested to slide up until the head is at the upper edge of the backrest and on the side next to the clinician. Note patient's head position in Figure 5-5.

C. Final Adjustment
Lower or raise the total chair until the patient's mouth is at the clinician's elbow level when the shoulder is relaxed.

D. Position of Clinician
Clinician's positions can be designated by the hours of a clock around the patient's head. Noon, or 12:00, is at the top, over the patient's forehead as shown in Figure 5-5.

E. Flexibility of Clinician's Position
Traditionally right-handed clinicians treat primarily from the right side of the patient and

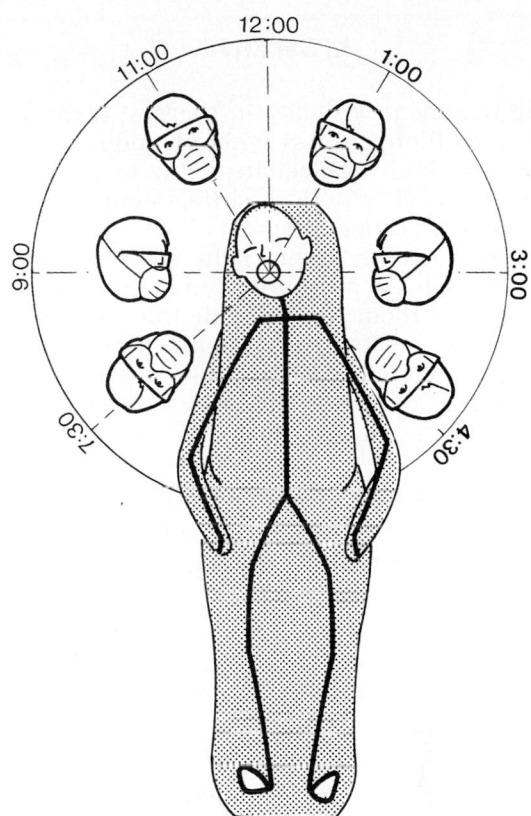

FIGURE 5-5 Range of Positions for Clinician. The patient's head is placed at the upper edge of the backrest or headrest at the convenience of the clinician.

left-handed clinicians from the left side. However, flexibility of position around the patient's head is made possible by the easy movement of the clinician's stool and turning the patient's head. Visibility and accessibility contribute to a more thorough treatment.

F. Conclusion of Appointment
1. Raise backrest slowly.
2. Tilt chair forward.
3. Request that patient sit in an upright position briefly to avoid effects of postural hypotension.

G. Contraindications for Supine Position
Most patients can be treated in the standard supine position described. Examples of conditions that may contraindicate the use of a supine position include congestive heart disease and any condition associated with breathing difficulty, such as emphysema, severe asthma, or sinusitis. During the third trimester of pregnancy, some women would be uncomfortable. Chair position during pregnancy is described on pages 657 to 659.

Usually when positioning is questionable, the patient volunteers a request for position variation. Questions on the patient's history may reveal the need for adaptation.

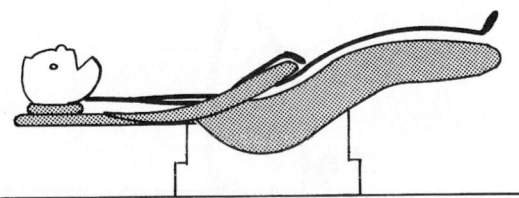

FIGURE 5-4 Dental Chair in Supine Position. For instrumentation in the maxillary arch, the patient is in supine position, with the back of the chair nearly parallel with the floor and the feet slightly higher than the head. For mandibular teeth, adjust the chair back to a 20° angle with the floor.

LIGHTING

During treatment, visibility in the oral cavity is prerequisite to thoroughness without undue trauma to the tissues. With inadequate light, inefficiency increases and leads to prolonged treatment time, which reduces patient cooperation.

The position of the dental light or lights and the intensity of the beam affect the illumination. A study of the treatment room can be made that includes measurement of the total light at the patient's face in working position. Selection of a light that meets certain standards can assure intensity sufficient for good visibility and yet safe for the eyes.

I. DENTAL LIGHT: SUGGESTED FEATURES

A. The light should be readily adjustable both vertically and horizontally and the beam capable of being focused.

B. The size must be small enough so that it may be brought close to the treatment area without being in the way, blocking the room light, or being a hazard for movement of people in its vicinity.

C. Intensity of room light should be sufficient to prevent a marked contrast between it and the illuminating beam of the dental light. An all-luminous ceiling contributes to evenly distributed room lighting.

II. DENTAL LIGHT: LOCATION

A. *Attachment.* The most versatile arrangement is a ceiling-mounted light on a track, which permits the light to move over a range from behind a supine patient's head to a position in front of the patient's chin.

B. *Dual Lighting.* With a supine patient position in a contoured chair, advantages to the use of two operating lights have been demonstrated.

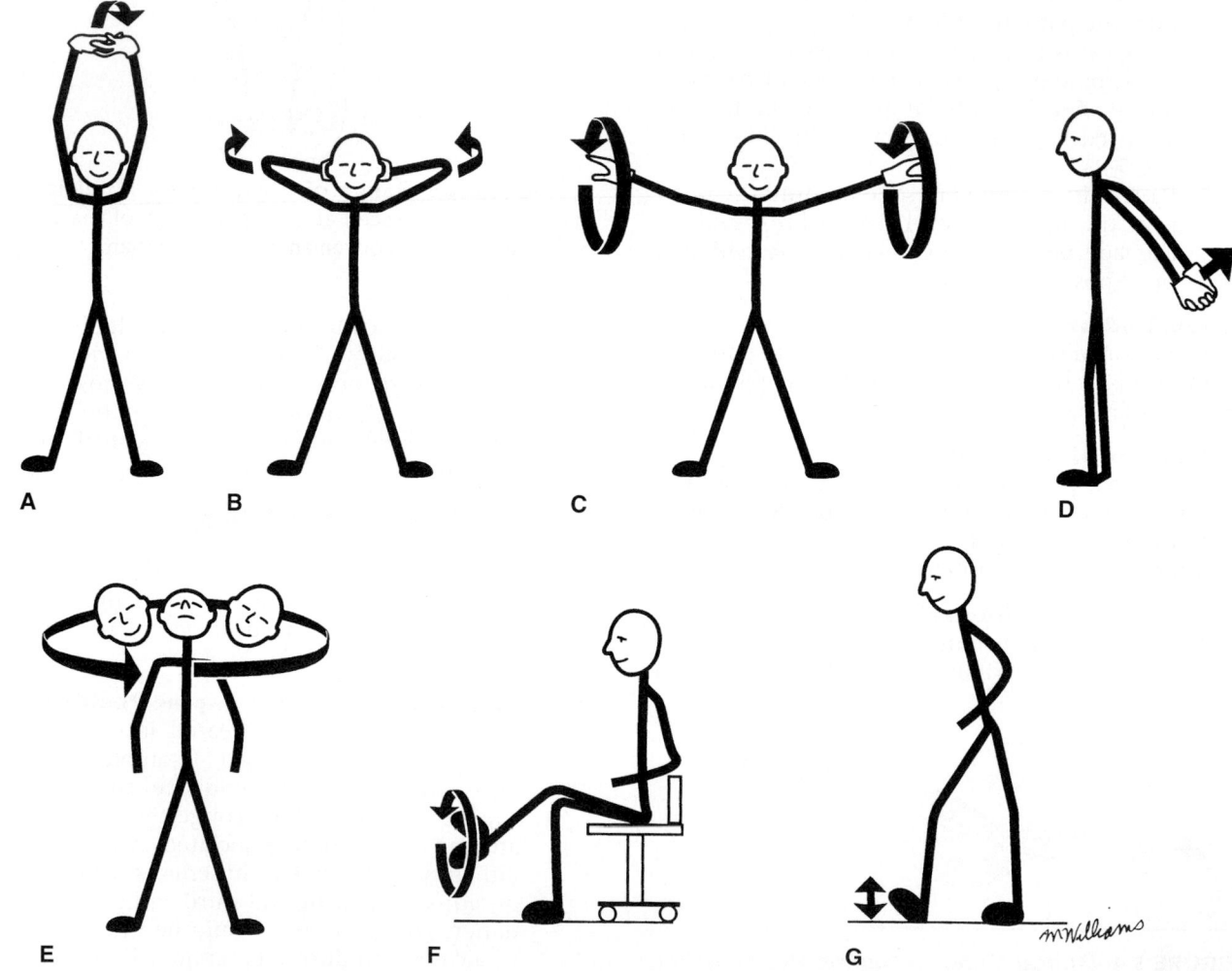

FIGURE 5-6 Exercises to Relieve Tension and Improve Posture. (A) Stretch up and pull back. **(B)** Head up, elbows push back. **(C)** Circle from the shoulders. Small circles, then gradually larger. **(D)** Clasp hands, pull back, head up. **(E)** Hang the arms and shoulders loose. Circle head to right, then left, 5 to 10 times each. **(F)** Cross leg and circle ankle: right 10 times, then left. Other leg too. **(G)** Foot up and down, heel on ground. Pull the muscles in the back of the leg. Next, the other foot.

One light directed from the front of the patient may be attached to the dental unit; the other light is mounted on a ceiling track as just described.

III. DENTAL LIGHT: ADJUSTMENT

A. The area being treated should be seen clearly without having to assume body positions that are harmful if held over long periods.

B. Direct the light first on the napkin under the patient's chin, then rotate the light up to the mouth to avoid flashing light in the patient's eyes.

RELATED OCCUPATIONAL PROBLEMS

Dental hygienists are at risk for developing a variety of physical ailments when inappropriate chair positioning and instrument handling continue over a long period of time. Many of the problems come under the category of cumulative trauma. Cumulative trauma is described and illustrated on pages 528 to 530.

Prevention of occupational problems of the back, shoulders, and conditions related to cumulative trauma is based on following good principles and practices of posture and stretching exercises to counteract the repetitive activities used during dental hygiene instrumentation. A few of the exercises that can be used during practice hours are shown in Figure 5-6. Other exercises particularly for the hands and shoulders are shown in Figure 32-22 on page 531.

FOUR-HANDED DENTAL HYGIENE

I. POSITIONS

A. Assistant is seated with eye level 4 to 6 inches above the clinician's eye level and facing toward the head of dental chair (Figure 5-7).

B. When an assistant participates, the patient's oral cavity must be accessible and visible to both clinician and dental assistant.

C. Instruments and other essential materials are kept within arm's length, and the portable cabinet with sterilized prepared tray is in front of the dental assistant.

II. PROCEDURES

A. Four-handed dentistry procedures are practiced with instrument transfers and evacuation.[3,4]

B. Benefits to a dental hygiene practice are multiplied when a dental hygiene assistant is trained to participate in the patient activities that do not require a dental hygiene license.[5,6]

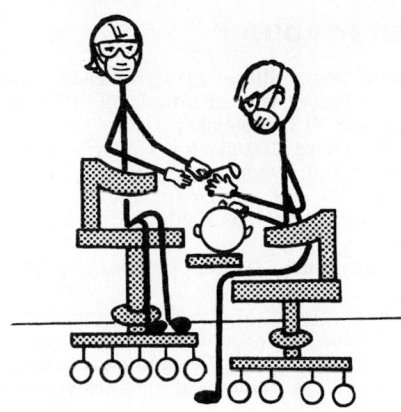

FIGURE 5-7 Clinician with Assistant. The dental assistant is seated with eye level 4 to 6 inches higher than that of the clinician. The sterile tray is placed on a portable cabinet in front of the assistant within easy reach for passing instruments.

TECHNICAL HINTS

I. Orientation of patients, particularly previous patients, is important when changes in equipment and treatment procedures are introduced.

II. Keep body contact at a minimum. A good clinician does not lean on the patient, rest the forearms on the patient's shoulders, or rest the hands on the patient's face or forehead. Unnecessary contact can be unpleasant to certain patients, and more importantly, it contributes to cross-contamination.

FACTORS TO TEACH THE PATIENT

I. Specific instruction on the components of a dental chair or other equipment that will be of concern to the patient to prevent embarrassment or adverse reactions.

II. How certain chair positions needed during scaling relate to the sites around the teeth where more calculus forms.

REFERENCES

1. **Sinnett,** G.M. and Wuehrmann, A.H.: The Dental Operatory of the Future, in Peterson, S., ed.: *The Dentist and His Assistant,* 3rd ed. St. Louis, The C.V. Mosby Co., 1972, pp. 392–401.
2. **Tatro,** D.E.: Ergonomics for the Dental Hygienist, *J. Pract. Hyg., 6,* 35, January/February, 1997.
3. **Sinnett,** G.M., McDevitt, E.J., Robinson, G.E., and Wuehrmann, A.H.: Four-handed Dentistry: A New Mobile Dental Cabinet Design, *J. Am. Dent. Assoc., 78,* 305, February, 1969.
4. **Torres,** H.O., Ehrlich, A., Bird, D., and Dietz, E.: *Modern Dental Assisting,* 5th ed. Philadelphia, W.B. Saunders, 1995, pp. 279–292.
5. **Blitz,** P. and Wright, V.: It Takes Two, *RDH, 14,* 18, September, 1994.
6. **Quinn,** C.: The DHA, *RDH, 17,* 36, February, 1997.

SUGGESTED READINGS

Cunningham, M.A., Sharp, J.D., and Field, H.M.: Teaching Dental Students a Proper Way of Introducing Patients to Instructors, *J. Dent. Educ., 48,* 518, September, 1984.

Ettinger, R.: Office Design for Geriatric Patients, *DentalHygienistNews, 3,* 12, Fall, 1990.

Nield-Gehrig, J.S. and Houseman, G.A.: *Fundamentals of Periodontal Instrumentation,* 3rd ed. Baltimore, Williams & Wilkins, 1996, pp. 15–25.

Nunn, P.J. and Nunn T.D.: Perfect Posture, *RDH, 13,* 14, September, 1993.

Schoen, D.H. and Dean, M.-C.: *Contemporary Periodontal Instrumentation*. Philadelphia, W.B. Saunders Co., 1996, pp. 3–6.

Sunnell, S. and Maschak, L.: Preventing Back, Neck and Shoulder Pain, *Can. Dent. Hyg. (Probe), 30,* 216, November/December, 1996.

Occupational Problems

Barry, R.M., Woodall, W.R., and Mahan, J.M.: Postural Changes in Dental Hygienists, Four Year Longitudinal Study, *J. Dent. Hyg., 66,* 147, March–April, 1992.

Bramson, J.B., Smith, S., and Romagnoli, G.: Evaluating Dental Office Ergonomic Risk Factors and Hazards, *J. Am. Dent. Assoc., 129,* 174, February, 1998.

Liskiewicz, S.T. and Kerschbaum, W.E.: Cumulative Trauma Disorders: An Ergonomic Approach for Prevention, *J. Dent. Hyg., 71,* 162, Summer, 1997.

Seradge, H., Jia, Y.-C., and Owens, W.: *In Vivo* Measurement of Carpal Tunnel Pressure in the Functioning Hand, *J. Hand Surg., 20A,* 855, September, 1995.

Shevach, A., Berg, R.G., Berkey, D.B., and Mann, J.: Ergonomics and Health Considerations at Chairside. Team Members Must Deal With Occupational Risks, *Dent. Teamwork, 9,* 10, November–December, 1996.

Stevens, M.M.: Harmony in Hygiene. The Right Balance to Nutrition and Exercise Can Prolong Your Career, *RDH, 16,* 27, December, 1996.

ASSESSMENT

INTRODUCTION

The dental hygiene process of care is described in Chapter 1 and illustrated in Figure 1-1 (page 6). Assessment of the patient holds the key position in the subsequent dental hygiene diagnosis, identification of the individual needs of the patient, selecting the interventions to treat and bring health to oral tissues, and carrying out the clinical treatment needed.

After treatment, when the outcome is evaluated, reassessment reveals the success thus far and the continuing care needed. The process of care makes a full cycle.

Assessment includes the gathering, organizing, and analyzing of all data from observations, patient questioning, and clinical and radiographic examinations. Basically, it is a collection of all pertinent facts and materials to use during care planning and during all treatment as a guide. The chapters in this section, "Assessment," include descriptions for the preparation and assembling of materials for the care plan.

I. PARTS OF THE ASSESSMENT

A. Basic Procedures
1. Patient histories (personal, dental, and medical).
2. Determination of vital signs.
3. Extraoral and intraoral examination.
4. Radiographic survey.
5. Study casts.
6. Examination of the gingival and periodontal tissues, including clinical signs of disease involvement, probing depths and charting, and mobility evaluation.
7. Examination of the teeth to determine and record deposits, restorations, sealants, carious lesions, structural defects, pulp vitality, and occlusal factors.

B. Supplementary Procedures
In addition to the basic assessments, other procedures are selected because of the individual needs of a patient. Selection of procedures may be influenced by the age group to which the patient belongs.

Certain procedures may be for an emergency examination. For example, if during the intraoral examination of the oral mucosa a suspicious lesion was found for which a biopsy was indicated, such a diagnostic procedure would take precedence over any other.

Assessment may include some or all of the following:
1. Photographs.
2. Biopsy or cytologic smear.
3. Laboratory tests for suspected systemic conditions, such as bleeding tendencies, sickle cell anemia, or diabetes.
4. Special consultations with or referrals to medical specialists.

C. Assessment for the Preventive Care Plan
Built into the sequence of clinical procedures is the initiation of steps for arresting the disease processes and control of etiologic factors. The patient must learn methods to prevent episodes of recurrence of disease.

Assessment for the preventive care plan will include analysis of the patient's history of dental caries and periodontal infections, and the measures used for self-care. Assessment includes learning about the attitudes of the patient and the values placed on maintenance of oral health and the prevention of disease. Assessment will include gathering information about at least the following:
1. Current bacterial plaque score.
2. Personal bacterial plaque removal methods; frequency, implements used.
3. Use of tobacco.
4. Dietary factors.
5. Fluoride history and current use.
6. Pit and fissure sealants.
7. Regularity of continuing care and the frequency of maintenance appointments.

II. PURPOSES

An efficiently conducted assessment can benefit the patient and provide an overall perspective from which a patient-oriented dental hygiene care program can be formulated. Basic objectives are to:
A. Organize information and materials for use while making the diagnosis and outlining the treatment plan for the patient.
B. Aid in
   1. Planning dental hygiene preventive care and instruction for the patient.
   2. Guiding instrumentation during dental hygiene appointments.
   3. Correlating dental hygiene care with dental care.
C. Provide a permanent, documented, continuing record of the patient's oral and general health for
   1. Evaluating the response to treatment, which may be compared with future observations at maintenance appointments.
   2. Protecting the practice in case of misunderstandings or evidence in legal matters should questions arise.
D. Increase the scope of contribution of the dental hygienist to comprehensive patient care by the dental health team.

EXAMINATION PROCEDURES

A specific objective of patient examination as a part of the total assessment is the recognition of deviations from normal that may be signs and symptoms of disease. The importance of careful, thorough examination cannot be overstressed. Concentration and attention to detail are necessary in order that each slight deviation from normal may be entered on the record. Signs and symptoms of disease are the deviations from normal that must be recorded.

I. SIGNS AND SYMPTOMS

A. Sign
A *sign* is any abnormality that may be indicative of a deviation from normal or of disease that is discovered by a professional person while examining a patient. A sign is an objective symptom.

Examples of signs are changes in color, shape, or consistency of a tissue not observable by the patient. Other signs are findings revealed by the use of a probe, explorer, radiograph, or vitality tester of the dental pulp.

B. Symptom
A *symptom* is also any departure from the normal that may be indicative of disease. Symptoms may be subjective or objective.
1. *Subjective Symptom.* Symptom observed by the patient. Examples are pain, tenderness, or itching.
2. *Objective Symptom.* Symptom observed by the professional person during an examination. As just described, objective symptoms are frequently called *signs*.

C. Pathognomonic Signs and Symptoms
Some signs and symptoms are general and may occur during various disease states. An increase in body temperature, for example, accompanies many infections.

Other signs and symptoms are *pathognomonic,* which means that the sign or symptom is unique to a particular disease and can be used to distinguish that disease or condition from other diseases or conditions.

II. TYPES OF EXAMINATION

A. Complete
A complete examination means that a thorough, comprehensive study is made with all the parts listed on page 82.

B. Screening
Screening implies a brief examination. Screening may be used for initial assessment and classification. In a community health program, a survey of a population made to single out people with a particular condition is called screening.

C. Limited
A limited examination is usually made for an emergency. It may be used in the management of acute conditions.

D. Follow-up
A follow-up examination is a type of limited examination. It is used to observe the effects of treatment after a period of time during which the tissue or lesion can recover and heal. Indications of the need for additional or alternate treatment are apparent at a follow-up examination.

E. Maintenance
An examination is made after a specified period of time following the completion of treatment and the restoration to health. A maintenance examination is a complete reassessment from which a new care plan is derived.

III. EXAMINATION METHODS

A patient is examined by various visual, tactile, manual, and instrumental methods. General types are defined briefly here, and other specific methods are found throughout the book as they apply to a certain area under consideration.

A. Visual Examination
1. *Direct Observation.* Visual examination is made in a systematic order to note surface appearance (color, contour, size) and to observe movement and other evidence of function.
2. *Radiographic Examination.* The use of radiographs can reveal deviations from the normal not noticeable by direct observation.
3. *Transillumination.* A strong light directed through a soft tissue or a tooth to enhance examination is especially useful for detecting irregularities of the teeth and locating calculus.

B. Palpation
Palpation is examination using the sense of touch through tissue manipulation or pressure on an area with the fingers or hand. The method used depends on the area to be investigated. Types of palpation are described on page 118.

C. Instrumentation
Examination instruments, such as the explorer and probe, are used for specific examination of the teeth and periodontal tissues. They are described in detail on pages 204 to 212 and 215 to 217.

D. Percussion

Percussion is the act of tapping or striking a surface or tooth with the fingers or an instrument. Information about the status of health of the part is determined either by the response of the patient or by the sound. For example, a metal mirror handle may be used to tap each tooth successively. When a tooth is known to be painful to movement, percussion should be avoided.

E. Electrical Test

An electrical pulp vitality tester is used to detect the presence or absence of vital pulp tissue. The technique for use is described on pages 249 to 251.

F. Auscultation

Auscultation is the use of sound. An example is the sound of clicking or snapping of the temporomandibular joint when the jaw is moved.

TOOTH NUMBERING SYSTEMS

The three tooth designation systems in general use are the *Universal* or *Continuous Numbers 1 through 32* as adopted by the American Dental Association;[1] the *F.D.I. Two-Digit,* adopted by the Fédération Dentaire Internationale;[2] and the *Palmer* or *Quadrant Numbers 1 through 8.*[3,4] *Because different systems are used in dental offices and clinics, it is necessary to be familiar with all of them.*

I. CONTINUOUS NUMBERS 1 THROUGH 32

This tooth numbering method is referred to as the *universal* or *ADA* system.

A. Permanent Teeth

Start with the right maxillary third molar (number 1) and follow around the arch to the left maxillary third molar (16); descend to the left mandibular third molar (17); and follow around to the right mandibular third molar (32). Figure III-1 shows the crowns of the teeth with the corresponding numbers.

B. Primary or Deciduous Teeth

Use continuous upper case letters A through T in the same order as described for the permanent teeth: right maxillary second molar (A) around to left maxillary second molar (J); descend to left mandibular second molar (K), and around to the right mandibular second molar (T).

II. F.D.I. TWO-DIGIT

The *F.D.I.* system is also called the *International.*

A. Permanent Teeth

Each tooth is numbered by the quadrant (1 to 4) and by the tooth within the quadrant (1 to 8).
1. *Quadrant Numbers*
   1 = Maxillary right
   2 = Maxillary left
   3 = Mandibular left
   4 = Mandibular right

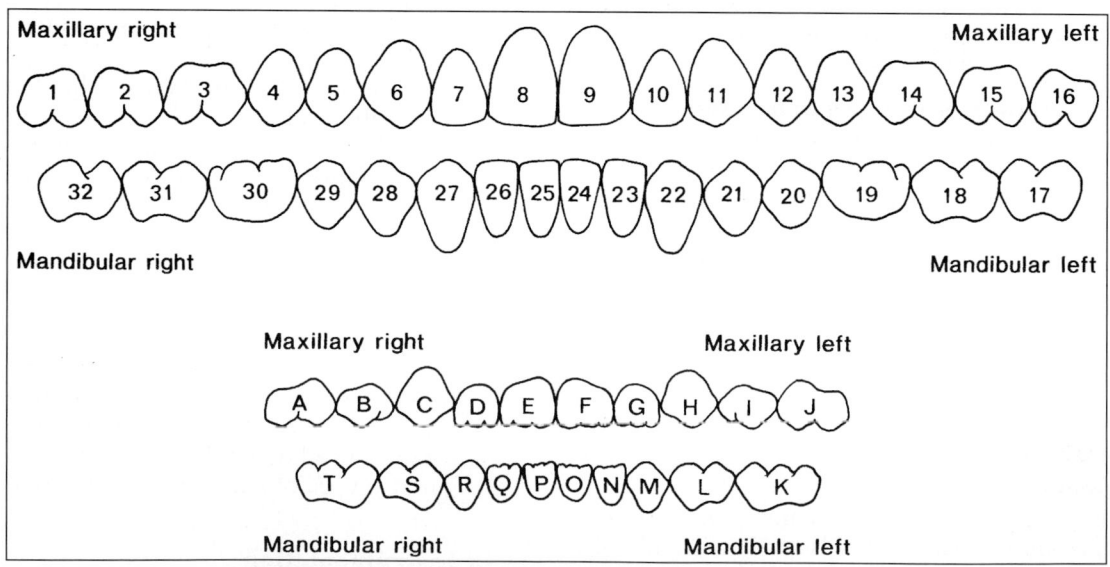

■ **FIGURE III-1 Universal Tooth Numbering (American Dental Association).** *Above,* permanent dentition designated by numbers 1 through 32, starting at the maxillary right with 1 and following around to maxillary left third molar (number 16) to the left mandibular third molar (number 17) and around to the right mandibular third molar (number 32). *Below,* primary teeth are designated by letters in the same sequence.

```
                        PERMANENT TEETH
Q-1                                                    Q-2
Maxillary right                                 Maxillary left

 18   17   16   15   14   13   12   11  │  21   22   23   24   25   26   27   28

 48   47   46   45   44   43   42   41  │  31   32   33   34   35   36   37   38

Mandibular right                                Mandibular left
Q-4                                                    Q-3


                        PRIMARY TEETH
            Q-5                        Q-6
            Maxillary right           Maxillary left

             55   54   53   52   51  │  61   62   63   64   65

             85   84   83   82   81  │  71   72   73   74   75

            Mandibular right          Mandibular left
            Q-8                              Q-7
```

FIGURE III-2 International Tooth Numbering (Fédération Dentaire Internationale). Each quadrant is numbered 1 through 4, with number 1 on maxillary right, number 2 on maxillary left, number 3 on mandibular left, number 4 on mandibular right. Each tooth in a quadrant is numbered 1 through 8 from the central incisor. Quadrants of the primary dentition are numbered from 5 through 8. It is a 2-digit system.

2. *Tooth Numbers Within Each Quadrant.* Start with number 1 at the midline (central incisor) to number 8, third molar. Figure III-2 shows each tooth number in the four quadrants.
3. *Designation.* The digits are pronounced separately. For example, "two-five" (25) is the maxillary left second premolar, and "four-two" (42) is the mandibular right lateral incisor.

B. Primary or Deciduous Teeth

Each tooth is numbered by quadrant (5 to 8) to continue with the permanent quadrant numbers. The teeth are numbered within each quadrant (1 to 5).
1. *Quadrant Numbers*
   5 = Maxillary right
   6 = Maxillary left
   7 = Mandibular left

8 = Mandibular right
2. *Tooth Numbers Within Each Quadrant.* Number 1 is the central incisor, and number 5 is the second primary molar.
3. *Designation.* The digits are pronounced separately. For example, "eight-three" (83) is the mandibular right primary canine, and "six-five" (65) is the maxillary left second primary molar.

III. QUADRANT NUMBERS 1 THROUGH 8

Names to identify this method are the *Palmer System* or *Set-square.*

A. Permanent Teeth

With number 1 for each central incisor, the teeth in each quadrant are numbered to 8, the third molar (Figure III-3). To identify individual teeth, horizontal and vertical lines are drawn to

```
                        PERMANENT TEETH
Maxillary right                                   Maxillary left

 8│  7│  6│  5│  4│  3│  2│  1│ │ │1   │2   │3   │4   │5   │6   │7   │8

 8│  7│  6│  5│  4│  3│  2│  1│ │ │1   │2   │3   │4   │5   │6   │7   │8
Mandibular right                                  Mandibular left


                        PRIMARY TEETH
Maxillary right                                   Maxillary left

 E│  D│  C│  B│  A│ │ │A   │B   │C   │D   │E

 E│  D│  C│  B│  A│ │ │A   │B   │C   │D   │E
Mandibular right                                  Mandibular left
```

FIGURE III-3 Palmer System Tooth Numbering. Each permanent tooth is designated by number 1 through 8, starting at the central incisor of each quadrant. Quadrants are designated by horizontal and vertical lines. Primary teeth are identified by the letters A through E, starting at the central incisor.

indicate the quadrant. For example, the left maxillary first premolar is |4, the right mandibular first and second molars are $\overline{76}$|. An entire quadrant may be represented by the use of the letter Q, for example, the maxillary right quadrant is Q|.

B. Primary or Deciduous Teeth

Upper case letters A through E are used instead of the numbers. Examples are the mandibular left canine $\overline{C}$| and the maxillary right first primary molar D|.

REFERENCES

1. **American Dental Association:** System of Tooth Numbering and Radiograph Mounting, Approved by the American Dental Association House of Delegates, October, 1968.

2. **Fédération Dentaire Internationale:** Two-digit System of Designating Teeth, *Int. Dent. J., 21,* 104, March, 1971.
3. **American Dental Association:** Proceedings of Dental Societies, *Dent. Cosmos, 12,* 522, October, 1870.
4. **Palmer,** C.: Palmer's Dental Notation, *Dent. Cosmos, 33,* 194, 1891.

SUGGESTED READINGS

American Academy of Periodontology: *Current Procedural Terminology for Periodontics and Insurance Reporting Manual,* 7th ed. Chicago, American Academy of Periodontology, 1995, 64 pp.

Carranza, F.A. and Newman, M.G.: *Clinical Periodontology,* 8th ed. Philadelphia, W.B. Saunders Co., 1996, pp. 344–361.

Peck, S. and Peck, L.: A Time for Change of Tooth Numbering Systems, *J. Dent. Educ., 57,* 643, August, 1993.

Peck, S. and Peck, L.: Tooth Numbering Progress, *Angle Orthodont., 66,* 83, Number 2, 1996.

Villa Vigil, M.A., Arenal, A.A., and Gonzalez, M.A.R.: Notation of Numerical Abnormalities by an Addition to the F.D.I. System, *Quintessence Int., 20,* 299, April, 1989.

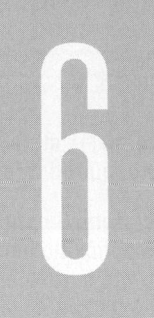

Personal, Dental, and Medical Histories

For safe, scientific dental and dental hygiene care, a meaningful, complete patient history is an essential part of the complete assessment. The history directs and guides steps to be taken in preparation for, during, and following appointments.

The history is needed before oral examination procedures with periodontal probe and explorer are carried out. The use of instruments that would manipulate the soft tissue around the teeth is contraindicated until after it has been determined whether antibiotic premedication is required.

When a question exists about the medical history as described by the patient, or when an unusual or abnormal condition is observed, consultation with the patient's physician or referral for examination of the patient who does not have a physician is mandatory. Even emergency treatment, such as for the relief of pain, should be postponed tentatively or kept to a minimum until the patient's status is determined.

I. SIGNIFICANCE

The significance of the history cannot be overestimated. Oral conditions reflect the general health of the patient. Dental procedures may complicate or be complicated by existing pathologic or physiologic conditions elsewhere in the body. General health factors influence response to treatment, such as tissue healing, and thereby influence the outcomes that may be expected from oral care.

The state of the patient's health is constantly changing. Therefore, the history represents only the period in the patient's life during which the history was made. With successive appointments, the history must be reviewed and considered along with other

BOX 6-1 KEY WORDS AND ABBREVIATIONS: Personal, Medical, and Dental Histories

Allergy (ăl′er-jē): state of abnormal and individual hypersensitivity acquired through exposure to a particular allergen.

Antibiotic premedication (ăn-″tĭ-bī-ŏt′ik): provision of an effective antibiotic before invasive clinical procedures that can create a transient bacteremia, which, in turn, can cause infective endocarditis or other serious infection.

Bacteremia (băk″tĕr-ē′mē-ah): presence of microorganisms in the blood stream.

Drug interaction: a change in the effect of one drug when a second drug is introduced concomitantly; the change may be desirable, adverse, or inconsequential.

Forensic (fō-rĕn′zik): pertaining to or applied in legal proceedings.

Forensic dentistry: dentolegal science; the relation and application of dental facts to legal problems, as in using the teeth for identifying the dead.

Hematogenous (hē″mah-toj′ĕ-nŭs): produced or derived from blood; disseminated through the blood stream.

Immunocompromised (ĭm″ū-nō-kŏm′prō-mīzd): when the immune response is attenuated by administration of immunosuppressive drugs, by irradiation, by malnutrition, or by certain disease processes.

Informed consent: a medicolegal document that holds providers responsible for ensuring that patients understand the risks and benefits of a procedure or medication before it is administered.

OTC: over the counter; nonprescription drug; pertains to distribution of drugs directly to the public without prescription.

PDR: *Physicians' Desk Reference*; contains current information about the actions, side effects, and interactions of drugs; a new edition is published annually.

Premedication: preliminary medication; may be for the purpose of allaying apprehension, preventing bacteremia, or otherwise facilitating the clinical procedure.

SBE: subacute bacterial endocarditis, now called infective endocarditis.

---

new findings. Key words relating to the preparation and use of the histories are defined in Box 6-1.

II. PURPOSES OF THE HISTORY

Carefully prepared personal, medical, and dental histories are used in comprehensive patient care to

A. Provide information pertinent to the etiology and diagnosis of oral conditions and the total patient care plan.

B. Reveal conditions that necessitate precautions, modifications, or adaptations during appointments to ensure that dental and dental hygiene procedures will not harm the patient and that emergency situations will be prevented.

C. Aid in the identification of possible unrecognized conditions for which the patient should be referred for further diagnosis and treatment.

D. Permit appraisal of the general health and nutritional status, which, in turn, contributes to the prognosis of success in patient care and instruction.

E. Give insight into emotional and psychological factors, attitudes, and prejudices that may affect present appointments as well as continuing care.

F. Document records for reference and comparison over a series of appointments for periodic follow-up.

G. Furnish evidence in legal matters should questions arise.[1]

HISTORY PREPARATION

The general methods in current use for obtaining a health history are the *interview*, the *questionnaire*, or a combination of the two. There are several systems for obtaining the history.

I. SYSTEMS

A. Preappointment Information

Basic information obtained prior to the initial assessment appointment can save time and facilitate the process. A brief telephone screening interview can help to determine potential medical problems and need for premedication, and it can identify medically compromised or physically challenged patients for whom modifications in routine care may be needed.

B. Brief History

A brief history of vital items is obtained at the initial visit; a complete history is obtained at a succeeding appointment.

1. Purposes of brief history are to prepare for emergency care and to learn of any condition that may contraindicate instrumentation.

2. Brief history may be in the form of a questionnaire; an interview for follow-up provides opportunity for individual evaluation.

C. Self-history

Because a self-history can be prepared at home,

the history form may be mailed to the patient in advance or given at the first appointment to complete and bring in at the second appointment. Such a form might include some checking, as in a questionnaire, and some space to allow free expression by the patient.

D. Complete History

Complete history is made at the initial visit and may be a combination of interview and questionnaire.

II. RECORD FORMS

A. Basic History Forms

Many varying forms are in current use. Forms are available commercially or from the American Dental Association (ADA),[2] but many dentists and dental hygienists prefer to develop their own and have a form printed to their specifications.

B. Characteristics of an Adequate Form

The number of items or questions included is not necessarily indicative of the value of the form. The extensive and involved form may be as practical or impractical as the brief checklist that permits no detailed description. Success in use depends on function and a clear common understanding of the meaning of the recorded information to all who refer to it.

Some characteristics of an adequate form are that it should

1. Provide for conventional notation of important details in a logical sequence.
2. Permit quick identification of special needs of a patient when the history is reviewed prior to each appointment.
3. Allow ample space to record the patient's own words whenever possible in the interview method, or for self-expression by the patient on a questionnaire.
4. Have space for notes concerning attitudes and knowledge as stated or displayed by the patient during the history-taking or other later appointments.
5. Be of a size consistent with the complete patient record forms for filing and ready availability.

C. Supplementary Forms

A second questionnaire for specialized topics is needed to determine details. The basic questionnaire reveals whether the topic applies to the individual, and if the answer is positive, additional information is requested.

For example, simple questions may appear on the basic questionnaire to show the use of tobacco. Completion of another questionnaire such as Figure 27-2 (page 435) provides details of the type of tobacco used and frequency.

III. INTRODUCTION TO THE PATIENT

The patient needs to realize why the information requested in the histories is essential before treatment can be undertaken. Dental personnel must convey the idea that oral health and general health are interrelated, without creating undue alarm concerning potential ill effects or harmful sequelae from required treatment.

For building rapport, children may participate in their history preparation, but most of the information will need to be supplied by a parent. The signature of the responsible adult on the record is needed.

IV. LIMITATIONS OF A HISTORY

Many patients cannot or will not provide complete or, in certain cases, correct information when answering medical or dental history questions. There may be problems related to the method of obtaining the histories, how the questions are worded, or an inadvertent lack of neutrality in the attitude of the person preparing the history. Some patients may have difficulty in comprehending a self-administered test, or there may be a language barrier.

Where the questionnaire is completed may influence answers. A crowded reception area where other patients can see the form and the checks made does not provide sufficient privacy.

Another reason for inaccuracy or incompleteness is that patients may not understand the relationship between certain diseases or conditions and dental treatment. Information may seem irrelevant, so it is withheld. Occasionally, a patient will not want to tell about a condition that may be embarrassing to discuss. The patient may fear refusal of treatment, particularly if such had been a previous experience in other dental practices.

THE QUESTIONNAIRE

Positive findings on a completed questionnaire need supplementation in a personal interview. A questionnaire by itself cannot be expected to satisfy the overall purposes of the history, but it can be adapted best to phases of the personal history, some aspects of the dental history, and factual information in the medical history.

I. TYPES OF QUESTIONS

The health questionnaire available from the American Dental Association (Figure 6-1) provides useful examples of questions essential to patient evaluation.[2]

A. System-oriented

Direct questions or topics that check whether the patient has had a disease of, for example, the digestive system, respiratory system, or urinary system may be used. The questions may contain references to body parts, for example,

ADA. Health History Form

Medical Alert	Condition	Premedication	Allergies	Anaest.		Date

Name_____
Last   First   Middle

Home Phone ( )_____ Business Phone ( )_____

Address _____
P.O. Box or Mailing address

City_____ State_____ Zip Code_____

Occupation_____

Height_____ Weight_____ Date of Birth ___/___/___ Sex ☐ M ☐ F

Emergency Contact _____ Relationship _____ Phone ( )_____

If you are completing this form for another person, what is your relationship to that person? _____
Name   Relationship

For the following questions, please (X) whichever applies, your answers are for our records only and will be kept confidential in accordance with applicable laws. Please note that during your initial visit you will be asked some questions about your responses to this questionnaire and there may be additional questions concerning your health. This information is vital to allow us to provide appropriate care for you. This office does not use this information to discriminate.

Dental Information

Yes	No	Don't Know		Yes	No	Don't Know	
☐	☐	☐	Do your gums bleed when you brush?	☐	☐	☐	Have you ever had orthodontic (braces) treatment?
☐	☐	☐	Are your teeth sensitive to cold, hot, sweets or pressure?	☐	☐	☐	Do you have headaches, earaches or neck pains?
☐	☐	☐	Have you had any periodontal (gum) treatments?	☐	☐	☐	Do you wear removable dental appliances?
☐	☐	☐	Have you had a serious/difficult problem associated with any previous dental treatment? If so, explain				

How would you describe your current dental problem?_____

Date of your last dental exam _____ Date of last dental x-rays _____

What was done at that time?_____

How do you feel about the appearance of your teeth? _____

Medical Information

Yes	No	Don't Know	
☐	☐	☐	Are you in good health?
☐	☐	☐	Has there been any change in your general health within the past year?

Do you have any of the following diseases or problems: **If you answer yes to any of the 3 items below, please stop and return this form to the receptionist.**

Yes	No	Don't Know	
☐	☐	☐	**Active Tuberculosis**
☐	☐	☐	**Persistent cough greater than a 3 week duration**
☐	☐	☐	**Cough that produces blood**
☐	☐	☐	Are you now under the care of a physician? If so, what is/are the condition(s) being treated? _____

_____ Date of last physical examination _____

Physician(s) _____
NAME   PHONE   ADDRESS   CITY/STATE/ZIP

_____
NAME   PHONE   ADDRESS   CITY/STATE/ZIP

Yes	No	Don't Know	
☐	☐	☐	Have you had any serious illness, operation, or been hospitalized in the past 5 years? If so, what was the illness or problem? _____
☐	☐	☐	Are you taking or have you recently taken any medicine(s) including non-prescription medicine? If so, what medicine(s) are you taking?

Prescribed _____

Over the counter _____

Natural or herbal preparations _____

Yes	No	Don't Know	
☐	☐	☐	Are you taking, or have you taken, any diet drugs such Pondimin (fenfluramine), Redux (dexphenfluramine) or phen-fen (phentermine)?
☐	☐	☐	Do you drink alcoholic beverages? If yes, how much alcohol did you drink in the last 24 hours? _____ In the past month? _____
			If yes, _____ # of drinks per day for _____ # of years
☐	☐	☐	Are you alcohol and/or drug dependent? If so, have you received treatment? (Check one) ☐ Yes ☐ No
☐	☐	☐	Do you use drugs or other substances for recreational purposes? If yes, please list_____
			Frequency of use (daily, weekly, etc.) _____ Number of years of recreational drug use _____
☐	☐	☐	Do you use tobacco (smoking, snuff, chew)? If so, how interested are you in stopping? (Check one) ☐ Very ☐ Somewhat ☐ Not interested
☐	☐	☐	Do you wear contact lenses?

Allergies Are you allergic to or have you had a reaction to: (Please fill out both columns)

Yes	No	Don't Know		Yes	No	Don't Know	
☐	☐	☐	Local anesthetics	☐	☐	☐	Latex
☐	☐	☐	Aspirin	☐	☐	☐	Iodine
☐	☐	☐	Penicillin or other antibiotics	☐	☐	☐	Hay fever/seasonal
☐	☐	☐	Barbiturates, sedatives, or sleeping pills	☐	☐	☐	Animals
☐	☐	☐	Sulfa drugs	☐	☐	☐	Food (Specify)_____
☐	☐	☐	Codeine or other narcotics	☐	☐	☐	Other (Specify)_____

To yes responses, specify type of reaction _____

Please complete both sides

FIGURE 6-1 Health History Form. From American Dental Association, Council on Dental Practice. Reprinted with permission.

(Women Only)

☐	☐	☐	Are you pregnant?
☐	☐	☐	Nursing?
☐	☐	☐	Taking birth control pills?

☐	☐	☐	Have you had an orthopedic total joint (hip, knee, elbow, finger) replacement? If so when was this operation done? _____
☐	☐	☐	Have you had any complications or difficulties with your prosthetic joint?
☐	☐	☐	Has a physician or previous dentist recommended that you take antibiotics prior to your dental treatment? If so, what antibiotic and dose?

Name of physician or dentist*_____ Phone _____

NOTE TO PATIENT: A new report (July 1997) prepared and endorsed by the American Dental Association and the American Academy of Orthopaedic Surgeons has recommended that antibiotic prophylaxis before dental treatment is not indicated for most dental patients with artificial orthopedic prosthetic joints. This office will be glad to discuss this report with you and provide a copy of it to you and your orthopedic surgeon/physician.

Please (X) if you have or had any of the following diseases or problems.

Yes	No	Don't Know		Yes	No	Don't Know		Yes	No	Don't Know	
☐	☐	☐	Abnormal bleeding	☐	☐	☐	Disease, drug, or radiation-induced immunosurpression	☐	☐	☐	Neurological disorders. If yes, specify _____
☐	☐	☐	AIDS or HIV infection	☐	☐	☐	Diabetes. If yes, specify below:	☐	☐	☐	Osteoporosis
☐	☐	☐	Anemia				○ Type I (Insulin dependent)	☐	☐	☐	Persistent swollen glands in neck
☐	☐	☐	Arthritis				○ Type II	☐	☐	☐	Respiratory problems. If yes, specify below:
☐	☐	☐	Rheumatoid arthritis	☐	☐	☐	Dry mouth				○ Emphysema,
☐	☐	☐	Asthma	☐	☐	☐	Eating disorder. If yes, specify _____				○ Bronchitis, etc.
☐	☐	☐	Blood transfusion If yes, date _____	☐	☐	☐	Epilepsy	☐	☐	☐	Severe headaches
☐	☐	☐	Cancer/Chemotherapy/radiation treatment	☐	☐	☐	Fainting spells or seizures	☐	☐	☐	Severe or rapid weight loss
				☐	☐	☐	G.E. reflux	☐	☐	☐	Sexually transmitted disease
☐	☐	☐	Cardiovascular disease. If yes, specify below:	☐	☐	☐	Glaucoma	☐	☐	☐	Sinus trouble
			○ Angina	☐	☐	☐	Hemophilia	☐	☐	☐	Sleep disorder
			○ Arteriosclerosis	☐	☐	☐	Hepatitis, jaundice or liver disease	☐	☐	☐	Sores or ulcers in the mouth
			○ Artificial heart valves	☐	☐	☐	Recurrent infections	☐	☐	☐	Stroke
			○ Coronary insufficiency				Indicate type of infection	☐	☐	☐	Systemic lupus erythematosus
			○ Coronary occlusion				_____	☐	☐	☐	Thyroid problems
			○ Damaged heart valves	☐	☐	☐	Kidney problems	☐	☐	☐	Tuberculosis
			○ Heart attack	☐	☐	☐	Low blood pressure	☐	☐	☐	Ulcers
			○ Heart murmur	☐	☐	☐	Mental health disorders. If yes, specify below:	☐	☐	☐	Excessive urination
			○ High blood pressure				_____	☐	☐	☐	Do you have any disease, condition, or problem not listed above that you think I should know about? Please explain.
			○ Inborn heart defects				_____				
			○ Mitral valve prolapse								
			○ Pacemaker								
			○ Rheumatic heart disease								
☐	☐	☐	Chest pain upon exertion	☐	☐	☐	Malnutrition				
☐	☐	☐	Chronic pain	☐	☐	☐	Migraines				
☐	☐	☐	Persistent diarrhea	☐	☐	☐	Night sweats				

NOTE: Both doctor and patient are encouraged to discuss any and all relevant patient health issues prior to treatment.
I certify that I have read and understand the above. I acknowledge that my questions, if any, about inquiries set forth above have been answered to my satisfaction. I will not hold my dentist, or any other member of his/her staff, responsible for any action they take or do not take because of errors or omissions that I may have made in the completion of this form.

_____
Signature of Patient/Legal Guardian   Date

For completion by dentist

Comments on patient interview concerning health history_____
_____
_____

Significant findings from questionnaire or oral interview _____
_____
_____

Dental management considerations _____

_____   _____
Signature of Dentist   Date

Health History Update: On a regular basis the patient should be questioned about any medical history changes, date and comments notated, along with signature.

Date	Comments	Signature of patient and dentist
_____	_____	_____
_____	_____	_____
_____	_____	_____
_____	_____	_____

■ **FIGURE 6-1** (CONTINUED)

the stomach, lungs, kidneys. Questions can then be directed to the specific disease state and the dates and duration.

B. Disease-oriented

A typical set of questions for the patient to check may start with "Do you have, or have you had, any of the following diseases or problems?" A listing under that question contains such items as diabetes, asthma, or rheumatic fever arranged alphabetically or grouped by systems or body organs.

Follow-up questions can determine dates of illness, severity, and outcome.

C. Symptom-oriented

In the absence of previous or current disease states, questions may lead to a suspicion of a condition, which, in turn, can provide an opportunity to recommend and encourage the patient to schedule an examination by a physician. Examples of the symptom-oriented questions are "Are you thirsty much of the time?" "Does your mouth frequently become dry?" or "Do you have to urinate (pass water) more than six times a day?" Positive answers could lead to tests for diabetes detection.

II. ADVANTAGES OF A QUESTIONNAIRE

A. Broad in scope; useful during the interview to identify positive areas that need additional clarification.
B. Time-saving.
C. Consistent; all selected questions are included, and none is omitted because of time or other factors.
D. Patient has time to think over the answers; not under pressure, nor under the eyes of the interviewer.
E. Patient may write information that might not be expressed directly in an interview.
F. Legal aspects of a written record with patient's signature.

III. DISADVANTAGES OF A QUESTIONNAIRE (IF USED ALONE WITHOUT A FOLLOW-UP INTERVIEW)

A. Impersonal; no opportunity to develop rapport.
B. Inflexible; no provision for additional questioning in areas of specific importance to an individual patient.

THE INTERVIEW

In long-range planning for the patient's health, much more is involved than asking questions and receiving answers. The rapport established at the time of the interview contributes to the continued cooperation of the patient.

I. PARTICIPANTS

The interviewer is alone with the patient or parent of the child patient. The history should never be taken in a reception area when other patients are present.

II. SETTING

A. A consultation room or office is preferred; the patient should be away from the atmosphere of the treatment room, where thoughts may be on the techniques to be performed.
B. Treatment room may be the only available place where privacy is afforded.
   1. Seat patient comfortably in upright position.
   2. Turn off running water and dental light, and close the door.
   3. Sit on clinician's stool to be at eye level with the patient.

III. POINTERS FOR THE INTERVIEW

Interviewing involves communication between individuals. Communication implies the transmission or interchange of facts, attitudes, opinions, or thoughts, through words, gestures, or other means. Through tactful but direct questioning, communication can be successful, and the patient will give such information as is known. Frequently, the patient is unaware of a health problem.

The attitude of the dental personnel should be one of friendly understanding, reassurance, and acceptance. Genuine interest and willingness to listen when a patient wishes to describe symptoms or complaints not only aids in establishing the rapport needed, but frequently provides insight into the patient's real attitudes and prejudices. By asking simple questions at first, and more personal questions later after rapport has developed, the patient will be more relaxed and frank in answering.

Self-confidence and gentle efficiency on the part of the interviewer help to give the patient a feeling of confidence. Skill is required, because tact, ingenuity, and judgment are taxed to the fullest in the attempt to obtain both accurate and complete information from the patient.

IV. INTERVIEW FORM

The interviewer may use a structured form with places to check and fill in. Another method is to record on blank sheets from questions created from a guide list of essential topics. Either may involve reference to the positive or negative answers on a previously completed questionnaire.

Familiarity with the items on the history permits the interviewer to be direct and informal without reading from a fixed list of topics, a method that may lack the personal touch necessary to gain the patient's confidence. When appropriate, the patient's own words are recorded.

V. ADVANTAGES OF THE INTERVIEW

A. Personal contact contributes to development of rapport for future appointments.

B. Flexibility for individual needs; details obtained can be adapted for supplementary questioning.

VI. DISADVANTAGES OF INTERVIEW

A. Time-consuming when not prefaced with questionnaire.

B. Unless a list is consulted, items of importance may be omitted.

C. Patient may be embarrassed to talk about personal conditions and may hold back significant information.

ITEMS INCLUDED IN THE HISTORY

Information obtained by means of the history is directly related to how the goals for patient care can and will be accomplished. In Tables 6-1, 6-2, and 6-3, items are listed with possible medications and other treatments the patient may have or has had, along with suggested considerations for appointment procedures.

In specialized practices, objectives may require increased emphasis on certain aspects. The age group most frequently served would influence the material needed. Parental history and pre- and postnatal information may take on particular significance for the treatment of a small child; in a pedodontist's practice, a special form could be devised to include all essential items.

Insight and awareness shown while preparing the patient history depend on background knowledge of the manifestations of systemic diseases and the medications for various conditions. Objectives for the items to include in the various parts of the history are listed here.

I. PERSONAL HISTORY (Table 6-1)

The basic objectives in gathering personal information about the patient are

A. Data essential for appointment planning and business aspects.

B. Approval of care of a minor and other legal aspects.

C. For consultation with the patient's physician relative to interrelations between general and oral health.

II. DENTAL HISTORY (Table 6-2)

The dental history should contribute to knowledge of

A. The immediate problem, chief complaint, cause of present pain, or discomfort of any kind in the oral cavity.

B. The previous dental hygiene and dental care as described by the patient, including preventive care, periodontal treatments, and the extent of restorative and prosthetic replacement, as well as any adverse effects.

C. The attitude of the patient toward oral health and care of the mouth as may be indicated by previous periodic dental and dental hygiene treatments and family history of oral care.

D. The personal daily care exercised by the patient as evidence of knowledge of the purposes of continuing care and of the value placed on the teeth and their supporting structures.

III. MEDICAL HISTORY (Table 6-3)

Objectives of the medical history are to determine whether the patient has or has had any conditions in the following categories:

A. **Conditions That May Complicate Certain Kinds of Dental and Dental Hygiene Treatment**

Examples. Lowered resistance to infection; uncontrolled hypertension; or systemic disease that requires treatment before stressful dental procedures, particularly surgery, can be carried out.

B. **Diseases That Require Special Precautions or Premedication Prior to Treatment**

Example. Antibiotic coverage for patient with a history of rheumatic fever or congenital heart defect, to prevent infective endocarditis.

C. **Conditions Under Treatment by a Physician That Require Medicating Drugs That May Influence or Contraindicate Certain Procedures**

Examples. Anticoagulant therapy requires consultation with physician; antihypertensive drugs may alter the choice of local anesthetic used.

D. **Allergic or Untoward Reactions**

Examples. Latex hypersensitivity; medication or material for which there was a previous adverse reaction.

E. **Diseases and Drugs With Manifestations in the Mouth**

Examples. Hematologic disorders; phenytoin-induced gingival overgrowth; infectious diseases such as herpesvirus.

F. **Communicable Diseases That Endanger the Dental Personnel**

Examples. Active tuberculosis; viral hepatitis; herpes; syphilis.

G. **Physiologic State of the Patient**

Examples. Pregnancy; puberty; menopause; birth control pills.

(text continues on page 101)

TABLE 6-1 Items for the Personal History

Items to Record in Patient History	Record Notes	Considerations for Appointment Procedures
1. Name 　Addresses: residence and business 　Telephone numbers 　Sex 　Marital status 　For child: name of parent or guardian 　For parent: age and sex of children	Accurate recording necessary for business aspects of dental practice	Aids in establishing rapport Instruction applicable to entire family Advice concerning fluorides for children
2. Birthdate	Whether of age or a minor Oral conditions related to age changes; diseases, healing, and other possible characteristics	Informed consent of parent or guardian necessary for care of minor or person with a mental handicap; signature must be obtained Approach to patient instruction
3. Birthplace and residence in early years	Presence of fluoride in drinking water Food and eating patterns Conditions endemic to certain areas	Effects of fluoride on teeth Instruction in dietary needs adapted to cultural practices
4. Occupation: present and former 　Spouse's occupation 　For children: parent's occupation	May be a factor in etiology of certain diseases, dental stains, occlusal wear May affect diet, oral habits, general health	Instruction applied to specific needs Dexterity in use of self-care devices related to dexterity gained from occupation Influence on oral care of entire family For child: which parent will supervise and assist child in oral care
5. Physician	Name, address, and telephone number For consultation	Consultation indicated: 　(1) when disease symptoms are suspected but patient does not state 　(2) in an emergency 　(3) Medication/premedication
6. Referred by and address	To whom to send referral acknowledgment and appreciation	Contribution to rapport with patient Patient referred by another patient may have concept of the office procedures

TABLE 6-2 Items for the Dental History

Items to Record in the History	Record Notes	Considerations for Appointment Procedures
1. Reason for present appointment	Chief complaint in patient's own words Pain or discomfort Onset, symptoms, duration of an acute condition	Need for immediate treatment Attitude toward dentistry and preventive care
2. Previous dental appointments	Date of last treatment Services performed Regularity	Patient knowledge concerning regular dental care Cooperation anticipated
3. Anesthetics used	Local, general Adverse reactions	Choice of anesthetic

(continued)

TABLE 6-2 Items for the Dental History (Continued)

Items to Record in the History	Record Notes	Considerations for Appointment Procedures
4. Radiation history	Type, number, dates of dental and medical radiographs Therapeutic radiation Availability of dental radiographs from previous dentist Amount of exposure considered with exposure for medical purposes	Amount of exposure; limitations Patient's appreciation for need and use of radiographs
5. Family dental history	Parental tooth loss or maintenance	Attitude toward saving teeth and preventive dentistry

6. Previous treatment
 	
  a. periodontal
 	
  b. orthodontic
 	
  c. endodontic
  d. prosthodontic
  e. other
	Type of treatment; frequency of maintenance appointments
	Whether referred to specialist
	History of acute infection (necrotizing ulcerative gingivitis)
	Surgery; posttreatment healing
	Age during treatment; completion date
	Previous problem
	Habit correction
	Dates, etiology
	Types of prostheses
	Extent of restorations
	Tooth loss
	Implants
		Attitude toward specialized care
		Previous familiarity with role of dental hygienist
		Attitude toward self-care and disease control
		
		For current treatment, consultation with orthodontist needed to determine instructions
		
		Periodic recheck
		Care of prostheses and abutment teeth
		Understanding prevention

7. Injuries to face or teeth	Causes and extent Fractured teeth or jaws	Limitation of opening Special care during healing
8. Temporomandibular joint	History of injury, discomfort, disease, dislocation Previous treatment	Effect on opening; accessibility during instrumentation
9. Habits	Clenching, bruxism Mouth breathing Biting objects; fingernails, pipe stem, thread, other Cheek or lip biting Patient awareness of habits	Tension of patient Instruction relative to effects of habits
10. Tobacco use	Form of tobacco, amount used Frequency Knowledge of effects on oral tissues	Instruction concerning oral effects Tobacco cessation program Periodontal risk Dental stains; dentifrice selection
11. Fluorides	Systemic, topical, dates Residence during tooth development years Amount of fluoride in drinking water	Current preventive procedures and need for reevaluation

12. Plaque control procedures	Toothbrushing: current procedures
	  type of brush (manual or powered)
	  texture of filaments
	  frequency of use
	  age of brush; frequency of having a new brush
	Dentifrice
	  name
	  how selected; reason
	Additional cleansing devices and frequency of use
	  dental floss
	  water irrigation
	  implants care
	Mouthrinse or other agents: frequency, purpose
	Source of instruction in care of oral cavity
		Present practice and previous instruction
		New instruction needed; reception by patient
		Relation of techniques to prevention of dental caries and periodontal infections
		Supervision of child by parent: current practices
		Problems of habit change

TABLE 6-3 Items for the Medical History

Item to Record in History	Record Notes	Medications and Treatment Modalities	Considerations for Appointment Procedures
1. General health and appearance	Disabilities Overall impression of well-being Patient's appraisal of own health		Response, cooperation, and attitude to expect during appointments
2. Medical examination	Date most recent examination Reason for the examination Tests performed; results Anticipated surgery	New prescriptions received Previous prescriptions continued	Verification with physician for added information Need for superior state of oral health in advance of surgery 1. When long recovery is expected and patient may miss maintenance appointments 2. Prior to transplant, heart surgery, or prosthesis
3. Major illnesses, hospitalizations, surgeries	Causes of illness Type and duration of treatment Anesthetics used Convalescence Course of healing: normal, not normal	Medications, treatments	Influence of illnesses on health and care of the oral cavity Anesthetic choice Expected outcome from gingival treatment
4. Age factors	Problems of health in different age groups Geriatric: multiple disease entities; patient may need to bring the containers for identification of their medications	See individual medical problem Update drug regimen at each appointment	Effects on dental and dental hygiene procedures and personal care
5. Height and weight	Weight changes over past years or months Obesity Undernourishment Child growth pattern	Diet pills Substance abuse	Marked weight change may be a symptom of undiagnosed disease; suggest referral for medical examination Influence on dietary instructions for oral health
6. Medications prescribed by physician	Reasons: relation to dental care Frequency Patient's regularity of taking Sugar content of liquid medicines, effect on dental caries (also true of over-the-counter [OTC] items)	List all drugs by name Ask patient for drugs, medicine, injections, tonics, vitamins, patches, pills, capsules, to get a complete answer Dosage; route of administration	Consultation with physician concerning adjustments in dosage for dental or dental hygiene appointments Indications for premedication Side effects of drugs
7. Self-medication	Type, frequency OTC preparations Substance abuse	Pain relievers Sleeping tablets Cough syrup Antacids Cathartics Vitamins Diet pills	Information not revealed by patient could complicate treatment Lack of interest in oral health, only pain relief Drug side effects
8. Family medical history	Predisposition to certain diseases (example: diabetes) History of diseases that occur in the family	Cultural beliefs about medications	May help patient seek medical examination when symptom suggests possible disease

(continued)

TABLE 6-3 Items for the Medical History (Continued)

Item to Record in History	Record Notes	Medications and Treatment Modalities	Considerations for Appointment Procedures
9. Daily diet	Recommendations of patient's physicians, past and present Vitamin supplements Appetite Regularity of meals Food likes and dislikes	Vitamin supplements	Instructions to be given relative to oral health Prognosis for healing after treatment Need for dietary review and analysis

10. Alcohol consumption	Frequency
	Amount
	Substance abuse
		Recovering alcoholic:
		  May be taking disulfiram,
		  Must avoid all alcohol-containing preparations, including commercial mouthrinses
			Excessive use: effect on anesthesia; increased healing time
			Poor nutritional state is common; lack of oral care
			Avoid alcohol-containing mouthrinse
			May result in poor patient cooperation

11. Allergies	Determine substances to which the patient is allergic
	  Latex
	  Anesthetics
	  Penicillin
	  Medicaments
	  Foods
	  Iodine
		Antihistamines
		Inhalers
		Decongestants
		Steroids
			Preparation for emergency
			Xerostomia
			Avoid use of substances to which the patient is allergic
			Consider allergies when planning dietary recommendations

12. Arthritis	Joint pain Immobility Temporomandibular joint involvement	Aspirin Nonsteroidal anti-inflammatory drugs Corticosteroids Total joint replacements	Antibiotic premedication: consult physician if treated with chemotherapeutic agent Dental chair adjustment
13. Blood disorder	Type and duration of disease Leukemia: remission, thrombocytopenia	Vitamins Minerals: iron (iron-deficiency anemia) Folic acid supplement (sickle cell anemia) Antineoplastic drugs	Consultation with physician Need for high level of oral health Antibiotic premedication Immunosuppression Increased bleeding Oral lesions
14. Bleeding	Bleeding associated with previous dental appointments History of disorder with coagulation problem History of transfusions or other blood products Check use of aspirin (relation to bleeding tendency) Laboratory tests for bleeding time, coagulation may be needed	Anticoagulant medication Hemophilia factor replacement	Emergency prevention through preappointment precautions May need to apply direct pressure or hemostatic agent after scaling Special measures for hemophilia
15. Cancer	Head and neck radiation effects on oral cavity, salivary glands Dental and dental hygiene therapy updated before start of surgery, radiation therapy, or immunosuppression Blood count prior to dental and dental hygiene therapy	Radiation therapy Fluoride therapy: daily topical application Antineoplastic drugs, alkylating agents, antimetabolites, antibiotics, plant alkaloids, steroids	Antibiotic premedication Bleeding; infection; poor healing response Avoid trauma to tissues Effect on oral radiographic survey: prevention of overexposure Dental caries: preventive measures Xerostomia: substitute saliva

(continued)

TABLE 6-3 Items for the Medical History (Continued)

Item to Record in History	Record Notes	Medications and Treatment Modalities	Considerations for Appointment Procedures
16. Cardiovascular diseases	Consultation with physician Refer for examination when patient seems unsure of problem	Cardiac glycosides Antiarrhythmics Antianginals Antihypertensives Anticoagulants	Minimize stress Premedication for stress Ascertain that medications have been taken Monitor vital signs
Congenital heart disease Rheumatic heart disease	Susceptibility to infective endo-carditis Type of problem; date of rheumatic fever	 Antibiotic (prevent recurrence of rheumatic fever)	Antibiotic premedication required
Hypertension	Symptom of other disease state Monitoring blood pressure for each appointment Anesthesia: limit epinephrine or omit as recommended by physician	Diuretics Antiadrenergic agents Vasodilators Angiotensin-converting enzyme inhibitors Calcium channel–blocking agent	Postural hypotension (raise dental chair slowly) Xerostomia: saliva substitute and fluoride rinse may be needed Gingival hyperplasia
Angina pectoris	Prepare for symptoms: have ready amyl nitrite inhalant or nitroglycerin tablets or spray	Amyl nitrite, nitroglycerin, or other antianginal drugs	Allay fears and prevent stress Morning appointment
Heart diseases	History of disease symptoms of fatigue, short-ness of breath or cough Consult with physician	Glycosides (digitalis) Anticoagulants Antiarrhythmic drugs Pacemaker	Monitor vital signs Short, more frequent appointments Change dental chair slowly Patient with breathing problem (sleeps with two or more pil-lows) may need semi-upright position Bleeding tendency associated with anticoagulant Check use of ultrasonic (pace-maker)
Surgically corrected cardiovascular lesions	Type, date of surgery Consultation with physician Before surgical procedure, when possible: the patient needs complete oral evaluation and corrective dental work done, with motivation to high level of oral personal care daily	No tobacco use Anticoagulants Cyclosporine Nifedipine	Antibiotic premedication vital for synthetic valves or other replacements, indefinitely Gingival bleeding can be expected Gingival enlargement
Cerebrovascular accident (stroke)	Date of onset; residual disabilities Speech, vision, mental function	No tobacco; low-salt diet Anticoagulants Antihypertensives Vasodilator Steroid Anticonvulsant	Gingival bleeding likely when anticoagulants are used Adapt procedures for physical disability
17. Communicable diseases	History of diseases; immunizations Present disease; communicability Residence or extended trips in countries with high endemic incidence of certain diseases Risk group factor	Immunizations Drug therapy for current infection	Appointment postponement

(continued)

TABLE 6-3 Items for the Medical History (Continued)

Item to Record in History	Record Notes	Medications and Treatment Modalities	Considerations for Appointment Procedures
17. Communicable diseases *(continued)* Hepatitis B	Jaundice history Clarification of type of hepatitis Laboratory clearance	Vaccine for HBV	Precautions against percutaneous injury
Tuberculosis	Active or passive Cough Duration of disease	Isoniazid Rifampin Pyrazinamide	Length of treatment: infectivity diminished after few months of treatment
Sexually transmitted Infections (STIs)	May not obtain history of STIs Oral and pharyngeal lesions may be indicators of disease	Antibiotics	Infectiousness diminishes with antibiotic therapy for gonorrhea and syphilis Refer to physician and postpone treatment when lesions or other signs suggest infection Caution for risk from previously treated diseases
Herpes	Lesions can be transmitted readily	Nondefinitive; symptomatic and palliative treatment Acyclovir	Postpone routine care when oral lesions are present
HIV infection AIDS	Risk group identification Oral manifestations	Wide variety of opportunistic infections and complications require variety of drugs	Oral lesions Complete sterilization and barrier procedures as for all communicable diseases
18. Diabetes Mellitus	Uncontrolled: requires antibiotic premedication Undiagnosed: excess thirst, appetite, and urination Family incidence: help in finding susceptible undiagnosed Severe advanced diabetes: complications (vision, kidney, cardiovascular, nervous system)	Insulin Diet control Hypoglycemics	Prepare for emergency: insulin; apple juice; frosting Appointment time related to insulin therapy and mealtime Need frequent maintenance appointments Periodontal disease accelerated Referral for tests for suspected undiagnosed
19. Ears	Deafness or degree of hearing impairment Infections, ringing, dizziness, balance	Treatment for infection Hearing aid	Adaptations for communication and plaque control instruction
20. Endocrine	Age-group relations to certain conditions Growth, development Menstruation, menopause	Thyroid hormone supplement Antithyroid Estrogen/progestin Oral contraceptives Corticosteroids	Emphasis on high level of plaque control Any patient taking steroids may need antibiotic premedication for appointments Monitor blood pressure
21. Epilepsy	Type, frequency of seizures precipitating factors Preparation for emergency seizure	Anticonvulsant Sedative	Minimize stress Medications make patient drowsy, less alert Valproic acid requires bleeding time before treatment

(continued)

TABLE 6-3 Items for the Medical History (Continued)

Item to Record in History	Record Notes	Medications and Treatment Modalities	Considerations for Appointment Procedures
22. Eyes	Disturbance of vision Purpose for corrective eyeglasses or contact lenses Manifestations of systemic disease	Eyedrops (for example, glaucoma)	Avoid epinephrine if glaucoma Protective eyewear during appointment Adaptations for communication with limited sight
23. Gastrointestinal	Nature and treatment of the disease Diet restriction prescribed by physician	Antacids Antidiarrheal Laxatives Antispasmodics	Patient instruction in accord with prescribed diet and medication Xerostomia
24. Kidney	Renal disease; kidney stones Hemodialysis: hypertension, anemia, hepatitis carrier Transplant: hypertension, hepatitis	Salt restriction Many drugs are nephrotoxic Immunosuppressive drugs (cyclosporine)	Antibiotic premedication Monitor blood pressure Bleeding tendency Poor healing Susceptibility to infection Limited stress tolerance
25. Liver	History of jaundice, hepatitis Impaired drug metabolism Cirrhosis: history of alcoholism	 Nutritional emphasis Abstinence from alcohol	Laboratory test for hepatitis Bleeding problems
26. Mental, psychiatric	Emotional problems hinder oral care	Antipsychotic drugs Antianxiety drugs Tranquilizers Antidepressants Antiparkinsonism drugs	Limited stress tolerance Xerostomia (side effect) Avoid mouthrinse containing alcohol
27. Physical activity	Overall health consciousness	Good health habits Regular exercise	Contribute to cooperative attitude in maintaining oral health
28. Physical disabilities	Extent, cause, duration Type of treatment related to individual condition Consultation with physician or medical specialist	Pain reliever Muscle relaxant Anticonvulsant	Adjustment of physical arrangements Wheelchair accessibility and transfer Adaptations of techniques and instruction Consult for antibiotic premedication for certain conditions: for example: prosthetic joint replacement, shunt
29. Pregnancy	Month, parturition date Possible oral manifestations History of previous pregnancies Iron deficiency anemia	Iron Folic acid Multivitamins	Adjust physical position for comfort Frequent appointments for maintaining high level of oral hygiene
30. Respiration	Breathing problems Persistent cough Cough up blood Chest pain Precipitation of asthmatic attack	Codeine cough syrup Antihistamine Bronchial dilator Expectorant Decongestant Steroid	Dental chair position Ultrasonic and air-powder polisher contraindicated Anesthesia choice: nitrous oxide contraindicated No aerosol agents

REVIEW OF HISTORY

Updating the history at each maintenance appointment is essential. Changes in health status revealed by interim medical examinations or evidenced by reported illness or hospitalizations must be recorded and considered during continuing treatment.

Following a review of the previously recorded history, questions can be directed to the patient to compare the present condition with the previous one and to determine at least the following:

A. Interim illnesses; changes in health.
B. Visits to physician; reasons and results.
C. Laboratory tests performed and the results; blood, urine, or other analyses.
D. Current medications.
E. Changes in the oral soft tissues and the teeth observed by the patient.

IMMEDIATE APPLICATIONS OF PATIENT HISTORIES

Together with information from all other parts of the diagnostic work-up, the patient histories are essential for the preparation of the dental hygiene care plan. Care planning for an individual patient is described on pages 322 to 328.

Immediate evaluation of the histories is necessary before proceeding to complete the assessment.

The list that follows is not intended to be exhaustive, but rather suggestive. From these items, the dental personnel should be alerted to precautions that may be needed.

I. MEDICAL CONSULTATION

Dentist and physician need to consult relative to the patient's current therapy and medications or to elements of the patient's past health status that could influence present dental treatment needs.[3]

A. Telephone or Personal Contact
Immediate consultation may be needed so that urgent treatment may proceed. Follow-up in writing is essential, because without legal record of the advice or decision, a misunderstanding could result.

B. Written Request
A letter of formal request is the preferred procedure. A prepared form can be developed with spaces for filling in the specific questions, and with space in the lower half for the physician or the assistant completing confidential information from the patient's medical record to provide the necessary directions.

C. Referrals
1. Patient should be referred for medical examination when signs of a possible disease condition are apparent.

2. Patient should be referred for laboratory tests when recent test results are not available or follow-up tests are needed.

II. RADIATION

When a patient is receiving radiation therapy or has had recent radiation for other purposes, a conference with the physician or oncologist involved is recommended to discuss the quantity of radiation to be received from any necessary dental radiographs. No apparent rationale exists for precluding a properly justified dental radiographic examination because of a history of radiation therapy.[4]

III. PROPHYLACTIC PREMEDICATION

Patients at risk for infective endocarditis must have antibiotic premedication prior to any tissue manipulation that could create a bacteremia. All tissue manipulation, particularly the use of instruments subgingivally, must be withheld until the risk has been determined, the condition has been discussed with the patient's physician, and the prescription has been obtained and taken appropriately. Infective endocarditis is described on pages 850 to 852.

Table 6-4 shows the specific regimen for antibiotic selection and prescription. The timing objective is to have adequate concentrations in the blood during, and immediately following, the actual instrumentation.

At-risk patients already taking an antibiotic for other health conditions require additional antibiotic prophylaxis prior to dental and dental hygiene instrumentation. The recommendation is to administer a different class of antibiotic rather than to increase the dose of the current antibiotic.[5]

AMERICAN HEART ASSOCIATION GUIDELINES

The American Heart Association and the American Dental Association recommend that certain risk patients have antibiotic premedication for all dental hygiene procedures likely to induce gingival bleeding.[5] The list below specifies the cardiac conditions involved, which includes mitral valve prolapse. The flowchart in Figure 6-2 shows a clinical approach for selecting the patients with mitral valve prolapse who will need antibiotic premedication. Medical evaluation is needed to confirm whether there is mitral regurgitation and therefore a need for premedication. More detail about mitral valve prolapse is described on page 850 in Chapter 58.

I. CARDIAC-RELATED CONDITIONS WHERE PROPHYLAXIS IS RECOMMENDED

High Risk Category
Prosthetic cardiac valves, including bioprosthetic and homograft valves
Previous infective endocarditis
Complex cyanotic congenital heart disease

TABLE 6-4 Prophylactic Regimens for Dental, Oral, Respiratory Tract, or Esophageal Procedures

Situation	Agent	Regimen Adult	Regimen Child*
Standard general prophylaxis	Amoxicillin	2.0 g orally 1 hour before procedure	50 mg/kg orally 1 hour before procedure
Unable to take oral medications	Ampicillin	2.0 g IM or IV[†]	50 mg/kg IM or IV within 30 minutes before procedure
Allergic to penicillin	Clindamycin	600 mg 1 hour before procedure	20 mg/kg orally 1 hour before procedure
	or Cephalexin[‡] or Cefadroxil	2.0 g 1 hour before procedure	50 mg/kg orally 1 hour before procedure
	or Azithromycin or Clarithromycin	500 mg 1 hour before procedure	15 mg/kg orally 1 hour before procedure
Allergic to penicillin and unable to take oral medications	Clindamycin	600 mg IV within 30 minutes before procedure	20 mg/kg IV within 30 minutes before procedure
	or Cefazolin[‡]	1.0 g IM or IV within 30 minutes before procedure	25 mg/kg IM or IV within 30 minutes before procedure

*Total children's dose should not exceed adult dose.
[†]IM = intramuscularly; IV = intravenously.
[‡]Cephalosporins should not be used in individuals with immediate-type hypersensitivity reaction (urticaria, angioedema, or anaphylaxis) to penicillin.

Surgically constructed systemic pulmonary shunts or conduits

Moderate Risk Category
Most other congenital cardiac malformations
Acquired valvular dysfunction (eg, rheumatic heart disease)
Hypertrophic cardiomyopathy
Mitral valve prolapse with regurgitation and/or thickened leaflets

II. CARDIAC CONDITIONS WHERE PROPHYLAXIS IS NOT RECOMMENDED

Negligible Risk Category: (Individuals with these conditions are at no greater risk for infective endocarditis than the general population.)

Isolated ostium secundum atrial septal defect
Surgical repair of atrial septal defect, ventricular septal defect, or patent ductus arteriosus (without residua beyond six months)
Previous coronary artery bypass graft surgery
Mitral valve prolapse without valvular dysfunction
Previous Kawasaki disease without valvular dysfunction
Previous rheumatic fever without valvular dysfunction
Cardiac pacemaker (intravascular and epicardial) and implanted defibrillators

III. INDIVIDUALS WITH TOTAL JOINT REPLACEMENT[6]

The risk of endocarditis is much greater in mouths with ongoing periodontal infection than when the periodontal tissues are healthy. When it is known that a person will have surgery for total joint arthroplasty, all possible effort should be made to complete the treatment necessary to bring periodontal tissues to a healthy, maintainable state before the joint replacement.

Patients listed below must be considered for antibiotic prophylaxis. The most critical period for bacteremias to cause hematogenous seeding is up to 2 years following the surgery for joint replacement. Other patients such as those with pins, plates, or screws do not require antibiotic prophylaxis for reason of the pin, plate, or screw, but other health factors must always be considered for all patients.

A. Patients at Potential Increased Risk of Hematogenous Total Joint Infection
1. *Immunocompromised/immunosuppressed patients*
   a. Inflammatory arthropathies; rheumatic arthritis; systemic lupus erythematosus
   b. Disease-, drug-, or radiation-induced immunosuppression
2. *Other Patients*
   a. Type I diabetes (insulin-dependent)
   b. First 2 years following joint replacement
   c. Previous prosthetic joint infections

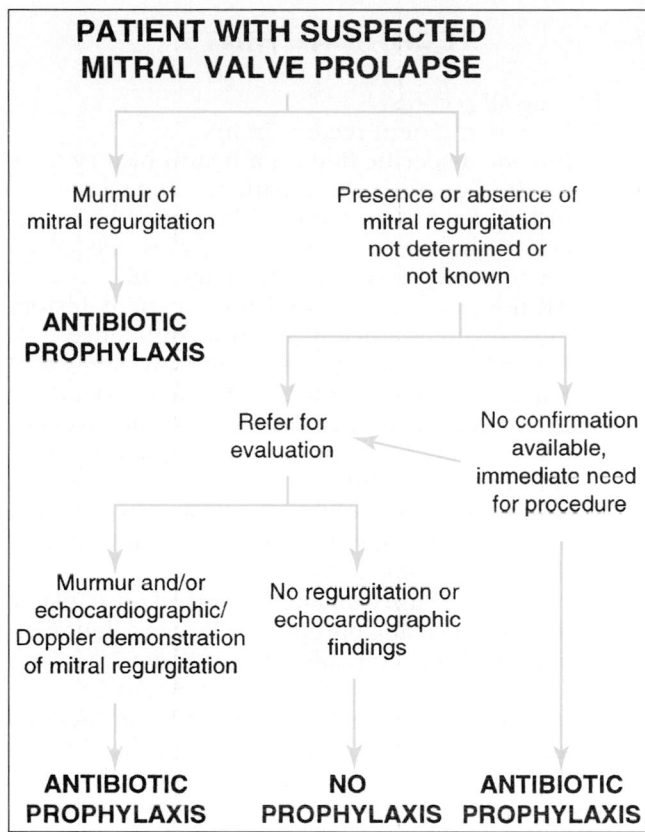

PATIENT WITH SUSPECTED MITRAL VALVE PROLAPSE

Murmur of mitral regurgitation

Presence or absence of mitral regurgitation not determined or not known

ANTIBIOTIC PROPHYLAXIS

Refer for evaluation

No confirmation available, immediate need for procedure

Murmur and/or echocardiographic/ Doppler demonstration of mitral regurgitation

No regurgitation or echocardiographic findings

ANTIBIOTIC PROPHYLAXIS

NO PROPHYLAXIS

ANTIBIOTIC PROPHYLAXIS

FIGURE 6-2 Determination of Need for Antibiotic Prophylaxis in Patient with Mitral Valve Prolapse.

d. Malnourishment
e. Hemophilia

B. Suggested Antibiotic Prophylaxis Regimens

1. *Standard Prophylaxis: Patients Not Allergic to Penicillin*
   Cephalexin, cephradine, or amoxicillin: 2 g orally 1 hour before procedure.
2. *Patients Not Allergic to Penicillin and Unable to Take Oral Medications*
   Cefazolin: 1 g, or ampicillin: 2 g, intramuscularly or intravenously 1 hour before procedure.
3. *Patients Allergic to Penicillin*
   Clindamycin: 600 mg orally 1 hour before procedure.
4. *Patients Allergic to Penicillin and Unable to Take Oral Medications*
   Clindamycin: 600 mg intravenously 1 hour before procedure.

IV. OTHER SYSTEMIC CONSIDERATIONS

Specific recommendations are impossible to define for all patients who may require antibiotic premedication. Each patient must be considered individually. Consultation with the patient's physician and the use of intelligent clinical judgment are necessary for the selection of patients who will benefit from antibiotics.

Routine use of antibiotic premedication is never indicated. In certain instances the patient is less at risk from the dental procedure than from the potential side effects of an antibiotic. Overuse of antibiotics can induce microbial resistance and, rarely, allergy or toxicity to the drug used.[7]

The following represent a partial list of patients requiring antibiotic premedication:

A. Reduced Capacity to Resist Infection
1. Corticosteroid or other immunosuppressive therapy
2. Chemotherapy (cancer treatments; certain treatments for arthritis)
3. Blood diseases (acute leukemia, agranulocytosis, sickle-cell anemia)
4. Human immunodeficiency virus infection[8]

B. Uncontrolled, Unstable Diabetes
Controlled stable diabetes can be treated as normal.

C. Facial Injuries
Grossly contaminated, traumatic facial injuries and compound fractures

D. Renal Disorders
Renal transplant and hemodialysis, glomerulonephritis, or other renal disorder[9]

E. Valvular Dysfunction
1. Cardiac transplant with valvular dysfunction[7]
2. Valvular heart disease resulting from use of fenfluramine and phentermine (appetite suppressants)[10,11]

F. Shunt
Ventriculoatrial shunt[12]

PROPHYLAXIS FOR DENTAL AND DENTAL HYGIENE PROCEDURES

Partial lists of procedures requiring and not requiring antibiotic prophylaxis are provided within the American Heart Association recommendations included here. The incidence and extent of a bacteremia is directly proportional to the degree of infection and inflammation in the tissues as well as the trauma produced by the clinical procedure.

Maintenance of healthy tissues by the patient through personal daily care and routine professional supervision are first in the prevention of bacteremias. Preprocedural rinsing with antimicrobial mouthrinse helps to reduce the incidence and severity of the bacteremias produced.

I. PROCEDURES FOR WHICH PROPHYLAXIS IS RECOMMENDED[5]

Dental extractions
Periodontal procedures including surgery, scaling and root planing, probing, recall maintenance

Dental implant placement and reimplantation of avulsed teeth

Endodontic (root canal) instrumentation or surgery beyond the apex

Subgingival placement of antibiotic fibers or strips

Initial placement of orthodontic bands but not brackets

Intraligamentary local anesthetic injections

Prophylactic cleaning of teeth or implants where bleeding is anticipated

II. PROCEDURES FOR WHICH PROPHYLAXIS IS NOT DEEMED NECESSARY

In all cases mentioned here, when bleeding is expected, prophylaxis is advised for susceptible individuals. Clinical judgment must be applied.

Restorative dentistry including restoration of carious teeth and replacement of missing teeth (with or without retraction cords).

Local anesthetic injections (non-intraligamentary)

Intracanal endodontic treatment; post placement build-up

Postsurgical suture removal

Placement of rubber dams

Placement of removable prosthodontic or orthodontic appliances

Taking of oral impressions

Fluoride treatments

Taking of oral radiographs

Orthodontic appliance adjustment

Shedding of primary teeth

ASA DETERMINATION

With the completion of the patient histories, an overall estimate of medical risk of a patient can be made. The **ASA Physical Status Classification System** was adopted by the American Society of Anesthesiologists in 1962[13] and describes five categories as follows:

ASA I: A patient without apparent systemic disease: a normal healthy patient.

ASA II: A patient with mild systemic disease.

ASA III: A patient with severe systemic disease that limits activity but is not incapacitating.

ASA IV: A patient with an incapacitating systemic disease that is a constant threat to life.

ASA V: A moribund patient not expected to survive 24 hours with or without care.

ASA E: Emergency of any variety: precede the ASA number with E to indicate the patient's physical status (for example, ASA E-III).

In a typical dental setting the ASA V category is omitted. In Table 21-2 (page 324) examples of the categories are given.

TECHNICAL HINTS

I. Date all records.

II. Keep permanent records in ink.

III. Provide a specific line on a health history form for the signature of the patient.[1] The completed history for a minor should be signed by a parent or guardian. A signature is also needed on the informed consent form (page 328).

IV. All information obtained for a patient history must be maintained in strictest confidence.

V. For patients with special health problems that require premedication, some type of coded tab can be used to alert all dental personnel to check the medical history prior to each appointment.

VI. Analyze the usefulness of items on the patient history form periodically, and plan for revision as scientific research reveals new information that must be applied.

VII. A medical history update wall plaque is available for posting in an appropriate place in a dental office or clinic. It reads: *Please Advise Us of Any Change in Your Medical History Since Your Last Visit.* It is available from the American Dental Association, Department of Salable Materials, 211 East Chicago Avenue, Chicago, Illinois 60611.

FACTORS TO TEACH THE PATIENT

I. The need for obtaining the personal, medical, and dental history prior to performance of dental and dental hygiene procedures, and the need for keeping the histories up to date.

II. The assurance that recorded histories are kept in strict professional confidence.

III. The relationship between oral health and general physical health.

IV. The interrelationship of medical and dental care.

V. All patients who require antibiotic premedication need special attention paid to (1) the importance of preventive dentistry, (2) the imperative need for regular dental care, and (3) the necessity for taking the prescribed prescription 1 hour before the appointment starts.

REFERENCES

1. **Robbins,** K.S.: Medicolegal Considerations, in Malamed, S.F.: *Medical Emergencies in the Dental Office,* 4th ed. St. Louis, The C.V. Mosby Co., 1993, pp. 91–101.

2. **American Dental Association:** Medical History Form (S-500), ADA Department of Salable Materials, 211 East Chicago Avenue, Chicago, IL 60611-2678.

3. **Chiodo,** G.T. and Rosenstein, D.I.: Consultation Between Dentists and Physicians, *Gen. Dent., 32,* 19, January–February, 1984.

4. **United States Department of Health and Human Services,** Food and Drug Administration, Center for Devices and Radiological Health: *Selection of Patients for X-Ray Examinations: Dental Radiographic Examinations.* Washington, D.C., Superintendent of Documents, HHS Publication FDA 88-8274, 1988, p. 10.

5. **Dajani,** A.S., Taubert, K.A., Wilson, W., Bolger, A.F., Bayer, A., Ferrieri, P., Gewitz, M.H., Shulman, S.T., Nouri, S., New-

burger, J.W., Hutto, C., Pallasch, T.J., Gage, T.W., Levison, M.E., Peter, G., and Zuccaro, G.: Prevention of Bacterial Endocarditis. Recommendations by the American Heart Association, *JAMA, 277,* 1794, June 11, 1997.

6. **American Dental Association and American Academy of Orthopaedic Surgeons:** Advisory Statement: Antibiotic Prophylaxis for Dental Patients With Total Joint Replacements, in *ADA Guide to Dental Therapeutics,* Chicago, ADA Publishing Co., 1998, pp. 547–551.

7. **Pallasch,** T.J. and Slots, J.: Antibiotic Prophylaxis and the Medically Compromised Patient, *Periodontology 2000, 10,* 107, 1996.

8. **Lockhart,** P.B. and Schmidtke, M.A.: Antibiotic Considerations in Medically Compromised Patients, *Dent. Clin. North Am., 38,* 381, July, 1994.

9. **DeRossi,** S.S. and Glick, M.: Dental Considerations for the Patient With Renal Disease Receiving Hemodialysis, *J. Am. Dent. Assoc., 127,* 211, February, 1996.

10. **Connolly,** H.M., Crary, J.L., McGoon, M.D., Hensrud, D.D., Edwards, B.S., Edwards, W.D., and Schaff, H.V.: Valvular Heart Disease Associated with Fenfluramine-Phentermine, *N. Engl. J. Med., 337,* 581, August 28, 1997.

11. **United State Centers for Disease Control and Prevention:** Cardiac Valvulopathy Associated With Exposure to Fenfluramine or Dexfenfluramine: U.S. Department of Health and Human Services Interim Public Health Recommendations, November, 1997, *MMWR, 46,* 1061, November 14, 1997.

12. **Little,** J.W., Falace, D.A., Miller, C.S., and Rhodus, N.L.: *Dental Management of the Medically Compromised Patient,* 5th ed. St. Louis, C.V. Mosby Co., 1997, pp. 74, 605.

13. **American Society of Anesthesiologists:** New Classification of Physical Status, *Anesthesiology, 24,* 111, January–February, 1963.

SUGGESTED READINGS

Biron, C.: Patients with Thyroid Dysfunctions Require Risk Management Before Dental Procedures, *RDH, 16, 42,* April, 1996.

DeRossi, S.S. and Glick, M.: Dental Considerations in Asplenic Patients, *J. Am. Dent. Assoc., 127,* 1359, September, 1996.

Drinnan, A.J.: Medical Conditions of Importance in Dental Practice, *Int. Dent. J., 40,* 206, August, 1990.

McClain, D.L., Bader, J.D., Daniel, S.J., and Sams, D.H.: Gingival Effects of Prescription Medications Among Adult Dental Patients, *Spec. Care Dentist., 11,* 15, January/February, 1991.

Miller, C.S., Kaplan, A.L., Guest, G.F., and Cottone, J.A.: Documenting Medication Use in Adult Dental Patients: 1987–1991, *J. Am. Dent. Assoc., 123,* 41, November, 1992.

Naylor, G.D., Hall, E.H., and Terezhalmy, G.T.: The Patient With Chronic Renal Failure Who Is Undergoing Dialysis or Renal Transplantation: Another Consideration for Antimicrobial Prophylaxis, *Oral Surg. Oral Med. Oral Pathol., 65,* 116, January, 1988.

Pyle, M.A., Faddoul, F.F., and Terezhalmy, G.T.: Clinical Implications of Drugs Taken By Our Patients, *Dent. Clin. North. Am., 37,* 73, January, 1993.

Schow, S.R.: Organ Transplant Patients and Immunosuppression, *DentalHygienistNews, 8,* 23, Number 3, 1995.

Smith, R.G. and Burtner, A.P.: Oral Side-effects of the Most Frequently Prescribed Drugs, *Spec. Care Dentist., 14,* 96, May/June, 1994.

Spolarich, A.E.: The Pharmacologic History, *Access, 9,* 33, March, 1995.

Spolarich, A.E.: Understanding Pharmacology. Basic Principles, *Access, 9,* 25, July, 1995.

Wynn, R.L.: The Top 20 Medications Prescribed in 1993, *Gen. Dent., 43,* 114, March–April, 1995.

History Forms

Cooper, M.D. and Winans, G.J.: Basics of a Good Medical History Form. How to Protect the Patient and Prepare the Staff, *Dent. Teamwork, 5,* 19, January–February, 1992.

deJong, K.J.M., Abraham-Inpijn, L., Oomen, H.A.P.C., and Oosting, J.: Clinical Relevance of a Medical History in Dental Practice: Comparison Between a Questionnaire and a Dialogue, *Community Dent. Oral Epidemiol., 19,* 310, October, 1991.

deJong, K.J.M., Borgmeijer-Hoelen, A., and Abraham-Inpijn, L.: Validity of a Risk-related Patient-administered Medical Questionnaire for Dental Patients, *Oral Surg. Oral Med. Oral Pathol., 72,* 527, November, 1991.

Fenlon, M.R. and McCartan, B.E.: Validity of a Patient Self-completed Health Questionnaire in a Primary Care Dental Practice, *Community Dent. Oral Epidemiol., 20,* 130, June, 1992.

Fine, J.I. and Kopriva, K.H.: The Health History. Interview and Communication Skills, *DentalHygienistNews, 7,* 7, Fall, 1994.

Flaitz, C.M., Vojir, C.P., Bradley, K.A., Casamassimo, P.S., and Kaplan D.W.: A Comparison of Parent and Adolescent Responses from Independent Health Histories, *Pediatr. Dent., 13,* 27, January/February, 1991.

Frese, P.A. and Scaramucci, M.K.: Medical History Update, *Dentalhygienistnews, 4,* 9, Spring, 1991.

Jolly, D.E.: Evaluation of the Medical History, *Anesth. Prog., 42,* 84, Numbers 3/4, 1995.

Levy, S.M. and Jakobsen, J.R.: A Comparison of Medical Histories Reported by Dental Patients and Their Physicians, *Spec. Care Dentist., 11,* 26, January/February, 1991.

McDaniel, T.F., Miller, D., Jones, R., and Davis, M.: Assessing Patient Willingness to Reveal Health History Information, *J. Am. Dent. Assoc., 126,* 375, March, 1995.

Miller, D.L.: Medical History Evaluation and Alterations for Care, in Hodges, K.O., ed.: *Concepts in Nonsurgical Periodontal Therapy.* Albany, N.Y.: Delmar, 1998., pp. 29–48.

Minden, N.J. and Fast, T.B.: Evaluation of Health History Forms Used in U.S. Dental Schools, *Oral Surg. Oral Med. Oral Pathol., 77,* 105, January, 1994.

Minden, N.J. and Fast, T.B.: The Patient's Health History Form: How Healthy Is It? *J. Am. Dent. Assoc., 124,* 95, August, 1993.

Prisant, L.M. and Doll, N.C.: Hypertension. The Rediscovery of Combination Therapy, *Geriatrics, 52,* 28, November, 1997.

Thibodeau, E.A. and Rossomando, K.J.: Survey of the Medical History Questionnaire, *Oral Surg. Oral Med. Oral Pathol., 74,* 400, September, 1992.

Woolley, R.J., Klein, H.G., and Eisenman, D.: Value of Routine Inquiry About Blood Donation, (Correspondence) *N. Engl. J. Med., 322,* 132, January 11, 1990.

Prophylactic Antibiotics

Barco, C.T.: Prevention of Infective Endocarditis: A Review of the Medical and Dental Literature, *J. Periodontol., 62,* 510, August, 1991.

Bender, I.B. and Barkan, M.J.: Dental Bacteremia and Its Relationship to Bacterial Endocarditis: Preventive Measures, *Compend. Cont. Educ. Dent., 10,* 472, September, 1989.

Biron, C.R.: Despite Diligent Staff, Infective Endocarditis Surfaces During Periodontal Treatment, *RDH, 17,* 42, March, 1997.

Carroll, G.C. and Sebor, R.J.: Dental Flossing and Its Relationship to Transient Bacteremia, *J. Periodontol., 51,* 691, December, 1980.

Felder, R.S., Nardone, D., and Palac, R.: Prevalence of Predisposing Factors for Endocarditis Among an Elderly Institutionalized Population, *Oral Surg. Oral Med. Oral Pathol., 73,* 30, January, 1992.

Friedlander, A.H. and Yoshikawa, T.T.: Pathogenesis, Management, and Prevention of Infective Endocarditis in the Elderly Dental Patient, *Oral Surg. Oral Med. Oral Pathol., 69,* 177, February, 1990.

Glick, M.: Intravenous Drug Users: A Consideration for Infective Endocarditis in Dentistry? (Editorial) *Oral Surg. Oral Med. Oral Pathol., 80,* 125, August, 1995.

Hobson, R.S. and Clark, J.D.: Management of the Orthodontic Patient At Risk from Infective Endocarditis, *Brit. Dent. J., 178,* 289, April 22, 1995.

Luce, E.B., Presti, C.F., Montemayor, I., and Crawford, M.H.: Detecting Cardiac Valvular Pathology in Patients With Systemic Lupus Erythematosus, *Spec. Care Dentist., 12,* 193, September/October, 1992.

McLaughlin, J.O.: The Incidence of Bacteremia After Orthodontic Banding, *Am. J. Orthod. Dentofac. Orthop., 109,* 639, June, 1996.

Tzukert, A.A., Leviner, E., and Sela, M.: Prevention of Infective Endocarditis: Not By Antibiotics Alone, *Oral Surg. Oral Med. Oral Pathol., 62,* 385, October, 1986.

7

Vital Signs

Determination of four vital signs, the *body temperature, pulse and respiratory rate*, and *blood pressure*, is considered standard procedure in patient care. Table 7-1 summarizes the normal values of the four basic vital signs for adolescents and adults.

Adding a fifth new vital sign, the smoking status, gives the opportunity to introduce early in the encounter with the patient the significance of smoking to general and oral heath. The fact that smoking is the number one preventable cause of illness and death more than justifies including smoking status as a vital sign.[1] Figure 7-1 illustrates a suggested vital sign stamp for convenient recording of all five signs.

Recording vital signs contributes to the proper systemic evaluation of a patient in conjunction with the complete medical history. Dental hygiene care planning and appointment sequencing are directly influenced by the findings.

When vital signs are not within normal range, the patient should be informed and referral made for medical evaluation and treatment. Key words related to the vital signs are defined in Box 7-1.

BODY TEMPERATURE

While preparing the patient history and making the extraoral and intraoral examinations, the need for taking the temperature may become apparent, or the dentist may have requested the procedure in conjunction with current oral disease. When the temperature is to be taken along with the other vital signs, the pulse and respiratory rates are determined while the thermometer is in the patient's mouth.

A temperature above the normal range can indicate the presence of infection. Patients can have an elevated body temperature from oral causes, such as necrotizing ulcerative gingivitis, an apical or periodontal abscess, or acute pericoronitis. Determination of the temperature of a patient with an oral infection may be necessary for diagnosis and treatment planning.

For the protection of the health of the personnel in the dental office or clinic, to prevent loss of working time because of illness, and for the protection of sub-

TABLE 7-1 Adult Vital Signs

Vital Sign	Values of Significance in Dental and Dental Hygiene Appointments	
Body temperature (oral)	Normal 37.0°C (98.6°F) Normal range 35.5° to 37.5°C (96.0° to 99.5°F)	
Pulse Rate	Normal range 60 to 100 per minute	
Respiration	Normal range 14 to 20 per minute	

Blood Pressure Category	Systolic mmHg	Diastolic mmHg
Normal	<130	<85
High normal	130–139	85–89
Hypertension		
Stage 1	140–159	90–99
Stage 2	160–179	100–109
Stage 3	180–209	110–119

*Data from *The Sixth Report of the Joint National Committee on Prevention, Detection, Evaluation, and Treatment of High Blood Pressure.* National Institutes of Health, National Heart, Lung, and Blood Institute, Publication 98-4080, November, 1997.

sequent patients who may be indirectly exposed, it is important to detect the presence of a systemic, contagious condition. Screening for elevated temperature among patients may have particular significance during certain seasons or epidemics. When a definite increase in temperature is found, the patient can be dismissed by the dentist to prevent further contamination of the office or clinic. The patient should be advised to seek medical care.

I. MAINTENANCE OF BODY TEMPERATURE

A. Normal
1. *Adult.* The normal average temperature is 37.0°C (98.6°F) as illustrated in Figure 7-2. The normal range is from 35.5° to 37.5°C (96.0° to 99.5°F). Over 70 years of age, the average temperature is slightly lower (36.0°C, 96.8°F).
2. *Children.* There is no appreciable difference between boys and girls. Average temperatures are as follows:
   a. First year: 37.3°C (99.1°F).
   b. Fourth year: 37.5°C (99.4°F).
   c. Fifth year: 37°C (98.6°F).
   d. Twelfth year: 36.7°C (98.0°F).

B. Temperature Variations
1. *Fever (pyrexia).* Values over 37.5°C (99.5°F).
2. *Hyperthermia.* Values over 41.0°C (105.8°F).

VITAL SIGNS

NAME _____ DATE_____
Blood Pressure _____
Pulse _____
Temperature _____
Respiratory Rate _____
Smoking Status Current Former Never
(please circle)

▪ **FIGURE 7-1 Vital Signs Stamp for a Patient's Record.** (Adapted from Fiore, M.C.: The New Vital Sign. Assessing and Documenting Smoking Status, *JAMA*, 266, 3183, December 11, 1991.)

3. *Hypothermia.* Values below 35.5°C (96.0°F).

C. Factors That Alter Body Temperature
1. *Time of Day.* Highest in late afternoon and early evening; lowest during sleep and early morning.
2. *Temporary Increase.* Exercise, hot drinks, smoking, or application of external heat.
3. *Pathologic States.* Infection, dehydration, hyperthyroidism, myocardial infarction, or tissue injury from trauma.
4. *Decrease.* Starvation, hemorrhage, or physiologic shock.

II. METHODS OF DETERMINING TEMPERATURE

A. Oral
Most commonly used.
1. *Indications for Use.* An oral thermometer is used for the patient who
   a. Can follow instructions.
   b. Can keep the mouth closed to hold the thermometer.
   c. Will not bite or otherwise break the thermometer (which could happen with small children or confused patients of any age).
   d. Has no mouth injuries or problems breathing through the nose.
2. *Contraindications.* The oral thermometer can-

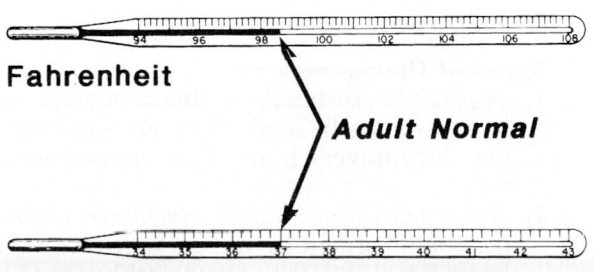

Fahrenheit

Adult Normal

Centigrade

▪ **FIGURE 7-2 Thermometers.** Centigrade and Fahrenheit thermometers compared. Adult normal temperature is shown at 37.0° Centigrade and 98.6° Fahrenheit.

BOX 7-1 KEY WORDS: Vital Signs

Anoxia (ah-nŏk'sē-ah): oxygen deficiency; a reduction of oxygen in the tissues can lead to deep respirations, cyanosis, increased pulse rate, and impairment of coordination.

Apnea (ăp'nē-ah): temporary cessation of breathing; absence of spontaneous respirations.

Auscultation (aws"kūl-tā-shun): listening for sounds produced within the body; may be performed directly or with a stethoscope.

Bradycardia (brăd"ē-kar'dē-ah): unusually slow heartbeat evidenced by slowing of the pulse rate.

Core temperature: the temperature of the deep tissues of the body; remains relatively constant; contrasts with body surface temperature, which rises and falls in response to environment.

Diastole (dī-as'tō-lē): the phase of the cardiac cycle in which the heart relaxes between contractions and the two ventricles are dilated by the blood flowing into them; **diastolic pressure** is the lowest blood pressure.

Diurnal (dī-er'nal): pertaining to or occurring during the daytime or period of light.

Hypertension (hī"per-ten'shun): systolic blood pressure of 140 mmHg or greater and diastolic blood pressure of 90 mmHg or greater.

Hyperthermia (hī"per-ther'mē-ah): higher-than-normal body temperature.

Hypothermia (hī"pō-ther'mē-ah): lower-than-normal body temperature.

Korotkoff sounds (kō-rŏt-kŏf'): the sounds heard during the determination of blood pressure; sounds originating within the blood passing through the vessel or produced by vibratory motion of the arterial wall.

Normotensive (nŏr"mō-tĕn'sĭv): normal tension or tone; of or pertaining to having normal blood pressure.

Pulse pressure (pŭls): the difference between systolic and diastolic blood pressure; normally 30 to 40 mmHg.

Pyrexia (pī-rĕk'sē-ah): an abnormal elevation of the body temperature above 37.0°C (98.6°F).

Stethoscope (stĕth'ō-skōp): instrument used to hear and amplify the sounds produced by the heart, lungs, and other internal organs.

Systole (sĭs'tō-lē): the contraction, or period of contraction, of the heart, especially the ventricles, during which blood is forced into the aorta and the pulmonary artery; **systolic pressure** is the highest, or greatest, pressure.

Tachycardia (tăk"ĭ-kahr'dē-ah): unusually fast heartbeat; at a rate greater than 100 beats per minute.

---

not be used for a patient who is unconscious, confused, irrational, or restless; for infants or small children; or for a patient with a very dry mouth.

B. Rectal
Generally applicable when the oral thermometer is contraindicated.

C. External
Axillary and groin positions are the least accurate, but occasionally, the oral or rectal method is impossible to use.

D. Types of Thermometers
1. *Disposable.* Disposable thermometers are most frequently used. They are most effective for universal infection control procedure.
2. *Mercury-Column Clinical Thermometer.* Consists of a bulb containing mercury, which, when heated by the body temperature, expands and rises in the hollow center of the glass stem. The bulb of the oral thermometer is usually tapered, whereas the bulb of the rectal thermometer is blunted and round.
3. *Electronic.* Electronic thermometers require

less time for taking the temperature, are more easily cared for because of their disposable tips, and decrease the possibility of cross-contamination.

E. Comparison of Readings
Rectal readings are about 1° above oral readings, and oral readings are about 1° above axillary or groin readings.

III. PROCEDURE

A. Equipment
Clinical thermometer, tissues, clock or watch with second hand, sheath.

B. Prepare Patient
1. Tell patient what is to be done.
2. Wait 15 minutes for the patient who has just had a hot or cold beverage or has smoked within 10 minutes, because the surface temperature of the oral mucosa can alter the accuracy of the thermometer reading.

C. Prepare the Thermometer
1. Hold the thermometer only by the stem, never by the bulb.
2. Wipe with a tissue.

3. Check the reading: it must be below 35.6°C (96°F).
4. Shake down the mercury level if not already below 35.6°C (96°F). The thermometer maintains the highest temperature previously registered and remains there until the force of shaking lowers the mercury level.
   a. Move away from furniture or other hard objects to prevent accidental forceful contact of the thermometer.
   b. Grasp stem firmly and shake with a firm, even, downward motion one or two times.
   c. Recheck the reading and reshake if indicated.
5. Place the thermometer into a thermometer sheath (a disposable cover available from a medical supply) to prevent contact with the patient's oral microflora. Figure 7-3 illustrates the procedure for preparation of a sheath.

D. Take the Temperature
1. Insert the bulb under the patient's tongue, with the stem outside the mouth.
2. Instruct patient to hold the thermometer gently with the lips, to avoid biting, and to breathe through the nose.
3. Observe watch or other timer, and remove thermometer after 3 clocked minutes.

E. Read and Record
1. Stand with back to light source and hold the thermometer by the stem at eye level to read.
2. Roll the thermometer slowly between the fingers to find the solid column of mercury.
3. Read at the point where the mercury ends. Each long line represents a degree of temperature, and short lines between are at two-tenths (0.2) of a degree.
4. Retake the temperature when the reading is unusually high or low.
   a. Reshake the mercury column down.
   b. Watch the patient to make certain that the thermometer is in position during the 3 minutes.
5. Record date, time of day, and temperature on the patient's record.

F. Care of the Thermometer
1. *Disposable Thermometer Sheath.* Remove and dispose in waste.
2. *Conventional*
   a. Wash with soap and slightly warm water; rinse with clear cool water; dry. Hot water can raise the temperature and force the mercury to break the thermometer.
   b. Soak in disinfectant solution, completely covered.
   c. Rinse with water and dry before placing in container or using again. Container should be sterilizable.

IV. CARE OF PATIENT WITH TEMPERATURE ELEVATION

A. Temperature Over 41.0°C (105.8°F)
1. Treat as medical emergency.
2. Transport to a hospital for medical care.

B. Temperature 37.6° to 41.0°C (99.6°C to 105.8°F)
1. Check possible temporary or factitious cause, such as hot beverage or smoking, and observe patient while repeating the determination.

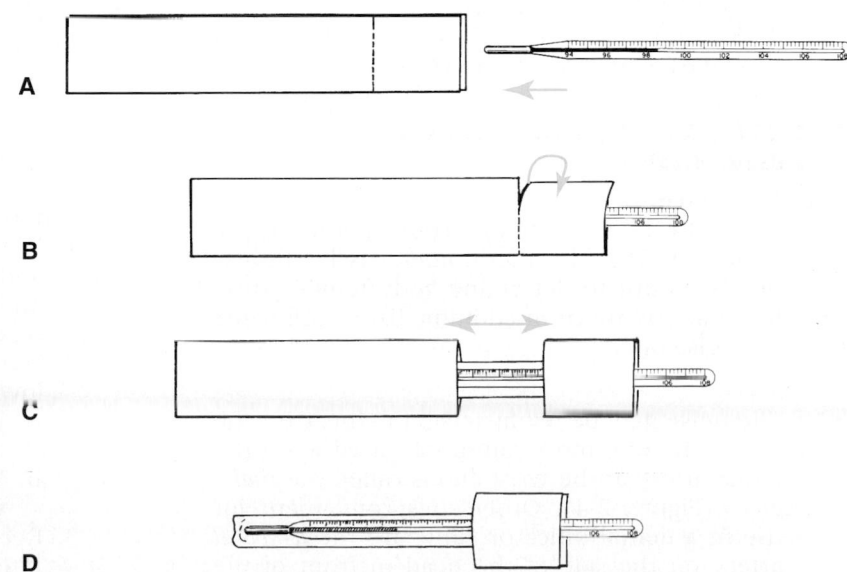

FIGURE 7-3 Thermometer Sheath. (A) Insert the thermometer gently to the bottom of the sheath. **(B)** Tear at dotted line by twisting. **(C)** Pull apart, holding by the small section of cover. **(D)** Sheathed thermometer is ready for insertion under patient's tongue.

2. Review the dental and medical history.
3. Provide no elective oral care when there are signs of respiratory infection or other possible communicable disease.

PULSE

The pulse is the intermittent throbbing sensation felt when the fingers are pressed against an artery. It is the result of the alternate expansion and contraction of an artery as a wave of blood is forced through the heart. The pulse rate or heart rate is the count of the heartbeats. Irregularities of strength, rhythm, and quality of the pulse should be noted while counting the pulse rate.

I. MAINTENANCE OF NORMAL PULSE

A. Normal Pulse Rates
1. *Adults.* There is no absolute normal. The adult range is 60 to 100 beats per minute, slightly higher for women than for men.
2. *Children.* The pulse or heart rate falls steadily during childhood.
   a. *In utero*—150 beats per minute (bpm).
   b. At birth—130 bpm.
   c. Second year—105 bpm.
   d. Fourth year—90 bpm.
   e. Tenth year—70 bpm.

B. Factors That Influence Pulse Rate
An unusually fast heartbeat (over 100 beats per minute in an adult) is called *tachycardia;* an unusually slow beat (below 50) is *bradycardia.*
1. *Increased Pulse.* Caused by exercise, stimulants, eating, strong emotions, extremes of heat and cold, and some forms of heart disease.
2. *Decreased Pulse.* Caused by sleep, depressants, fasting, quieting emotions, and low vitality from prolonged illness.
3. *Emergency Situations.* Listed in Tables 61-5 and 61-6, pages 910 to 916.

II. PROCEDURE FOR DETERMINING PULSE RATE

A. Sequence
The pulse rate is obtained conveniently at the same time that the thermometer is in the patient's mouth to determine body temperature. Respirations are counted immediately following the pulse rate.

B. Sites
The pulse may be felt at several points over the body. The one most commonly used is on the radial artery at the wrist and is called the *radial pulse* (Figure 7-4). Other sites convenient for use in a dental office or clinic are the *temporal* artery on the side of the head in front of the

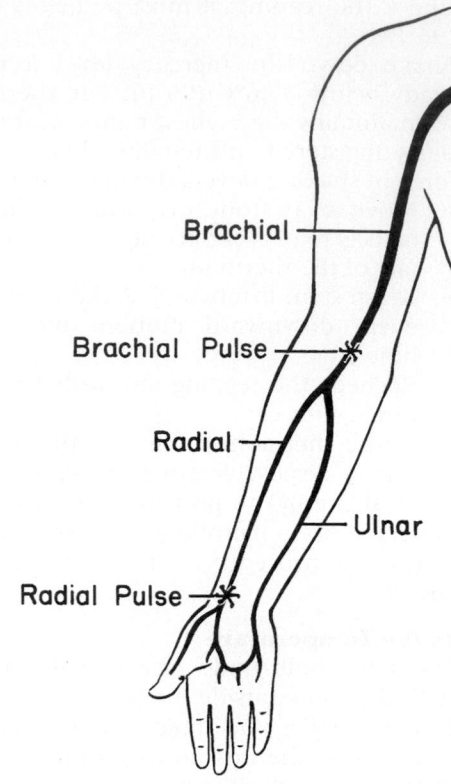

FIGURE 7-4 Arteries of the Arm. Note location of radial pulse. The brachial pulse may be felt just before the brachial artery branches into the radial and ulnar arteries.

ear, or the *facial* artery at the border of the mandible.

The carotid pulse is used during cardiopulmonary resuscitation (pages 903 to 904 and Figure 61-7) for an adult, and the brachial pulse is used for an infant.

C. Prepare the Patient
1. Tell the patient what is to be done.
2. Have the patient in a comfortable position with arm and hand supported, palm down.
3. Locate the radial pulse on the thumb side of the wrist with the tips of the first three fingers (Figure 7-5). Do not use the thumb because it contains a pulse that may be confused with the patient's pulse.

D. Count and Record
1. When the pulse is felt, exert light pressure and count for 1 clocked minute. Use the second hand of a watch or clock. Check with a repeat count.
2. While taking the pulse, observe the following:
   a. Rhythm: regular, regularly irregular, irregularly irregular.
   b. Volume and strength: full, strong, poor, weak, thready.
3. Record on patient's record the date, pulse rate, other characteristics.

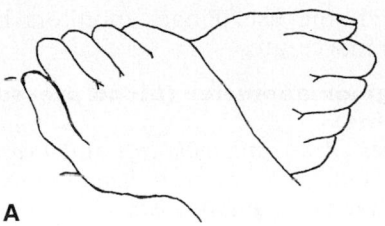

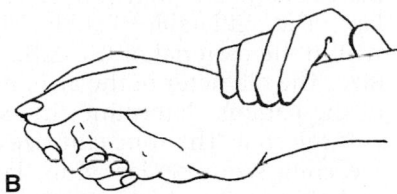

FIGURE 7-5 Determination of Pulse Rate. (A) Correct position of hands. **(B)** The tips of the first three fingers are placed over the radial pulse located on the thumb side of the ventral surface of the wrist.

    4. A pulse rate over 90 should be considered abnormal for an adult and over 120 abnormal for a child.

RESPIRATION

The function of respiration is to supply oxygen to the tissues and to eliminate carbon dioxide. Variations in normal respirations may be shown by such characteristics as the rate, rhythm, depth, and quality and may be symptomatic of disease or emergency states.

I. MAINTENANCE OF NORMAL RESPIRATIONS

A respiration is one breath taken in and let out.

A. Normal Respiratory Rate
    1. *Adults.* The adult range is from 14 to 20 per minute, slightly higher for women.
    2. *Children.* The respiratory rate decreases steadily during childhood. Averages are
        a. First year—30 per minute.
        b. Second year—25 per minute.
        c. Eighth year—20 per minute.
        d. Fifteenth year—18 per minute.

B. Factors That Influence Respirations
    Many of the same factors that influence pulse rate also influence the number of respirations. A rate of 12 per minute or fewer is considered subnormal for an adult; over 28 is accelerated; and rates over 60 are extremely rapid and dangerous.
    1. *Increased Respiration.* Caused by work and exercise, excitement, nervousness, strong emotions, pain, hemorrhage, shock.
    2. *Decreased Respiration.* Caused by sleep, certain drugs, pulmonary insufficiency.
    3. *Emergency Situations.* Listed in Tables 61-5 and 61-6, pages 910 to 916.

II. PROCEDURES FOR OBSERVING RESPIRATIONS

A. Determine Rate
    1. Make the count of respirations immediately after counting the pulse.
    2. Maintain the fingers over the radial pulse.
    3. Respirations must be counted so that the patient is not aware, as the rate may be voluntarily altered.
    4. Count the number of times the chest rises in 1 clocked minute. It is not necessary to count both inspirations and expirations.

B. Factors to Observe
    1. *Depth.* Describe as shallow, normal, or deep.
    2. *Rhythm.* Describe as regular (evenly spaced) or irregular (with pauses of irregular lengths between).
    3. *Quality.* Describe as strong, easy, weak, or labored (noisy). Poor quality may have an effect on body color; for example, a bluish tinge of the face or nailbeds may mean an insufficiency of oxygen.
    4. *Sounds.* Describe deviant sounds made during inspiration, expiration, or both.
    5. *Position of Patient.* When the patient assumes an unusual position to secure comfort during breathing or prefers to remain seated upright, mark records accordingly.

C. Record
    Record all findings on the patient's record.

BLOOD PRESSURE

Information about the patient's blood pressure is essential during dental and dental hygiene appointments because special adaptations may be needed. Blood pressure readings most usually are recorded with the medical history and other assessment data. Readings taken at the start of an appointment can be significantly higher than at the end of treatment.[2]

To establish a baseline reading and determine the need for patient referral for medical attention, several readings are needed, especially at the close of appointments when the patient is relaxed.

Screening for blood pressure in dental offices has been shown to be an effective health service for all ages since many patients are unaware that they have hypertension. Cardiovascular diseases are described in Chapter 58, and the causes, predisposing factors, and treatment of hypertension are reviewed on pages 852 to 854. That information can be a helpful introduction and is recommended for reading in conjunction with this section on the techniques for obtaining blood pressure.

I. COMPONENTS OF BLOOD PRESSURE

Blood pressure is the force exerted by the blood on the blood vessel walls. When the left ventricle of the heart contracts, blood is forced out into the aorta and travels through the large arteries to the smaller arteries, arterioles, and capillaries. The pulsations extend from the heart through the arteries and disappear in the arterioles. During the course of the cardiac cycle, the blood pressure is changing constantly.

A. Systolic Pressure
Systolic pressure is the peak or the highest pressure. It is caused by ventricular contraction. The normal systolic pressure is less than 130 mmHg.

B. Diastolic Pressure
Diastolic pressure is the lowest pressure. It is the effect of ventricular relaxation. The normal diastolic pressure is less than 85 mmHg.

C. Pulse Pressure
The pulse pressure is the difference between the systolic and the diastolic pressures. The normal or safe difference is less than 45 mmHg.

II. BLOOD PRESSURE CLASSIFICATION

Table 7-1 (page 107) includes the classification for blood pressure in adolescents and adults. Normal average blood pressure in mmHg at younger ages is as follows:[3]

Age	Mean Systolic	Mean Diastolic
3 years	108	70
6 years	114	74
12 years	122	78

III. FACTORS THAT INFLUENCE BLOOD PRESSURE

A. Maintenance of Blood Pressure
Blood pressure depends on
1. Force of the heart beat (energy of the heart).
2. Peripheral resistance; condition of the arteries; changes in elasticity of vessels, which may occur with age.
3. Volume of blood in the circulatory system.

B. Factors That Increase Blood Pressure
1. Exercise, eating, stimulants, and emotional disturbance.
2. Use of oral contraceptives; blood pressure increases with age and length of use.

C. Factors That Decrease Blood Pressure
1. Fasting, rest, depressants, and quiet emotions.
2. Such emergencies as fainting, blood loss, shock (see Tables 61-5 and 61-6, pages 910 to 916).

IV. EQUIPMENT FOR DETERMINING BLOOD PRESSURE

The mercury sphygmomanometer is the preferred instrument. A recently calibrated aneroid manometer or a validated electronic device can be used and are practical for home use. Finger monitors have been shown to be inaccurate.

A. Sphygmomanometer (blood pressure machine)
Consists of an *inflatable cuff* and *two tubes,* one connected to the *pressure hand control bulb* and the other to the *pressure gauge.*
1. *Cuff*
   a. Material. The cuff is made of a nonelastic material and is fastened by a Velcro overlap. The inflatable bladder is located within the material of the cuff.
   b. Size. The diameter of the arm, not the age of the patient, determines the size of the cuff selected. The four cuff sizes available are child size, regular adult, large adult, and thigh. The thigh size is needed for grossly obese persons.
   c. Dimension. The cuff width that is used should be 20% greater than the diameter of the arm to which it is applied (Figure 7-6). It should cover approximately two-thirds of the upper arm.
      When a cuff is too narrow, the blood pressure reading is too high; when the cuff is too wide, the reading is too low.[4]
2. *Mercury Manometer*
   a. Gauges are marked with long lines at each 10 mmHg, with shorter lines at 2-mm intervals between each long line.
   b. The level of the column of mercury of the manometer should be at eye level for accurate reading and must not be tilted.

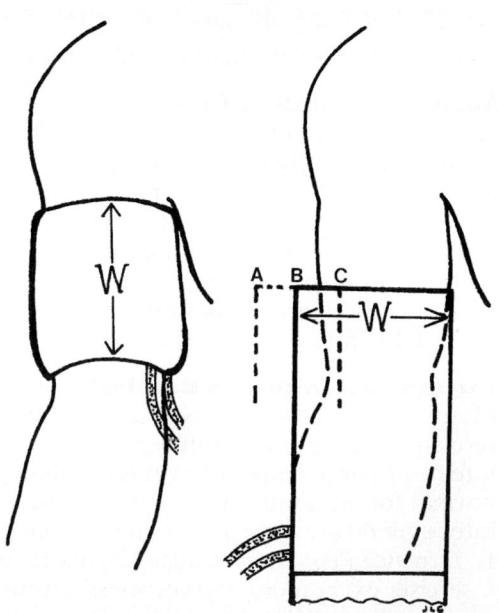

■ **FIGURE 7-6 Selection of Cuff Size.** The correct width (W) is 20% greater than the diameter of the arm where applied. **(A)** Too wide. **(B)** Correct width. **(C)** Too narrow.

B. Stethoscope (a listening aid that magnifies sound)

Consists of an *endpiece* that is connected by tubes to carry the sound to the *earpieces*.

1. *Types of Endpieces.* Bell-shaped or flat (diaphragm); the bell shape is used for medical examinations, particularly for chest examination.
2. *Care of Earpieces.* Clean by rubbing with gauze sponge moistened in disinfectant.

V. PROCEDURE FOR DETERMINING BLOOD PRESSURE

A. Prepare Patient

1. Tell patient briefly what is to be done. Detailed explanations should be avoided because they may excite the patient and change the blood pressure.
2. Seat patient comfortably, with the arm slightly flexed, with palm up, and with the whole forearm supported on a level surface at the level of the heart.
3. Use either arm unless otherwise indicated, for example, by a handicap. Repeat blood pressure determinations should be made on the same arm, because the difference between arms may be as much as 10 mmHg.
4. Take pressure on bare arm, not over clothing. A tight sleeve should be loosened.

B. Apply Cuff

1. Apply the completely deflated cuff to the patient's arm, supported at the level of the heart. It has been shown that when the arm rests on the arm of a dental chair, higher than the heart, the diastolic pressure shows a small but significant increase.[5]
2. Place the portion of the cuff that contains the inflatable bladder directly over the brachial artery. The cuff may have an arrow to show the point that should be placed over the artery. The lower edge of the cuff is placed 1 inch above the antecubital fossa (Figure 7-7). Fasten the cuff evenly and snugly.
3. Adjust the position of the gauge for convenient reading but so that the patient cannot see the mercury.
4. Palpate 1 inch below the antecubital fossa to locate the brachial artery pulse (Figure 7-4). The stethoscope endpiece is placed over the spot where the brachial pulse is felt.
5. Position the stethoscope earpieces in the ears, with the tips directed forward.

C. Locate the Radial Pulse (Figures 7-4 and 7-5)

Hold the fingers on the pulse.

D. Inflate the Cuff

1. Close the needle valve (air lock) attached to

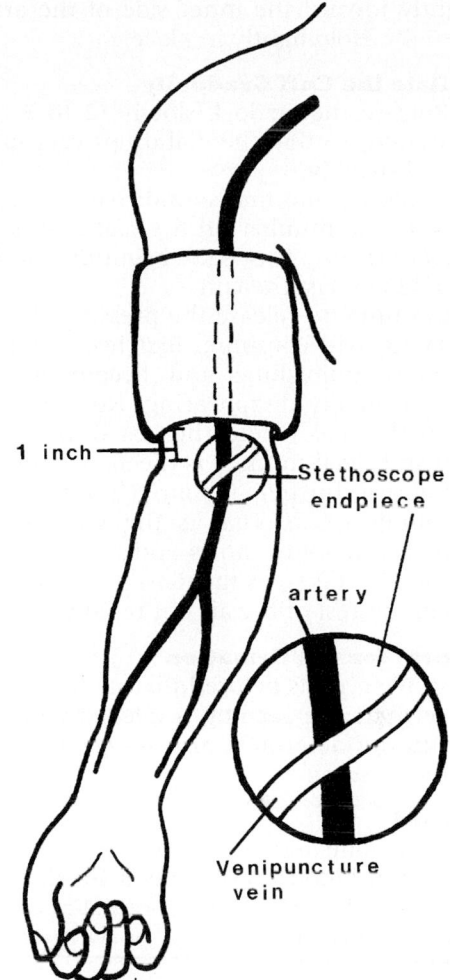

FIGURE 7-7 Blood Pressure Cuff in Position. The lower edge of the cuff is placed approximately 1 inch above the antecubital fossa. The stethoscope endpiece is placed over the palpated brachial artery pulse point approximately 1 inch below the antecubital fossa and slightly toward the inner side of the arm.

the hand control bulb firmly but so it may be released readily.
2. Pump to inflate the cuff until the radial pulse stops. Note the mercury level at which the pulse disappears.
3. Look at the dial, and pump to 20 or 30 mmHg beyond where the radial pulse was no longer felt. This is the maximum inflation level (MIL). It means that the brachial artery is collapsed by the pressure of the cuff and no blood is flowing through.

Unless the MIL is determined, the level to which the cuff is inflated will be arbitrary. Excess pressure can be very uncomfortable for the patient.

E. Position the Stethoscope Endpiece

Place the endpiece over the palpated brachial artery, 1 inch below the antecubital fossa, and slightly toward the inner side of the arm (Figure 7-7). Hold lightly in place.

F. Deflate the Cuff Gradually

1. Release the air lock slowly (2 to 3 mm per second) so that the dial drops very gradually and steadily.
2. Listen for the first sound: *systole* ("tap tap"). Note the number on the dial that is the *systolic pressure*. This is the beginning of the flow of blood past the cuff.
3. Continue to release the pressure slowly. The sound will continue, first becoming louder, then diminishing and becoming muffled, until finally disappearing. Note the number on the dial where the last distinct tap was heard. That number is the *diastolic pressure*.
4. Release further (about 10 mm) until all sounds cease. That is the second diastolic point. In some clinics and hospitals, the last sound is taken as the diastolic pressure.
5. Let the rest of the air out rapidly.

G. Repeat for Confirmation

Wait 30 seconds before inflating the cuff again. More than one reading is needed within a few minutes to determine an average and ensure a correct reading.

H. Record

1. Write date and arm used.
2. Record blood pressure as a fraction, for example, 120/80. When both diastolic points are recorded, they can be written as 120/80/72.

VI. BLOOD PRESSURE FOLLOW-UP CRITERIA[6]

Table 7-2 provides a summary of recommendations at each level of blood pressure findings. Dental personnel have an obligation to advise and *refer for further evaluation*. Diagnosis of hypertension would never be made or treatment started on the basis of an isolated reading.

When the blood pressure is within normal range (130/85), it should be rechecked within 2 years. Rechecking within 1 year rather than 2 years is recommended for persons at increased risk for hypertension. The risks include family history, weight gain, obesity, African American, use of oral contraceptives, smoking, and excessive alcohol consumption.

Consultation with a patient's physician is indicated prior to dental or dental hygiene treatment when the blood pressure is in a moderate or higher category (Table 7-1).

TECHNICAL HINTS

I. When a patient's sleeve is drawn back for blood pressure determination, observe the sleeve and the arm for small blood stains or ev-

TABLE 7-2 Recommendations for Follow-up Based on Initial Set of Blood Pressure Measurements for Adults

Initial Blood Pressure (mmHg)*		Follow-Up Recommended
Systolic	Diastolic	
<130	<85	Recheck in 2 years
130–139	85–89	Recheck in 1 year†
140–159	90–99	Confirm within 2 months†
160–179	100–109	Evaluate or refer to source of care within 1 month
≥180	≥110	Evaluate or refer to source of care immediately or within 1 week depending on clinical situation

*If the systolic and diastolic categories are different, follow recommendation for the shorter time follow-up (for example, 160/85 mmHg should be evaluated or referred to source of care within 1 month).
†Provide advice about lifestyle modifications.

idence of an injection, which may reveal an IV drug user. The patient may request, even insist, that a particular arm be used. When suspicion of drug abuse has been previously aroused because of physical observation or items in a medical history, determine the blood pressure on both arms to permit observation. Tell the patient that the pressure should always be measured on both sides.

II. Proficiency in determination of the vital signs is essential for monitoring during emergency treatment (Chapter 61).

III. Sources of Materials

National High Blood Pressure Education Program
High Blood Pressure Information Center
120/80 National Institutes of Health
Bethesda, MD 20205
American Heart Association
7320 Greenville Avenue
Dallas, TX 75231

FACTORS TO TEACH THE PATIENT

I. How vital signs can influence dental and dental hygiene appointments.
II. The importance of having a blood pressure determination at regular intervals.
III. For patient diagnosed as hypertensive, encourage regular continuing use of prescription drugs for control of high blood pressure.

REFERENCES

1. **Fiore**, M.C.: The New Vital Sign. Assessing and Documenting Smoking Status, *JAMA, 266*, 3183, December 11, 1991.
2. **Nichols**, C.: Dentistry and Hypertension, *J. Am. Dent. Assoc., 128*, 1557, November, 1997.
3. **United States National High Blood Pressure Education Program:** *The Fifth Report of the Joint National Committee on Detection, Evaluation, and Treatment of High Blood Pressure,* Washington, D.C., National Institutes of Health, National Heart, Lung, and Blood Institute, N.I.H. Publication No. 93-1088, January, 1993, 49 pp.
4. **Geddes**, L.A. and Whistler, S.J.: The Error in Indirect Blood Pressure Measurement with the Incorrect Size of Cuff, *Am. Heart J., 96*, 4, July, 1978.
5. **Beck,** F.M., Weaver, J.M., Blozis, G.G., and Unverferth, D.V.: Effect of Arm Position and Arm Support on Indirect Blood Pressure Measurements Made in a Dental Chair, *J. Am. Dent. Assoc., 106*, 645, May, 1983.
6. **United States National High Blood Pressure Education Program:** *The Sixth Report of the Joint National Committee on Prevention, Detection, Evaluation, and Treatment of High Blood Pressure,* Washington, D.C., National Institutes of Health, National Heart, Lung, and Blood Institute, N.I.H. Publication No. 98-4080, November, 1997.

SUGGESTED READINGS

Cline, N.V. and Springstead, M.C.: Monitoring Blood Pressure. Five Minutes Critical to Quality Patient Care, *J. Dent. Hyg., 66*, 363, October, 1992.

Fast, T.B.: Physical Evaluation and Monitoring Devices in Dental Practice, *Gen. Dent., 41*, 242, June, 1993.

Malamed, S.F.: *Medical Emergencies in the Dental Office,* 4th ed. St. Louis, Mosby, 1993, pp. 27–36.

Martin, C., Moore, D., Templin, K., and Moore, J.: Electronic Blood Pressure Screening: Fast, Easy, and Essential, *Access, 12*, 33, January, 1998.

Nesselroad, J.M., Flacco, V.A., Phillips, D.M., and Kruse, J.: Accuracy of Automated Finger Blood Pressure Devices, *Fam. Med., 28*, 189, March, 1996.

Nunn, P.J.: The Life You Save May Be Your Patient's, *RDH, 14*, 44, April, 1994.

Raab, F.J., Schaffer, E.M., Guillaume-Cornelissen, G., and Halberg, F.: Interpreting Vital Sign Profiles for Maximizing Patient Safety During Dental Visits, *J. Am. Dent. Assoc., 129*, 461, April, 1998.

Yeatts, D.E., Wood, A.J. and McCarter, W.J.: Fevers in Children, *ASDC J. Dent. Child, 61*, 249, July–August, 1994.

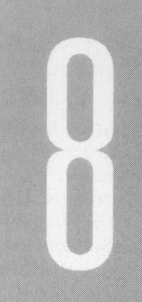

Extraoral and Intraoral Examination

A careful overall observation of each patient and a thorough examination of the oral cavity and adjacent structures are essential to total assessment prior to care planning. A variety of lesions may be observed for which the patient may or may not report subjective symptoms. Recognition, treatment, and follow-up of specific lesions may be of definite significance to the present and future general and oral health of the patient.

Despite the occurrence of many seemingly minor lesions, the danger of oral malignancies remains a definite possibility. Every effort must be made to detect potentially cancerous lesions early.

Each area of the mucous membrane must be examined, and minor deviations from normal must be given prompt attention. A life may depend on an oral examination. Routine examination for each new patient and at each maintenance appointment provides a realistic approach to the control of oral disease.

The oral tissues are sensitive indicators of the general health of the individual. Changes in these structures may be the first indication of subclinical disease processes in other parts of the body.

Prerequisite to the recognition of deviations from the normal appearance of the oral cavity is knowledge and understanding of the normal morphology, anatomy, and physiology of the oral cavity and the surrounding area. Box 8-1 defines terms used for extraoral and intraoral examination.

OBJECTIVES

A thorough examination is essential to the total care of the patient. The dental hygienist will:
   I. Observe the patient overall, as well as in all areas in and about the oral cavity, and record those areas that appear to deviate from normal and that may be evidence of disease.

BOX 8-1 KEY WORDS: Extraoral/Intraoral Examination

Aphtha (af'thah): a little white or reddish ulcer.

Crust: outer scablike layer of solid matter formed by drying of a body exudate or secretion.

Cyst (sĭst): a closed, epithelia-lined sac, normal or pathologic, that contains fluid or other material.

Dorsal (dor'sal): back surface; opposite of ventral.

Epidermis (ĕp"ĭ der'mĭs): outermost and nonvascular layers of the skin composed of basal layer, spinous layer, granular layer, and horny layer.

> **Corium** (kō'rē-um): the dermis or true skin just beneath the epidermis; well supplied with nerves and blood vessels.

Erosion (e-rō'zhun): soft tissue slightly depressed lesion in which the epithelium above the basal layer is denuded.

Erythema (ĕr"ĭ-thē'mah): red area of variable size and shape; reaction to irritation, radiation, or injury.

Exophytic (ĕk'sŏ-fĭt'ĭk): growing outward.

Exostosis (ĕk"sŏs-tō-sĭs): a benign bony growth projecting from the surface of bone.

Fissure (fĭsh'er): a narrow slit or cleft in the epidermis; where infected ulceration, inflammation, and pain can result.

Forensic (fō-rĕn'zĭk): pertaining to or used in legal proceedings.

Idiopathic (ĭd"ē-ō-păth'ĭk): of unknown etiology.

Indurated (ĭn'du-rāt"ed): hardened; abnormally hard.

Lymphadenopathy (lĭm-făd"ĕ-nŏp'ah-thē): disease of the lymph nodes; regional lymph node enlargement.

Morphology (mōr-fŏl'ō-jē): science that deals with form and structure.

Palpation (păl-pā'shun): perceiving by sense of touch.

Papilla (pah-pĭl'ah): small, nipple-shaped projection or elevation (**papillary:** adjective).

Patch: circumscribed flat lesion larger than a macule; differentiated from surrounding epidermis by color and/or texture.

Pedunculated (pē-dŭng'kū-lāt"ed): elevated lesion attached by a thin stalk.

Petechia (pe-tĕ'ke-ah): hemorrhagic spot of pinpoint to pinhead size.

Polyp (pŏl'ĭp): any growth or mass protruding from a mucous membrane.

Pseudomembrane (soo"dō-mĕm'brān): a loose membranous layer of exudate containing microorganisms, precipitated fibrin, necrotic cells, and inflammatory cells produced during an inflammatory reaction on the surface of a tissue.

Punctate (pŭnk'tāt): marked with points or punctures differentiated from the surrounding surface by color, elevation, or texture.

Purulent (pyū'roo-lent): containing, forming, or discharging pus.

Rubefacient (roo"bĕ-fā'shent): reddening of the skin.

Scar (skahr): cicatrix; mark remaining after healing of a wound or healing following a surgical intervention.

Sclerosis (sklĕ-rō'sĭs): induration or hardening.

Sessile (sĕs'ĭl): elevated lesion with a broad base.

Temporomandibular disorder (TMD): a collective term that includes a wide range of disorders of the masticatory system characterized by one or more of the following: pain in the preauricular area, temporomandibular joint (TMJ), and muscles of mastication, with limitation or deviation in mandibular motion and TMJ sounds during mandibular function.

Torus (tō'rus): bony elevation or prominence usually located on the midline of the hard palate (torus palatinus) and the lingual surface of the mandible in the premolar area (torus mandibularis).

Trismus (trĭz'mus): motor disturbance of the trigeminal nerve, especially spasm of the masticatory muscles with difficulty in opening the mouth.

Ventral (ven'tral): anterior or inferior surface; opposite of dorsal.

Verruca (vĕ-roo'kah): a wartlike growth.

II. Screen each patient at each appointment to detect lesions that may be pathologic, particularly those that may be cancerous.

III. Recognize a need for postponement of the current appointment because of evidence of communicable disease or in deference to the need for urgent medical consultation and/or treatment.

IV. Prevent the development of advanced, irreversible, or untreatable oral disease by early recognition of initial lesions.

V. Identify suspected conditions that require additional testing and refer for medical evaluation.

VI. Identify extraoral and intraoral deviations from normal for which dental hygiene care and instruction may need special adaptations.

VII. Provide a means of comparison of individual oral examinations over a series of maintenance appointments, and thus determine the effects of dental and dental hygiene care and the success of patient instruction.

VIII. Provide information for continuing records of the patient's diagnosis and treatment plan for legal purposes.

COMPONENTS OF EXAMINATION

The current concept of patient care is that the total patient is being treated, not only the oral cavity, and particularly not only the teeth and their immediately surrounding tissues. The examination is, therefore, all-inclusive to detect any physical, mental, or psychological influences of the whole patient on the oral health.

Thorough examination becomes a routine part of each patient appointment so that treatment for the control and prevention of oral diseases will be effective.

I. PREPARATION FOR EXAMINATION

A. Review the patient's health histories and other parts of the records.
B. Examine radiographs on viewbox.
C. Explain the procedures to be performed.

II. METHODS OF EXAMINATION

The various examination methods were defined on page 83. The extraoral and intraoral examination is accomplished primarily by direct visual observation and palpation, but other methods may also be used.

A. Direct Observation

Patient position, optimum lighting, and effective retraction for accessibility and visibility contribute to the accuracy and completeness of the examination.

B. Palpation

Types of palpation include the following:
1. *Digital.* Use of a single finger. Example: index finger applied to inner border of the mandible beneath the canine–premolar area to determine the presence of a torus mandibularis.

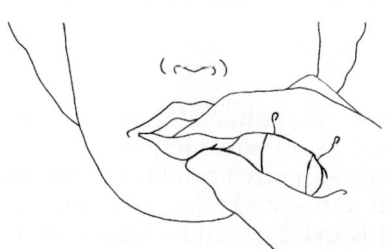

FIGURE 8-1 Bidigital Palpation. Palpation of the lip to illustrate the use of a finger and thumb of the same hand.

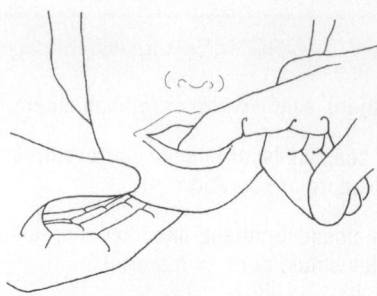

FIGURE 8-2 Bimanual Palpation. Examination of the floor of the mouth by simultaneous palpation with fingers of each hand in apposition.

2. *Bidigital.* Use of finger and thumb of the same hand. Example: palpation of the lips (Figure 8-1).
3. *Bimanual.* Use of finger or fingers and thumb from each hand applied simultaneously in coordination. Example: index finger of one hand palpates on the floor of the mouth inside, while a finger or fingers from the other hand press on the same area from under the chin externally (Figure 8-2).
4. *Bilateral.* The two hands are used at the same time to examine corresponding structures on opposite sides of the body. Comparisons may be made. Example: fingers placed beneath the chin to palpate the submandibular lymph nodes (Figure 8-3).

SEQUENCE OF EXAMINATION

A recommended order for examination is outlined in Table 8-1, in which factors to consider during appointments are related to the actual observations made and recorded. The sequence presented in Table 8-1 is adapted from *Detecting Oral Cancer* available from the National Institutes of Health.[1]

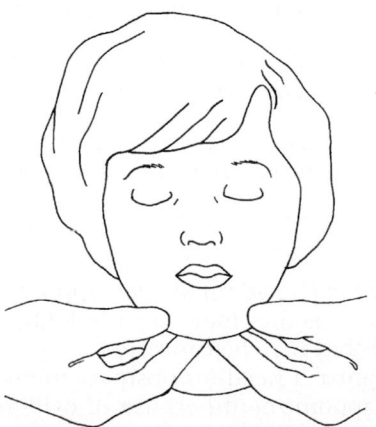

FIGURE 8-3 Bilateral Palpation. Bilateral palpation is used to examine corresponding structures on opposite sides of the body.

TABLE 8-1 Extraoral and Intraoral Examination

Order of Examination	To Observe	Indication and Influences on Appointments
1. Overall appraisal of patient	Posture, gait General health status; size Hair; scalp Breathing; state of fatigue Voice, cough, hoarseness	Response, cooperation, attitude toward treatment Length of appointment
2. Face	Expression: evidence of fear or apprehension Shape: twitching; paralysis Jaw movements during speech Injuries; signs of abuse	Need for alleviation of fears Evidence of upper respiratory or other infections Enlarged masseter muscle (related to bruxism)
3. Skin	Color, texture, blemishes Traumatic lesions Eruptions, swellings Growths	Relation to possible systemic conditions Need for supplementary history Biopsy or other treatment Influences on instruction in diet
4. Eyes	Size of pupil (Figure 8–11) Color of sclera Eyeglasses (corrective) Protruding eyeballs	Dilated pupils or pinpoint may result from drugs, emergency state (Tables 61–5 and 61-6, pages 910–916) Eyeglasses essential during instruction Hyperthyroidism

5. Nodes (palpate) (Figure 8–4)
    a. Pre- and postauricular
    b. Occipital
    c. Submental; submandibular
    d. Cervical chain
    e. Supraclavicular
	Adenopathy; lymphadenopathy
	Induration
		Need for referral
		Medical consultation
		Coordinate with intraoral examination

6. Temporomandibular joint (palpate) (Figure 8–5)	Limitations or deviations of movement Tenderness; sensitivity Noises: clicking, popping, grating	Disorder of joint; limitation of opening Discomfort during appointment and during personal plaque control

7. Lips
    a. Observe closed, then open
    b. Palpate (Figure 8–1)
	Color, texture, size
	Cracks, angular cheilosis
	Blisters, ulcers
	Traumatic lesions
	Irritation from lip-biting
	Limitation of opening; muscle elasticity; muscle tone
	Evidences of mouthbreathing
	Induration
		Need for further examination: referral
		Immediate need for postponement of appointment when a lesion may be communicable or could interfere with procedures
		Care during retraction
		Accessibility during intraoral procedures
		Patient instruction: dietary, special plaque control for mouthbreather

8. Breath odor	Severity Relation to oral hygiene, gingival health	Possible relation to systemic condition Alcohol use history; special needs

9. Labial and buccal mucosa, left and right examined systematically
    a. Vestibule
    b. Mucobuccal folds
    c. Frena
    d. Opening of Stensen's duct
    e. Palpate cheeks
	Color, size, texture, contour
	Abrasions, traumatic lesions, cheekbite
	Effects of tobacco use
	Ulcers, growths
	Moistness of surfaces
	Relation of frena to free gingiva
	Induration
		Need for referral, biopsy, cytology
		Frena and other anatomic parts that need special adaptation for radiography or impression tray
		Avoid sensitive areas during retraction

10. Tongue
    a. Dorsal surface
    b. Lateral borders
    c. Base of tongue (retract)
        (Figure 8–6)
	Shape: normal asymmetric
	Color, size, texture, consistency
	Fissures; papillae
	Coating
	Lesions: elevated, depressed, flat
	Induration
		Need for referral, biopsy, cytology
		Need for instruction in tongue cleaning

(continued)

119

TABLE 8-1 Extraoral and Intraoral Examination (Continued)

Order of Examination	To Observe	Indication and Influences on Appointments

11. Floor of mouth
  a. Ventral surface of tongue
  b. Palpate (Figure 8–2)
  c. Duct openings
  d. Mucosa, frena
  e. Tongue action
	Varicosities
	Lesions: elevated, flat, depressed, traumatic
	Induration
	Limitation or freedom of movement of tongue
	Frena; tongue-tie
		Large muscular tongue influences retraction, gag reflex, accessibility for instrumentation
		
		Film placement problems

12. Saliva	Quantity; quality (thick, ropy) Evidences of dry mouth; lip wetting Tongue coating	Reduced in certain diseases, by certain drugs Special dental caries control program Influence on instrumentation Need for saliva substitute
13. Hard palate	Height, contour, color Appearance of rugae Tori, growths, ulcers	Need for referral, biopsy, cytology Signs of tongue thrust, deviate swallow Influence on radiographic film placement
14. Soft palate, uvula	Color, size, shape Petechiae Ulcers, growths	Referral, biopsy, cytology Large uvula influences gag reflex
15. Tonsillar region, throat	Tonsils: size and shape Color, size, surface characteristics Lesions, trauma	Referral, biopsy, cytology Enlarged tonsils encourage gag reflex Throat infection, a sign for appointment postponement

I. SYSTEMATIC SEQUENCE FOR EXAMINATION

The advantages of following a routine order for examination include the following:

  A. Minimal possibility of overlooking an area and missing details of importance.

  B. Increased efficiency and conservation of time.

  C. Maintenance of a professional atmosphere, which inspires the patient's confidence.

II. STEPS FOR THOROUGH EXAMINATION (TABLE 8-1)

A. Extraoral

  1. Observe patient during reception and seating to note physical characteristics and abnormalities, and make an overall appraisal.

  2. Observe head, face, eyes, and neck, and evaluate the skin of the face and neck.

  3. Palpate the salivary glands and lymph nodes. Figure 8-4 shows the location of the major lymph nodes of the face, oral regions, and neck.

  4. Observe mandibular movement and palpate the temporomandibular joint (Figure 8-5). Relate to items from questions in the medical/dental history.[2,3]

B. Intraoral

  1. Make a preliminary examination of the lips and intraoral mucosa, using a mouth mirror or a tongue depressor.

  2. View and palpate lips, labial and buccal mucosa, and mucobuccal folds.

  3. Examine and palpate the tongue, including the dorsal and ventral surfaces, lateral borders, and base. Retract to observe posterior third, first to one side then the other (Figure 8-6). The papillae of the tongue are shown in Figure 11-2, page 188.

  4. Observe mucosa of the floor of the mouth. Palpate the floor of the mouth (Figure 8-2).

  5. Examine hard and soft palates, tonsillar

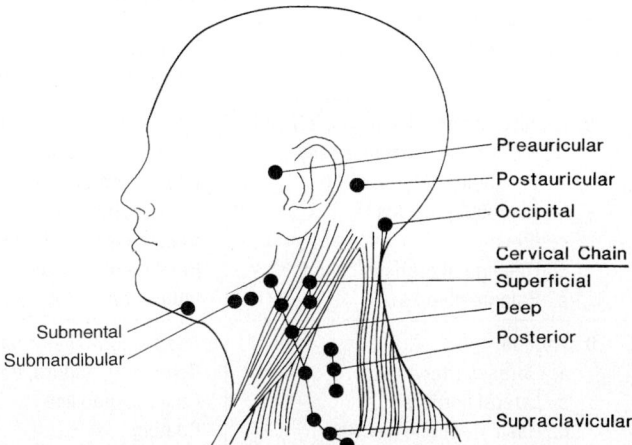

FIGURE 8-4 Lymph Nodes. The location of the major lymph nodes into which the vessels of the facial and oral regions drain.

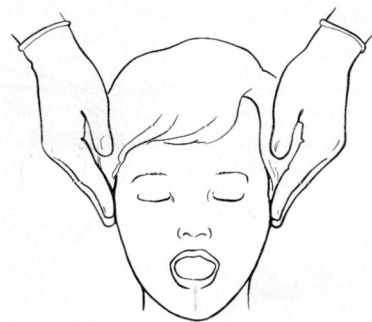

FIGURE 8-5 Assessment of the Temporomandibular Joint. The joint is palpated as the patient opens and closes the mouth.

areas, and pharynx. Use mirror to observe oropharynx, nasopharynx, and larynx.

6. Note amount and consistency of the saliva and evidences of dry mouth.

DOCUMENTATION OF FINDINGS

I. RECORDS

A. Record Form

1. Contains adequate space for complete descriptions of lesions observed; not merely a check sheet.

2. Contains spaces for successive examinations at follow-up and maintenance appointments.

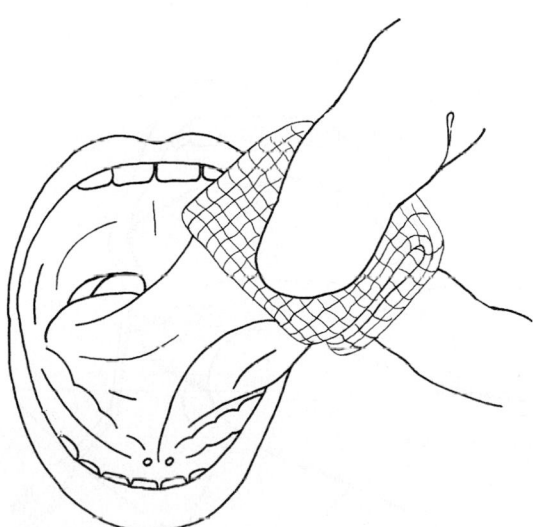

FIGURE 8-6 Examination of the Tongue. To observe the posterior third of the tongue and the attachment to the floor of the mouth, hold the tongue with a gauze sponge, retract the cheek and move the tongue out, first to one side and then the other, as each section of the mucosa is carefully examined.

B. Information to Record

A complete description of each finding includes the location, extent, size, color, surface texture or configurations, consistency, morphology, and history.

II. HISTORY

Questions directed to the patient provide necessary information in the management of an oral lesion. Because alarming the patient must be avoided, judgment is needed for selecting the appropriate time to obtain the history of a lesion.

A. Whether the lesion is known or not known to the patient.

B. If known, when first noticed; if recurrence, previous date.

C. Duration; changes in size and appearance.

D. Symptoms.

III. LOCATION AND EXTENT

When a lesion is first seen, its location is noted in relation to adjacent structures. A printed diagram of parts of the oral cavity drawn into the record form can be a valuable aid for marking the location (Figure 8-7). Descriptive words to define the location and extent include the following:

A. *Localized.* Lesion limited to a small focal area.

B. *Generalized.* Involves most of an area or segment.

C. *Single Lesion.* One lesion of a particular type with a distinct margin.

D. *Multiple Lesions.* More than one lesion of a particular type. Lesions may be

1. Separate. Discrete, not running together; may be arranged in clusters.

2. Coalescing. Close to each other with margins that merge.

IV. PHYSICAL CHARACTERISTICS

A. Size and Shape

Record length and width in millimeters. The height of an elevated lesion may be significant. Use a probe to measure as shown in Figure 8-8.

B. Color

Red, pink, white, and red and white are the most commonly seen. Other more rare lesions may be blue, purple, gray, yellow, black, or brown.

C. Surface Texture

A lesion may have a smooth or an irregular surface. The texture may be papillary, verrucous or wartlike, fissured, corrugated, or crusted. Other descriptive terms are defined in Box 8-1 with the key words.

D. Consistency

Lesions may be soft, spongy, resilient, hard, or indurated.

Draw outlines of abnormalities in proper locations

MUCOSAL ABNORMALITIES

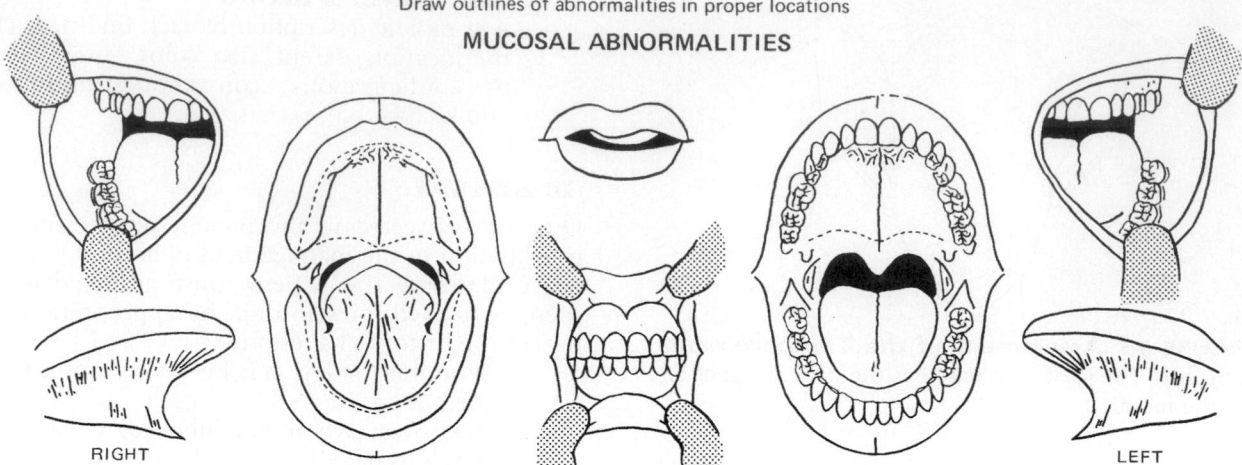

RIGHT LEFT

FIGURE 8-7 Record Form for Clinical Findings. As part of a clinical examination record form, deviations from normal can be drawn to show the location and relative size. (Courtesy, University of Southern California School of Dentistry.)

MORPHOLOGIC CATEGORIES[4]

Most lesions can be classified readily as *elevated, depressed,* or *flat* as they relate to the normal level of the skin or mucosa. Tables 8-2, 8-3, and 8-4 break down the terms used for describing lesions in each category.

I. ELEVATED LESIONS (Table 8-2)

An elevated lesion is above the plane of the skin or mucosa. Elevated lesions are considered *blisterform* or *nonblisterform.*

A. Blisterform

Blisterform lesions contain fluid and are usually soft and translucent. They may be vesicles, pustules, or bullae.

1. *Vesicle.* A vesicle is a small (1 cm or less in diameter), circumscribed lesion with a thin surface covering. It may contain serum or mucin and appear white.
2. *Pustule.* A pustule may be more or less than 5 mm in diameter. It contains pus. Pus gives the pustule a yellowish color.
3. *Bulla.* A bulla is large (more than 1 cm). It is filled with fluid, usually mucin or serum, but may contain blood. The color depends on the fluid content.

B. Nonblisterform

Nonblisterform lesions are solid and do not contain fluid. They may be papules, nodules, tumors, or plaques. Papules, nodules, and tumors are also characterized by the base or attachment. As shown in Figure 8-9, the *pedunculated* lesion is attached by a narrow stalk or pedicle, whereas the *sessile* lesion has a base as wide as the lesion itself.

1. *Papule.* A papule is a small (pinhead to 5 mm in diameter), solid lesion that may be pointed, rounded, or flat-topped.
2. *Nodule.* A nodule is larger than a papule (greater than 5 mm but less than 1 cm).
3. *Tumor.* A tumor is 2 cm or greater in width. In this context, "tumor" means a general swelling or enlargement and does not refer to neoplasm, either benign or malignant.
4. *Plaque.* A plaque is a slightly raised lesion with a broad, flat top. It is usually larger than 5 mm in diameter, with a "pasted on" appearance.

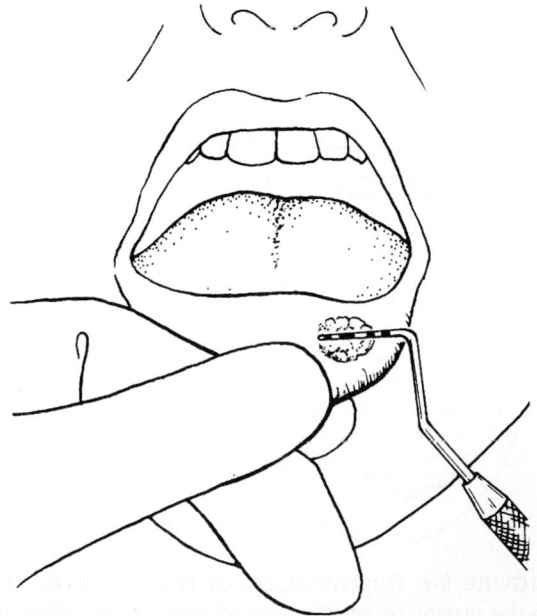

FIGURE 8-8 Use of Probe to Measure a Lesion. In addition to the exact location, the width and length of a lesion should be recorded. Using the probe provides a convenient method.

TABLE 8-2 Description of Elevated Soft Tissue Lesions

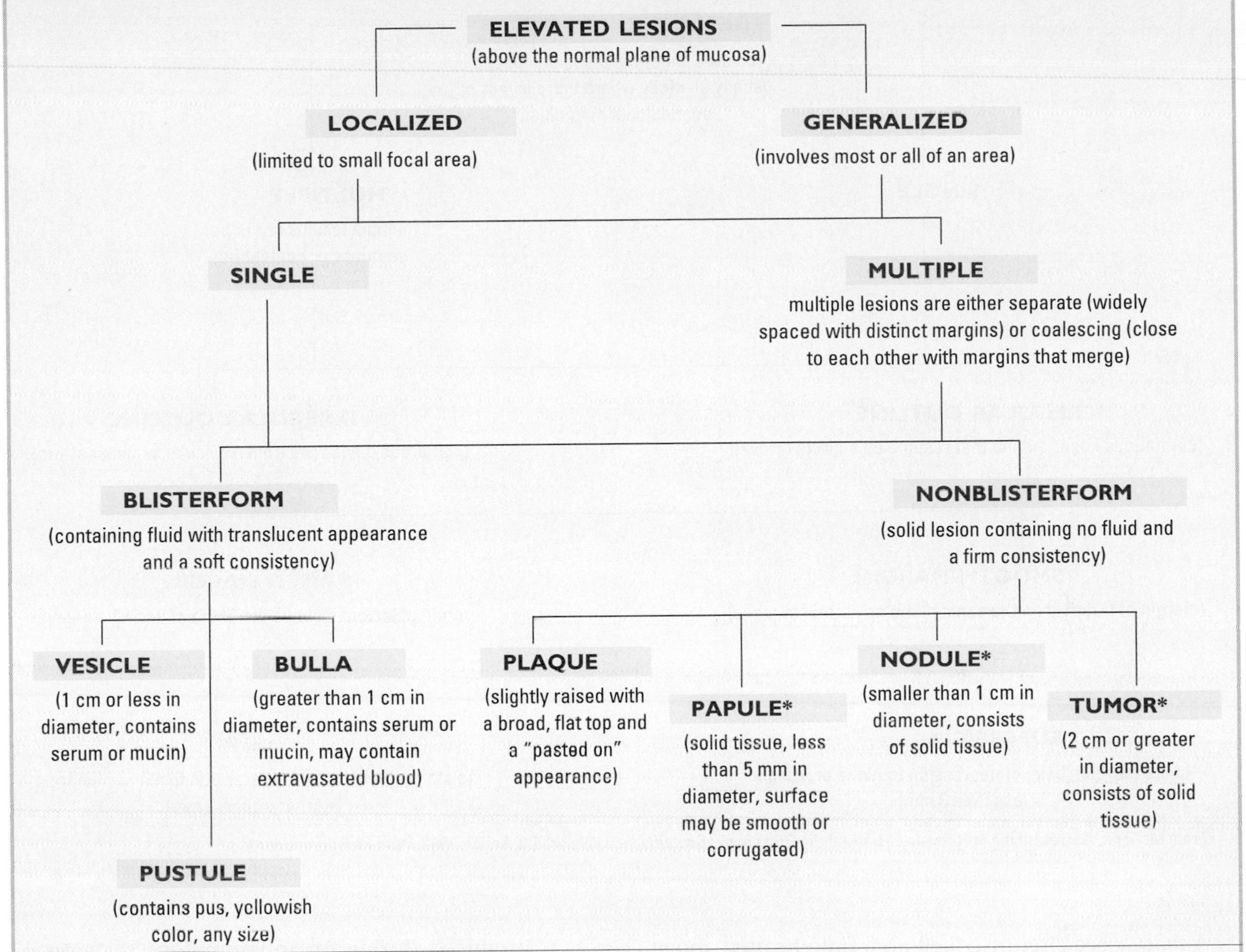

ELEVATED LESIONS
(above the normal plane of mucosa)

LOCALIZED
(limited to small focal area)

GENERALIZED
(involves most or all of an area)

SINGLE

MULTIPLE
multiple lesions are either separate (widely spaced with distinct margins) or coalescing (close to each other with margins that merge)

BLISTERFORM
(containing fluid with translucent appearance and a soft consistency)

NONBLISTERFORM
(solid lesion containing no fluid and a firm consistency)

VESICLE
(1 cm or less in diameter, contains serum or mucin)

BULLA
(greater than 1 cm in diameter, contains serum or mucin, may contain extravasated blood)

PLAQUE
(slightly raised with a broad, flat top and a "pasted on" appearance)

PAPULE*
(solid tissue, less than 5 mm in diameter, surface may be smooth or corrugated)

NODULE*
(smaller than 1 cm in diameter, consists of solid tissue)

TUMOR*
(2 cm or greater in diameter, consists of solid tissue)

PUSTULE
(contains pus, yellowish color, any size)

*May be pedunculated (on a stem or stalk) or sessile (base or attachment is the greatest diameter of the lesion)
(From McCann, A.: Describing Soft Tissue Lesions of the Oral Cavity, *DentalHygienistNews, 5,* 9, Spring, 1992. Used with permission.)

II. DEPRESSED LESIONS (Table 8-3)

A depressed lesion is below the level of the skin or mucosa. The outline may be regular or irregular, and there may be a flat or raised border around the depression. The depth is usually described as superficial or deep. A deep lesion is greater than 3 mm deep.

A. Ulcer

Most depressed lesions are ulcers and represent a loss of continuity of the epithelium. The center is often gray to yellow, surrounded by a red border. An ulcer may result from the rupture of an elevated lesion (vesicle, pustule, or bulla).

B. Erosion

An erosion is a shallow, depressed lesion that does not extend through the epithelium to the underlying tissue.

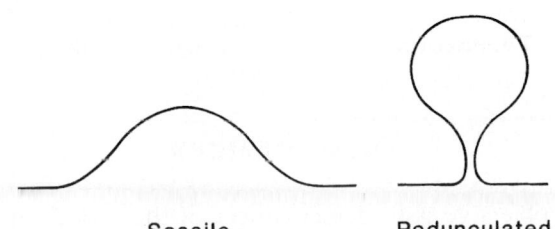

Sessile   Pedunculated

■ **FIGURE 8-9 Attachment of Nonblisterform Lesions.** The *sessile* lesion has a base as wide as the lesion itself; the *pedunculated* lesion is attached by a narrow stalk or pedicle.

III. FLAT LESIONS (Table 8-4)

A flat lesion is on the same level as the normal skin or oral mucosa. Flat lesions may occur as single or multiple lesions and have a regular or irregular form.

TABLE 8-3 Description of Depressed Soft Tissue Lesions

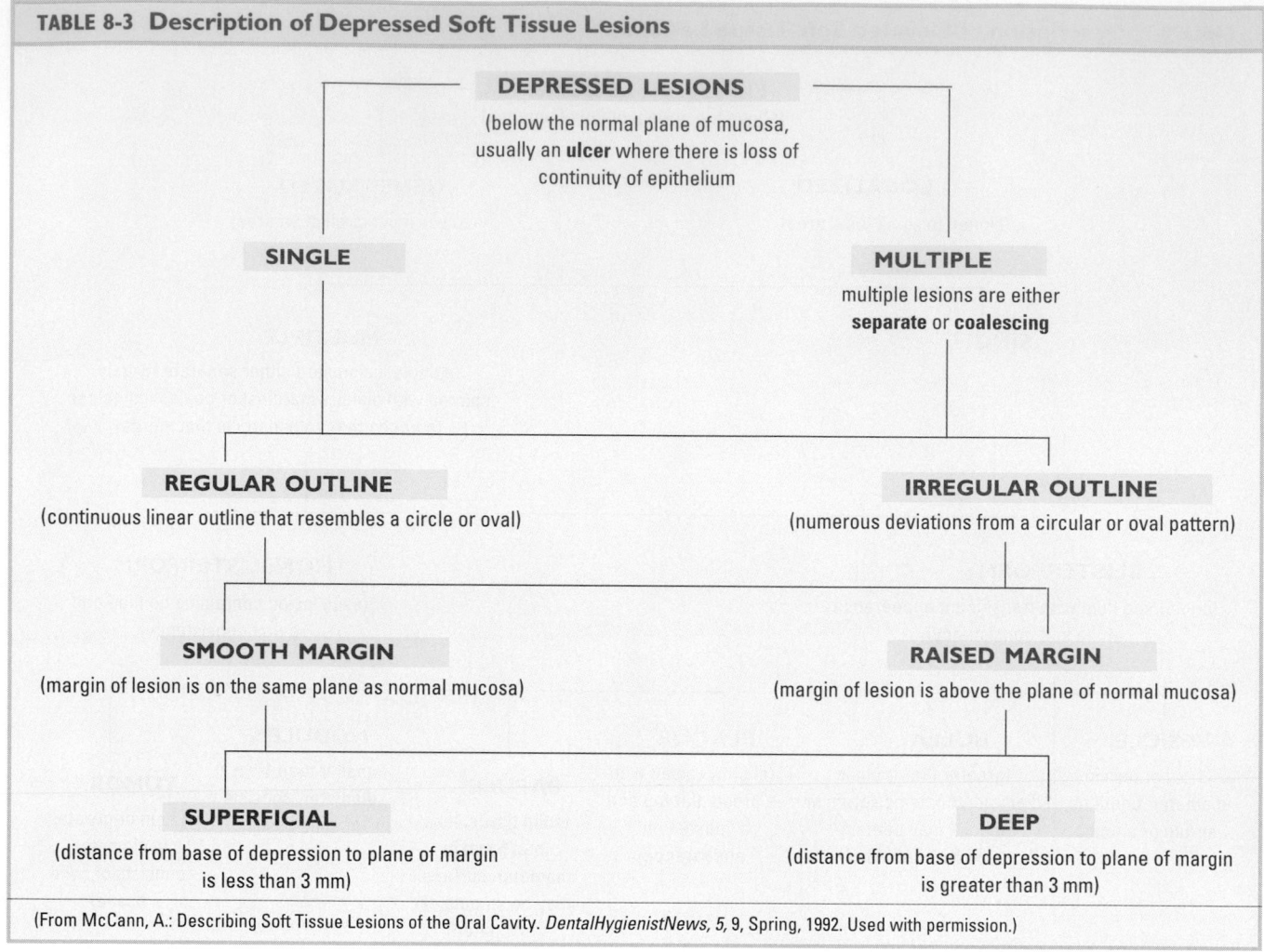

DEPRESSED LESIONS

(below the normal plane of mucosa, usually an **ulcer** where there is loss of continuity of epithelium

SINGLE

MULTIPLE

multiple lesions are either **separate** or **coalescing**

REGULAR OUTLINE

(continuous linear outline that resembles a circle or oval)

IRREGULAR OUTLINE

(numerous deviations from a circular or oval pattern)

SMOOTH MARGIN

(margin of lesion is on the same plane as normal mucosa)

RAISED MARGIN

(margin of lesion is above the plane of normal mucosa)

SUPERFICIAL

(distance from base of depression to plane of margin is less than 3 mm)

DEEP

(distance from base of depression to plane of margin is greater than 3 mm)

(From McCann, A.: Describing Soft Tissue Lesions of the Oral Cavity. *DentalHygienistNews, 5,* 9, Spring, 1992. Used with permission.)

A *macule* is a circumscribed area not elevated above the surrounding skin or mucosa. It may be identified by its color, which contrasts with the surrounding normal tissues.

IV. OTHER DESCRIPTIVE TERMS

A. Crust: an outer layer, covering, or scab that may have formed from coagulation or drying of blood, serum, or pus, or a combination. A crust may form after a vesicle breaks; for example, the skin lesion of chicken pox is first a macule, then a papule, then a vesicle, and then a crust.

B. Erythema: red area of variable size and shape.

C. Exophytic: growing outward.

D. Indurated: hardened.

E. Papillary: resembling a small, nipple-shaped projection or elevation.

F. Petechiae: minute hemorrhagic spots of pinhead to pinpoint size.

G. Pseudomembrane: a loose membranous layer of exudate, containing organisms, precipitated fibrin, necrotic cells, and inflammatory cells, produced during an inflammatory reaction on the surface of a tissue.

H. Polyp: any mass of tissue that projects outward or upward from the normal surface level.

I. Punctate: marked with points or dots differentiated from the surrounding surface by color, elevation, or texture.

J. Torus: bony elevation or prominence usually found on the midline of the hard palate (torus palatinus) and the lingual surface of the mandible (torus mandibularis) in the premolar area.

K. Verrucous (verrucose): rough, wartlike.

ORAL CANCER

The objective is to detect cancer of the mouth at the earliest possible stage. Discovered later, when a cancer extends into adjacent structures and to the lymph nodes of the neck, the prognosis is less favorable.

Because the early lesions are generally symptomless, they may go unnoticed and unreported by the

TABLE 8-4 Description of Flat Soft Tissue Lesions

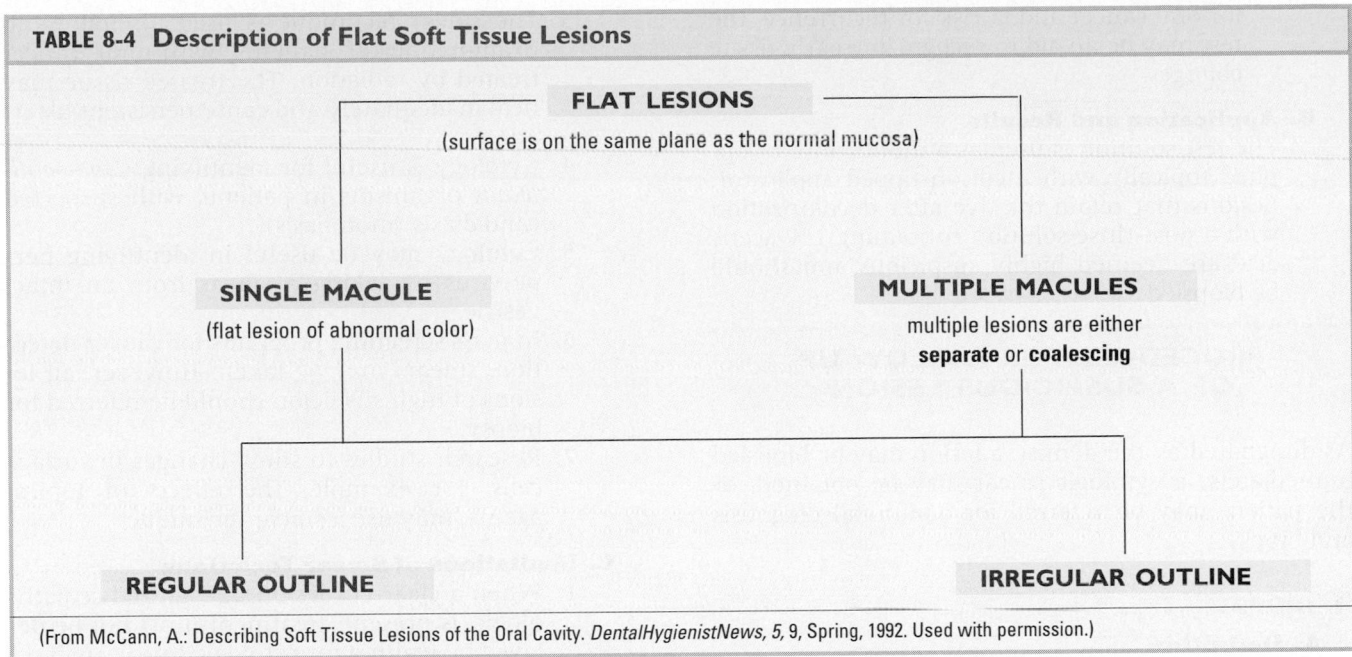

(From McCann, A.: Describing Soft Tissue Lesions of the Oral Cavity. *DentalHygienistNews*, *5*, 9, Spring, 1992. Used with permission.)

patient. Observation by the dentist or dental hygienist, therefore, is the principal method for the control of oral cancer. The first step in accomplishing this task is to examine the entire face, neck, and oral mucous membrane of each patient at the initial examination and at each maintenance appointment (Table 8-1).

It is necessary to know how to conduct the oral examination, where oral cancer occurs most frequently, what an early cancerous lesion may look like, and what to do when such a lesion is found. In addition to the early lesions of oral cancers, the oral manifestations of neoplasms elsewhere in the body as well as the oral manifestations of chemotherapy can be recognized (Chapter 49, pages 730 to 732).

I. LOCATION

Neoplasms may arise at any site in the oral cavity. The most common sites are the floor of the mouth, lateral parts of the tongue, the lower lip, and the soft palate complex.

Although patients may be instructed in self-examination to watch for changes in oral tissues, it is difficult for persons to see their own tissues, particularly the entire floor of the mouth and base of the tongue, by the usual mirror and lighting systems available in a private home. Self-examination should be routinely supplemented with professional examination.

II. APPEARANCE OF EARLY CANCER

Early oral cancer takes many forms and may resemble a variety of common oral lesions. All types should be looked at with suspicion. Five basic forms are listed here.

A. White Areas
These may vary from a filmy, barely visible change in the mucosa to heavy, thick, heaped-up areas of dry white keratinized tissue. Fissures, ulcers, or areas of induration in a white area are most indicative of malignancy.

Leukoplakia is a white patch or plaque that cannot be scraped off or characterized as any other disease. It may be associated with physical or chemical agents and the use of tobacco.

B. Red Areas
Lesions of red, velvety consistency, sometimes with small ulcers, should be identified.

The term *erythroplakia* is used to designate lesions of the oral mucosa that appear as bright red patches or plaques that cannot be characterized as any specific disease.

C. Ulcers
Ulcers may have flat or raised margins. Palpation may reveal induration.

D. Masses
Papillary masses, sometimes with ulcerated areas, occur as elevations above the surrounding tissues. Other masses may occur below the normal mucosa and may be found only by palpation.

E. Pigmentation
Brown or black pigmented areas may be located on mucosa where pigmentation does not normally occur.

III. DIAGNOSTIC AID: TOLUIDINE BLUE[5]

A. Uses
1. *Initial Examination.* To identify mucosal changes that may be malignant.[6]
2. *Maintenance.* For patients previously treated

for oral cancer and at risk for recurrence, the test may be an aid in recognizing early tissue changes.[7]

B. Application and Results

The test solution is used as a mouthrinse or applied topically with a cotton-tipped applicator. Lesions that retain the dye after decolorization with a post-rinse solution containing 1% acetic acid are deemed highly suspicious and should be biopsied.

PROCEDURE FOR FOLLOW-UP OF A SUSPICIOUS LESION

As designated by the dentist, a lesion may be biopsied immediately, a cytologic smear may be obtained, or the patient may be referred for additional diagnosis and biopsy.

I. BIOPSY

A. Definition

Biopsy is the removal and examination, usually by microscope, of a section of tissue or other material from the living body for the purposes of diagnosis. A biopsy is either *excisional,* when the entire lesion is removed, or *incisional,* when a representative section from the lesion is taken.

B. Indications for Biopsy[8,9]

1. Any unusual oral lesion that cannot be identified with clinical certainty must be biopsied.
2. Any lesion that has not shown evidence of healing in 2 weeks should be considered malignant until proven otherwise.
3. A persistent, thick, white, hyperkeratotic lesion and any mass (elevated or not) that does not break through the surface epithelium should be biopsied.
4. Any tissue surgically removed should be submitted for microscopic examination.

II. CYTOLOGIC SMEAR

A. Definition

The cytologic smear technique is a diagnostic aid in which surface cells of a suspicious lesion are removed for microscopic evaluation.

B. Indications for Smear Technique[8]

1. In general, a lesion for which a biopsy is not planned may be examined by smear. An exception is a keratotic lesion that is not suitable for exfoliative cytology.
2. A lesion that looks like potential cancer should be examined by smear if the patient refuses to have a biopsy specimen taken. A positive report from a smear should convince the patient of the need for treatment or biopsy.

3. The smear technique is used for follow-up examination of patients with oral cancer treated by radiation. The treated tissue may heal inadequately and cause persistent ulceration.
4. Cytology is useful for identifying *Candida albicans* organisms in patients with suspected candidiasis (moniliasis).
5. Cytology may be useful in identifying herpesvirus by taking a smear from an intact vesicle.
6. In mass screening programs for cancer detection, smears may be taken. However, all lesions of high suspicion should be referred for biopsy.
7. Research studies to show changes in surface cells, for example, the effects of topical agents, may use a smear technique.

C. Limitations of Smear Technique

1. When a clear-cut lesion, recognized as pathologic, is present, treatment must not be delayed by waiting for cytologic smear analysis.
2. The smear detects only surface lesions.
3. It is difficult or impossible to scrape deep enough to obtain representative cells from a heavily keratinized lesion.
4. Except for candidiasis, treatment cannot be determined by smear technique results only. After a positive smear, a biopsy is needed for definitive diagnosis.
5. Because research has shown that the smear technique is not diagnostically reliable (there can be "false negatives," which turn out to be positive biopsies), a negative report should not be considered conclusive.

EXFOLIATIVE CYTOLOGY

Stratified squamous epithelial cells are constantly growing toward the surface of the mucous membrane, where they are exfoliated. Exfoliated cells and cells beneath them are scraped off, and when these cells are prepared on a slide, changes in the cells can be detected by staining and studying them microscopically. The malignant cells stain differently from normal cells and take on unusual, abnormal forms.

I. PROCEDURE

A. Materials

Gauze sponges
Glass microscopic slides with frosted end
Plain lead pencil
Paper clips
Blade to scrape lesion (flexible metal spatula)
Fixative (70% alcohol)
Protective mailing container
History form or data sheet

B. Steps

1. *Prepare Materials.* Write the patient's name on the frosted ends of two glass slides (two for each lesion) in pencil, and place a paper clip on the end of one slide to prevent contact between the slides when packaged for mailing to the laboratory.
2. *Prepare the Lesion.* Irrigate the surface to remove debris. Wipe the surface gently with a wet gauze sponge as needed to remove debris or blood. Do not dry.
3. *Scrape the Lesion.* Use a flexible metal spatula. Scrape the entire surface of the lesion firmly several times (all strokes in the same direction) (Figure 8-10A). When a wooden tongue depressor is used, it must be wet before taking the sample so the material will not be absorbed into the wood. For intact vesicles, carefully rupture the vesicle so the fluid flows onto the glass slides.
4. *Smear the Glass Slide.* Spread the collected material on the glass slide. Start at the center of the clear end of the slide and smear evenly across the surface. Cover an area approximately 20 mm wide. Handle all glass slides by their edges to prevent fingerprints or other contamination (Figure 8-10B).
5. *Fix the Cells.* Immediately, to prevent drying of the cells, place the slide on a flat surface and flood with generous drops of 70% alcohol or use prepared commercial fixative spray.
6. *Obtain Second Smear.* Duplicate previous smear technique. Apply fixing agent immediately.
7. *Complete the Fixation.* Leave slides for 30 minutes. After 20 minutes, tip the slide to let remaining alcohol run off. Air dry where dust or other foreign material cannot contaminate the smear.
8. *Prepare History or Data Sheet.* Basic information includes the following:
   a. Dentist. Name and address.
   b. Patient. Name and address.
   c. Lesion. Description (size, color, location, shape, consistency, and duration).
   d. Other. Additional related clinical findings or pertinent history.
9. *Prepare for Mailing.* Wrap slides to prevent breakage. Pack with the history or data sheet. Mailing containers, provided by most laboratories list specific instructions.

II. LABORATORY REPORT

The pathologist makes the microscopic examination and classifies the specimen in one of the following categories:

Unsatisfactory: Slide is inadequate for diagnosis. The specimen may have been too thick or thin, or the cells may have dried before fixation. Another smear should be made promptly.

Class I: Normal.

Class II: Atypical, but not suggestive of malignant cells.

Class III: Uncertain (possible for cancer).

Class IV: Probable for cancer.

Class V: Positive for cancer.

III. FOLLOW-UP

A. Report of Class IV or V
Refer for biopsy.

B. Report of Class III
Re-evaluate clinical findings; biopsy usually indicated.

C. Report of Class I or II
1. The patient must not be dismissed until the lesion has healed.
2. When lesion persists, the dentist either re-evaluates the clinical findings and requests a repeat cytologic smear or performs a biopsy.

D. Negative Report
Either biopsy or smear requires careful follow-up when a negative report is obtained for an oral lesion that appears suspicious by clinical examination. False-negative reports are possible; that is, a malignancy may be present, but the sample examined in the smear or biopsy may not have included cancerous cells.

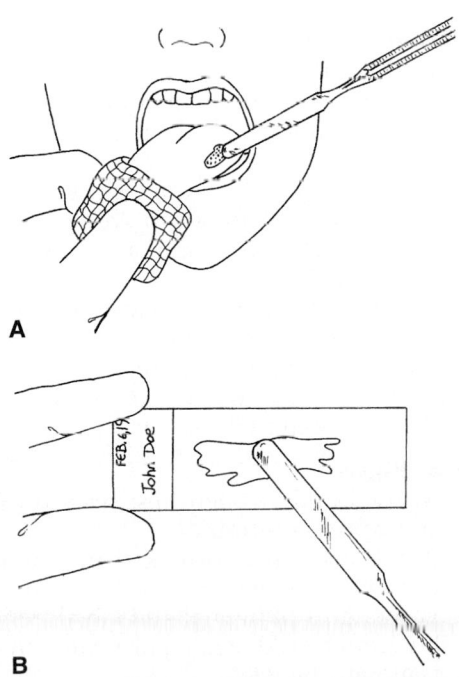

A

B

■ **FIGURE 8-10 Oral Cytology Technique. (A)** Tongue is held out with gauze sponge while a metal spatula is used to scrape a lesion. **(B)** Collected material is spread evenly on a glass slide. See text for details.

SPECIAL APPLICATIONS FOR THE EXTRAORAL AND INTRAORAL EXAMINATION

In Part VI of this book, many types of patients with special needs for adapted techniques are described. Some of them have general physical and oral characteristics that can be identified during an extraoral and intraoral examination. Facial and oral tissue examinations for pathology apply to all patients.

With certain patients, the recognition of particular characteristics has another dimension, which may have social and legal implications. One example is the group of intraoral and extraoral signs that may reveal a person who is a victim of abuse or neglect. The physical or emotional abuse, neglect, or exploitation of older adults has become a problem of growing significance.[10]

Another patient who may not be identified by questions from a medical and dental history is a substance abuser. A variety of treatment problems are related to the care of a patient who misuses drugs. Identification of the patient's addiction can be essential to successful treatment. Characteristics for recognition of certain special patients are described here.

FAMILY ABUSE AND NEGLECT

Recognition of a person who has been abused or neglected is a responsibility of the entire dental team. There is a need to be aware of the problem of family abuse, to be able to identify and report suspected cases, and to document the injuries observed for future reference and comparison.

Family abuse may be physical, emotional, or sexual abuse; neglect; or financial exploitation. There are many forms of abuse, including abuse and neglect of children; abuse and neglect of senior adults; abuse of women, particularly spouse violence; and dating violence. Those at risk are women, children, older adults, and people with disabilities.

During the extraoral and intraoral examination, various findings may lead to a suspicion of abuse. Head, facial, or oral trauma occurs in many abuse cases. Some of the patients may be seen in dental offices or clinics, whereas others are taken to a hospital emergency clinic because other serious bodily injuries have been inflicted.

I. RECOGNITION OF CHILD ABUSE

Children ranging from infants through teenagers are involved. Several thousands a year die as a result of the severe physical damage inflicted, whereas others suffer permanent brain damage or physical deformities.

A. Definitions

Maltreatment of children may be categorized as abuse and neglect.

1. *Abuse.* Abuse refers to nonaccidental physical, sexual, or emotional acts against a child by a parent or caregiver that are beyond the acceptable norms of child care. Characteristically, the injury is more severe than might be expected from the explanation provided by the parent or caregiver.
2. *Neglect.* Child neglect can be defined as the failure of a parent or other person legally responsible for the child to provide for basic needs at an adequate level of care. Basic needs include food, clothing, health care, safety, and education.
3. *Dental Neglect.* Dental neglect is the willful failure of parent or guardian to seek and follow through with treatment necessary to ensure a level of oral health essential for adequate function and freedom from pain and infection.[11]

B. General Signs

Recognition of signs of suspected neglect or abuse is the first step toward protection of the child. As the child enters the reception area and then goes into the treatment room, identifiable characteristics may be displayed that are suggestive of abuse.

1. *Behavioral.* An abused child may be very fearful and cry excessively, show no fear at all, or appear unhappy and withdrawn. The child may act differently when the parent is present than when alone, which may provide clues to the type of relationship that exists. Frequently, evidence exists of developmental delays, including those of language or motor skills.
2. *Overall appearance.*
   a. Failure to thrive; malnutrition.
   b. Uncleanliness and other signs of lack of care.
   c. Clothing with long sleeves and long pants, even in warm weather, may suggest that bruises and lacerations are being covered.
3. *Wounds.* Abrasions and lacerations of varying degrees of healing inconsistent with explanations given by the parent.
4. *Signs of Trauma.* Burns; bite marks; trauma to the eyes, external ears, or neck.

C. Oral Signs

1. Bruised and swollen lips; scars on lips may show previous trauma.
2. Abrasions at the corners of the mouth, such as from a gag tied around the head.
3. Lacerations of lingual and labial frena, possibly from forced feeding or related to external traumatic blows.
4. Teeth
   a. Avulsed, fractured, darkened.
   b. Radiographic signs of fractures in different degrees of healing.

5. Jaw fracture.
6. Tongue injuries; evidence of scarring and recent healing.
7. Signs of dental neglect.
   a. Untreated disease, including rampant dental caries, pain, inflammation, bleeding gingiva.
   b. Lack or irregularity of professional care. Appointments may have been primarily for tooth removal.

D. Parental Attitude

Parents who abuse their children are frequently immature and not prepared to accept the responsibilities of parenting. On the other hand, they may have been abused by their own parents. Drug abuse and alcoholism are sometimes involved.

Child abuse is very complex. A few of the possible parental attitudes and behavior patterns are mentioned here.

1. Disinterest or denial in relationship to the child; may be critical, scolding, or belittling in front of others, including dental personnel.
2. Lack of interest in proposed dental and dental hygiene treatment plan, with a tendency to want only pain relief for the child. Such an attitude may not be shown toward other children in the family.
3. Unavailable for consultation. Does not usually accompany the child for dental appointments, but sends the child with another sibling.
4. Provides inconsistent information about the sources and causes of damaged teeth, bruises, or other signs of trauma.

II. RECOGNITION OF ABUSE OF ELDERLY PERSONS[12]

Abuse may be physical, emotional, sexual, or financial, as well as neglect of the needs of the individual. Maltreatment occurs more often when the family member who is the caretaker abuses alcohol or drugs, was a victim of abuse when growing up, or has a mental illness. Abuse or neglect is more likely when the elderly person has a history of being abused, has physical or medical disabilities, or has financial problems and may be dependent on the caregiver.

A. General Signs
1. *Physical*. Slapping, hitting, and striking with objects lead to cuts, abrasions, skeletal fractures, and burns.
2. *Psychological*. Humiliation, intimidation, threatening of institutionalization, abandonment.
3. *Neglect*. Dehydration and malnutrition, poor personal care, withholding treatment or medication.

B. Oral and Facial Signs
1. Lip trauma, bruising

2. Fractured mandible or maxilla; fractured teeth or dentures
3. Eye injuries; hair loss; lines on throat suggestive of choking
4. Neglect of oral hygiene and professional care

III. REPORTING

Professional people have a particular responsibility to report suspected child abuse to the proper authorities. In certain states, the failure to report can lead to legal involvement. The failure to recognize and act in behalf of the child may be dangerous, even fatal, for the child involved. Telephone numbers for specific reporting should be kept current and readily available.

SUBSTANCE ABUSE[13]

It is usually not possible to determine from a patient's medical and dental histories whether the patient uses alcohol and/or unprescribed drugs regularly, perhaps to the level of dependency. The general categories of the drugs of abuse are listed with examples in Table 8-5, along with their "street" names. When a history is being prepared, more information may be obtained about drug use if the common street names of products are used.

Problems related to the use of alcohol and alcoholism are considered in Chapter 57.

Patients who use drugs recreationally may "premedicate" themselves when a stressful situation, such as a dental appointment, is anticipated. Because the day-to-day use of drugs varies, questioning at each appointment may be necessary to prevent complications. Certain precautions must be taken during patient care.

When no information is provided by the patient, awareness by dental personnel of the characteristics that suggest the possible use of drugs is important. A few of the common features that may aid in general identification are included in this section.

I. DEFINITIONS

A. Drug
A drug is a chemical substance used for diagnosis, prevention, or treatment of disease. Drugs are classified by biochemical action, physiologic effect, or the organ system involved.

B. Substance Abuse
Substance or drug abuse is the regular use of a drug other than for its accepted medical purpose or in doses greater than those considered appropriate.

C. Chemical Dependence
Dependence refers to the interaction between a drug and the individual when there is a compulsion to take the drug to obtain its effects and/or to avoid the discomforts of withdrawal.

TABLE 8-5 Categories of Substances of Abuse with Street Names

Drug Category	Examples	Street Names

Opioids
    Analgesics
	Heroin
	
	Morphine
		H, Horse, junk, smack, Harry, chip, skag, hard or heavy
		    goods
		M, white stuff, Miss Emma, hocus, monkey

Central nervous system depressants
    Sedative-hypnotics
    Antianxiety
	Barbiturates
	
	Alcohol
	Diazepam (Valium)
		Goofball, barbs, peanuts, downers, candy, yellows, yellow
		    jackets, reds, red birds, red devils, blue devils, blue
		    heavens, double trouble

Central nervous system stimulants	Amphetamines Cocaine Freebase cocaine	Bennies, peaches, splash, speed, crystal, uppers C, coke, Charlie, Cadillac, gold dust, stardust, joy powder, snow Crack
Hallucinogen	LSD (d-lysergic acid diethylamide) Mescaline	Acid, cubes, cupcake, blue dragon, sunshine Big chief, buttons, mesc
Phencyclidines	Phencyclidine Ketamine	Hog, angel dust, peace pill, PCP PCE
Cannabinoids	Marijuana Hashish	Grass, pot, hemp, Mary Jane, weed Cigarettes: joint, reefer, roach Hash, soles
Inhalants	Acetone (paint thinner, model cement) Benzene (adhesives, gasoline) Ethyl acetate (paint thinner) Nitrous oxide (anesthetic, propellant)	

D. Physical Dependence

Physical dependence results when the drug becomes necessary for continued body functioning. An altered physiologic state has developed from repeatedly increasing drug concentrations.

E. Psychologic Dependence

Psychologic dependence refers to the state of mind in which the individual believes the drug is required for maintaining well-being.

F. Tolerance

The state of tolerance means that increased amounts of the drug are needed to achieve the same effect.

G. Withdrawal (Abstinence) Syndrome

A group of signs and symptoms, both physiologic and psychologic, occurs on abrupt discontinuation of drug use.

II. RECOGNITION

There are many addictive drugs, each with characteristic effects on the user. Specific identification is usually difficult or impossible without information from the patient. Physical and behavioral factors that are common signs of drug abuse follow.

A. General Signs

1. Personal appearance
   a. Careless in appearance with apparent lack of interest in dress and personal hygiene, particularly a person who previously was neatly groomed.
   b. Wears long sleeves to cover needle marks.
   c. May have small blood stains on clothes or skin left from previous injections.
   d. Dramatic weight loss.
2. Eyes
   a. Wears sunglasses to conceal dilated or constricted pupils and eye redness, or to avoid bright light because of eye sensitivity.
   b. Pupils dilated (amphetamine, LSD, cocaine, marijuana) (Figure 8-11).
   c. Pupils constricted (heroin, morphine, methadone).
   d. Red, inflamed, bloodshot (marijuana).
3. Needle marks on arms. These may be noted when sleeve is raised to determine the blood pressure.
4. Unusual behavior
   a. Sneezing; itching.
   b. Tendency to gaze into space; moodiness.
   c. Drowsiness; yawning; may sleep long hours.
   d. Appearance of intoxication without odor of alcohol; slurred speech.

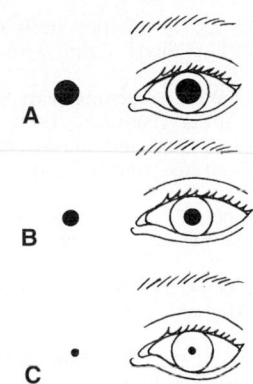

FIGURE 8-11 Examination of the Pupils. (A) Dilated; occurs in shock, heart failure, and other emergencies, and in the use of hallucinogens and amphetamines. **(B)** Normal. **(C)** Pinpoint; occurs in use of morphine and related drugs, heroin, barbiturates. (Adapted from *American National Red Cross, Standard First Aid and Personal Safety.*)

  e. Changes in habits, attitudes, and efficiency, or irregular attendance at appointments by a previously conscientious, regular patient.
  5. Possession of pills, capsules.
  6. Hallucinations or convulsions; indicate need for immediate medical emergency care.

B. Oral Characteristics
  1. Poor oral hygiene; lack of personal care or interest in care; diet high in cariogenic substances.
  2. Higher incidence of periodontal infections than peers. Gingival lesions may result from direct application of cocaine.[14,15]
  3. High dental caries incidence with open rampant carious lesions and tooth loss; few if any restorations. The abuse of analgesic drugs, which reduce pain, helps the addict to become indifferent to pain.
  4. Drug-induced xerostomia may relate to high incidence of dental caries.

III. APPOINTMENT FACTORS

A. Drug Effects
  Possible drug interactions should be checked. For example, epinephrine-containing products should not be used when treating habitual marijuana or cocaine users.[16] Methadone masks the effects of narcotics, so other drugs must be used for pain relief.

B. Prophylactic Antibiotic Premedication[17]
  For addicts who inject their drugs, antibiotic premedication has been advised. People who abuse intravenous substances frequently share needles and syringes. Therefore, a greater risk for bacteremia exists. See pages 101 to 104 for the regimen.
  Many intravenous drug abusers use prophy-

lactic antibiotics regularly to prevent infections. Specific history questions can be directed to obtain this information.

TECHNICAL HINTS

  I. Addicts frequently use dentists to obtain prescriptions for various pain-relieving drugs. A person with a toothache who refuses to have the tooth removed can obtain a prescription for pain relief. Prescription pads should be kept out of sight, as addicts have been known to steal a pad and forge the dentist's signature.
  II. Drugs kept in the dental office or clinic should be locked in a place inaccessible and unknown to patients to prevent theft.
  III. When treating a patient who is recovering from substance abuse, pain management should be coordinated with the primary physician.

FACTORS TO TEACH THE PATIENT

  I. Reasons for a careful extraoral and intraoral examination at each maintenance appointment.
  II. A method for self-examination. Examination should include the face, neck, lips, gingiva, cheeks, tongue, palate, and throat. Any changes should be reported to the dentist and the dental hygienist.
  III. The Warning Signs of Oral Cancer
    A. A swelling, lump, or growth anywhere; with or without pain.
    B. White scaly patches, or red velvety areas.
    C. Any sore that does not heal promptly (within 2 weeks).
    D. Numbness or tingling.
    E. Excessive dryness or wetness.
    F. Prolonged hoarseness, sore throats, persistent coughing, or the feeling of a "lump in the throat."
    G. Difficulty with swallowing.
    H. Difficulty in opening the mouth.
  IV. General dietary and nutritional influences on the health of the oral tissues.
  V. How the oral cavity tends to reflect the general health.

REFERENCES

  1. *Detecting Oral Cancer. A Guide for Dentists.* National Institute of Dental Research, Building 31, Room 2C35, 31 Center Drive MSC 2290, Bethesda, MD 20892-2290.
  2. **Coakley,** M.C.: Temporomandibular Joint Dysfunction (TMJ): The Role of the Dental Hygienist, *J. Dent. Hyg., 62,* 521, November/December, 1988.
  3. **McNeill,** C., Mohl, N.D., Rugh, J.D., and Tanaka, T.T.: Tem-

poromandibular Disorders: Diagnosis, Management, Education, and Research, *J. Am. Dent. Assoc., 120,* 253, March, 1990.

4. **McCann,** A.L. and Wesley, R.K.: A Method for Describing Soft Tissue Lesions of the Oral Cavity, *Dent. Hyg., 61,* 219, May, 1987.

5. **OraScan, Zila, Inc.,** 5227 North 7th Street, Phoenix, AZ 85014-2800.

6. **Warnakulasuriya,** K.A.A.S. and Johnson, N.W.: Sensitivity and Specificity of OraScan® Toluidine Blue Mouthrinse in the Detection of Oral Cancer, *J. Oral Pathol. Med., 25,* 97, March, 1996.

7. **Epstein,** J.B., Oakley, C., Millner, A., Emerton, S., van der Meij, E., and Le, N.: The Utility of Toluidine Blue Application as a Diagnostic Aid in Patients Previously Treated for Upper Oropharyngeal Carcinoma, *Oral Surg. Oral Med. Oral Pathol. Oral Radiol. Endod., 83,* 537, May, 1997.

8. **Sandler,** H.C. and Stahl, S.S.: Exfoliative Cytology as a Diagnostic Aid in the Detection of Oral Neoplasms, *J. Oral Surg., 16,* 414, September, 1958.

9. **Sabes,** W.R.: *The Dentist and Clinical Laboratory Procedures.* St. Louis, Mosby, 1979, pp. 109–113.

10. **Denham,** D. and Gillespie, J.: *Family Violence Handbook for the Dental Community.* Mental Health Division and Health Service Systems Division, Health Services Directorate, Health Canada, December, 1994.

11. **American Academy of Pediatric Dentistry**: Oral Health Policies, Definition of Dental Neglect, *Pediatr. Dent., 18,* 25, Special Issue, Number 6, 1996.

12. **Lachs,** M.S. and Pillemer, K.: Abuse and Neglect of Elderly Persons, *N. Engl. J. Med., 332,* 437, February 16, 1995.

13. **Kittelson,** L: Substance Abuse, in American Dental Association: *ADA Guide to Dental Therapeutics.* Chicago, ADA Publishing Co., 1998, pp. 517–526.

14. **Dello Russo,** N.M. and Temple, H.V.: Cocaine Effects on Gingiva (Letters to the Editor), *J. Am. Dent. Assoc., 104,* 13, January, 1982.

15. **Yukna,** R.A.: Cocaine Periodontitis, *Int. J. Periodontics Restorative Dent., 11,* 73, No. 1, 1991.

16. **Lee,** C.Y.S., Mohammad, H., and Dixon, R.A.: Medical and Dental Implications of Cocaine Abuse, *J. Oral Maxillofac. Surg., 49,* 290, March, 1991.

17. **Glick,** M.: Intravenous Drug Users: A Consideration for Infective Endocarditis in Dentistry? *Oral Surg. Oral Med. Oral Pathol., 80,* 125, August, 1995.

SUGGESTED READINGS

Abdel-Salam, M., Mayall, B.H., Chew, K., Silverman, S., and Greenspan, J.S.: Which Oral White Lesions Will Become Malignant? An Image Cytometric Study, *Oral Surg. Oral Med. Oral Pathol., 69,* 345, March, 1990.

Allen, C.M.: Diagnosing and Managing Oral Candidiasis, *J. Am. Dent. Assoc., 123,* 77, January, 1992.

Bottomley, W.K., Brown, R.S., and Lavigne, G.J.: A Retrospective Survey of the Oral Conditions of 981 Patients Referred to an Oral Medicine Private Practice, *J. Am. Dent. Assoc., 120,* 529, May, 1990.

Cataldo, E.: The Early Warning Signs of Oral Cancer, *DentalHygienistNews, 7,* 15, Spring, 1994.

Cormier, L. and Lavelle, C.L.B.: The Dental Hygienist's Role in Screening for Oral Cancer, *Canad. Dent. Hyg. Assoc./Probe, 29,* 53, March/April, 1995.

DeMattei, R. and Aubertin, M.: Dental Hygiene Screening Reveals Childhood Neck Mass, *J. Dent. Hyg., 70,* 225, November–December, 1996.

Epstein, J.B. and Scully, C.: Assessing the Patient at Risk for Oral Squamous Cell Carcinoma, *Spec. Care Dentist., 17,* 120, July/August, 1997.

Evans, D.E. and Haring, J.I.: Sentry Duty: On Guard for Oral Cancer, *RDH, 16,* 30, November, 1996.

Flaitz, C.M. and Coleman, G.C.: Differential Diagnosis of Oral Enlargements in Children, *Pediatr. Dent., 17,* 294, July/August, 1995.

Hays, G.L., Lippman, S.M., Flaitz, C.M., Brown, R.S., Pang, A.,

Devoll, R., and Hong, W.K.: Co-carcinogenesis and Field Cancerization: Oral Lesions Offer First Signs, *J. Am. Dent. Assoc., 126,* 47, January, 1995.

Johnson, N.: Oral Cancer Screening (Part 5 in Oral Cancer Series), *FDI World, 7,* 14, January/February, 1998.

Jones, A.C., Migliorati, C.A., and Stewart, C.M.: Oral Cytology: Indications, Contraindications, and Technique, *Gen. Dent., 43,* 74, January–February, 1995.

Layfield, L.L. Shopper, T.P., and Weir, J.C.: A Diagnostic Survey of Biopsied Gingival Lesions, *J. Dent. Hyg., 69,* 175, July–August, 1995.

Muzyka, B.C. and Glick, M.: A Review of Oral Fungal Infections and Appropriate Therapy, *J. Am. Dent. Assoc., 126,* 63, January, 1995.

Price, S.S. and Lewis, M.W.: Body Piercing Involving Oral Sites, *J. Am. Dent. Assoc., 128,* 1017, July, 1997.

Robinson, H.B.G. and Miller, A.S.: *Colby, Kerr, and Robinson's Color Atlas of Oral Pathology,* 5th ed. Philadelphia, J.B. Lippincott Co., 1990, pp. 85–124.

Williamson, G.F. and Summerlin, D.-J.: Evaluating Oral Lesions. A Systematic Approach With Exercises, *J. Dent. Hyg., 66,* 264, July–August, 1992.

Zimmers, P.L. and Gobetti, J.P.: Head and Neck Lesions Commonly Found in Musicians, *J. Am. Dent. Assoc., 125,* 1487, November, 1994.

Temporomandibular Disorder

Ash, M.M.: *Oral Pathology, An Introduction to General and Oral Pathology for Hygienists,* 6th ed. Philadelphia, Lea & Febiger, 1992, pp. 293–306.

Dworkin, S.F.: Perspectives on the Interaction of Biological, Psychological and Social Factors in TMD, *J. Am. Dent. Assoc., 125,* 856, July, 1994.

Greene, C.S.: Managing TMD Patients: Initial Therapy is the Key, *J. Am. Dent. Assoc., 123,* 43, June, 1992.

Harriman, L.P., Snowdon, D.A., Messer, L.B., Rysavy, D.M., Ostwald, S.K., Lai, C.-H., and Soberay, A.H.: Temporomandibular Joint Dysfunction and Selected Health Parameters in the Elderly, *Oral Surg. Oral Med. Oral Pathol., 70,* 406, October, 1990.

Okeson, J.P.: Current Terminology and Diagnostic Classification Schemes, *Oral Surg. Oral Med. Oral Pathol., 83,* 61, January, 1997.

Pertes, R.A. and Cohen, H.V.: Guidelines for Clinical Management of Temporomandibular Disorders: Part 1, *Compend. Cont. Educ. Dent., 13,* 268, April, 1992.

Truelove, E.L., Sommers, E.E., LeResche, L., Dworkin, S.F., and von Korff, M.: Clinical Diagnostic Criteria for TMD. New Classification Permits Multiple Diagnoses, *J. Am. Dent. Assoc., 123,* 47, April, 1992.

Family Abuse

Chiodo, G.T., Tilden, V.P., Limandri, B.J., and Schmidt, T.A.: Addressing Family Violence Among Dental Patients: Assessment and Intervention, *J. Am. Dent. Assoc., 125,* 69, January, 1994.

Dym, H.: The Abused Patient, *Dent. Clin. North Am., 39,* 621, July, 1995.

Gibson-Howell, J.C.: Domestic Violence Identification and Referral, *J. Dent. Hyg., 70,* 74, March–April, 1996.

Jorgensen, J.E.: A Dentist's Social Responsibility to Diagnose Elder Abuse, *Spec. Care Dentist., 12,* 113, May/June, 1992.

Kelly, M.A., Grace, E.G., and Wisnom, C.: Abuse of Older Persons: Detection and Prevention by Dental Professionals, *Gen. Dent., 40,* 30, January–February, 1992.

Kempe, C.H., Silverman, F.N., Steele, B.F., Droegemueller, W., and Silver, H.K.: The Battered Child Syndrome, *JAMA, 181,* 17, July 7, 1962.

McNeese, M.C. and Hebeler, J.R.: The Abused Child. A Clinical Approach to Identification and Management, *CIBA Clinical Symposia, 29,* No. 5, 1977, 36 pp.

Mouden, L.D. and Bross, D.G.: Legal Issues Affecting Dentistry's Role in Preventing Child Abuse and Neglect, *J. Am. Dent. Assoc., 126,* 1173, August, 1995.

Mouden, L.D. and Smedstad, B.: Reporting Child Abuse and Neglect. The Dental Hygienist's Role, *DentalHygienistNews, 8,* 15, Number 4, 1995.

Mouden, L.D.: The Hygienist's Role in Recognizing and Reporting Child Abuse and Neglect, *J. Pract. Hyg., 5,* 25, March/April, 1996.

Ochs, H.A., Neuenschwander, M.C., and Dodson, T.B.: Are Head, Neck and Facial Injuries Markers of Domestic Violence? *J. Am. Dent. Assoc., 127,* 757, June, 1996.

Substance Abuse

Duxbury, A.J.: Ecstasy: Dental Implications, *Br. Dent. J., 175,* 38, July 10, 1993.

Kapila, Y.L. and Kashani, H.: Cocaine-associated Rapid Gingival Recession and Dental Erosion. A Case Report, *J. Periodontol., 68,* 485, May, 1997.

Leshner, A.I.: Molecular Mechanisms of Cocaine Addiction, *N. Engl. J. Med., 335,* 128, July 11, 1996.

Meltzer, L: Substance Abuse and Chemical Dependency, *Access, 10,* 31, August, 1996.

Mendelson, J.H. and Mello, N.K.: Management of Cocaine Abuse and Dependence, *N. Engl. J. Med., 334,* 965, April 11, 1996.

Mitchell-Lewis, D.A., Phelan, J.A., Kelly, R.B., Bradley, J.J., and Lamster, I.B.: Identifying Oral Lesions Associated with Crack Cocaine Use, *J. Am. Dent. Assoc., 125,* 1104, August, 1994.

O'Connor, P.G., Selwyn, P.A., and Schottenfeld, R.S.: Medical Care for Injection-drug Users with Human Immunodeficiency Virus Infection, *N. Engl. J. Med., 331,* 450, August 18, 1994.

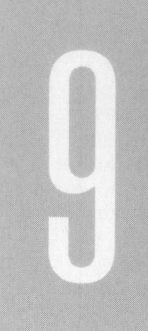

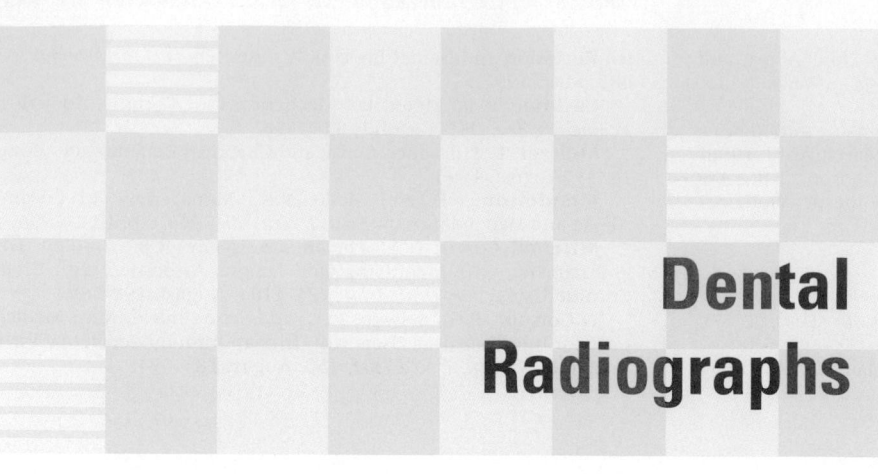

Dental Radiographs

Radiographs are essential adjuncts to other means of assessment when planning the complete care program for a patient. They provide the clinician with an important diagnostic tool that can be used to detect lesions, diseases, conditions of teeth and supporting structures; to localize foreign objects; to assess growth and development; to demonstrate changes and progress of a condition over time.[1]

The dentist is responsible for determining the need for radiographs. Designation of the number and types of dental exposures must be made selectively only after a review of the patient's health history and a complete clinical examination.[2] A history of oral and body exposures to radiation is needed. Excessive dental exposure to low levels of ionizing radiation cannot be justified.[3]

The objective in radiography is to use procedures that require the least amount of radiation exposure possible to produce radiographs of the greatest interpretive value. The first consideration is to limit the number of exposures to those that have been determined necessary. Quality assurance then can be accomplished by application of known safety measures for the patient and the clinician and by following precise steps for exposure and processing.

This chapter provides a summary of terminology and fundamentals of x-ray production. Procedures are included for film exposure and processing, safety factors, analysis of the completed radiographs, and suggestions for patient instruction.

Selected terms used in the study of radiography are listed and defined in Box 9-1. Other terms are described throughout the chapter.* Table 9-1 provides a list of universally used abbreviations.

ORIGIN AND CHARACTERISTICS OF X RAYS

I. HISTORY

Wilhelm C. Roentgen first discovered x rays in 1895. They were called *x rays* after the mathematical symbol *"x"* for an unknown. Professor Roentgen used a Hittorf-Crookes tube to determine if cathode rays produced were strong enough to penetrate the glass wall.[4] It was not until 1913 that William D. Coolidge designed a tube in which electricity was used instead of gas. Modern x-ray tubes have the same principles of construction as those of the Coolidge tube. The development of the science of radiology and radiography is a tribute to the early researchers and their efforts.

*Definitions in this chapter are taken from or adapted from and in accord with the *Glossary of Maxillofacial Radiology,* 3rd ed., prepared by the American Academy of Oral and Maxillofacial Radiology, 1990.

TABLE 9-1 Abbreviations Used in Radiography

ALARA	As Low as Reasonably Achievable
Gy	gray
HVL	half value layer
kVp	kilovolt peak
mA	milliampere
mAi	milliampere impulse
mAs	milliampere second
mGy	milligray
MPD	maximum permissible dose
mSv	millisievert
PID	position-indicating device
R	roentgen
rad	radiation absorbed dose
rem	roentgen equivalent man
Sv	sievert
XCP	extension cone paralleling

II. DEFINITION AND CHARACTERISTICS

X-ray energy is electromagnetic ionizing radiation of very short wavelengths, resulting from the bombardment of a material (usually tungsten) by highly accelerated electrons in a high vacuum. Electric and magnetic fields positioned at right angles to one another produce the electromagnetic energy.

The various types of energy in the electromagnetic spectrum have similar attributes; the properties of x rays are listed in Table 9-2.

HOW X RAYS ARE PRODUCED

Essential to x-ray production are (1) a source of electrons, (2) a high voltage to accelerate the electrons, and (3) a target to stop the electrons. The parts of the tube and the circuits within the machine are designed to provide these elements.

I. THE X-RAY TUBE (Figure 9-1)

A. Protective Tube Housing

Heavy metal enclosure that houses the x-ray tube and reduces the primary radiation to permissible exposure levels.

B. X-Ray Tube

A highly vacuated glass tube surrounded by

BOX 9-1 KEY WORDS: Radiography

Ammeter: an instrument for measuring electric current in amperes.

Attenuation (ah-ten"ū-ā'shun): the process by which a beam of radiation is reduced in intensity when passing through some material; the combination of absorption and scattering processes leads to a decrease in flux density of the beam when projected through matter.

Circuit: the complete path of an electric current including the source of electrical energy.

Cassette (kah-set'): a light-tight container in which x-ray films are placed for exposure to x radiation; usually backed with lead to reduce the effect of backscatter radiation; may be made of cardboard or of metal with an exposure side of Bakelite, aluminum, or magnesium and containing an intensifying screen(s).

Cone-cut: An error of technique that results when the PID is not angled for the beam of radiation to cover completely the film being exposed.

Intensifying screen: a card or plastic sheet coated with fluorescent material positioned singly or in pairs in a cassette to contact the film; when the cassette is exposed to x radiation, the visible light from the fluorescent image on the screen adds to the latent image produced directly by x radiation.

Impulse: the burst of radiation generated during a half cycle of alternating current; film exposure time is measured in impulses.

Irradiation (ĭ-rā"dē-ā'shun): the exposure to radiation; one speaks of radiation therapy and of irradiation of a body part.

Latent image: the invisible change produced in an x-ray film emulsion by the action of x radiation or light from which the visible image is subsequently developed and fixed chemically.

Panoramic radiography: an extraoral radiographic technique used to examine the maxillary and mandibular jaws on a single film.

Penumbra (pĕ-nŭm'brah): the secondary shadow that surrounds the periphery of the primary shadow; in radiography, it is the blurred margin of an image detail (geometric unsharpness).

Photoelectric effect: the ejection of bound electrons by an incident photon such that the whole energy of the photon is absorbed and transitional or characteristic x-ray emissions are produced.

Photon (fō'ton): a finite bundle of energy of visible light or electromagnetic radiation.

Radiation: the emission and propagation of energy through space or a material medium in the form of waves or particles. Types of radiation are defined in Box 9-2.

Radiograph: a visible image on a radiation-sensitive film emulsion produced by chemical processing after exposure of the film emulsion to ionizing radiation that has passed through an area, region, or substance of interest.

Radiography: the art and science of making radiographs.

Radiologic health: the art and science of protecting human beings from injury by radiation, as well as of promoting better health through beneficial applications of radiation.

Radiology: that branch of science that deals with the use of radiant energy in the diagnosis and treatment of disease.

Rare earth: commonly used to refer to intensifying screens that contain rare earth elements; it may also refer to a screen-film system used for x-ray imaging; the systems are considered "fast" exposure systems.

Rectification: conversion of alternating current (AC) to direct current (DC); a **rectifier** changes AC to DC.

Soma (sō'mah): the entire body with the exclusion of germ cells. Somatic (so-măt'ik): adj.

Subtraction radiography: a photographic or digital method of eliminating background anatomic structures from the final image, thus bringing out the differences between the pre- and postprocedure radiographic images.

Digital subtraction radiography: a radiographic image subtraction method in which the pre- and postprocedure radiographic images are digitized into the computer memory; these images are subtracted from each other within the computer memory, and the resultant subtracted image is displayed on the monitor.

Tomography: a radiographic technique used to image a selected plane of tissue while blurring structures that are outside of the selected plane.

Xeroradiography (zē"rō-rā"dē-og'rah-fē): a dry process that produces prints of x-ray images by means of a selenium plate, which records an image through the radiation-induced discharge of a positive electrostatic potential.

TABLE 9-2 Properties of X Rays

CHARACTERISTIC

- invisible
- no mass
- no weight

TRAVEL

- in straight line; can be scattered
- at the speed of light

WAVELENGTHS

- have short wavelengths, high frequency
- hard x rays: short wavelengths, high penetration
- soft x rays: relatively longer wavelengths; relatively less penetrating; more likely to be absorbed into the tissue

PENETRATION

- pass through matter, or
- absorbed by matter, depending on atomic structure of matter

CAUSES

- ionization
- fluorescence of certain crystals
- biologic changes in living cells

PRODUCES

- an image on photographic film

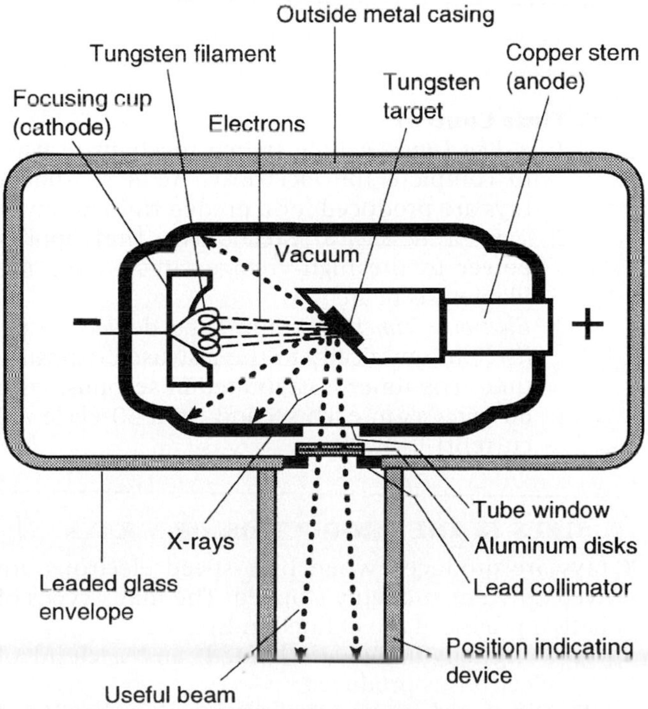

FIGURE 9-1 X-Ray Tube. High-speed electrons flowing from cathode to anode hit the tungsten target, create x-ray photons. X rays exit through the tube window and position indicating device.

a specially refined oil with high insulating powers.

C. Cathode (−)
1. Tungsten filament, which is heated to generate a cloud of electrons.
2. Molybdenum cup around the filament to focus the electrons toward the anode.

D. Anode (+)
1. Copper stem containing a tungsten button, the target, positioned opposite the cathode at an angle.
2. Focal spot (tungsten target), the part of the target on the anode bombarded by the focused electron stream when the tube is energized.

E. Aperture
Where the useful beam emerges from the tube; covered with a permanent seal of glass or aluminum.

F. Aluminum Disks
Thin (0.5 mm) sheets of aluminum placed at the aperture to filter out longer wavelength x rays.

G. Lead Diaphragm
A lead collimator with a hole to restrict the size of the x-ray beam.

H. Position-Indicating Device (PID)
Open-ended lead-lined cylinder that shapes and aims the x-ray beam.

II. CIRCUITS

A circuit is the complete path over which an electrical current may flow. Two circuits are used to produce x rays. Refer to Figure 9-2 to examine the electrical circuits in a dental x-ray machine.

A. Low-voltage filament circuit.

B. High-voltage cathode–anode circuit.

III. TRANSFORMERS

A transformer increases or decreases the incoming voltage.

A. Autotransformer
A voltage compensator that corrects minor variations in line voltage.

B. Filament Step-down Transformer
Decreases the line voltage to approximately 3 volts to heat the filament and form the electron cloud.

C. High-Voltage Step-up Transformer
Increases the current (110 volts) to 70 or 90 kVp (kilovoltage peak) to give electrons the required high speed to produce x-ray photons.

IV. MACHINE CONTROL DEVICES

Machines vary, but, in general, when operating an

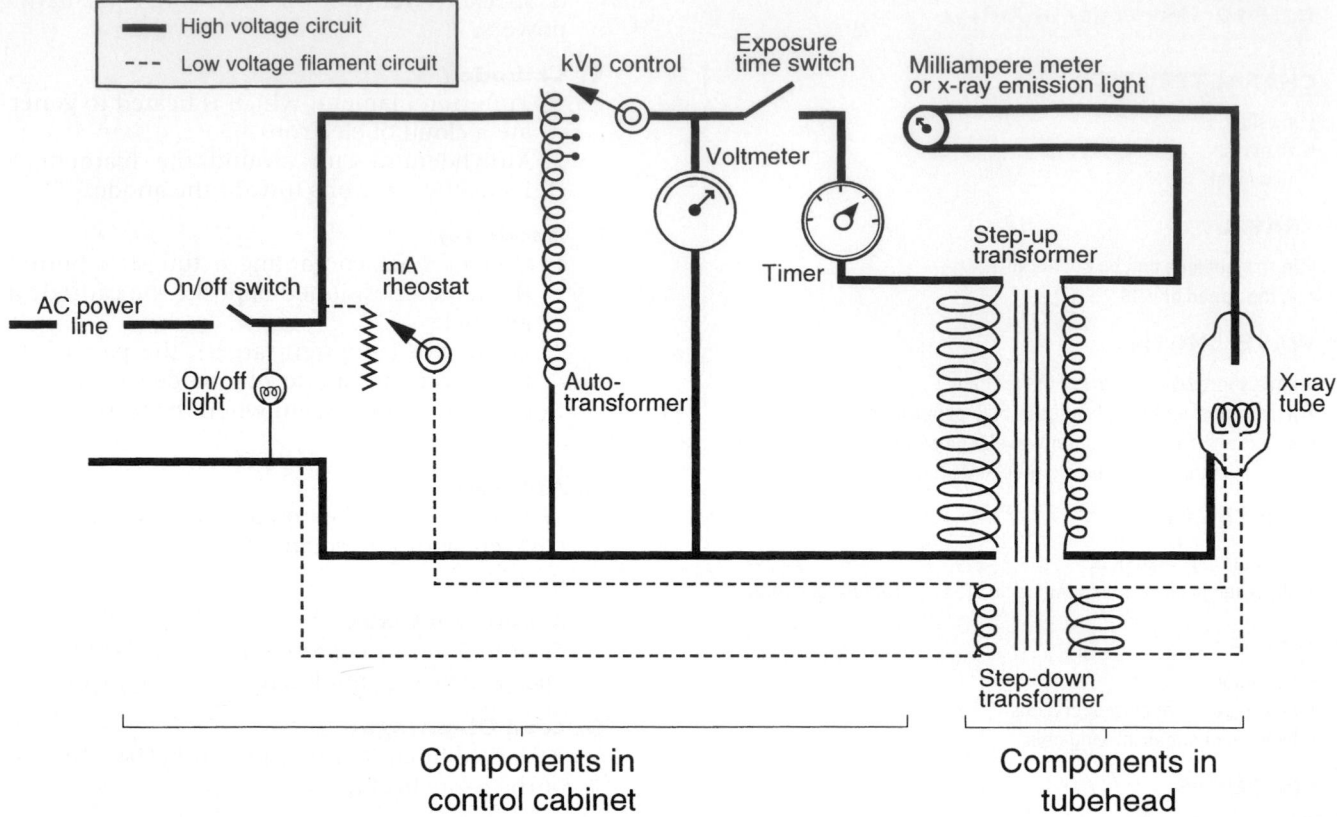

FIGURE 9-2 Dental X-Ray Machine Circuits. High- and low-voltage circuits in a dental x-ray machine demonstrating flow of electricity from on/off switch to the x-ray tubehead. (Adapted from Olson, S.S.: *Dental Radiography Laboratory Manual*, Philadelphia, W.B. Saunders, 1995, p. 40.)

x-ray machine, there are four factors to control: the line switch (to electrical outlet), the kilovoltage, the milliamperage, and the time.

A. Voltage Control

Voltage is the unit of measurement used to describe the force that pushes an electric current through a circuit.

1. *Circuit Voltmeter*. Registers line voltage before voltage is stepped up by the transformer (with alternating current, this is 110 volts), or may register the kilovoltage that results after step-up.

2. *kVp (Kilovoltage Peak) Selector*. Used to change the line voltage to a selected kilovoltage (70 to 90 kVp).

B. Milliamperage Control

1. *Ampere*. The unit of intensity of an electric current produced by 1 volt acting through a resistance of 1 ohm. A milliampere (mA) is 1/1000 of an ampere.

2. *Milliammeter*. Instrument used to select the actual current through the tube circuit during the time of exposure.

C. Time Control

1. *X-Ray Timer*. A time switch mechanism used to complete the electrical circuit so that x rays are produced for a predetermined time.

2. *Time-Delay Switch*. Mechanism that applies power to the high-voltage circuit once the filament is heated.

3. *Electronic Timer*. Vacuum tube device; resets itself automatically to the last-used exposure time. The timer is calibrated in seconds, with 60 *impulses* in each second (in a 60-cycle AC current).

V. STEPS IN THE PRODUCTION OF X RAYS

X rays are produced when high-speed electrons are slowed down or suddenly stopped. The many types of radiation produced are defined in Box 9-2.

A. Tungsten filament is heated, and a cloud of electrons is produced.

B. Difference in electrical potential is developed between the anode and the cathode.

C. Electrons are attracted to the anode from the cathode at high speed during the intervals of

BOX 9-2 KEY WORDS: Types of Radiation

Bremsstrahlung radiation (white radiation) (brĕm'strah-loong): a distribution of x rays from very low energy photons to those produced by the peak kilovoltage applied across an x-ray tube; bremsstrahlung means "braking radiation" and refers to the sudden deceleration of electrons (cathode rays) as they interact with highly positively charged nuclei, such as tungsten.

Characteristic radiation: the radiation produced by electron transitions from higher energy orbitals to replace ejected electrons of inner electron orbitals; the energy of the electromagnetic radiation emitted is unique or "characteristic" of the emitting atom.

Electromagnetic radiation: forms of energy propagated by wave motion as photons; the radiations differ widely in wavelength, frequency, and photo energy; examples are infrared waves, visible light, ultraviolent radiation, x rays, gamma rays, and cosmic radiation.

Gamma radiation: short-wavelength electromagnetic radiation of nuclear origin similar to x rays but usually of higher energy.

Leakage radiation: the radiation that escapes through the protective shielding of the x-ray unit tube head; it may be detected at the sides, top, bottom, or back of the tube head.

Primary radiation: all radiation coming directly from the target of the anode of an x-ray tube.

Scatter radiation: a form of secondary radiation that, during passage through a substance, has been deviated in direction; it may also have been modified by an increase in wavelength.

Backscatter: radiation deflected by scattering processes at angles greater than 90° to the original direction of the beam of radiation.

Coherent scattering (Thompson or unmodified): scattering of relatively low-energy x rays by elastic collisions without loss of photon energy.

Compton scatter radiation: the incident radiation that has sufficient energy to dislodge a bound electron, but attacks a loosely bound electron; the remaining radiation energy proceeds in a different direction as scatter radiation.

Secondary radiation: particles or photons produced by the interaction of primary radiation with matter.

Stray radiation: radiation that serves no useful purpose; it includes leakage, secondary, and scatter radiation.

---

the alternating current, when the anode is charged positive and the cathode negative. (During the alternating half of the cycle, the electrons are attracted back into the filament in a self-rectifying tube.)

D. Curvature of the molybdenum cup controls the direction of the electrons and causes them to be projected on the focal spot.

E. Reaction of the electrons as they strike the tungsten target results in loss of energy.
   1. Approximately 1% of the energy of electrons is converted to x-ray energy (larger percent at higher kilovoltages).
   2. Approximately 99% of the energy is converted to heat and is dissipated through the copper anode and oil of the protective tube housing.

F. Most high-speed electrons decelerate and come near or miss the target nuclei. These electrons lose kinetic energy, which is given off in the form of photons of electromagnetic radiation. The closer the high-speed electrons come to the nuclei, the greater will be the electrostatic attraction on the electrons. This causes a braking effect and results in Bremsstrahlung radiation.

G. *Characteristic radiation* results when a bombarding electron displaces an electron from a shell of the target atom, ionizing the atom. Another electron in an outer shell replaces the missing electron, causing a cascading effect. When the displaced electron is replaced, a photon is emitted, resulting in characteristic radiation. This only occurs above 70 kVp.

H. X rays leave the tube through the aperture to form the useful beam.

I. The beam is an emission of electromagnetic radiation.
   1. *Useful Beam.* The part of the primary radiation that is permitted to emerge from the tube head aperture and the accessory collimating devices.
   2. *Central Beam* (central ray). The center of the beam of x rays emitted from the tube.

COMPUTERIZED DIGITAL RADIOGRAPHY

Computerized digital radiography interfaces the dental x-ray machine and the computer to digitize the radiographic image so that it can be immediately displayed on the computer's monitor. Instead of using radiographic film, an image receptor plate or sensor is placed intraorally, and a traditional dental x-ray machine records the latent image onto the sensor.

Disposable sheaths are placed over the plate before it is positioned into a film holder. The sensor and film holder are then placed in the patient's mouth and exposed to radiation. A laser electronically processes the latent image in the sensor and then transmits the electronic signal to a computer screen where the image can be viewed. Besides reducing radiation to the patient, digital radiography eliminates the need for darkroom processing.[5]

CHARACTERISTICS OF AN ACCEPTABLE RADIOGRAPH

A *radiograph* is the visible image on a radiation-sensitive film emulsion. The image is produced by chemical processing after exposure of the film emulsion to ionizing radiation that has passed through an area, or, specifically for dentistry, through teeth or a part of the oral cavity. A *radiographic survey* refers to a series of radiographs.

Before making a radiograph, it is important to know the characteristics that will result in a finished radiograph of maximum value and will be truly useful for diagnosis. The basic essentials are the appearance of the image itself, the area covered, and the quality of the processed radiograph.

I. PARTS OF THE IMAGE

All parts of the image must be shown as close to their natural size and shape as possible with a minimum of distortion and superimposition.

II. AREA TO BE EXAMINED

The area being examined for assessment must be shown completely with sufficient surrounding tissue included for comparative interpretation.

III. QUALITY OF THE RADIOGRAPH

The quality depends on its density, contrast, and definition.

A. Radiolucency and Radiopacity

A radiograph has graduations from white to black that are referred to as radiopaque or radiolucent. For example, a dense material, such as a metallic restoration, prevents the passage of x rays and appears white on the processed radiograph. Soft tissue does not resist passage of x rays and, thus, appears black to gray.

1. *Radiopacity.* The appearance of light (white) images on a radiograph is a result of the lesser amount of radiation that penetrates the structures and reaches the film. A *radiopaque* structure inhibits the passage of x rays.
2. *Radiolucency.* The appearance of dark images on a radiograph is a result of the greater amount of radiation that penetrates the structures and reaches the film. A *radiolucent* structure permits the passage of radiation with relatively little attenuation by absorption.

B. Density

The density of a radiograph refers to the degree of darkening of the exposed and processed x-ray film. The term "background density" is used when referring to factors other than radiation that may have affected the appearance of the finished radiograph. Examples are exposure to white light and film used after its expiration date.

C. Contrast

Contrast means the visual differences in image density appearing between adjacent areas on a radiograph. Types of contrast are referred to as follows:

1. *Film Contrast.* A characteristic inherent in the type of film used.
2. *Long-Scale Contrast.* An increased range of grays between the blacks and whites on a radiograph. Higher voltages increase the range.
3. *Short-Scale Contrast.* A reduced range of grays between the blacks and whites on a radiograph. Lower kilovoltages decrease the range.
4. *Subject Contrast.* The relative difference in density and thickness of the components of the radiographed subject. Subject contrast relates to radiopacity and radiolucency.

D. Definition

Definition refers to the property of an image that pertains to the sharpness, distinctness, or clarity of outline. Inadequate definition may be related to movement of the patient, the film, or the tube head during exposure.

FACTORS THAT INFLUENCE THE FINISHED RADIOGRAPH

As the beam leaves the x-ray tube (Figure 9-1) it is collimated, filtered, and allowed to travel a designated source–film (or focal spot–film) distance before reaching the film of a selected speed. The quality or diagnostic usefulness of the finished radiograph, as well as the total exposure of the patient and clinician, are influenced by the *collimation, filtration, kilovoltage, milliampere seconds, source–film distance, and film speed.*

Film processing (pages 162 to 165) also influences directly the quality of the radiograph and indirectly the total exposure. Re-exposure would be necessary should the film be rendered inadequate during processing.

I. COLLIMATION

Collimation is the technique for controlling the size

and shape of the beam of radiation emitted through the aperture of the tube. A *collimator* is a diaphragm or system of diaphragms made of an absorbing material designed to define the dimensions and direction of a beam of radiation.

A. Purposes

1. Eliminate peripheral or more divergent radiation.
2. Minimize exposure to patient's face.
3. Minimize secondary radiation, which can fog the film and expose the bodies of patient and clinician.

B. Methods

1. *Diaphragm.* A diaphragm usually is made of lead with a central aperture of the smallest practical diameter for making radiographic exposure; it is located between the x-ray tube and the position-indicating device (PID).
   a. Recommended thickness of lead: ⅛ inch.
   b. Recommended size of aperture: to permit a diameter of the beam of radiation equal to 2¾ inches at the end of the PID next to the patient's face.
2. *Rectangular Collimation.* As shown in Figure 9-3, a patient receives far less unnecessary radiation with the use of a rectangular PID because the size of the beam is greatly reduced. When a rectangular collimeter is used, it should be approximately 1½ × 2 in. at the skin. A rectangular collimeter must be rotated to accommodate films positioned horizontally or vertically.
3. *Lead-Lined Cylindrical PID.*
   The PID was formerly called the "cone" or "plastic cone." Research has shown that the PID must be a lead-lined, open-ended cylinder to prevent secondary radiation.

C. Relation to Techniques

The dimensions of the largest periapical film are 1¼ × 1⅝ in.[2] Precise angulation techniques are required to eliminate "cone-cut" of film, particularly when rectangular collimation is used. "Cone-cut" refers to an error of technique that results when the PID is not angled for the beam of radiation to cover completely the film being exposed. The term "cone-cut" is still commonly used and is used in this chapter.

II. FILTRATION

Filtration is the insertion of absorbers or filters for the preferential attenuation of radiation from a primary beam of x radiation. Two different types of filters provide filtration in the dental x-ray machine.

A. Types of Filters

1. *Aluminum filters* remove low-energy x-ray photons from the x-ray beam.

2. *Rare earth filters* selectively remove both low- and high-energy photons from the x-ray beam. Examples of rare earth filters include samarium, erbium, yttrium, niobium, gadolinium, terbium-activated gadolinium oxysulfide, and thulium-activated lanthanum oxybromide.

B. Purpose

To minimize exposure of the patient's skin to unnecessary radiation that will not reach and expose the film.

C. Methods

1. *Inherent Filtration.* Includes the glass envelope encasing the x-ray tube and the glass window in the tube housing (Figure 9-1).
2. *Added Filtration.* Thin, commercially pure aluminum disks inserted between the lead diaphragm and the x-ray tube.
3. *Total Filtration.* The sum of inherent and added filtration.
   a. Recommended total is the equivalent of 0.5 mm (below 50 kVp); 1.5 mm (50 to 70 kVp); and 2.5 mm (over 70 kVp) of aluminum.
   b. Check the inherent filtration of the individual x-ray machine; then add a sufficient amount of commercially pure aluminum or rare earth elements to bring the total to the recommended level.

D. Disadvantage of Added Filtration

Some secondary radiation is produced that can scatter in all directions.

III. KILOVOLTAGE

Kilovoltage is the potential difference between the anode and cathode of an x-ray tube. The kilovoltage peak (kVp) refers to the crest value (in kilovolts) of the potential difference of a pulsating generator. When only one-half of the wave is used, the value refers to the useful half of the cycle.

A. Amount of Kilovoltage

Determines the quality of the x radiation.

1. Kilovoltage creates a difference in potential between the anode and the cathode for the production of x rays.
2. The higher the kilovoltage, the greater the acceleration of the electrons, and the greater the force with which they bombard the target results in a shorter wavelength of x rays.
3. The shorter the wavelength, the greater the penetrating power at the skin surface.

B. Use of High Kilovoltage (90 kVp)

1. Density of the finished radiograph increases with increased kilovoltage (other factors remaining constant).
2. To maintain the proper film density, the mil-

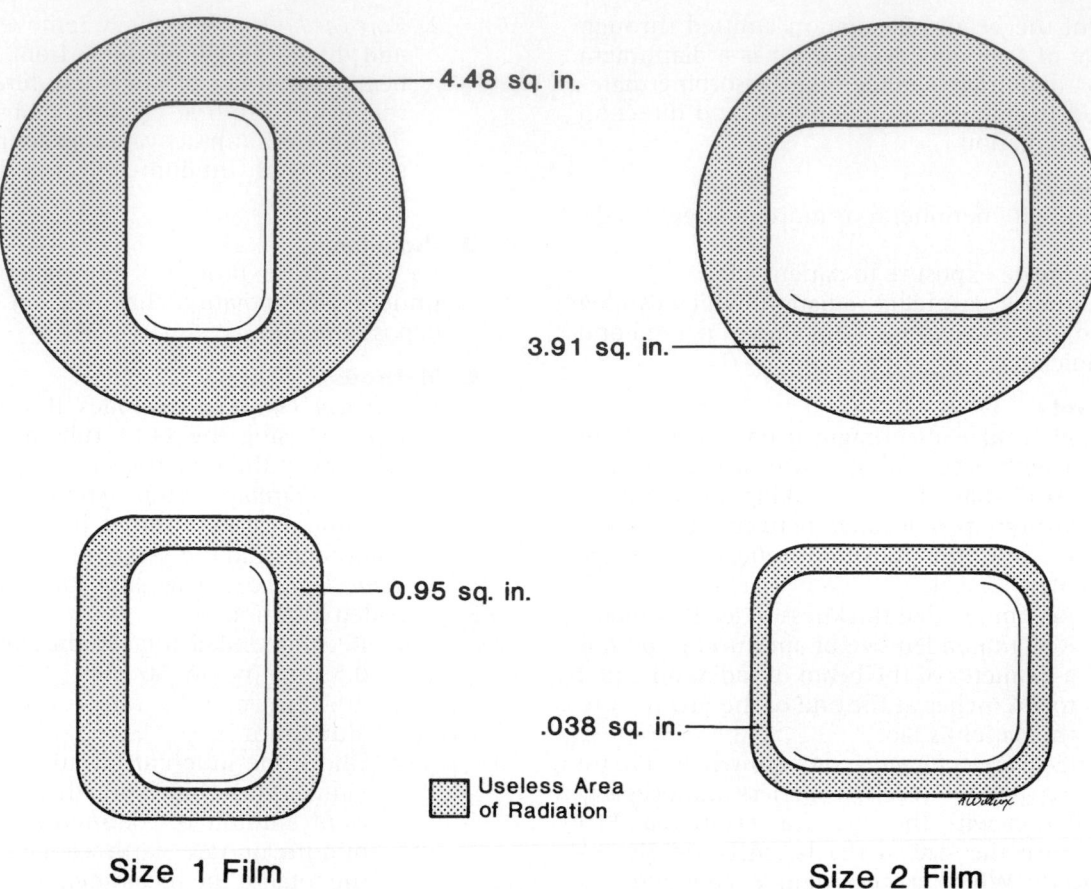

4.48 sq. in.

3.91 sq. in.

0.95 sq. in.

.038 sq. in.

☐ Useless Area
of Radiation

Size 1 Film

Size 2 Film

■ **FIGURE 9-3 Cylindrical and Rectangular Position-Indicating Devices.** The useless areas of radiation are greatly lessened when rectangular collimation is used. The patient can be spared exposure to excess radiation. (Redrawn from Shannon, S.A.: Rectangular Versus Cylindrical Collimation, *Dent. Hyg.*, *61*, 173, April, 1987; copyright 1987 by the American Dental Hygienists' Association.)

liampere seconds must be decreased as the kVp is increased.
3. Variation in contrast
   a. Low kilovoltage. High contrast, with sharp black-white differences in densities between adjacent areas, but small range of distinction between subject thicknesses recorded.
   b. High kilovoltage. Low contrast, with wide range of subject thicknesses recorded; greater range of densities from black to white (more gray tones), which, when examined under proper viewing conditions, provide more interpretive details.
4. Advantages
   a. Permits shorter exposure time.
   b. Reduces exposure to tissues lying in front of the film packet.
5. Disadvantages
   a. Increased radiation to tissues outside the edges of the film.
   b. More internal scattered radiation at 90

kVp than at 70 kVp once the primary beam has hit the film, but more scatter at the face with 70 kVp.

IV. MILLIAMPERE SECONDS

A. Milliamperage

The measure of the electron current passing through the x-ray tube; it regulates the heat of the filament, which determines the number of electrons available to bombard the target.

B. Quantity of Radiation

Quantity of radiation is expressed in milliampere seconds (mAs).
1. Definition: mAs is the milliamperes multiplied by the exposure time in seconds; mAi is the milliamperes multiplied by the exposure time in impulses.
2. Example: At 10 milliamperes for ½ second, the exposure of the film would be 5 mAs. At 10 milliamperes for 15 impulses, the exposure of the film would be 150 mAi.

C. Radiographic Density

Radiographic density increases with increased milliamperage and/or time of exposure (other factors remaining constant).

V. DISTANCE

Several distances are involved in x-ray film exposure. The object–film, the source–film, and the source–surface distances must be considered for film placement.

A. Object–Film Distance

The object–film distance refers to the distance between the object (tooth) and the film.

With the paralleling technique and the use of a film holder, the object–film distance is greater than it is for the bisecting-angle technique. A collimated beam and increased source–film distance compensate to preserve definition and film quality.

B. Source–Film Distance

The PID on the x-ray machine is designed to indicate the direction of the central axis of the x-ray beam and to serve as a guide in establishing desired source–surface and source–film distances. Techniques using 8- and 16-inch source–film distances are common.

The source–film distance is the sum total of the distance from the source to the PID within the tube housing, the length of the PID, and the distance from the end of the PID (at the face) to the film. Directions in technique call for lightly touching the skin with the end of the PID to standardize the source–film distance.

Principles related to source–film distance are as follows:

1. The intensity of the x-ray beam varies inversely as the square of the source–film distance. For example, if two films of the same speed were used, one at a 16-inch source–film distance and one at an 8-inch distance, with all other factors, such as kVp and mAs, remaining constant, the film at 16 inches would require four times the exposure (time) to maintain the same density in the finished radiograph.
2. The exposure decreases as the distance increases; when the distance is made twice as great, the radiation exposure to the patient is reduced to one-fourth.
3. To maintain film density when distance is increased, an increase in mAs, kVp, or film speed is required.

C. Advantages in the Use of an Extended Source–Film Distance

1. Definition or distinctness and clarity of detail improve (because the image is produced by the most central rays).
2. Enlargement or magnification of image decreases (because at shorter distances the outer, more divergent rays tend to enlarge or magnify the image).
3. Skin exposure of the patient is reduced.
4. Less tissue is within the primary beam of radiation, because less spreading of the x-ray beam occurs.

VI. FILMS

With optimum filtration, collimation, and fast film, the skin dose to the face can be reduced significantly. Within recent years, the manufacture of very slow speed films has been discontinued, the speed of many films has been doubled, and the use of higher speed films has gained increased acceptance by the dental profession.

A. Film Composition

A film is a thin, transparent sheet of cellulose acetate or similar material coated on one or both sides with an emulsion sensitive to radiation and light.

1. *Emulsion.* Gelatin containing a suspension of countless tiny crystals of silver halide salts (mostly silver bromide).
2. *Film Packet.* Sealed paper envelope that is small, lightproof, and moisture resistant, containing an x-ray film (or two) and a thin sheet of lead foil.
   a. Two-film packet: Useful for processing one film differently from the other to make diagnostic comparisons; for sending to specialist to whom patient may be referred; for legal evidence.
   b. Purpose of lead foil backing: To prevent exposure of the film by scattered radiation that could enter from back of packet, and to protect the patient's tissues lying in the path of the x ray.

B. Film Speed

Film speed or film emulsion speed refers to the sensitivity of the film to radiation exposure. The speed is the amount of exposure required to produce a certain image density. The smaller the grain size, the slower the film speed.

1. *Classification.* Films have been classified by the American National Standard Institute (ANSI) in cooperation with the American Dental Association (ADA). The ANSI/ADA Specification No. 22 designates 6 groups, A through F. Speed groups A, B, and C, the slowest, are associated with excess radiation exposure and are no longer used. Only film speeds D or faster are used for dental purposes. E-speed film can reduce the radiation exposure to the patient by as much as 50% over D-speed film.
2. *Choice.* E-speed film is recommended for use with rectangular collimation for marked reduction in radiation exposure.

EXPOSURE TO RADIATION

I. IONIZING RADIATION

Ionizing radiation is electromagnetic radiation (for example, x rays or gamma rays) or particulate radiation (for example, electrons, neutrons, protons) capable of ionizing air directly or indirectly.

The phenomenon of separation of electrons from molecules to change their chemical activity is called ionization. The organic and inorganic compounds that make up the human body may be altered by exposure to ionizing radiation. The biologic effects following irradiation are secondary effects in that they result from physical, chemical, and biologic action set in motion by the absorption of energy from radiation.

II. FACTORS THAT WOULD INFLUENCE THE BIOLOGIC EFFECTS OF RADIATION

   A. Quality of the radiation
   B. Chemical composition of the absorbing medium
   C. Sensitivity of tissues
   D. Total dose and dose rate
   E. Blood supply to the tissues
   F. Size of the area exposed
   G. Somatic versus genetic cells
     Radiation to the somatic tissues will affect the irradiated individual only, whereas radiation to the genetic tissues will affect offspring and possibly future generations.

III. EXPOSURE

A. Types of Exposure

Exposure is a measure of the x radiation to which a person or object, or a part of either, is exposed at a certain place; this measure is based on its ability to produce ionization.
1. *Threshold Exposure.* The minimum exposure that produces a detectable degree of any given effect.
2. *Entrance or Surface Exposure.* Exposure measured at the surface of an irradiated body, part, or object. It includes primary radiation and backscatter from the irradiated underlying tissue. The term skin exposure is used with reference to the exposure measured at the center of an irradiated skin surface area.
3. *Erythema Exposure.* The radiation necessary to produce a temporary redness of the skin.

B. Exposure Units[6]

The units of absorbed dose are expressed in joules/kilogram (1 rad = 0.01 J/kg). The units shown in Table 9-3 are the recommendations of the International Commission on Radiation Units and Measurements.

The unit of measurement is the *gray* (Gy). An absorbed dose of 1 gray is equal to 1 J/kg; therefore, an absorbed dose of 1 Gy is equal to 100 rad.

The unit of biologic equivalence is the *sievert* (Sv). 1 Sv = 100 rem.

C. Dose

The radiation dose is the amount of energy absorbed per unit mass of tissue at a site of interest. The kinds of doses are defined in Box 9-3.

D. Permissible Dose

The amount of radiation that may be received by an individual within a specified period without expectation of any significantly harmful result is called the *permissible dose.*

Assumptions on which permissible doses are calculated include the following:
1. No irradiation is beneficial.
2. There is a dose below which no somatic cellular changes can be produced.
3. Children are more susceptible than older people.
4. There is a dose below which, even though it is delivered before the end of the reproductive period, the probability of genetic effects is slight.

TABLE 9-3 Radiation Units

Definition	Traditional Unit	S.I. Unit*	Equivalent
Unit of radiation exposure	Roentgen (R)	Coulomb per kilogram (C/kg)	$1 \text{ R} = 2.58 \times 10^{-4} \text{ C/kg}$
Unit of absorbed dose	Rad	Gray (Gy)	100 rad = 1 Gy
Unit of dose equivalent	Rem	Sievert (Sv)	100 rem = 1 Sv
Unit of radioactivity	Curie (Ci)	Becquerel (Bq)	$1 \text{ Ci} = 3.7 \times 10^{10} \text{ Bq}$

*S.I. (System International) is from the French *Système International d'Unités.*

BOX 9-3 KEY WORDS AND ABBREVIATIONS: Types of Radiation Doses

Absorbed dose: the amount of energy imparted by ionizing radiation to a unit mass of irradiated material at a specific exposure point; the unit of absorbed dose is the gray (Gy).

Cumulative dose: the total dose resulting from repeated exposures to radiation of the same region or of the whole body.

Dose: the amount of energy absorbed per unit mass of tissue at a site of interest.

Dose equivalent: the product of absorbed dose and modifying factors, such as the quality factor, distribution factor, and any other necessary factors; different types of radiation cause differing biologic effects; the unit of dose equivalence is the sievert (Sv).

Dose rate: rate of exposure.

Erythema dose: the minimum quantity of x or gamma radiation that produces the appearance of redness (erythema).

Exit dose: the absorbed dose delivered by a beam of radiation to the surface through which the beam emerges from an object.

LD 50–30: the dose of radiation that is lethal for 50% of a large population in a specified period of time, usually 30 days.

Lethal dose: the amount of radiation that is, or could be, sufficient to cause death of an organism.

Maximum permissible dose: the maximum dose equivalent that a person (or specified parts of that person) is allowed to receive in a stated period of time; the dose of radiation that would not be expected to produce any significant radiation effects in a lifetime.

Skin dose (surface absorbed dose): the absorbed dose delivered by a radiation beam and backscatter at the point where the central ray passes through the superficial layer of the object.

Threshold dose: the minimum dose that produces a detectable degree of any effect.

E. Radiation Hazard

A condition under which persons might receive radiation in excess of the maximum permissible dose. Exposure would be a risk in an area where x-ray equipment is being used or where radioactive materials are stored.

F. National Council on Radiation Protection and Measurements[7]

1. *Limits for Dentists and Dental Personnel.* See Table 9-4.

2. *Limits for Patients.* Exposure to x radiation shall be kept to the minimum level consistent with clinical requirements. This limitation is determined by the professional judgment of the dentist.

3. *ALARA Concept.* Radiation exposures must be kept As Low As Reasonably Achievable. This concept is accepted and enforced by all regulatory agencies.

IV. SENSITIVITY OF CELLS

A. Factors Affecting Cell Sensitivity to Radiation

1. *Cell Differentiation.* Immature cells are most sensitive. Highly specialized cells are radioresistant.

2. *Mitotic Activity.* Rapidly reproducing cells are more sensitive; most sensitive when undergoing mitosis.

3. *Cell Metabolism.* Cells are more sensitive in periods of increased metabolism.

B. Radiosensitive and Radioresistant Tissues

1. Radiosensitive: a cell that is sensitive to radiation.

2. Radioresistant: a cell that is resistant to radiation.

3. Radiation sensitivity of tissues and organs: the relative sensitivities are shown in Table 9-5.

TABLE 9-4 Maximum Permissible Dose Equivalent Values (MPD)* to Whole Body, Gonads, Blood-Forming Organs, Lens of Eye

Average Weekly Exposure[†]	Maximum 13-week Exposure	Maximum Yearly Exposure	Maximum Accumulated Exposure[‡]
0.1 R	3 R	5 R	$5(N-18)$ R[§]

*Exposure of persons for dental or medical purposes is not counted against their maximum permissible exposure limits.

[†]Used only for the purpose of designating radiation barriers.

[‡]When the previous occupational history of an individual is not definitely known, it shall be assumed that the full dose permitted by the formula $5(N-18)$ has already been received.

[§]N = Age in years and is greater than 18. The unit for exposure is the roentgen (R).

TABLE 9-5 Radiation Sensitivity of Tissues and Organs

HIGH

Bone marrow
Reproductive cells
Intestines
Lymphoid tissue

MODERATELY HIGH

Oral mucosa
Skin

MODERATE

Growing bone
Growing cartilage
Small vasculature
Connective tissue

MODERATELY LOW

Salivary glands
Mature bone
Mature cartilage
Thyroid gland tissue

LOW

Liver
Optic Lens
Kidneys
Muscle
Nerve

C. **Tissue Reaction**
   1. *Latent Period.* Lapse between the time of exposure and the time when effects are observed. (May be as long as 25 years or relatively short, as in the case of the production of a skin erythema.)
   2. *Cumulative Effect*
      a. Amount of reaction depends on dose; reaction to radiation received in fractional doses is less than the reaction to one large dose.
      b. Partial or total repair occurs as long as destruction is not complete.
      c. Some irreparable damage may be cumulative as, little by little, more radiation is added (for example, hair loss, skin lesions, falling blood count).

RISK OF INJURY FROM RADIATION

The risk of injury from dental diagnostic radiation is extremely low; however, the more radiation received, the higher the chance of cellular injuries. With each exposure to radiation, cellular damage is followed by repair. The effects of radiation exposure are cumulative, and any cellular changes that are not repaired

result in damaged tissues. Most of the damage caused by dental diagnostic low-level radiation is repaired within the body cells.

RULES FOR RADIATION PROTECTION

Dental X-Ray Protection, prepared by the National Council on Radiation Protection and Measurements,[7] provides specific information about radiation barriers, film speed group rating, film badge service sources, x-ray equipment data, and operating procedure regulations.

In the application of procedures for protecting the clinician and the patient from excessive radiation, particular attention should be paid to unnecessary radiation that may result from the need for an unusual number of retakes because of inadequate technical procedures. Perfecting techniques contributes to the accomplishment of minimum exposure for maximum safety.

PROTECTION OF CLINICIAN

I. PROTECTION FROM PRIMARY RADIATION
   A. Stand behind a protective barrier.
   B. Avoid the useful beam of radiation.
   C. Never hand-hold the film during exposure.

II. PROTECTION FROM LEAKAGE RADIATION
   A. Do not hand-hold the tube housing or the PID of the machine during exposures.
   B. Test machine for leakage radiation.
   C. Wear monitoring device for testing exposure.

III. PROTECTION FROM SECONDARY RADIATION

The major sources of secondary radiation are the filter and the irradiated soft tissues of the patient. Formerly when a pointed plastic cone was used for the PID, the cone was a major source of scatter radiation. Other sources may be the leakage from the tube housing, or scatter from furniture and walls contacted by the primary beam. Methods of protection are related to these sources.

   A. **Minimization of Total X Radiation**
      1. Use high-speed films.
      2. Have x-ray machines tested frequently for x-ray output and leakage.
      3. Replace older x-ray machines with modern equipment.

   B. **Collimation of Useful Beam**
      Use diaphragms and lead-lined PIDs to collimate the useful beam to an area no larger than 2.75 inches in diameter at the patient's skin. Rectangular collimation has been shown to be

more effective than round (Figure 9-3, page 142).

C. Type of PID

Use a shielded (lead-lined) cylinder that is rectangular, long, and open-ended, or use some other form of rectangular collimation.

D. Position of Clinician While Making Exposures

The clinician shall stand behind the patient's head behind the major sources of secondary radiation to prevent direct exposure.

1. *Exposure of the Region of the Central Incisors.* Stand at a 45° angle to the path of the central ray. This position is approximately behind either the left or the right ear of the patient (Figure 9-4).
2. *Exposure of Other Regions.* Stand behind the patient's head and at an angle of 45° to the path of the central ray of the x-ray beam.

E. Distance

1. Safety increases with distance.
2. The correct position for the clinician is behind an appropriate radiation-resistant barrier wall, preferably with a leaded window to permit a view of the patient during exposures.
3. When protective barrier shielding is not available, the clinician shall stand as far as practical from the patient, at least 6 feet (2 meters)[8] in the zone between 90° and 135° to the primary central ray, as shown in Figure 9-4.

IV. MONITORING

Monitoring refers to the periodic or continuous determination of the amount of ionizing radiation or radioactivity present at a given location, usually for considerations of health protection.

The amount of x radiation that reaches the dental personnel can be measured economically with a film badge. Badges can be obtained from one of several laboratories. The film badge is worn on the clothing for 1, 2, or 4 weeks and is then returned by mail to the laboratory from which it was purchased. At the laboratory, the film in the badge is carefully processed and its exposure evaluated. The amount of radiation recorded by the film badge is a measure of the exposure of the wearer. The wearer is notified by mail of the amount of exposure.

PROTECTION OF PATIENT

I. FILMS

Use high-speed films.

II. COLLIMATION

Use diaphragms and an open-ended, shielded (lead-

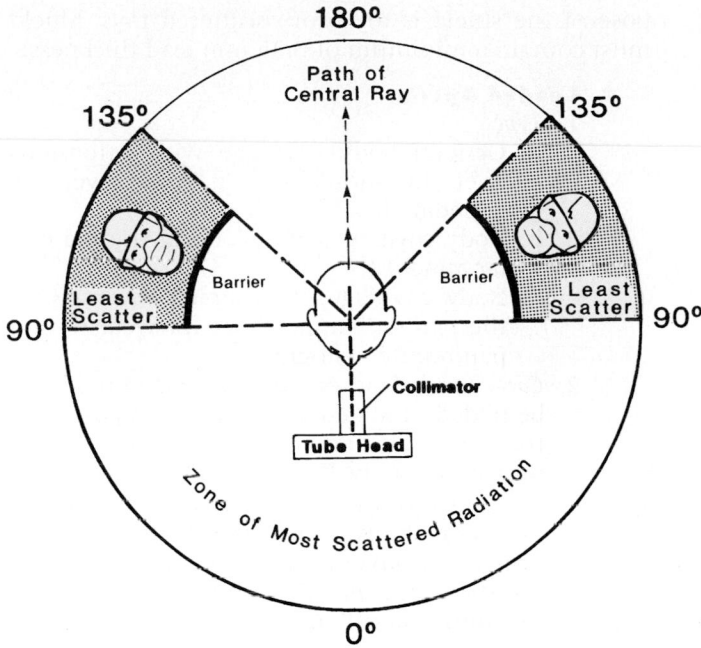

FIGURE 9-4 Safe Position for Clinician. While making an exposure, the clinician must stand behind the patient's head, between 90° and 135° from the primary beam.

lined), rectangular cylinder to collimate the useful beam.

III. FILTRATION

Use filtration of the useful beam to recommended levels (page 141).

IV. PROCESSING

Process films according to the manufacturer's directions. When a choice of two periods of development is offered, the exposure of the patient can be reduced if the longer development time is employed.

V. FILM SIZE

Use the largest intraoral film that can be placed skillfully in the mouth. Maximum coverage is provided in this manner with one exposure, whereas two exposures may be required if smaller films are used to examine the same area of the mouth. This factor is especially important when examining the mouths of children.

VI. TOTAL EXPOSURE

Do not expose the patient unnecessarily. There must be a good and valid reason for each exposure.

VII. PATIENT BODY SHIELDS

The use of leaded body shields for each patient is required by law in many states and countries. The purpose of the shield is to absorb scattered rays. Shield must contain a minimum of 0.25 mm lead thickness.

A. Leaded Apron

1. *Types*
   a. General body coverage with extensions over the shoulders and down over the gonadal area.
   b. Body coverage, with cervical thyroid collar attached.
   c. Body coverage, with added coverage for the patient's upper back for wear during panoramic radiography.
2. *Care.* Leaded aprons and collars should not be folded. If folded and creased, cracks eventually can develop and decrease the effective protection, as well as decrease the length of usefulness of the apron. A hanging device or hooks on the wall near the dental chair can provide a convenient arrangement for keeping the apron flat (Figure 9-5). Disinfecting the apron is facilitated.

B. Thyroid Cervical Collar

Thyroid cancer can result from long-term exposure of the gland to x rays.[9,10] The gland should be covered during dental radiographs throughout life. Figure 9-6 shows the position of a thyroid collar over the neckline of a body apron. The gland is positioned over the trachea approximately halfway between the chin and the clavicles.

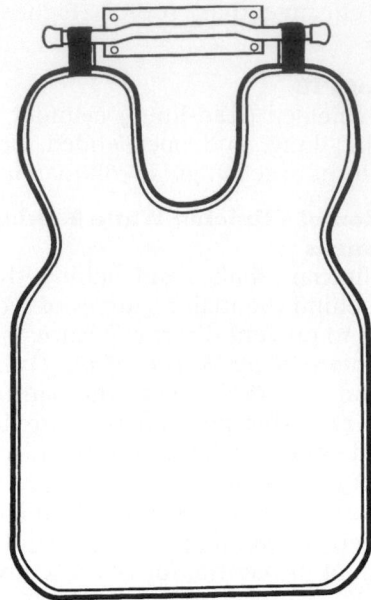

FIGURE 9-5 Care of Leaded Apron. The apron can be kept on hooks or a hanging device near the x-ray machine to prevent cracks and prolong the usefulness of the apron.

CLINICAL APPLICATIONS

I. ASSESSMENT FOR NEED OF RADIOGRAPHS

A. Review health history.
B. Prepare or review radiation exposure history.
   1. Medical diagnostic or therapeutic radiation.
   2. Dates of dental surveys and availability of previous radiographs.
C. Perform clinical examination.
D. Obtain dentist's prescription for number and type of radiographs. Refer to the *Guidelines for Prescribing Dental Radiographs* in Table 9-6.[2,11]

II. PREPARATION OF CLINIC FACILITY: INFECTION CONTROL ROUTINE (Pages 66 to 69)

A. Universal precautions should be followed for all radiographic equipment and materials.
B. Use barrier single-use plastic covers for all surfaces to be contacted, including x-ray machine controls.
C. Use disposable materials wherever possible.
D. Wear gloves or overgloves for handling of all radiographic materials.

III. PREPARATION OF CLINICIAN

A. Use full barrier protection that includes mask, protective eyewear, gloves.
B. Apply universal precautions throughout the radiographic procedure.

IV. PREPARATION OF PATIENT

A. Apply paper neck protection before positioning lead apron and thyroid collar.
B. Provide cup for holding removable dental prostheses.
C. For panoramic radiographs, ask patient to remove all jewelry and other metallic objects.
D. Provide antiseptic mouthrinse to lower bacterial contamination of radiographs and aerosols.

V. INTRAORAL EXAMINATION

A. Purpose

To determine necessary adaptations during film placement.

B. Factors of Particular Interest

1. Accessibility, determined by height and shape of palate, flexibility of muscles of orifice, floor of the mouth, possible gag reflex, size of tongue.
2. Position of teeth and edentulous areas.
3. Apparent size of teeth as compared with average size of teeth.
4. Unusual features, such as tori, sensitive areas of the mucous membranes.

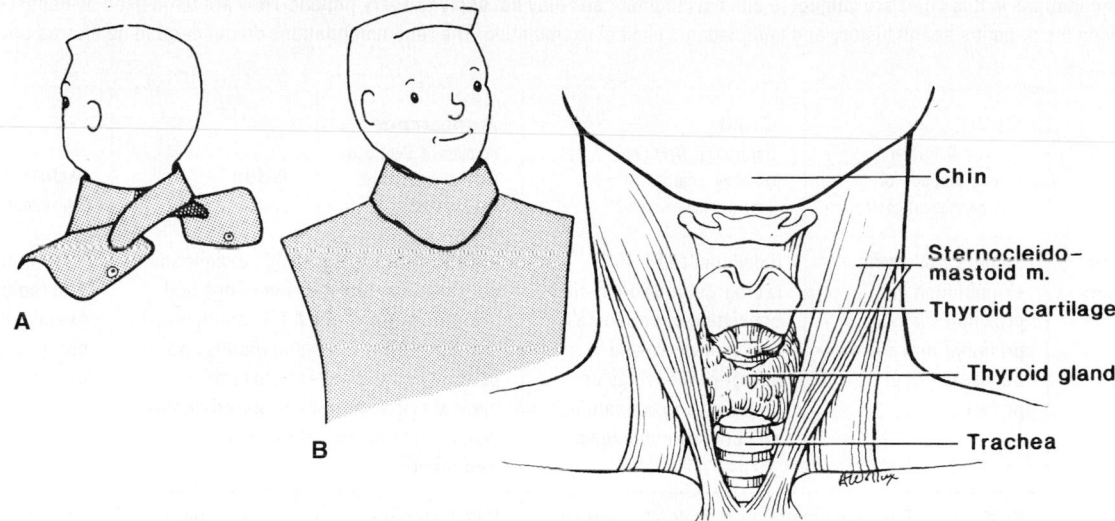

■ FIGURE 9-6 Thyroid Cervical Collar. (A) Thyroid collar in position, covering the neck and overlapping the leaded apron used for general body coverage. Velcro tabs facilitate overlap fastening at back of neck. Collars are available in child and adult sizes. **(B)** The thyroid gland is located over the trachea approximately half way between the chin and the clavicles. Drawing shows anatomic relationship to the sternocleidomastoid muscle.

VI. PATIENT COOPERATION: PREVENTION OF GAGGING

Gagging may be the result of psychological or physiologic factors. It may present some problem in the placement of all films for molar radiographs and may be initiated in the patient who ordinarily does not gag when techniques are carried out efficiently. Many of the factors related to the prevention of gagging may be applied for the comfort and cooperation of all patients.

A. Causes of Gagging

1. *Hypersensitive Oral Tissues.* Particularly common in posterior region of oral cavity.
2. *Anxiety and Apprehension*
   a. Fear of unknown, of the film touching a sensitive area.
   b. Previous unpleasant experiences with radiographic techniques.
   c. Failure to comprehend the clinician's instructions.
   d. Lack of confidence in the clinician.
3. *Techniques.* Film moved over the oral tissues or retained in the mouth longer than necessary.

B. Preventive Procedures

1. Inspire confidence in ability to perform the service.
2. Alleviate anxiety; explain procedures carefully. Smile and be cheerful.
3. Minimize tissue irritation.
   a. Request patient to swallow before opening for film placement.
   b. Place film firmly and positively without sliding the film over the tissue.

   c. Use a film holder on which the patient can bite to distract from the procedure.
   d. Instruct patient to breathe through the nose with quick, short breaths during film placement and to hold the breath during exposure.
   e. Use stick-on film cushions to make film placement more comfortable.
4. Use a premedicating agent prescribed by the dentist.
5. Use a topical anesthetic.
   a. Cold water or ice cube: hold in the mouth for a short time before film placement to dull the sensory nerve endings.
   b. Salt: Place one half teaspoonful on the tongue for an anesthetic effect; it may be swallowed or rinsed after radiographs are made.
   c. Prepared topical anesthetics: Apply in the form of an ointment with cotton swab or give patient a troche, or rinse to provide up to 20 minutes of surface anesthesia (pages 507 to 509).

PROCEDURES FOR FILM PLACEMENT AND ANGULATION OF RAY

The characteristics of the acceptable finished radiograph have been listed (page 140), and certain technical factors, including collimation, filtration, kilovoltage, milliampere seconds, distance, and films, have been described.

The image projected onto the film is a shadow of

TABLE 9-6 Guidelines for Prescribing Dental Radiographs

The recommendations in this chart are subject to clinical judgment and may not apply to every patient. They are to be used by dentist only after reviewing the patient's health history and completing a clinical examination. The recommendations do not need to be altered because of pregnancy.

Patient Category	Child Primary Dentition (before eruption of first permanent tooth)	Child Transitional Dentition following eruption of (first permanent tooth)	Adolescent Permanent Dentition (before eruption of third molars)	Adult Dentulous	Adult Edentulous
New Patient* All new patients to assess dental diseases and growth and development	Posterior bitewing examination if proximal surfaces of primary teeth cannot be visualized or probed	Individualized radiographic examination consisting of periapical/occlusal views and posterior bitewings or panoramic examination and posterior bitewings	Individualized radiographic examination consisting of posterior bitewings and selected periapicals. A full mouth intra-oral radiographic examination is appropriate when the patient presents with clinical evidence of generalized dental disease or a history of extensive dental treatment		Full mouth intra-oral radiographic examination or panoramic examination
Recall Patient* Clinical caries or high-risk factors for caries[†]	Posterior bitewing examination at 6-month intervals or until no carious lesions are evident		Posterior bitewing examination at 6–12 month intervals or until no carious lesions are evident	Posterior bitewing examination at 12–18 month intervals	Not applicable
No clinical caries and no high-risk factors for caries[†]	Posterior bitewing examination at 12–24 month intervals if proximal surfaces of primary teeth cannot be visualized or probed	Posterior bitewing examination at 12–24 month intervals	Posterior bitewing examination at 18–36 month intervals	Posterior bitewing examination at 24–36 month intervals	Not applicable
Periodontal disease or a history of periodontal treatment	Individualized radiographic examination consisting of selected periapical and/or bitewing radiographs for areas where periodontal disease (other than nonspecific gingivitis) can be demonstrated clinically.		Individualized radiographic examination consisting of selected periapical and/or bitewing radiographs for areas where periodontal disease (other than nonspecific gingivitis) can be demonstrated clinically		Not applicable
Growth and development assessment	Usually not indicated	Individualized radiographic examination consisting of a periapical/occlusal or panoramic examination	Periapical or panoramic examination to assess developing third molars	Usually not indicated	Usually not indicated

*Clinical Situations for Which Radiographs May Be Indicated Include:

A. Positive historical findings
  1. Previous periodontal or endodontic therapy
  2. History of pain or trauma
  3. Familial history of dental anomalies
  4. Postoperative evaluation of healing
  5. Presence of implants
B. Positive clinical signs/symptoms
  1. Clinical evidence of periodontal disease
  2. Large or deep restorations
  3. Deep carious lesions
  4. Malposed or clinically impacted teeth
  5. Swelling

6. Evidence of facial trauma
7. Mobility of teeth
8. Fistula or sinus tract infection
9. Clinically suspected sinus pathology
10. Growth abnormalities
11. Oral involvement in known or suspected systemic disease
12. Positive neurologic findings in the head and neck
13. Evidence of foreign objects
14. Pain and/or dysfunction of the temporo-mandibular joint

15. Facial asymmetry
16. Abutment teeth or fixed or removable partial prosthesis
17. Unexplained bleeding
18. Unexplained sensitivity of teeth
19. Unusual eruption, spacing, or migration of teeth
20. Unusual tooth morphology, calcification, or color
21. Missing teeth with unknown reason

[†]Patients at High Risk for Caries May Demonstrate Any of The Following:

1. High level of caries experience
2. History of recurrent caries
3. Existing restoration of poor quality
4. Poor oral hygiene
5. Inadequate fluoride exposure

6. Prolonged nursing (bottle or breast)
7. Diet with high sucrose frequency
8. Poor family dental health
9. Developmental enamel defects
10. Developmental disability

11. Xerostomia
12. Genetic abnormality of teeth
13. Many multisurface restorations
14. Chemo/radiation therapy

United States Food and Drug Administration, Center for Devices and Radiological Health: *Selection of Patients for X-ray Examinations: Dental Radiographic Examinations.* Washington, D.C., Government Printing Office, No. 017-015-00236-5.

TABLE 9-7 Principles of Shadow Casting

1. Place the film as parallel as possible to the object.

2. Use as small an effective focal spot as practical.

3. Use as long a target object distance as possible.

4. Use as short an object film distance as possible.

5. Aim the x-ray beam perpendicular to the film.

the teeth and the surrounding structures. The dental radiographer should follow as closely as possible the five principles of shadow casting, listed in Table 9-7, when exposing radiographs.

Basic intraoral procedures for periapical, bitewing, and occlusal radiographs are included in this chapter. The principles and uses of panoramic radiographs are also described.

Two fundamental periapical procedures are used in practice: the *paralleling* or right-angle and the *bisecting angle*. The principles for film placement are shown in Figure 9-7.

Clinicians vary in their application of the principles of the two techniques. Basically, the primary ray should pass through the region to be examined, and the film should be placed in relation to the teeth so that all parts of the image are shown as close to their natural size and shape as possible with a minimum of distortion in the finished radiograph.

As with other oral care, the development of a systematic, comfortable, smooth procedure saves time and energy for both patient and clinician. It increases the confidence of the patient, allows for consistency in technique, and leads to the production of good quality radiographs. A basic objective during radiographic technique is to minimize the length of time the film packet remains in the patient's mouth.

FILM SELECTION FOR INTRAORAL SURVEYS

I. PERIAPICAL SURVEYS

A. Area Covered
To obtain a view of the entire tooth and its periodontal supporting structures.

B. Films
1. *Child Size.* No. 0 (1.0) (22 × 35 mm) for primary teeth and small mouths.
2. *Anterior.* No. 1 (1.1) (24 × 40 mm) for anterior regions where width of arch makes positioning of standard film difficult or impossible.
3. *Standard.* No. 2 (1.2) (31 × 41 mm) may be used for all positions.

C. Number of Films Used in a Complete Survey
For the adult mouth, from 14 to 24 films may be used, depending on the clinician's preferences, objectives for showing specific areas, anatomy of the patient's mouth, and size of the films used. For children, see pages 160 to 161.

II. BITEWING (INTERPROXIMAL) SURVEYS

A. Area Covered
1. *Horizontal Bitewing Film.* To show the crowns of the teeth, proximal carious lesions, overhanging restorations, and the alveolar crest in a dentition with normal bone level to minimal bone loss. The horizontal bitewing is the film of choice in the presence of normal height alveolar bone.
2. *Vertical Bitewing Film.* To show the crowns of the teeth, proximal root caries, overhanging restorations, the alveolar bone level includ-

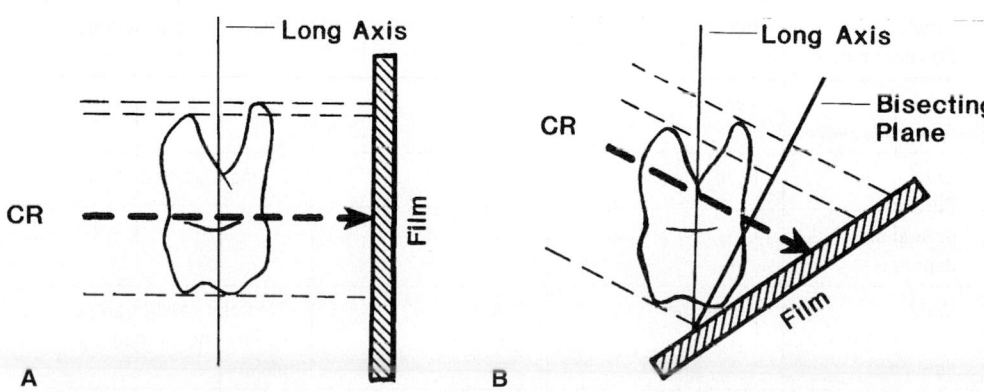

FIGURE 9-7 Comparison of Paralleling and Bisecting Angle Techniques. **(A)** Paralleling technique. The film is parallel with the long axis of the tooth and the central ray (CR) is directed perpendicularly both to the film and to the long axis of the tooth. **(B)** Bisecting angle technique. The central ray (CR) is directed perpendicularly to an imaginary line that bisects the angle formed by the film and the long axis of the tooth.

ing furcation involvement, and bony defects in a dentition with 5 mm or more of bone loss.

B. Films

The number and size of films used for bitewing surveys are determined by the size of the dental arch, number of teeth present, and patient tolerance. Refer to Table 9-8 for film size and number guidelines.

III. OCCLUSAL SURVEYS

A. Purpose

To show large areas of the maxilla, mandible, or floor of the mouth.

B. Film

No. 4 (57 × 76 mm) for use in self packet or in intraoral cassette.

C. Standard Film

No. 2 (31 × 41 mm) for child or individual areas of adult.

DEFINITIONS AND PRINCIPLES

I. PLANES

A. Sagittal or Median

The plane that divides the body in the midline into right and left sides.

B. Occlusal

The mean occlusal plane represents the mean curvature from the incisal edges of the central incisors to the tips of the occluding surfaces of the third molars. The occlusal plane of the premolars and first molar may be considered as the mean occlusal plane.

When it is specified in techniques that the occlusal plane of the teeth being radiographed shall be parallel to the floor, at least three head positions are involved for the maxillary: for anterior teeth, the head must be tipped forward; for premolars, held at the mean occlusal plane; and for molars, tipped back.

II. ANGULATION

A. Horizontal

The angle at which the central ray of the useful beam is directed within a horizontal plane. Inadequate horizontal angulation results in *overlapping* or *superimposition* of parts of adjacent teeth in the radiograph.

B. Vertical

The plane at which the central ray of the useful beam is directed within a vertical plane. Less vertical angulation than necessary results in *elongation*, and more angulation than necessary creates *foreshortening* of the image.

III. LONG AXIS OF A TOOTH

The long axis can be represented by an imaginary line passing longitudinally through the center of the tooth. Because of marked variations in tooth position and root curvature, estimation of the long axis of a

TABLE 9-8 Bitewing Film Surveys				
Patient	**Film Placement**	**Film Size**	**Number of Films**	**Region**
Adult Posterior survey	Horizontal or vertical	2	4	Premolars and molars
Adult Posterior survey	Horizontal	3	2	Premolars and molars
Adult Anterior survey	Vertical	1 or 2	3	Centrals, laterals, canines
Child Survey: permanent dentition	Horizontal	2	2	Premolars and molars
Child Survey: mixed dentition	Horizontal	1 or 2	2	Premolars and/or primary molars and permanent molars
Child Survey: all primary teeth	Horizontal	0	2	Primary molars

Film size is determined by size of dental arch and patient tolerance. Use largest film the patient will tolerate.

tooth is difficult. Clinically, it can be considered that the long axis of a posterior tooth is at right angles to the occlusal surface plane.

For single-rooted teeth, the long axis would ordinarily pass from the center of the incisal edge to the tip of the apex, but it is not possible to observe such a line during clinical examination. The line from the incisal edge to the cervical third on the labial surface must not be confused with the long axis.

PERIAPICAL SURVEY: PARALLELING TECHNIQUE

The paralleling or right-angle technique is based on the principles that *the film is placed as nearly parallel to the long axis of the tooth as the anatomy of the oral cavity permits, and the central ray is directed at right angles to the film*. In Figure 9-7A, the parallel relationship of the film with the long axis of the tooth and the right-angle direction of the central ray are shown.

The distance between the crown of the tooth and the film is increased to attain parallelism.

I. PATIENT POSITION

As long as the film is parallel to the long axis of the tooth and the central ray is directed at right angles to the film, the head may be in any position convenient to the clinician and comfortable for the patient. Slight modification of positioning may be needed for making radiographs in a supine position.

For the inexperienced clinician, horizontal angulation may be visualized more readily when the occlusal plane of the teeth being radiographed is parallel with the floor and the sagittal plane is perpendicular to the floor.

II. FILM PLACEMENT

A. Film Position and Angulation of the Central Ray
Instructions for film placement and angulation are included in this section.
1. *Basic Principles.* Principles for film placement and angulation of the central ray are shown in Figures 9-8 and 9-9. The image objective in the completed radiograph is also illustrated.
2. *Horizontal Angulation.* The central ray is directed approximately at the center of the film and through the interproximal area.
3. *Vertical Angulation.* The central ray is directed at a right angle to the film.

B. Film-Positioning Devices
The use of a film holder (film-positioning device) facilitates obtaining the correct angulation of the central ray. Lining up the PID with coordinating parts of the film holder sets the correct vertical and horizontal angulation so that the central ray is perpendicular to the film. An ex-

ample of a disposable film-positioning device is shown in Figure 9-10, and one that can be sterilized in Figure 9-11.
1. *Purposes.* The use of a beam-guiding, field-size-limiting, film-holding instrument provides important advantages, including dose reduction, film quality, and consistently adequate diagnostic radiographs without frequent retakes. Sanitation is improved, and lack of need for patient involvement in holding films is helpful.
2. *Characteristics.* An effective film-positioning device has such characteristics as the following:
   a. Adaptable to all necessary positions.
   b. Aids in reducing radiation exposure to patient. An example is shown by the position of the Precision film holder in Figure 9-11.
   c. Aids in alignment of x-ray beam.
   d. Weight and other properties do not hinder placement or holding.
   e. Comfortable for the patient.
   f. Simplicity of placement; minimal complexity for learning.
   g. Disposable or conveniently sterilized.
3. *Types*
   Several types of film holders are listed in Table 9-9. Examples of widely used types include the following:
   a. Styrofoam disposable filmholder
      A disposable bite block used with the paralleling or bisecting angle techniques (Figure 9-10).
   b. Precision film holder
      A stainless steel film holder that offers rectangular collimation for the paralleling technique. Figure 9-11 demonstrates how the stainless steel shield provides rectangular collimation to protect the patient from scatter radiation.
   c. Rinn X-C-P
      A plastic and stainless steel film holder with aiming devices that is used with the paralleling technique.

III. PARALLELING TECHNIQUE: FEATURES
A. Accuracy
The paralleling technique gives truer size and shape of dental structures with less distortion than when the bisecting-angle technique is used.
1. In Figures 9-8 and 9-9 an accurate crown/root ratio is shown with facial and lingual aspects in proper relation to each other.
2. Zygomatic bone can be shown in its normal position above the root apices of the molars and premolars.

B. Horizontal Ray Direction
No rays are directed toward the thyroid,

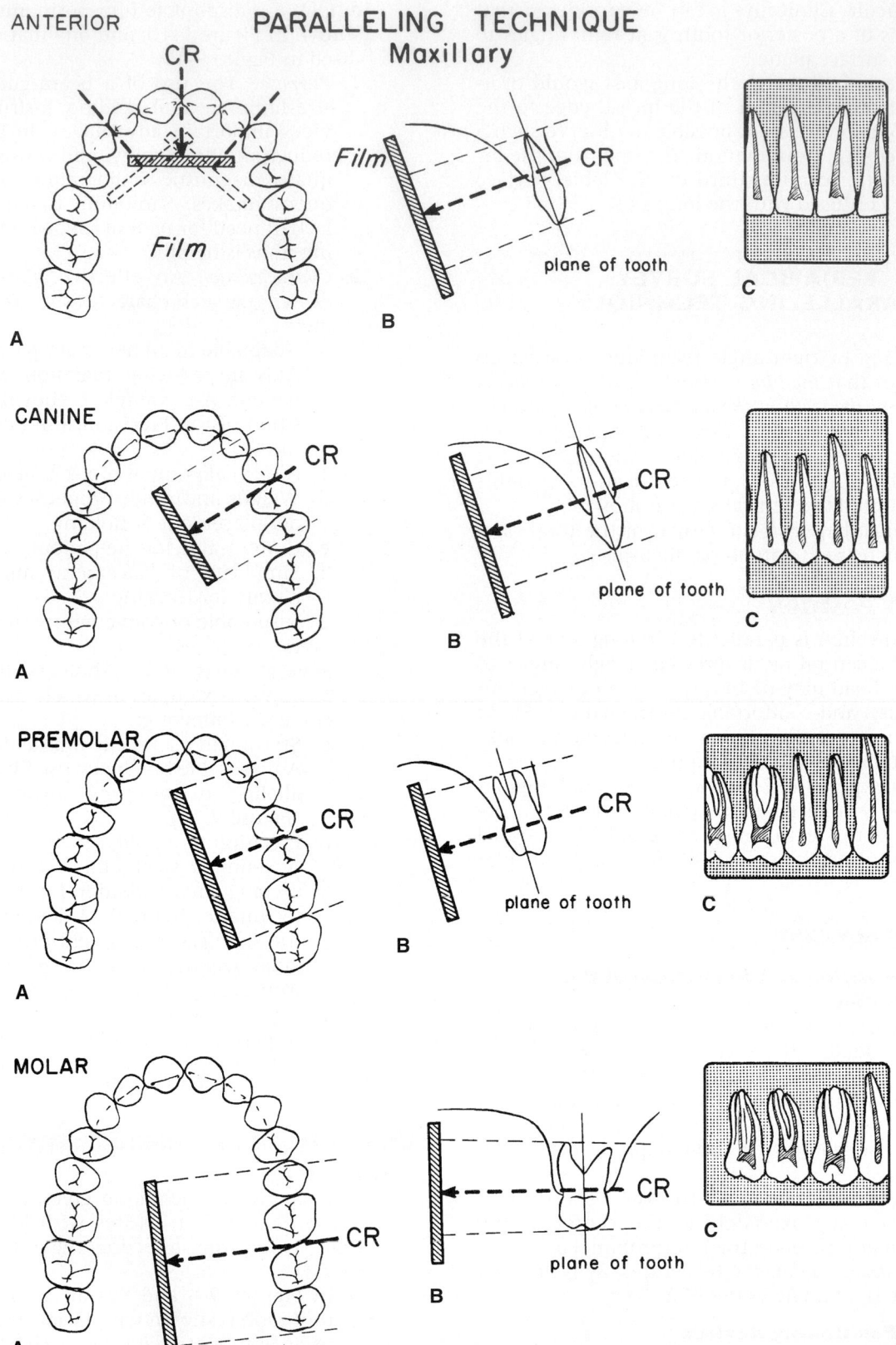

FIGURE 9-8 Paralleling Technique, Maxillary Arch. Film positioning for the major maxillary positions. **(A)** Horizontal angulation, with film placed parallel to the long axes of the teeth; central ray (CR) directed parallel with a line through the interproximal space. **(B)** Vertical angulation, with central ray (CR) directed at right angles to the film. **(C)** Image objective for the completed radiograph.

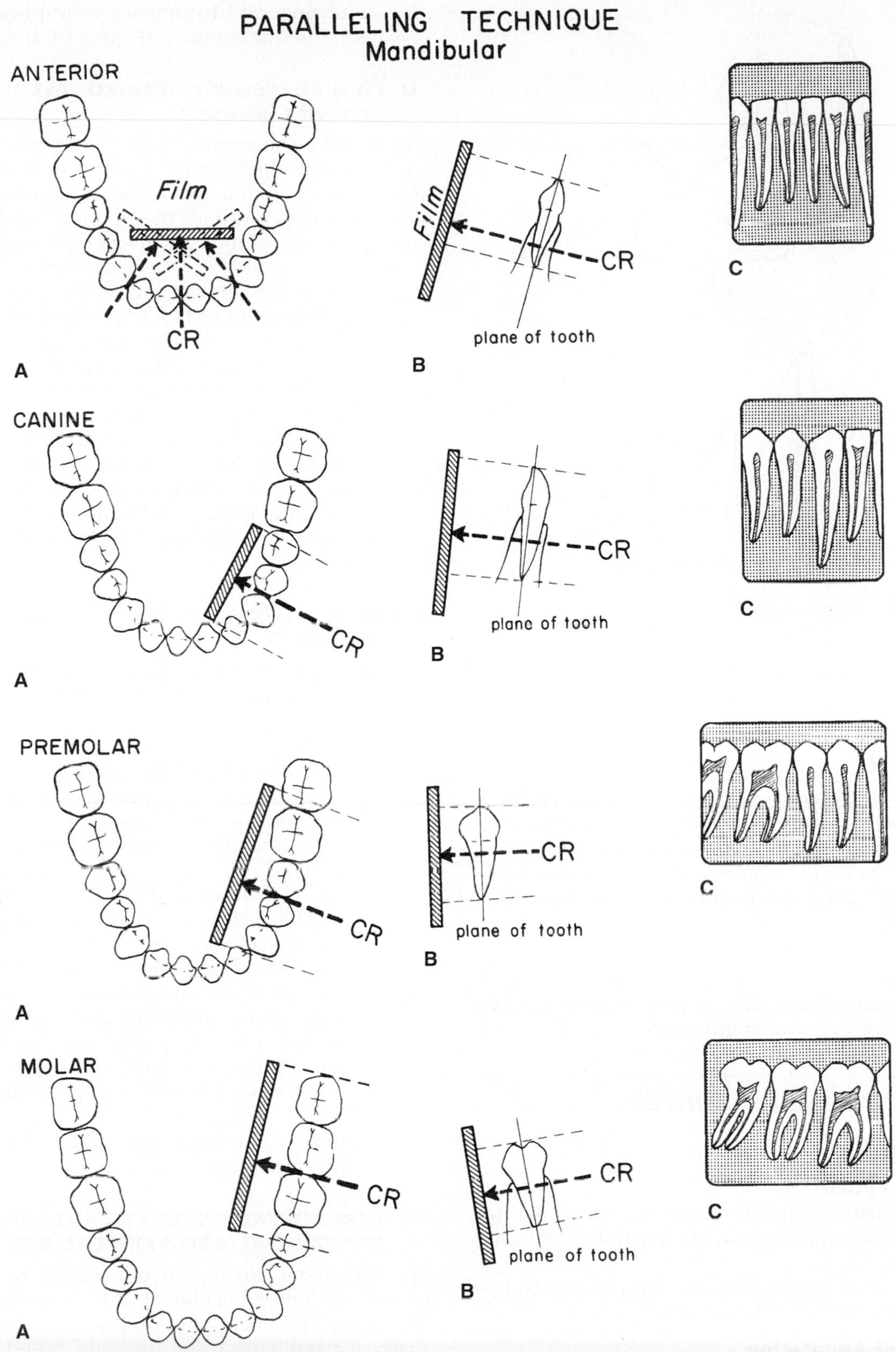

PARALLELING TECHNIQUE
Mandibular

ANTERIOR

A

Film

CR

B

Film

CR

plane of tooth

C

CANINE

A

CR

B

CR

plane of tooth

C

PREMOLAR

A

CR

B

CR

plane of tooth

C

MOLAR

A

CR

B

CR

plane of tooth

C

FIGURE 9-9 Paralleling Technique, Mandibular Arch. Film positioning for the major mandibular positions. **(A)** Horizontal angulation, with film placed parallel to the long axes of the teeth; central ray (CR) directed through the interproximal space. **(B)** Vertical angulation, with central ray (CR) directed at right angles to the film. **(C)** Image objective for the completed radiograph.

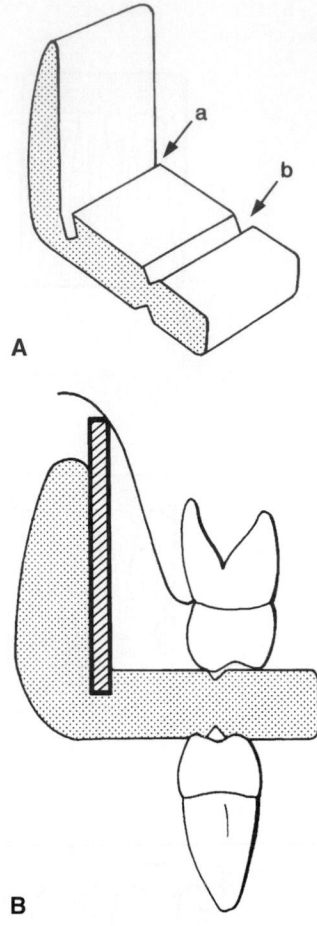

FIGURE 9-10 Styrofoam Disposable Film Holder.
(A) Empty holder to show: **a,** slot for insertion of the film, and **b,** break-off point to shorten the bite surface for use in the mandibular posterior positions. **(B)** Film placement for maxillary molar radiograph for patient with a high palatal vault.

whereas with the bisecting-angle technique, several maxillary radiographs require a relatively steep vertical angulation.

BITEWING SURVEY

I. PREPARATION

A. Patient Position
1. *Traditional.* Sagittal plane perpendicular to the floor and occlusal plane parallel with the floor.
2. *Patient in Supine Position.* The planes are reversed in their relation to the floor.

B. Vertical Angulation
Set at +8° to +10° for horizontal or vertical bitewings (Figure 9-12B).

C. Patient Instruction
Request patient to practice closing on posterior teeth prior to positioning film for posterior

bitewing, and to practice edge-to-edge closure for anterior bitewing (Figure 15-4, page 257).

II. FILM PLACEMENT: HORIZONTAL BITEWING SURVEY
Figure 9-12 shows in diagram form the position of the horizontal molar bitewing film in relation to the teeth, the horizontal and vertical angulation, and the image objective for both the premolar and the molar completed radiographs when standard film is used.
  A. *Molar* (standard film in horizontal position). Center the film on the second molar with the mesial border of film placed to include the distal half of mandibular second premolar. Distal surfaces of third molars can be examined clinically (see Figure 9-12A).
  B. *Premolar* (standard film in horizontal position). Center the film over the second premolar with the mesial border of film at midline of the mandibular canine to include the distal surfaces of maxillary and mandibular canines and a clear view of both the first and second premolars.

III. FILM POSITION: VERTICAL BITEWING SURVEY
  A. *Molar* (standard film in vertical position). Center of the film positioned over the middle of the second molar to include at least the distal portion of the first molar and the mesial portion of the third molar.
  B. *Premolar* (standard film in vertical position). Position the mesial border of film at midline of the mandibular canine to include the distal portion of maxillary and mandibular canines and a clear view of the first and second premolars. Figure 9-13 shows in diagram form the image objective for the vertical premolar bitewing, which includes the distal portion of the maxillary and mandibular canines, first and second maxillary and mandibular premolars, and the mesial portion of the first maxillary and mandibular molars.
  C. *Anterior.* Center of film at proximal space between the lateral and canine for the two canine/lateral bitewings; center of film at midline for central bitewing.

IV. HORIZONTAL ANGULATION (FOR HORIZONTAL AND VERTICAL BITEWINGS)
The horizontal angulation is adjusted to direct the central ray perpendicular to the center of the film. The central ray must pass through the interproximal space or parallel to a line through the interproximal spaces of the teeth of interest.

V. MAINTAIN FILM FLAT DURING EXPOSURE
Although slight curving of the film may be needed for certain patients, depending on the oral anatomy and

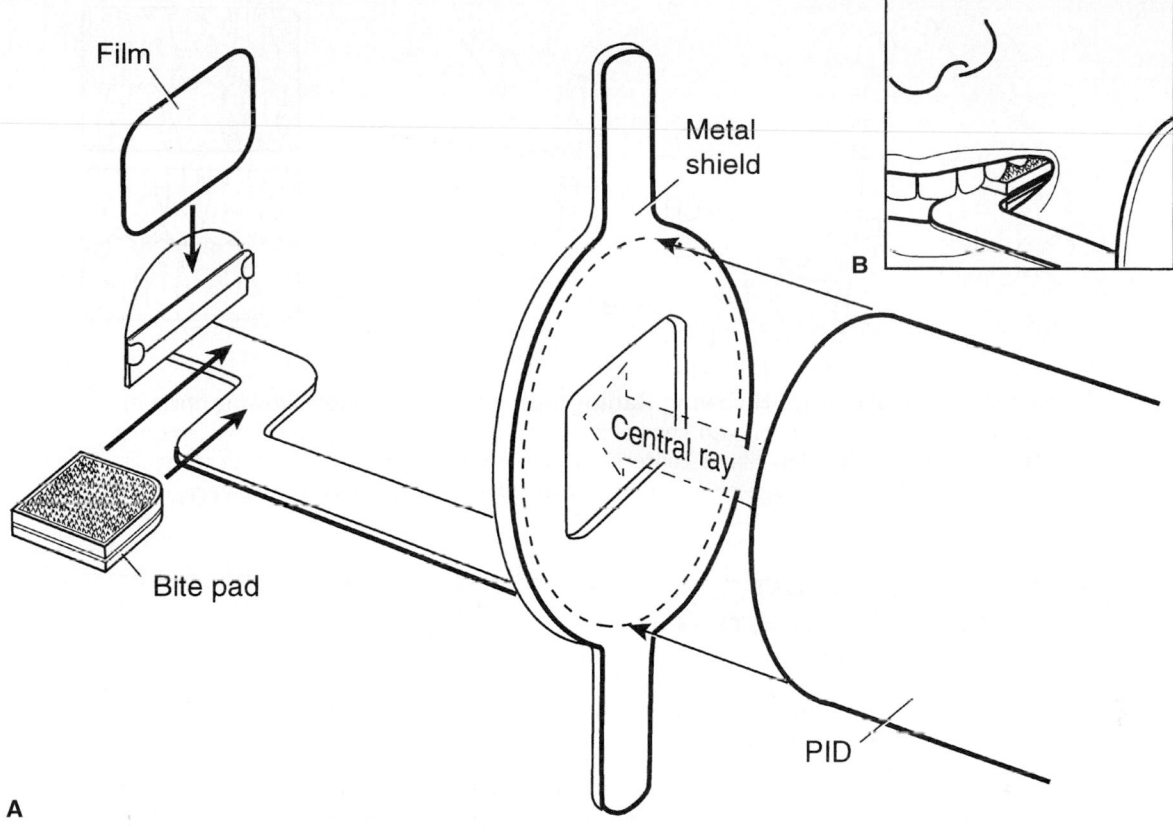

FIGURE 9-11 Collimating Film Holder. (A) Metal film holder with metal face plate that provides rectangular collimation of the primary beam. Offers dose reductions of approximately 60% to the facial tissues. **(B)** Shows placement of the film holder in the mouth.

tissue sensitivity, the basic rule is to keep the film as flat as possible to prevent distortion.

PERIAPICAL SURVEY: BISECTING-ANGLE TECHNIQUE

The bisecting-angle technique is based on the geometric principle that *the central ray is directed perpendicularly to an imaginary line that is the bisector of the angle*

TABLE 9-9 Film-Positioning Devices

FILM HOLDERS

Bite blocks, plastic or wooden
Styrofoam disposable film holder (Stabe)
Precision x-ray device
Snap-a-ray
X-C-P (Extension Cone Paralleling)
V.I.P. (Versatile Intraoral Positioner)
Hemostat with rubber bite block

SUPPLEMENTS

Removable denture for stabilization of film holder
Cotton roll to achieve parallelism

---

formed by the long axis of the tooth and the plane of the film. Figure 9-7B illustrates in diagram form the relationship of the long axis of the tooth, the film, and the bisector of the angle formed by these two.

I. PATIENT POSITION

A. Sagittal Plane
Perpendicular to the floor.

B. Occlusal Plane
Parallel with the floor.

II. FILM PLACEMENT AND POSITION

A. Center of Film
At center of teeth being radiographed. The exception to this rule is the maxillary canine film, which is placed slightly distal to accommodate film positioning.

B. Border of Film
Located ⅛ to ¼ inch beyond the occlusal or incisal surface.

C. Film Must Be Kept as Flat as Possible
A cotton roll may be used with the anterior and maxillary molar films to aid in accomplishing this goal.

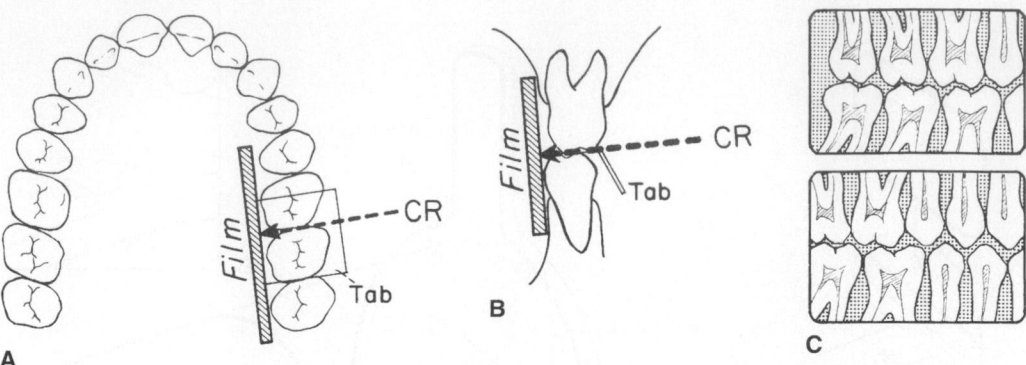

FIGURE 9-12 Horizontal Bitewing Radiograph. (A) Film position showing horizontal angulation for molar viewing, with central ray (CR) directed through the interproximal space to the center of the film. Film is centered over the second molar. **(B)** Vertical angulation set at +8 to +10°. **(C)** Image objective for molar (*above*) and premolar (*below*) regions.

III. DIRECTION OF THE CENTRAL RAY

A. Direct the Ray Through the Apical Third of the Teeth Being Radiographed

1. *Maxillary.* To determine location of the apices of the teeth, draw an imaginary line from the ala of the nose to the tragus of the ear; the apices are approximately at that level.
2. *Mandibular.* Apices are located approximately ½ inch above the lower border of the mandible.

B. Horizontal Angulation

The ray should pass through the interproximal space or parallel to a line through the interproximal space, at approximately the center of the area being radiographed.

C. Vertical Angulation

Bisect the angle formed by the film and the long axes of the teeth, and direct the ray perpendicular to this line.

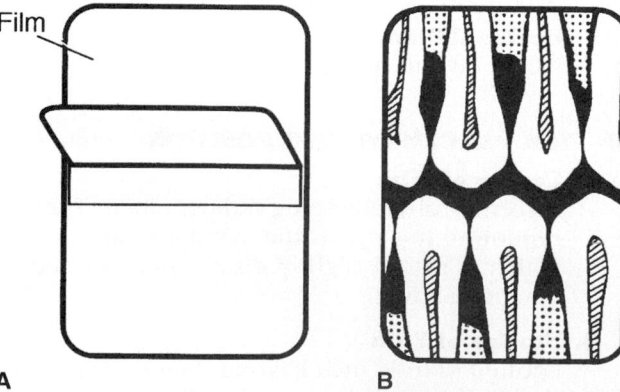

FIGURE 9-13 Vertical Bitewing Radiograph. (A) Vertical bitewing film with the tab positioned vertically over the center of the film. **(B)** Image objective of maxillary and mandibular premolar regions. Anterior edge of the film is placed behind the midline of the mandibular canine.

OCCLUSAL SURVEY

The central midline films for maxillary and mandibular arches are described in this section. A variety of positions for the occlusal films is possible, depending on the area to be examined.

I. USES

The purpose of the occlusal film is particularly important:

A. To observe areas that cannot be completely or conveniently shown on other films.

B. Where positioning periapical films is difficult or impossible.

C. To supplement the angulation provided by other films for such conditions as fractures, impacted teeth, or salivary duct calculi.

D. As a specific part of a complete survey for edentulous or very young patients.

II. MAXILLARY MIDLINE PROJECTION

A. Position of Patient's Head

The line from the tragus of the ear to the ala of the nose is parallel with floor.

B. Position of Film

The stippled side of the film packet is toward the palate; posterior border of film is brought back close to third molar region; film is held between the teeth with edge-to-edge closure.

C. Angulation

The PID is directed toward the bridge of the nose at a +65° angle.

D. Exposure

Consult chart of film manufacturer's specifications for exposure related to source–film distance, kilovoltage, and milliamperage. When a cassette is used, exposure time is reduced, an advantage in prevention of movement of the film.

III. MANDIBULAR MIDLINE PROJECTION

A. Position of Patient's Head
The head is tilted directly back.

B. Position of Film
The stippled side is toward the floor of the mouth, the posterior border of the film is in contact with the soft tissues of the retromolar area, and the film is held between the teeth in an edge-to-edge bite.

C. Angulation
For the incisal region, the PID is pointed at the tip of the chin at an angle of approximately −55°. For the floor of the mouth, the PID is directed from under the chin, perpendicular to the film.

D. Exposure
Consult chart of film manufacturer's specifications.

PANORAMIC RADIOGRAPHS

Panoramic radiography, or pantomography, refers to methods that produce continuous radiographs showing the maxillary and mandibular arches with adjacent structures on a single radiograph.

The panograph is a supplement to a periapical survey, but it is not a substitute because of less sharpness and detail in the panoramic radiograph. The derived benefit must be weighed against the additional exposure to a wide area of tissues outside the oral tissues.

I. PANORAMIC FILM AND TECHNIQUE

A panograph is a radiographic projection that is positioned outside the mouth during x-ray exposure and is used to examine the maxillary and mandibular jaws on a single film. The movement of the film and tube head produce an image through the process known as tomography. The prefix *tomo* means section; tomography is a radiographic technique that depicts one layer or section of the body in focus while surrounding structures in other planes are blurred. In a panoramic tomograph, the attempt is to radiograph the maxillary and mandibular dentitions in focus in one film. The film and tube head rotate around the patient's head in opposite directions.

A. Patient Position
Patient positioning depends on the panoramic unit and the patient's height.
1. Seated or standing.
2. The head is stabilized with a chin support or one of several types of head holders characteristic of each machine.
3. Position the patient to ensure that the Frankfort plane (orbitale to tragus of the ear) is parallel to the floor.

B. Cassette
1. Curved or flat.
2. Rigid or flexible.
3. Must be marked for the left or right side of the patient.
4. Contains calcium tungstate or rare earth intensifying screens that provide for reduced radiation exposure to the patient.

II. USES

There are numerous applications for panoramic radiographs. Routine use for patients seeking general oral care cannot be recommended as a substitute for a periapical survey.

A. Oral Pathology
The area surveyed increases with the use of a panoramic radiograph. Radiolucent or radiopaque areas outside the border of possibility in periapical views can be seen.

B. Edentulous Patient
A panoramic survey prepared prior to making complete dentures can usually provide sufficient information for most patients.

C. Patients at Risk for Stroke
Individuals at risk for a cerebrovascular accident can be identified by appropriate interpretation of panoramic films. Radiopaque calcifications of the carotid arteries seen on the panographs of asymptomatic patients have been correlated with the presence of atherosclerosis.[12]

D. Orthodontics
The overall view of growth and development at the beginning of orthodontic observation, diagnosis, and treatment, and during the treatment to assess periodic progress, can be helpful to the orthodontist.

E. Patients for Whom Intraoral Radiographs Cannot Be Used
Panoramic projections can be used for patients with disabilities that hinder cooperation, such as trismus, temporomandibular joint disorder, Parkinson's disease, facial paralysis, intermaxillary fixation, or facial trauma.

III. LIMITATIONS

Because definition and detail are inferior to those attained with periapical radiographs, and because distortion occurs, panoramic radiographs provide an overall, but not a detailed, view. They do not show proximal carious lesions except for large cavities, which can be seen by direct examination. They are also inadequate for examination of periodontal supporting structures.

A. Inferiority of Definition and Detail
Causes of poor definition are
1. Use of intensifying screens.
2. Increased object–film distance.
3. Movement of x-ray tube and film.

B. Distortion
1. Magnified images are produced because of increased film–object distance.
2. Overlapping. In periapical techniques, each film is angulated with the central ray so that when a tooth is out of line, adjustment is made to prevent overlapping. With panoramic technique, the head and teeth remain fixed, and the ray and film are positioned for the average only.

IV. PROCEDURES
Learning to use panoramic equipment is not difficult. Each machine has its own characteristics that can be learned readily from the manufacturer's instructions.

A. Patient Preparation
A thyroid shield cannot be used because of superimposition on the image. A special shield for panoramic radiography is available with coverage over the shoulders and part way down the back.

B. Film
Film sizes are usually either 5 × 12 or 6 × 12 in. Fast speed film should be used to minimize radiation.

C. Processing
Regular processing solutions are used for panoramic film. Special film holders for panoramic films are used during manual processing.

CHILD PATIENT SURVEY

For all ages, the frequency of making radiographic surveys, as well as the selection of type, size, and number of films to be used, is based on individual patient evaluation. The objective is to minimize exposure of children to radiation. Low levels of x radiation are associated with the induction of cancer, and growing tissues are more sensitive.

The need for radiographs in a healthy child is limited when the oral cavity appears free from disease as shown by direct clinical examination. This is especially true when teeth are spaced.

A specific rule of frequency for making complete surveys is not in keeping with current knowledge of radiation hygiene and safety. The aim for a young child is to make as thorough a clinical assessment of the teeth and the surrounding structures as possible. The real need for radiographs can then be determined.

I. INDICATIONS
With consideration for risk and benefit, six categories are suggested as indications for radiographs. Refer to Table 9-6 for guidelines.

A. Detection of congenital anomalies in the mixed dentition of children undergoing complete dental care or needing orthodontic treatment.
B. Detection of proximal surface dental caries when close contacts do not permit direct visual or explorer examination.
C. Third molar assessment.
D. Pulpal disease; infections.
E. Trauma to the teeth or jaws.
F. Periodontal assessment is needed when probing reveals periodontal pockets. Prepubertal periodontitis, although relatively rare, may be generalized or localized and may be evident as early as 4 years of age. Severe bone destruction is characteristic.[13,14]

II. PRIMARY DENTITION
When radiographs are indicated, various combinations of periapical, bitewing, occlusal, panoramic, and extraoral films are possible (refer to Table 9-6). Film size should be consistent with the size of the mouth, the cooperation of the patient, and the ability of the clinician. Examples of number and size of films for three effective surveys are listed here.
A. Occlusal views of anterior maxillary and mandibular arches (standard film) and posterior bitewings (child or adult anterior film); total of four films.
B. Occlusal views of anterior maxillary and mandibular and maxillary posterior (standard film), posterior bitewings (child or standard film), and extraoral lateral jaw films (5 × 7 in.[2]).
C. Periapical views for each posterior quadrant and one each for anterior (child-size film); total of six films.

III. MIXED DENTITION (6 TO 9 YEARS)
When a complete survey is determined necessary, 12 to 14 exposures using size 1 film are suggested. These include two posterior bitewings, four molar (to include first permanent and primary molars), four canine, and two or four incisor periapical views.

IV. TECHNIQUE WITH CHILDREN
A. Use of Leaded Apron and Thyroid Collar
Children are more susceptible than are adults to low-level radiation.

B. Orientation to Lessen Apprehension
1. For a young child's first visit to the dental office, the radiographic survey may be a necessary first procedure. When the child is not able to cooperate, the survey may be delayed until the second or even the third visit, except in an emergency.
2. Explain procedures carefully; rehearse to show what is to be done; repeat instructions with each film placement.

C. Sequence
Make the easiest, most comfortable exposures first (extraoral, panoramic, occlusal).

D. Periapical Films
Use film holder.

EDENTULOUS SURVEY

I. INDICATIONS

Periapical, occlusal, and panoramic surveys have been used alone and together for edentulous patients. Radiographic examination of an edentulous mouth is used frequently to detect residual pathologic conditions, foreign bodies, and retained teeth or root tips prior to denture construction.

The need for radiographs for edentulous patients should be reviewed in light of the patient's health history, as well as of the history of radiation exposure and of the clinical examination. Edentulous patients who previously have worn dentures and now need new dentures do not require radiographs routinely unless radiographs were not made for prior dentures.

II. PROCEDURES FOR SURVEY

The periapical series, usually of 14 to 16 films, has been considered to be the most complete and accurate for diagnosis.

A. Paralleling Technique
A film holder adjusted to provide a wider biting area is needed.
1. Turn the rubber bite block on a hemostat around. That way the broader dimension is in the vertical plane.
2. Film holder can be padded with cotton rolls.

B. Panoramic Radiograph
As shown in Table 9-6, a panoramic examination may be the choice for an edentulous patient. For the patient who has worn dentures for a long time without having a radiographic check, a definite advantage can be seen with the survey of a wider area than could be shown with a periapical survey.

PARACLINICAL PROCEDURES

Supplemental to the chairside clinical procedures are the processing of the films and the mounting of radiographs for diagnostic and clinical use. Standard procedures are outlined in the following sections.

INFECTION CONTROL

I. PRACTICE POLICY

Personnel of each office or clinic must work out a specific protocol appropriate to their facility and the type of processing used. A written policy is necessary for infection control during film exposure, processing, and mounting and during management of the completed radiographs throughout clinical treatment appointments.[15]

II. BASIC PROCEDURES

Prevention of cross-infection during film exposure was addressed on page 148 with other clinical applications. Additional procedures must be followed to prevent cross-contamination during transport to the darkroom and during the use of the processing equipment.[16,17]

A. Contamination of Films
Films become covered with contaminated saliva and should be confined to a disposable cup after exposure.

B. Gloves
1. Gloved hands fresh from contamination from the patient's mouth should not contact walls, doors, light switches, and other environmental surfaces when transporting a cup of contaminated exposed films to the darkroom.
2. Gloves are not needed to mount the films on hangers for a conventional system nor to feed the films into an automatic processor.

C. During Processing
1. The darkroom work area is prepared by the disinfection of all touch surfaces, and the counter is covered with clean paper.
2. Research has shown that bacteria on radiographic film can survive the processing procedures. Processing procedures may reduce the bacterial counts, but the potential for cross-contamination still exists.[18,19]

D. Waste
Dispose of film wrappers, cups, and contaminated gloves with contaminated waste. Lead foil should be disposed of according to environmental waste guidelines.

III. NO-TOUCH METHOD

A. With gloved hands and under appropriate safelight, pull open packets by their tabs or from their barrier envelopes as shown in Figure 9-14.
B. Allow films to drop out into a cup or onto the clean barrier-covered surface.
C. Take care not to touch the film. Remove gloves, wash hands, and place films on hangers being careful to touch the films by the edges only.
D. Dispose of waste properly.
E. Alternative no-touch method
1. Wear overgloves over powder-free treatment gloves and remove them after dropping film into the cup.

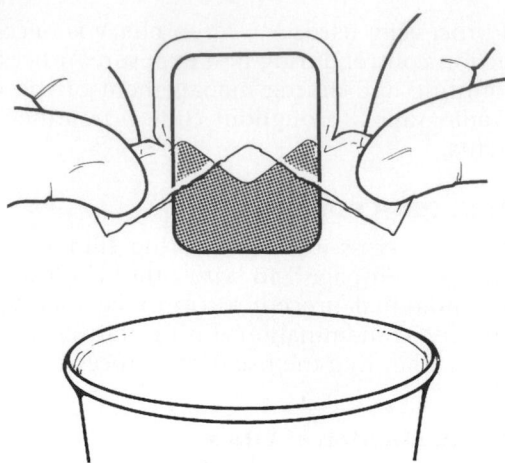

■ FIGURE 9-14 **Plastic Film Barrier.** Opening plastic film barrier using the no-touch method. Plastic film barriers placed over intraoral film are used to protect film from salivary contamination.

2. Films are then processed while wearing powder-free treatment gloves.

IV. FILM IMMERSION METHOD

A. Immerse plastic-coated films in 5.25% sodium hypochlorite solution for 30 seconds to 5 minutes.[17]
B. Remove and dry films thoroughly.
C. Remove gloves, wash and dry hands. Process films with ungloved hands.

V. DAYLIGHT LOADER METHOD

A. With powder-free regloved hands and exposed films in a paper cup, insert films in the daylight compartment.
B. Remove films from packets with the no-touch method, dropping films into a clean cup.
C. Remove gloves. Process films with ungloved hands, being careful to touch film by the edges only.
D. Remove ungloved hands from daylight loader. Don new gloves.
E. Disinfect daylight loader.

FILM PROCESSING

Film processing is the chemical transformation of the latent image, produced in a film emulsion by exposure to radiation, into a stable image visible by transmitted light.

I. STANDARD PROCEDURES

Standardization of processing procedure goes hand in hand with standardized exposure techniques if consistently acceptable radiographs are to be prepared. Processing should be treated as an exacting chemical operation in which each step has specific objectives for the finished product.

II. FILM SENSITIVITY

Fast and extra-fast-speed films are even more sensitive to variations in temperature, light, and processing chemicals than were the medium and slow films formerly in general use. Hence there is the need for fastidious attention to detail.

III. THE CHEMISTRY OF PROCESSING

A. Processing Chemicals
  In Table 9-10 the developer and fixer ingredients are listed with the chemicals involved and their specific reactions.

B. Chemical Reactions
  1. Development: selective reduction of affected silver halide salts to metallic silver grains.
  2. Fixation: the selective removal of unaffected silver halide crystals.
  3. Washing to remove the processing chemicals.

IV. HOW THE IMAGE IS PRODUCED

A. Film emulsion contains crystals of silver halides (bromide and iodide).
B. X-ray exposure changes the silver halides to silver and halide ions.
C. Developer reacts with the halide ions, leaving only the metallic silver in an arrangement corresponding with the radiolucency and radiopacity of the tissue being radiographed.
D. Fixer removes only those crystals of silver halide that were not affected by the action of the x rays. Fixer has no effect on the black metallic silver produced by the developer.
E. End result is a *negative*, showing various degrees of lightness and darkness (microscopic grains of black metallic silver).

ESSENTIALS OF AN ADEQUATE DARKROOM

The work area must be free from chemicals, water, dust, and other substances that could contaminate the film either by splashing or by direct contact should a film touch the bench. The processing room should not be used as a storage room nor for other dental procedures in which dust or fumes may be produced.

LIGHTING

I. DARKROOM COMPLETELY VOID OF WHITE LIGHT

A. Find and eliminate all possible light leaks.

TABLE 9-10 Processing Chemicals

Developer Ingredients	Chemical	Activity
Reducing agent	Hydroquinone and phenidone Elon	Converts exposed silver halide crystals to black metallic silver Generates gray tones in the image
Accelerator	Sodium carbonate or potassium hydroxide	Swells the emulsion and provides an alkaline medium
Restrainers	Potassium bromide and potassium iodide	Blocks the action of the reducing agent on the unexposed crystals
Preservative	Sodium sulfite	Slows the oxidation and breakdown of the developer
Solvent	Water	Mixes the chemicals
Fixer Ingredients		
Clearing agents	Ammonium thiosulfate or sodium thiosulfate	Removes all unexposed undeveloped silver halide crystals from emulsion
Acid or activator	Acetic acid Sulfuric acid	Stops development; neutralizes any remaining developer
Hardeners	Aluminum chloride Potassium alum	Toughens and shrinks the gelatin in the emulsion
Preservative	Sodium sulfite	Slows the oxidation of the fixer
Solvent	Water	Mixes the chemicals

B. Do not use fluorescent overhead light because of afterglow.

II. SAFELIGHT

Safelight is the illumination used in the darkroom that does not affect (fog) the film emulsion. By following the manufacturer's instructions, the correct safelighting can be used.

A 15-watt bulb or less is used in a light fixture 4 feet above the working surface, and a filter is selected for the light in accord with the type of film. Different films require different light filters.

A. Filter Type GBX-2 (red filter) is designed for both intraoral and extraoral film.
B. Filter Type ML-2 (orange filter) is for intraoral film only.

III. SAFELIGHTING TEST

A. Unwrap a film in totally dark darkroom.
B. Place film on work tabletop and place a coin on the film.
C. Turn on safelight and leave for maximum amount of time (such as 5 minutes) typical of that required when preparing a survey to be processed.
D. Turn off safelight, remove coin, process film.
E. Observe the radiograph; if any evidence exists of a light circle where the coin was placed, the darkroom safelight is excessive.

AUTOMATED PROCESSING

Automatic film processing refers to the use of equipment designed to transport film mechanically through a series of solutions under controlled conditions. Figure 9-15 illustrates the film being transported from the entry slot to the developer, the fixer, the water bath, the dryer, and the exit slot.

I. OBJECTIVES AND ADVANTAGES

Although cost and maintenance factors may be greater than those of a traditional darkroom procedure, an automated and/or rapid processing machine has advantages:

A. Conservation of time by dental personnel.
B. Finished radiographs in 5 to 8 minutes, depending on the machine used. Some have dryers.
C. Consistency of results through automated control of temperature and time.
D. Radiographs available for immediate use during diagnosis, which is particularly important in emergencies, during endodontic therapy, and in certain surgical procedures.

II. PRINCIPLES OF OPERATION

Manufacturer's instructions must be followed and routine care and cleaning attended to for maintenance of equipment.

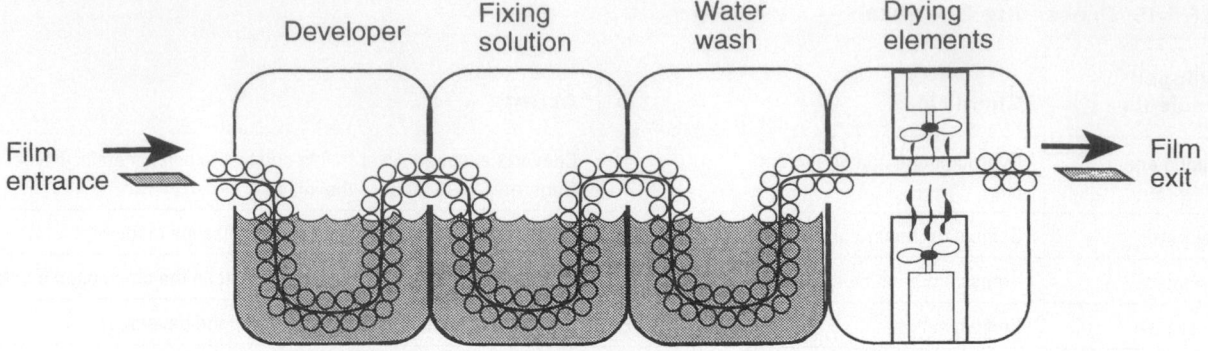

FIGURE 9-15 Automatic Processor. Diagram to show an automatic roller transport system that conveys the film over the rollers through the developer, fixer, water bath, and drying elements. (Adapted from Olson, S.S.: *Dental Radiography Laboratory Manual.* Philadelphia, W.B. Saunders, 1995, p. 86.)

A. Automated Film Transport
Rollers or tracks are used to carry the film through developing, fixing, washing, and finally forced drying. Certain machines produce wet films and do not have hot-air drying chambers. The various machines available are built to carry different sizes of film. Some machines may process only standard intraoral films, whereas others may also accommodate extraoral sizes.

B. High Temperature
Increased temperature decreases processing time. Special solutions are needed for the rapid processors, because with conventional solutions, the excess temperature causes deterioration and fogging of the film.

C. Care of Automatic Processor
The automatic processor requires meticulous routine maintenance.
1. A large sheet of special acetate or cleaning film is run through the roller-type processor daily to clean the rollers.
2. Depending upon usage and number of films processed, the processor should be scoured with a nylon pad weekly or bi-weekly.
3. Once a week the rollers are removed from roller-type processors and soaked in warm water for 10 to 20 minutes.
4. When the solutions are changed, a special cleaning solution is used to clean the racks and tanks.

D. Care of Automatic Processor Solutions
1. Solution levels must be checked at the beginning of each day and replenished according to manufacturer's specifications. Solutions must be replaced every 15 working days, depending upon film volume.
2. Failure to replenish solutions will cause non-diagnostic films.

3. Large films require more solution and would therefore necessitate more frequent change of the solutions.

MANUAL PROCESSING

The darkroom has three tanks of chemicals and water for processing by hand: the developing tank, fixing tank, and water bath. In most darkrooms, the developer is the left tank, the water bath is in the center tank, and the fixer is in the right tank. The fixer can be identified by a smell similar to vinegar and has a slippery feel to the touch.

I. MANUAL PROCESSING EQUIPMENT
A. Developer, water, fixer tanks, and stirring rods
B. Accurate, steel-based thermometer; timer
C. Safelights and white lights
D. Film hangers and drying rod for hangers, or electric dryer
E. Processing log

II. PROCESSING TEMPERATURE AND TIMES
The quality of the radiographic image depends greatly upon the processing time and temperature, with optimal developing conditions for manual processing being 68°F for 5 minutes.

Higher temperatures would produce films with excessive density; cooler temperatures, too little density. It is necessary to check the developer temperature and recommended time as outlined in Table 9-11.

III. STEPS FOR MANUAL PROCESSING
A. Check level and temperature of solutions; stir solutions.
B. Complete the processing log.
C. Turn on safelights and turn off the white lights.

TABLE 9-11 Processing Temperatures and Times*

Solution Temperature	Time in Developer (minutes)	Rinse Time (seconds)	Time in Fixer (minutes)	Wash Time (minutes)
65°F	6	30	2–4	10
68°F	5	30	2–4	10
70°F	4.5	30	2–4	10
72°F	4	30	2–4	10
75°F	3	30	2–4	10
80°F	2.5	30	2–4	10

*These times and temperatures are for D- or E-speed film and Kodak GBX fixer and developer.

D. Load films from the film packet or cassette onto hangers, making sure films are securely fastened.

E. Immerse film in the developer; activate timer.

F. When timer buzzes, rinse films in circulating water for 30 seconds.

G. Immerse the films in the fixer for the appropriate time.

F. Wash the films in circulating water for 10 minutes.

G. Dry films until they are no longer tacky.

ANALYSIS OF COMPLETED RADIOGRAPHS

The completed radiographs are mounted and examined at a viewbox with an adequate light source. Interpretation of radiographs is difficult and the determination of a pathologic condition requires keen evaluation. Attempting to base interpretation on inadequate, insufficient radiographs will result in guesswork rather than an accurate, timely diagnosis.

I. USE OF REFERENCE RADIOGRAPHS

The characteristics of acceptable finished radiographs (page 140) serve as the basis for analysis. Nothing less than the ideal should satisfy, and errors must be studied so that techniques can be improved for future surveys.

A. Available Ideal Radiographs
1. Tape an ideal periapical or bitewing radiograph to a viewbox for continuing reference and comparison.
2. Note changes in density, contrast, or other features so that techniques can be adjusted.

B. Complete Surveys
Examples of ideal surveys for periapical, bitewing, panoramic, edentulous, or other special radiographs can be maintained for study and review. New staff members can benefit by learning what is expected.

II. MOUNTING

A. Legibly mark the mount with the name of patient, age, date, name of dentist; printing is preferred.

B. Handle radiographs only by the edges with clean, dry hands.

C. Keep films clean and free from dust, liquids, or other contaminants.

D. Place a clean, dry towel or paper in front of the illuminator where mounting is to be done; arrange radiographs on this or mount one by one directly as they are removed from the hanger.

E. The embossed dot near the edge of the negative is the guide to mounting; the depressed side of the dot is on the lingual or palatal side.

F. Identify individual negatives by the teeth and other anatomic landmarks.

G. Approved mounting system is as follows: Looking at the teeth from outside the mouth, the teeth are viewed and mounted in the same manner as the approved numbering system (Figure III-1, page 84).

III. ANATOMIC LANDMARKS

A. Definition
An anatomic landmark is an anatomic structure, the image of which may serve as an aid in the localization and identification of the regions portrayed by a radiograph. The teeth are the primary landmarks.

B. Landmarks That May Be Seen in Individual Radiographs
1. *Maxillary Molar.* Maxillary sinus, zygomatic process, zygomatic (malar) bone, hamular

process, coronoid process of the mandible, maxillary tuberosity.

2. *Maxillary Premolar.* Maxillary sinus.
3. *Maxillary Canine.* Maxillary sinus, junction of the maxillary sinus and nasal fossa (Y-shaped, radiopaque).
4. *Maxillary Incisors.* Incisive foramen, nasal septum and fossae, anterior nasal spine (V-shaped), median palatine suture, symphysis of the maxillae.
5. *Mandibular Molar.* Mandibular canal, internal oblique line, external oblique ridge, mylohyoid ridge.
6. *Mandibular Premolar.* Mental foramen.
7. *Mandibular Incisors.* Lingual foramen, mental ridge, genial tubercles, symphysis of the mandible. Nutrient canals are seen most frequently in this radiograph.

IV. IDENTIFICATION OF INADEQUACIES IN RADIOGRAPHS

Table 9-12 outlines the more common inadequacies, their causes, and the keys to correction.

A. Causes
Inadequacies and errors may be related to any step in the entire procedure, including film placement, angulation, exposure, processing, and care and handling of the film.

B. Types
Errors appear as problems of improper density or contrast, incomplete or distorted images, fogging, artifacts, or stains.

1. *Distortion:* an inaccuracy in the size or shape of an object in the radiograph. Distortion is brought about by misalignment of the PID relative to the object. Vertical distortion produces elongation or foreshortening of the object.
2. *Fog:* a darkening of the whole or part of a radiograph by sources other than the radiation of the primary beam to which the film was exposed. Types of fog include chemical, light, and radiation.
3. *Artifact:* a blemish or an unintended radiographic image that can result from faulty manufacture, manipulation, exposure, or processing of an x-ray film.

V. INTERPRETATION

Radiographs are used in conjunction with clinical assessment for a complete care program. Periodic radiographs permit continuing evaluation. As part of the permanent record, radiographs help to document the oral condition for comparison as well as for legal purposes.

The quality of the radiographs determines their usability for diagnostic interpretation. Procedures for the preparation of radiographs must be perfected so that the radiographs have maximum interpretability with minimum radiation exposure of the patient.

A. Prerequisites for Interpretation
1. *Mounting.* Mount radiographs in an opaque mount to prevent light between each radiograph from creating glare and producing a blinding effect.
2. *Viewbox.* Use an adequately lighted viewbox. Dimmed room light improves visibility for contrasting radiolucent and radiopaque areas.

   Holding the radiographs up to view by window, room, or unit light is inadequate, and only gross interpretation can be accomplished. When a viewbox is larger than the mount used, cover the edges to block out peripheral light.
3. *Hand Magnifying Glass.* Examine radiographs on a viewbox through a magnifying glass. A viewbox is available with a built-on magnifying glass.

B. Systematic Examination
1. Observe one radiographic feature at a time. Examine all of the radiographs in a survey for that feature, rather than taking each radiograph separately to find everything. It is important to note comparisons for each change over the entire survey.
2. When examining a particular tooth, compare the appearance of that tooth in each radiograph in which it appears, including bitewings. At different angulations, different findings may become apparent.

C. Coordination With Clinical Examination
A description of radiographic examination of the teeth may be found on pages 248 to 249 and of the periodontal tissues on pages 219 to 221. Correlation of radiographic findings with the clinical examination, using probe and explorer, is basic to an understanding of the true oral condition of the patient.

TECHNICAL HINTS

I. CHECK GOVERNMENTAL RADIATION PROTECTION LAWS
Many states have regulations concerning x-ray unit registration, inspection, safety requirements, and limitations for use of x rays.

II. RECORD IN PATIENT'S PERMANENT RECORD

A. Radiation Exposure History
Inquire whether the patient is receiving or has recently received radiation treatment. It may be necessary to minimize the number of expo-

TABLE 9-12 Analysis of Radiographs: Causes of Inadequacies

	Inadequacy	Cause: Factors in Correction
Image	Elongation	Insufficient vertical angulation
	Foreshortening	Excessive vertical angulation
	Superimposition (overlapping)	Incorrect horizontal angulation (central ray not directed through interproximal space)
	Partial image	Cone-cut (incorrect direction of central ray or incorrect film placement) Incompletely immersed in processing tank Film touched other film or side of tank during processing
	Blurred or double image	Patient, tube, or packet movement during exposure Film exposed twice
	Stretched appearance of trabeculae or apices	Bent film
	No image	Machine malfunction from time-switch to wall-plug Failure to turn on the machine Film placed in fixer before developer
Density	Too dark	Excessive exposure Excessive developing Developer too warm Unsafe safelight Accidental exposure to white light (may be completely black)
	Too light	Insufficient exposure Insufficient development or excessive fixation Solutions too cool Use of old, contaminated, or poorly mixed solutions Film placement: leaded side toward teeth Film used beyond expiration date
Fog	Chemical fog	Imbalance or deterioriation of processing solutions
	Light fog	Unintentional exposure to light to which the emulsion is sensitive, either before or during processing (1) Unsafe safelight (2) Darkroom leak (3) Holding unprocessed films too close to the safelight too long
	Radiation fog	Improper storage of unused film Film exposed prior to processing
Reticulation	(puckered or pebbly surface)	Sudden temperature changes during processing, particularly from warm solutions to very cold water
Artifacts	Dark lines	Bent or creased film Static electricity (1) Film removed from wrapper with excessive force (2) Wrapper sticking to film when opened with wet fingers, or if there was excessive moisture from patient's mouth Fingernail used to grasp film during placement on hanger
	Herringbone pattern (light film)	Packet placed in mouth backwards with foil next to teeth

(continued)

TABLE 9-12 Analysis of Radiographs: Causes of Inadequacies (Continued)

	Inadequacy	Cause: Factors in Correction
Discoloration	Stains and spots	Unclean film hanger Spatterings of developer, fixer, dust Finger marks Insufficient rinsing after developing before fixing Splashing dry negatives with water or solutions Air bubbles adhering to surface during processing (insufficient agitation) Overlap of film on film in tanks or while drying Paper wrapper stuck to film (film not dried when removed from patient's mouth)
	At later date after storage of completed radiographs	Incomplete processing or rinsing Storage in too warm a place Storage near chemicals

sures. A consultation with the patient's physician is recommended (page 101).

B. Radiation Services Exposure Record

A continuing record for each patient is kept to show the date, number of exposures, and the area.

C. Patient Signature

When a patient refuses to have radiographs made, record such in the patient's permanent record. Obtain patient's signature to a statement indicating such refusal in the event a legal issue should arise.

III. OWNERSHIP

Radiographs were once thought to be the property of the dental office; however, this is no longer always the case.[20] Patients have a right to a copy of their records and radiographs. When possible, a duplicate set can be made by using a two-film packet. If that is not possible, the original series must be duplicated so that the originals can be kept with the patient's complete record and the duplicated series given to the patient.

IV. FILM STORAGE

Film should always be stored in a clean, cool, dry place between 50° to 70°F at 30% to 50% humidity. It should not be stored in a refrigerator. Keep in lead-lined container. Watch expiration dates. Store oldest film in front for next use. Purchase as needed, not in excess quantity.

V. DISPOSAL OF LIQUID CHEMICALS

Fixer is considered an environmentally hazardous waste material and must be disposed of according to governmental regulations.

FACTORS TO TEACH THE PATIENT

I. WHEN THE PATIENT ASKS ABOUT THE SAFETY OF RADIATION

Patients ask questions about safety factors, and occasionally, a patient may refuse to have any radiographs made. The patient must be reassured with confidence, instructed as to why radiographs are necessary at this time, and informed about how modern equipment and techniques are in accord with radiation standards.

A. Adapt the answer to the patient. Certain patients have more fear; others have more knowledge about x rays. The clinician who expresses confidence aids in allaying fears. Hesitation increases the patient's doubt.

B. Radiographs are essential to diagnosis and treatment. Without the information provided, the clinician can only guess at conditions not visible clinically.

C. The benefits resulting from the intelligent use of x rays outweigh any possible negative effects.

D. Modern x-ray machines are equipped for safety. For the patient who will understand, details about filtration, collimation, film speed, and short exposure times can be explained.

II. EDUCATIONAL FEATURES IN DENTAL RADIOGRAPHS

A. Position of unerupted permanent teeth in relation to primary teeth.

B. Detection of early carious lesions not visible by clinical examination.

C. Effects of loss of teeth and the importance of having replacements.

D. Periodontal changes and other pathologic conditions appropriate to an individual patient.

REFERENCES

1. **Haring**, J.I. and Lind, L.J.: *Dental Radiography, Principles and Techniques.* Philadelphia, W.B. Saunders, 1996, p.5.
2. **United States Department of Health and Human Services,** Public Health Service, Food and Drug Administration, Center for Devices and Radiological Health: *Selection of Patients for X-ray Examinations: Dental Radiographic Examinations.* (HHS Publication FDA 88-8273). Washington, D.C., Government Printing Office, 1987.
3. **United States National Research Council:** *Health Effects of Exposure to Low Levels of Ionizing Radiation. BEIR-V,* Washington, D.C., National Academy Press, 1990.
4. **Jacobsohn**, P.H. and Fedran, R.J.: Making Darkness Visible: The Discovery of X-ray and Its Introduction to Dentistry, *J. Am. Dent. Assoc., 126,* 1359, October, 1995.
5. **Saxe**, M.J.C. and West, D.J.: Incorporating Digital Imaging into Dental Hygiene Practice, *J. Dent. Hyg., 71,* 71, March–April, 1997.
6. **International Commission on Radiation Units and Measurements** (ICRU): *Radiation Quantities and Units.* ICRU Report No. 33, Washington, D.C., 1980.
7. **National Council on Radiation Protection and Measurements:** *Dental X-Ray Protection.* Washington, D.C., NCRP Report No. 35, 1970.
8. **Haring** and Lind: op. cit., p.72.
9. **White**, S.C.: 1992 Assessment of Radiation Risk from Dental Radiography, *Dentomaxillofac. Radiol., 21,* 118, August, 1992.
10. **Horner**, K.: Review Article: Radiation Protection in Dental Radiology, *Br. J. Radiol., 67,* 1041, November, 1994.
11. **Lusk**, L.T.: Radiographic Selection Criteria, *Access, 8,* 59, March, 1994.
12. **Friedlander**, A.H. and Gratt, B.M.: Panoramic Dental Radiography as an Aid in Detecting Patients at Risk for Stroke, *J Oral Maxillofac. Surg., 52,* 1257, December, 1994.
13. **Cogen**, R.B, Wright, J.T., and Tate, A.L.: Destructive Periodontal Disease in Healthy Children, *J. Periodontol., 63,* 761, September, 1992.
14. **Watanabe**, K.: Prepubertal Periodontitis: A Review of Diagnostic Criteria, Pathogenesis, and Differential Diagnosis, *J. Periodont. Res., 25,* 31, January, 1990.
15. **American Academy of Oral and Maxillofacial Radiology:** Infection Control Guidelines for Dental Radiographic Procedures, *Oral Surg. Oral Med. Oral Pathol., 73,* 248, February, 1992.
16. **American Dental Association:** Infection Control Recommendations for the Dental Office and Dental Laboratory, *J. Am. Dent. Assoc., 127,* 672, May, 1996.
17. **Wyche**, C.J.: Infection Control Protocols for Exposing and Processing Radiographs, *J. Dent Hyg., 70,* 122, May–June, 1996.
18. **Bachman**, C.E., White, J.M., Goodis, H.E., and Rosenquist, J.W.: Bacterial Adherence and Contamination During Radiographic Processing, *Oral Surg. Oral Med. Oral Pathol., 70,* 669, November, 1990.
19. **Stanczyk**, D.A., Paunovich, E.D., Broome, J.C., and Fatone, M.A.: Microbiologic Contamination During Dental Radiographic Film Processing, *Oral Surg. Oral Med. Oral Pathol., 76,* 112, July, 1993.
20. **Mauriello**, S.M., Overman, V.P., and Platin, E.: *Radiographic Imaging for the Dental Team.* Philadelphia, J.B. Lippincott, 1995, pp. 403–404.

SUGGESTED READINGS

Bohay, R.N., Stephens, R.G., and Kogon, S. L.: Survey of Radiographic Practices of General Dentists for the Dentate Adult Patient, *Oral Surg. Oral Med. Oral Pathol. Oral Radiol. Endod., 79,* 526, April, 1995.

Flack, V.F., Atchison, K.A., Hewlett, E.R., and White, S.C.: Relationships Between Clinician Variability and Radiographic Guidelines, *J. Dent. Res., 75,* 775, February, 1996.

Hausmann, E. and Allen, K.: Reproducibility of Bone Height Measurements Made on Serial Radiographs, *J. Periodontol., 68,* 839, September, 1997.

Kandemir, S.: The Radiographic Investigation of the Visibility of Secondary Caries Adjacent to the Gingiva in Class II Amalgam Restorations, *Quintessence Int., 28,* 387, June, 1997.

Law, A.N., Bollen, A.-M., and Chen, S.-K.: Detecting Osteoporosis Using Dental Radiographs: A Comparison of Four Methods, *J. Am. Dent. Assoc., 127,* 1734, December, 1996.

Ludlow, J.B., Platin, E., Delano, E.O., and Clifton, L.: The Efficacy of Caries Detection Using Three Intraoral Films Under Different Processing Conditions, *J. Am. Dent. Assoc., 128,* 1401, October, 1997.

Lyman, S. and Boucher, L. J.: Radiographic Examination of Edentulous Mouths, *J. Prosthet. Dent., 64,* 180, August, 1990.

Peterson, C.A., Mauriello, S.M., Overman, V.P., Platin, E., and Tangen, C.M.: Effects of Beam Collimation on Image Quality, *J. Dent. Hyg., 71,* 61, March–April, 1997.

Dental Implants

Pham, A.N., Fiorellini, J.P., Paquette, D., Williams, R.C., and Weber, H.P.: Longitudinal Radiographic Study of Crestal Bone Levels Adjacent to Non-submerged Dental Implants, *J Oral. Implantol., 20,* 26, Number One, 1994.

Reddy, M.S., Mayfield-Donahoo, T., Vanderven, F.J.,and Jeffcoat, M.K.: A Comparison of the Diagnostic Advantages of Panoramic Radiography and Computed Tomography Scanning for Placement of Root Form Dental Implants, *Clin. Oral Implants Res., 5,* 229, December, 1994.

Infection Control

Glass, B.J.: Infection Control in Dental Radiology, Current and Future, *NY State Dent. J., 60,* 42, April, 1994.

Hubar, J.S., Oeschger, M.P., and Reiter, L.T.: Effectiveness of Radiographic Film Barrier Envelopes, *Gen. Dent., 42,* 406, September–October, 1994.

Jefferies, D., Morris, J.W., and White, V.P.: KVP Meter Errors Induced by Plastic Wrap, *J. Dent. Hyg., 65,* 91, February, 1991.

Wolfgang, L.: Analysis of a New Barrier Infection Control System for Dental Radiographic Film, *Compend. Cont. Educ. Dent. 13,* 68, January, 1992.

Technique

Bohay, R.N., Kogon, S.L., and Stephens, R.G.: A Survey of Radiographic Techniques and Equipment Used by a Sample of General Dental Practitioners, *Oral Surg. Oral Med. Oral Pathol., 78,* 806, December, 1994

Dubrez, B., Jacot-Descombes, S., and Cimasoni, G.: Reliability of a Paralleling Instrument for Dental Radiographs, *Oral Surg. Oral Med. Oral Pathol. Oral Radiol. Endod., 80,* 358, September, 1995.

Pepelassi, E.A. and Diamanti-Kipioti, A.: Selection of the Most Accurate Method of Conventional Radiography for the Assessment of Periodontal Osseous Destruction, *J. Clin. Periodontol., 24,* 557, August, 1997.

Potter, B.J., Shrout, M.K., and Harrell, J.C.: Reproducibility of Beam Alignment Using Different Bite-wing Radiographic Techniques, *Oral Surg. Oral Med. Oral Pathol. Oral Radiol. Endod., 79,* 532, April, 1995.

Rushton, V.E. and Horner, K.: A Comparative Study of Radiographic Quality with Five Periapical Techniques in General Dental Practice, *Dentomaxillofac. Radiol., 23,* 37, February, 1994.

Radiation Exposure Control

Atchison, K.A., White, S.C., Flack, V.F., and Hewlett, E.R.: Assessing the FDA Guidelines for Ordering Dental Radiographs, *J. Am. Dent. Assoc., 126,* 1372, October 1995.

Atchison, K.A., White., S.C., Flack, V.F., Hewlett, E.R., and Kinder, S.A.: Efficacy of the FDA Selection Criteria for Radiographic Assessment of the Periodontium, *J. Dent. Res., 74,* 1424, July, 1995.

Avendanio, B., Frederiksen, N.L., Benson, B.W., and Sokolowski, T.W.: Effective Dose and Risk Assessment from Detailed Narrow Beam Radiography, *Oral Surg. Oral Med. Oral Pathol. Oral Radiol. Endod., 82*, 713, December, 1996.

Freeman, J. P. and Brand, J.W.: Radiation Doses of Commonly Used Dental Radiographic Surveys, *Oral Surg. Oral Med. Oral Pathol., 77*, 285, March, 1994.

Hayakawa, Y., Fujimori, H., and Kuroyanagi, K.: Absorbed Doses with Intraoral Radiography. Function of Various Technical Parameters, *Oral Surg. Oral Med. Oral Pathol., 76*, 519, October 1993.

Kogon, S., Bohay, R., and Stephens, R.: A Survey of the Radiographic Practices of General Dentists for Edentulous Patients, *Oral Surg. Oral Med. Oral Pathol. Oral Radiol. Endod., 80*, 365, September, 1995.

Rushton, V.E., Horner, K., and Worthington, H.V.: Factors Influencing the Frequency of Bitewing Radiography in General Dental Practice, *Community Dent. Oral Epidemiol., 24*, 272, August, 1996.

White, S.C., Atchison, K.A., Hewlett, E.R., and Flack V.F.: Efficacy of FDA Guidelines for Ordering Radiographs for Caries Detection, *Oral Surg. Oral Med. Oral Pathol., 77*, 531, May, 1994.

Computerized Digital Radiography

Hausmann, E., Allen, K., Loza, J., Buchanan, W., and Cavanaugh, P.F.: Validation of Quantitative Digital Subtraction Radiography Using the Electronically Guided Alignment Device/Impression Technique, *J Periodontol., 67*, 895, September, 1996.

Jean, A., Epelboin, Y., Rimsky, A., Soyer, A., and Ouhayoun, J.P.: Digital Image Ratio: A New Radiographic Method for Quantifying Changes in Alveolar Bone. Part I: Theory and Methodology, *J. Periodontal Res., 31*, 161, April, 1996.

Jean, A., Soyer, A., Epelboin, Y., and Ouhayoun, J.P.: Digital Image Ratio: A New Radiographic Method for Quantifying Changes in Alveolar Bone. Part II: Clinical Application, *J Periodontal Res., 31*, 533, November, 1996.

Shrout, M. K., Russell, C.M., Potter, B.J., Powell, B. J., and Hildebolt, C.F.: Digital Enhancement of Radiographs: Can It Improve Caries Diagnosis?, *J Am. Dent. Assoc., 127*, 469, April, 1996.

Vandre, R.H. and Webber, R.L.: Future Trends in Dental Radiology, *Oral Surg. Oral Med. Oral Pathol. Oral Radiol. Endod., 80*, 471, October, 1995.

Pediatric Radiography

Bimstein, E.: Radiographic Diagnosis of the Normal Alveolar Bone Height in the Primary Dentition, *J Clin. Pediatr. Dent., 19*, 269, Summer, 1995.

Bohay, R.N., Stephens, R.G., and Kogon, S.L.: Radiographic Examination of Children. A Survey of Prescribing Practices of General Dentists, *Oral Surg. Oral Med. Oral Pathol. Oral Radiol. Endod., 79*, 641, May, 1995.

Sjödin, B., Matsson, L., Unell, L., and Egelberg, J.: Marginal Bone Loss in the Primary Dentition of Patients With Juvenile Periodontitis, *J. Clin. Periodontol., 20*, 32, January, 1993.

Thomson-Lakey, E.M.: Dental Radiographs for the Child Patient, *DentalHygienistNews, 6*, 19, Fall, 1993.

Panoramic

Friedlander, A.H.: Identification of Stroke-prone Patients by Panoramic and Cervical Spine Radiography, *Dentomaxillofac. Radiol., 24*, 160, August, 1995.

Friedlander, A.H. and Baker J.D.: Panoramic Radiography: An Aid in Detecting Patients at Risk of a Cerebrovascular Accident, *J. Am. Dent. Assoc., 125*, 1598, December, 1994.

Leite, L., Webber, R.L., Weems, R.A., and Greer, D.F.: Evaluation of Off-axis Projection Geometry in Dental Panoramic Radiography, *Oral Surg. Oral Med. Oral Pathol., 77*, 183, February, 1994.

Molander, B., Ahlqwist, M., and Gröndahl, H.-G.: Image Quality in Panoramic Radiography, *Dentomaxillofac. Radiol., 24*, 17, February, 1995.

Molander, B.: Panoramic Radiography in Dental Diagnostics, *Swed. Dent. J.,* Supplement, 119, 1996, pp. 1–25.

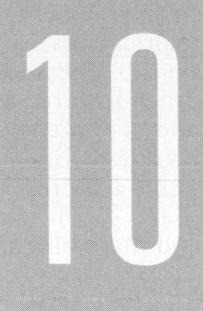

Study Casts

CHAPTER OUTLINE

As reproductions of the teeth, gingiva, and adjacent structures, study casts can be useful and frequently indispensable adjuncts in the care of a patient. Accurate and esthetically acceptable casts have a special use as visual aids for patient instruction.

The study casts, radiographs, and clinical examination with recordings and chartings, together with the medical and dental histories, are utilized in the diagnosis, total care planning, treatment, and subsequent maintenance.

I. PURPOSES AND USES OF STUDY CASTS

A. To serve as a permanent record of the patient's present condition.

B. To give sharper delineation to and corroboration of the observations made during the oral examination.

C. To observe normal conditions and the variations of and departures from the normal at the outset of treatment and, by comparison with subsequent periodic casts, to compare and evaluate certain aspects of treatment.

D. During charting of the teeth, to note missing teeth; anomalies of size, shape, or number; partial eruption; tooth positions, such as drifting, tilting, rotation, and open or closed spacing; and other factors.

E. During examination of the occlusion, to observe the static relations (Angle's classification, malrelations of groups of teeth, and malpositions of individual teeth; pages 255 to 259) and other features, such as wear patterns and the effects of premature loss of teeth.

F. During periodontal charting, to record anatomic features, such as the position, size, and shape of the gingiva and interdental papillae and the position of frena.

G. To be an effective visual aid to use when the oral conditions are explained and the dental and dental hygiene care plans are presented; to enable the patient to visualize and understand the need for the specific care outlined.

H. To serve as a guide to clinical treatment procedures.

I. To supplement clinical observations when the bacterial plaque control program for the patient's daily self-care is explained.

II. STEPS IN THE PREPARATION OF STUDY CASTS

Terms used to describe study casts and their preparation are defined in Box 10-1.

Procedures described in this chapter are as follows:

A. Clinical Procedures
1. Assemble materials and equipment.
2. Prepare the patient.
3. Select and prepare the impression trays.
4. Make the mandibular impression.
5. Make the maxillary impression.
6. Make the interocclusal record for occluding the casts.

B. Paraclinical Procedures
1. Assemble materials and equipment.
2. Prepare the impressions for pouring.
3. Pour the casts.
4. Trim and finish the casts.
5. Polish the casts.

CLINICAL PREPARATION

I. ASSEMBLE MATERIALS AND EQUIPMENT
A. Coverall (plastic drape), towel, and mouthrinse.
B. Impression trays
   1. Perforated type generally used; small, medium, and large sizes are available.
   2. Trays for use in the patient's mouth must

BOX 10-1 KEY WORDS: Study Casts*

Alginate (ăl'gĭ-nāt): an aqueous impression material used for recording minimal detail such as for study casts.

Cast (model): a positive life-size reproduction of the teeth and adjacent tissues usually formed by pouring dental plaster or stone into a matrix or impression.

   Diagnostic or study cast: used in the study of a patient's oral condition in preparation for treatment planning and patient instruction.

   Master cast: used to fabricate a dental restoration or prosthesis.

Centric occlusion or **habitual occlusion** (o-kloo'zhun): the usual maximum intercuspation or contact of the teeth of the opposing arches.

Dental plaster: the beta form of calcium sulfate hemihydrate; a fibrous aggregate of fine crystals with capillary pores that are irregular in shape and porous in character; also referred to as plaster of Paris.

Dental stone: the alpha form of calcium sulfate hemihydrate with physical properties superior to those of the beta form (dental plaster); the alpha form consists of cleavage fragments and crystals in the form of rods and prisms and is therefore more dense than the beta form.

Impression (ĭm-presh'un): a negative imprint of an oral structure used to produce a positive replica of the structure; used as a permanent record or in the production of a dental restoration or prosthesis; usually identified by the type of material used, such as "hydrocolloid impression," "alginate impression," or "rubber base impression."

Interocclusal record: a registration of the positional relationship of the opposing teeth or dental arches made in a plastic material, such as a soft baseplate wax; also called the **maxillomandibular relationship record** or "wax-bite."

Occlusal plane: the average plane established by the incisal and occlusal surfaces of the teeth; generally not actually a plane, but the planar mean of the curvature of those surfaces.

Polish: to make smooth and glossy usually by friction; the act or process of making a casting smooth and glossy.

Prosthesis (prŏsthē'sĭs): an artificial replacement of an absent part of the human body; a therapeutic device to improve or alter function.

---

*Definitions in this chapter are taken or adapted from and in accord with *The Glossary of Prosthodontic Terms,* 6th ed. Academy of Prosthodontics Foundation. 1993.

be disposable or clean, shiny, and sterilized metal.

C. Mixing bowl: clean, dry, flexible rubber or plastic with smooth, unscratched surface. Reserve separate bowls for each dental material: one always for impression material, another kept only for plaster or stone.

D. Spatula: clean, dry, stiff, with a smooth, rounded end that reaches every part of the bowl without scraping or cutting its surface.

E. Saliva ejector.

F. Dental materials
1. Soft utility wax for preparation of tray rim.
2. Alginate: irreversible hydrocolloid with manufacturer's measuring device.
3. Soft baseplate wax for interocclusal record.

G. Water thermometer.

II. CLINICIAN PREPARATION

Universal precautions should be observed for all clinic procedures. A mask should always be worn when handling powder forms of dental materials to prevent inhalation.

III. PREPARE THE PATIENT

A. Antibiotic Premedication
Impression making can be planned for an appointment when the patient who is at risk for bacteremia is protected and has received antibiotic coverage for other procedures. The medical and dental histories must be reviewed for all possible precautionary needs.

B. Explain the Procedure to be Performed
The need for, and uses of, study casts are explained as with any procedure not familiar to the patient. The reactions of patients who have had an impression made previously may range from indifference to dread, and the conversation and approach can be directed accordingly.

C. Position the Patient
Position the patient upright for maximum visibility and accessibility and to minimize gagging. Stabilize the patient's head on the headrest.

D. Receive Removable Prostheses
Provide a container with water in which the patient can place removable oral prostheses.

E. Provide Preprocedural Mouthrinse
1. To aid in the removal of saliva and debris and lessen the numbers of surface microorganisms.
2. To lower the surface tension; aids in preventing bubbles in the impression.
3. To provide a pleasant taste and feeling for the patient.
4. To distract an anxious patient while the trays are being prepared.

F. Examine the Oral Cavity
Note facially displaced teeth, height of palate, undercut areas, mandibular tori, and other factors that may influence the size or preparation of the impression tray and the procedures to be carried out during impression making.

G. Free the Mouth of Debris
When excess, tenacious debris is present, plaque control instruction should be initiated or continued so that debris and plaque can be removed during brushing by the patient.

H. Dry the Teeth
Use a cotton roll or compressed air stream to remove saliva from the teeth to prevent irregularities in the surface of the study cast.

I. Prevent Gagging
1. General approach
   When the radiographic survey has been made for the new patient prior to the study casts, the clinician will have already determined whether precautions to prevent gagging are needed. With all patients, a calm approach, an exhibition of confidence, a direct and efficient procedure, and a gentle handling of the patient's oral tissues increase rapport and contribute to a satisfactory result. Suggestions are listed on page 149.
2. Technique considerations
   a. Avoid excessive impression material in the tray.
   b. Seat the maxillary tray from posterior to anterior as described on page 178.
   c. Instruct patient to breathe deeply through the nose before the tray is inserted and to continue after insertion; bring head forward.

THE INTEROCCLUSAL RECORD (WAX BITE)

I. PURPOSES
A. To relate the maxillary and mandibular casts correctly. Many, if not most, maxillary and mandibular casts orient to each other readily in only one position, but when such problems as open bite, crossbite, edentulous areas, and end-to-end or edge-to-edge relations interfere with direct occlusion of the casts, a wax bite is needed.

B. To place between the casts during trimming and storage to prevent breakage of teeth.

II. PROCEDURE
A. Request patient to practice opening and closing on the posterior teeth to assure that the habitual position can be obtained.

B. Ask patient to rinse with cold water.

C. Shape a double layer of soft baseplate wax in the form of the arch, warm slightly over a gas burner or soften in warm water, and place over the maxillary occlusal surfaces.

D. Guide patient to close in habitual occlusion; press the wax against the facial surfaces of the teeth to shape it accurately to the arch.

E. Remove carefully to prevent distortion; chill in cold water.

PREPARATION OF IMPRESSION TRAYS

I. SELECTION OF PROPER SIZE AND SHAPE

A. Width

1. Objective is to allow an adequate thickness of impression material on the facial and lingual surfaces of each tooth to provide strength and rigidity to the impression.

2. Tray flanges may be spread to accommodate for extra width in the molar regions, particularly lingual to the mandibular molars in the mylohyoid region.

3. When a tooth is in prominent labio-, bucco-, or linguoversion, a minimum thickness of ⅛ to ¼ inch is suggested, but even then, the fragility of the impression material in that area is increased.

4. The tray that is too wide may appear in correct relation to the facial surfaces but may impinge on the lingual or palatal cusps of molars.

B. Length

1. Objective is to allow coverage of the retromolar area of the mandible and the tuberosity of the maxilla.

2. Anteriorly there should be at least ¼ inch clearance labial to the most protruded incisor without impingement on lingual or palatal gingiva.

II. MAXILLARY TRAY TRY-IN

A. Position of Clinician
At side back of patient.

B. Retraction

1. With index finger of nondominant hand, retract the patient's lip and cheek.

2. At the same time, use the side of the tray to distend the other side of the patient's mouth to gain entry (Figure 10-1).

C. Insertion

1. With a rotary motion, insert the tray.

2. Orient the tray beneath the arch and center it by using the tray handle and the midline (usually between the central incisors and in line with the middle of the nose) as guides for positioning.

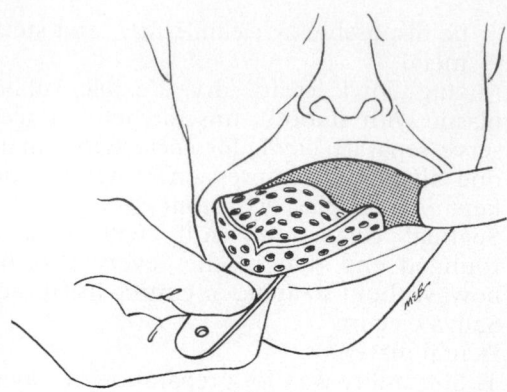

■ FIGURE 10-1 Maxillary Tray Insertion. The patient's lip and cheek are retracted with the fingers of the nondominant hand while the side of the tray is used to distend the other lip and cheek to gain entry. The tray is inserted with a rotary motion. The procedure for the mandibular tray is similar.

3. Bring the front of the tray to a position ¼ inch labial to the most labially inclined incisor.

4. Seat the tray by bringing the posterior up before the anterior; retract the lip as the anterior is brought into place.

D. Evaluation of the Tray Size

1. Lower the front of the tray while holding the posterior border in place (Figure 10-2).

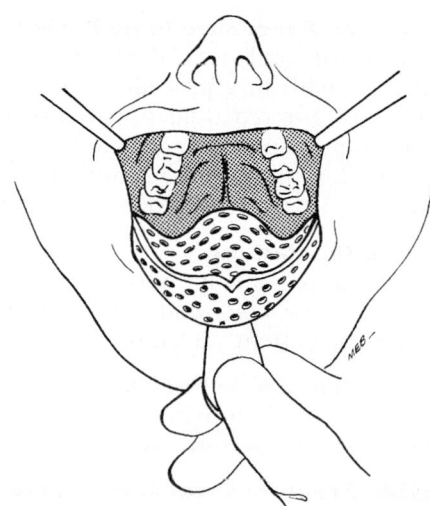

■ FIGURE 10-2 Selection of Impression Tray. Adequate coverage is determined as the posterior border of the tray is held in position while the front of the tray is lowered to observe the relationship of the posterior border to the maxillary tuberosity areas to be covered by the impression. The mandibular tray position is examined by lifting the tray to observe coverage of the retromolar areas.

2. Examine the relationship of the posterior border to the most posterior molars and the tuberosity areas to determine whether the coverage will be ample.

3. Move the tray up and down to observe the relation to the facial surfaces of all teeth, malaligned teeth, protuberances, and other features and thus to assay the space allowed for the impression material.

III. MANDIBULAR TRAY TRY-IN

A. Position of Clinician
At side front of patient.

B. Retraction
1. With index and middle fingers of nondominant hand, retract the patient's lip and cheek.
2. At the same time, use the side of the tray to distend the side of the mouth to gain entry, similar to the procedure illustrated in Figure 10-1 for the maxillary tray.

C. Insertion
1. With a rotary motion, insert the tray.
2. Orient the tray over the dental arch and center it by using the tray handle and the midline (usually between the central incisors and in line with the center of the chin) as guides for positioning.
3. Bring the tray rim to about ¼ inch anterior to the most labially positioned incisor; instruct the patient to raise the tongue to permit the lingual flange of the tray to pass by the lateral borders of the tongue without interference.
4. As the tray is lowered, retract the cheeks in the posterior regions to make certain the buccal mucosa is not caught beneath the edge of the tray; hold the lip out to ascertain that there is clearance to the base of the vestibule.

D. Evaluation of Tray Size
1. Lift the tray handle while keeping the posterior border of the tray in position, similar to the procedure illustrated in Figure 10-2 for the maxilla, to determine whether the coverage will be ample posteriorly to include the retromolar areas, and laterally to allow for ¼-inch thickness of impression material on the facial and lingual aspects of the teeth.
2. Reselect larger or smaller trays as indicated and repeat try-in. When in doubt, use the larger tray rather than the smaller.

IV. APPLICATION OF WAX RIM AROUND BORDERS OF TRAYS (BEADING)

A. Purposes
1. To prevent the metal tray rims from causing discomfort to the soft tissues.

2. To seat the vestibular periphery firmly into position with reduced pressure on the displaced tissues.
3. To prevent penetration of the incisal or occlusal surfaces through the impression material and thus to prevent a defective cast.
4. To provide a slight undercut at the rim as an aid in the retention of the alginate in the tray during placement and removal.
5. To create a posterior palatal seal to aid in preventing excess material from passing into the throat.

B. Procedure
1. *Application of Wax.* Attach a strip of soft utility wax firmly around the entire periphery of each tray (Figure 10-3).
2. *Mandibular Tray.* Add extra layers from canine to canine labially, and notch the wax to fit about the labial frenum.
3. *Maxillary Tray*
   a. Add extra layers as needed to extend the tray into the vestibule above the anterior teeth, and notch the wax to fit about the labial frenum (Figure 10-4).
   b. Apply extra thickness across the posterior palatal seal area.
   c. When a patient has a high palatal vault, apply extra wax to support the impression material in that area.
4. *Try-in.* Try the rimmed trays in the mouth; examine by retraction of the lips and cheeks and by use of a mouth mirror for lingual areas, hold the tray in position.
5. *Characteristics of the Completed Molding.* When the tray is held firmly, all borders of the wax should contact the mucous membrane and displace the soft tissue outward and upward. The teeth do not touch the tray.

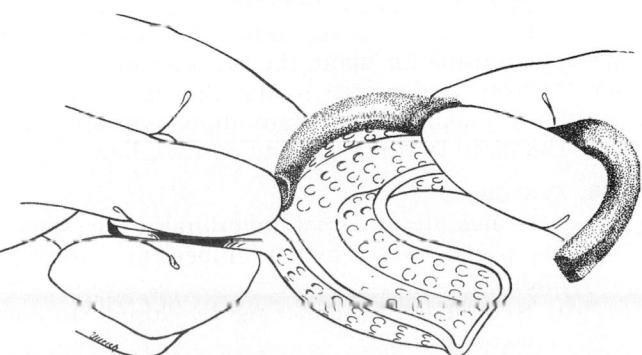

FIGURE 10-3 Beading the Tray. A strip of soft utility wax is applied around the periphery of each tray.

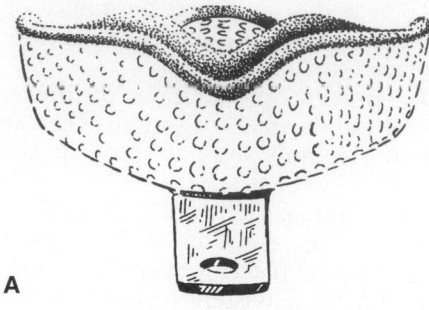

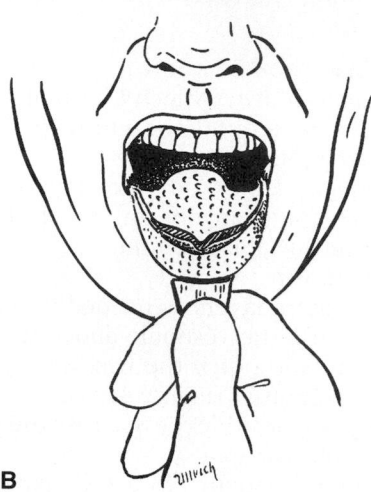

■ FIGURE 10-4 **Check the Beading Wax. (A)** Tray with double layer of beading wax about the labial frenum. The extra wax extends the tray, protects the soft tissue from the metal rim, and provides a more complete impression of the area. **(B)** Try-in after beading. The wax should contact all borders of the mucous membrane, displace the soft tissue outward, and prevent the teeth from contacting the tray.

THE IMPRESSION MATERIAL

I. FACTORS RELATED TO THE IMPRESSION MATERIAL THAT CONTRIBUTE TO A SATISFACTORY IMPRESSION

Texts on dental materials should be reviewed for complete information about the irreversible hydrocolloids.[1,2] Properties related to the clinical procedures essential to making an accurate impression are listed here. The manufacturer's directions are followed.

A. Powder
The alginate material deteriorates on standing, particularly at higher temperatures and humidity.
1. Keep metal container tightly closed; store in a cool place.
2. Use individually sealed packages to eliminate the problems of heat and moisture.
3. Individual package may be refrigerated in hot weather, provided the powder is used

immediately on opening. If left exposed, water condenses on the powder. The bulk container cannot be refrigerated for that reason.

B. Water
Temperature controls gelation time.
1. At room temperature, 20° to 21°C (68° to 70°F), an ideal gelation time between 3 to 4 minutes provides adequate working time.
2. Temperature of the water should be measured with a thermometer at the time of mixing.
3. For control in hot, humid weather, use cooler water and refrigerate the bowl and spatula.

C. Strength and Quality
The strength and quality of the finished impression depend on the following factors:
1. Powder/water ratio accurately weighed and measured.
2. Spatulation (1 minute) to allow chemical reactions to proceed uniformly.
3. Holding the impression material in position for an optimum period in accord with manufacturer's specifications. The elasticity of most alginates improves with time; therefore, a superior reproduction can be obtained by waiting. Distortion can result when the impression is left in the mouth too long.

D. Surface Accuracy
The cast must be poured promptly to prevent loss of water from the impression. Permanent distortion can result.

II. MIXING THE IMPRESSION MATERIAL
Follow manufacturer's specifications precisely; total time lapse for mixing and insertion is approximately 2 minutes.
   A. Place measured water 20° to 21°C (68° to 70°F, measured with a thermometer) in a clean, dry mixing bowl.
   B. Sprinkle measured powder (from individually sealed package or premeasured from large container) into the water.
   C. Quickly incorporate the powder and water, using a clean, dry, stiff spatula.
   D. Mix for 1 minute (clocked) vigorously, incorporating powder into the water, until a smooth, creamy mix is obtained.

III. TRAY PREPARATION
The mandibular impression is made first to introduce the patient to the procedure in an area where discomfort or gagging may be the least likely.

A. Working Time
The working time is 30 seconds.

B. Filling the Tray
1. Fill the tray from one end to the other, being careful not to trap air bubbles.
2. Adapt the material to the tray thoroughly; press slightly through the perforations in the tray.
3. Do not overload; fill to a level just below the edge of the wax rim.
4. Wet index finger with cold water and pass lightly over the surface of the impression material; smooth the surface and make a slight indent where the teeth will insert.

C. Excess Material
Quickly gather the excess material from the bowl and bring the material on the spatula near to patient to use for precoating.

THE MANDIBULAR IMPRESSION

I. PRECOAT POTENTIAL AREAS OF AIR ENTRAPMENT

The precoat prevents air bubbles in the finished impression.
A. Take a small amount of impression material from the spatula onto the index finger.
B. Apply quickly with a positive pressure to
  1. Undercut areas, such as distal surfaces of teeth adjacent to edentulous areas; cervical areas of erosion or abrasion; and gingival surfaces of fixed partial dentures.
  2. Vestibular areas, particularly anterior areas about the frena.
  3. Occlusal surfaces.

II. STEPS FOR INSERTION OF TRAY

A. Follow mandibular tray try-in (page 175). In summary, the procedure is as follows.
  1. From 8 o'clock position (4 o'clock if left-handed), retract lip and cheek with fingers of nondominant hand.
  2. Use side of tray to distend the other lip and cheek.
  3. Rotate the tray into position, center it over the teeth, and introduce the tray ¼ inch anterior to the facial surface of the most anterior incisor.
  4. Instruct patient to raise the tongue while tray is lowered; retract cheeks and lip to clear the way for impression material to reach the base of the vestibule.
B. Seat the tray directly downward with a slight vibratory motion to aid in filling all crevices between the teeth.
C. Instruct the patient to extrude the tongue briefly to mold the lingual borders of the impression.
D. Apply equal bilateral pressure firmly, holding the middle fingers over the premolar regions and using the thumbs to support the mandible; or, if equal pressure can be maintained with one hand, place an index finger over the patient's premolar area on one side and the middle finger over the opposite side, with the thumb under the edge of the mandible for stabilization. Mold cheeks around the tray.
E. When the impression tray is held with one hand or when assistance is available, slip the saliva ejector in over the tray and then remove it before the tray is removed.
F. When the leftover material on the spatula has lost its surface stickiness (tackiness), hold the impression in position 2 more clocked minutes.

III. THE COMPLETED IMPRESSION

A. Removal of Impression
1. Hold tray with thumb and fingers.
2. Retract cheek and lip with fingers and release the edge of the impression by depressing the buccal mucosa.
3. Do not rock the impression back and forth to release it because these movements may cause permanent distortion of the final impression.
4. Remove the impression with a gentle jerk or snap.

B. Rinse
Rinse under cool running water to remove saliva, blood, and bacteria. Rinse carefully to prevent splashing contaminated saliva or blood over surroundings.

C. Examine and Evaluate the Impression
Observe surface detail, proper extension over retromolar area, and peripheral roll (rounded border of the impression) generally.

D. Repeat Procedure When Necessary
Correct mistakes rather than be satisfied with a substandard impression.

E. Storage
Wrap mandibular impression in a wet towel while making the maxillary impression.

THE MAXILLARY IMPRESSION

I. PREPARATION

A. Request Patient to Rinse
To clear particles left from the mandibular impression and to relax the oral muscles.

B. Examine the Maxillary Teeth
Examine for particles of mandibular impression material and remove. Request patient to use mouthrinse.

C. Prepare the Alginate
Fill the tray as described previously for the mandibular impression.

D. Precoat Undercut Areas

Precoat undercut areas, vestibular areas, and occlusal surfaces (see procedure for mandibular impression).

II. STEPS FOR INSERTION OF TRAY

A. Follow maxillary tray try-in (page 174). In summary, the procedure is as follows:
1. From 11 o'clock position (1 o'clock if left-handed), retract lip with fingers of non-dominant hand.
2. Use side of tray to distend the lip and cheek.
3. Insert the tray with a rotary motion; center it over the teeth by using the small gap in the red wax border to relate to the labial frenum.
4. Introduce the material to the teeth so the wax rim is ¼ inch facial to the most anterior incisor.
B. Seat the tray from posterior to anterior to direct the impression material forward and thus prevent irritation to the soft palate area.
C. Retract the lip and bring the tray to place with a slight vibratory motion to allow the material to flow into crevices and proximal areas.
D. The middle finger of each hand is placed over the premolar region to support and guide the tray; the index fingers and thumbs hold the lip out.
E. Request the patient to form a tight "O" with the lips to mold the impression material.
F. Maintain equal pressure on each side of the tray throughout the setting of the alginate. If assistance is available or if the pressure to hold the tray can be maintained with one hand, a saliva ejector can be inserted.
G. When the leftover material on the spatula has lost its surface stickiness, hold the impression in place for 2 more clocked minutes.

III. THE COMPLETED IMPRESSION

A. Remove Impression

Hold the tray handle with the thumb and fingers of the dominant hand, and retract the opposite lip and cheek with the fingers of the other hand. Elevate the cheek over the edge of the impression to break the seal, and remove the impression with a sudden jerk.

B. Rinse

Rinse under cool running water to remove saliva, blood, and bacteria. Rinse carefully to prevent dissemination of contaminated saliva and blood.

C. Examine

Examine surface detail and proper extension to include tuberosity areas and a complete reproduction of the height of the vestibule.

D. Repeat Procedure When Necessary

Repeat procedure rather than be satisfied with a substandard impression.

E. Disinfection

Proceed with disinfection for maxillary and mandibular casts.

DISINFECTION OF IMPRESSIONS[3,4]

To prevent cross-contamination during laboratory procedures, impressions should be disinfected in an approved disinfectant after rinsing. The dimensional stability of some impression materials may be affected by certain disinfectants, so research and manufacturer's information must be heeded.

When impressions are to be sent to a laboratory, they should be isolated in a package. A sealable plastic bag can be used.

I. DISINFECTANTS

Iodophor (1:213) and sodium hypochlorite (1:10) have been tested and are effective with no distortion of an alginate impression when used for 10 to 15 minutes before pouring.

II. PROCEDURE

A. Apply universal precautions; wear protective gloves, eyewear, and mask to handle contaminated impressions and to protect against chemical disinfectants.
B. Immerse to assure maximum contact of the agent with all undercut areas. Impression then can be placed in the solution in a sealable plastic bag for 10 to 15 minutes.
C. Discard disinfectant solution and rinse the impression under running water.

PARACLINICAL PROCEDURES

Supplemental to the chairside clinical procedures is the laboratory work involved in the production of the study casts from the impressions. These duties may be the responsibility of the dental laboratory technician or other dental team member.

The most frequent error in the use of the alginates for impressions is delay in pouring the cast. Undue dehydration or water loss from the alginate causes permanent distortion, an uneven surface, and hence an inaccurate cast. Regard for the sensitive properties of the dental materials, precision and practice in laboratory procedures, and pride in the production of neat, smooth, well-proportioned study casts determine the finished product's appearance, usefulness, and accuracy.

I. EQUIPMENT AND MATERIALS

A. Mixing bowl: clean, dry, flexible rubber or plastic, with smooth, unscratched surface. Separate bowls are reserved for each dental material.
B. Spatula: clean, dry, stiff, metal with a smooth,

rounded end that can reach every part of the bowl without scraping or cutting its surface.

C. Plaster knife: sharp.

D. Vibrator with protective covering.

E. Mechanical mixer.

F. Model-base formers, glass or ceramic slab, waxed paper or other nonabsorbent material.

G. Dental materials
1. Baseplate wax (and wax spatula).
2. White dental stone.

H. Water at room temperature, with measuring container.

I. Model trimmer.

J. Compass or dividers.

K. Plastic ruler.

L. Waterproof sandpaper.

M. Soap solution.

II. PREPARATION OF THE IMPRESSIONS

A. Rinse impressions under cool running water to remove residual disinfection that may affect the plaster or stone surface after pouring; shake out excess water gently and apply gentle blast of compressed air.

B. Create an artificial floor of the mouth in the mandibular impression to facilitate pouring and trimming of the cast.
1. Trim the lingual impression material all around so that the height is consistent from the occlusal and incisal surfaces to the base of the impression.
2. Using alginate
    a. Mix a small portion of alginate.
    b. Hold the mandibular impression upright in the nondominant hand, with the middle and ring fingers extended from under the tray into the tongue area.
    c. Apply alginate over the fingers to form a flat bridge slightly above the lingual flanges of the impression.
    d. Smooth the surface with a finger moistened with cool water; hold until the alginate sets.
    e. When assisted at the chair, the floor of the mandibular impression can be made while the maxillary impression is being held for setting. There is usually sufficient alginate mixed with that for the maxillary impression to use for this purpose.
3. Using baseplate wax
    a. Cut a piece of baseplate wax to the shape of the lingual periphery of the impression.
    b. Seal into place with a warm spatula, taking care that no heat is applied to the anatomic portions of the impression.
    c. Cool under running water.

MIXING THE STONE

I. FACTORS RELATED TO DENTAL STONE THAT CONTRIBUTE TO THE SUCCESSFUL CAST

Texts on dental materials should be reviewed for complete information about gypsum products.[5,6] Some pertinent properties are listed here as reference points.

A. **Dental Stone**
   Sensitive to changes in the relative humidity of the atmosphere.
   1. Store in airtight container; close soon after use; do not let water enter the container.
   2. Keep the spoon or scoop (used to remove the powder) clean and dry.

B. **Water**
   Controls the strength, rigidity, and hardness of the cast.
   1. *Temperature*. Generally, cooler water decreases the setting time and warmer water increases it.
   2. *Quantity*. Follow manufacturer's proportions exactly. Increasing the water over the specifications prolongs the setting time and reduces the strength.

C. **Spatulation**
   Prolonged or very rapid mixing can hasten the chemical reaction and shorten the setting time.

II. THE MIX

A. Measure the water and powder by the manufacturer's specifications.
   1. White stone is generally preferred for study casts. Plaster produces a cast more susceptible to breakage.
   2. Ratio of 30 to 40 mL water to 100 g stone.

B. Place measured water (room temperature) in a clean, dry mixing bowl.

C. Sift in the powder gradually to prevent air trapping and to allow each particle to become wet.

D. Wait briefly until all powder is wet, then vibrate to release large bubbles.

E. Use vacuum mixer (follow manufacturer's directions).

F. The result is a smooth, homogeneous, creamy mix.

POURING THE CAST

The finished cast has two connected parts, the anatomic portion and the base or art portion (see Figure 10-6, page 182).

I. POURING THE ANATOMIC PORTION

A. Shake water out of the impression.

B. Hold the impression tray by the handle and press handle against the vibrator.

C. With a small amount of stone mix on the end of the spatula, start at one posterior corner and allow the mix to flow through the impression. Use small amounts and vibrate continually.

1. Tip the impression so the material passes into the tooth indentations and flows slowly down the side, across the occlusal surface or the incisal edge, and up the other side of the impression of each tooth.

2. Air is trapped when the process is hurried or when too large a quantity of mix is poured in at one time without attentive control of the flow.

D. When all tooth indentations are covered, add larger amounts of mix to fill the impression slightly over the periphery. Vibrate.

II. ONE-STEP METHOD FOR FORMING THE BASE OF THE CAST

A. Fill rubber model-base former with the remainder of the mix, or form a mass of stone on a glass or ceramic slab or other nonabsorbent surface (waxed paper on a smooth surface). Add excess stone at the heel areas.

B. Invert the poured impression onto the base.

1. Use a slight back-and-forth motion to secure the two parts together.

2. Avoid the common error of inverting the impression before the stone is firm. The mix can flow out of the impression.

C. Adjust tray to proper position

1. Occlusal plane (at premolars) should be parallel with the base of the model-base former or tabletop.

2. Midline (anterior as judged by handle of impression tray) centered at the midline of the model-base former.

3. Accommodate position so that a tooth in labio- or buccoversion does not protrude over the trimming line of the art portion (see Figure 10-6).

D. Add stone on peripheral and heel areas to provide a smooth surface; remove excess so that wax periphery of the tray is visible. When excess stone above the edge of the tray rim is permitted to set, the tray is difficult to separate, and the use of a knife to carve the excess from the tray may damage the cast.

E. Final set occurs within 1 hour. Separate 1 hour after pouring to preserve the accuracy and prevent damage to the surface of the cast.

III. OTHER METHODS FOR FORMING THE BASE OF THE CAST

A. Two-Step or Double-Pour

Both maxillary and mandibular impressions are poured and left upright (see "Pouring the Anatomic Portion," page 179). Stone is then prepared separately for the bases, and the model-base formers are filled or the mass is placed on the smooth nonabsorbent surface.

The impression is inverted and held on the surface of the new stone while the sides and periphery are shaped and smoothed. An advantage to this method is that there is no danger of inverting the poured impression too soon. If the cast is turned before it starts to set, the unset stone can fall away from the occlusal and incisal portions and leave bubbles in strategic places.

B. Boxing Technique

The object is to form a wall around the impression before pouring to provide a shape for the base as well as to prevent the need for inverting the poured impression. A strip of utility (beading) wax is attached slightly below the periphery of the impression and completely around the impression. Boxing wax or baseplate is applied around the strip of utility wax and attached to it by means of a warm spatula at a height that allows for proper thickness of the final cast, about ½ inch. Care must be taken not to displace the impression dimensionally nor to touch the anatomic portions with the warm spatula. Pouring is carried out as described previously.

Work-model formers with side walls to provide the boxing effect are available. Such a mold has a slot through the rubber where the handle of the impression tray can be inserted.

IV. SEPARATION OF THE IMPRESSION AND THE CAST

A. Objective is to remove tray and impression material without breaking the teeth.

B. When model-based former is used, remove it first.

C. Cut away stone from the periphery to free the margin of the tray.

D. Remove the tray by itself.

E. Cut the impression material along the line of the occlusal surfaces and peel off the impression material (with care not to scratch the stone cast during cutting).

F. Direct removal is possible when the teeth are in reasonably normal alignment; remove the tray and the impression material with a straight pull after first releasing the anterior portion by a slight downward and forward movement. When this method is used, do not apply lateral pressures or rock the tray back and forth, because the teeth are broken easily by such forces.

G. Trimming is started promptly, or if delayed, the cast must be thoroughly soaked in water before trimming.

TRIMMING THE CASTS

The exact proportions of the study casts and the steps required to accomplish the trimming and finishing depend on several factors, including the measurements of the patient's dental arches, the positions of the teeth, and the preferences of the dentist. Development of a routine, systematic procedure for trimming can lead to the production of consistent, attractive, and useful diagnostic casts.

I. USE OF MODEL TRIMMER

The method described here depends on the use of a precision-type model trimmer. No specific directions are provided for the use of angulators that are available to fit on the table of the model trimmer to give average set angles for trimming the margins of the casts; when these are available, usually directions are supplied by the manufacturer.

When a mechanical model trimmer is not available, greater skill must be developed to produce well-proportioned and smooth casts. The use of the model-base formers or a boxing method can be developed to a higher degree of precision. Trimming with a plaster knife must be started as soon as the impression is separated. Plaster files are available to aid in cutting the borders of the base.

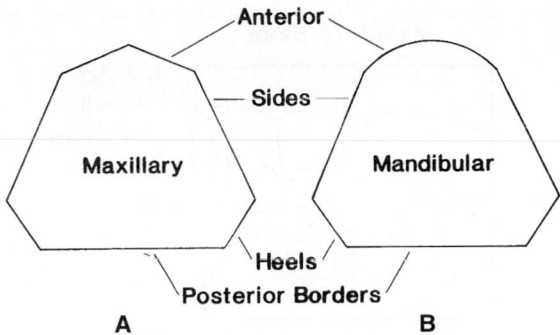

FIGURE 10-5 Base Shapes for Finished Study Casts. Maxillary and mandibular casts are trimmed at the labeled areas. See text for procedures.

II. OBJECTIVES: CHARACTERISTICS OF THE FINISHED CASTS

Before the step-by-step description of the trimming procedure, an outline of the characteristics of the finished casts is provided as an overall guide. Table 10-1 lists the criteria for each cast feature.

III. PRELIMINARY STEPS TO TRIMMING THE CAST

A. Casts must be wet; soak at least 5 minutes.

TABLE 10-1 Criteria for an Acceptable Cast

Cast Feature	Criteria	Figure Number
Overall base shape	See Figure 10-5 with labels	10-5
Proportions	⅓ art portion ⅔ anatomic portion	10-6A
Bases	Mean occlusal plane of the related casts – parallel with both bases Bases are parallel with each other	10-6A

Posterior borders	(1) At right angle with bases
	 (2) Stand on the posterior borders: the casts rest together in natural intercuspation
	 (3) Posterior borders are perpendicular
	    (a) to median line from the incisors through palate
	    (b) to middle of tongue
		10-6B
		 10-6B
		
		 10-7A
		 10-7B

Sides	Symmetrical angulation with posterior border and heel cuts Parallel with line through the occlusal grooves of the premolars of each side	10-7 10-10A
Heels	½-inch cuts parallel with the mesiodistal plane of the opposite canine	10-10B
Anterior	Maxillary: pointed with the cuts extending from canine area Mandibular: arc shape	10-11A 10-11B
Borders	Posterior: includes retromolar area and tuberosity Sides: ¼ to 5⁄16 inch from protuberance over premolars and molars; anatomy of mucobuccal fold included Anterior: ¼ to 5⁄16 inch from the most protruded tooth or from depth of the mucobuccal fold, whichever is most facial	10-7 10-11
Surfaces of the cast	Smooth and polished with air bubbles removed or filled	

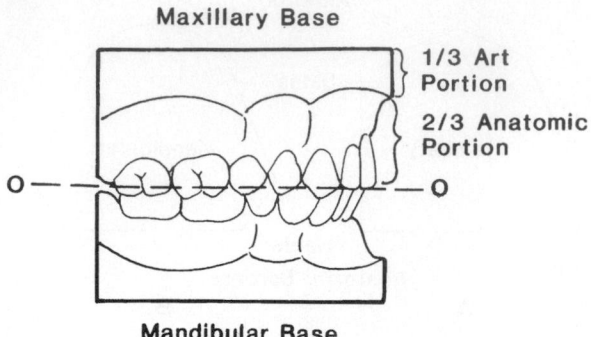

Maxillary Base

1/3 Art Portion

2/3 Anatomic Portion

O ———— O

Mandibular Base

A

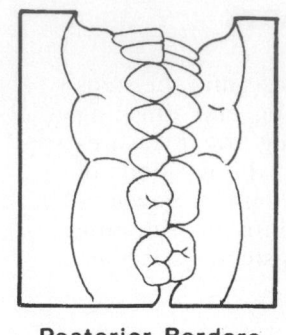

Posterior Borders

B

▦ **FIGURE 10-6 Finished Study Casts. (A)** Proportions and planes. The *art* portion is one third and the anatomic portion two thirds of the total height of the cast. Note parallelism of the maxillary and mandibular bases with the mean occlusal plane (0—0). **(B)** Posterior borders are at right angles to the bases. When the maxillary and mandibular casts are placed on their posterior borders, the teeth intercuspate exactly.

  B. Remove bubbles of stone on or about the teeth with a small sharp instrument; use care not to scar the cast.
  C. Level down excess stone that is distal to the retromolar area and tuberosity so casts may be occluded. Do not shorten the cast anteriorly to posteriorly at this time.
  D. Trim casts conservatively on the sides to make a smooth surface for marking.

IV. TRIMMING THE BASES

A. Objectives
  1. To make bases parallel with the mean occlusal plane and to each other.
  2. To make correct proportions for the height of the casts; art portion one-third and anatomic portion two-thirds (Figure 10-6A).

B. Mandibular Cast Is Trimmed First
  1. Measure the greatest height of the anatomic portion (usually this is from the tip of the canine to the depth of the vestibule) with a plastic ruler (Figure 10-8).
  2. Divide by two to obtain the height of the art portion.
  3. Add the measured height of the anatomic portion to the height of the art portion for the total height of the cast. Set compass or dividers at this measurement.
  4. Place the cast teeth down on a flat surface

and mark a line around the art portion at the height calculated in step 3. This line should be parallel with the occlusal plane (line 0–0 in Figure 10-8). Trim the cast at the line.

C. Maxillary Cast Base
  1. Measure the greatest depth of the anatomic portion (usually at the canine) and divide by two to obtain the height of the art portion.
  2. Relate the two casts (use the wax bite if necessary) and place the mandibular base on the flat surface.
  3. Measure from the base of the mandibular cast to the highest point of the maxillary anatomic portion (usually in the vestibule over the canine), and add this figure to the height of the maxillary art portion calculated in step 1 above.
  4. Set the compass at this measurement, and mark a line around the maxillary cast at the total height. The line must be parallel with the base of the mandibular cast and with the occlusal plane. Trim.

V. POSTERIOR BORDERS

  A. *Select the longest cast to trim first* by measuring from the incisors to points distal to the retromolar and tuberosity areas.
  B. On the longest cast, place the tip of the com-

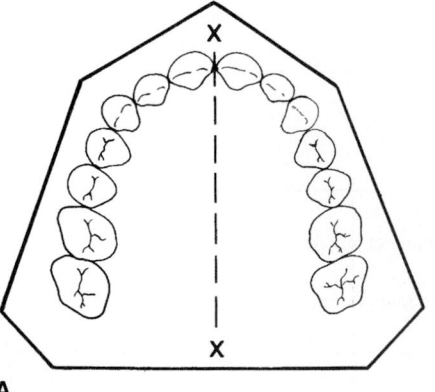

X

X

A

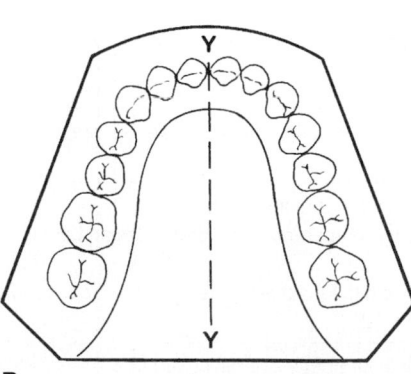

Y

Y

B

▦ **FIGURE 10-7 Occlusal Views of Finished Casts. (A)** Maxillary. **(B)** Mandibular. The posterior border is perpendicular to the median line from the incisors through the palate (X—X) and the middle of the tongue (Y—Y). The tuberosity of the maxilla and the retromolar areas of the mandible are preserved.

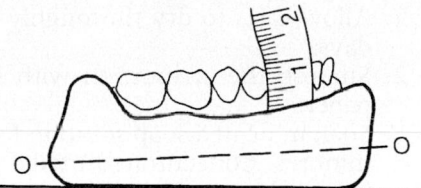

■FIGURE 10-8 **Trimming the Base.** Measure the anatomic portion at its greatest height, which is usually from the tip of the canine to the depth of the vestibule. Note ruler in position. One half of the measurement is the height of the art portion. The trimming line (0—0) is parallel with the mean occlusal plane. See text for details.

pass at the gingival border behind the midline anteriorly (usually this is between the central incisors) and mark an arc ¼-inch distal to the tuberosity (if the maxillary cast) or retromolar area (if the mandibular cast) on each side.

C. Intersect the arc with a line through the central grooves of the molars (Figure 10-9A).

D. Connect the two points across the back of the cast (0–0 in Figure 10-9A). Check that this line is perpendicular to the median line from the incisors through the palate or the tongue (X–Y in Figure 10-9B).

E. With the base of the cast flat on the model trimmer table, trim on the line marked for the posterior border.

F. For the shorter cast, relate the two casts with the wax bite and place flat on the base of the first trimmed cast. Bring them carefully to the cutting surface of the model trimmer, and trim

until the two posterior borders are even and parallel.

G. Check by placing the casts on their posterior borders and bringing them together. They should relate in their natural intercuspation (Figure 10-6B).

VI. SIDES AND HEELS

A. *Select the widest cast to trim first;* casts are usually widest at the molar region.

B. Mark with ruler two symmetrical lines ¼ inch buccal from the buccal bony prominence at the premolar regions and parallel with lines through the central grooves of the premolars (Figure 10-10A).

1. Check that the lines form equal angles with the posterior border.

2. Before trimming, make certain that the lines when cut would not remove any vestibular anatomy.

3. Trim the sides with the base flat on the model trimmer table.

C. Mark trimming lines for the heels; cuts are ½-inch wide and parallel with a line through the mesiodistal plane of the opposite canine (Figure 10-10B). Trim with base flat on the model trimmer table.

D. Relate the opposite cast with the wax bite, and trim the sides and heels to match the previously trimmed cast.

VII. ANTERIOR

The maxillary cast is trimmed to a point, and the mandibular cast is rounded (Figure 10-5).

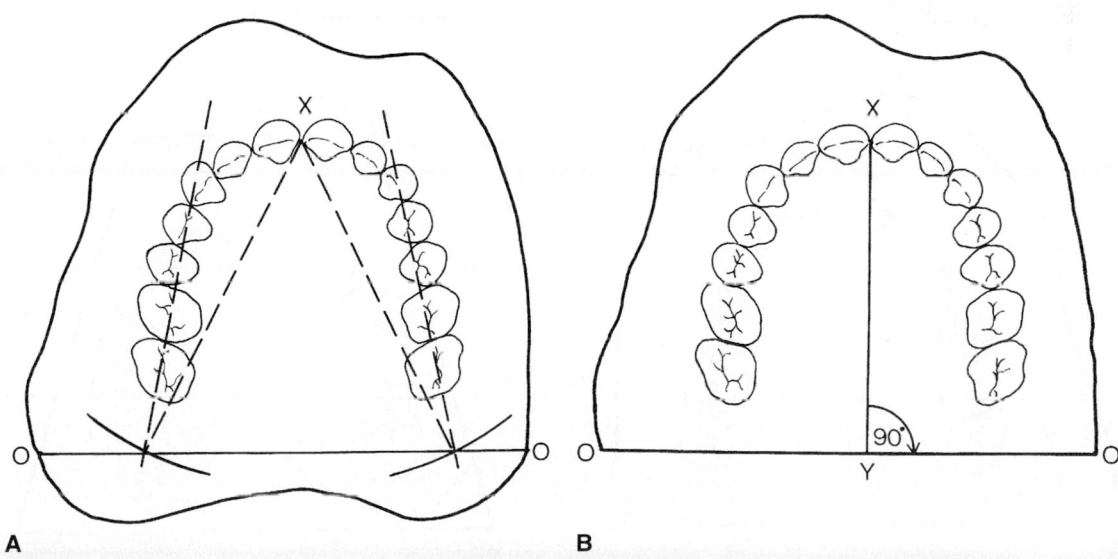

A   **B**

■FIGURE 10-9 **Trim Line for Posterior Borders. (A)** On the longest cast, use a compass to draw arcs from the anterior midline point (X) to 1/4 inch distal to the tuberosity (maxilla) or retromolar area (mandible). Intersect the arc with a line through the central grooves of the molars and connect the two points across the cast (0—0). **(B)** Check that the 0—0 line is perpendicular to the median line from the incisors through the palate or tongue (X—Y) before trimming.

A. Maxillary

1. A ruler can be used to draw guidelines for trimming on each side of the midline to the canine areas. Note the broken lines in Figure 10-11A. The lines should be ¼ inch labial to the depth of the mucobuccal fold (vestibule) or to the most labially inclined tooth.
2. Before trimming, check that both sides of the cast are the same length from the intersection of the front cut to the heels.

B. Mandibular

1. Sketch the shape of an arc from canine to canine to conform generally with the curvature of the anterior teeth and approximately ¼ inch labial to the depth of the mucobuccal fold or the most labially inclined or positioned tooth (Figure 10-11B).
2. Before trimming, check that both sides of the cast are the same length from the intersection of the front cut to the heels.

VIII. FINISHING AND POLISHING

A. Trim rough edges and margins of both casts and the lingual portion of the mandibular cast to even off irregularities and make the depth of the vestibule visible. Remaining bubbles are removed.

B. Use waterproof sandpaper and a plaster smoothing stone to remove marks left by the model trimmer on the art portion. Sandpaper is not used on the anatomic portion.

C. Fill any holes in the wet casts with stone applied with a spatula to the flat surfaces of the art portion or a camel's hair brush to the anatomic portion. Smooth off excess.

D. Finish and polish

1. Allow casts to dry thoroughly for 2 to 3 days.
2. Smooth the art portion with fine sandpaper.
3. Soak in heated soap solution for 30 to 60 minutes. Concentrated model gloss soap is available commercially.
4. Rub with chamois, cotton, or a soft cloth.
5. Talc or baby talcum powder with olive oil may be used, followed by rubbing with a chamois or soft cloth.

TECHNICAL HINTS

I. Safety Factors
A. Use protective eyewear and mask while handling powdered dental materials or using a model trimmer. Goggles are indicated for laboratory procedures (see Figure 3-2, page 47).
B. Do not agitate powders unnecessarily during mixing. Inhaled dust particles can cause serious irritation to the respiratory system.
II. Label each cast with the patient's name and the date. These may be inscribed into the posterior border of the cast before soaping and polishing.
III. Boxes of an appropriate size are available commercially for storage of one or more pairs of casts.
IV. Record in the patient's permanent data file the size of impression tray used. When casts are made periodically for follow-up, time is saved both in the sterilization of all sizes for try-in

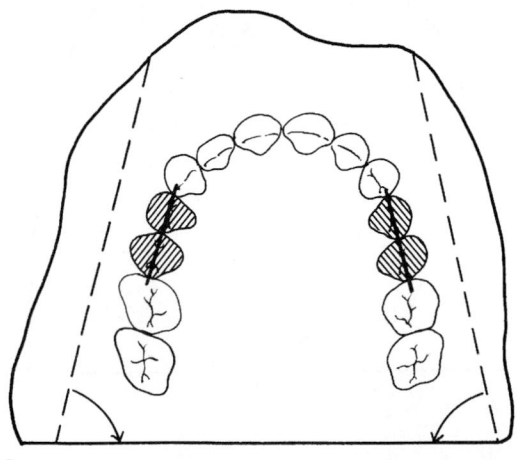
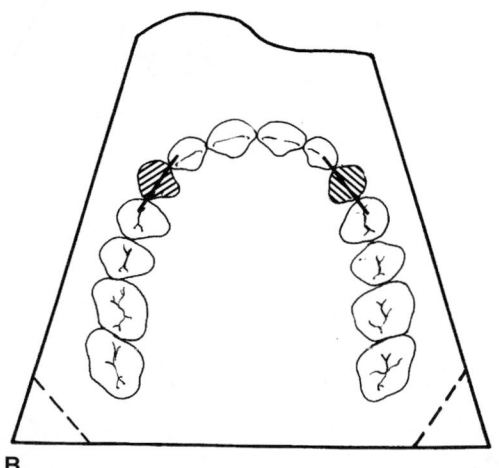

A **B**

■ **FIGURE 10-10 Trim Lines for Sides and Heels. (A)** On the widest cast, the trim lines for the sides are drawn parallel with lines through the central grooves of the premolars. The two symmetrical lines form equal angles with the posterior border of the cast. **(B)** Mark trim lines for heels 1/4 inch wide and parallel with lines through the mesiodistal plane of the opposite canine. The lines are symmetrical with each other and form equal angles with the posterior border.

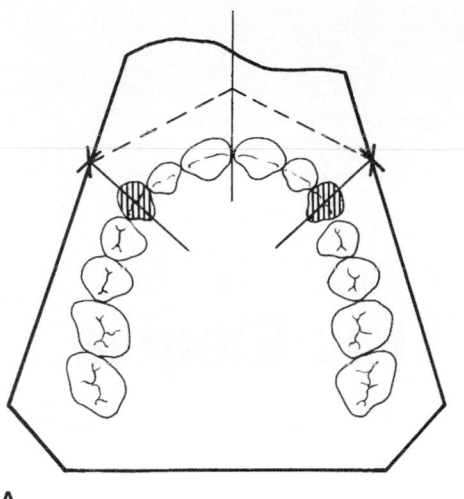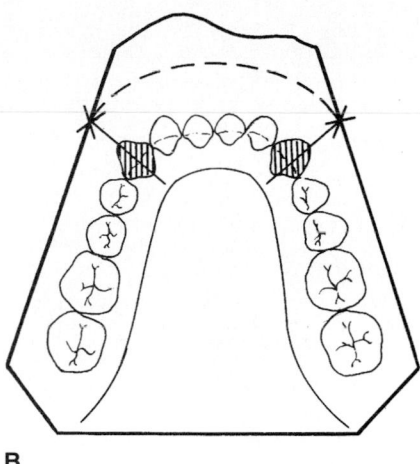

■ FIGURE 10-11 Trim Lines for Anterior. (A) Maxillary lines are drawn from opposite the middle of each canine to meet in a point at the midline and approximately 1/4 inch labial to the most labially positioned tooth. **(B)** Mandibular line forms an arc drawn from the middle of each canine approximately 1/4 inch labial to the most labially positioned tooth.

A   **B**

and in the preparation of the wax rim in advance of the patient's appointment.

V. Make duplicate cast for the permanent record when the dentist uses the original for the design of a prosthesis or fabrication of a secondary impression tray. The duplicate cast is made by taking a laboratory impression of the original and pouring it in the same manner as the original.

VI. To care for the model trimmer following its use, allow motor to run until clear water is flowing through and all particles of stone or plaster have been washed away.

VII. Replace scratched mixing bowls.

VIII. Sterilize aluminum impression trays. Clean completely to prepare for sterilization.

FACTORS TO TEACH THE PATIENT

I. Importance and purposes of study casts. Reasons for comparative casts following treatment or at a later date.

II. Use the casts of other patients to show effects of treatment or what can happen if the prescribed treatment is not carried out.

III. Areas that present difficulty in the bacterial plaque control program:
   A. Show anatomy of gingiva and teeth.
   B. Demonstrate use of plaque removal devices on the patient's own study casts.

REFERENCES

1. **Craig,** R.G. and Ward, M.L., eds.: *Restorative Dental Materials,* 10th ed. St. Louis, Mosby, 1997, pp. 281–289.
2. **Anusavice,** K.J.: *Phillips' Science of Dental Materials,* 10th ed. Philadelphia, W.B. Saunders Co., 1996, pp. 111–137.
3. **American Dental Association,** Council on Scientific Affairs and Council on Dental Practice: Infection Control Recommendations for the Dental Office and the Dental Laboratory, *J. Am. Dent. Assoc., 127,* 672, May, 1996.
4. **Thouati,** A., Deveaux, E., Iost, A., and Behin, P.: Dimensional Stability of Seven Elastomeric Impression Materials Immersed in Disinfectants, *J. Prosthet. Dent., 76,* July 8, 1996.
5. **Craig** and Ward: op. cit., pp. 333–346.
6. **Anusavice:** op. cit., pp. 185–208.

SUGGESTED READINGS

Andrieu, S.C. and Springstead, M.C.: A Simplified Guide To Taking Accurate Alginate Impressions and Trimming Diagnostic Study Casts, *J. Practical Hygiene, 1,* 11, September, 1992.

Berry, T.G. and Berry, J.C.: Preparation of Study Models, in Woodall, I.R.: *Comprehensive Dental Hygiene Care,* 4th ed., St. Louis, Mosby, 1993, pp. 312–335.

Ehrlich, A., Torres, H.O., and Bird, D.: *Essentials of Dental Assisting,* 2nd ed. Philadelphia, W.B. Saunders Co., 1996, pp. 201–212.

Pratten, D.H. and Novetsky, M.: Detail Reproduction of Soft Tissue: a Comparison of Impression Materials, *J. Prosthet. Dent., 65,* 188, February, 1991.

Infection Control

Chia, W.K., Stevens, L., and Basford, K.E.: Dimensional Change of Impressions on Sterilization, *Aust. Dent. J., 35,* 23, February, 1990.

del Pilar Rios, M., Morgano, S.M., Stein, R.S., and Rose, L.: Effects of Chemical Disinfectant Solutions on the Stability and Accuracy of the Dental Impression Complex, *J. Prosthet. Dent., 76,* 356, October, 1996.

Gerhardt, D.E. and Williams, H.N.: Factors Affecting the Stability of Sodium Hypochlorite Solutions Used to Disinfect Dental Impressions, *Quintessence Int., 22,* 587, July, 1991.

King, B.B., Norling, B.K., and Seals, R.: Gypsum Compatibility of Antimicrobial Alginates After Spray Disinfection, *J. Prosthodont., 3,* 219, December 1994.

Mitchell, D.L., Hariri, N.M., Duncanson, M.G., Jacobsen, N.L., and McCallum, R.E.: Quantitative Study of Bacterial Colonization of Dental Casts, *J. Prosthet. Dent., 78,* 518, November, 1997.

Peutzfeldt, A. and Asmussen, E.: Effect of Disinfecting Solutions on Surface Texture of Alginate and Elastomeric Impressions, *Scand. J. Dent. Res., 98,* 74, February, 1990.

Samaranayake, L.P., Hunjan, M., and Jennings, K.J.: Carriage of Oral Flora on Irreversible Hydrocolloid and Elastomeric Impression Materials, *J. Prosthet. Dent., 65,* 244, February, 1991.

Touyz, L.Z.G. and Rosen, M.: Disinfection of Alginate Impression Material Using Disinfectants as Mixing and Soak Solutions, *J. Dent., 19,* 255, August, 1991.

Verran, J., Kossar, S., and McCord, J.F.: Microbial Study of Selected Risk Areas in Dental Technology Laboratories, *J. Dent., 24,* 77, January/March, 1996.

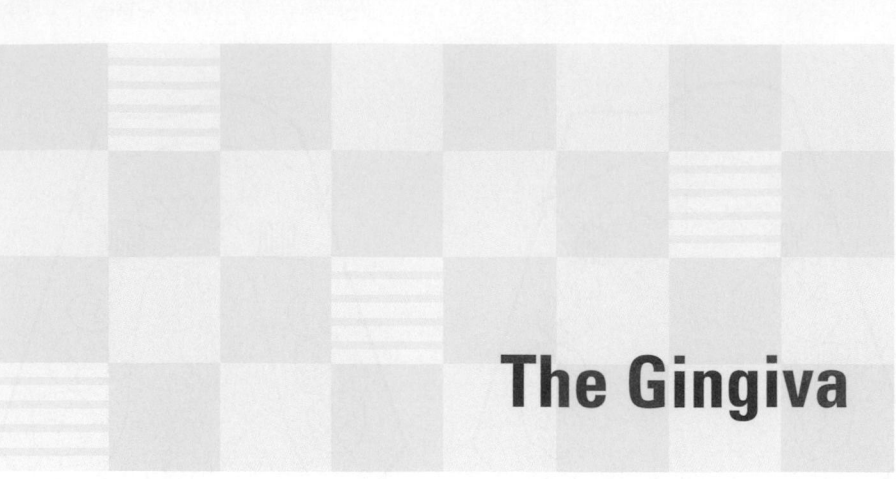

The Gingiva

The true test of successful treatment, the real evaluation of the effects of scaling and related instrumentation, is the *health* of the gingival tissues. The objective of all treatment is to bring the diseased gingiva to a state of health that can be maintained by the patient. To do this, the first objective is to learn to recognize normal healthy tissue; to observe certain characteristics of color, texture, and form; to test for bleeding; and to apply this knowledge to the treatment and supervision of the patient's gingiva until health is attained.

An outline of the clinical features of the periodontal tissues in health and disease is included in this chapter. Key words are defined in Box 11-1.

OBJECTIVES

The ultimate objective is to apply knowledge and skill in examination and assessment of the periodontal tissues to patient care so that each patient attains and maintains optimum oral health. The dental hygienist must know when the treatment provided by dental hygiene services is definitive in restoring health and when additional treatment is needed. The patient can be properly informed so that complete treatment can be provided.

Specific objectives are to be able to
  I. Recognize normal periodontal tissues.
  II. Know the clinical features of the periodontal tissues that must be examined for a complete assessment.
  III. Recognize the markers that are the basic signs of periodontal infections and classify them by type and degree of severity.
  IV. Identify the dental hygiene treatment and instruction needed.
  V. Outline the patient's preventive program.

THE TREATMENT AREA

The treatment procedures are applied directly to the teeth, the gingiva, and the gingival sulcus. Detailed knowledge and understanding of the anatomy and normal clinical appearance of the hard and soft oral

BOX 11-1 KEY WORDS: Gingiva and Periodontium

Attachment apparatus: the cementum, periodontal ligament, and the alveolar bone.

Clinical attachment level: the probing depth measured from a fixed point, such as the cementoenamel junction.

Desmosome (dĕz'mō-sōm): cell junction; consists of a dense plate near the cell surface that relates to a similar structure on an adjacent cell, between which are thin layers of extracellular material.

Epithelium (ĕp"ĭ-thē'lē-um)

   Oral: the tissue serving as a liner for the intraoral mucosal surfaces.

   Squamous (skwā'mus): composed of a layer of flat, scale-like cells; or may be stratified.

Exudate (eks'ū-dāt): material, such as fluid, cells, and cellular debris, that has escaped from blood vessels and is deposited in tissues or on tissue surfaces, usually as a result of inflammation.

Fibroblast (fĭ'brō-blǎst): fiber-producing cell of the connective tissue; a flattened, irregularly branched cell with a large oval nucleus that is responsible in part for the production and remodeling of the extracellular matrix.

Fibrosis (fĭ'brō'sĭs): a fibrous change of the mucous membrane, especially the gingiva, as a result of chronic inflammation; fibrotic gingiva may appear outwardly healthy, thus masking underlying disease.

Hemidesmosome (hĕm'ē dez'mō-sōm): half of a desmosome that forms a site of attachment between junctional epithelial cells and the tooth surface.

Hyperkeratosis (hī"per-kĕr"ah-tō'sĭs): abnormal thickening of the keratin layer (stratum corneum) of the epithelium.

Hyperplasia (hī"per-plā'zah): abnormal increase in volume of a tissue or organ caused by formation and growth of new normal cells.

Hypertrophy (hī"-per'trō-fē): increase in size of tissue or organ caused by an increase in size of its constituent cells.

Keratinization (kĕr"ah-tin"ĭ-zā'shun): development of a horny layer of flattened epithelial cells containing keratin.

Marker: identifier; symptoms or signs by which a particular condition can be recognized; for example, clinical and microbiologic markers are used to identify gingival and periodontal infections.

Mastication (măs"tĭ-kā'shun): act of chewing.

Nonkeratinized mucosa: lining mucosa in which the stratified squamous epithelial cells retain their nuclei and cytoplasm.

Periodontium (pĕr"ē-ō-dŏn'shē-um): tissues surrounding and supporting the teeth; in two sections are the **gingival unit**, composed of the free and attached gingiva and the alveolar mucosa, and the **attachment apparatus,** which includes the cementum, periodontal ligament, and alveolar process.

Probing depth: the distance from the gingival margin to the location of the periodontal probe tip inserted for gentle probing at the attachment.

Pus (pŭs): a fluid product of inflammation that contains leukocytes, degenerated tissue elements, tissue fluids, and microorganisms.

Sharpey's fibers: penetrating connective tissue fibers by which the tooth is attached to the adjacent alveolar bone; the fiber bundles penetrate cementum on one side and alveolar bone on the other.

Stippling (stĭp'lĭng): the pitted, orange peel appearance frequently seen on the surface of the attached gingiva.

Suppuration (sŭp"ū-rā'shun): formation of pus.

Taste bud: receptor of taste on tongue and oropharynx; goblet-shaped cells oriented at right angles to the surface of the epithelium.

---

tissues are prerequisite to meaningful examination and treatment.

I. THE TEETH

A. Clinical Crown

The part of the tooth above the attached periodontal tissues. It can be considered the part of the tooth where clinical treatment procedures are applied (Figure 11-1).

B. Clinical Root

The part of the tooth below the base of the gingival sulcus or periodontal pocket. It is the part of the root to which periodontal fibers are attached.

C. Anatomic Crown

The part of the tooth covered by enamel.

D. Anatomic Root

The part of the tooth covered by cementum.

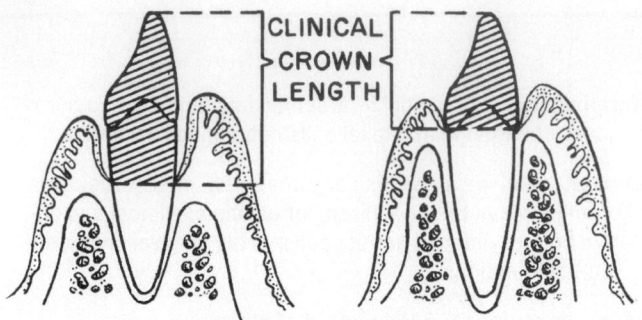

FIGURE 11-1 Clinical Crown. The clinical crown is the part of the tooth that is above the attached periodontal tissue. *Left,* When the periodontal pocket depth is increased, the clinical crown extends to a position at which the clinical crown length is greater than the clinical root length. The clinical root is that part of the tooth with attached periodontal tissues. *Right,* When the clinical attachment level is at the cementoenamel junction, the clinical crown and the anatomic crown are the same.

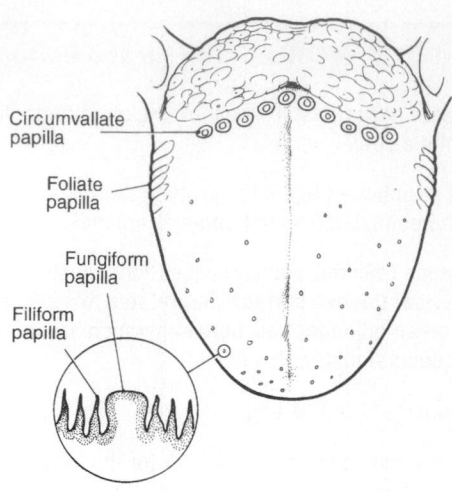

FIGURE 11-2 Papillae of the Tongue. Dorsal surface of a human tongue shows the four types of papillae. Inset enlargement shows the shape of filiform and fungiform papillae.

II. ORAL MUCOSA

The lining of the oral cavity, the oral mucosa, is a mucous membrane composed of connective tissue covered with stratified squamous epithelium. There are three divisions or categories of oral mucosa.

A. Masticatory Mucosa
1. Covers the *gingiva* and the *hard palate,* the areas used most during the mastication of food.
2. Except for the free margin of the gingiva, the masticatory mucosa is firmly attached to underlying tissues.
3. The epithelial covering is generally keratinized.

B. Lining Mucosa
1. Covers the *inner surfaces of the lips and cheeks, the floor of the mouth, the under side of the tongue, the soft palate, and the alveolar mucosa.*
2. These tissues are not firmly attached to underlying tissue.
3. The epithelial covering is not generally keratinized.

C. Specialized Mucosa
1. Covers the *dorsum* (upper surface) *of the tongue.* It is composed of many papillae; some contain taste buds.
2. The distribution of the four types of papillae is shown in Figure 11-2.
   a. Filiform. Threadlike keratinized elevations that cover the dorsal surface of the tongue; they are the most numerous of the papillae.
   b. Fungiform. Mushroom-shaped papillae interspersed among the filiform papillae on the tip and sides of the tongue. They are redder than the filiform papillae

and contain variable numbers of taste buds. The inset enlargement in Figure 11-2 shows the comparative shape and size of the filiform and fungiform papillae.
   c. Circumvallate (vallate). The 10 to 14 large round papillae arranged in a "V" between the body of the tongue and the base. Taste buds line the walls.
   d. Foliate. Vertical grooves on the lateral posterior sides of the tongue; also contain taste buds.

III. THE PERIODONTIUM

The periodontium is the functional unit of tissues that surrounds and supports the tooth. The four parts are the gingiva, periodontal ligament, cementum, and bone; the last three make up the attachment apparatus.

A. Periodontal Ligament
The periodontal ligament is the fibrous connective tissue that surrounds and attaches the roots of teeth to the alveolar bone.

The ligament is located in the periodontal space between the cementum and the alveolar bone. It is composed of connective tissue cells and intracellular substance. The fibers that are inserted into the cementum on one side and the alveolar bone on the other are called *Sharpey's fibers.*

The two general groups of fibers are the *gingival groups* (around the cervical area within the gingival tissues) and the *principal fiber groups* (surrounding the root).[1]
1. *Gingival Fiber Groups* (Figure 11-3)
   a. **Dentogingival fibers** (free gingival). From the cementum in the cervical re-

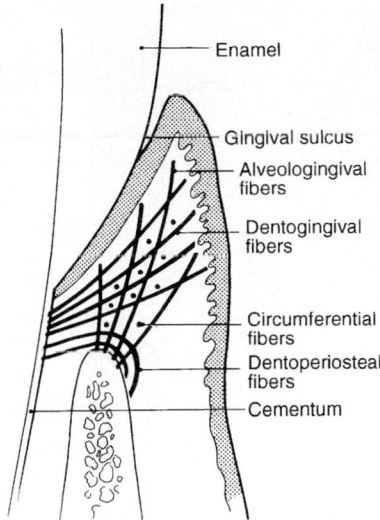

FIGURE II-3 Gingival Fiber Groups. Cross-section of the gingiva shows the relation of the gingival fiber groups to the gingival sulcus, the free gingiva, the cementum, and the alveolar bone.

gion into the free gingiva to give support to the gingiva.

b. **Alveologingival fibers** (attached gingival). From the alveolar crest into the free and attached gingiva to provide support.

c. **Circumferential fibers** (circular). Continuous around the neck of the tooth to help to maintain the tooth in position.

d. **Dentoperiosteal fibers** (alveolar crest). From the cervical cementum over the alveolar crest to blend with fibers of the periosteum of the bone.

e. **Transseptal fibers.** From the cervical area of one tooth across to an adjacent tooth (on the mesial or distal only) to provide resistance to separation of teeth (Figure 11-4).

2. *Principal Fiber Groups* (Figure 11-4)

The five principal groups of collagen fibers are named for their location on the root and for their direction. They are also called the dentoalveolar fiber groups.

a. **Apical fibers.** From the root apex to adjacent surrounding bone to resist vertical forces.

b. **Oblique fibers.** From the root above the apical fibers obliquely toward the occlusal to resist vertical and unexpected strong forces.

c. **Horizontal fibers.** From the cementum in the middle of each root to adjacent alveolar bone to resist tipping of the tooth.

d. **Alveolar crest fibers.** From the alveolar crest to the cementum just below the cementoenamel junction to resist intrusive forces.

e. **Interradicular fibers.** From cementum between the roots of multirooted teeth to the adjacent bone to resist vertical and lateral forces.

B. Cementum

The cementum is a thin layer of calcified connective tissue that covers the tooth from the cementoenamel junction to, and around, the apical foramen.

1. *Functions*

a. To seal the tubules of the root dentin.

b. To provide attachment for the periodontal fiber groups.

2. *Characteristics*

a. Thickness is 50 to 200 μm about the apex; 30 to 60 μm about the cervical area.

b. Vascular and nerve connections are missing; therefore, cementum is insensitive.

c. Relationship of enamel and cementum at the cervical area is shown in Figure 13-2, page 229.

C. Alveolar Bone

The alveolar bone consists of the lamina dura, which surrounds the tooth socket, and the supporting bone. When teeth are lost, the alveolar bone is resorbed. The bone functions to support the teeth and provide attachment for the periodontal ligament fibers.

D. Gingiva

The part of the masticatory mucosa that surrounds the necks of the teeth and is attached to the teeth and the alveolar bone.

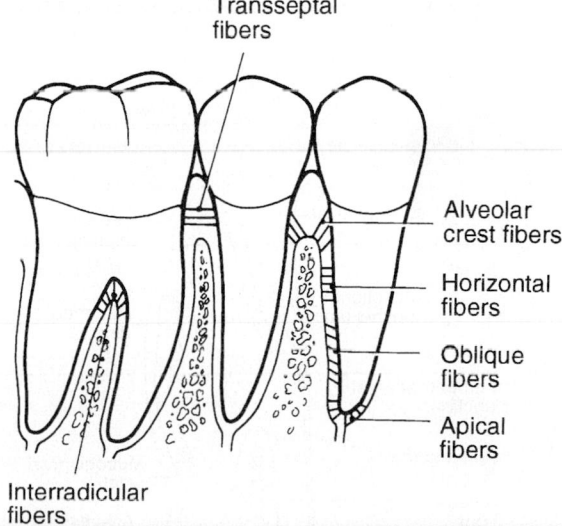

FIGURE II-4 Principal Fiber Groups of the Periodontium. The five principal groups (apical, oblique, horizontal, alveolar crest, and interradicular) are shown. The transseptal fibers of the gingival fibers groups are also shown as they span across from the cervical area of one tooth to the neighboring tooth.

THE GINGIVA AND RELATED STRUCTURES

The gingiva is made up of the free gingiva, the attached gingiva, and the interdental gingiva or interdental papilla.

I. FREE GINGIVA (MARGINAL GINGIVA)

In health the free gingiva is closely adapted around each tooth. It connects with the attached gingiva at the free gingival groove and attaches to the tooth at the coronal portion of the junctional epithelium (Figure 11-5).

A. Free Gingival Groove

1. The free gingival groove is a shallow linear groove that demarcates the free from the attached gingiva. Generally, about one-third of the teeth show a visible gingival groove when the gingiva is healthy.[2]
2. In the absence of inflammation and pocket formation, the gingival groove runs somewhat parallel with and about 0.5 to 1.5 mm from the gingival margin,[3] and it is approximately at the level of the bottom of the gingival sulcus.

B. Oral Epithelium (outer gingival epithelium, Figure 11-6)

1. Covers the free gingiva from the gingival groove over the gingival margin.
2. Composed of keratinized stratified squamous epithelium.

C. Gingival Margin (gingival crest, margin of the gingiva, or free margin, Figure 11-5)

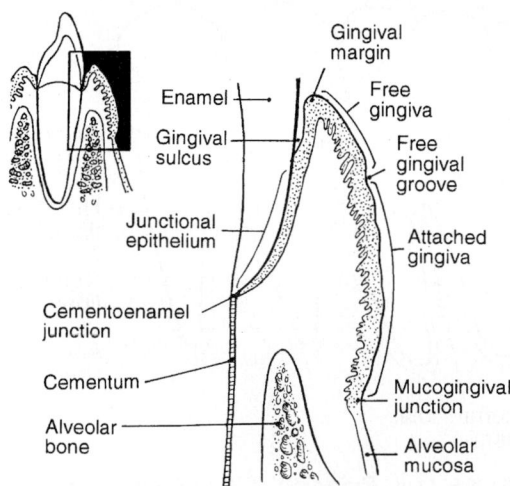

FIGURE 11-5 Parts of the Gingiva. Cross-sectional diagram shows the parts of the gingiva and adjacent tissues of a partially erupted tooth. Note that the junctional epithelium in on the enamel.

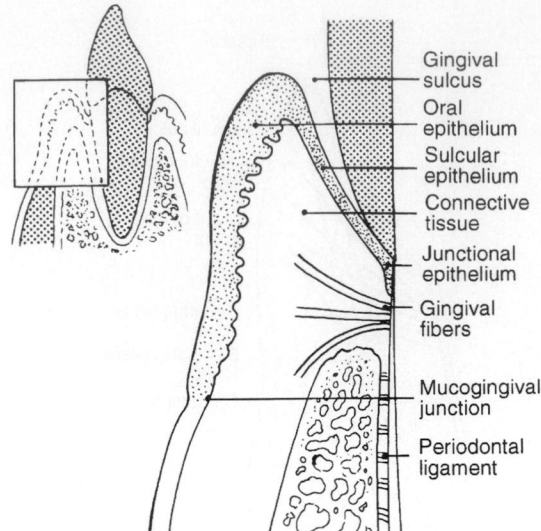

FIGURE 11-6 The Gingival Tissues. Cross-sectional diagram shows the histologic relationships of the oral, sulcular, and junctional epithelia and the connective tissue.

1. This is the edge of the gingiva nearest the incisal or occlusal surface.
2. Marks the opening of the gingival sulcus.

II. GINGIVAL SULCUS (CREVICE)

A. Location

The crevice or groove between the free gingiva and the tooth.

B. Boundaries (Figure 11-6)

1. *Inner.* Tooth surface. May be the enamel, cementum, or part of each, depending on the position of the junctional epithelium.
2. *Outer.* Sulcular epithelium.
3. *Base.* Coronal margin of the attached tissues. The base of the sulcus or pocket is also called the "probing depth," the "depth of the sulcus," or the "bottom of the pocket."

C. Sulcular Epithelium

The continuation of the oral epithelium covering the free gingiva. Sulcular epithelium is not keratinized.

D. Depth of Sulcus

Healthy sulci are shallow and may be only 0.5 mm. The average depth of the healthy sulcus is about 1.8 mm.[4]

E. Gingival Sulcus Fluid (sulcular fluid, crevicular fluid)

1. A serumlike fluid that seeps from the connective tissue through the epithelial lining of the sulcus or pocket.
2. Occurrence is slight to none in a normal sulcus; increased with inflammation. It is part of the local defense mechanism and is able to

transport many substances including, endotoxins, enzymes, antibodies, and certain systemically administered drugs.

III. JUNCTIONAL EPITHELIUM (ATTACHMENT EPITHELIUM)

A. Description

The junctional epithelium is a cufflike band of stratified squamous epithelium that is continuous with the sulcular epithelium and completely encircles the tooth. It is triangular in cross section, is widest at the junction with the sulcular epithelium, and narrows down to the width of a few cells at the apical end.

The junctional epithelium is not keratinized. It has two basement membranes: one adjacent to the connective tissue and one adjacent to the tooth surface.

B. Size

The junctional epithelium may be up to 15 or 20 cells in thickness where it joins the sulcular epithelium and tapers down to 1 or 2 cells in thickness at the apical end. The length ranges from 0.25 to 1.35 mm.

C. Position

1. As the tooth erupts, the attachment is on the enamel; during eruption, the epithelium migrates toward the cementoenamel junction (Figure 11-7).
2. At full eruption, the attachment is usually on the cementum, where it becomes firmly attached (Figure 11-7D).
3. With wear of the tooth on the incisal or occlusal surface and with periodontal infections, the attachment migrates along the root surface (Figure 11-7E).

D. Relation of Crest of Alveolar Bone to the Attached Gingival Tissue

The distance between the base of the attachment and the crest of the alveolar bone is approximately 1.0 to 1.5 mm. This distance is maintained in disease when the epithelium moves along the root surface and bone loss occurs.

E. Attachment of the Epithelium to the Tooth Surface

The junctional epithelium or attachment epithelium provides a seal at the base of the sulcus. The attachment, or connecting interface between the tooth and the tissue, is accomplished by hemidesmosomes and the basal lamina of the junctional epithelium.

IV. INTERDENTAL GINGIVA (INTERDENTAL PAPILLA)

A. Location

In health, the interdental gingiva occupies the interproximal area between two adjacent teeth. The tip and lateral borders are continuous with the free gingiva, whereas other parts are attached gingiva.

B. Shape

1. *Varies With Spacing or Overlapping of the Teeth.* The interdental gingiva may be flat or saddle-shaped when wide spaces are between the teeth, or it may be tapered and narrow when the teeth are crowded or overlapped.
2. *Between Anterior Teeth.* Pointed, pyramidal.
3. *Between Posterior Teeth*
   a. Flatter than anterior papillae, because of wider teeth, wider contact areas, and flattened interdental bone.
   b. Two papillae, one facial and one lingual, connected by a col, are found when teeth are in contact.

C. Col

1. A col is the depression between the lingual or palatal and facial papillae that conforms to the proximal contact area (Figure 11-8).
2. The center of the col area is not usually keratinized, and thus is more susceptible to in-

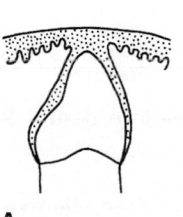 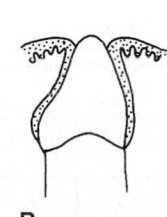 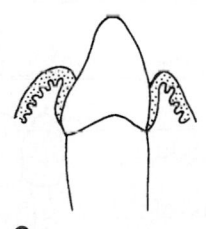 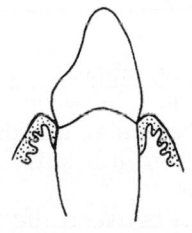 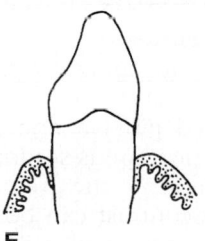

A   B   C   D   E

■ **FIGURE 11-7 Tooth Eruption and the Gingiva. (A)** Before eruption, the oral epithelium covers the tooth. **(B)** As the tooth emerges, the reduced epithelium joins the oral epithelium as the gingival sulcus is formed. **(C)** Partial eruption with the junctional epithelium along the enamel. **(D)** Eruption complete, with junctional epithelium at the cementoenamel junction. **(E)** From disease or other cause, the attachment migrates along the root surface, exposing the cementum.

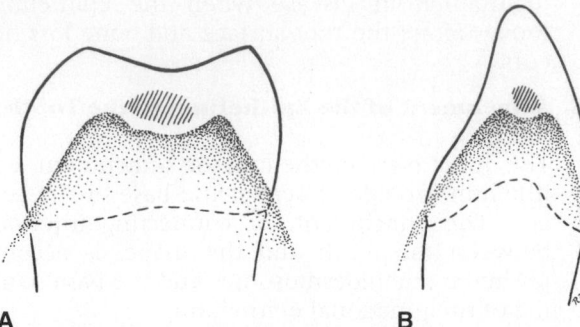

A   **B**

▪ FIGURE 11-8 **Col.** A col is the depression between the lingual or palatal and the facial papillae under the contact area. The contact area is represented by the striped lines. **(A)** Mesial of mandibular molar to show wide col area. **(B)** Mesial of mandibular incisor to show a narrow col. The col deepens when gingival enlargement occurs.

fection. Most periodontal infection begins in the col area.

V. ATTACHED GINGIVA

A. Extent
1. The attached gingiva is continuous with the oral epithelium of the free gingiva and is covered with keratinized stratified squamous epithelium.
2. Maxillary palatal gingiva is continuous with the palatal mucosa.
3. The attached gingiva of the mandibular facial and lingual gingiva and maxillary facial gingiva is demarcated from the alveolar mucosa by the mucogingival junction.

B. Attachment
Firmly bound to the underlying cementum and alveolar bone.

C. Shape
Follows the depressions between the eminences of the roots of the teeth.

VI. MUCOGINGIVAL JUNCTION

A. Appearance
The mucogingival junction appears as a line that marks the connection between the attached gingiva and the alveolar mucosa. The anterior line is scalloped, but it is fairly straight posterior to the premolars.

A contrast can be seen between the pink of the keratinized, stippled, attached gingiva and the darker alveolar mucosa.

B. Location
A mucogingival line is found on the facial surface of all quadrants and on the lingual surface of the mandibular arch. There is no alveolar mucosa on the palate. The palatal tissue is firmly attached to the bone of the roof of the mouth.

The three mucogingival lines are facial mandibular, lingual mandibular, and facial maxillary. In Figure 11-9, the facial maxillary and mandibular mucogingival junctions are shown in relation to the attached gingiva and the alveolar mucosa.

VII. ALVEOLAR MUCOSA

A. Description
Movable tissue loosely attached to the underlying bone. It has a smooth, shiny surface with nonkeratinized, thin epithelium. Underlying vessels may be seen through the epithelium.

B. Frena (singular: frenum or frenulum)
1. *Description.* a frenum is a narrow fold of mucous membrane that passes from a more fixed to a movable part, for example, from the attached gingiva at the mucogingival junction to the lip, cheek, or undersurface of the tongue. A frenum serves to check undue movement.
2. *Locations*
   a. Maxillary and mandibular anterior frena. At midlines between central incisors. Figure 11-9 shows diagrammatically the location of the anterior frena.
   b. Lingual frenum. From undersurface of the tongue.
   c. Buccal frena. In the canine–premolar areas, both maxillary and mandibular.
3. *Attachment of Frena in Relation to the Attached Gingiva*
   a. Closely associated with the mucogingival junction.
   b. When the attached gingiva is narrow or missing, the frena may pull on the free gingiva and displace it laterally. A "tension test" is used to locate frenal attachments and check the adequacy of the attached gingiva (page 211).

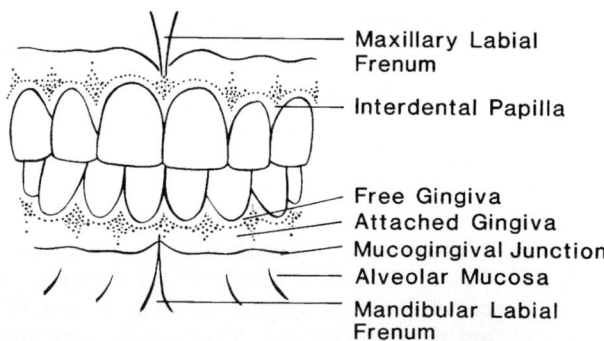

— Maxillary Labial Frenum
— Interdental Papilla
— Free Gingiva
— Attached Gingiva
— Mucogingival Junction
— Alveolar Mucosa
— Mandibular Labial Frenum

▪ FIGURE 11-9 **Parts of the Gingiva.** The mucogingival junction for each arch is shown in relation to the attached gingiva, alveolar mucosa, and labial anterior frena.

THE RECOGNITION OF GINGIVAL AND PERIODONTAL INFECTIONS

I. THE CLINICAL EXAMINATION

The recognition of normal gingiva, gingival infections, and deeper periodontal involvement depends on a disciplined, step-by-step examination. A basic examination performed to recognize the signs and effects of inflammation includes information about at least the following markers:

- Gingival tissue changes (color, size, shape, surface texture, position)
- Bleeding and exudate
- Mucogingival involvement (adequate width of attached gingiva)
- Probing depths; pocket formation (attachment levels)
- Furcation involvement
- Bacterial plaque (and calculus) present
- Mobility of teeth
- Radiographic evidence

It is also necessary to know the extent of the disease. *Gingival infections* are confined to the gingiva, whereas *periodontal infections* include all parts of the periodontium, namely, the gingiva, periodontal ligament, bone, and cementum.

II. SIGNS AND SYMPTOMS

Patients may or may not have specific symptoms to report because periodontal infections are insidious in development. Symptoms the patient notices or feels may include bleeding gingiva, sometimes only while brushing, sometimes with drooling at night, or sometimes spontaneously. Other possible symptoms are sensitivity to hot and cold, tenderness or discomfort while eating or some pain after eating, food retained between the teeth, unpleasant mouth odors, chronic bad taste, or a feeling that the teeth are loose. Most of these are symptoms of advanced disease.

III. CLINICALLY NORMAL

The terms "clinically normal" or "clinically healthy" may be used to designate gingival tissue that is characterized by the following: a shade of pale or coral pink varied by complexion and pigmentation; a knife-edged gingival margin that adapts closely around the tooth; stippling; firmness; and minimal sulcus depth with no bleeding when probed. Although "normal" varies with anatomic, physiologic, and other factors, general characteristics form a baseline for a contrast in the recognition of inflammation.

IV. CAUSES OF TISSUE CHANGES

Disease changes produce alterations in color, size, position, shape, consistency, surface texture, bleeding readiness, and exudate production.

To understand the changes that take place in the gingival tissues during the transition from health to disease, it is necessary to have a clear picture of what bacterial plaque is, the role of plaque microorganisms in the development of disease, and the inflammatory response by the body.

When the products of the plaque microorganisms cause breakdown of the intercellular substances of the sulcular epithelium, injurious agents can pass into the connective tissue, where an inflammatory response is initiated. An inflammatory response means that there is increased blood flow, increased permeability of capillaries, and increased collection of defense cells and tissue fluid. The changes produce the tissue alterations, such as in color, size, shape, and consistency, that are described in the next section.

V. DESCRIPTIVE TERMINOLOGY

The degree of severity and distribution of a change should be noted when examining the gingiva. When a deviation from normal affects a single area, it can be designated by the number of the adjacent tooth and the surface of the tissue involved, namely, facial, lingual, mesial, or distal. Teeth numbering systems are described on pages 84 to 86.

A. Severity

Severity is expressed as slight, moderate, or severe.

B. Distribution

Terms used for describing distribution are as follows:

1. *Localized:* The gingiva is involved only about a single tooth or a specific group of teeth.
2. *Generalized:* The gingiva is involved about all or nearly all of the teeth throughout the mouth. A condition may also be generalized throughout a single arch, the maxillary or mandibular.
3. *Marginal:* A change that is confined to the free or marginal gingiva. This is specified as either localized or generalized.
4. *Papillary:* A change that involves a papilla but not the rest of the free gingiva around a tooth. A papillary change may be localized or generalized.
5. *Diffuse:* Spread out, dispersed; affects gingival margin, attached gingiva, and interdental papillae; may extend into alveolar mucosa. A diffuse condition is more frequently localized, rarely generalized.

VI. EARLY RECOGNITION OF TISSUE CHANGES

Marked changes, such as moderate to severe generalized redness, enlargement, sponginess, deep pockets, and definite mobility, are relatively easy to detect even with limited experience, provided there is good light and accessibility for vision. In contrast, when changes are subtle, localized about one or a few teeth, and of a lesser degree of severity, more skillful application of knowledge is needed.

Early recognition and treatment of gingival and periodontal infections prevents neglect of conditions that can develop into severe disease. Treatment is less

TABLE 11-1 Examination of the Gingival Clinical Markers

	Appearance in Health	Changes in Disease Clinical Appearance	Causes for Changes

Color	Uniformly pale pink or coral pink	Acute: bright red	Inflammation
			   capillary dilation
			   increased blood flow

	Variations in pigmentation related to complexion, race	Chronic: bluish pink, bluish red pink	Vessels engorged Blood flow sluggish Venous return impaired Anoxemia Increased fibrosis
		Attached gingiva: color change may extend to the mucogingival line	Deepening of pocket, mucogingival involvement

Size	Not enlarged
	
	Fits snugly around the tooth
		Enlarged	Edematous:
			   inflammatory fluid
			   cellular exudate
			   vascular engorgement
			   hemorrhage
			Fibrotic: new collagen fibers

Shape (contour)	Marginal gingiva:
	   knife-edged, flat,
	   follows a curved line about
	   the tooth
	Papillae:
	  (1) normal contact: papilla is
	      pointed and pyramidal; fills
	      the interproximal area
	
	  (2) space (diastema) between
	      teeth; gingiva is flat or
	      saddle shaped
		Marginal gingiva:
		   rounded
		   rolled
		
		Papillae:
		   bulbous
		   flattened
		   blunted
		   cratered
			Inflammatory changes:
			   edematous or fibrous
			
			Bulbous with gingival enlargement
			   (see edematous and fibrotic, above)
			
			Cratered in necrotizing ulcerative
			   gingivitis

Consistency	Firm
	
	Attached gingiva firmly bound down
		Soft, spongy: dents readily when
		   when pressed with probe
		Associated with red color, smooth
		   shiny surface, loss of stippling,
		   bleeding on probing
			Edematous: fluid between cells in
			   connective tissue

		Firm, hard: resists probe pressure Associated with pink color, stippling, bleeding only in depth of pocket	Fibrotic: collagen fibers

(continued)

complicated, and the success of treatment and recovery to healthy tissue is predictable when early recognition makes early treatment possible.

THE GINGIVAL EXAMINATION

The examination of the gingiva includes evaluation of color, size, shape, consistency, surface texture, position, mucogingival junctions, bleeding, and exudate.

These are summarized in Table 11-1, which is a clinical reference chart.

I. COLOR

A. Signs of Health
1. *Pale Pink.* Darker in people with darker complexions.
2. *Factors Influencing Color*
   a. Vascular supply.
   b. Thickness of epithelium.

TABLE 11-1 Examination of the Gingival Clinical Markers (Continued)

	Appearance in Health	Changes in Disease Clinical Appearance	Causes for Changes
Surface texture	Free gingiva: smooth Attached gingiva: stippled	Acute condition: smooth, shiny gingiva Chronic: hard, firm, with stippling, sometimes heavier than normal	Inflammatory changes in the connective tissue; edema, cellular infiltration Fibrosis
Position of Gingival Margin	Fully erupted tooth: margin is 1–2 mm above cementoenamel junction, at or slightly below the enamel contour	Enlarged gingiva: margin is higher on the tooth, above normal, pocket deepened Recession: margin is more apical; root surface is exposed	Edematous or fibrotic Junctional epithelium has migrated along the root; gingival margin follows
Position of Junctional Epithelium	During eruption along the enamel surface (Figure 11-7) Fully erupted tooth: the junctional epithelium is at the cemento-enamel junction	Position determined by use of probe, is on the root surface	Apical migration of the epithelium along the root
Mucogingival Junctions	Make clear demarcation between the pink, stippled, attached gingiva and the darker alveolar mucosa with smooth shiny surface	No attached gingiva: (1) Color changes may extend full height of the gingiva; muco-gingival line obliterated (2) Probing reveals that the bottom of the pocket extends into the alveolar mucosa (3) Frenal pull may displace the gingival margin from the tooth	Apical migration of the junctional epithelium Attached gingiva decreases with pocket deepening Inflammation extends into alveolar mucosa
Bleeding	No spontaneous bleeding or upon probing	Spontaneous bleeding Bleeding on probing: bleeding near margin in acute condition; bleeding deep in pocket in chronic condition	Degeneration of the sulcular epithelium with the formation of pocket epithelium Blood vessels engorged Tissue edematous
Exudate	No exudate on pressure	White fluid, pus, visible on digital pressure Amount not related to pocket depth	Inflammation in the connective tissue Excessive accumulation of white blood cells with serum and tissue makes up the exudate (pus)

c. Degree of keratinization.

d. Physiologic pigmentation: melanin pigmentation occurs frequently in African Americans, Orientals, Indians, and Caucasians of Mediterranean countries.

B. Changes in Disease

1. *In Chronic Inflammation.* Dark red, bluish red, magenta, or deep blue.
2. *In Acute Inflammation.* Bright red.
3. *Extent.* Deep involvement can be expected when diffuse color changes extend into the attached gingiva, or from the marginal gingiva to the mucogingival junction, or through into alveolar mucosa.

II. SIZE

A. Signs of Health

1. *Free Gingiva.* Flat, not enlarged; fits snugly around the tooth.
2. *Attached Gingiva*

a. Width of attached gingiva varies among patients and among teeth for an individual, from 1 to 9 mm.[5]

b. Wider in maxilla than mandible; broadest zone related to incisors, narrowest at the canine and premolar regions.

B. Changes in Disease

1. *Free Gingiva and Papillae.* Become enlarged. May be localized or limited to specific areas or generalized throughout the gingiva. The col deepens as the papillae increase in size.

2. *Attached Gingiva.* Decreases in amount as the pocket deepens. Measurement of the amount of attached gingiva is described on page 212 and in Figure 12-10.

C. Enlargement From Drug Therapy

Certain drugs used for specific systemic therapy cause gingival enlargement as a side effect. Examples of such drugs are phenytoin, cyclosporine, and nifedipine. They are described on page 234 along with other factors contributing to disease development.

III. SHAPE (FORM OR CONTOUR)

A. Signs of Health

1. *Free Gingiva*
   a. Follows a curved line around each tooth; may be straighter along wide molar surfaces.
   b. The margin is knife-edged or slightly rounded on facial and lingual gingiva; closely adapted to the tooth surface.

2. *Papillae*
   a. Teeth with contact area. Facial and lingual gingiva are pointed or slightly rounded papillae with a col area under the contact (Figure 11-8).
   b. Spaced teeth (with diastemata). Interdental gingiva is flat or saddle shaped (Figure 13-4D, page 232).

B. Changes in Disease

1. *Free Gingiva.* Rounded or rolled.
2. *Papillae.* Blunted, flattened, bulbous, cratered (Figure 11-10).
3. *Festoon ("McCall's festoon").* An enlargement of the marginal gingiva with the formation of a lifesaver-like gingival prominence. Frequently, the total gingiva is very narrow, with associated apparent recession as shown in Figure 11-10D.
4. *Clefts*
   a. "Stillman's cleft" (Figure 11-11). A localized recession may be V-shaped, apostrophe-shaped, or form a slitlike indentation. It may extend several millimeters toward the mucogingival junction or even to or through the junction.
   b. Floss cleft. A cleft created by incorrect floss positioning appears as a vertical

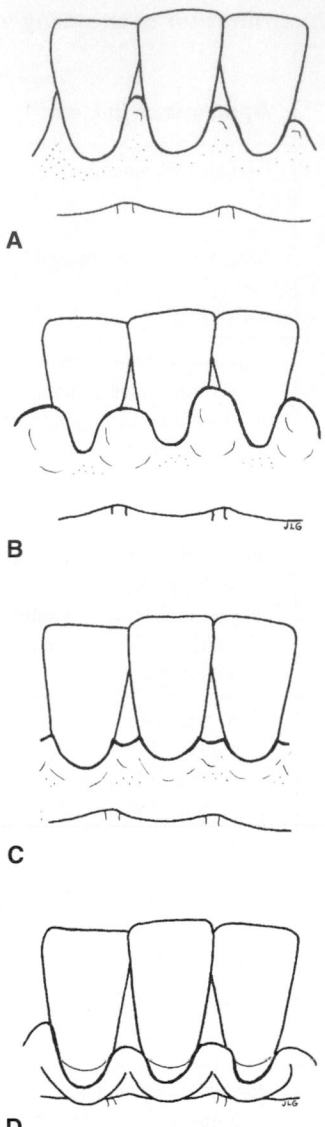

A

B

C

D

■ **FIGURE 11-10 Gingival Shape or Contour. (A)** Blunted papillae. **(B)** Bulbous papillae. **(C)** Cratered papillae. **(D)** Rolled, lifesaver-shaped "McCall's festoons."

linear or V-shaped fissure in the marginal gingiva.[6] It usually occurs at one side of an interdental papilla. The injury can develop when dental floss is curved repeatedly in an incomplete "C" around the line angle so the floss is pressed across the gingiva. Correct flossing positioning is shown in Figure 24-1 on page 374.

IV. CONSISTENCY

A. Signs of Health

1. Firm when palpated with the side of a blunt instrument (probe).
2. Attached gingiva is bound down firmly to the underlying bone.

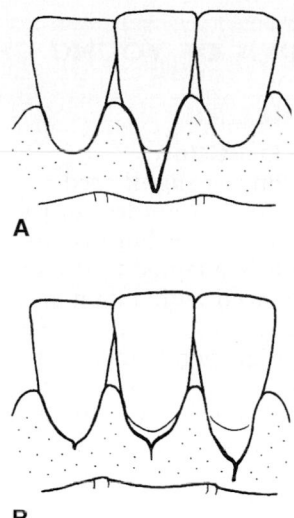

A

B

■ **FIGURE 11-11 Gingival Clefts. (A)** V-shaped Stillman's cleft. **(B)** Slit-like Stillman's clefts of varying degrees of severity in relation to the mucogingival junction.

B. Changes in Disease

1. *To Determine Consistency.* Gently press side of probe on free gingiva. Soft, spongy gingiva dents readily; firm, hard tissue resists.
2. *Soft, Spongy Gingiva.* Related to acute stages of inflammation with increased infiltration of fluid and inflammatory elements. The tissue appears red, may be smooth and shiny with loss of stippling, has marginal enlargement, and bleeds readily on probing.
3. *Firm, Hard Gingiva.* Related to chronic inflammation with increased fibrosis. The tissue may appear pink and well stippled. Bleeding, when probed, usually occurs only in the deeper part of a pocket, not near the margin.
4. *Retraction of the Margin Away From the Tooth.* Normally, the free gingiva fits snugly about the tooth. When the margin tends to hang slightly away or is readily displaced with a light air blast, the gingival fibers that support the margin have been destroyed (Figure 11-3).

V. SURFACE TEXTURE

A. Signs of Health

1. *Free Gingiva.* Smooth.
2. *Attached Gingiva.* Stippled (minutely "pebbled" or "orange peel" surface).
3. *Interdental Gingiva.* The free gingiva is smooth; the center portion of each papilla is stippled.

B. Changes in Disease

1. *Inflammatory Changes.* May be loss of stippling, with smooth, shiny surface.
2. *Hyperkeratosis.* May result in a leathery, hard, or nodular surface.

3. *Chronic Disease.* Tissue may be hard and fibrotic, with a normal pink color and normal or deep stippling.

VI. POSITION

The *actual* position of the gingiva is the level of the attached periodontal tissue. It is not directly visible but can be determined by probing.

The *apparent* position of the gingiva is the level of the gingival margin or crest of the free gingiva that is seen by direct observation.

A. Signs of Health

For the fully erupted tooth in an adult, the apparent position of the gingival margin is normally at the level of, or slightly below, the enamel contour or prominence of the cervical third of a tooth.

B. Changes in Disease

1. *Effect of Gingival Enlargement.* When the gingiva enlarges, the gingival margin may be high on the enamel, partly or nearly covering the anatomic crown.
2. *Effect of Gingival Recession*
   a. Definition. Recession is the exposure of root surface that results from the apical migration of the junctional epithelium (Figure 11-12).
   b. Actual recession. The actual recession is shown by the position of the attachment level. The "receded area" is from the cementoenamel junction to the attachment.
   c. Visible recession. The visible recession is the exposed root surface that is visible on

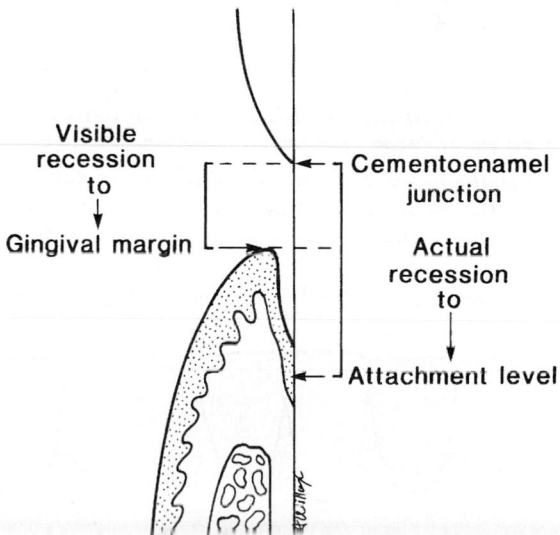

■ **FIGURE 11-12 Gingival Recession.** *Left,* Clinically visible recession of the gingival margin with root surface apparent to the eye. *Right,* The actual recession exposes the root surface as the periodontal attachment migrates along the root surface.

clinical examination. It is seen from the gingival margin to the cementoenamel junction.

  d. Localized recession (Figure 11-13). A localized recession may be narrow or wide, deep or shallow. The root surface is denuded, and the visible recession may extend to or through the mucogingival junction.

  e. Measurement. Both actual and visible recession can be measured with a probe from the cementoenamel junction. Total recession is the actual and visible positions added together.

VII. BLEEDING

A. Signs of Health
  1. No bleeding spontaneously or on probing.
  2. Healthy tissue does not bleed.

B. Changes in Disease
  1. Bleeding occurs spontaneously or when probed.
  2. Sulcular epithelium becomes diseased *pocket epithelium*. The ulcerated pocket wall bleeds readily on gentle probing. Development of inflammation and pocket formation is described on page 227.

VIII. EXUDATE

A. Signs of Health
There is no exudate except slight gingival sulcus fluid (page 190). Gingival sulcus fluid cannot be seen by direct observation.

B. Changes in Disease
  1. *Suppuration.* Formation or secretion of pus.
  2. *White Fluid* (pus and subgingival bacterial plaque). May appear at the entrance to the pocket or may be squeezed out of the pocket by light finger pressure on the external wall of the pocket.
  3. *Amount of Exudate.* Related to the severity of the acute inflammation, not to the depth of the pocket.

THE GINGIVA OF YOUNG CHILDREN[7,8]

I. SIGNS OF HEALTH

A. Primary Dentition
  1. *Color.* Pink or slightly red.
  2. *Shape.* Thick, rounded, or rolled.
  3. *Consistency.* Less fibrous than adult gingiva; not tightly adapted to the teeth; may be easily displaced with a light air jet.
  4. *Surface Texture.* May or may not have stippling; high percentage of patients has shiny gingiva.
  5. *Attached Gingiva.* Width of attached gingiva in children ages 3 to 5: between 1 and 6 mm.[5]
  6. *Interdental Gingiva*
      a. Anterior: diastemata are frequently present and the papillae are flat or saddle shaped.
      b. Posterior: col between facial and lingual papillae when teeth are in contact (Figure 11-8).

B. Mixed Dentition
  1. Constant state of change related to exfoliation and eruption.
  2. Free gingiva may appear rolled or rounded, slightly reddened, shiny, and with a lack of firmness.
  3. The gingiva covers a varying portion of the anatomic crown, depending on the stage of eruption (Figure 11-7).

II. CHANGES IN DISEASE
Examination of the periodontal tissues of a child is not different from that of an adult. A complete examination is necessary, including probing around each tooth.

Gingivitis occurs frequently in children but is usually reversible without leaving permanent damage.

Although relatively rare, periodontitis can occur in primary dentition. Prepubertal periodontitis is described on page 228, in Table 13-2.

Mucogingival problems occur in children.[9,10] The

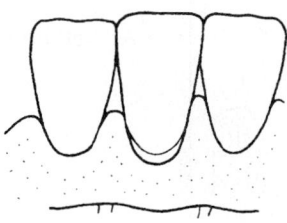 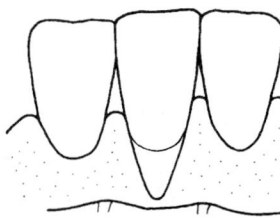 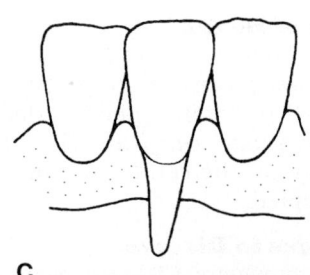

A   **B**   **C**

■ **FIGURE 11-13 Localized Recession.** A single tooth may show narrow or wide, deep or shallow recession. **(A)** Wide, shallow. **(B)** Wide, deep, with narrow attached gingiva. **(C)** Narrow, deep, with missing attached gingiva.

recognition of deficiencies of attached gingiva has particular significance for the child who will need orthodontic treatment.

THE GINGIVA AFTER PERIODONTAL SURGERY

The characteristics of "normal healthy gingiva" take on different dimensions for the patient who has completed treatment for pockets, bone loss, and other signs of a periodontal infection. The junctional epithelium is apical to the cementoenamel junction. After healing, the sulcus depth may be within normal range and no bleeding should occur when probed.

Depending on the exact treatment performed, examination shows changes from the initial evaluation. For example, where the initial examination showed a deficiency of attached gingiva with frenal pull, mucogingival surgery may have been designed and treatment satisfactorily completed to create new attached gingiva. With each maintenance appointment, a thorough, careful examination is necessary to control factors that may permit recurrence of disease.

FACTORS TO TEACH THE PATIENT

I. Characteristics of normal healthy gingiva.
II. The significance of bleeding; healthy tissue does not bleed.
III. Relationship of findings during a gingival examination to the personal daily care procedures for infection control.
IV. The special attention needed for an area of gingival recession to prevent abrasion, inflammation, and further involvement.
V. How the method of brushing, stiffness of toothbrush filaments, abrasiveness of a dentifrice, and pressure applied during brushing can be factors in gingival recession.
VI. Teach the warning signs of periodontal disease*
   1. Gums that bleed when you brush your teeth.
   2. Gums that are red, swollen, or tender.
   3. Gums that have pulled away from the teeth.
   4. Pus between the teeth and gums when the gums are pressed.
   5. Permanent teeth that are loose or separating.
   6. Any change in the way your teeth fit together when you bite.
   7. Any changes in the fit of your partial dentures.
   8. Bad breath.

*From *Gum Disease: The Warning Signs.* American Dental Association, Department of Salable Materials, 211 E. Chicago Avenue, Chicago, IL 60611.

REFERENCES

1. **Avery,** J.K. and Steele, P.F.: *Essentials of Oral Histology and Embryology. A Clinical Approach.* St. Louis, Mosby, 1992, pp. 131–134.
2. **Ainamo,** J. and Löe, H.: Anatomical Characteristics of Gingiva. A Clinical and Microscopic Study of the Free and Attached Gingiva, *J. Periodontol., 37,* 5, January–February, 1966.
3. **Orban,** B.: Clinical and Histologic Study of the Surface Characteristics of the Gingiva, *Oral Surg. Oral Med. Oral Pathol., 1,* 827, September, 1948.
4. **Bhaskar,** S.N., ed.: *Orban's Oral Histology and Embryology,* 11th ed. St. Louis, Mosby, 1991, pp. 323–325.
5. **Bowers,** G.M.: A Study of the Width of Attached Gingiva, *J. Periodontol., 34,* 201, May, 1963.
6. **Hallman,** W.W., Waldrop, T.C., Houston, G.D., and Hawkins, B.F.: Flossing Clefts. Clinical and Histologic Observations, *J. Periodontol., 57,* 501, August, 1986.
7. **Carranza,** F.A. and Newman, M.G.: *Clinical Periodontics,* 8th ed. Philadelphia, W.B. Saunders Co., 1996, pp. 276–280.
8. **Casamassimo,** P.S.: Periodontal Conditions, in Pinkham, J.R., ed.: *Pediatric Dentistry: Infancy Through Adolescence,* 2nd ed. Philadelphia, W.B. Saunders Co., 1994, pp. 353–357, 607–615.
9. **Maynard,** J.G. and Ochsenbein, C.: Mucogingival Problems, Prevalence and Therapy in Children, *J. Periodontol., 46,* 543, September, 1975.
10. **Andlin-Sobocki,** A., Marcusson, A., and Persson, M.: 3-Year Observations on Gingival Recession in Mandibular Incisors in Children, *J. Clin. Periodontol., 18,* 155, March, 1991.

SUGGESTED READINGS

Ainamo, A., Ainamo, J., and Poikkeus, R.: Continuous Widening of the Band of Attached Gingiva From 23 to 65 Years of Age, *J. Periodont. Res., 16,* 595, November, 1981.

Carranza, F.A. and Newman, M.G.: *Clinical Periodontics,* 8th ed. Philadelphia, W.B. Saunders Co., 1996, pp. 12–29.

Fedi, P.F., and Vernino, A.R.: *The Periodontic Syllabus,* 3rd ed. Baltimore, Williams & Wilkins, 1995, pp. 1–12.

Grant, D.A., Stern, I.B., and Listgarten, M.A., eds.: *Periodontics,* 6th ed. St. Louis, Mosby, 1988, pp. 3–75.

Hassell, T.M.: Tissues and Cells of the Periodontium, *Periodontology 2000, 3,* 9, 1993.

Hempton, T.J., Wilkins, E., and Lancaster, D.: Evaluation of Attached Tissue Aids in Treatment of Recession, *RDH, 16,* 34, June, 1996.

Hicks, M.J., Uldricks, J.M., Whitacre, H.L., Anderson, J., and Moeschberger, M.L.: a National Study of Periodontal Assessment by Dental Hygienists, *J. Dent. Hyg., 67,* 82, February, 1993.

Hoag, P.M. and Pawlak, E.A.: *Essentials of Periodontics,* 4th ed. St. Louis, Mosby, 1990, pp. 1–18.

Mariotti, A.: The Extracellular Matrix of the Periodontium: Dynamic and Interactive Tissues, *Periodontology 2000, 3,* 39, 1993.

Melfi, R.C.: *Permar's Oral Embryology and Microscopic Anatomy,* 9th ed. Philadelphia, Lea & Febiger, 1994, pp. 227–242.

Serino, G., Wennström, J.L., Lindhe, J., and Eneroth, L.: The Prevalence and Distribution of Gingival Recession in Subjects with a High Standard of Oral Hygiene, *J. Clin. Periodontol., 21,* 57, January, 1994.

Vacek, J.S., Gher. M.E., Assad, D.A., Richardson, A.C., and Giambarresi, L.I.: The Dimensions of the Human Dentogingival Junction, *Int. J. Periodont. and Restorative Dent., 14,* 155, Number 2, 1994.

Gingiva of Children

American Academy of Periodontology, Committee on Research, Science and Therapy: Position Paper: Periodontal Diseases of Children and Adolescents, *J. Periodontol., 67,* 57, January, 1996.

Andlin-Sobocki, A.: Changes of Facial Gingival Dimensions in

Children. A 2-year Longitudinal Study, *J. Clin. Periodontol., 20,* 212, March, 1993.

Andlin-Sobocki, A. and Bodin, L.: Dimensional Alterations of the Gingiva Related to Changes of Facial/Lingual Tooth Position in Permanent Anterior Teeth of Children. A 2-year Longitudinal Study. *J. Clin. Periodontol., 20,* 218, March, 1993.

Bimstein, E. and Eidelman, E.: Longitudinal Changes in the Width of Attached Gingiva in Children, *Pediatr. Dent., 10,* 22, March, 1988.

Bimstein, E., Machtei, E., and Eidelman, E.: Dimensional Differences in the Attached and Keratinized Gingiva and Gingival Sulcus in the Early Permanent Dentition: A Longitudinal Study, *J. Pedod., 10,* 247, Spring, 1986.

Bimstein, E., Matsson, L., Soskolne, A.W., and Lustman, J.: Histologic Characteristics of the Gingiva Associated with the Primary and Permanent Teeth of Children, *Pediatr. Dent., 16,* 206, May/June, 1994.

Keszthelyi, G.: The Width of Plaque-free Zones on Primary Molars With Attachment Loss, *J. Clin. Periodontol., 18,* 94, February, 1991.

Keszthelyi, G. and Szabo, I.: Attachment Loss in Primary Molars, *J. Clin. Periodontol., 14,* 48, January, 1987.

Saario, M., Ainamo. A., Mattila, K., and Ainamo, J.: The Width of Radiologically-defined Attached Gingiva Over Permanent Teeth in Children, *J. Clin. Periodontol., 21,* 666, November, 1994.

Saario, M., Ainamo. A., Mattila, K., Suomalainen, K., and Ainamo, J.: The Width of Radiologically-defined Attached Gingiva Over Deciduous Teeth, *J. Clin. Periodontol., 22,* 895, December, 1995.

Tenenbaum, H. and Tenenbaum, M.: A Clinical Study of the Width of the Attached Gingiva in the Deciduous, Transitional and Permanent Dentitions, *J. Clin. Periodontol., 13,* 270, April, 1986.

12

Examination Procedures

Parts of the gingival and dental examinations are made by direct *visual* observation, while other parts require *tactile* using a probe and an explorer. These two types of instruments, assisted by a mouth mirror, are key instruments in patient examination and assessment. Considerable skill is required for accurate and efficient probing and exploring.

General principles of instrumentation are described in Chapter 32, pages 512 to 543. Study that chapter for basic descriptions of instrument parts, grasp, finger rests, and strokes. Box 12-1 contains definitions for key words used in or associated with this chapter.

I. PRECAUTION

A probe or an explorer should not be applied to the teeth and gingiva until an initial review of information from the patient history has been made. The immediate application of information from the history was outlined on page 101. Of particular significance is knowledge of a patient's susceptibility to bacteremia. Patients at risk must receive prophylactic antibiotic premedication before instrumentation (pages 101 to 104).

II. BASIC SET-UP

All tray arrangements need a basic set-up composed of a mouth mirror, probe, explorer, and cotton pliers. Wrapping these together for sterilizing increases efficiency. The packet should be labeled "basic set-up." Other packets can contain special instruments, such as a furcation probe, to use for supplemental examinations.

THE MOUTH MIRROR

I. DESCRIPTION

A. Parts

The mirror has three parts: the handle, shank, and working end, which is the mounted mirror or mirror head. Instrument parts are described on page 514.

B. Mirror Surfaces

1. *Plane (Flat).* May produce a double image.
2. *Concave.* Magnifying.
3. *Front Surface.* The reflecting surface is on the front of the lens rather than on the back as with plane or magnifying mirrors. The front surface eliminates "ghost" images.

C. Diameters

Diameters vary from ⅝ to 1¼ inches. In addition, special examination mirrors are available in 1½- to 2-inch diameters.

D. Attachments

Mirrors may be threaded plain stem or cone socket to be joined to a handle. Because mirrors tend to become scratched, replacement of the working end is possible without purchasing new handles.

E. Handles

1. Thicker handles contribute to a more comfortable grasp and greater control.
2. Wider mirror handles are especially useful for mobility determination (page 218).

BOX 12-1 KEY WORDS: Instruments of Examination

Calibration (kăl″ĭ-brā′shun): determination of the accuracy of an instrument by measurment of its variation from a standard; (calibration between examiners, see Box 19-1).

Clinical attachment level: probing depth as measured from the cementoenamel junction (or other fixed point) to the location of the probe tip at the coronal level of attached periodontal tissues.

Explorer: a slender stainless steel instrument with a fine flexible, sharp point used for examination of the surfaces of the teeth to detect irregularities.

Fremitus (frĕm′ĭ-tus): a vibration perceptible by palpation.

Periodontometer (pĕr″ē-ō-dŏn-tŏm′ē ter): instrument used to measure mobility.

Probe (prōb): smooth, slender instrument usually round in diameter with a rounded tip designed for examination of the teeth and soft tissues; except for a few probes made only for blunt examination, probes are calibrated in millimeter increments to facilitate recordings for comparison with periodic assessments.

Probing depth: the distance from the gingival margin to the location of the periodontal probe tip at the coronal border of attached periodontal tissues.

Tactile (tăk′tĭl): pertaining to the touch.

Tactile discrimination: the ability to distinguish relative degrees of roughness and smoothness, for example, on a tooth surface, using an explorer or a periodontal probe; also called tactile sensitivity.

Tension test: application of tension at the mucogingival junction by retracting cheek, lip, and tongue to tighten the alveolar mucosa and test for the presence of attached gingiva; area of missing attached gingiva is revealed when the alveolar mucosa and frena are connected directly to the free gingiva.

F. Disposable Mirrors
1. May be plastic in one piece or may be a handle with replaceable head for professional use; may have front surface.
2. Take-home mirrors for patient instruction. Patient may observe lingual and posterior aspects. One type of mirror has a light attachment.

II. PURPOSES AND USES

The mouth mirror is used to provide:

A. Indirect Vision
This is particularly needed for distal surfaces of posterior teeth and lingual surfaces of anterior teeth.

B. Indirect Illumination
Reflection of light from the dental overhead light to any area of the oral cavity can be accomplished by adapting the mirror.

C. Transillumination
Reflection of light through the teeth.
1. Mirror is held to reflect light from the lingual aspect while facial surfaces of the teeth are examined.
2. Mirror is held for indirect vision on the lingual while light from the overhead dental light passes through the teeth. Translucency of enamel can be seen clearly, whereas dental caries or calculus deposits appear opaque.

D. Retraction
The mirror is used to protect or prevent interference by the cheeks, tongue, or lips.

III. PROCEDURE FOR USE

A. Grasp
Use modified pen grasp with finger rest on a tooth surface wherever possible to provide stability and control.

B. Retraction
1. Use a water-based lubricant on dry or cracked lips and corners of mouth.
2. Adjust the mirror position so that the angles of the mouth are protected from undue pressure of the shank of the mirror.
3. Insert and remove mirror carefully to avoid hitting the teeth, because this can be very disturbing to the patient.

C. Maintain Clear Vision
1. Warm mirror with water, rub along buccal mucosa to coat mirror with thin transparent film of saliva, and request patient to breathe through the nose to prevent condensation of moisture on the mirror. Use a detergent or other means for keeping a clear surface.
2. Discard scratched mirrors.

IV. CARE OF MIRRORS

A. Dismantle mirror and handle for sterilization.
B. Examine carefully after ultrasonic cleaning or scrubbing with brush prior to sterilization to assure removal of debris around back, shank, and rim of reflecting surface.
C. Handle carefully during sterilization procedures to prevent other instruments from scratching the reflecting surface.
D. Consult manufacturer's specifications for sterilizing or disinfecting procedures that may cloud the mirror, particularly the front surface type.

INSTRUMENTS FOR APPLICATION OF AIR

I. PURPOSES AND USES

With appropriate, timely application of air to clear saliva and debris and/or dry the tooth surfaces, the following can be accomplished:

A. Improve and Facilitate Examination Procedures
1. Make a thorough, more accurate examination.
2. Dry supragingival calculus to facilitate exploring and scaling. Small deposits may be light in color and not visible until they are dried. Dried calculus appears chalky and presents a contrast to tooth color.
3. Deflect the free gingival margin for observation into the subgingival area. Subgingival calculus usually appears dark.
4. Make identification of areas of demineralization and carious lesions easier.
5. Recognize location and condition of restorations, particularly tooth-color restorations.

B. Improve Visibility of the Treatment Area During Instrumentation
1. Dry area for finger rest to provide stability during instrumentation.
2. Facilitate positive scaling techniques.
3. Minimize appointment time.
4. Evaluate complete removal of supragingival calculus after instrumentation.

C. Prepare Teeth and/or Gingiva for Certain Procedures
Examples are to dry surfaces for:
1. Application of caries-preventive agents.
2. Make impression for study cast.
3. Apply topical anesthetic.

II. COMPRESSED AIR SYRINGE

A. Description
1. *Air Source.* Air compressor with tubing attachment to syringe.

2. *Air Tip.* Has angled working end that can be turned for maxillary or mandibular application. Tip may be disposable or removable for sterilization.

B. Procedure for Use

1. Use palm grasp about the handle of the syringe; place thumb on release lever or on button on handle.
2. Test the air flow so that the strength of flow can be controlled.
3. Make controlled, relatively short, gentle applications of air.
4. Supplement air drying with use of saliva ejector and folded gauze sponge placed in vestibule.

C. Precautions

1. Avoid sharp blasts of air on sensitive cervical areas of teeth or open carious lesions. Such areas may be dried by blotting with a gauze sponge or cotton roll to avoid causing discomfort.
2. Avoid applying air directly into a pocket. Subgingival plaque may be forced into the tissues and a bacteremia created.
3. Avoid forceful application of air, which can direct saliva and debris out of the oral cavity, contaminate the working area and clinician, and create aerosols (page 18). Air directed toward the posterior region of the patient's mouth may cause coughing.
4. Avoid startling the patient; forewarn when air is to be applied.

PROBE

Early in patient examination, the patient's periodontal disease status must be determined. Treatment planning varies depending on whether the condition is gingivitis, which may be reversible, or periodontitis with periodontal pockets, bone loss, and root surface involvement, which may require more extensive therapy.

Two general types of probes available are the traditional or standard manual probes and the controlled force or automated probes. Automated probes were developed and researched in an attempt to overcome the problems in obtaining consistent readings with traditional probes.

Factors that influence probe determinations are described on page 207. Included are variations in pressure (probing force) used, diameter, and other physical features, and the inconsistent depth or penetration during application.

A probe is used to make the initial assessment, followed by a detailed evaluation to determine the extent and degree of severity of disease and tissue destruction for specific treatment planning. During treatment, the probe is applied to assess progress.

After treatment, use of the probe helps to determine completion of professional services as recognized by the health status of the tissues. At each maintenance appointment, a re-evaluation with the probe is needed to ensure continued self-care by the patient and to identify early disease changes that require additional professional treatment.

I. PURPOSES AND USES

A probe is used to

A. Assess the Periodontal Status for Preparation of a Treatment Plan

1. Classify the disease as gingivitis or periodontitis by determining whether bone loss has occurred and whether the pockets are gingival or periodontal (Figure 13-1, page 229). A systematic screening method can be used (PSR, pages 295 to 297).
2. Determine the extent of inflammation in conjunction with the overall gingival examination. Bleeding on probing is an early sign of inflammation in the gingiva.

B. Make a Sulcus and Pocket Survey

1. Examine the shape, topography, and dimensions of sulci and pockets.
2. Measure and record probing depths.
3. Evaluate tooth-surface pocket wall.
   a. Chart calculus location and severity.
   b. Record other root surface irregularities discerned by the probe.
4. Determine clinical attachment level (pages 209 to 210).

C. Make a Mucogingival Examination

1. Determine relationship of gingival margin, attachment level, and mucogingival junction.
2. Measure the width of the attached gingiva (Figure 12-10, page 212).

D. Make Other Gingival Determinations

1. Evaluate gingival bleeding on probing and prepare a gingival bleeding index (pages 305 and 306).
2. Measure the extent of visible gingival recession (Figure 11-12, page 197).
3. Determine the consistency of the gingival tissue.

E. Guide Treatment

1. Determine gingival characteristics, including probing depth, bleeding, and consistency (all determined using a probe), to provide a basis for patient instruction as part of the total treatment.
2. Define probing depth of sulcus or pocket for application of instruments for scaling and root planing, and define depth for use of an explorer for evaluation of these procedures.
3. Detect anatomic configuration of roots, subgingival deposits, and root irregularities that

TABLE 12-1 Types of Probes

Probe Markings (mm)	Examples	Description
Marks at 1-2-3-5-7-8-9-10	Williams University of Michigan with Williams marks Glickman Merritt A and B	Round, tapered (available with color-code) Round, narrow diameter, fine Round, with longer lower shank Round, single bend to shank
Marks at 3-3-2	University of Michigan O Premier O Marquis M-1	Round, fine, tapered, narrow diameter

Marks at
  3-6-9-12
  3-6-8-11
  (and other variations)
	Hu-Friedy QULIX
	Marquis
	Nordent
		Round, tapered, fine
		Color-coded

Marks at each mm to 15	Hu-Friedy PCPUNC 15	Round Color-coded at 5-10-15
Marks at 3.5-5.5-8.5-11.5	WHO Probe (World Health Organization)	Round, tapered, fine, with ball end Color-coded (Figure 19-1, page 296)
No marks	Gilmore Nabors 1N, 2N	Tapered, sharper than other probles Curved, with curved shank for furcation examination

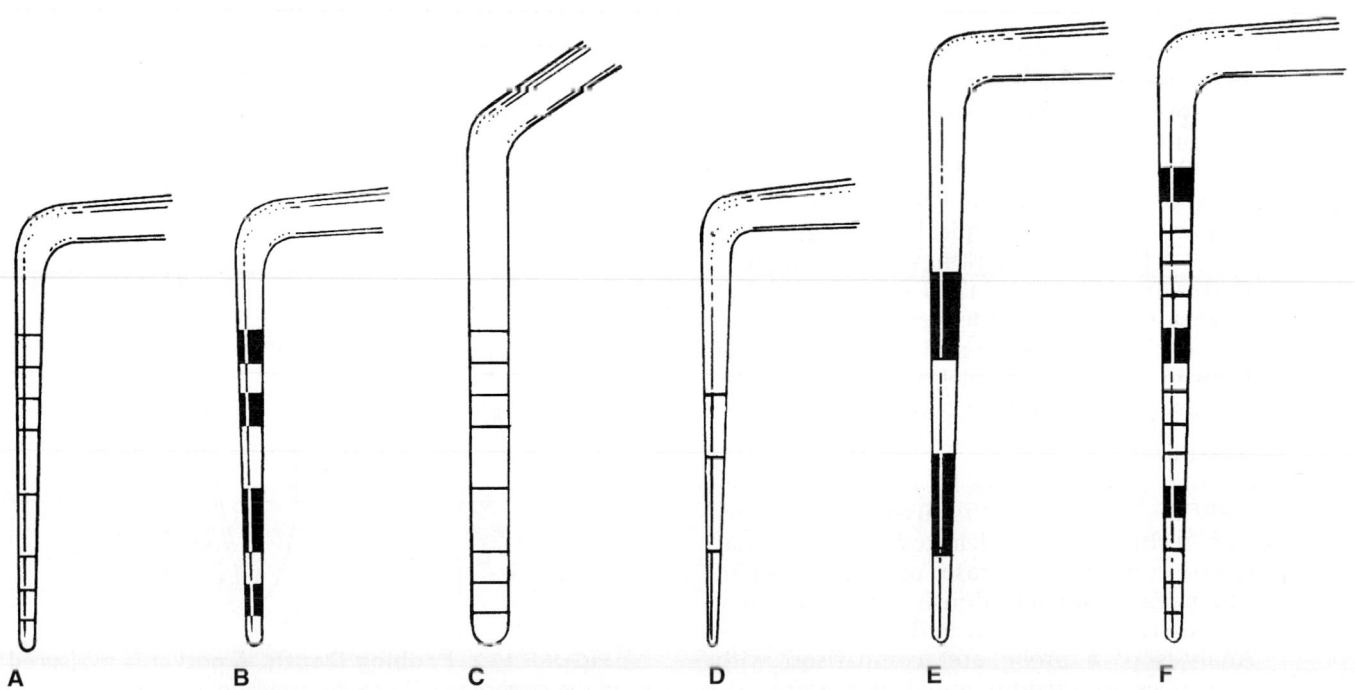

FIGURE 12-1 Examples of Probes. Names and calibrated markings shown are **(A)** Williams (1-1-1-2-2-1-1-1), **(B)** Williams, color-coded, **(C)** Goldman-Fox (1-1-1-2-2-1-1-1), **(D)** Michigan O (3-3-2), **(E)** Hu-Friedy or Marquis Color-coded (3-3-3-3 or 3-3-2-3) and **(F)** Hu-Friedy PCPUNC 15 (each millimeter to 15), color coded at 5-10-15. See Table 12-1 for additional data on probes.

A   B   C   D   E   F

complicate instrumentation. For this, the probe is used in conjunction with the explorer.

F. Evaluate Success and Completeness of Treatment

1. Evaluate post-treatment tissue response to professional treatment on an immediate, short-term basis, as well as at periodic maintenance examinations.
2. Evaluate patient's self-treatment through therapeutic disease control procedures.
3. Signs of health revealed by probing
   a. No bleeding; healthy tissue does not bleed.
   b. Reduced probing depth; comparison of pre- and post-treatment probing depth.
   c. Tissue is firm as shown by application of the probe to the surface of the free gingiva.

II. DESCRIPTION

A probe is a slender instrument with a smooth, rounded tip designed for examination of the depth and topography of an area. It has three parts: the handle, the angled shank, and the working end, which is the probe itself.

A. Materials

1. Stainless steel.
2. Plastic, for screenings and titanium implant probing (Figure 26-8, page 421).

B. Characteristics

1. *Straight Working End*
   a. Tapered, round, flat, or rectangular in cross section with a smooth rounded end.
   b. Calibrated in millimeters at intervals specific for each kind of probe; some have color coding. Figure 12-1 shows a comparison of a few typical markings; Table 12-1 lists probe markings with examples.
2. *Curved Working End.* Paired furcation probes have a smooth, rounded end for investigation of the topography and anatomy around roots in a furca. Examples are the Nabers 1N and 2N probes (Figure 12-8).

C. Selection

The probe chosen for use by a clinician is frequently the instrument first used when a particular technique was learned, or one that provides comfort and ease of manipulation. Another reason for selection is that consistency in reading can be accomplished.

Analysis of a probe and comparison with other probes are recommended. Important features to be considered in probe selection are

1. *Adaptability.* The probe should be adaptable around the complete circumference of each tooth, both posterior and anterior, so that no millimeter of probing depth can be ne-

glected. Flat probes require more attention to adaptation and are useful primarily on facial and lingual surfaces.
2. *Markings.* Markings should be easy to read so that probing depth can be readily identified and measured, and no disease area is overlooked. Color coding contributes to readability.

GUIDE TO PROBING

The information in Chapters 11 and 13 concerning the gingival examination, the normal tissues, and the development and types of pockets should be studied in conjunction with this outline of probing procedures.

A pocket is a diseased gingival sulcus. The use of a probe is the only accurate, dependable method to locate, assess, and measure sulci and pockets.

I. POCKET CHARACTERISTICS

A. A pocket is measured from the base of the pocket (top of attached periodontal tissue) to the gingival margin. Figure 12-2 shows two probing depths beneath gingival margins that are at the same level.
B. The pocket (or sulcus) is continuous around the entire tooth, and the entire pocket or sulcus must be measured. "Spot" probing is inadequate.
C. The depth varies around an individual tooth; probing depth rarely measures the same all around a tooth or even around one side of a tooth.

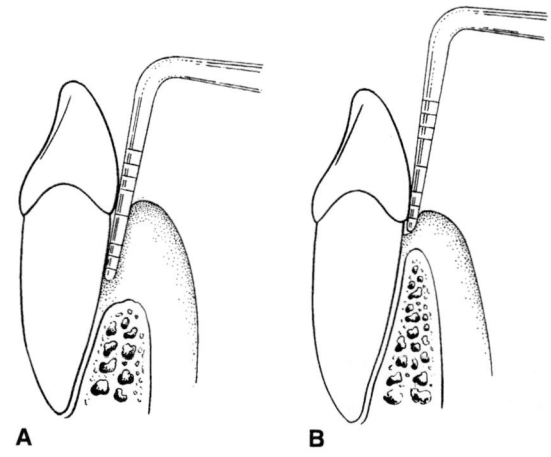

A   **B**

■ **FIGURE 12-2 Probing Depth.** A pocket is measured from the gingival margin to the attached periodontal tissue. Shown is the contrast of probe measurements with gingival margins at the same level. **(A)** Deep periodontal pocket (7 mm) with apical migration of attachment. **(B)** Shallow pocket (2 mm) with the attachment near the cemento-enamel junction.

1. The level of attached tissue assumes a varying position around the tooth.
2. The gingival margin varies in its position on the tooth.
D. Proximal surfaces must be approached by entering from both the facial and lingual aspects of the tooth.
   1. Gingival and periodontal infections begin in the col area more frequently than in other areas (Figure 11-8, page 192).
   2. Probing depth may be deepest directly under the contact area because of crater formation in the alveolar bone (Figure 12-3).
E. Anatomic features of the tooth-surface wall of the pocket influence the direction of probing. Examples are concave surfaces, anomalies, shape of cervical third, and position of furcations.

II. EVALUATION OF TOOTH SURFACE

During the movement of the probe, calculus and tooth surface irregularities can be felt and evaluated. The information obtained is used to plan the scaling and root planing appointments. The root surface in a pocket is described on page 229.

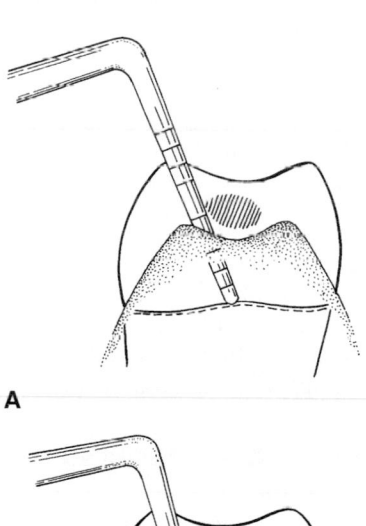

A

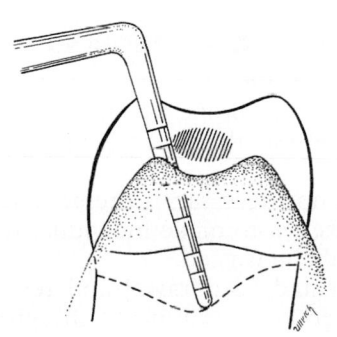

B

FIGURE 12-3 Proximal Surface Probing. (A) Probe must be applied more than half way across from facial to overlap with probing from the lingual. **(B)** Probe in area of crater formation. Probing is usually deeper on the proximal surface under the contact area than on the facial or lingual surfaces.

III. FACTORS THAT AFFECT PROBE DETERMINATIONS

The general objectives of probing are accuracy and consistency so that recordings are dependable for comparison with future probings as well as with colleagues in practice together. At the same time, patient discomfort and trauma to the tissues must be minimal. Probing is influenced by many factors, such as those that follow:

A. Severity and Extent of Periodontal Disease
With application of a light pressure, the probe passes along the tooth surface to the attached tissue level. Diseased tissue offers less resistance, so that with increased severity of inflammation, the probe inserts to a deeper level.[1] Average levels show that the probe is stopped as follows:
   1. *Normal Healthy Tissue.* The probe is at the base of the sulcus or crevice, at the coronal end of the junctional epithelium.
   2. *Gingivitis and Early Periodontitis.* The probe tip is within the junctional epithelium.
   3. *Advanced Periodontitis.* Probe tip penetrates through the junctional epithelium to reach attached connective tissue fibers.

B. The Probe Itself
   1. *Calibration.* Must be accurately marked.
   2. *Thickness.* A thinner probe slips through a narrow pocket more readily.
   3. *Readability.* Aided by the markings and color-coding.

C. Technique
   1. *Grasp.* Appropriate for maximum tactile sensitivity.
   2. *Finger Rest.* Placed on nonmobile tooth with uniformity.

D. Placement Problems
   1. *Anatomic Variations.* Tooth contours, furcations, contact areas, anomalies.
   2. *Interferences.* Calculus, irregular margins of restorations, fixed dental prostheses.
   3. *Accessibility, Visibility.* Obstructed by tissue bleeding, limited opening by patient, macroglossia.

E. Application of Pressure
Consistent pressure is accomplished by consistent grasp and finger rest in addition to keen tactile sensitivity.

PROBING PROCEDURES

I. PROBE INSERTION

A. Grasp probe with modified pen grasp (pages 520 to 521).
B. Establish finger rest on a neighboring tooth, preferably in the same dental arch.

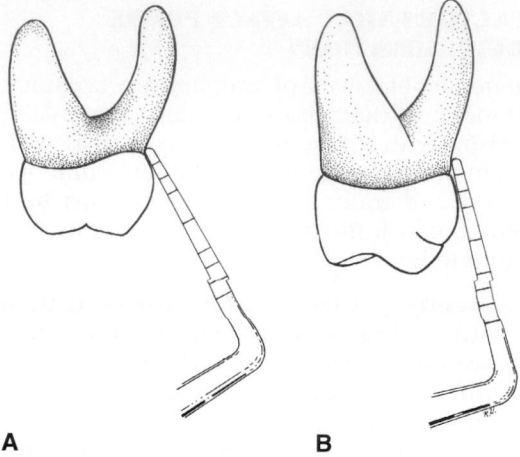

A   **B**

■ **FIGURE 12-4 Primary and Permanent Maxillary Molars. (A)** Accentuated convexity of the cervical third and widespread roots of the primary molar complicate probe placement. Probe may encounter the root. **(B)** Permanent tooth with less convexity of the cervical third and roots that are less widely spread.

C. Hold side of instrument tip flat against the tooth near the gingival margin. The cervical third of a primary tooth is more convex (Figure 12-4).

D. Gently slide the tip under the gingival margin.
1. *Healthy or Firm Fibrotic Tissue.* Insertion is more difficult because of the close adaptation of the tissue to the tooth surface; underlying gingival fibers are strong and tight.
2. *Spongy, Soft Tissue.* Gingival margin is loose and flabby because of the destruction of underlying gingival fibers. Probe inserts readily, and bleeding can be expected on gentle probing.

II. ADVANCE PROBE TO BASE OF POCKET

A. Hold side of probe tip flat against the tooth surface. Widespread roots of primary molars may make this probe position difficult unless the tissue is unduly distended by the probe (Figure 12-4).

B. Slide the probe along the tooth surface vertically down to the base of the sulcus or pocket.
1. Maintain contact of the side of the tip of the probe with the tooth.
   a. Gingival pocket. Side of probe is on enamel.
   b. Periodontal pocket. Side of probe is on the cemental or dentinal surface when inserted to a level below the cemento-enamel junction.
2. As the probe is passed down the side of the tooth, roughness may be felt. Evaluation of the topography and nature of the tooth surface is important to instrumentation.
3. When obstruction by hard bulky calculus deposit is encountered, lift the probe away

from tooth and follow over the edge of the calculus until the probe can move vertically into the pocket again.

4. The base of the sulcus or pocket feels soft and elastic (compared with the hard tooth surface and calculus deposits), and with slight pressure, the tension of the attached periodontal tissue at the base of the pocket can be felt.

C. Use only the pressure needed to detect by tactile means the level of the attached tissue, whether junctional epithelium or deep connective tissue fibers. A light pressure of 10 g, or of no more than 20 g, is ample.

D. Position probe for reading.
1. Bring the probe to position as nearly parallel with the long axis of the tooth as possible for reading the depth.
2. Interference of the contact area does not permit placing the probe parallel for the measurement directly beneath the contact area. Hold the side of shank of the probe against the contact to minimize the angle (Figure 12-3).

III. READ THE PROBE

A. Measurement for a probing depth is made from the gingival margin to the attached periodontal tissue.

B. Count the millimeters that show on the probe above the gingival margin and subtract the number from the total number of millimeters marked on the particular probe being used. A comparison of pocket measurement using probes with different calibrations is shown in Figure 12-5.

C. When the gingival margin appears at a level between probe marks, use the higher mark for the final reading.

D. Dry the area being probed to improve visibility for specific reading.

IV. CIRCUMFERENTIAL PROBING

A. Probe Stroke

Maintain the probe in the sulcus or pocket of each tooth as the probe is moved in a walking stroke.
1. It is not necessary to remove the probe and reinsert it to make individual readings. Time would be wasted.
2. Repeated withdrawal and reinsertion cause unnecessary trauma to the gingival margin and hence increase post-treatment discomfort.

B. Walking Stroke

1. Hold the side of the tip against the tooth at the base of the pocket.
2. Slide the probe up (coronally) about 1 to 2 mm and back to the attachment in a "touch

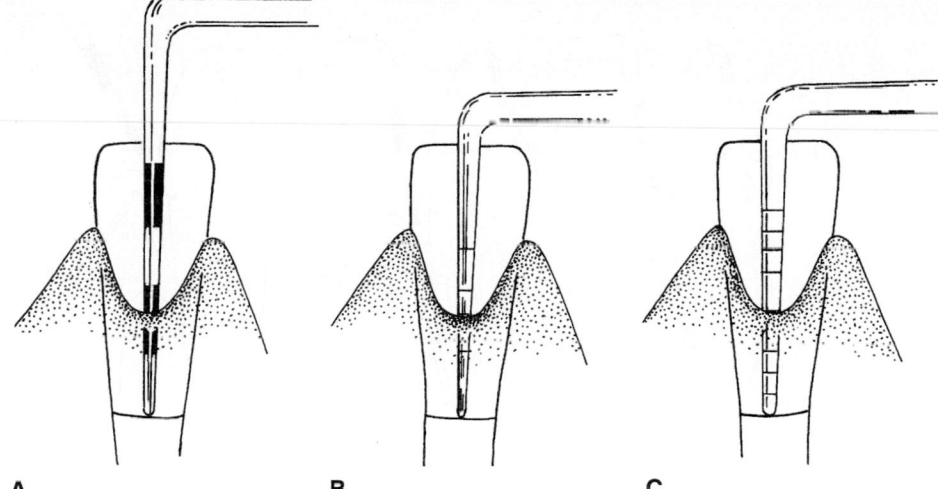

FIGURE 12-5 Comparison of Probe Readings. Measurement of same 5-mm pocket with 3 different probes. **(A)** Color-coded, **(B)** Michigan O, **(C)** Williams.

. . . touch . . . touch . . ." rhythm (Figure 12-6).
3. Observe probe measurement at the gingival margin at each touch.
4. Advance millimeter by millimeter along the facial and lingual surfaces into the proximal areas.

V. ADAPTATION OF PROBE FOR INDIVIDUAL TEETH

A. Molars and Premolars
1. Orient the probe at the distal line angle for both facial and lingual application.
2. Insert probe at the distal line angle and probe in a distal direction; adapt the probe around the line angle, probe across the distal surface until the side of the probe contacts

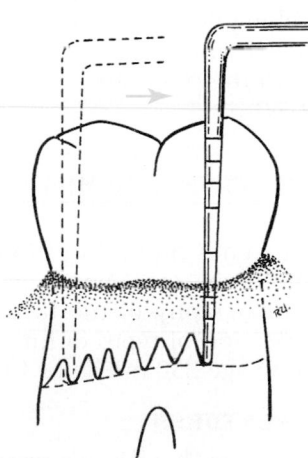

FIGURE 12-6 Probe Walking Stroke. The side of the tip of the probe is held in contact with the tooth. From the base of the pocket, the probe is moved up and down in 1- to 2-mm strokes as it is advanced in 1-mm steps. The attached periodontal tissue at the base of the pocket is contacted on each down stroke to identify probing depth in each area.

the contact area, then slant the probe to continue under the contact area.
3. Note the probing depth and slide the probe back to the distal line angle. Proceed in the mesial direction around the mesial line angle and across the mesial surface.

B. Anterior Teeth
1. Initial insertion may be at the distal line angle or from the midline of the facial or lingual surfaces.
2. Proceed around the distal line angle and across the distal surface; reinsert and probe the other half of the tooth.

C. Proximal Surfaces
1. Continue the walking stroke around each line angle and onto the proximal surface.
2. Roll the instrument handle between the fingers to keep the side of the probe tip adapted to the tooth surface at line angles and as the tooth contour varies.
3. Continue the strokes under the contact area. Overlap strokes from facial surface with strokes from lingual surface to assure full coverage (Figure 12-3). Make sure that the col area under each contact has been thoroughly examined.

CLINICAL ATTACHMENT LEVEL

Attachment level refers to the position of the periodontal attached tissues at the base of a sulcus or pocket. It is measured from a fixed point to the attachment, whereas the probing depth is measured from a changeable point (the crest of the free gingiva) to the attachment (Figure 12-7A).

I. RATIONALE

A loss of attachment occurs in disease as the junctional epithelium migrates toward the apex. Stability

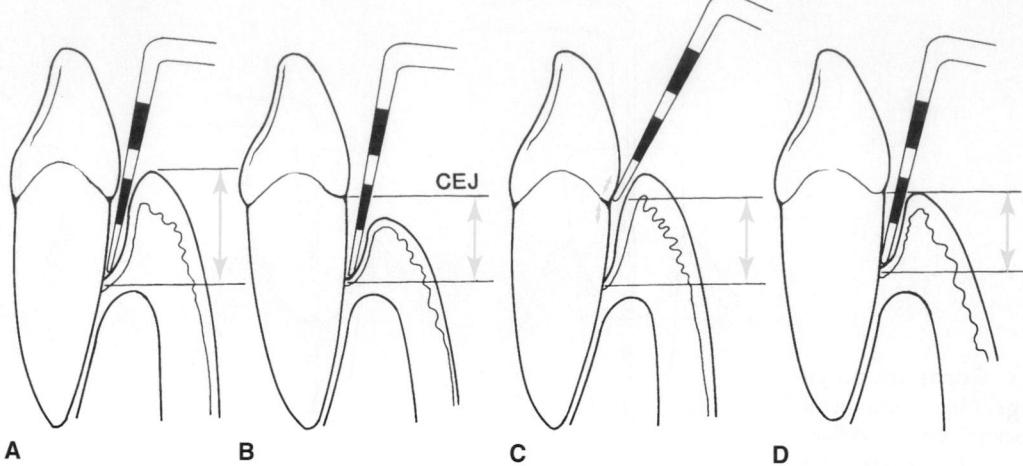

A   **B**   **C**   **D**

▢ **FIGURE 12-7 Clinical Attachment Level. (A)** Probing depth: the pocket is measured from the gingival margin to the attached periodontal tissue. **(B)** Clinical attachment level in the presence of gingival recession is measured directly from the cementoenamel junction (CEJ) to the attached tissue. **(C)** Clinical attachment level when the gingival margin covers the cementoenamel junction: first the cementoenamel junction is located as shown, and then the distance to the cementoenamel junction is measured and subtracted from the probing depth. **(D)** The clinical attachment level is equal to the probing depth when the gingival margin is at the level of the cementoenamel junction.

of attachment is characteristic in health, and treatment procedures may be aimed to obtain a gain of attachment.

Evaluation can be made of the outcome of periodontal treatment and the stability of the attachment during maintenance examinations. When periodontal disease is active, pocket formation and migration of the attachment along the cemental surface continue.

II. PROCEDURE

A. Selecting a Fixed Point
1. Cementoenamel junction is usually used.
2. Margin of a permanent restoration.
3. For animal research, a notch may be made in the tooth; in human research studies, a template or splint may be made for each patient.

B. Measuring in the Presence of Visible Recession
1. Cementoenamel junction is visible directly.
2. Measure from the cementoenamel junction to the attachment (Figure 12-7*B*).
3. The clinical attachment level is greater than the probing depth when there is visible recession.

C. Measuring When the Cementoenamel Junction Is Covered by Gingiva
1. Slide the probe along the tooth surface, into the pocket, until the cementoenamel junction is felt (Figure 12-7*C*).
2. Remove the calculus when it covers the cementoenamel junction.

3. Measure from the gingival crest to the cementoenamel junction.
4. Subtract the millimeters from cementoenamel junction to gingival crest from the total probing depth to the attachment.
5. Probing depth is greater than the clinical attachment level when the cementoenamel junction is covered by free gingiva.

D. Measuring When the Free Gingival Margin Is Level With the Cementoenamel Junction
1. Apply the probe as has been described.
2. The probing depth equals the clinical attachment level when the free gingival margin is level with the cementoenamel junction (Figure 12-7*D*).

FURCATIONS EXAMINATION

When a pocket extends into a furcation area, special adaptation of the probe must be made to determine the extent and topography of the furcation involvement. The classification of types of furcation involvement is shown on page 230 in Figure 13-3.

I. ANATOMIC FEATURES

A. Bifurcation (teeth with two roots)
1. *Mandibular Molars.* The furcation area is accessible for probing from the facial and lingual surfaces (Figure 12-8).
2. *Maxillary First Premolars.* The furcation area is accessible from the mesial and distal aspects, under the contact area.
3. *Primary Mandibular Molar.* Widespread roots.

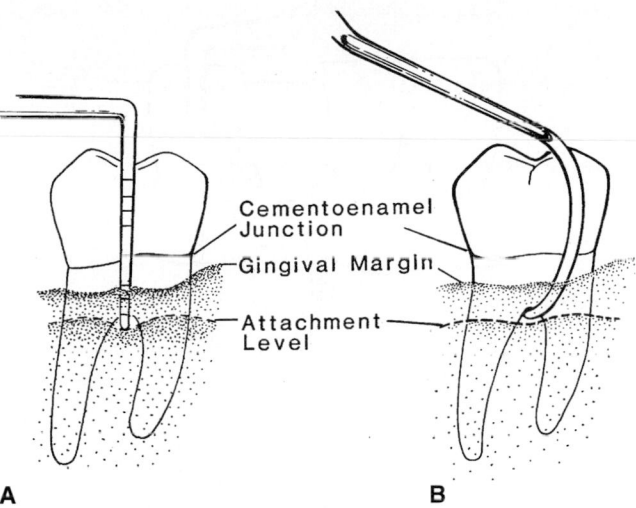

Cementoenamel Junction

Gingival Margin

Attachment Level

A   B

FIGURE 12-8 Furcation Examination. (A) Williams probe inserted into bifurcation in area of gingival recession shows probing depth of 3 mm. **(B)** Nabers furcation probe used to examine the topography of the furcation area.

B. Trifurcation (teeth with three roots)

1. *Maxillary Molars.* A palatal root and two buccal roots, the mesiobuccal and the distobuccal roots. Access for probing is from the mesial, buccal, and distal surfaces.
2. *Maxillary Primary Molars.* Widespread roots (Figure 12-4, page 208).

II. EXAMINATION METHODS

A. Early Furcation
1. Measure probing depth.
2. Examine the area by adapting the probe closely to the tooth surface and moving the end of the probe over the anatomic curvatures of the roots. An example is shown in Figure 33-1C, page 549.
3. Check radiograph for signs of furcation involvement (Figure 12-18, page 220).

B. Points of Access
Measure probing depths at points of access for each bifurcation or trifurcation area. Position of gingival margin will vary. Figure 12-8A shows apparent recession and 3-mm pocket in bifurcation.

C. Probe Adaptation
Use probe in diagonal or horizontal position to examine between roots when there is gingival recession or a flexible, short, soft pocket wall that permits access.

D. Use of Furcation Probe
Use a furcation probe, such as a Nabers 1N or 2N, to examine advanced furcation (Figure 12-8B).

E. Complications
Anatomic variations that complicate furcation examination are fused roots; anomalies, such as extra roots; or low or high furcations (Figure 33-2, page 549).

MUCOGINGIVAL EXAMINATION

I. TENSION TEST[2]

A. Purposes
1. To detect adequacy of the width of the attached gingiva.
2. To locate frenal attachments and their proximity to the free gingiva.
3. To identify promptly the mucogingival junction.

B. Procedures
1. *Facial*
   a. Retract cheeks and lips laterally by grasping the lips with the thumbs and index fingers. Watch at the mucogingival junction.
   b. Move the lips and cheeks up and down and across, creating tension at the mucogingival junction.
   c. Follow around from the molar areas on the right to molar areas on the left, both maxillary and mandibular.
2. *Lingual (Mandible)*
   a. Hold a mouth mirror to tense the mucosa of the floor of the mouth, gently retracting the side of the tongue, so that the mucogingival junction is clearly visible.
   b. Request patient to move the tongue to the left, to the right, and up to touch the palate.

C. Observations
1. Blanching at the mucogingival junction.
2. Frenal attachments.
3. Area(s) of apparent recession where there is very little keratinized gingiva and the base of the sulcus or pocket is near the mucogingival junction (Figure 11-13B, page 198).
4. Area where color, size, loss of stippling, smooth shininess, or other characteristic indicates the need for careful probing to determine the amount of attached gingiva.
5. Area where tension pulls the free gingiva away from the tooth, thereby indicating no attached gingiva.

II. GINGIVAL TISSUE EXAMINATION

When inflammation is present and a pocket extends to or through the mucogingival junction, a streak of color (red, bluish-red) that shows the inflammatory changes from the gingival margin to the mucogingival junction may be apparent. When such an area does not pull away during a tension test or does not permit passage of a probe through to the alveolar mucosa, the area should be noted in the record for examination after elimination of inflammation.

III. PROBING

When a pocket extends to or beyond the mucogingival junction, the probe may pass through the pocket directly into the alveolar mucosa (Figure 12-9). Mucogingival involvement is present.

IV. MEASURE THE AMOUNT OF ATTACHED GINGIVA

A. Place the probe on the external surface of the gingiva and measure from the mucogingival junction to the gingival margin to determine the width of the total gingiva (Figure 12-10A).
B. Insert the probe and measure probing depth (Figure 12-10B).
C. Subtract the probing depth from the total gingival measurement to get the width of the attached gingiva.
D. Record findings.

PERIODONTAL CHARTING

Charting of findings while using the probe is a part of the complete periodontal record. The summary of periodontal observations and records may be found on page 318.

The procedure described here assumes the use of a chart form with outline drawings of teeth with both facial and lingual root drawings. The exact procedure and format are entirely the choice of the individual dentist. A composite chart that includes dental as well as periodontal findings is frequently used.

In the preparation of the charting, contrasting colors should be used. For example, when red is used to

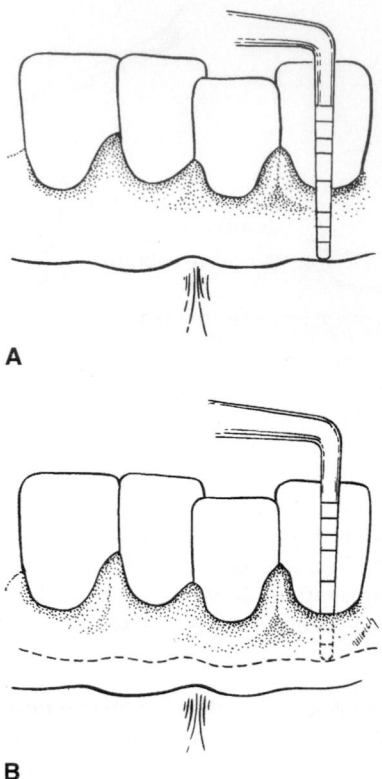

A

B

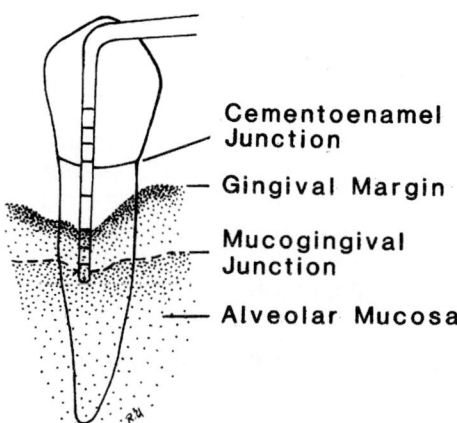

FIGURE 12-9 **Mucogingival Examination.** Probe in position for measuring probing depth where attached gingiva is missing. Absence of attached gingiva permits the probe to pass through the mucogingival junction into the alveolar mucosa.

Labels in figure:
- Cementoenamel Junction
- Gingival Margin
- Mucogingival Junction
- Alveolar Mucosa

FIGURE 12-10 **Measuring Attached Gingiva. (A)** Measure the total gingiva by laying the probe over the surface of the gingiva and measuring from the free margin to the mucogingival junction. **(B)** Measure the probing depth. Dotted line represents the base of the pocket. Subtract the probing depth (B) from the total gingiva (A) to obtain the width of attached gingiva. The area illustrated shows 2 mm of attached gingiva.

chart dental caries on a composite charting, red would not be a good color selection for drawing the gingival margin because of possible interference with a drawing of a Class V carious lesion (Table 14-3, page 241). One procedure for a relatively simple charting system is described here.

I. TEETH IDENTIFICATION

Mark missing, unerupted, or impacted teeth. When radiographs and study casts are available before the recording of clinical findings is scheduled, these markings can be made in advance of the patient's appointment.

II. DRAW GINGIVAL LINES

A. Gingival Margin

1. Draw the outline of the position and contour of the gingival margin on the chart form as it appears in relation to the teeth both facial and lingual.
2. Prepare in advance of the patient's appointment when new study casts are available.

B. Mucogingival Lines
1. *General Procedures*
   a. Use contrasting color to that used for drawing the gingival margin line.
   b. Draw on the facial aspect for all quadrants; draw the lingual line only on mandibular chart.
2. *Three Methods.* For all, draw the gingival margin line first.
   a. Draw the lines directly, estimating distances between the gingival margin and the mucogingival junction.
   b. Measure with probe.
      i. Measure the total gingiva from gingival margin to mucogingival junction at the center of each tooth (facial and lingual). Write the millimeters on the tooth crown in light pencil to be erased later.
      ii. Place a dot on the tooth chart at the point of millimeters measured from the margin; connect the dots in a relatively straight line representing the mucogingival junction for the molars and premolars and in a scalloped line for the anterior teeth, in keeping with the actual appearance.
   c. Study casts. When parts or all of the mucogingival lines show clearly on the casts, the drawing can be made in advance of the patient's appointment.

III. RECORD PROBING DEPTHS
A. Record all diseased pockets of any depth.
B. Record deepest millimeter measurement for each of the six areas around a tooth as shown in Figure 12-11. Areas numbered 1, 3, 4, 6 extend from the line angle to under the contact area.
C. Supplement the six recordings with additional readings to show particular areas of

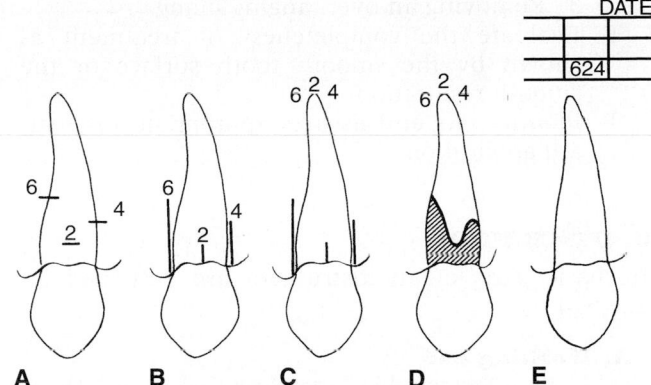

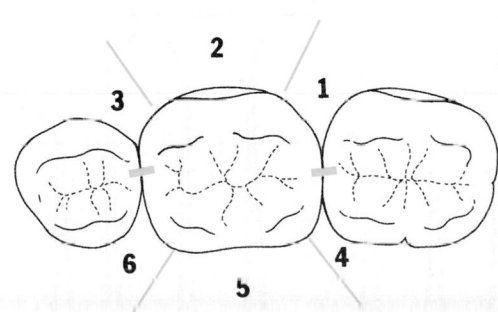

FIGURE 12-11 Charting Probing Depths. The pocket/sulcus is measured completely around each tooth. Record the deepest measurement for each of the 6 areas around the tooth. Areas 1, 3, 4, and 6 extend from the line angle to under the contact area.

FIGURE 12-12 Methods for Charting Probing Depths. (A), (B) Chart forms with free-hand lines that designate relative depths. **(C)** Numeric notations written at the apex of each tooth. **(D)** A continuous line that defines the entire pocket and that can be shaded. **(E)** Multiple spaces over the apex of each tooth, used to record the probing depths. Each row can be dated, thus allowing comparisons of measurements at successive follow-up and maintenance examinations.

unusually deep pockets, furcation involvement, or mucogingival involvement.
D. Record on the charting form. Figure 12-12 shows five possible methods for recording the millimeter depth.

IV. RECORD SPECIAL DISEASE PROBLEMS
Furcation involvement, mucogingival involvement, and frenal pull must be recorded either by a special symbol or by writing directly on the chart or in the record. See Figure 20-2 (page 317) for a suggested method of charting.

EXPLORERS

I. GENERAL PURPOSES AND USES
An explorer is used to
A. Detect, by tactile sense, the texture and character of the tooth surface.
B. Examine the supragingival tooth surfaces for calculus, demineralized and carious lesions, defects or irregularities in the surfaces and margins of restorations, and other irregularities that are not apparent to direct observation. An explorer is used to confirm direct observation.
C. Examine the subgingival tooth surfaces for calculus, demineralized and carious lesions, diseased altered cementum, and other cemental changes that can result from periodontal pocket formation.
D. Define the extent of instrumentation needed and guide techniques for
   1. Scaling and root planing.
   2. Finishing a restoration.

3. Removing an overhanging filling.

E. Evaluate the completeness of treatment as shown by the smooth tooth surface or the smooth restoration.

F. Identify pits and fissures appropriate for sealant application.

II. DESCRIPTION

The basic parts of an instrument are described on page 514.

A. Working End

1. Slender, wirelike, metal *tip* that is circular in cross section and tapers to a fine sharp *point*.
2. Design
   a. Single. A single instrument may be universal and adaptable to any tooth surface, or it may be designed for specific groups of surfaces. In Figure 12-13, Nos. 2 through 7, 17, 18, 20, and 23 are single instruments.
   b. Paired. Paired instruments are mirror images of each other, curved to provide access to contralateral tooth surfaces. In Figure 12-13, Nos. 9 and 10, 11 and 12, 13 and 14, and 21 and 22 are paired.
   c. Design of a balanced instrument. Middle of working end should be centered over the long axis of the handle (Figure 12-14). Figure 32-1 (p. 514) shows a balanced curet.

B. Shank

1. *Straight, Curved, or Angulated.* Whether a shank is straight, curved, or angulated depends on the use and adaptation for which the explorer was designed. In Figure 12-13, compare the straight shanks of Nos. 2, 5, 6, 7, 13, and 14 with the others in the series, which are not straight. A curved shank may facilitate application of the instrument to

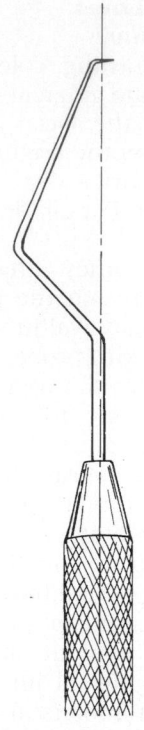

FIGURE 12-14 Balanced Explorer Design. With the middle of the tip centered over the long axis of the handle (shown by broken line from tip), the explorer can be positioned in a sulcus or pocket with ease and does not cause trauma to the gingival tissue. Shown is the balanced TU-17 explorer.

proximal surfaces, particularly of posterior teeth.

2. *Flexibility.* The slender, wirelike explorers have a degree of flexibility that contributes to increased sensitivity.

C. Handle

1. *Weight.* For increased acute tactile sensitivity, a lightweight handle is more effective.

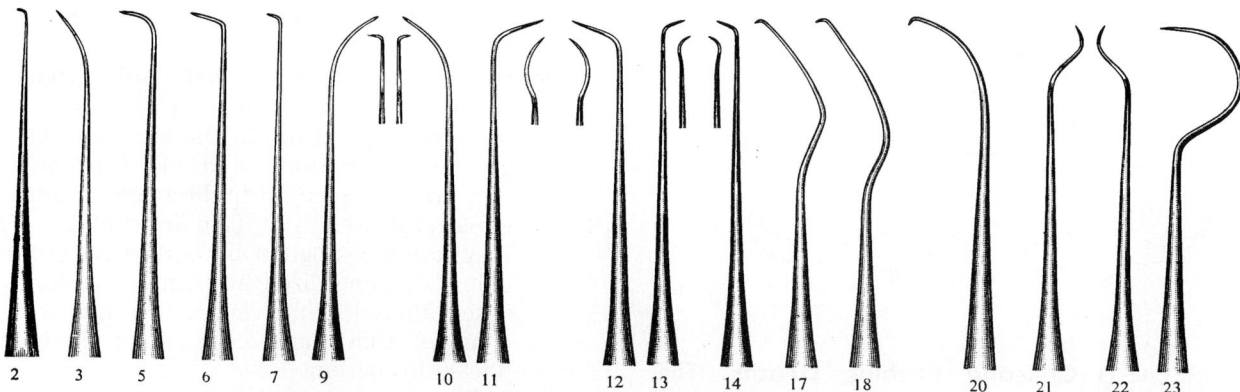

FIGURE 12-13 Explorers. This series from Nos. 2 through 23 shows standard shapes of explorer tips. Nos. 2 through 7, 17, 18, 20, and 23 are single instruments. Nos. 9 and 10, 11 and 12, 13 and 14, and 21 and 22 are paired instruments. (Courtesy of the S.S. White Company, Philadelphia, PA.)

2. *Diameter.* A wider diameter with serrations for friction while grasping can prevent finger cramping from too tight a grasp. With a lighter grasp, tactile sensitivity can be increased.

D. Construction
1. *Single-ended.* A single-ended instrument has one working end on a separate handle.
2. *Double-ended.* A double-ended instrument has two working ends, one on each end of a common handle. Most paired instruments are available double-ended. Other double-ended instruments combine two single instruments, for example, two unpaired explorers or an explorer with a probe.

III. PREPARATION OF EXPLORERS

Sharpen and retaper a dull explorer tip (page 541). With the explorer tip sharp and tapered, the following can be expected:
 A. Increased tactile sensitivity with less pressure required.
 B. Prevention of unnecessary trauma to the gingival tissue, because less pressure allows greater control.
 C. Decreased instrumentation time with increased patient comfort.

IV. SPECIFIC EXPLORERS AND THEIR USES

A variety of explorers is available as shown by the examples in Figure 12-13. The function of each type is related to its adaptability to specific surfaces of teeth at particular angulations. Certain explorers can be used effectively for detection of dental caries in pits and fissures, and others are designed to be adapted to examine proximal surfaces for calculus or dental caries. By other criteria, some can be used subgingivally, whereas others cannot be adapted subgingivally without inflicting damage to the sulcular epithelium. Therefore, such explorers are limited to supragingival adaptation only.

A. Subgingival Explorer
1. *Names and Numbers.* Orban No. 20, TU-17, pocket explorer.
2. *Shape.* The pocket explorer has an angulated shank with a short tip (Figure 12-14). The tip should be measured to assure that it is less than 2 mm. A longer tip cannot be adapted to the line angles of narrow roots.
3. *Features for Subgingival Root Examination*
   a. Back of tip can be applied directly to the attached periodontal tissue at the base of the pocket without lacerating. When a straight or sickle explorer is directed toward the base of the pocket, the sharp tip can pass into the epithelium without resistance.
   b. The short tip can be adapted to rounded tooth surfaces and line angles. Long tips of other explorers have a tangential rela-

tionship with the tooth and cause distention and trauma to sulcular or pocket epithelium.
   c. Narrow short tip can be adapted at the base where the pocket narrows without undue displacement of the pocket soft tissue wall.
4. *Supragingival Use of No. TU-17.* It may be adapted to all surfaces and is especially useful for proximal surface examination. It is not readily adaptable to pits and fissures.

B. Sickle or Shepherd's Hook (No. 23 in Figure 12-13)
1. *Use.* Examining pits and fissures and supragingival smooth surfaces; examining surfaces and margins of restorations and sealants.
2. *Adaptability*
   a. Difficult to apply to proximal surfaces because the wide hook can contact an adjacent tooth and the straight long section of the tip can pass over a small proximal carious lesion.
   b. Not adaptable for deep subgingival exploration. When the point is directed to the base of a pocket, trauma to the attachment area can result. In the attempt to prevent such damage, the clinician may not explore to the base of the pocket, thus providing incomplete service.

C. Pigtail or Cowhorn (Nos. 21 and 22 in Figure 12-13)
1. *Use.* Proximal surfaces for calculus, dental caries, or margins of restorations.
2. *Adaptability.* As paired, curved tips, they are applied to opposite tooth surfaces.

D. Straight (Nos. 2, 6, 7 in Figure 12-13)
1. *Use.* Supragingival, for pits and fissures, tooth irregularities of smooth surfaces, and surfaces and margins of restorations and sealants.
2. *Adaptability*
   a. For pit and fissure caries, the explorer tip is held parallel with the long axis of the tooth and applied straight into a pit.
   b. Not adaptable deep in subgingival area. Straight shanked instruments or those with long tips cannot be adapted readily in the apical portion of the pocket near the attached tissue or on line angles.

BASIC PROCEDURES FOR USE OF EXPLORERS

Development of ability to use an explorer and a probe is achieved first by learning the anatomic features of each tooth surface and the types of irregularities that may be encountered on the surfaces. The second step is repeated practice of careful and deliberate techniques for application of the instruments.

The objective is to adapt the instruments in a routine manner that relays consistent comparative information about the nature of the tooth surface. Concentration, patience, attention to detail, and alertness to each irregularity, however small it may seem, are necessary.

I. USE OF SENSORY STIMULI

Both explorers and probes can transmit tactile stimuli from tooth surfaces to the fingers. A fine explorer usually gives a more acute sense of tactile discrimination to small irregularities than does a thicker explorer. Probes vary in diameter; the narrow types may provide greater sensitivity.

II. TOOTH SURFACE IRREGULARITIES

Three basic tactile sensations must be distinguished when probing or exploring. These may be grouped as normal tooth surface, irregularities created by excess or elevations in the surface, and irregularities caused by depressions in the tooth surface. Examples of these are listed here.

A. Normal
1. *Tooth Structure.* The smooth surface of enamel and root surface that has been planed; anatomic configurations, such as cingula, furcations.
2. *Restored Surfaces.* Smooth surfaces of metal (gold, amalgam) and the softer feeling of plastic; smooth margin of a restoration.

B. Irregularities: Increases or Elevations in Tooth Surface
1. *Deposits.* Calculus.
2. *Anomalies.* Enamel pearl; unusually pronounced cementoenamel junction.
3. *Restorations.* Overcontoured, irregular margins (overhang).

C. Irregularities: Depressions, Grooves
1. *Tooth Surface.* Demineralized or carious lesion, abrasion, erosion, pits such as those caused by enamel hypoplasia, areas of cemental resorption on the root surface.
2. *Restorations.* Deficient margin, rough surface (Figure 40-1, page 624).

III. TYPES OF STIMULI

During exploring and probing, distinction of irregularities can be made through auditory and tactile means.

A. Tactile
Tactile sensations pass through the instrument to the fingers and hand and to the brain for registration and action. Tactile sensations, for example, may be the result of catching on an overcontoured restoration, dropping into a carious lesion, hooking the edge of a restoration or

lesion, encountering an elevated deposit, or simply passing over a rough surface.

B. Auditory
As an explorer or probe moves over the surface of enamel, cementum, a metallic restoration, a plastic restoration, or any irregularity of tooth structure or restoration, a particular surface texture is apparent. With each contact, sound may be created. The clean smooth enamel is quiet; the rough cementum or calculus is scratchy or noisy. Sometimes a metallic restoration may "squeak" or have a metallic "ring." With experience, differentiations can be made.

SUPRAGINGIVAL PROCEDURES

I. USE OF VISION

Supragingival exploration for defects of the tooth surface differs from subgingival in that, when a surface is dried, much of the actual exploration is performed to confirm visual observation. The exceptions are the proximal areas near and around contact areas that cannot be directly observed.

Unnecessary exploration should be avoided. With adequate light and a source of air, proper retraction, and use of mouth mirror, dried supragingival calculus can generally be seen as either chalky white or brownish-yellow in contrast to tooth color. A minimum of exploration can confirm the finding.

II. FACIAL AND LINGUAL SURFACES
A. Adapt the side of tip with the point always on the tooth surface.
B. Move the instrument in short walking strokes over the surface being examined, or direct the tip gently into a suspected carious lesion.
C. Avoid deliberate exploration of cervical third areas where there is recession or where the patient has previously exhibited sensitivity. If a sensitive area must be dried, avoid an air blast, and blot with a gauze sponge or a cotton roll. Methods for desensitization are described on page 600.

III. PROXIMAL SURFACES
A. Lead with the tip onto a proximal surface, rolling the handle between the fingers to assure adaptation around the line angle. Keep the side of the point of the explorer in contact with the tooth surface at all times.
B. Explore under the proximal contact area when there is recession of the papilla and the area is exposed. Overlap strokes from facial and lingual surfaces to ensure full coverage.

SUBGINGIVAL PROCEDURES

I. ESSENTIALS FOR DETECTION OF TOOTH SURFACE IRREGULARITIES

A. Definite but light grasp.

B. Consistent finger rest with light pressure.

C. Definite contact of the instrument with the tooth.

D. Light touch as the instrument is moved over the tooth surface.

II. STEPS

A. With the tip in contact with the tooth supragingivally, hold the lower shank (the part of the shank that is next to the tip) parallel with the long axis of the tooth. Gently slide the tip under the gingival margin into the sulcus or pocket.

B. Keep the point in contact with the tooth at all times to prevent unnecessary trauma to the pocket or sulcular epithelium. Adapt the tip closely to the tooth surface by applying the side of the point.

C. Slide the explorer tip over the tooth surface to the base of the pocket until, with the back of the tip, the resistance of the soft tissue of the attached periodontal tissue is felt (Figure 12-15*A*). Calculus deposits may obstruct direct passage of the instrument to the base of the pocket. Lift the tip slightly away from the tooth surface and follow over the deposit to proceed to the base of the pocket.

D. Use a "walking" stroke, vertical or diagonal (oblique).

1. Lead with the tip. Move it ahead as the instrument progresses (Figure 12-15*B*).

2. Length of stroke depends on the depth of a pocket.

   a. Shallow pocket. The stroke may extend the entire depth, from the base of the pocket to just beneath the gingival margin.

   b. Deep pocket. Controlled strokes 2- to 3-mm long can provide more acute sensitivity to the surface and allow improved adaptation of the instrument. A deep pocket should be explored in sections. One should first explore the apical area next to the base of the pocket, then move up to a higher section, overlapping for full coverage.

3. Do not remove the explorer from the pocket for each stroke on a particular surface because

   a. Trauma to the gingival margin caused by repeated withdrawal and reinsertion can cause the patient post-treatment discomfort.

   b. Concentration on the texture of the tooth surface is interrupted.

   c. More time is consumed.

E. Proximal surface

1. Lead with tip of instrument; do not "back into" an area.

2. Continue the strokes around the line

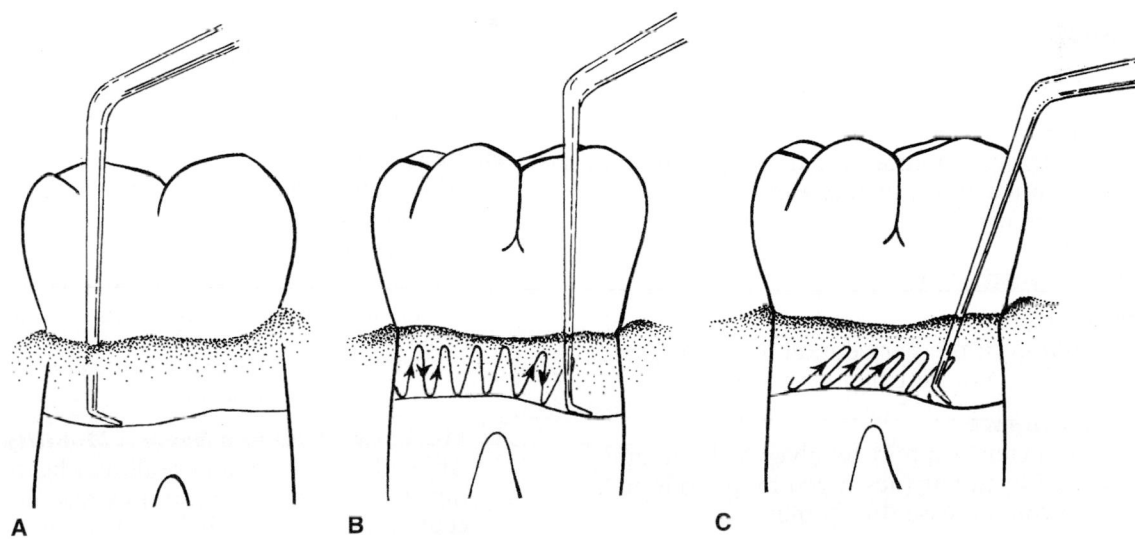

■FIGURE 12-15 **Use of Subgingival Explorer. (A)** The lower shank (next to tip) is held parallel with the long axis of the tooth. The explorer is passed into the pocket and lowered until the back of the working tip meets resistance from the attached periodontal tissue at the base of the pocket. **(B)** Vertical walking stroke. With the side of the tip in contact with the tooth surface at all times, the explorer is moved over the surface. **(C)** Diagonal walking stroke. Complete exploration of the surface is needed; therefore, groups of strokes are overlapped.

angle. Roll the instrument handle between the fingers to keep the tip closely adapted as the tooth contour changes.

3. Continue strokes under the contact area. Overlap strokes from facial and lingual aspects for full coverage.

RECORD FINDINGS

I. SUPRAGINGIVAL CALCULUS

A. Distribution

Supragingival calculus is generally localized. It is most commonly confined to the lingual surfaces of the mandibular anterior teeth and the facial surfaces of the maxillary first and second molars, opposite the openings to the salivary ducts (page 279).

B. Amount

Slight, moderate, heavy.

II. SUBGINGIVAL CALCULUS

A. Distribution

Subgingival calculus can be either localized or generalized.

B. Amount

Slight, moderate, heavy.

III. OTHER IRREGULARITIES OF TOOTH SURFACE

Note on the chart or in the record any other deviation from normal detected while using the explorer.

MOBILITY EXAMINATION

Because of the nature and function of the periodontal ligament, teeth have a slight normal mobility. Mobility can be considered abnormal or pathologic when it exceeds normal. Increased mobility can be an important clinical sign of disease.

I. CAUSES OF MOBILITY

A. Inflammation

Inflammation in the periodontal ligament leads to degeneration or destruction of the fibers.

B. Loss of Support

Loss of sufficient support by alveolar bone and periodontal ligament (destroyed by periodontal infection) can increase the mobility.

C. Trauma From Occlusion

Injury to the periodontal tissues can result from occlusal forces (page 261).

II. PROCEDURE FOR DETERMINATION OF MOBILITY

A. Position the patient for clear visibility with maximum light and ready accessibility through convenient retraction.

B. Stabilize the head. Motion of the head, lips, or cheek can interfere with a true evaluation of tooth movement.

C. Use two single-ended metal instruments with wide blunt ends, held with a modified pen grasp. Use of wooden tongue depressors or plastic mirror handles is not recommended because of their flexibility. Testing with the fingers without the metal instruments can be misleading because the soft tissue of the fingertips can move and give an illusion of tooth movement.

D. Apply specific, firm finger rests (fulcrums). A standardized finger rest pressure contributes increased consistency to the determinations. The teeth may be dried with air or sponge to prevent slipping of the instruments or the finger on the finger rest.

E. Apply the blunt ends of the instruments to opposite sides of a tooth, and rock the tooth to test horizontal mobility. Keep both instrument ends on the tooth as pressure is applied first from one side and then the other.

F. Test vertical mobility (depression of the tooth into its socket) by applying, on the occlusal or incisal surface, pressure with one of the mirror handles.

G. Test each primary abutment tooth of a fixed partial denture.

H. Move from tooth to tooth in a systematic order.

III. RECORD DEGREE OF MOVEMENT

A. Scale

N, 1, 2, 3 or I, II, III are frequently used, sometimes with a + to indicate mobility between numbers.

B. Recording

Although subjective, interpretation may be considered as follows.[3]

N = normal, physiologic
1 = slight mobility, greater than normal
2 = moderate mobility, greater than 1 mm displacement
3 = severe mobility, may move in all directions, vertical as well as horizontal.

C. The Letter N Means *Normal Mobility*

All teeth that have a periodontal ligament have normal mobility. No tooth has zero mobility except in a condition, such as ankylosis, in which there is no periodontal ligament.

D. Chart Form

A chart form should provide for a place to record mobility. Preferably more than one place should be reserved so that comparative readings may be recorded at successive maintenance appointments (Figure 20-2, page 317).

FREMITUS

I. DEFINITION

Fremitus means palpable vibration or movement. In dentistry it refers to the vibratory patterns of the teeth. A tooth with fremitus has excess contact, possibly related to a premature contact. Usually, the tooth also demonstrates some degree of mobility because the excess contact forces the tooth to move. The test is used in conjunction with occlusal analysis and adjustment.

Because fremitus depends on tooth contact, determination is made only on the maxillary teeth.

II. PROCEDURE FOR DETERMINATION OF FREMITUS

A. Seat the patient upright with the head stabilized against the headrest.
B. Press an index finger on each maxillary tooth at about the cervical third (Figure 12-16).
C. Request the patient to "click the back teeth" repeatedly.
D. Start with the most posterior maxillary tooth on one side, and move the index finger tooth by tooth around the arch.
E. Record by tooth number the teeth where vibration is felt and the teeth where actual movement is noted. The degree recorded may be subjective, but the following range has been suggested.

   N = normal (without vibration or movement).
   + = One-degree fremitus; only slight vibration can be felt.

+ + = Two-degree fremitus; the tooth is clearly palpable but movement is barely visible.
+ + + = Three-degree fremitus; movement is clearly observed visually.

RADIOGRAPHIC EXAMINATION

Radiographs provide essential information to aid and supplement clinical findings. During other phases of the examination, and especially during probing, the mounted radiographs should be on a viewbox for viewing in conjunction with examination. When the radiographs have not been processed at the time of probing, areas of special confirmation can be marked on the record for review at the next appointment.

For observing evidence of periodontal involvement, periapical radiographs are needed. Horizontal bitewing radiographs do not show the complete periodontal tissues that extend around the roots. When bone loss is moderate to severe, the crest of the bone may be seen in a vertical bitewing survey (Figure 9-13, page 158).

Principles for use of radiographs were described on pages 166 to 168. The need for mounted radiographs free from errors of technique and viewed on an adequately lighted viewbox cannot be overemphasized. A magnifying reading glass is of special assistance when studying periodontal findings.

RADIOGRAPHIC CHANGES IN PERIODONTAL INFECTIONS

I. BONE LEVEL

A. Normal Bone Level

The crest of the interdental bone appears from 1.0 to 1.5 mm from the cementoenamel junction (Figure 12-17).

B. Bone Level in Periodontal Disease

The height of the bone is lowered progressively as the inflammation is extended and bone is resorbed.

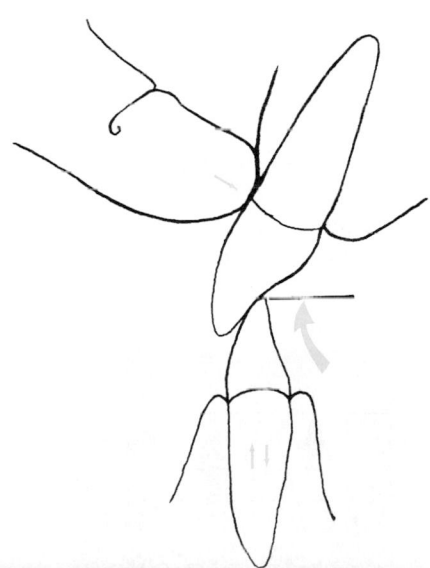

FIGURE 12-16 Fremitus. With the patient seated upright and the head stabilized against the headrest, an index finger is placed firmly over the cervical third of each maxillary tooth in succession starting with the most posterior tooth on one side and moving around the arch. The patient is requested to click the posterior teeth.

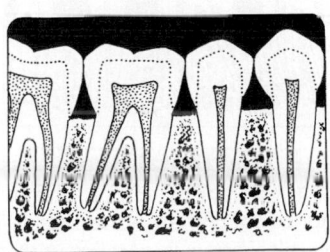

FIGURE 12-17 Normal Bone Level. Drawing of a radiograph to show normal bone level, 1 to 1.5 mm from the cementoenamel junction.

II. SHAPE OF REMAINING BONE

A. Horizontal

1. When the crest of the bone is parallel with a line between the cementoenamel junctions of two adjacent teeth, the term "horizontal bone loss" is used (Figures 12-18 and 12-19).

2. When inflammation is the sole destructive factor, the bone loss usually appears horizontal.

3. When the amount of remaining bone is fairly evenly distributed throughout the dentition, the condition is described as *generalized* horizontal bone loss. It may be designated either by millimeters from the position of the normal bone level or by percentage. When making estimates, referral to the table of average root lengths can be helpful (Appendix 2, Tables A-1 and A-2).

4. When bone loss is confined to specific areas, the condition is described as *localized* horizontal bone loss.

B. Angular or Vertical

1. Reduction in height of crestal bone that is irregular; the bone level is not parallel with a line joining the adjacent cementoenamel junctions (Figure 12-20); bone loss is greater on the proximal surface of one tooth than on the adjacent tooth.

2. Angular bone loss is more commonly localized; rarely generalized.

3. When inflammation and trauma from occlusion are combined in causing the destruction and irregular shape of the bone, the bone may appear with "angular defects" or with "vertical bone loss."

III. CRESTAL LAMINA DURA

A. Normal

White, radiopaque; continuous with and connects the lamina dura about the roots of two

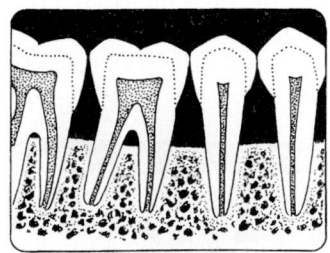

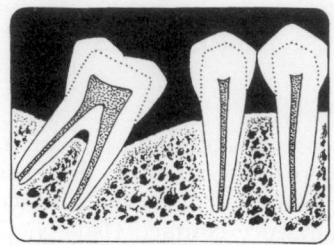

FIGURE 12-19 Horizontal Bone Loss. Second molar has drifted mesially into the space created when the first molar was removed. Note that the level of the crestal bone is parallel with a line between the cementoenamel junctions of the second premolar and the tipped second molar.

adjacent teeth; covers the interdental bone (Figure 12-18).

B. Evidence of Disease

The crestal lamina dura is indistinct, irregular, radiolucent, fuzzy (Figure 12-20, mesial of first molar).

IV. FURCATION INVOLVEMENT

A. Normal

Bone fills the area between the roots (Figure 12-17).

B. Evidence of Disease

Radiolucent area in the furcation.

1. Early furcation involvement may appear as a small radiolucent black dot or as a slight thickening of the periodontal ligament space. It can be confirmed by probing. Early furcation involvement is shown in the second molar in Figure 12-18.

2. Furcation involvement of maxillary molars may become advanced before radiographic evidence can be seen. Superimposition of the palatal root may mask a small area of involvement. When the proximal bone level in the radiograph appears at the level where

FIGURE 12-18 Horizontal Bone Loss. Bone level in periodontal disease is more than 1 to 1.5 mm from the cementoenamel junction. When bone loss is horizontal, the crest of the alveolar bone is parallel with a line between the cementoenamel junctions of adjacent teeth. Note early furcation involvement in the second molar and moderate furcation involvement in the first molar.

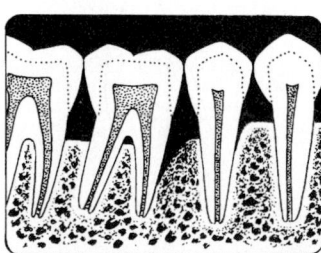

FIGURE 12-20 Angular or Vertical Bone Loss; Mesial of the First Molar. The level of the crestal bone between the second premolar and the first molar is not parallel with a line between the cementoenamel junctions of the same teeth.

the furcation is normally located, furcation involvement should be suspected and probed for confirmation.

3. Maxillary first premolar furcation involvement cannot be seen in a radiograph except at an unusual angulation or unusual position of the tooth. With correct vertical and horizontal angulation, the roots are superimposed.

4. Furcations may show at one angulation but not at another; variations in technique can obscure a furcation involvement. All furcations must be carefully probed.

V. PERIODONTAL LIGAMENT SPACE

A. Normal

The periodontal ligament is connective tissue and, hence, appears radiolucent in a radiograph. It appears as a fine black radiolucent line next to the root surface. On its outer side is the lamina dura, the bone that lines the tooth socket and appears radiopaque (Figure 12-21).

B. Evidence of Disease

Widening or thickening.

1. *Angular Thickening or Triangulation.* The space is widened only near the coronal third, near the crest of the interdental bone.

2. *Complete Periodontal Ligament Thickened Along an Entire Side of a Root to the Apex, or Around the Root* (Figure 12-21). When viewed at different angulations (in the various radiographs of a complete survey), the ligament space may reveal varying thicknesses, thus showing that the disease involvement is not consistent around the entire root or that other structures are superimposed.

EARLY PERIODONTAL DISEASE

The real preventive service is to recognize *early signs* of periodontal involvement so that treatment can be initiated to arrest the disease and prevent more severe

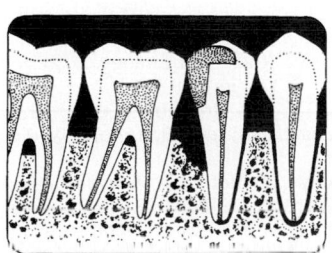

FIGURE 12-21 Periodontal Ligament Space. First and second molars have a normal periodontal ligament space, which appears as a fine black line about the roots. The first premolar shows thickening of the ligament space about the entire root, and the second premolar has thickening only about the mesial surface of the root.

involvement, which could lead to tooth loss. The recognition of severe bone loss, advanced furcation involvement, and marked thickening of the periodontal ligament space is not difficult after a basic understanding has been gained. The difficult part is to watch carefully for incipient, often isolated indications of early periodontal disease. These changes can be seen in all age groups, from young children to elderly patients.

I. EARLIEST SIGNS

The earliest signs of periodontal involvement are not evident in a radiograph. Only after the inflammation has extended from the soft tissue (gingivitis) to the supporting periodontal tissues and bone resorption has become sufficient does radiographic evidence appear.

II. INITIAL BONE DESTRUCTION

A. The usual interproximal pathway of inflammation from gingivitis to periodontitis is directly from the inflamed gingival connective tissue into the crest of the interdental bone (pages 225 to 226).

B. Initial bone destruction most frequently occurs at the crest of the interdental bone in the crestal lamina dura.

III. RADIOGRAPHIC EVIDENCE

A. Crestal lamina dura may appear slightly irregular, fuzzy, and radiolucent. At this stage it is best examined with a hand magnifying glass.

B. Angular thickening of the periodontal ligament space (triangulation) may also be apparent.

OTHER RADIOGRAPHIC FINDINGS

Any other radiographic findings that may be related directly or indirectly to periodontal involvement and its contributing factors should be noted in the record. Certain findings have a direct relation to dental hygiene care and instruction, particularly local factors that contribute to food impaction or plaque retention.

I. CALCULUS

Gross deposits, primarily those on proximal surfaces, may be seen in radiographs. Observing these may be helpful, but the probe and explorer are needed to define the exact location and extent.

The density and contrast of the radiograph influence whether or not calculus is seen. Because all deposits are not visible, the use of radiographs has very limited value for specific calculus detection.

II. OVERHANGING RESTORATIONS

Some proximal overhanging margins may be seen in radiographs. The use of an explorer is necessary to detect irregular margins and to examine all proximal margins that do not reveal irregularities in the radiographs. Superimposition can mask an overhanging margin. Types of irregularities of restorations are described on pages 624 to 626.

III. DENTAL CARIES

Clinical and radiographic identification of carious lesions is described on pages 248 and 249. Certain findings should be noted for their relationship to the periodontal tissues.

    A. Large carious lesions may leave open contact areas that permit food impaction and hence damage to the periodontal tissues.

    B. Carious lesions, either enamel or root caries, hold plaque and provide a rough surface for retention of food debris and bacterial plaque.

    C. Root caries and demineralization may interfere with techniques of root planing and require instruction in remineralization procedures.

IV. RELATIONSHIP TO POCKETS

Radiographs do not show pockets; soft tissue does not show in a radiograph. Because a pocket is measured from the gingival margin to the base of the pocket, both of which are soft tissue, pockets cannot be seen in a radiograph. Probing is necessary to identify pockets.

TECHNICAL HINTS

    I. Use topical anesthetic to help to alleviate discomfort while probing.

    II. Avoid the most common errors in probing:

        A. Not passing the probe to the full pocket depth.

        B. Not measuring around the entire tooth and therefore missing pockets. This error most commonly applies to proximal surface probing. The probe must be passed more than halfway across from the facial aspect to overlap with the probe used on the lingual aspect, which should also be passed more than halfway across.

    III. Check the markings on a new probe by measuring on a standard millimeter ruler.

    IV. When bleeding is readily elicited on probing or exploring and tooth surfaces are obscured so that examination is complicated, initiate toothbrushing and other appropriate disease control methods. Explain the problem to the patient, and outline a specific home care routine designed to reduce gingival inflammation. Postpone the complete examination for 1 week, after which the gingival condition should be improved.

    V. Replace mirror heads frequently. Scratched mirrors obscure vision and delay procedures.

    VI. Handle explorers and probes carefully. Because the tips are pliable and relatively fragile, precautions must be taken against breakage or bending (pages 59 and 60).

FACTORS TO TEACH THE PATIENT

    I. The need for a careful, thorough examination if treatment is to be complete and effective.

    II. Information about the instruments and how their use makes the examination complete. Examples are the complete radiographic survey, probing 360° around each tooth, and exploring each subgingival tooth surface.

    III. Why bleeding can occur when probing. Healthy tissue does not bleed.

    IV. Relation of probing depth measurements to normal sulci.

    V. Significance of mobility.

REFERENCES

1. **Listgarten**, M.A.: Periodontal Probing: What Does it Mean?, *J. Clin. Periodontol.*, 7, 165, June, 1980.
2. **Kopczyk**, R.A. and Saxe, S.R.: Clinical Signs of Gingival Inadequacy: The Tension Test, *ASDC J. Dent. Child.*, 41, 352, September–October, 1974.
3. **Miller**, S.C.: *Textbook of Periodontia*, 3rd ed. Philadelphia, The Blakiston Co., 1950, p. 125.

SUGGESTED READINGS

Armitage, G.C.: Clinical Evaluation of Periodontal Diseases, *Periodontology 2000*, 7, 39, 1995.

Armitage, G.C.: Periodontal Diseases: Diagnosis, *Annals of Periodontology*, 1, 54–96, November, 1996.

Daly, C., Mitchell, D., Grossburg, D., Highfield, J., and Stewart, D.: Bacteraemia Caused by Periodontal Probing, *Austr. Dent. J.*, 42, 77, April, 1997.

Eickholz, P.: Reproducibility and Validity of Furcation Measurements as Related to Class of Furcation Invasion, *J. Periodontol.*, 66, 984, November, 1995.

Giargia, M. and Linde, J.: Tooth Mobility and Periodontal Disease, *J. Clin. Periodontol.*, 24, 785, November, 1997.

McKechnie, L.B.: Root Morphology in Periodontal Therapy, *DentalHygienistNews*, 6, 3, Winter, 1993.

Nield-Gehrig, J.S. and Houseman, G.A.: *Fundamentals of Periodontal Instrumentation*, 3rd ed. Baltimore, Williams & Wilkins, 1996, pp. 215–245.

Papaioannou, W., Bollen, C.M.L., vanEldere, J., and Quirynen, M.: The Adherence of Periodontopathogens to Periodontal Probes: A Possible Factor in Intra-oral Transmission? *J. Periodontol.*, 67, 1164, November, 1996.

Strassler, H.E.: Perio Charting Systems, *RDH*, 12, 23, January, 1992.

Svärdstrom, G. and Wennström, J.L.: Prevalence of Furcation Involvements in Patients Referred for Periodontal Treatment, *J. Clin. Periodontol.*, 23, 1093, December, 1996.

Waerhaug, J.: The Furcation Problem. Etiology, Pathogenesis, Diagnosis, Therapy and Prognosis, *J. Clin. Periodontol.*, 7, 73, April, 1980.

Probing

Aguero, A., Garnick, J.J., Keagle, J., Steflik, D.E., and Thompson, W.O.: Histological Location of a Standardized Periodontal Probe in Man, *J. Periodontol., 66,* 184, March, 1995.

Clerehugh, V., Abdcia, R., and Hull, P.S.: The Effect of Subgingival Calculus on the Validity of Clinical Probing Measurements, *J. Dent., 24,* 329, September, 1996.

Lang, N.P., Nyman, S., Senn, C., and Joss, A.: Bleeding on Probing as It Relates to Probing Pressure and Gingival Health, *J. Clin. Periodontol., 18,* 257, April, 1991.

Mayfield, L., Bratthall, G., and Attström, R.: Periodontal Probe Precision Using 4 Different Periodontal Probes, *J. Clin. Periodontol., 23,* 76, February, 1996.

Pattison, A.M. and Pattison, G.L.: *Periodontal Instrumentation,* 2nd ed. Norwalk, CT, Appleton & Lange, 1992, pp. 17–24.

Reddy, M.S., Palcanis, K.G., and Geurs, N.C: A Comparison of Manual and Controlled-force Attachment-level Measurements, *J. Clin. Periodontol., 24,* 920, December, 1997.

Samuel, E.D., Griffiths, G.S., and Petrie, A.: In Vitro Accuracy and Reproducibility of Automated and Conventional Periodontal Probes, *J. Clin. Periodontol., 24,* 340, May, 1997.

Villata, L. and Baelum, V.: Reproducibility of Attachment Level Recordings Using an Electronic and a Conventional Probe, *J. Periodontol., 67,* 1292, December, 1996.

Zappa, U., Grosso, L., Simona, C., Graf, H., and Case, D.: Clinical Furcation Diagnoses and Interradicular Bone Defects, *J. Periodontol., 64,* 219, March, 1993.

Temperature Probe

Fedi, P.F. and Killoy, W.J.: Temperature Differences at Periodontal Sites in Health and Disease, *J. Periodontol., 63,* 24, January, 1992.

Haffajee, A.D., Socransky, S.S., and Goodson, J.M.: Subgingival Temperature (I). Relation to Baseline Clinical Parameters, *J. Clin. Periodontol., 19,* 401, July, 1992.

Haffajee, A.D., Socransky, S.S., and Goodson, J.M.: Subgingival Temperature (II). Relation to Future Periodontal Attachment Loss, *J. Clin. Periodontol., 19,* 409, July, 1992.

Haffajee, A.D., Socransky, S.S., Smith, C., Dibart, S., and Goodson, J.M.: Subgingival Temperature (III). Relation to Microbial Counts, *J. Clin. Periodontol., 19,* 417, July, 1992.

Kung, R.T.V., Ochs, B., and Goodson, J.M.: Temperature as a Periodontal Diagnostic, *J. Clin. Periodontol., 17,* 557, September, 1990.

Perdok, J.F., Lukacovic, M., Majeti, S., Arends, J., and Busscher, H.J.: Sulcus Temperature Distributions in the Absence and Presence of Oral Hygiene, *J. Periodont. Res., 27,* 97, March, 1992.

Radiographs

Åkesson, L., Håkansson, J., and Rohlin, M.: Comparison of Panoramic and Intraoral Radiography and Pocket Probing for the Measurement of the Marginal Bone Level, *J. Periodontol., 19,* 326, May, 1992.

Carranza, F.A. and Newman, M.G.: *Clinical Periodontology,* 8th ed. Philadelphia, W.B. Saunders Co., 1996, pp. 362–369.

Hausmann, E., Allen, K., and Clerehugh, V.: What Alveolar Crest Level on a Bite-wing Radiograph Represents Bone Loss?, *J. Periodontol., 62,* 570, September, 1991.

Hausmann, E., Allen, K., Norderyd, J., Ren, W., Shibly, O., and Machtei, E.: Studies on the Relationship Between Changes in Radiographic Bone Height and Probing Attachment, *J. Clin. Periodontol., 21,* 128, February, 1994.

Herzog, A. and Paarmann, C.: Enhancing Accurate Assessment of Periodontal Disease by Improving Radiographic Interpretation, *Can. Dent. Hyg. (Probe), 31,* 130, July/August, 1997.

13

Disease Development and Contributing Factors

Early in the process of case assessment in preparation for care planning, the presence and severity of periodontal infection must be determined. Is the patient's disease limited to the gingival tissue without loss of periodontal attachment? Does the patient have bone loss, pocket formation, or other signs of periodontitis?

Table 13-1 shows the clinical case types. The case type designation for a patient is determined by first noting the gingival markers by direct observation (see Table 11-1, pages 194 and 195), and then using the probe and studying the radiographs. The probe is utilized for many parts of the examination, one of which is assessment of the gingival and periodontal probing depths.

When the disease is limited to the gingiva, the possibility of reversal of the infection is considered first in the care planning objectives. Can the patient be guided to learn new habits of self-treatment through daily infection control supplemented by periodic professional scaling? On the other hand, if there is apical positioning of the periodontal attachment with alveolar bone loss and other indications of periodontitis, can conservative procedures of *nonsurgical periodontal therapy* provide sufficient professional treatment? Is more complex periodontal therapy required?

Individual differences and the particular clinical features of each patient must be recognized. The oral tissues need treatment that can bring them to a state of maximum health that can be maintained by the patient.

Except in cases of advanced periodontitis, the need for additional treatment after initial nonsurgical periodontal therapy is rarely possible to predict. A reassessment of the treated tissues must be built into the care plan. The patient must be given a clear understanding of the purpose of such a re-evaluation.

In this chapter, gingival and periodontal pockets and their development are described. Local and systemic risk factors for the initiation and progression of gingival and periodontal diseases are outlined. Key words are defined in Box 13-1.

TABLE 13-1 Periodontal Case Types

CASE TYPE I—GINGIVAL DISEASE

Inflammation of the gingiva characterized clinically by changes in color, gingival form, position, surface appearance, and presence of bleeding and/or exudate.

CASE TYPE II—EARLY PERIODONTITIS

Progression of the gingival inflammation into the deeper periodontal structures and alveolar bone crest, with slight bone loss. There is usually a slight loss of connective tissue attachment and alveolar bone.

CASE TYPE III—MODERATE PERIODONTITIS

A more advanced stage of the preceding condition, with increased destruction of the periodontal structures and noticeable loss of bone support, possibly accompanied by an increase in tooth mobility. There may be furcation involvement in multirooted teeth.

CASE TYPE IV—ADVANCED PERIODONTITIS

Further progression of periodontitis with major loss of alveolar bone support usually accompanied by increased tooth mobility. Furcation involvement in multirooted teeth.

CASE TYPE V—REFRACTORY PERIODONTITIS

Includes those patients with multiple disease sites that continue to demonstrate attachment loss after appropriate therapy. These sites presumably continue to be infected by periodontal pathogens no matter how thorough or frequent the treatment provided. Also includes those patients with recurrent disease at single or multiple sites.

From American Academy of Periodontology: *Current Procedural Terminology for Periodontics and Insurance Reporting Manual,* 7th ed. Chicago, 1995, p. 15.

DEVELOPMENT OF GINGIVAL AND PERIODONTAL INFECTIONS

The stages of development of gingivitis are divided into the *initial lesion,* the *early lesion,* and the *established lesion.*[1] With an accumulation of bacterial plaque on the cervical tooth surface adjacent to the gingival margin, an inflammatory reaction is set up, and the natural defense mechanisms respond. Plaque formation is described in Chapter 16 (page 267).

I. THE INITIAL LESION

A. Inflammatory Response to Bacterial Plaque
Occurs within 2 to 4 days.
1. Migration and infiltration of white blood cells into the junctional epithelium and gingival sulcus.
2. Increased flow of gingival sulcus fluid.
3. Early breakdown of collagen; fluid fills the spaces in the connective tissue.

B. Clinical Appearance
No clinical evidence of change appears in the earliest phases.

II. THE EARLY LESION

A. Increased Inflammatory Response
1. Bacterial plaque becomes older and thicker (7 to 14 days; time reflects individual differences).
2. Infiltration of fluid, lymphocytes, and neutrophils with a few plasma cells into the connective tissue.
3. Breakdown of collagen fiber support to the gingival margin.
4. Epithelium proliferates and epithelial extensions and rete ridges are formed.

B. Clinical Appearance
1. Early signs of gingivitis become apparent with slight gingival enlargement; will become an established lesion if undisturbed.
2. Early gingivitis is reversible when plaque is controlled and inflammation is reduced. Healthy tissue may be restored.
3. Susceptibility of individuals varies; time before lesion becomes established varies.

III. THE ESTABLISHED LESION

A. Progression From the Early Lesion
1. Fluid and leukocyte migration into tissues and sulcus increase; plasma cells are related to areas of chronic inflammation.
2. Formation of *pocket epithelium.*
   a. Proliferation of the junctional and sulcular epithelium continues in an attempt to wall out the inflammation.
   b. Pocket epithelium is more permeable;

BOX 13-1 KEY WORDS: Disease Development

Cicatrix (sĭk'ah-trĭks): the fibrous tissue left after the healing of a wound; cicatricial: adj.

Collagen (kŏl'ah-jen): white fibers of the connective tissue.

Collagenase (kōl-lăj'e-nās): enzyme that catalyzes the degradation (hydrolysis) of collagen.

Desquamation (dĕs"kwah-mā'shun): shedding of the outer epithelial layer of the stratified squamous epithelium of skin or mucosa.

Diastema (dī"h-stē'mah): a space or abnormal opening; as a dental term, it is a space between two adjacent teeth in the same dental arch.

Edema (ĕ-dē'mah): an accumulation of excessive fluid in cells, tissues, or a serous cavity.

Enzyme (ĕn'zīm): a protein secreted by body cells that acts as a catalyst to induce chemical changes in other substances, but remains unchanged itself.

Food impaction: forceful wedging of food into the periodontium by occlusal forces.

Gingivitis (jĭn"gĭ-vī'tĭs): inflammation of the gingival tissues.

Iatrogenic (ī-ăt"rō-gĕn'ĭk): resulting from treatment by a professional person.

Infiltration (ĭn"fĭl-trā'shun): the diffusion or accumulation in a tissue or cells of substances not normal to it or in amounts in excess of normal.

Lesion (lē'zhun): any pathologic or traumatic discontinuity of tissue or loss of function of a part; broad term including wounds, sores, ulcers, tumors, and any other tissue damage.

Nonsurgical periodontal therapy: includes bacterial plaque removal and plaque control (by patient); supra- and subgingival scaling; root planing; and the adjunctive use of chemotherapeutic agents for control of bacterial infection, desensitizing hypersensitive exposed root surfaces, and dental caries prevention as related to the health of the periodontium.

Periodontitis (pĕr"ē-ō-dŏn-tī'tĭs): inflammation in the periodontium affecting gingival tissues, periodontal ligament, cementum, and supporting bone.

Permeable (per'mē-ah-b'l): permitting passage of a fluid.

Refractory (rē-frăk'tō-rē): not readily responsive to treatment.

Toxin (tŏk'sĭn): a poison; protein produced by certain animals, higher plants, and pathogenic bacteria.

Bacterial toxin: poison produced by bacteria; includes exotoxins, endotoxins, and toxic enzymes.

Xerostomia (zē'rō-stō'mē-ah): dryness of the mouth from a lack of normal secretions.

---

areas of ulceration of the lining epithelium develop.
  c. Early pocket formation.
3. Collagen destruction continues; connective tissue fiber support lost.
4. Progression to early periodontal lesion may occur, or some established lesions may remain stable for extended periods of time.

B. Clinical Appearance
Clear evidence of inflammation is present with marginal redness, bleeding on probing, and spongy marginal gingiva. Later, chronic fibrosis develops.

IV. THE ADVANCED LESION
A. Extension of Inflammation
1. Bacteria from supragingival plaque enter the sulcus and provide the source for subgingival plaque bacteria.
2. Plaque microorganisms produce irritants.
3. Alveolar bone destruction
  a. Inflammation spreads through the loose connective tissue along (beside) the blood vessels to the alveolar bone.[2]
  b. Most commonly, the inflammation enters the bone through small vessel channels in the alveolar crest.
  c. Inflammation spreads through the bone marrow and out into the periodontal ligament.

B. Progressive Destruction of Connective Tissue
1. Connective tissue fibers below the junctional epithelium are destroyed; the epithelium migrates along the root surface.
2. Coronal portion of junctional epithelium becomes detached.
3. Exposed cementum where Sharpey's fibers were attached becomes altered by inflammatory products of bacteria and the sulcus fluid.
4. Diseased cementum contains a thin superficial layer of endotoxins from the bacterial breakdown.
5. Without treatment, the pocket becomes progressively deepened.

C. Characteristics of the Advanced Lesion

1. Pocket formation, mobility, bone loss; all signs of periodontitis.
2. Persistence of the chronic inflammatory process; plasma cells predominate (see plasma cell, Figure 59-1, page 867).
3. Junctional epithelium continues to migrate; lesion extends through connective tissue.
4. Periods of inactivity alternating with periods of activity can be expected.

V. CLASSIFICATION

Periodontal disease is not a single pathologic entity. It is a term used to describe a variety of inflammatory and degenerative diseases that affect the supporting structures of the teeth. A widely used system for classifying the types and severity of periodontal disease has been prepared by the American Academy of Periodontology as shown in Table 13-2.[3]

GINGIVAL AND PERIODONTAL POCKETS

A pocket is a diseased sulcus. The area of the sulcus and the pocket is the treatment area where calculus collects and instrumentation for nonsurgical periodontal therapy is applied (see Figure 11-1, page 188).

It is the presence or absence of infection that distinguishes a pocket from a sulcus and the level of attachment on the tooth that distinguishes a gingival pocket from a periodontal pocket. A pocket has an *inner wall, the tooth surface,* and an *outer wall, the sulcular epithelium or pocket epithelium* of the free gingiva. The two walls meet at the base of the pocket.

The base of the pocket is the coronal margin of the attached periodontal tissues. Histologically, the base of a healthy sulcus is the coronal border of the junctional epithelium, whereas the base of a pocket (diseased sulcus) may be at the coronal border of the connective tissue attachment.

Pockets are divided into *gingival* and *periodontal* types to clarify the degree of anatomic involvement. They are then further categorized by their position in relation to the alveolar bone, that is, whether their pocket base is suprabony or intrabony (Figure 13-1).

I. GINGIVAL POCKET

A. Definition: A pocket formed by gingival enlargement without apical migration of the junctional epithelium (Figure 13-1*B*).
B. The margin of the gingiva has moved toward the incisal or occlusal without the deeper periodontal structures becoming involved.
C. The tooth wall is enamel.
D. During eruption, the base of the sulcus is at various levels along the enamel. The base of the sulcus of a fully erupted tooth is near

the cementoenamel junction (see Figure 11-7, page 191).
E. All gingival pockets are suprabony; that is, the base of the pocket is coronal to the crest of the alveolar bone.

II. PERIODONTAL POCKET

A. Definition: A pocket formed as a result of disease or degeneration that caused the junctional epithelium to migrate apically along the cementum.
B. The periodontal deeper structures (attachment apparatus) are involved, that is, the cementum, periodontal ligament, and bone.
C. The tooth wall is cementum or partly cementum and partly enamel.
D. The base of the pocket is on cementum at the level of attached periodontal tissue.
E. Periodontal pockets may be suprabony or intrabony.
  1. *Suprabony:* Pocket in which the base of the pocket is coronal to the crest of the alveolar bone (Figure 13-1*C*).
  2. *Intrabony:* Pocket in which the base of the pocket is below or apical to the crest of the alveolar bone (Figure 13-1*D*). "Intra" means located within the bone. The term "infrabony" is used in some texts. "Infra" means under or beneath.

TOOTH SURFACE POCKET WALL

I. TOOTH STRUCTURE INVOLVED

A sulcus or a pocket has a gingival side, which is the sulcular epithelium, and a tooth side. In gingival pockets, the tooth surface wall is enamel, whereas in periodontal pockets, the tooth surface wall is either cementum or a combination of cementum and enamel.

The positions of the periodontal attachment and the gingival margin determine whether the tooth surface wall is cementum or enamel. Pockets may be the same depth when measured with a probe, but because of the location of the attachment on the tooth surface, the tooth surface pocket wall varies (see Figure 12-2, page 206).

II. CONTENTS OF A POCKET

A. Pocket Size

A pocket is narrow, and the pocket epithelial lining is adjacent to and follows the contour of the tooth. When calculus deposits are present, the pocket wall follows the contour of the calculus. The firmness of the free gingiva is influential in confining and shaping the subgingival calculus deposit.

Access of the opening of the pocket to the oral cavity provides an opportunity for bacterial plaque to collect. The deeper the pocket, the

---

TABLE 13-2 Classification of Gingival and Periodontal Diseases

GINGIVAL DISEASES

I. **Plaque-associated gingivitis**
   A. Chronic gingivitis.
   B. Acute necrotizing ulcerative gingivitis (NUG).
   C. Gingivitis associated with systemic conditions or medications. (These forms of gingivitis are plaque associated, but the clinical presentation and therapeutic approaches may be modified by the systemic factors.)
      1. Hormone-influenced gingivitis (for example, pregnancy gingivitis).
      2. Drug-induced gingivitis (for example, phenytoin- or cyclosporine-induced gingivitis).
      3. Linear gingival erythema in **HIV+** individuals (formerly HIV-G).

II. **Gingival manifestations of systemic diseases and mucocutaneous lesions**
   A. Bacterial, viral, or fungal (for example, acute herpetic gingivostomatitis).
   B. Blood dyscrasias (for example, acute monocytic leukemia).
   C. Mucocutaneous diseases (for example, lichen planus, cicatricial pemphigold).

PERIODONTAL DISEASES

I. **Periodontitis**
   A. Adult periodontitis.
   B. Early-onset periodontitis—age of onset is usually prior to 35 years; rapid rate of progression of tissue destruction; manifestation of defects in host defense; composition of the associated flora different from that of adult periodontitis.
      1. Prepubertal—may be generalized or localized; onset between eruption of the primary dentition and puberty; may affect the primary and the mixed dentition; characterized by severe gingival inflammation, rapid bone loss, tooth mobility, and tooth loss.
      2. Juvenile—may be generalized or localized; onset during the circumpubertal period; familial distribution; relative paucity of microbial plaque; less acute signs of inflammation than would be expected based upon the severity of destruction; presence of abnormalities in leukocyte chemotaxis and bactericidal activity.
      3. Rapidly progressive—most of the teeth are affected; the extent of clinical signs of inflammation may be less than expected; the age of onset is usually in the early 20s through the mid-30s.
   C. Periodontitis associated with systemic disease (for example, diabetes, HIV infection)—several systemic diseases appear to predispose the affected individuals to periodontitis, which may be of the early-onset type.
   D. Necrotizing ulcerative periodontitis—severe and rapidly progressive disease that has a distinctive erythema of the free gingiva, attached gingiva, and alveolar mucosa; extensive soft tissue necrosis; severe loss of periodontal attachment; deep pocket formation is usually not evident.
   E. Refractory periodontitis—destructive periodontal disease(s) in patients who demonstrate attachment loss at one or more sites, despite well-executed therapeutic treatment and patient efforts to stop the progression of disease; characterized by additional attachment loss after repeated attempts to control the infection with conventional periodontal therapy. This diagnosis is not appropriate in patients with recurrent progressive periodontitis after many years of supportive therapy.
   F. Peri-implantitis—in a manner similar to the pathogenesis of periodontal disease around natural teeth, a periodontitis-like process, peri-implantitis can affect dental implants.

II. **Mucogingival conditions**—deviation from the normal anatomic relationship between the gingival margin and the mucogingival junction, where the anatomy and position of the periodontal tissues do not allow the control of inflammation, or which are associated with progressive recession and loss of attachment. Common mucogingival conditions are recession, absence or reduction of keratinized tissue, and probing depths extending beyond the mucogingival junction.

III. **Occlusal trauma**—an injury to the attachment apparatus as a result of excessive occlusal forces.
   A. Primary occlusal trauma—trauma resulting from excessive occlusal forces applied to a tooth or teeth with normal supporting structures.
   B. Secondary occlusal trauma—trauma that occurs when normal occlusal forces are applied to the attachment apparatus of a tooth or teeth with inadequate support.

Based on American Academy of Periodontology: *Current Procedural Terminology for Periodontics and Insurance Reporting Manual,* 7th ed. Chicago, American Academy of Periodontology, 1995, pp. 1–2.

---

less it can be cleaned by toothbrushing or other plaque control devices.

B. Substances Found
Subgingival plaque is described in Chapter 16. Table 16-2 (page 268) lists content and features of subgingival plaque and the periodontal pocket.

The following may be inside a pocket in contact with the tooth surface on one side and with the surface of the pocket epithelium on the other side.
1. Microorganisms and their products: enzymes, endotoxins, and other metabolic products.
2. Gingival sulcus fluid.

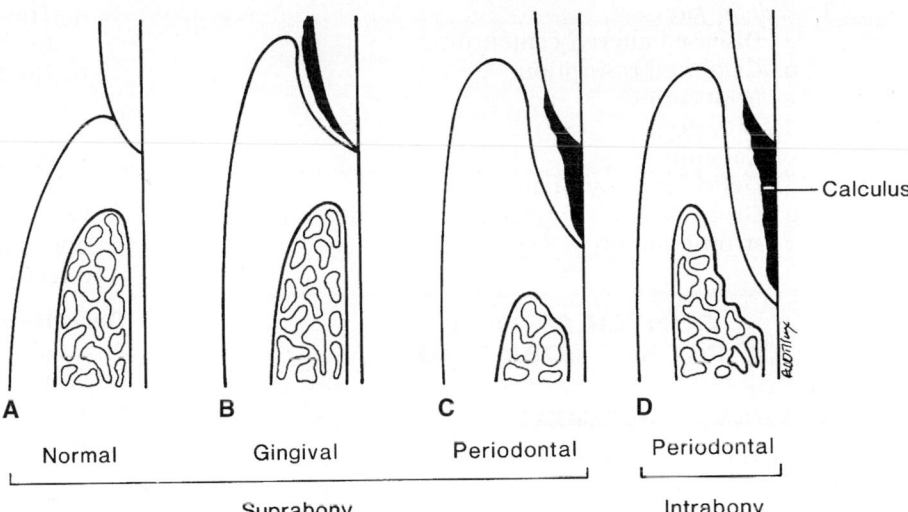

FIGURE 13-1 Types of Pockets. (A) Normal relationship of the gingival tissue and the cementoenamel junction in a fully erupted tooth. **(B)** Gingival pocket showing attachment at the cementoenamel junction and the pocket formed by enlarged gingival tissue. There is no bone loss. **(C)** Periodontal pocket showing attachment on cementum with root surface exposed. Gingival tissue has enlarged. **(D)** Periodontal intrabony pocket with the bottom of the pocket within the bone. See the text for further description of each type of pocket.

3. Desquamated epithelial cells.
4. Leukocytes, the numbers of which increase with increased inflammation in the tissues.
5. Purulent exudate made up of living and broken down leukocytes, living and dead microorganisms, and serum.

III. NATURE OF THE TOOTH SURFACE

Knowledge of the characteristics and quality of the tooth surface pocket wall is of prime importance in instrumentation. During the examination of the tooth surface with probe and explorer, the various irregularities that can occur must be differentiated. The manner in which the irregularities came into existence is important for interpretation and understanding.

A. Pocket Development Factors

1. The pocket deepens as a result of continuing action of the irritants and destructive agents from bacterial plaque.
2. The periodontal ligament fibers become detached, and the junctional epithelium migrates apically.
3. The cementum becomes exposed to the open pocket and the oral fluids.
4. Physical, structural, and chemical changes alter the cementum.
5. Surface changes occur as a result of the exchange of minerals with oral fluids and exposure to plaque bacteria and their products. On different surfaces of the same teeth or different teeth in the same mouth, any of the following can occur:[4]
   a. Hypermineralization of the surface cementum increases with time.
   b. Demineralization.
   c. Calculus formation.
   d. Bacterial plaque and debris collection.

B. Tooth Surface Irregularities

Surface irregularities are detected supragingi-

vally by drying the surface with air and observing under adequate direct or indirect light; an explorer is used as needed.

Subgingivally, examination is dependent, for the most part, on tactile and auditory sensitivity transmitted by a probe and an explorer. Causes of surface roughness include the following:

1. *Enamel Surface*
   a. Structural defects: cracks and grooves.
   b. Dental caries, demineralization.
   c. Calculus deposits and heavy stain deposits.
   d. Erosion, abrasion.
   e. Pits and irregularities from hypoplasia.
2. *Cementoenamel Junction.* Cementum overlaps enamel in 60% to 65% of teeth, cementum and enamel meet directly in 30%, and a small zone of dentin may be between the cementum and enamel in 5% to 10%.[5] The relationships of enamel and cementum at the cementoenamel junction are shown in Figure 13-2.

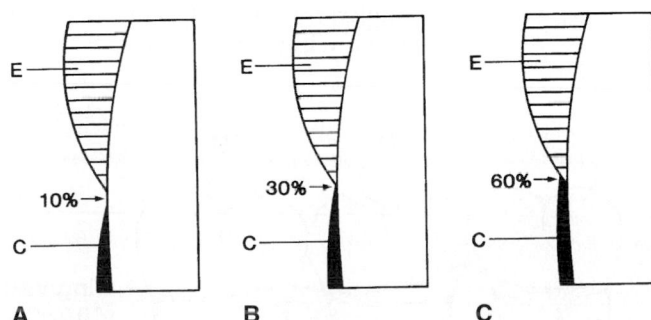

FIGURE 13-2 Cementoenamel Junction. The possible relationships of the enamel and the cementum of the cementoenamel junction. **(A)** The cementum and the enamel do not meet and there is a small zone of dentin exposed in 10% of teeth. **(B)** The cementum meets the enamel in approximately 30% of teeth. **(C)** The cementum overlaps the enamel in about 60% of teeth.

3. *Root Surface*
   a. Diseased altered cementum.
   b. Cemental resorption.
   c. Root caries.
   d. Abrasion.
   e. Calculus.
   f. Deficient or overhanging filling.
   g. Grooves from previous incomplete instrumentation.

COMPLICATIONS OF POCKET FORMATION

I. FURCATION INVOLVEMENT

Furcation involvement means that the clinical attachment level and bone loss have extended into the furcation area, or furca, the area between the roots of a multirooted tooth.

A. Types of Furcations

Furcation involvement is usually classified by the amount of a furcation that has been exposed by periodontal bone destruction.

The four general classes, as shown in Figure 13-3, are as follows:
1. *Class I:* Early, beginning involvement. A probe can enter the furcation area, and the anatomy of the roots on either side can be felt by moving the probe from side to side (see Figure 33-1C, page 549).
2. *Class II:* Moderate involvement. Bone has been destroyed to an extent that permits a probe to enter the furcation area but not to pass through between the roots.
3. *Class III:* Severe involvement. A probe can be passed between the roots through the entire furcation.
4. *Class IV:* Same as Class III, with exposure resulting from gingival recession, especially after periodontal therapy.

B. Clinical Observations
1. When the gingiva over the furcation has not receded, the following may be seen:

   a. The furcation is covered by the gingival tissue pocket wall.
   b. No differences in color, size, or other tissue changes may exist to differentiate the area from adjacent gingiva, but when color changes do exist, they provide clues to supplement probe examination.
2. When the gingiva over a molar buccal furcation is receded, the root division may be seen directly (Figure 13-3, Class IV).

C. Detection
A suggested procedure for probing furcations is described on pages 210 to 211. Radiographic examination of furcation areas may be studied on page 220.

II. MUCOGINGIVAL INVOLVEMENT

A pocket that extends to or beyond the mucogingival junction and into the alveolar mucosa is described as *mucogingival involvement.* There is no attached gingiva in the area, and a probe can be passed through the pocket and beyond the mucogingival junction into the alveolar mucosa (see Figure 12-9, page 212).

A. Significance of Attached Gingiva
1. *Functions of Attached Gingiva*
   a. Give support to the marginal gingiva.
   b. Withstand the frictional stresses of mastication and toothbrushing.
   c. Provide attachment or a solid base for the movable alveolar mucosa for the action of the cheeks, lips, and tongue.
2. *Barrier to Passage of Inflammation.* Without attachment, inflammation from a pocket area can extend to the alveolar mucosa. The junctional epithelium (epithelial attachment) acts as a barrier to keep infection outside the body.

   With destruction of the connective tissue and periodontal ligament fibers under the junctional epithelium, the epithelium migrates along the root. A pocket is created.

   In mucogingival involvement, the bottom of the pocket extends into the alveolar mu-

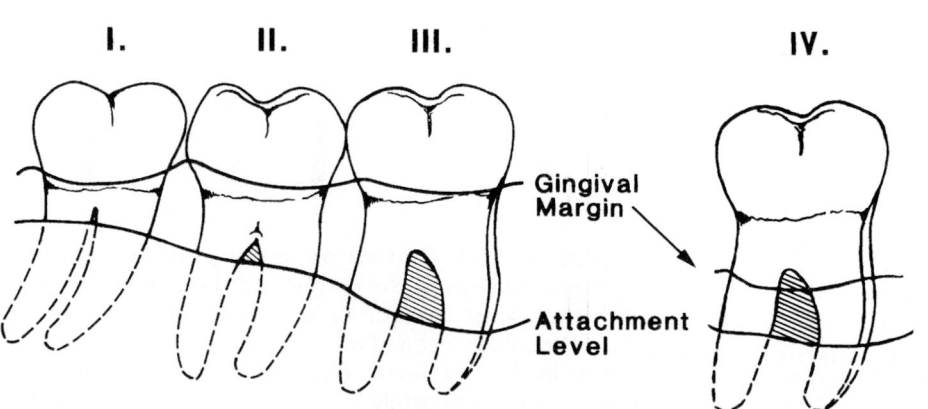

I.　　**II.**　　**III.**　　　　　**IV.**

Gingival Margin

Attachment Level

▢ **FIGURE 13-3 Classification of Furcations. (I)** Early, beginning involvement. **(II)** Moderate involvement, in which the furcation can be probed but not through and through. **(III)** Severe involvement, when the bone between the roots is destroyed and a probe can be passed through. **(IV)** Same as III, with clinical exposure resulting from gingival recession.

cosa. There, the unconfined inflammation can spread more rapidly in the loose connective tissue.

B. Clinical Observations

Color changes, tension test, and probe measurements are used during assessment of the mucogingival areas. These are described on page 211.

1. *Width of Attached Gingiva.* A narrow zone of gingiva from gingival margin to mucogingival junction, caused by recession or occurring naturally without recession, is more susceptible to developing mucogingival involvement because there is less attached gingiva at the start.

2. *Base of Pocket at Mucogingival Junction.* When the probe measures only 1 to 2 mm and there is no bleeding on probing, but the tip of the probe is at the mucogingival junction, the area should be charted and re-evaluated at each successive maintenance review. A patient with such an area needs specific instruction in plaque control procedures for preventive maintenance.

   When an area of minimal attached gingiva (1 to 2 mm) is placed under stress by restorative, prosthetic, or orthodontic treatment procedures, an assessment should be made of the need for periodontal treatment to increase the zone of attached gingiva.

LOCAL CONTRIBUTING FACTORS IN DISEASE DEVELOPMENT

Microbial plaque is the primary etiologic factor in the development of gingival and periodontal diseases. A variety of other factors predispose some patients to the retention of bacterial deposits and hence to the development of disease in the soft tissues.

Factors described in this section relate to microbial plaque retention. Although loose debris can be cleared away by self-cleansing, bacterial plaque adheres firmly to the tooth surface and cannot be removed completely by self-cleansing. Retentive areas relate to rough surfaces of teeth and restorations, tooth contour and position, and gingival size, shape, and position.

Iatrogenic causes, that is, factors created by professionals during patient treatment or neglect of treatment, are significant. Other factors such as mastication, saliva, the tongue, cheeks, lips, oral habits, and personal plaque control procedures contribute.

The patient's study casts can be especially useful for observing the physical factors. Irregularities, contour, position, malocclusion, and contact areas of the teeth, as well as features of the gingiva, may be partially or wholly noted. Problem areas can be explained to the patient by demonstration on the study casts. Changes in the patient's habits and daily personal care routine must be encouraged.

I. FACTORS INVOLVED

Complicating and risk factors to disease development may be etiologic, predisposing, or contributing. They are delineated as follows:

1. *Etiologic Factor:* A factor that is the actual cause of a disease or condition.
2. *Predisposing Factor:* A factor that renders a person susceptible to a disease or condition.
3. *Contributing Factor:* A factor that lends assistance to, supplements, or adds to a condition or disease.
4. *Risk Factor:* An exposure that increases the probability that disease will occur.

Etiologic, predisposing, and contributing factors may be local or systemic, defined as follows:

1. *Local Factor:* A factor in the immediate environment of the oral cavity or specifically in the environment of the teeth or periodontium.
2. *Systemic Factor:* A factor that results from or is influenced by a general physical or mental disease or condition.

II. DENTAL FACTORS

A. Tooth Surface Irregularities

Pellicle and plaque microorganisms attach to defective or rough surfaces, including the following:

1. Pits, grooves, cracks.
2. Calculus.
3. Exposed altered cementum with irregularities (pages 229 to 230).
4. Dental caries and demineralization.
5. Iatrogenic
   a. Rough or grooved surfaces left after scaling.
   b. Inadequately contoured and polished dental restorations (Figure 13-4B).

B. Tooth Contour

Altered shape may interfere with self-cleansing mechanisms and make personal care procedures difficult.

1. Congenital abnormalities
   a. Extra or missing cusps.
   b. Bell-shaped crown with prominent facial and lingual contours tends to provide deeper retentive area in cervical third.
2. Teeth with flattened proximal surfaces have faulty contact with adjacent teeth, thus permitting debris to wedge between.
3. Occlusal and incisal surfaces altered by attrition interrupt normal excursion of food during chewing. Marginal ridges have worn down.
4. Areas of erosion and abrasion (see Figure 14-8, page 245).

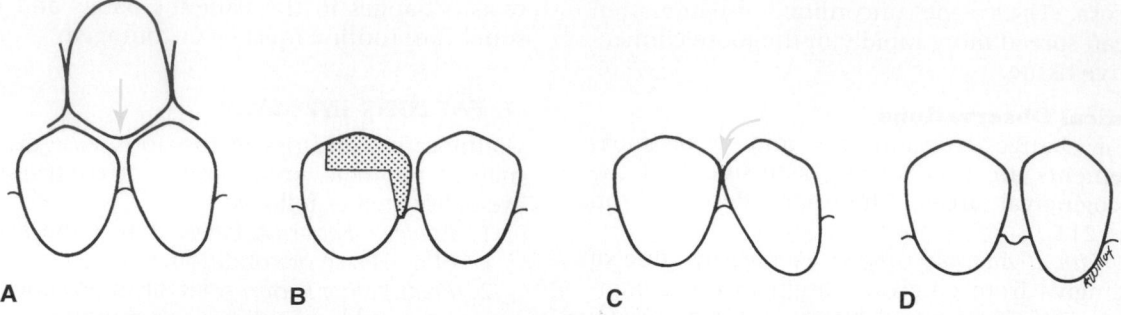

◼ **FIGURE 13-4 Effect of Tooth Position. (A)** Food impaction area, shown by plunger cusp (with arrow) directing pressure between lower teeth with open contact area. **(B)** Inadequate restoration without proximal contact and with overhang. **(C)** Tipped tooth leaving irregular marginal ridge relation. **(D)** Natural open contact (diastema) with saddle-shaped gingival margin.

5. Carious lesions.
6. Heavy calculus deposits; plaque retained on rough surface.
7. Overcontoured and undercontoured restorations (see Figure 40-1, page 624).

C. Tooth Position
1. Malocclusion: Irregular alignment of a single tooth or groups of teeth leaves areas conducive to collection of microorganisms for plaque formation.
   a. Crowded or overlapped (Figure 16-5, page 272).
   b. Rotated.
   c. Deep anterior overbite
      i. Mandibular teeth force food particles against maxillary lingual surface (see Figure 15-10, page 257).
      ii. Lingual inclination of mandibular teeth allows maxillary teeth to force food particles against mandibular facial gingiva.
2. Tooth adjacent to edentulous area may be inclined or migrated; contact missing.
3. Opposing tooth missing; tooth may extrude beyond the line of occlusion.
4. Related to eruption
   a. Incomplete eruption: below line of occlusion.
   b. Partially erupted impacted third molar.
5. Lack of function or use of teeth eliminates or decreases effectiveness of natural cleansing.
   a. Lack of opposing teeth.
   b. Open bite.
   c. Marked maxillary anterior protrusion.
   d. Crossbite with limited lateral excursion.
   e. Unilateral chewing.
6. Food impaction
   a. Created by the combined effect of tooth contour, missing proximal contact, proximal carious lesions, irregular marginal ridge relationship.

   b. Inclination related to loss of adjacent tooth, and a plunger cusp from the opposite arch (Figure 13-4A).
7. Defective contact area
   a. Restoration margin is faulty, and the contact area is missing, improperly located, or unnaturally wide (Figure 13-4B).
   b. Inclined tooth with irregular marginal ridge relation (Figure 13-4C).

D. Dental Prostheses
1. Orthodontic appliances provide retentive areas.
2. Fixed partial denture with deficient margin of an abutment tooth or an unusually shaped pontic (see Figures 26-1 and 26-2, pages 413 and 414).
3. Removable partial denture with inadequately adapted clasps.

III. GINGIVA

A. Position
Deviations from normal provide retentive areas.
1. Receded: depressed area is left at cemento-enamel junction.
2. Enlarged: extended to or over the height of contour.
3. Reduced height of interdental papilla leaves open interdental area.
4. Tissue flap over occlusal surface of erupting tooth.
5. Periodontal pocket
   a. Free gingiva cannot adhere to tooth.
   b. Shape of pocket conducive to bacterial plaque collection.
   c. Depth of pocket not available to toothbrush and cleaning aids.
   d. Calculus provides rough retentive surface.

B. Size and Contour
1. Deviation of shape of enlarged gingiva: rolled, bulbous, cratered.

2. Combination with presence of irregular restorations or dental prosthesis can result in marked plaque retention.

C. Effect of Mouth Breathing

Dehydration of oral tissues in anterior region leads to changes in size, shape, surface texture, and consistency.

IV. OTHER FACTORS

A variety of factors may predispose or contribute to the progression of periodontal infections. Some of the items listed here may have an indirect effect, whereas others have a direct effect on the oral tissues.

A. Personal Oral Care

1. *Neglect:* Neglect can lead to generalized bacterial plaque accumulation and disease promotion.
2. *Faulty Plaque Control Techniques:* Incorrect use of brush, abrasive dentifrice, and the effects of other harmful, detrimental procedures are described on pages 366 to 367.
3. *Awareness of Oral Cleanliness:* Cleansing habits, including both self-cleansing mechanisms and mechanical plaque removal, depend in part on an individual's perception and feeling of debris through taste and tongue activity.

B. Diet and Eating Habits

1. Soft foods tend to adhere more than fibrous, firm foods.
2. Cariogenic food selection.
3. Masticatory deficiencies limit diet selection. Missing teeth, ill-fitting partial dentures, and various occlusal deficiencies alter diet selection and eating habits.

SELF-CLEANSING MECHANISMS

The teeth, by their anatomy, alignment, and occlusion, function with the gingiva, tongue, cheeks, and saliva in a relationship called the self-cleansing mechanism of the oral cavity. A summary of the natural self-cleansing mechanisms during and following mastication is included here.

The following steps are described for food particles, but the same processes apply to any substances that enter the mouth and influence oral cleanliness and the formation of deposits on the teeth.

I. FOOD ENTERS THE MOUTH

Food is carried by the tongue, assisted by the lips and cheeks, to the occlusal surfaces for grinding.
  A. Salivary flow increases as a result of sensory reflex stimulation.
  B. Saliva begins lubrication of food and oral tissues.

II. THE TEETH ARE BROUGHT TOGETHER FOR CHEWING

The food moves over the occlusal surfaces.
  A. Marginal ridges tend to force particles toward occlusal surfaces, away from the proximal region.
  B. Contact areas prevent interdental entrance.

III. FOOD IS FORCED OUT BY PRESSURE OF BITE

Food passes over the smooth facial and lingual surfaces.
  A. Embrasures provide spillways for the escape of particles.
  B. Cervical enamel ridges deflect particles away from the free gingiva onto the attached gingiva.
  C. Gingival crest prevents retention of particles by its position at a point below the height of contour of the cervical enamel ridge, by its knife-edge shape, and by its close adherence to the tooth surface.
  D. Interdental papilla fills the interproximal area and prevents particles from entering.

IV. FOOD PARTICLES ARE BROUGHT BACK BY THE TONGUE TO THE OCCLUSAL SURFACES FOR ADDITIONAL CHEWING

The process is repeated until the food is ready for swallowing.
  A. Salivary flow continues to be stimulated by repeated masticatory movements.
  B. Saliva moistens food and oral mucosa and thus reduces the adhering capacity of the food.

V. FOOD PARTICLES REMAINING ON THE TEETH ARE REMOVED

  A. Tip of tongue explores and attempts to dislodge remaining particles.
  B. Lips and cheeks in conjunction with tongue aid in natural rinsing process by forcing saliva over and between the teeth.
  C. Saliva continues to flow in increased amounts during rinsing and swallowing of particles, then gradually returns to its normal flow.

RISK FACTORS FOR PERIODONTAL DISEASES

Identification of risk factors for periodontal disease can provide significant insight for the assessment and care planning for an individual patient. The various periodontal pathogenic microorganisms do not affect all people with the same degree of severity. It is clear that host factors play a significant role.

Risk factors are included as part of care planning in Chapter 21, pages 322 to 323. Certain risk factors are related to lifestyle, habits, treatable systemic diseases, and other controllable factors. On the other hand, factors derived from genetic predisposition, congenital immunodeficiencies, or other systemic conditions require a greater effort for the control of periodontal problems.

Many periodontal risk factors have been identified, and a few examples will be described in this section. A list of outstanding articles from the literature is provided in the Suggested Readings at the close of this chapter.

I. EFFECT OF CERTAIN DRUGS

Medications for specific systemic conditions can lead to gingival enlargement.[6,7] The enlarged tissue encourages bacterial plaque retention, thus increasing the potential for periodontal infections.

A. *Phenytoin-Induced Gingival Enlargement.* Phenytoin is a drug used to control seizures (pages 804 to 806).

B. *Cyclosporine-Induced Gingival Enlargement.* Cyclosporine is an immunosuppressant drug used for patients with organ transplants to prevent rejection.

C. *Nifedipine-Induced Gingival Enlargement.* Nifedipine is used in the treatment of angina and ventricular arrhythmias.

II. TOBACCO

A. Smokers, especially cigarette users, have increased bone loss. An association between periodontal disease and tobacco use has been shown (pages 429 to 430).[8,9]

B. Users of smokeless tobacco products experience oral effects, including predisposition to oral cancer. Periodontal lesions with severe recession and root exposure occur where the quid is held.[10]

III. DIABETES[11]

A. Increased susceptibility to periodontal infections (page 888).

B. Periodontal treatment improves the metabolic control of diabetes.

C. Patient with well-controlled diabetes and healthy periodontal tissues is not at greater risk for susceptibility to infections, including periodontal.

IV. OTHER SYSTEMIC CONDITIONS

A. Osteoporosis[12]

1. Many risk factors for osteoporosis are also risk factors for periodontitis including cigarette smoking, nutritional deficiencies, corticosteroid use, and immune dysfunction.

2. Greater periodontal attachment loss in patients with osteoporosis.

3. Loss of alveolar bone results from osteopenia.

B. Psychosocial Factors

1. Higher levels of social strain are found in patients with periodontal infections.[13]

2. Stress is considered a factor in the etiology of necrotizing ulcerative gingivitis (pages 578 to 579).

FACTORS TO TEACH THE PATIENT

I. What a pocket is and how it forms.

II. How a pocket is measured with a probe and that, until the sulci and pockets are probed, it is not possible to tell whether disease is present and how far it has progressed. Probing depth must be checked regularly all around every tooth to be sure nothing is developing insidiously.

III. Factors that contribute to disease development and progression.

IV. What a risk factor is, and the importance of planning personal and professional care to include risk factor problems.

REFERENCES

1. **Page,** R.C. and Schroeder, H.E.: Structure and Pathogenesis, in Schluger, S., Yuodelis, R., Page, R.C., and Johnson, R.H.: *Periodontal Diseases,* 2nd ed. Philadelphia, Lea & Febiger, 1990, pp. 185–207.

2. **Weinmann,** J.P.: Progress of Gingival Inflammation Into the Supporting Structures of the Teeth, *J. Periodontol., 12,* 71, July, 1941.

3. **American Academy of Periodontology:** *Current Procedural Terminology for Periodontics and Insurance Reporting Manual,* 7th ed. Chicago, American Academy of Periodontology, 1995, pp. 1–2, 15.

4. **Selvig,** K.A.: Biological Changes at the Tooth-saliva Interface in Periodontal Disease, *J. Dent. Res., 48,* 846, September–October, 1969.

5. **Bhaskar,** S.N., ed.: *Orban's Oral Histology and Embryology,* 11th ed. St. Louis, Mosby, 1991, p. 192.

6. **Fattore,** L., Stablein, M., Bredfeldt, G., Semla, T., Moran, M., and Doherty-Greenberg, J.M.: Gingival Hyperplasia: A Side Effect of Nifedipine and Diltiazem, *Spec. Care Dentist., 11,* 107, May/June, 1991.

7. **Payne,** J.B.: The Facts About Gingival Hyperplasia, *Dent. Teamwork, 5,* 22, September–October, 1992

8. **Akef,** J., Weine, F.S., and Weissman, D.P.: The Role of Smoking in the Progression of Periodontal Disease: A Literature Review, *Compend. Cont. Educ. Dent., 13,* 526, June, 1992.

9. **Haber,** J., Wattles, J., Crowley, M., Mandell, R., Joshipura, K., and Kent, R.L.: Evidence for Cigarette Smoking as a Major Risk Factor for Periodontitis, *J. Periodontol., 64,* 16, January, 1993.

10. **Johnson,** R. and Herzog, A.: Oral Effects of Smokeless Tobacco Use, *Dent. Hyg., 61,* 354, August, 1987.

11. **American Academy of Periodontology,** Committee on Research, Science and Therapy: Position Paper: Diabetes and Periodontal Diseases, *J. Periodontol., 70,* 935, August, 1999.

12. **Wactawski-Wende,** J., Grossi, S.G., Trevisan, M., Genco, R.J., Tezal, M., Dunford, R.G., Ho, A.W., Hausman, E., Hreshchyshyn, M.M.: The Role of Osteopenia in Oral Bone Loss and Periodontal Disease, *J. Periodontol., 67,* 1076, October, Supplement, 1996.

13. **Moss,** M.E., Beck, J.D., Kaplan, B.H., Offenbacher, S., Weintraub, J.A., Koch, G.G., Genco, R.J., Machtei, E.E., and Tedesco, L.A.: Exploratory Case-control Analysis of Psychoso-

cial Factors and Adult Periodontitis, *J. Periodontol.,* 67, 1060, October, Supplement, 1996.

SUGGESTED READING

Atack, N.E., Sandy, J.R., and Addy, M.: Periodontal and Microbial Changes Associated with the Placement of Orthodontic Appliances. A Review, *J. Periodontol.,* 67, 78, February, 1996.

Gagnon, F., Knoernschild, K.L., Payant, L., Tompkins, G.R., Litaker, M.S., and Schuster, G.S.: Endotoxin Affinity for Provisional Restorative Resins, *J. Prosthodont.,* 3, 228, December, 1994.

Kornman, K.S. and Löe, H.: The Role of Local Factors in the Etiology of Periodontal Diseases, *Periodontology 2000,* 2, 83, 1993.

Leknes, K.N., Lie, T., and Selvig, K.A.: Root Grooves: A Risk Factor in Periodontal Attachment Loss, *J. Periodontol.,* 65, 859, September, 1994.

Tatakis, D.N.: The Inflammatory Response in Periodontitis, *DentalHygienistNews,* 8, 5, Special Issue, Spring, 1995.

Risk Factors

Alpagot, T., Wolff, L.F., Smith, Q.T., and Tran, S.D.: Risk Indicators for Periodontal Disease in a Racially Diverse Urban Population, *J. Clin. Periodontol.,* 23, 982, November, 1996.

Clarke, N.G. and Hirsch, R.S.: Personal Risk Factors for Generalized Periodontitis, *J. Clin. Periodontol.,* 22, 136, February, 1995.

Daniel, M.A. and Van Dyke, T.E.: Alterations in Phagocyte Function and Periodontal Infection, *J. Periodontol.,* 67, 1070, October, Supplement, 1996.

Goulding, M.: Risk Assessment for Periodontal Disease, *Can. Dent. Hyg. Assoc./Probe,* 30, 100, May/June, 1996.

Michalowicz, B.S.: Genetic and Heritable Risk Factors in Periodontal Disease, *J. Periodontol.,* 65, 479, Supplement, May, 1994.

Offenbacher, S., Katz, V., Fertik, G., Collins, J., Boyd, D., Maynor, G., McKaig, R., and Beck, J.: Periodontal Infection as a Possible Risk Factor for Preterm Low Birth Weight, *J. Periodontol.,* 67, 1103, October, Supplement, 1996.

Page, R.C. and Beck, J.D.: Risk Assessment for Periodontal Diseases, *Internat. Dent. J.,* 47, 61, April, 1997.

Schutte, D.W. and Donley, T.G.: Determining Periodontal Risk Factors in Patients Presenting for Dental Care, *J. Dent. Hyg.,* 70, 230, November–December, 1996.

Drug-Induced Gingival Enlargement

Bredfeldt, G.W.: Phenytoin-induced Hyperplasia Found in Edentulous Patients, *J. Am. Dent. Assoc.,* 123, 61, June, 1992.

Daley, T.D., Wysocki, G.P., and Mamandras, A.H.: Orthodontic Therapy in the Patient Treated with Cyclosporine, *Am. J. Orthod. Dentofacial Orthop.,* 100, 537, December, 1991.

Hefti, A.F., Eshenaur, A.E., Hassell, T.M., and Stone, C.: Gingival Overgrowth in Cyclosporine A Treated Multiple Sclerosis Patients, *J. Periodontol.,* 65, 744, August, 1994.

Karpinia, K.A., Matt, M., Fennel, R.S., and Hefti, A.F.: Factors Affecting Cyclosporine-induced Gingival Overgrowth in Pediatric Renal Transplant Recipients, *Pediatr. Dent.,* 18, 450, November/December, 1996.

Montebugnoli, L., Bernardi, F., and Magelli, C.: Cyclosporine-A-induced Gingival Overgrowth in Heart Transplant Patients. A Cross-sectional Study, *J. Clin. Periodontol.,* 23, 868, September, 1996.

Seymour, R.A., Thomason, J.M., and Ellis, J.S.: The Pathogenesis of Drug-induced Gingival Overgrowth, *J. Clin. Periodontol.,* 23, 165, March, 1996.

Somacarrera, M.L., Lucas, M., and Acero, J.: Reversion of Gingival Hyperplasia in a Heart Transplant Patient Upon Interruption of Cyclosporine Therapy, *Spec. Care Dentist.,* 16, 18, January/February, 1996.

Thomason, J.M., Seymour, R.A., and Rice, N.: The Prevalence and Severity of Cyclosporin and Nifedipine-induced Gingival Overgrowth, *J. Clin. Periodontol.,* 20, 36, January, 1993.

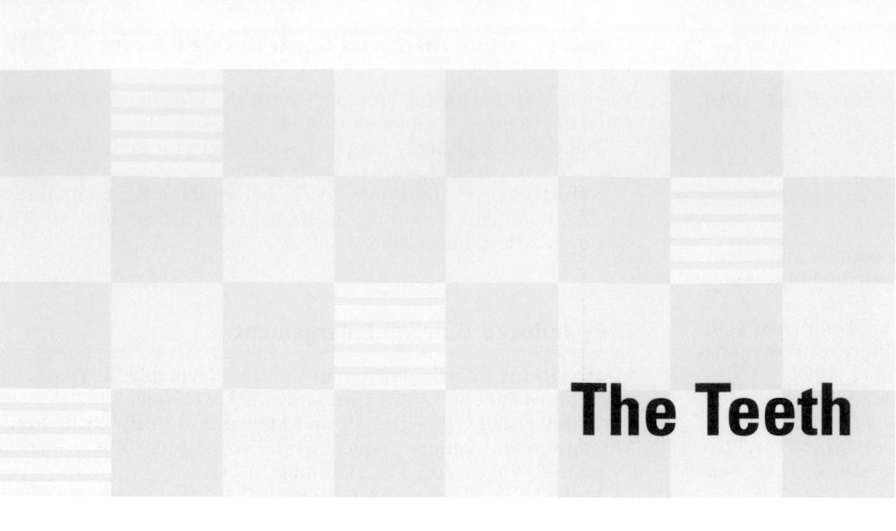
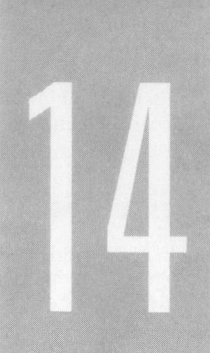

The Teeth

Clinical examination of the teeth is essential prior to treatment to provide guidelines for treatment planning, instrumentation, instruction, and follow-up evaluation. In general, patients may tend to be more concerned about their teeth than about their gingiva. The reasons may be related to personal appearance; degree of information, which may be greater about teeth than gingiva; and sensitivity and pain associated with ailments of the teeth.

Background study of histology, dental anatomy, and oral pathology is essential to this phase of clinical practice. Key words are defined in Box 14-1.

With information from the patient's personal and dental histories (see Tables 6-1 and 6-2, pages 94 and 95) and a thorough clinical and radiographic examination, the objectives are to:

A. Prepare a charting and provide a record of deviations from the normal.
B. Identify the treatment and counseling needed in relation to the teeth for the particular patient.
C. Outline the patient's preventive program (pages 324 and 333 to 335).
D. Utilize the specific data during treatment for instrument selection and adaptation.

BOX 14-1 KEY WORDS AND ABBREVIATIONS: Teeth

Accessory root canal: a secondary canal extending from the pulp to the surface of the root; frequently found near the apex of a root but may occur higher and provide a connection to a periodontal pocket.

Amelogenesis (am″ē-lō-jen′ĕ-sis): production and development of enamel.

Avulsion (ah-vul′-shun): the tearing away or forcible separation of a structure or part. **Tooth avulsion** is the traumatic separation of a tooth from the alveolus.

Bruxism (bruk′sĭzm): an oral habit of grinding, clenching, or clamping the teeth; involuntary, rhythmic, or spasmodic movements outside the chewing range; may damage teeth and attachment apparatus.

Cariogenic (kăr″ē-ō-jen′ik): adj. conducive to dental caries.

Carious (kă′rē-us): adj. used to define a **carious lesion.**

Cementicle (sĕ-men′tĭ-kel): a calcified spherical body, composed of cementum, lying free within the periodontal ligament, attached to the cementum or imbedded within the cementum.

Dental caries (kăr′ēz): disease of the mineralized structures of the teeth characterized by demineralization of the hard components and dissolution of the organic matrix.

Arrested caries: carious lesion that has become stationary and does not show a tendency to progress further; frequently has a hard surface and takes on a dark brown or reddish-brown color.

Primary caries: occurs on a surface not previously affected; also called initial caries; early lesion may be referred to as incipient caries.

Rampant caries: widespread formation of chalky white areas and incipient lesions that may increase in size over a comparatively short time.

Recurrent caries: occurs on a surface adjacent to a restoration; may be a continuation of the original lesion; also called secondary caries.

Dentition (den-tĭsh′un): the natural teeth in the dental arch.

Primary (deciduous) dentition: the first teeth; normally will be shed and replaced by permanent teeth.

Permanent dentition: the natural 32 teeth that serve throughout life.

Mixed dentition: combination of primary and permanent teeth between ages 6 and 12 when primary teeth are being replaced; starts with the eruption of the first permanent tooth.

Succedaneous (suk″sĕ-dā′nē-us): the permanent teeth that erupt into the positions of exfoliated primary teeth.

Edentulous (ē-den′tū-lus): without teeth; referred to as partially edentulous when some, but not all, teeth are missing.

Electrolyte (ē-lek′trō-līt): a conductor; a substance that, in solution, dissociates into electrically charged particles (ions) and thus is capable of conducting an electric current.

Etiology (ē″tē-ol′ĕ-jē): the science or study of the cause of a disease or disorder.

Exfoliation (eks-fō″lē-ā′shun): loss of primary teeth following physiologic resorption of root structure.

Facet (făs′et): a small flattened surface on a hard body, such as a tooth; a wear facet can result from attrition or repeated parafunctional contact.

Hypoplasia (hī″pō-plā′zhah): incomplete development or underdevelopment of a tissue or organ.

Enamel hypoplasia: incomplete or defective formation of the enamel of either primary or permanent teeth. The result may be an irregularity of tooth form, color, or surface.

Idiopathic (id″ē-ō-path′ik): denoting a condition of unknown cause.

Incipient (in-sip′ē-ent): beginning; coming into existence.

pH: the symbol of hydrogen ion concentration expressed in numbers corresponding to the acidity or alkalinity of an aqueous solution; the range is from 14 (pure base) to 0 (pure acid); neutral is at 7.0.

Critical pH: the pH at which demineralization occurs; for enamel, pH 4.5 to 5.5; for cementum, pH 6.0 to 6.7.

Resorption (rē-sorp′shun): removal of bone or tooth structure; gradual dissolution of the mineralized tissue; may be internal or external; occurs during exfoliation of a primary tooth and from the pressure of orthodontic treatment.

THE DENTITIONS

Formation of the primary teeth begins *in utero*. Table 14-1 shows the weeks *in utero* when each primary tooth begins to mineralize and the average months after birth when the enamel is completely formed before the date of eruption.

Mineralization of the permanent teeth starts at birth and continues into adolescence. The chronology of development and eruption appears in Table 14-2. Roots normally are completed by 3 years after eruption.

The mixed dentition, when primary teeth are being exfoliated and permanent teeth move in to take their places, occurs between the ages of 6 and 12 years. Figure 14-1 illustrates the mixed dentition of a child approximately 6 years of age.

DENTAL CARIES

The World Health Organization has defined dental caries as a "localized, post-eruptive, pathologic process of external origin involving softening of the hard tooth tissue and proceeding to the formation of a cavity."[1] Dental caries is a preventable disease.

I. DEVELOPMENT OF DENTAL CARIES

Requirements for the development of a carious lesion are microorganisms; carbohydrate, primarily sucrose; and a susceptible tooth surface. Figure 28-1 (page 443) is a diagram that shows four overlapping circles to illustrate the essential factors in the process of dental caries initiation.

Bacterial plaque may contain numerous types of acid-forming bacteria. Mutans streptococci have been specifically implicated. The role of bacterial plaque and the factors involved in dental caries initiation are described in Chapter 16, pages 272 to 274.

II. CLASSIFICATION OF CAVITIES

A. G.V. Black's Classification[2]

The standard method for classifying dental caries was developed by Dr. G.V. Black, a noted dental educator who divided the categories into classes according to surfaces of the teeth; each class is represented by a Roman numeral. The categories customarily are used for carious lesions, cavity preparations, and finished restorations. Table 14-3 defines and illustrates the classifications.

B. Nomenclature by Surfaces

1. *Simple Cavity:* Involves one tooth surface. *Example:* occlusal cavity.
2. *Compound Cavity:* Involves two tooth surfaces. *Example:* mesio-occlusal cavity, referred to as an "M-O" cavity.
3. *Complex Cavity:* Involves more than two tooth surfaces. *Example:* mesio-occlusal-distal, referred to as an "M-O-D" cavity.

TABLE 14-1 Tooth Development and Eruption: Primary Teeth

		Hard Tissue Formation Begins (weeks in utero)	Enamel Completed (months after birth)	Eruption (months)	Root Completed (year)
Maxillary	Central incisor	14	1½	10 (8–12)	1½
	Lateral incisor	16	2½	11 (9–13)	2
	Canine	17	9	19 (16–22)	3¼
	First molar	15½	6	16 (13–19 boys) (14–18 girls)	2½
	Second molar	19	11	29 (25–33)	3
Mandibular	Central incisor	14	2½	8 (6–10)	1½
	Lateral incisor	16	3	13 (10–16)	1½
	Canine	17	9	20 (17–23)	3¼
	First molar	15½	5½	16 (14–18)	2¼
	Second molar	18	10	27 (23–31 boys) (24–30 girls)	3

From Lunt R. C. and Law, D.B., A Review of the Chronology of Eruption of Deciduous Teeth. *J. Am. Dent. Assoc. 89,* 872. October, 1974.

TABLE 14-2 Tooth Development and Eruption: Permanent Teeth

		Hard Tissue Formation Begins	Enamel Completed (years)	Eruption (years)	Root Completed (years)
Maxillary	Central incisor	3–4 mo	4–5	7–8	10
	Lateral incisor	10 mo	4–5	8–9	11
	Canine	4–5 mo	6–7	11–12	13–15
	First premolar	1½–1¾ yr	5–6	10–11	12–13
	Second premolar	2–2¼ yr	6–7	10–12	12–14
	First molar	at birth	2½–3	6–7	9–10
	Second molar	2½–3 yr	7–8	12–13	14–16
	Third molar	7–9 yr	12–16	17 21	18–25
Mandibular	Central incisor	3 4 mo	4–5	6–7	9
	Lateral incisor	3–4 mo	4–5	7–8	10
	Canine	4–5 mo	6–7	9–10	12–14
	First premolar	1¾–2 yr	5–6	10–12	12–13
	Second premolar	2¼–2½ yr	6–7	11–12	13–14
	First molar	at birth	2½–3	6–7	9–10
	Second molar	2½–3 yr	7–8	11–13	14–15
	Third molar	8 10 yr	12–16	17–21	18–25

From Ash, M.M.: *Wheeler's Dental Anatomy, Physiology, and Occlusion,* 7th ed. Philadelphia, W.B. Saunders Co., 1993, page 25.

ENAMEL CARIES

I. STEPS IN THE FORMATION OF A CAVITY

A. Phase I: Incipient Lesion
1. *Subsurface Demineralization:* Acid products from cariogenic bacterial plaque pass through microchannels (pores) of the enamel.
2. *Visualization:* Area of demineralization is not visible by clinical observation during initial changes; thin layer of enamel remains over the surface.
3. *First Clinical Evidence:* White spot appears with no breakthrough to enamel surface; with time, area may turn brown from food, beverages, or tobacco use.
4. *Remineralization:* Low concentrations of fluoride applied frequently during the early phase can provide sources for uptake by the demineralized zone. The porous demineralized area readily takes up fluoride from dentifrice, mouthrinse, fluoridated drinking water, and all possible sources. Figure 29-3 (page 459) shows examples of levels of concentration of fluoride in surface enamel and in a white spot area.

B. Phase II: Untreated Incipient Lesion
1. *Breakdown of Enamel Over the Demineralized Area (White Spot):* Visible to observation and irregular to application of an explorer.
2. *Progression of Carious Lesion:* Follows general direction of enamel rods.
3. *Spread of Carious Lesion:* Spreads at dentino-enamel junction; continues along the dentinal tubules (Figure 14-2).

II. TYPES OF DENTAL CARIES (DESCRIBED BY LOCATION)

A. Pit and Fissure
Caries begins in a minute fault in the enamel.
1. Pit or fissure irregularity occurs where three or more lobes of the developing tooth join; closure of the enamel plates is imperfect. *Examples:* occlusal pits of molars and premolars.
2. Occurs at the endings of grooves of the teeth. *Example:* the buccal groove of a mandibular molar.

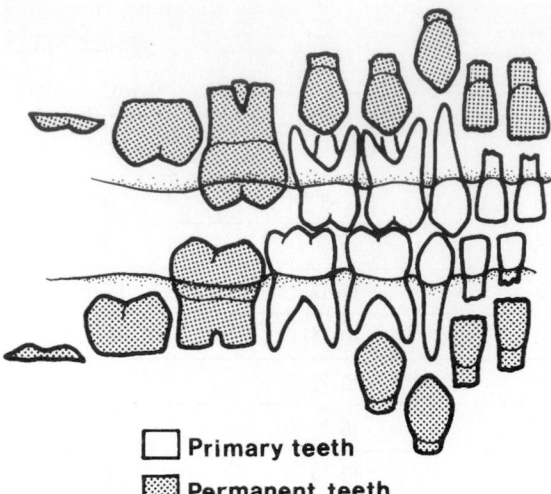

☐ **Primary teeth**
▨ **Permanent teeth**

■ **FIGURE 14-1 Mixed Dentition at Approximately Age 6 Years.** The average child has 20 primary teeth in place and root resorption of the incisors has started as the developing permanent incisors move into position. The first permanent molars are partially erupted.

B. Smooth Surface

Caries begins in smooth surfaces where there is no pit, groove, or other fault. It occurs in areas where bacterial plaque collects, such as proximal tooth surfaces, cervical thirds of teeth, and other difficult-to-clean areas.

EARLY CHILDHOOD CARIES[3,4]

Baby bottle tooth decay is a form of rampant caries found in very young children who routinely have been given a nursing bottle when going to sleep or who have experienced prolonged at-will breast-feeding. Other names for the same condition are nursing

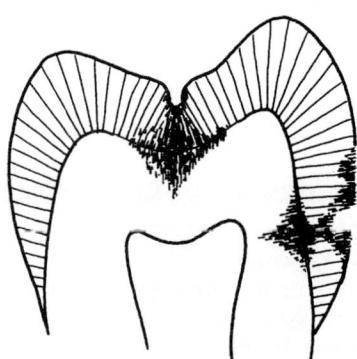

■ **FIGURE 14-2 Dental Caries.** Cones of dental caries in a pit and fissure and on a smooth tooth surface. Dental caries follows the general direction of the enamel rods, spreads at the dentinoenamel junction, and then continues along the dentinal tubules.

bottle mouth, baby bottle syndrome, baby bottle caries, and prolonged nursing habit.

I. ETIOLOGY

A. Microbiology

High levels of mutans streptococci have been cultured from the saliva and bacterial plaque from the teeth of children with baby bottle tooth decay.[5,6] Lactobacilli also were found in large numbers in the plaque.

B. Risk Factors

The risk factors are listed in Table 14-4. Teaching the parents about the cause and effects of baby bottle tooth decay must be a significant part of anticipatory guidance (see Table 43-3, page 661).

C. Predisposing Factors

1. Nursing bottle that contains sweetened milk or other fluid sweetened with sucrose.
2. Pacifier dipped or filled with a sweet agent, such as honey.
3. Prolonged at-will breast-feeding.

II. EFFECTS

Maxillary anterior teeth and primary molars are the first to be affected (Figure 14-3). As the baby falls asleep, pools of sweet liquid can collect about the teeth. While the sucking is active, the liquid passes beyond the teeth. The nipple covers the mandibular anterior teeth; hence, they are rarely affected.

III. RECOGNITION

Children should be seen for an examination no later than 6 months after eruption of the first tooth.[7] Demineralization may be noted along the cervical third of the maxillary anterior teeth. The source of the problem may be detected and preventive procedures initiated through parental counseling.

At a later stage the lesions appear dark brown. Eventually, the crowns may be destroyed to the gum line, abscesses may develop, and the child may suffer severe pain and discomfort.

ROOT SURFACE CARIES

Root surface caries is a soft, progressive lesion of cementum and dentin that involves bacterial infection and invasion. It is also called cemental caries, cervical caries, or radicular caries.

The incidence of root caries increases with age, but not because of age. Gingival recession is necessary for root caries, and gingival recession is related to periodontal conditions that lead to recession.

I. STEPS IN THE FORMATION OF A CAVITY

A. Gingival recession exposes the cemental sur-

TABLE 14-3 Dental Caries Charting: Classification of Cavities

Classification: Location	Appearance	Method of Examination

Class I.
Cavities in pits or fissures
  a. Occlusal surfaces of premolars and molars
  b. Facial and lingual surfaces of molars
  c. Lingual surfaces of maxillary incisors
		Direct or indirect visual
		Exploration
		Radiographs not useful

Class II.
Cavities in proximal surfaces of premolars and molars
		Early caries: by radiographs only
		Moderate caries not broken through from proximal to occlusal:
		  1. Visual by color changes in tooth and loss of translucency
		  2. Exploration from proximal
		Extensive caries involving occlusal: direct visual

Class III.
Cavities in proximal surfaces of incisors and canines that do not involve the incisal angle
		Early caries: by radiographs or transillumination
		Moderate caries not broken through to lingual or facial:
		  1. Visual by tooth color change
		  2. Exploration
		  3. Radiograph
		Extensive caries; direct visual

Class IV. Cavities in proximal surfaces of incisors or canines that involve the incisal angle		Visual Transillumination
Class V. Cavities in the cervical 1/3 of facial or lingual surfaces (not pit or fissure)		Direct visual: dry surface for vision Exploration to distinguish demineralization: whether rough or hard and unbroken Areas may be sensitive to touch
Class VI. Cavities on incisal edges of anterior teeth and cusp tips of posterior teeth		Direct visual May be discolored

face. Caries does not form in the root surface while periodontal fibers are still attached.

B. Dental caries starts near the cementoenamel junction. Cementum is very thin and is soon destroyed; dentin is invaded.

C. Enamel is not involved except by extension or when it is undermined. Root caries occurs in a mildly acidic environment. If the pH were lower, enamel would also become carious. The critical pH for enamel is 4.5 to 5.0; for cementum, 6.0 to 6.7.[8]

D. Mutans streptococci and lactobacilli are pri-

TABLE 14-4 Risk Factors: Nursing Bottle Tooth Decay

- Use of sugar-containing liquids in a nursing bottle
- Child put to bed and to sleep with a bottle
- Baby falling asleep while feeding with breast or bottle; milk or sweet bottle contents pools around the teeth
- Breast and bottle feeding that persists beyond beginning of the first primary tooth eruption
- Weaning from bottle not started early enough
- Infant not learning to drink from a cup by first birthday
- Medications containing high percentage of sucrose; made into a syrup formula to disguise unpleasant flavor of drug, given several times each day (eg, child with HIV infection)
- Inappropriate fluoride supplementation
- Oral hygiene measures not implemented by time of eruption of first tooth
- Inadequate professional anticipatory guidance about preventive measures
- Health of parents' (primary caregiver's) teeth and periodontal tissues; lack of adequate care to prevent transmission.

mary organisms associated with root caries. Antibody levels to *Streptococcus mutans* are elevated.[9,10]

E. Effects

Root caries incidence has been shown to be directly related to the fluoride concentration in the drinking water.[11] Lifelong residence in a community with near-optimum levels of fluoride in the water was shown to be associated with at least an average of 30% decrease in the incidence of root caries compared with that associated with lifelong residence in a nonfluoridated community.[12]

II. CLINICAL RECOGNITION

Root caries lesions are described as soft, leathery, or hard. Active lesions are soft or leathery, whereas inactive or arrested lesions are hard.

A. Soft, shallow, ill-defined lesion.
B. Increases laterally to coalesce with other small lesions and eventually may extend completely around the tooth with undermining of the enamel (Figure 14-4).
C. Yellowish, light brown, dark brown to black.
D. Leathery in texture when explored (active lesion).
E. Arrested root caries displays cavitation and discoloration, but it is hard to the touch of the explorer.

III. RISK FACTORS FOR ROOT SURFACE CARIES

The risk factors are shown in Table 14-5. Prevention and control of root caries depend on control of the risk factors.

NONCARIOUS DENTAL LESIONS

ENAMEL HYPOPLASIA

I. DEFINITION

Enamel hypoplasia is a defect that occurs as a result of a disturbance in the formation of the organic enamel matrix.

II. TYPES AND ETIOLOGY

A. **Hereditary**
Enamel is partly or wholly missing. An example is amelogenesis imperfecta, which is described on page 289.

B. **Systemic (Environmental)**
Factors that may contribute to enamel hypoplasia during tooth development include severe

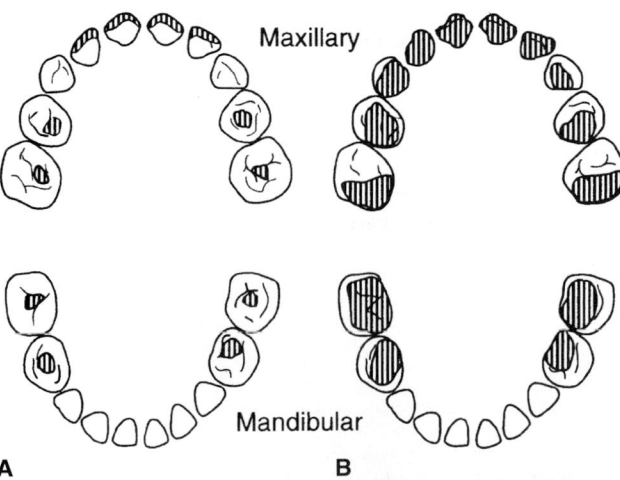

A   **B**

■ **FIGURE 14-3 Baby Bottle Tooth Decay. (A)** Earliest caries affects the maxillary anterior teeth followed by the molars as they erupt. **(B)** Severe extensive lesions develop in all except the mandibular anterior teeth. Protection for the mandibular incisors and canines is provided by the tongue during the sucking process.

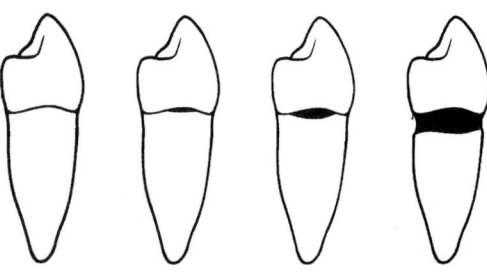

■ **FIGURE 14-4 Root Surface Caries.** A root surface lesion starts near the cementoenamel junction after gingival recession has exposed the root surface. The lesion is progressive, undermines the enamel, and may eventually surround the cervical third of the cementum. (Drawn after Banting, D.W. and Courtright, P.N.: Distribution and Natural History of Carious Lesions on the Roots of the Teeth, *Can Dent. Assoc. J.*, 41, 45, January, 1975.)

TABLE 14-5 Risk Factors: Root Caries

- Periodontal infection: Root surfaces exposed
  All factors that contribute to bone loss and attachment loss
- Microorganisms: Caries-producing
  Potential transmission
- Local/Behavioral
  Inadequate personal hygiene
  Bacterial plaque accumulations
  Poor compliance
- Diet: Frequent use of cariogenic foods
- Low fluoride exposure
  Outside fluoridated community water supply
  Insufficient daily self-application (dentifrice, mouthrinse, frequency)
- Xerostomia
  Medications with side effect
  Radiation to head/neck
  Salivary gland dysfunction
- History of dental caries
  Many restorations: coronal and root
  Overhanging margins, open contact areas, and other plaque traps
  Poor compliance for dental care
- Prosthetic devices
  Inadequate plaque removal daily
  Overdentures, clasps, provide plaque retentive areas
- Tobacco use: Sugar content of smokeless tobacco

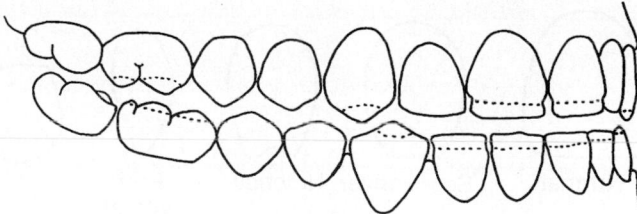

FIGURE 14-5 Enamel Hypoplasia. Chronologic hypoplasia, usually in the form of grooves or pits, appears in the enamel at a level corresponding with the stage of development of the teeth. For this patient, the disturbance in enamel development occurred at approximately 10 months of age.

nutritional deficiency, particularly rickets; fever-producing diseases, such as measles, chicken-pox, and scarlet fever; congenital syphilis; hypoparathyroidism; birth injury; prematurity; Rh hemolytic disease; fluorosis; or idiopathy.

C. Local
A single tooth can be affected; trauma or periapical inflammation about a primary tooth can injure the adjacent developing permanent tooth.

III. APPEARANCE

A. Hereditary
May appear brown (page 289).

B. Systemic
Called also "chronologic hypoplasia" because the lesions are found in areas of those teeth where the enamel was forming during the systemic disturbance.
1. *Single Narrow Zone* (smooth or pitted): Disturbance lasted a short period of time (Figure 14-5).
2. *Multiple:* Disturbance to the ameloblast occurred over a period of time, or several times.
3. *Teeth Most Frequently Affected:* First molars, incisors, canines, because the disturbances generally occur during the first year when those teeth are mineralizing (Table 14-2).

C. Hypoplasia of Congenital Syphilis
Transmission of syphilis from mother to fetus after the 16th week of pregnancy may alter the

development of the tooth germs. Figure 14-6 illustrates tooth forms that may result. The mesiodistal width may be reduced, and incisors are frequently narrowed at the incisal third.

Other conditions may also cause similar variations of tooth form.

D. Local Enamel Hypoplasia
A single tooth with a yellow or brown intrinsic stain.

ATTRITION

I. DEFINITION
Attrition is the wearing away of a tooth as a result of tooth-to-tooth contact (Figure 14-7).

II. OCCURRENCE

A. Location
May be found on occlusal, incisal, and proximal surfaces.

B. Age Factor
Increases with age, and more attrition is seen in men than in women of comparable age.

III. ETIOLOGY

A. Bruxism
Predisposing factors may be psychologic, tension, or occlusal interferences.

B. Usage
Wear of surfaces on each other. Predisposing factors may be coarse foods, chewing tobacco, or abrasive dusts associated with certain occupations.

IV. APPEARANCE

A. Initial Lesion
Small polished facet on a cusp tip or ridge, or slight flattening of an incisal edge.

B. Advanced
Gradual reduction in cusp height, flattening of occlusal plane (Figure 14-7).

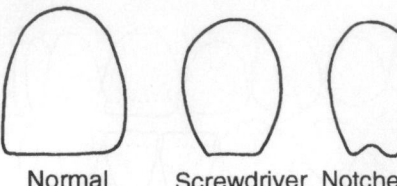

Normal

Screwdriver Notched
Hutchinson's incisors

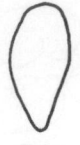

Peg
lateral

Normal

Mulberry
molar

■ **FIGURE 14-6 Crown Forms of Enamel Hypoplasia.** Hutchinson's incisors and mulberry molars are typical crown forms that result from congenital syphillis. The central incisors are narrowed at the incisal third, and the lateral incisors may be conical or peg-shaped.

C. Staining of Exposed Dentin
May occur; stain usually is brown.

D. Radiographic
The pulp chamber and canals may be narrowed and sometimes obliterated as the result of formation of secondary dentin.

EROSION

I. DEFINITION

Erosion is the loss of tooth substance by a chemical process that does not involve known bacterial action.

II. OCCURRENCE

A. Location
Facial or lingual surfaces, depending on cause.

B. Usually Involves Several Teeth

III. ETIOLOGY

The lesions are caused by some form of chemical dissolution.

A. May Be Idiopathic (Unknown)

B. Chronic Vomiting
Acid of chronic vomiting affects lingual surfaces, particularly anterior teeth.
1. Pregnancy.
2. Eating disorder, such as bulimia (page 832).

C. Extrinsic
1. *Industrial.* Workers' teeth can be exposed to atmospheric acids.
2. *Dietary.* Facial surfaces are most frequently affected.
   a. Carbonated beverages or lemon juice used frequently.
   b. Lemons or other citrus fruit sucked frequently.

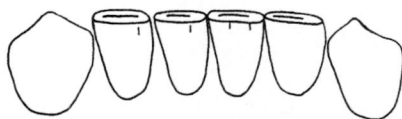

■ **FIGURE 14-7 Attrition.** Attrition of the incisal surfaces of mandibular anterior teeth has extended to expose the dentin. Dentin usually appears as a brown line or ring.

IV. APPEARANCE

A. Smooth, shallow, hard, shiny (in contrast to dental caries, in which appearance is soft and discolored).
B. Shape varies from shallow saucer-like depressions to deep wedge-shaped grooves; margins are not sharply demarcated.
C. May progress to involve the dentin and stimulate secondary dentin.
D. May occur in combination with dental caries, calculus, or dental restorations.[13]

ABRASION

I. DEFINITION

Abrasion is the mechanical wearing away of tooth substance by forces other than mastication.

II. OCCURRENCE

A. Location
Exposed root surfaces.

B. Other Types
At incisal edge.

III. ETIOLOGY

The lesion originates from a mechanical abrasive activity. The action of microorganisms is not essential for the development of abrasion. Dental caries may occur in the abraded area as a secondary lesion.

A. Abrasive Agent
The most common cause is an abrasive dentifrice applied with vigorous horizontal toothbrushing (Figure 14-8).

B. Other Types
Abrasion may occur at the incisal or occlusal surfaces.
1. Opening bobby pins may leave a small notch in one incisal edge. People with this habit usually utilize the same tooth each time.
2. Occupational causes include, for example, tacks held by carpenters, pins by dressmakers.
3. Pipe held between teeth; usually held in the same place over many years.

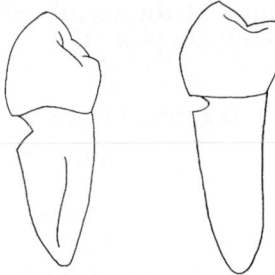

FIGURE 14-8 Abrasion. Profile view of the facial surface of mandibular premolars shows shape of abrasion on the root. Note that the area of abrasion undermines the enamel.

IV. APPEARANCE

A. V or wedge shaped with hard, smooth, shiny surface and clearly defined margins.

B. Except for incisal biting habits, the lesions occur initially on exposed cementum, then extend into the dentin.

FRACTURES OF TEETH

Trauma to the face may involve fractured bones and teeth in addition to soft tissue injuries. Fractured jaws and methods of treatment are described in Chapter 48, pages 712 to 719.

I. CAUSES OF TOOTH FRACTURES

A. Automobile, bicycle, and diving accidents.

B. Contact sports when mouth protectors are not worn.

C. Blows incurred while fighting.

D. Falls.

II. DESCRIPTION

A. Line of Fracture
1. Horizontal.
2. Diagonal.
3. Vertical.

B. Radiographic Signs of Recent Trauma
1. Widened periodontal ligament space.
2. Radiolucent fracture line.
3. Radiopaque areas where fracture segments overlap.
4. Tooth displacement.

III. CLASSIFICATION: WORLD HEALTH ORGANIZATION[14]

Classification provided by the World Health Organization is numbered as a special section of the International Classification of Diseases. Both primary and permanent dentitions are included. Figure 14-9 illustrates fractures of a central incisor.

873.60 Fracture of enamel of tooth only. Includes chipping and incomplete fractures (cracks).

873.61 Fracture of crown of tooth without pulpal involvement.

873.62 Fracture of crown with pulpal involvement.

873.63 Fracture of root of tooth.

873.64 Fracture of crown and root of tooth with or without pulpal involvement.

873.65 Fracture of tooth, unspecified.

873.66 Luxation (dislocation) of tooth. This category may involve concussion, subluxation, and luxation. A tooth with concussion is sensitive to percussion but is not loosened or displaced. Loosening without displacement is subluxation, and loosening with displacement is luxation.

873.67 Intrusion or extrusion of tooth. Intrusion into the alveolar bone is usually accompanied by

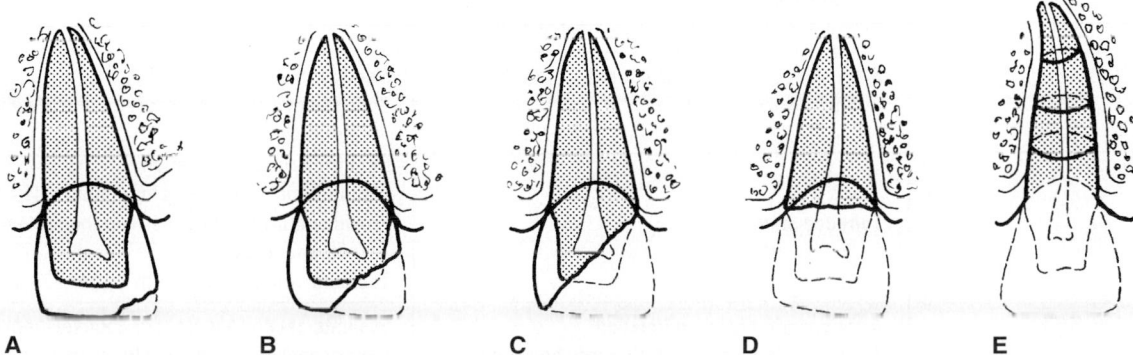

A   B   C   D   E

FIGURE 14-9 Fractures of Teeth. (A) Enamel fracture. **(B)** Crown fracture without pulpal involvement. **(C)** Crown fracture with pulpal involvement. **(D)** Fracture of crown and root near neck of tooth. **(E)** Root fractures involving cementum, dentin, and the pulp may occur in the apical, middle, or coronal third of the root.

fracture of the alveolar socket. Extrusion from the socket is a partial displacement.

873.68 Avulsion of tooth. Avulsion is the complete displacement of the tooth out of its socket. The emergency care for a tooth forcibly displaced may be found in Table 61-6 (page 916).

CLINICAL EXAMINATION OF THE TEETH

Following is a list of major factors to observe when examining the teeth. Several of these are described in other chapters, for which page references are noted. Information about hypoplasia, attrition, erosion, abrasion, dental caries, and tooth vitality is included in this chapter. Table 14-6 lists factors to observe during the examination of the teeth and suggests relationships to appointment procedures.

I. GENERAL CHARACTERISTICS

A. Number of teeth; eruption pattern (Tables 14-1 and 14-2).
B. Anomalies of size, form, number.
C. Replacements, such as restorations for individual teeth and groups of teeth (fixed and removable).

II. DEPOSITS (TABLE 16-1, PAGE 265)

A. Calculus.
B. Bacterial plaque.
C. Materia alba and food debris.

TABLE 14-6 Examination of the Teeth		
Feature	**To Observe**	**Dental Hygiene Implication**
Morphology	Number of teeth (missing teeth verified by radiographic examination) Size, shape Arch form Position of individual teeth Injuries: fractures of the crown (root fractures observed in radiographs	Selection and adaptation of instruments Areas prone to dental caries initiation, particularly the difficult-to-reach areas during plaque control Pulp test for vitality may be indicated
Development	Anomalies and developmental defects Pits and white spots	Distinguish hypoplasia and dental fluorosis from demineralization Identify pits for sealants
Eruption	Sequence of eruption: normal, irregular Unerupted teeth observed in radiographs	Care in using floss in the col area where the epithelium is usually less mature in young children Orthodontic needs Procedures for preservation of primary teeth

Deposits
  Food debris
  Plaque
  Calculus
    Supragingival
    Subgingival
	Overall evaluation of self-care and plaque-control measures
	Relation of appearance of teeth to gingival health
	Extent and location of plaque, debris, and calculus
	Calculus and the tooth surface pocket wall
		Need for instruction and guidance
		Frequency of follow-up and maintenance appointments

Stains
  Extrinsic
 	
  Intrinsic
	Extrinsic: colors relate to causes
	Intrinsic: dark, grayish
	
	Tobacco stain
		Need for test for pulp vitality
		Stain removal procedures; selection of polishing agent
		Dentifrice recommendation
		Plaque-control emphasis for plaque-related stains
		Provide information concerning the oral effects of tobacco use
		Tobacco cessation program (pages 436 to 438)

Regressive Changes	Attrition: primary and permanent Abrasion: physical agents that may be a cause Erosion	Evaluate causes and treat or counsel for prevention Dietary analysis: for finding foods that may be related Selection of nonabrasive dentifrice Habit evaluation

(continued)

TABLE 14-6 Examination of the Teeth (Continued)

Feature	To Observe	Dental Hygiene Implication
Exposed Cementum	Relation to gingival recession, pocket formation Areas of narrow attached gingiva Hypersensitivity	Special care areas where only slight attached gingiva remains Nonabrasive dentifrice advised Measures to prevent root-surface caries Care during instrumentation Indication for application of desensitizing agent
Dental Caries	Areas of demineralization Carious lesions (proximal lesions observed in radiographs) Arrested caries Root caries	Charting Treatment plan Preventive program for caries control, fluoride, dietary factors Follow-up and frequency of maintenance
Restorations	Contour of restorations, overhangs Proximal contact (see separate heading later in this table) Surface smoothness Staining	 Chart and correct inadequate margins Selection of instruments and polishing agents Dentifrice selection to prevent discoloration
Factors Related to Occlusion Tooth wear	Facets; worn-down cusp tips Health of supporting structures; observation of radiographs for signs of trauma from occlusion	Need for study of bruxism and other parafunctional habits
Proximal contacts	Use of floss to find open contact areas Areas of food retention	Chart inadequate contacts for corrective measures Use of floss by patient
Mobility	Degree; comparison of chartings Possible causes	Need for reduction of inflammatory factors that may be related Dentist will identify and treat factors related to trauma from occlusion
Classification	Position of teeth Angle's classification	Relationship to orthodontic treatment needs
Habits	Nail or object biting; lip or cheek biting Observe effects on lip, cheek, teeth Tongue thrust; reverse swallow	Guidance for habit correction when indicated
Edentulous Areas	Radiographic evaluation for impacted, unerupted teeth, retained root tips, other deviations from normal	Supplemental fulcrum selection during instrumentation Applied plaque-control procedures for abutment teeth

Replacement for Missing Teeth
  Dentures
  Partial dentures
  Implants
	Teeth and tissue that support a prosthesis
	Cleanliness of a prosthesis
	Factors that contribute to food and debris retention
		Preventive measures for harm to supporting teeth and soft tissues
		Instruction in personal care of fixed and removable dentures; use of floss under fixed partial denture; other appropriate care

Saliva	Amount and consistency Dryness of mouth	Relation to instruction for prevention of dental caries: more caries can be expected in a dry mouth Use of saliva substitute; fluoride

III. COLOR

    A. Intrinsic stains (pages 289 to 290).
    B. Extrinsic stains (pages 286 to 289).

IV. DEVELOPMENTAL DEFECTS

    A. Enamel hypoplasia.
    B. Amelogenesis imperfecta; dentinogenesis imperfecta (page 289).

V. REGRESSIVE CHANGES

    A. Attrition.
    B. Erosion.
    C. Abrasion.

VI. OCCLUSION (PAGES 254 TO 262)

    A. Proximal contact relation: areas of food impaction.
    B. Mobility (page 218).

VII. DENTAL CARIES AND DEMINERALIZATION

VIII. VITALITY OF PULP

IX. TOOTH FRACTURES

RECOGNITION OF CARIOUS LESIONS

Both visual and exploratory means are used to identify dental caries.

I. PREPARATION

Dry each tooth or group of teeth with compressed air and carefully inspect each surface, first visually, and then with an explorer as necessary to confirm visual findings.

II. VISUAL EXAMINATION: ENAMEL CARIES

Characteristic changes in the color and translucency of tooth structure may be observed. Such changes either are definite signs of dental caries progress or may lead the examiner to suspect dental caries, which can then be checked further with an explorer. Variations in color and translucency include the following:

    A. Chalky white areas of demineralization.
    B. Grayish-white discoloration of marginal ridges caused by dental caries of the proximal surface underneath.
    C. Grayish-white color spreading from margins of restorations caused by lesions of secondary dental caries.
    D. In relation to an amalgam restoration, dental caries appears translucent in outer portion and white and opaque adjacent to the amalgam.
    E. Open carious lesions may vary in color from yellowish brown to dark brown.
    F. Discoloration is generally less severe when dental caries progresses rapidly than when it progresses slowly.
    G. Dull, flat white, opaque areas under direct light show loss of translucency, particularly of the enamel.
    H. Dark shadow on a proximal surface may be shown by transillumination. This type of observation is especially useful for anterior teeth and unrestored posterior teeth.

III. EXPLORATORY EXAMINATION

A. Smooth Surface Caries

    1. *Technique.* Adapt the side of the tip of the explorer closely to the tooth surface as described on page 217. Examine for hardness versus softness, roughness versus smoothness, and continuity of tooth surface versus breaks in continuity.
    2. *Restorations.* Follow the margins of all restorations around with an explorer. Overhanging margins may or may not appear in the radiographs, depending on superimposition. Types of overhangs are described on page 624. Chart all irregularities of existing restorations.

B. Pit and Fissure Caries

When a pit or fissure is discolored, one cannot determine visually whether dental caries is present except when a large obvious cavity can be seen. An obvious cavity should not be explored.

    1. Direct the explorer tip so that it can pass straight into the pit or fissure. When the tip is not positioned correctly, caries in a small narrow pit can go undetected.
    2. Explorer catches when dental caries is present and softening of tooth structure is evident.

IV. RADIOGRAPHIC EXAMINATION

During the clinical examination, information revealed by radiographs is utilized for supplementation and confirmation. Neither clinical nor radiographic examination is complete without the other. A few principal items to be seen in a radiographic examination of the teeth are

Anomalies
Impactions
Fractures
Internal and root resorption
Dental caries
Periapical radiolucencies

A. Technique Principles

Periapical radiographs usually provide sufficient information concerning the teeth, but panoramic, extraoral, or occlusal radiographs may be needed for detecting or defining anomalies and pathologic lesions outside the scope of periapical radiographs. Bitewing radiographs or periapical radiographs made by a paralleling technique with no overlapping are most satisfactory for dental caries detection.

Principles for examination were described on pages 165 to 168. Mounted radiographs on an adequately lighted viewbox are a necessity during charting and treatment procedures. For the detection of early carious lesions, a hand-held magnifying glass can be of invaluable assistance.

B. Detection of Dental Caries

Radiographs are not needed for facial, lingual, or occlusal carious lesions because they are accessible and best observed by exploration and direct vision. Because of superimposition of other parts of the tooth, facial, lingual, and occlusal carious lesions need to be fairly well advanced before they are definitely discernible in a radiograph.

1. *Proximal Caries.* Proximal surface lesions may be missed if radiographs are not used. Clinical skills for caries discernment need to be perfected, however, to prevent excess exposure of a patient to unnecessary radiation.
   a. Proximal lesions. Properly angulated radiographs with no overlapping are required for the detection of small lesions that involve the enamel or extend slightly into the dentin.
   b. Proximal overhanging restorations. An overhanging filling or dental caries under that filling may be present, even if none can be seen in the radiograph because of superimposition. An explorer must be passed around the complete margin to confirm the condition.
2. *Root Caries*
   a. Location. Most root carious lesions occur in the vicinity of and just beneath the cementoenamel junction.
   b. Appearance. Root caries appears as a saucer-shaped lesion in a radiograph. It may appear to undermine the enamel, or it may be located beneath an overhanging filling.

TESTING FOR PULPAL VITALITY

Any tooth suspected of being nonvital must be tested for pulpal vitality or degree of vitality. The two basic types of pulp testing are thermal and electric.

Such testing is particularly significant prior to treatment involving periodontal surgery, any restorative procedures, and orthodontic appliance placement. Diagnosis of vitality is made not only on the basis of a pulp test, but also on consideration of all data from the patient history and clinical and radiographic examinations.

A tooth may become nonvital from bacterial causes, particularly invasion of the pulp from dental caries or periodontal disease. Physical causes may be mechanical or thermal injuries. Examples of mechanical injuries are trauma, such as a blow, or iatrogenic dental procedures, such as cavity preparation or too-rapid orthodontic movement.

I. OBSERVATIONS THAT SUGGEST LOSS OF VITALITY

A. Clinical

1. Discoloration of a tooth crown (intrinsic stains, pages 289 to 290).
2. Fracture (part of the crown may be missing, Figure 14-9).
3. Large carious lesion or large restoration.
4. Fistula with opening into the oral cavity over the apical region of a tooth.

B. Radiographic

1. Apical radiolucency, which may indicate a granuloma, cyst, or abscess.
2. Bone loss with a widened periodontal ligament space extending to the apex.
3. Fractured root.
4. Large carious lesion or restoration that appears closely related to the pulp chamber.

II. RESPONSE TO PULP TESTING

A. Rationale

Pulp testing is based on the knowledge that a stimulus can create pain to which a patient can react. The pulp tester, therefore, determines the conduction of stimuli to the sensory receptors. The vitality of the pulp depends on its blood supply and not on its nerve supply. For that reason, a positive or negative pulp test may not always show the true condition of the pulp.

B. Factors That Influence a Patient's Response to a Pulp Test

1. *Degree of Pulpal Degeneration or Inflammation.* A necrotic pulp gives no response at all, whereas an acutely or chronically inflamed pulp responds at varying degrees between no response and full normal response.
2. *Pain Threshold.* The pain threshold is the lowest intensity of pain caused by a threshold stimulus. A threshold stimulus is the minimum stimulus necessary to induce patient response.
3. *Reaction to Pain.* May vary with a patient's attitude, age, sex, emotional security, fatigue, drugs used, as well as the size of the pulp and thickness of the dentin, particularly the amount of secondary dentin.
4. *Nerve Transmission Blocks.* Injuries or lesions of nerves, and anesthetics.
5. *Adjacent Metal.* Restorations or continuous bridgework.

C. Responses

An electric tester reveals only whether a pulp is vital or nonvital. Using thermal testing may show the following:

1. No response: necrotic pulp

2. Lingering pain after removal of stimulus: irreversible pulpitis
3. Pain subsides promptly: reversible pulpitis

III. THERMAL PULP TESTING

Cold or hot stimuli may be used. For all methods, a control test is performed on a healthy tooth on the opposite side of the arch. Inform the patient in advance about the procedure and what to expect.

A. Cold Test

1. *Materials.* Cold testing may be accomplished with an air blast, cold drink, ice stick, ethyl chloride in a spray or on a cotton swab, or a carbon dioxide dry-ice stick. Isolate the test teeth and dry with a gauze sponge.
2. *Preparation of ice stick.* Small icicles may be prepared by freezing water in anesthetic needle covers.
3. *Dry-ice stick.* Made from carbon dioxide and delivered using a special holder with a plunger.

B. Heat Test

1. *Temporary stopping.* Warm temporary stopping (gutta-percha). Apply to a tooth dried with cotton sponge.
2. *Water.* Warm to hot water. Isolate tooth and bathe in very warm water.

IV. ELECTRICAL PULP TESTER

A. Types

1. *Battery-operated*
   a. Advantages: Hand held so a clinician can work alone; portable.
   b. Disadvantage: Battery can run down. Some types have a light to indicate current in circuit.
2. *Plug-in*
   a. Advantage: More dependable than battery-operated.
   b. Disadvantage: Not self-contained; requires house-current plug.
   c. Newer models have grounding connection for patient to hold.

B. Precaution

The application of an electrical current to a patient with a cardiac pacemaker or any electronic life-support device by the use of a pulp tester, ultrasonic scaler, desensitizing equipment, or electrosurgical instrument may interfere with the function of the life-support device and may constitute a serious health hazard.[15] A review of the patient history and consultation with the patient's cardiologist are necessary prior to application of a pulp tester.

C. Preparation and Use of Equipment

Manufacturer's instructions are provided for each pulp tester and should be followed carefully. When the tester rheostat is separate from the applicator tip, an assistant is needed.

Consistency of procedures is essential to obtain consistent readings. The same pulp tester should be used for a particular patient at continuing comparative tests. Notes in a patient's record can indicate specific directions for that patient.

D. General Procedures

1. Assemble equipment.
2. Explain briefly to the patient what is to be done, but avoid detailed description, which could create anxiety or apprehension.
3. Dry the teeth to be tested to prevent the current from passing to the gingiva; isolate with cotton rolls and insert a saliva ejector, or use rubber dam.
4. Moisten the end of the tip of the tester with a small amount of toothpaste. Another electrolyte (conductor) may be used if its consistency allows it to remain where placed and prevents it from flowing over the tooth surface.
5. Instruct the patient to signal when a sensation is felt; suggest raising a hand or making a sound.
6. Apply tester tip. The patient lightly holds the handle to complete the circuit.
   a. Apply first to at least one tooth other than the one in question, preferably an adjacent tooth and the same tooth on the contralateral side. Such a procedure determines a normal response for the patient.
   b. Place *without pressure* but with definite contact on sound tooth structure in a consistent location on the middle or gingival third. The middle third of the crown of a single-rooted tooth and the middle third of each cusp of a multirooted tooth are frequently used (Figure 14-10).

E. Readings

1. Avoid contact with gingival or other soft tissues. A low-resistance circuit can be formed, thus allowing the circuit to by-pass the tooth.
2. Avoid contact with metallic restorations. The metal forms a more rapid conductor than does tooth structure. When approximal restorations are in contact, the circuit can be transmitted across to the adjacent tooth. The reading obtained would not pertain to the tooth in question (Figure 14-11). A nonconductive clear plastic matrix strip may be inserted to separate the two metallic restorations.
3. Test each tooth at least twice. Average the readings.
4. Record on patient's record the average number at which a minimal stimulus induced a response. Record for all teeth tested, not only the tooth in question.

F. Reasons for False-Negative Responses[15]

1. Patient premedicated with analgesics, tranquilizers, narcotics, or alcohol.
2. Recently traumatized tooth.

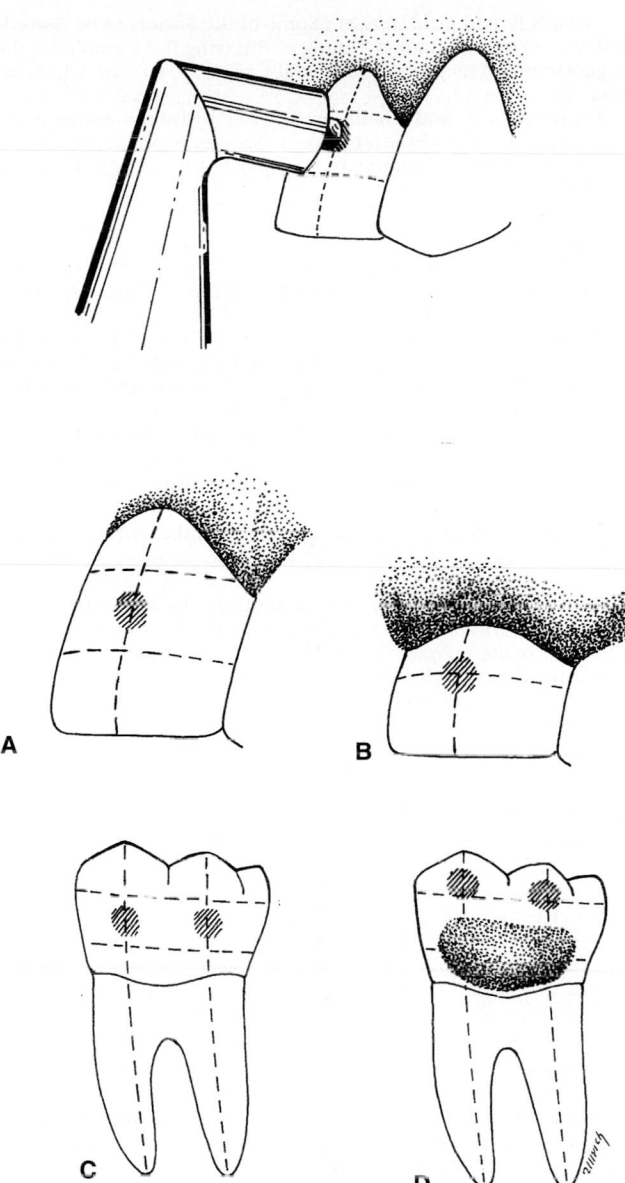

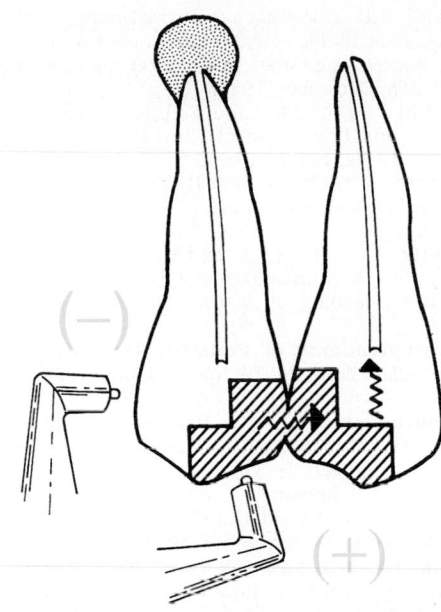

FIGURE 14-11 **Use of Pulp Tester.** False-positive response can result when the tester is placed on a metallic restoration. The current can be transmitted across a contact area to give a reading for the adjacent tooth rather than for the tooth in question. (Redrawn from Antel, J. and Christie, W.J.: Electrical Pulp Testing, *Can. Dent. Assoc. J.* 45, 597, November, 1979.)

dentin before there is evidence from the external surface.

III. Why radiographs may be used to detect proximal incipient caries.

IV. Reasons for preservation of primary teeth.

V. Frequency of complete oral examination in relation to a continuing preventive program.

VI. Preventive measures for control and prevention of tooth abrasion, such as dentifrice selection and correction of brush selection and use.

VII. Dietary factors related to erosion.

VIII. Methods for prevention of dental caries, such as fluorides, plaque prevention and control, and control of cariogenic foods in the diet.

IX. Methods for prevention of nursing caries. Nothing but plain water should be used in bedtime or naptime nursing bottles. Avoid the use of a sweetener on a pacifier. Use of a cup for milk or juice by the baby's first birthday.

X. Medicines or vitamin preparations made with heavy syrup (sucrose) have been shown to cause dental caries. Parents must learn to clean children's teeth after sugar exposures.[16]

XI. Discuss accident prevention procedures, such as always wearing a mouthguard for contact sports and wearing seat belts.

FIGURE 14-10 **Pulp Tester in Position. (A)** Correct contact point for tip of pulp tester is within the middle third of the crown. Avoid contact with gingiva or restorations. **(B)** Adjustment of position of contact point because of gingival enlargement. **(C)** Contact points on multirooted tooth. Place tip of pulp tester in the middle third over each root. **(D)** Adjustment of position of contact points because of large Class V restoration.

3. Pulp canal narrow and calcified.
4. Newly erupted tooth with incomplete closure at the apex; immature tooth.

FACTORS TO TEACH THE PATIENT

I. The cause and process of enamel or root caries formation and development for the patients at risk.

II. A description of the hardness of the enamel and of why a cavity is sometimes larger in the

REFERENCES

1. **World Health Organization:** *The Etiology and Prevention of Dental Caries.* WHO Technical Report Series, No. 494, Geneva, World Health Organization, 1972, 19 pp.

2. **Blackwell,** R.E.: *G.V. Black's Operative Dentistry,* Volume II, 9th ed. Milwaukee, Medico-Dental Publishing Co., 1955, pp. 1–4.
3. **Ripa,** L.W.: Nursing Caries: A Comprehensive Review, *Pediatr. Dent., 10,* 268, December, 1988.
4. **Brice,** D.M., Blum, J.R., and Steinberg, B.J.: The Etiology, Treatment, and Prevention of Nursing Caries, *Compend. Cont. Educ. Dent., 17,* 92, January, 1996.
5. **Van Houte,** J., Gibbs, G., and Butera, C.: Oral Flora of Children With "Nursing Bottle Caries," *J. Dent. Res., 61,* 382, February, 1982.
6. **Berkowitz,** R.G., Turner, J., and Hughes, C.: Microbial Characteristics of the Human Dental Caries Associated With Prolonged Bottle-feeding, *Arch. Oral Biol., 29,* 949, Number 11, 1984.
7. **American Academy of Pediatric Dentistry:** Oral Health Policies, *Pediatr. Dent., 20,* 72, Special Issue, Number 6, November, 1998.
8. **Hoppenbrouwers**, P.M.M., Driessens, F.C.M., and Borggreven, J.M.P.M.: The Mineral Solubility of Human Tooth Roots, *Arch. Oral Biol., 32,* 319, Number 5, 1987.
9. **van Houte**, J., Lopman, J., and Kent, R.: The Predominant Cultivable Flora of Sound and Carious Human Root Surfaces, *J. Dent. Res., 73,* 1727, November, 1994.
10. **Zambon**, J.J. and Kasprzak, S.A.: The Microbiology and Histopathology of Human Root Caries, *Am. J. Dent., 8,* 323, December, 1995.
11. **Burt,** B.A., Ismail, A.I., and Eklund, S.A.: Root Caries in an Optimally Fluoridated and a High-fluoride Community, *J. Dent. Res., 65,* 1154, September, 1986.
12. **Stamm,** J.W., Banting, D.W., and Imrey, P.B.: Adult Root Caries Survey of Two Similar Communities With Contrasting Natural Water Fluoride Levels, *J. Am. Dent. Assoc., 120,* 143, February, 1990.
13. **Sognnaes,** R.F., Wolcott, R.B., and Xhonga, F.A.: Dental Erosion. 1. Erosion-like Patterns Occurring in Association with Other Dental Conditions, *J. Am. Dent. Assoc., 84,* 571, March, 1972.
14. **World Health Organization:** *Application of the International Classification of Diseases to Dentistry and Stomatology,* ICD-DA, 2nd ed. Geneva, World Health Organization, 1978, pp. 88–89.
15. **Cohen,** S. and Burns, R.C., eds.: *Pathways of the Pulp,* 7th ed. St. Louis, Mosby, 1998, pp. 13–14.
16. **Rekola,** M.: *In vivo* Acid Production From Medicines in Syrup Form, *Caries Res., 23,* 412, November–December, 1989.

SUGGESTED READINGS

Anderson, M.H., Molvar, M.P., and Powell, L.V.: Treating Dental Caries as an Infectious Disease, *Oper. Dent., 16,* 21, January–February, 1991.

Choksi, S., Brady, J.M., Dang, D.H., and Rao, M.S.: Detecting Approximal Dental Caries with Transillumination: A Clinical Evaluation, *J. Am. Dent. Assoc., 125,* 1098, August, 1994.

Hirsch, J.M., Livian, G., Edward, S., and Noren, J.G.: Tobacco Habits Among Teenagers in the City of Göteborg, Sweden and Possible Association With Dental Caries, *Swed. Dent. J., 15,* 117, No. 3, 1991.

Ismail, A.I.: The Role of Early Dietary Habits in Dental Caries Development, *Spec. Care Dentist., 18,* 40, January/February, 1998.

Lagerlöf, F. and Oliveby, A.: Caries-protective Factors in Saliva, *Adv. Dent. Res., 8,* 229, July, 1994.

Massler, M. and Schour, I.: *Atlas of the Mouth,* 2nd ed. Chicago, American Dental Association, Plates 7–16.

McCabe, R.P., Adamkiewicz, V.W., and Pekovic, D.D.: Invasion of Bacteria in Enamel Carious Lesions, *J. Can. Dent. Assoc., 57,* 403, May, 1991.

Newbrun, E.: Preventing Dental Caries: Current and Prospective Strategies, *J. Am. Dent. Assoc., 123,* 68, May, 1992.

Newbrun, E.: Preventing Dental Caries: Breaking the Chain of Transmission, *J. Am. Dent. Assoc., 123,* 55, June, 1992.

Öhrn, K., Crossner, C.-G., Borgesson, L., and Taube, A.: Accuracy of Dental Hygienists in Diagnosing Dental Decay, *Community Dent. Oral Epidemiol., 24,* 182, June, 1996.

Pitts, N.B. and Kidd, E.A.M.: Some of the Factors to be Considered in the Prescription and Timing of Bitewing Radiography in the Diagnosis and Management of Dental Caries, *J. Dent., 20,* 74, April, 1992.

Tappuni, A.R. and Challacombe, S.J.: Distribution and Isolation Frequency of Eight Streptococcal Species in Saliva From Predentate and Dentate Children and Adults, *J. Dent. Res., 72,* 31, January, 1993.

Nursing Caries

Alaluusua, S.: Transmission of Mutans Streptococci, *Proc. Finn. Dent. Soc., 87,* 443, Number 4, 1991.

Barnes, G.P., Parker, W.A., Lyon, T.C., Drum, M.A., and Coleman, G.C.: Ethnicity, Location, Age, and Fluoridation Factors in Baby Bottle Tooth Decay and Caries Prevalence of Head Start Children, *Public Health Rep., 107,* 167, March–April, 1992.

Bowen, W.H., Pearson, S.K., Rosalen, P.L., Miguel, J.C., and Shih, A.Y.: Assessing the Cariogenic Potential of Some Infant Formulas, Milk and Sugar Solutions, *J. Am. Dent. Assoc., 128,* 865, July, 1997.

Caufield, P.W., Cutter, G.R., and Dasanayake, A.P.: Initial Acquisition of Mutans Streptococci by Infants: Evidence for a Discrete Window of Infectivity, *J. Dent. Res., 72,* 37, January, 1993.

Crall, J.J., Edelstein, B., and Tinanoff, N.: Relationship of Microbiological, Social, and Environmental Variables to Caries Status in Young Children, *Pediatr. Dent., 12,* 233, July–August, 1990.

Kamp, A.A.: Well-baby Dental Examinations: A Survey of Preschool Children's Oral Health, *Pediatr. Dent., 13,* 86, March–April, 1991.

Kaste, L.M., Marianos, D., Chang, R., and Phipps, K.R.: The Assessment of Nursing Caries and Its Relationship to High Caries in the Permanent Dentition, *J. Public Health Dent., 52,* 64, Winter, 1992.

Smith, D.J., Anderson, J.M., King, W.F., van Houte, J., and Taubman, M.A.: Oral Streptococcal Colonization of Infants, *Oral Microbiol. Immunol., 8,* 1, February, 1993.

Veerkamp, J.S.J. and Weerheijm, K.L.: Nursing-bottle Caries: The Importance of a Developmental Perspective, *ASDC J. Dent. Child., 62,* 381, November–December, 1995.

Yiu, C.K. and Wei, S.H.Y.: Management of Rampant Caries in Children, *Quintessence Int., 23,* 159, March, 1992.

Root Caries

Beighton, D., Lynch, E., and Heath, M.R.: A Microbiological Study of Primary Root-caries Lesions With Different Treatment Needs, *J. Dent. Res., 72,* 623, March, 1993.

Faine, M.P., Allender, D., Baab, D., Persson, R., and Lamont, R.J.: Dietary and Salivary Factors Associated With Root Caries, *Spec. Care Dentist., 12,* 177, July/August, 1992.

Fejerskov, O.: Recent Advancements in the Treatment of Root Surface Caries, *Int. J. Dent., 44,* 139, April, 1994.

Galan, D. and Lynch, E.: Prevention of Root Caries in Older Adults, *J. Can. Dent. Assoc., 60,* 422, May, 1994.

Hicks, M.J., Flaitz, C.M., and Garcia-Godoy, F.: Root Surface Caries Formation: Effect of In Vitro APF Treatment, *J. Am. Dent. Assoc., 129,* 449, April, 1998.

Hunt, R.J., Eldredge, J.B., and Beck, J.D.: Effect of Residence in a Fluoridated Community on the Incidence of Coronal and Root Caries in an Older Adult Population, *J. Public Health Dent., 49,* 138, Summer, 1989.

Katz, R.V.: Clinical Signs of Root Caries: Measurement Issues From an Epidemiologic Perspective, *J. Dent. Res., 69,* 1211, May, 1990.

Keltjens, H., Schaeken, T., and van der Hoeven, H.: Preventive Aspects of Root Caries, *Int. Dent. J., 43,* 143, April, 1993.

Krasse, B. and Fure, S.: Root Surface Caries: A Problem for Periodontally Compromised Patients, *Periodontology 2000, 4,* 139, 1994.

Mitchell, T.L. and Forgay, M.G.E.: Root Surface Caries: Implications for Dental Hygienists, *Can. Dent. Hyg./Probe, 21,* 31, March, 1987.

Sumney, D.L. and Jordan, H.V.: Characterization of Bacteria

Isolated from Human Root Surface Carious Lesions, *J. Dent. Res., 53,* 343, March–April, 1974.

Syed, S.A., Loesche, W.J., Pape, H.L., and Grenier, E.: Predominant Cultivable Flora Isolated From Human Root Surface Caries Plaque, *Infect. Immun., 11,* 727, April, 1975.

van der Veen, M.H., Tsuda, H., Arends, J., and ten Bosch, J.J.: Evaluation of Sodium Fluorescein for Quantitative Diagnosis of Root Caries, *J. Dent. Res., 75,* 588, January, 1996.

Vehkalahti, M. and Paunio, I.: Association Between Root Caries Occurrence and Periodontal State, *Caries Res., 28,* 301, July–August, 1994.

Wilkins, E.M.: Root Caries: The Problem and the Protocol. First of Two Parts, *DentalHygienistNews, 3,* 2, Fall, 1990; Second of Two Parts, *DentalHygienistNews, 4,* 6, Winter, 1991.

Noncarious Dental Lesions

Bishop, K., Kelleher, M., Briggs, P., and Joshi, R.: Wear Now? An Update on the Etiology of Tooth Wear, *Quintessence Int., 28,* 305, May, 1997.

Ellwood, R.P. and O'Mullane, D.: Enamel Opacities and Dental Esthetics, *J. Public Health Dent., 55,* 171, Summer, 1995.

Gabai, Y., Fattal, B., Rahamin, E., and Gedalia, I.: Effect of pH Levels in Swimming Pools on Enamel of Human Teeth, *Am. J. Dent., 1,* 241, December, 1988.

Gallien, G.S., Kaplan, I., and Owens, B.M.: A Review of Noncarious Dental Cervical Lesions, *Compend. Cont. Educ. Dent., 15,* 1366, November, 1994.

Grippo, J.O. and Simring, M.: Dental "Erosion" Revisited, *J. Am. Dent. Assoc., 126,* 619, May, 1995.

Harrison, J.L. and Roeder, L.B.: Dental Erosion Caused by Cola Beverages, *Gen. Dent., 39,* 23, January–February, 1991.

Järvinen, V.K., Rytömaa, I.I., and Heinonen, O.P.: Risk Factors in Dental Erosion, *J. Dent. Res., 70,* 942, June, 1991.

Krutchkoff, D.J., Eisenberg, E., O'Brien, J.E., and Ponzillo, J.J.: Cocaine-induced Dental Erosions (Correspondence), *N. Engl. J. Med., 322,* 408, February 8, 1990.

Lussi, A., Jaeggi, T., and Jaeggi-Schärer, S.: Prediction of the Erosive Potential of Some Beverages, *Caries Res., 29,* 349, September–October, 1995.

Owens, B.M. and Gallien, G.S.: Noncarious Dental "Abfraction" Lesions in an Aging Population, *Compend. Cont. Educ. Dent., 16,* 552, June, 1995.

Whittington, B.R. and Durward, C.S.: Survey of Anomalies in Primary Teeth and Their Correlation with the Permanent Dentition, *N. Zeal. Dent. J., 92,* 4, March, 1996.

Pulp Testing

Butel, E.M. and DiFiore, P.M.: Pulp Testing While Avoiding Dangers of Infection and Cross-contamination, *Gen. Dent., 39,* 42, January–February, 1991.

Certosimo, A.J. and Archer, R.D.: A Clinical Evaluation of the Electric Pulp Tester as an Indicator of Local Anesthesia, *Oper. Dent., 21,* 25, January–February, 1996.

Penna, K.J. and Sadoff, R.S.: Simplified Approach to Use of Electrical Pulp Tester, *NYSDJ, 61,* 30, January, 1995.

The Occlusion

Occlusion is the relationship of the teeth in the mandibular arch to those in the maxillary arch as they are brought together. The occlusion is examined and recorded as part of the oral examination. Knowledge of the occlusion of each patient can contribute significantly to complete care and instruction. Recognition of malocclusion assists in the referral of patients to the orthodontist, gives many valuable points of reference for patient instruction, and determines necessary adaptations in techniques. Box 15-1 defines key words relating to occlusion and occlusal factors.

Recognizing a patient's occlusion and understanding the oral health problems of malocclusion can aid in accomplishing the following:

A. Providing information for the comprehensive assessment and planning dental hygiene care.

B. Planning personalized instruction in relation to such factors as oral habits, masticatory efficiency, personal oral care procedures, and predisposing factors to dental and periodontal infections.

C. Adapting techniques of instrumentation to malpositioned teeth or groups of teeth.

D. Planning the frequency of maintenance appointments for professional care on the basis of deposit retention areas, particularly those that are difficult to reach in routine personal care.

E. Providing the general features of malocclusion to consider when orthodontic referral is discussed with the patient.

STATIC OCCLUSION

Static occlusal relationships are seen when the jaws are closed in centric relation. The static occlusion can be efficiently observed in occluded study casts and seen directly in the oral cavity when the lips and cheeks are retracted. Classification of malocclusion and the variations that occur with each category are described here.

I. NORMAL (IDEAL) OCCLUSION

The ideal mechanical relationship between the teeth of the maxillary arch and the teeth of the mandibular arch is as follows:

BOX 15-1 KEY WORDS: Occlusion

Ankylosis (ang"kĭ-lō'sis): union or consolidation of two similar or dissimilar hard tissues previously adjacent but not attached.

> **Dental ankylosis:** rigid fixation of a tooth to the surrounding alveolus as a result of ossification of the periodontal ligament; prevents eruption and orthodontic movement.

Centric occlusion (ŏ-kloo'zhun): the maximum intercuspation or contact of the teeth of the opposing arches; also called habitual occlusion.

Centric relation: the most unstrained, retruded physiologic relation of the mandible to the maxilla from which lateral movements can be made.

Cephalometer (sef"ah-lom'ĕ-ter): an orienting device for positioning the head for radiographic examination and measurement.

Cephalometric analysis (sef"ah-lō-met'rik): the process of evaluating dental and skeletal relationships by way of measurements obtained directly from the head or from cephalometric radiographs and tracings made from the radiographs.

Cephalostat (sef'ah-lō-stat"): a head-holding instrument used to obtain cephalometric radiographs; head is held in a precisely defined position relative to the film and to the central ray of the x-ray source.

Diastema (dī-ă'stē-mah): a space between two adjacent teeth in the same arch.

Occlusal guard: a removable dental appliance usually made of plastic that covers a dental arch and is designed to minimize the damaging effects of bruxism and other oral habits; also called bite guard, mouth guard, or night guard.

Occlusal prematurity: any contact of opposing teeth that occurs before the desirable intercuspation.

Orthodontic and dentofacial orthopedics: the specialty area of dentistry concerned with the diagnosis, supervision, guidance, and treatment of the growing and mature dentofacial structures; includes conditions that require movement of teeth and the treatment of malrelationships and malformations of the craniofacial complex.

Orthopedics (or"-thō-pē'diks): correction of abnormal form or relationship of bone structures; may be accomplished surgically (orthopedic surgery) or by the application of appliances to stimulate changes in the bone structure through natural physiologic response (orthopedic therapy); orthodontic therapy is orthopedic therapy.

Parafunctional: abnormal or deviated function, as in bruxism.

Pathologic migration: the movement of a tooth out of its natural position as a result of periodontal infection; contrasts with **mesial migration,** which is the physiologic process maintained by tooth proximal contacts in the normal dental arches.

Tongue thrust: the infantile pattern of suckle-swallow movement in which the tongue is placed between the incisor teeth or alveolar ridges; may result in an anterior open bite, deformation of the jaws, and abnormal function.

Trauma from occlusion: injury to the periodontium that results from occlusal forces in excess of the reparative capacity of the attachment apparatus; also called occlusal traumatism.

A. All teeth in maxillary arch are in maximum contact with all teeth in mandibular arch in a definite pattern.

B. Maxillary teeth slightly overlap the mandibular teeth on the facial surfaces.

II. MALOCCLUSION

Any deviation from the physiologically acceptable relationship of the maxillary arch and/or teeth to the mandibular arch and/or teeth.

III. TYPES OF FACIAL PROFILES (Figure 15-1)

A. Mesognathic

Having slightly protruded jaws, which give the facial outline a relatively flat appearance (straight profile).

B. Retrognathic

Having a prominent maxilla and a mandible posterior to its normal relationship (convex profile).

C. Prognathic

Having a prominent, protruded mandible and normal (usually) maxilla (concave profile).

IV. MALRELATIONS OF GROUPS OF TEETH

A. Crossbites

1. *Posterior.* Maxillary or mandibular posterior teeth are either facial or lingual to their normal position. This condition may occur bilaterally or unilaterally (Figure 15-2).
2. *Anterior.* Maxillary incisors are lingual to the mandibular incisors (Figure 15-3).

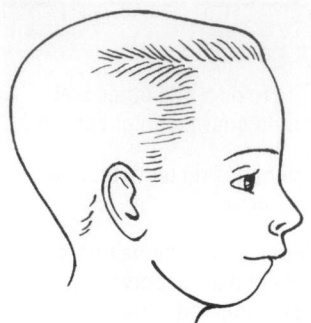

RETROGNATHIC

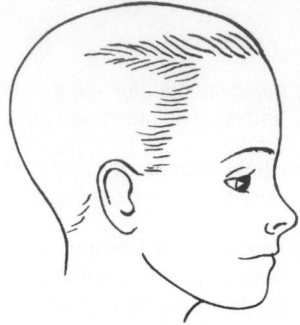

MESOGNATHIC

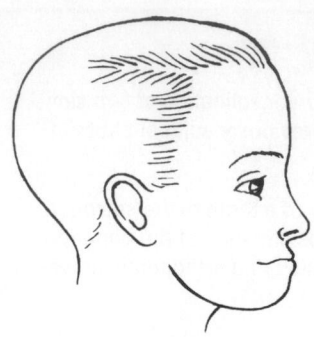

PROGNATHIC

▪ **FIGURE 15-1 Types of Facial Profiles.**

B. Edge-To-Edge Bite

Incisal surfaces of maxillary teeth occlude with incisal surfaces of mandibular teeth instead of overlapping as in normal occlusion (Figure 15-4).

C. End-to-End Bite

Molars and premolars occlude cusp-to-cusp as viewed mesiodistally (Figure 15-5).

D. Open Bite

Lack of occlusal or incisal contact between certain maxillary and mandibular teeth because either or both have failed to reach the line of occlusion. The teeth cannot be brought together, and a space remains as a result of the arching of the line of occlusion (Figure 15-6).

E. Overjet

The horizontal distance between the labioincisal surfaces of the mandibular incisors and the linguoincisal surfaces of the maxillary incisors (Figure 15-7). One way to measure the amount of overjet is to place the tip of a probe on the labial surface of the mandibular incisor and, holding it horizontally against the incisal edge of the maxillary tooth, read the distance in millimeters.

F. Underjet

Maxillary teeth are lingual to mandibular teeth. The horizontal distance between the labioincisal surfaces of the maxillary incisors and the linguoincisal surfaces of the mandibular incisors (Figure 15-8).

G. Overbite

Overbite, or vertical overlap, is the vertical distance by which the maxillary incisors overlap the mandibular incisors.

1. *Normal Overbite.* An overbite is considered normal when the incisal edges of the maxillary teeth are within the incisal third of the mandibular teeth, as shown in Figure 15-9 in side view and in Figure 15-11A in anterior view.
2. *Moderate Overbite.* An overbite is considered

moderate when the incisal edges of the maxillary teeth appear within the middle third of the mandibular teeth (Figure 15-11B).

3. *Deep (Severe) Overbite.* An overbite is considered deep (severe) when the incisal edges of the maxillary teeth are within the cervical third of the mandibular teeth (Figure 15-11C). When in addition the incisal edges of the mandibular teeth are in contact with the maxillary lingual gingival tissue, the overbite is called very deep. A side view of very deep overbite is shown in Figure 15-10.
4. *Clinical Examination of Overbite.* Normal, moderate, and severe anterior overbite are observed directly when the teeth are closed in occlusion. With the posterior teeth closed together, the lips can be retracted and the teeth observed as in Figure 15-11. The degree of anterior overbite is judged by the position of the incisal edge of the maxillary teeth: normal (slight), within the incisal third of the mandibular incisors; moderate overbite, within the middle third; and severe overbite, within the cervical third.

    By placing a mouth mirror under the incisal edge of the maxillary teeth, one can sometimes see the mandibular teeth in contact with the maxillary palatal gingiva. When contact is not visible, an examination of the lingual gingiva may reveal teeth prints or at least enlargement and redness from the contact.

V. MALPOSITIONS OF INDIVIDUAL TEETH

A. Labioversion

A tooth that has assumed a position labial to normal.

B. Linguoversion

Position lingual to normal.

C. Buccoversion

Position buccal to normal.

D. Supraversion

Elongated above the line of occlusion.

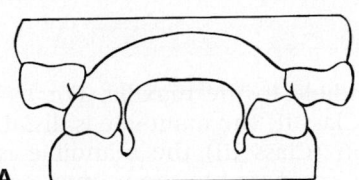 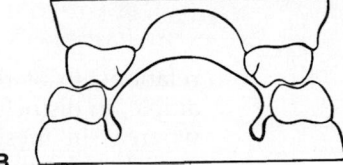 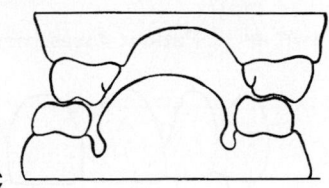

FIGURE 15-2 Posterior Crossbite. (A) Mandibular teeth lingual to normal position. **(B)** Mandibular teeth facial to normal position. **(C)** Unilateral crossbite: right side, normal; left side, mandibular teeth facial to normal position.

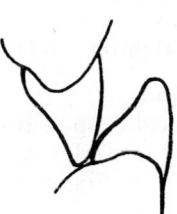

FIGURE 15-3 Anterior Crossbite. Maxillary anterior teeth are lingual to the mandibular anterior teeth. Anterior crossbite occurs in Angle's Class III malocclusion.

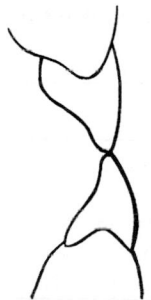

FIGURE 15-4 Edge-to-Edge Bite. Incisal surfaces occlude.

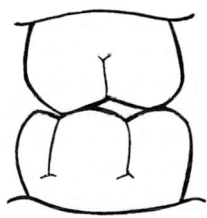

FIGURE 15-5 End-to-End Bite. Molars in cusp-to-cusp occlusion as viewed from the facial.

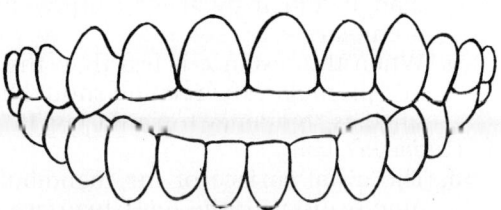

FIGURE 15-6 Open Bite. Lack of incisal contact. Posterior teeth in normal occlusion.

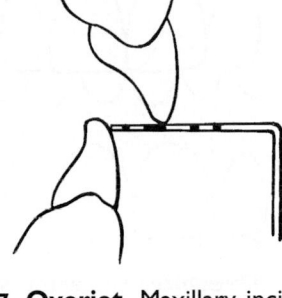

FIGURE 15-7 Overjet. Maxillary incisors are labial to the mandibular incisors. Measurable horizontal distance is evident between the incisal edge of the maxillary incisors and the incisal edge of the mandibular incisors. A periodontal probe can be used to measure for recording the distance.

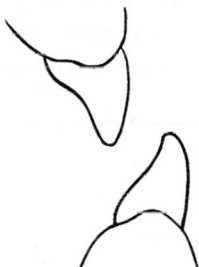

FIGURE 15-8 Underjet. Maxillary incisors are lingual to the mandibular incisors. Measurable horizontal distance is evident between the incisal edges of the maxillary incisors and the incisal edges of the mandibular incisors.

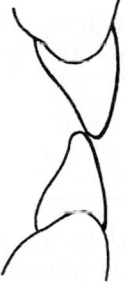

FIGURE 15-9 Normal Overbite. Profile view to show position of incisal edge of maxillary tooth within the incisal third of the facial surface of the mandibular incisor.

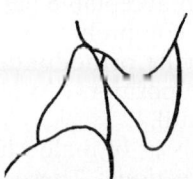

FIGURE 15-10 Deep (Severe) Anterior Overbite. Incisal edge of maxillary tooth is at the level of the cervical third of the facial surface of the mandibular anterior tooth. See the facial view in Figure 15-11C.

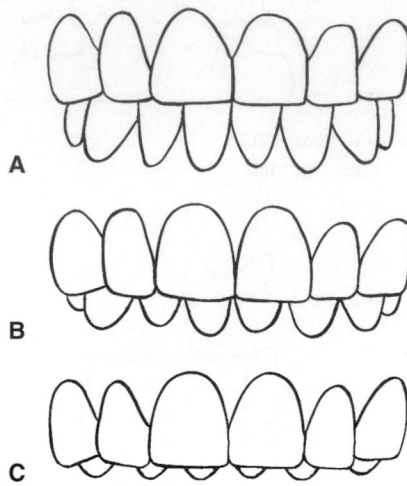

FIGURE 15-11 Overbite, Anterior View. (A) Normal overbite: incisal edges of the maxillary teeth are within the incisal third of the facial surfaces of the mandibular teeth. **(B)** Moderate overbite: incisal edges of maxillary teeth are within the middle third of the facial surfaces of the mandibular teeth. **(C)** Severe overbite: the incisal edges of the maxillary teeth are within the cervical third of the facial of the mandibular teeth. When the incisal edges of the mandibular teeth are in contact with the maxillary lingual gingival tissue, the overbite is considered very severe. See the profile view in Figure 15-10.

E. Torsiversion
Turned or rotated.

F. Infraversion
Depressed below the line of occlusion, for example, primary tooth that is submerged or ankylosed.

DETERMINATION OF THE CLASSIFICATION OF MALOCCLUSION

The determination of the classification of occlusion is based upon the principles of Edward H. Angle, presented in the early 1900s. He defined normal occlusion as "the normal relations of the occlusal inclined planes of the teeth when the jaws are closed"[1] and based his system of classification upon the relationship of the first permanent molars.

Although authorities have since agreed that the maxillary first permanent molars do not occupy a fixed position in the dental arch, Angle's system serves to provide an acceptable basis for a useful classification. A more comprehensive picture of malocclusion is made by the orthodontist, who studies the relationships of the position of the teeth to the jaws, the face, and the skull.

Three general classes of malocclusion are described in the following sections. These are designated by Roman numerals. Because the mandible is movable and the maxilla is stationary, the classes describe the relationship of the mandible to the maxilla. For example, in distoclusion (Class II) the mandible is distal, whereas in mesioclusion (Class III) the mandible is mesial to the maxilla, as compared to the normal position.

I. NORMAL (IDEAL) OCCLUSION (Figure 15-12)

A. Facial Profile
Mesognathic (Figure 15-1).

B. Molar Relation
The mesiobuccal cusp of the maxillary first permanent molar occludes with the buccal groove of the mandibular first permanent molar.

C. Canine Relation
The maxillary permanent canine occludes with the distal half of the mandibular canine and the mesial half of the mandibular first premolar.

II. MALOCCLUSION

A. Class I or Neutroclusion (Figure 15-12)
1. *Facial Profile:* Same as normal occlusion.
2. *Molar Relation:* Same as normal occlusion.
3. *Canine Relation:* Same as normal occlusion.
4. *Malposition of Individual Teeth or Groups of Teeth*
5. *General Types of Conditions That Frequently Occur in Class I:*
   a. Crowded maxillary or mandibular anterior teeth.
   b. Protruded or retruded maxillary incisors.
   c. Anterior crossbite.
   d. Posterior crossbite.
   e. Mesial drift of molars resulting from premature loss of teeth.

B. Class II or Distoclusion (Figure 15-12)
1. *Description:* Mandibular teeth posterior to normal position in their relation to the maxillary teeth.
2. *Facial Profile:* Retrognathic; maxilla protrudes; lower lip is full and often rests between the maxillary and mandibular incisors; the mandible appears retruded or weak (Figure 15-1, retrognathic).
3. *Molar Relation*
   a. The buccal groove of the mandibular first permanent molar is distal to the mesiobuccal cusp of the maxillary first permanent molar by at least the width of a premolar.
   b. When the distance is less than the width of a premolar, the relation should be classified as "tendency toward Class II."
4. *Canine Relation*
   a. The distal surface of the mandibular canine is distal to the mesial surface of the maxillary canine by at least the width of a premolar.
   b. When the distance is less than the width

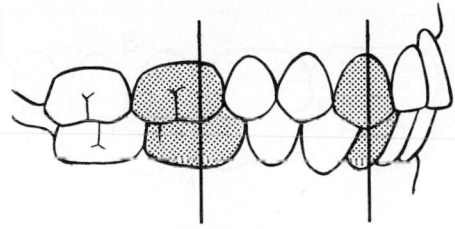

Normal (Ideal) Occlusion

Molar relationship: mesiobuccal cusp of maxillary first permanent molar occludes with the buccal groove of the mandibular first permanent molar.

Malocclusion

Class I: Neutroclusion. Molar relationship same as Normal, with malposition of individual teeth or groups of teeth.

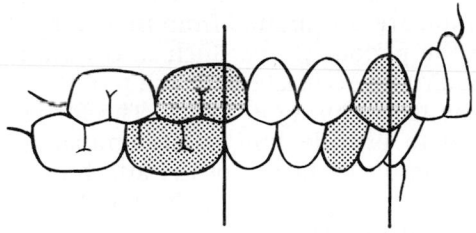

Class II: Distoclusion.

Molar relationship: buccal groove of the mandibular first permanent molar is distal to the mesiobuccal cusp of the maxillary first permanent molar by at least the width of a premolar.

Division 1: mandible is retruded and all maxillary incisors are protruded.

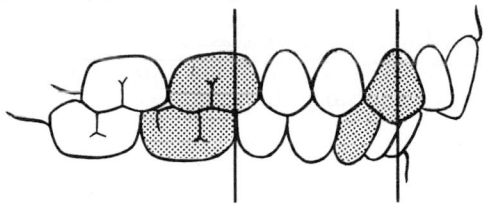

Class II: Distoclusion.

Division 2: mandible is retruded and one or more maxillary incisors are retruded.

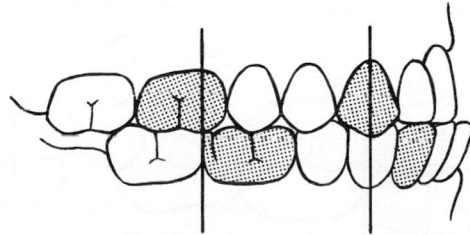

Class III: Mesioclusion.

Molar relationship: buccal groove of the mandibular first permanent molar is mesial to the mesiobuccal cusp of the maxillary first permanent molar by at least the width of a premolar.

■ FIGURE 15-12 Normal Occlusion and Classification of Malocclusion.

of a premolar, the relation should be classified as "tendency toward Class II."

5. *Class II, Division 1*
   a. Description: The mandible is retruded and all maxillary incisors are protruded.
   b. General types of conditions that frequently occur in Class II, Division 1 malocclusion: Deep overbite, excessive overjet, abnormal muscle function (lips), short mandible, or short upper lip.
6. *Class II, Division 2*
   a. Description: The mandible is retruded, and one or more maxillary incisors are retruded.
   b. General types of conditions that frequently occur in Class II, Division 2 malocclusion: Maxillary lateral incisors protrude while both central incisors retrude, crowded maxillary anterior teeth, or deep overbite.
7. *Subdivision:* One side is Class I, the other side is Class II (may be Division 1 or 2).

C. Class III or Mesioclusion (Figure 15-12)
1. *Description:* Mandibular teeth are anterior to normal position in relation to maxillary teeth.
2. *Facial Profile:* Prognathic; lower lip and mandible are prominent (Figure 15-1).
3. *Molar Relation*
   a. The buccal groove of the mandibular first permanent molar is mesial to the mesiobuccal cusp of the maxillary first permanent molar by at least the width of a premolar.
   b. When the distance is less than the width of a premolar, the relation should be classified as "tendency toward Class III."
4. *Canine Relation*
   a. The distal surface of the mandibular canine is mesial to the mesial surface of the maxillary canine by at least the width of a premolar.
   b. When the distance is less than the width of a premolar, the relation should be classified as "tendency toward Class III."
5. *General Types of Conditions That Frequently Occur in Class III Malocclusion:*
   a. True Class III: Maxillary incisors are lingual to mandibular incisors in an anterior crossbite (Figure 15-3).
   b. Maxillary and mandibular incisors are in edge-to-edge occlusion.
   c. Mandibular incisors are very crowded, but lingual to maxillary incisors.

OCCLUSION OF THE PRIMARY TEETH[2]

I. NORMAL (IDEAL)

A. Primary Canine Relation
Same as permanent dentition.

1. *With Primate Spaces**
   a. Mandibular: Between mandibular canine and first molar (Figure 15-13*A*).
   b. Maxillary: Between maxillary lateral incisor and canine (Figure 15-13*B*).
2. *Without Primate Spaces.* Closed arches.

B. Second Primary Molar Relation

The mesiobuccal cusp of the maxillary second primary molar occludes with the buccal groove of the mandibular second primary molar.

1. *Variations in Distal Surfaces Relationships.* Terminal step.
   a. The distal surface of the mandibular primary molar is mesial to that of the maxillary, thereby forming a mesial step (Figure 15-14*A*).
   b. Morphologic variation in molar size; maxillary and mandibular primary molars have approximately the same mesiodistal width.
2. *Variation.* Terminal plane.
   a. The distal surfaces of the maxillary and mandibular primary molars are on same vertical plane (Figure 15-14*B*).
   b. The maxillary molar is narrower mesiodistally than the mandibular molar (occurs in many patients).
3. *Effects on Occlusion of First Permanent Molars*
   a. Terminal step: First permanent molar erupts directly into proper occlusion (Figure 15-14*A*).
   b. Terminal plane: First permanent molars erupt end to end. With mandibular primate space, early mesial shift of primary molars into the primate space occurs, and the permanent mandibular molar shifts into proper occlusion. Without primate spaces, late mesial shift of permanent mandibular molar into proper occlusion occurs, following exfoliation of second primary molar (Figure 15-14*B*).

II. MALOCCLUSION OF THE PRIMARY TEETH

Same as permanent dentition.

FUNCTIONAL OCCLUSION

In contrast to static occlusion, which pertains to the relationship of the teeth when the jaws are closed, functional occlusion consists of all contacts during

---

****Primate space:** a diastema or gap in the tooth row occasionally observed in the human primary dentition. It is characteristic of nearly all species of primates except man. The maxillary primate spaces accommodate the mandibular canines, and the mandibular primate spaces accommodate the maxillary canines when the teeth are in occlusion. As a reduction in the length of canines accompanied man's evolution, the canines no longer protruded beyond the occlusal level. The diastema (primate space) was no longer functional.

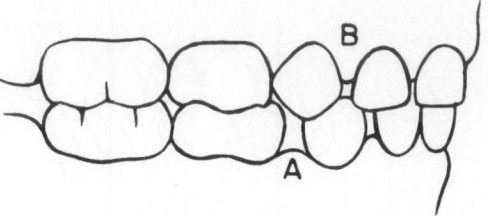

☐ **FIGURE 15-13 Primary Teeth With Primate Spaces. (A)** Mandibular primate space between canine and first molar. **(B)** Maxillary primate space between the lateral incisor and the canine.

chewing, swallowing, or other normal action. Functional occlusion is associated with performance.

The pressures or forces created by the muscles of mastication are transmitted from the teeth, after contact, to the periodontium. Such forces are necessary to maintain the occlusal relationship of the teeth and guide the teeth during eruption. The forces are also necessary to provide functional stimulation for the preservation of the health of the attachment apparatus, namely, the periodontal ligament, the cementum, and the alveolar bone.

I. TYPES OF OCCLUSAL CONTACTS

A. Functional Contacts

Functional contacts are the normal contacts that are made between the maxillary teeth and the mandibular teeth during chewing and swallowing. Each contact is momentary, so the total contact time is only a few minutes each day.

B. Parafunctional Contacts

Parafunctional contacts are those made outside the normal range of function.

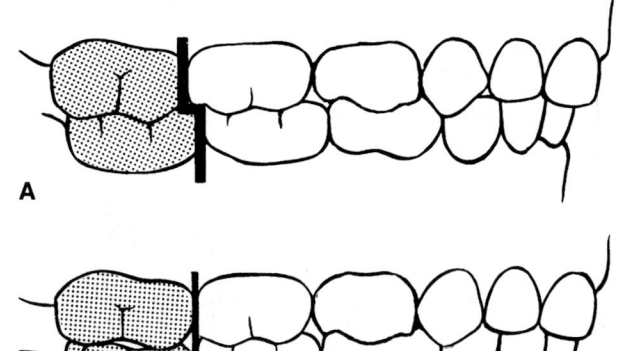

☐ **FIGURE 15-14 Eruption Patterns of the First Permanent Molars. (A)** Terminal step. The distal surface of mandibular second primary molar is mesial to the distal surface of the maxillary primary molar. **(B)** Terminal plane. The distal surfaces of the mandibular and maxillary second primary molars are on the same vertical plane; permanent molars erupt in end-to-end occlusion.

1. They result from occlusal habits and neuroses.
2. They are potentially injurious to the periodontal supporting structures, but only in the presence of bacterial plaque and inflammatory factors.
3. They create wear facets and attrition on the teeth. A facet is a shiny, flat, worn spot on the surface of a tooth, frequently on the side of a cusp.
4. They can be divided into the following:
   a. Tooth-to-tooth contacts: Bruxism, clenching, tapping.
   b. Tooth-to-hard-object contacts: Nail biting; occupational use of such objects as tacks or pins; use of smoking equipment, such as a pipe stem or hard cigarette holder.
   c. Tooth-to-oral-tissues contacts: Lip or cheek biting.

II. PROXIMAL CONTACTS

Proximal contacts serve to stabilize the position of teeth in the dental arches and to prevent food impaction between the teeth. Attrition or wear of the teeth occurs at the proximal contacts.

A. Drifting
When proximal contact is lost, teeth can drift into spaces created by unreplaced missing teeth. There is also a natural tendency for mesial migration of teeth toward the midline. In the absence of disease, the surrounding periodontal tissues adapt to repositioned teeth (see Figure 12-19, page 220, and Figures 25-5 and 25-6, pages 398 and 399).

B. Pathologic Migration
With destruction of the supporting structures of a tooth as a result of periodontal infection, and with a force to move a tooth weakened by disease and bone loss, migration of the tooth can result. *Pathologic migration occurs when disease is present; in contrast, drifting is migration with a healthy periodontium.*

TRAUMA FROM OCCLUSION

Periodontal tissue injury caused by repeated occlusal forces that exceed the physiologic limits of tissue tolerance is called *trauma from occlusion*. Other names are periodontal traumatism, occlusal traumatism, and periodontal trauma.

I. TYPES OF TRAUMA FROM OCCLUSION

A. Primary
When the excessive occlusal force is exerted on a tooth with normal bone support, *primary trauma from occlusion* results. An example is the effect of a new restoration placed above the line of occlusion.

B. Secondary
When the excessive occlusal force is exerted on a tooth with bone loss and inadequate alveolar bone support, and the ability of the tooth to withstand occlusal forces is impaired, *secondary trauma from occlusion* results. When a tooth has lost the support of the surrounding bone, even the pressures of what are usually considered normal occlusal forces may create lesions of trauma from occlusion.

II. EFFECTS OF TRAUMA FROM OCCLUSION

The attachment apparatus (periodontal ligament, cementum, and alveolar bone) has as its main purpose the maintenance of the tooth in the socket in a functional state. In a healthy situation, occlusal pressures and forces during chewing and swallowing are readily dispersed or absorbed and no unusual effects are produced.

A. Excess Forces
When the forces of occlusion are greater than can be taken care of by the attachment apparatus, damage can result. Circulatory disturbances, tissue destruction from crushing under pressure, bone resorption, and other pathologic processes are initiated.

B. Relation to Inflammatory Factors
1. *Trauma from occlusion does not cause gingivitis, periodontitis, or pocket formation.* The steps in the development of inflammatory disease and pockets were outlined on pages 225 to 227.
2. In the presence of inflammatory disease, the existing periodontal destruction may be aggravated or promoted by trauma from occlusion.

III. METHODS OF APPLICATION OF EXCESS PRESSURE

To understand the nature of the occlusal forces that can cause periodontal trauma from occlusion, it is helpful to recognize types of tooth contacts that can overburden a tooth or group of teeth.[3]

A. Individual Teeth That Touch Before Full Closure
The contact is premature and may put excessive force on an individual tooth.

B. Two or Only a Few Teeth in Contact During Movement of the Jaw
The teeth involved receive a disproportionate amount of force.

C. Initial Contacts on Inclined Planes of Cusps
Following the initial contact, when the teeth are brought together in a closed position, there

may be excess pressure on the teeth where initial contact was made.

D. Heavy Forces Not in a Vertical or Axial Direction

Normal occlusal relationships imply a direct cusp-to-fossa position during closure, with the force of occlusion in a vertical direction toward the tooth apex and parallel with the long axis. When pressures are exerted laterally or horizontally, excess force is placed on the periodontal attachment apparatus.

E. Increased Frequency, Intensity, and Duration of Contacts

In the presence of parafunctional habits, such as bruxism, clenching, tapping, or biting objects, many more than the usual number of tooth contacts are made each day, and the intensity and duration are altered.

IV. RECOGNITION OF SIGNS OF TRAUMA FROM OCCLUSION

No one clinical or radiographic finding clearly defines the presence of trauma from occlusion. Diagnosis of the condition is complex. The possible observations listed as follows should be looked for specifically and recorded for evaluation and correlation with the patient history and all other clinical determinations.

A. Clinical Findings That May Occur in Trauma From Occlusion

1. Tooth mobility.
2. Fremitus.
3. Sensitivity of teeth to pressure and/or percussion.
4. Pathologic migration.
5. Wear facets or atypical occlusal wear.
6. Open contacts related to food impaction.
7. Neuromuscular disturbances in the muscles of mastication. In severe cases muscle spasm can occur.
8. Temporomandibular joint symptoms.

B. Radiographic Findings

Characteristics that may occur in trauma from occlusion include:

1. Widened periodontal ligament spaces, particularly angular thickening (triangulation). This finding frequently occurs in conjunction with tooth mobility.
2. Angular (vertical) bone loss in localized areas (see Figure 12-20, page 220).
3. Root resorption.
4. Furcation involvement.
5. Thickened lamina dura. Although related to occlusal forces, thickened lamina dura should not be considered a detrimental or destructive effect of trauma from occlusion. It may be a defense reaction to strengthen tooth support against occlusal forces. Thickened lamina dura is frequently associated with teeth that have undergone orthodontic treatment.

TECHNICAL HINTS

I. Observe the facial profile as the patient enters and is seated in the dental chair to estimate the classification of occlusion before examination of the teeth.
II. Avoid mention of a dentofacial deformity that would make the patient feel self-conscious.
III. Avoid suggesting to the patient or a parent the possible procedures the orthodontist may use in treatment because complications become known only after the complete diagnosis.
IV. Closing to centric relation can be performed most effectively by instructing the patient to curl the tongue and to try to hold the tip of the tongue as far back as possible while closing.
V. When a small child has difficulty in occluding, the clinician may firmly but gently press the cushions of the thumbs on the mucous membrane over the pterygomandibular raphe, holding the thumbs between the cheek and buccal surfaces of the teeth as the patient is requested to close.
VI. Prepare mouth guards for patients in active sports.
VII. Study the occlusion of the patient with removable dentures with the dentures in place in the mouth.

FACTORS TO TEACH THE PATIENT

I. Interpretation of the *general* purposes of orthodontic care (function and esthetics) to patients referred by the dentist to an orthodontist.
   A. Dependence of masticatory efficiency on the occlusion of the teeth.
   B. Influence of masticatory efficiency on food selection in the diet.
   C. Influence of masticatory efficiency and diet on the nutritional status of the body and oral health.
II. Interpretation of the dentist's suggestions for the correction of oral habits.
III. The space-maintaining function of the primary teeth in prevention of malocclusion of permanent teeth.
IV. The role of malocclusion as a predisposing factor for bacterial plaque retention in the formation of dental caries and periodontal infections.
V. Bacterial plaque removal methods for reducing dental calculus and soft deposit retention in areas where teeth are crowded, displaced, or otherwise not in normal occlusion.
VI. The relation of the occlusion and the position

of the teeth to the patient's personal oral care procedures.

A. Selection of the proper type of toothbrush.
B. Application of thorough toothbrushing method or methods.
C. Use of dental floss.

VII. Specific reasons for frequency of maintenance examinations when related to malocclusion and while in the process of having orthodontic therapy.

REFERENCES

1. **Angle,** E.H.: *Malocclusion of the Teeth,* 7th ed. Philadelphia, S.S. White, 1907.
2. **Baume,** L.J.: Physiological Tooth Migration and Its Significance for the Development of the Occlusion, I. The Biogenetic Course of the Deciduous Dentition, *J. Dent. Res., 29,* 123, April, 1950; II. The Biogenesis of the Accessional Dentition, *J. Dent. Res., 29,* 331, June, 1950; III. The Biogenesis of the Successional Dentition, *J. Dent. Res., 29,* 338, June, 1950; IV. The Biogenesis of Overbite, *J. Dent. Res., 29,* 440, August, 1950.
3. **Allen,** D.L., McFall, W.T., and Jenzano, J.W.: *Periodontics for the Dental Hygienist,* 4th ed. Philadelphia, Lea & Febiger, 1987, pp. 85–86.

SUGGESTED READINGS

Baker, I.M.: Record Taking in the Orthodontic Office, *Dent. Assist., 60,* 25, March/April, 1991.

Brezniak, N. and Wasserstein, A.: Root Resorption After Orthodontic Treatment: Part 1. Literature Review, *Am. J. Orthod. Dentofacial Orthop., 103,* 62, January, 1993.

Bresniak, N. and Wasserstein, A.: Root Resorption After Orthodontic Treatment: Part 2. Literature Review, *Am. J. Orthod. Dentofacial Orthop., 103,* 138, February, 1993.

Burden, D.J., Garvin, J.W., and Patterson, C.C.: Pilot Study of an Orthodontic Treatment Need Learning Package for General Dental Practitioners, *Br. Dent. J., 179,* 300, October 21, 1995.

Dyer, G.S., Harris, E.F., and Vaden, J.L.: Age Effects on Orthodontic Treatment: Adolescents Contrasted With Adults, *Am. J. Orthod. Dentofacial Orthop., 100,* 523, December, 1991.

Fink, D.F. and Smith, R.J.: The Duration of Orthodontic Treatment, *Am. J. Orthod. Dentofacial Orthop., 102,* 45, July, 1992.

Finkbeiner, R.L., Nelson, L.S., and Killebrew, J.: Case Reports. Accidental Orthodontic Elastic Band-induced Periodontitis: Orthodontic and Laser Treatment, *J. Am. Dent. Assoc., 128,* 1565, November, 1997.

Khan, R.S. and Horrocks, E.N.: A Study of Adult Orthodontic Patients and Their Treatment, *Br. J. Orthod., 18,* 183, August, 1991.

Machen, D.E.: Legal Aspects of Orthodontic Practice: Risk Management Concepts. Oral Hygiene Assessment: Plaque Accumulation, Gingival Inflammation, Decalcification, and Caries, *Am. J. Orthod. Dentofacial Orthop., 100,* 93, July, 1991.

Martinez-Canut, P., Carrasquer, A., Magan, R., and Lorca, A.: A Study on Factors Associated with Pathologic Tooth Migration, *J. Clin. Periodontol., 24,* 492, July, 1997.

Massler, M.: Oral Habits: Development and Management, *J. Pedod., 7,* 109, Winter, 1983.

Newman, G.V.: Limited Orthodontics for the Older Population: Multidisciplinary Modalities, *Am. J. Orthod. Dentofacial Orthop., 101,* 281, March, 1992.

Ngan, P. and Fields, H.W.: Open Bite: A Review of Etiology and Management, *Pediatr. Dent., 19,* 91, March/April, 1997.

Robinson, H.B.G. and Miller, A.S.: *Color Atlas of Oral Pathology,* 5th ed. Philadelphia, J.B. Lippincott Co., 1990, pp. 52, 83–84, 93, 95.

Roe, S.: Treatment Recommendations for Nonnutritive Sucking Habits, *J. Pract. Hyg., 7,* 11, January/February, 1998.

Torres, H.O., Ehrlich, A., Bird, D., and Dietz, E.: *Modern Dental Assisting,* 5th ed. Philadelphia, W.B. Saunders Co., 1995, pp. 535–559.

Bacterial Plaque and Other Soft Deposits

Dental caries and gingival and periodontal infections are caused by microorganisms in microbial or bacterial plaques. Disease-producing microorganisms attach to the tooth surfaces and colonize. They bring about carious lesions of the enamel and root surfaces, in pits and fissures, and on smooth surfaces (pages 239 to 242). They also bring about inflammatory changes in the periodontium that can lead to destruction of tissues and loss of attachment. The morphologic forms of bacteria are shown in Figure 16-1.

During the clinical examination of the teeth and surrounding soft tissues, the soft and hard deposits that accumulate on the teeth and within the sulci or pockets must be recognized and assessed. From the findings, an initial care plan can be formulated based on the individual needs of the patient. Key words are defined in Box 16-1.

The soft deposits are acquired pellicle or cuticle, bacterial plaque, materia alba, and food debris, each of which is an entity, and the terms should not be interchanged. The hard, calcified deposit on teeth is dental calculus, which is described in Chapter 17. A classification with definitions of the dental deposits is presented in Table 16-1.[1]

ACQUIRED PELLICLE

The acquired pellicle is a tenacious membranous layer that is amorphous, acellular, and organic and that forms over exposed tooth surfaces, as well as over restorations and dental calculus. Its thickness, which varies from 0.1 to 0.8 μm, usually is greater near the gingiva.

I. FORMATION

Within minutes after all external material has been removed from the tooth surfaces with an abrasive, the acquired pellicle begins to form. It is composed

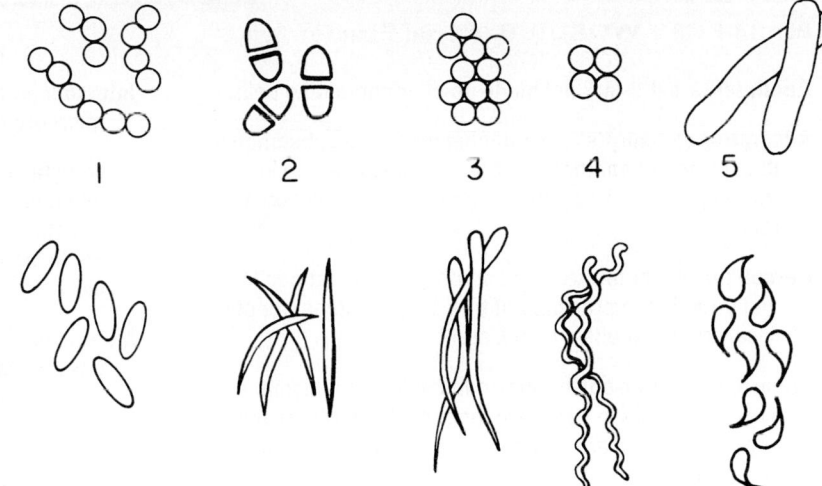

FIGURE 16-1 Morphologic Forms of Bacteria. (1) Streptococci. (2) Diplococci. (3) Staphylococci. (4) Sarcina. (5) Bacilli. (6) Coccobacilli. (7) Fusiform bacilli. (8) Filamentous bacilli. (9) Spirochetes. (10) Vibrios. (From Hammond, B.: Bacterial structure and function, in Schuster, G.S., ed.: *Oral Microbiology and Infectious Disease,* 2nd student ed. Toronto, B.C. Decker, 1988, p. 23.)

TABLE 16-1 Tooth Deposits

Category	Tooth Deposit	Description	Derivation
Nonmineralized	Acquired pellicle	Translucent, homogeneous, thin, unstructured film covering and adherent to the surfaces of the teeth, restorations, calculus, and other surfaces in the oral cavity	Supragingival: saliva Subgingival: gingival sulcus fluid
	Microbial (bacterial) plaque	Dense, organized bacterial systems embedded in an intermicrobial matrix that adhere closely to the teeth, calculus, and other surfaces in the oral cavity Water irrigation removes only the outer layer of loose organisms	Colonization of oral micro-organisms
	Materia alba	Loosely adherent, unstructured, white or grayish-white mass of oral debris and bacteria that lies over bacterial plaque Vigorous rinsing and water irrigation can remove materia alba	Incidental accumulation
	Food debris	Unstructured, loosely attached particulate matter Self-cleansing activity of tongue and saliva and rinsing vigorously remove debris	Food retention following eating
Mineralized	Calculus	Calcified bacterial plaque; hard, tenacious mass that forms on the clinical crowns of the natural teeth and on dentures and other appliances	Plaque mineralization
	a. supragingival	Occurs coronal to the margin of the gingiva; is covered with bacterial plaque	Supragingival: source of minerals is saliva
	b. subgingival	Occurs apical to the margin of the gingiva; is covered with bacterial plaque	Subgingival: source of minerals is gingival sulcus fluid

Adapted from Schroeder, H. E.: *Formation and Inhibition of Dental Calculus.* Vienna, Hans Huber, 1969, pp. 14–15.

BOX 16-I KEY WORDS: Bacterial Plaque

Acellular (ā-sel′ū-lar): not made up of or containing cells.

Adsorption (ad-sorp′shun): attachment of one substance to the surface of another; the action of a substance in attracting and holding other materials or particles on its surface.

Aerobe (ar′ōb): heterotrophic microorganism that can live and grow in the presence of free oxygen; some are obligate, others facultative; *adj.* aerobic.

Anaerobe (an-a′er-ōb): heterotrophic microorganism that lives and grows in complete (or almost complete) absence of oxygen; some are obligate, others facultative; *adj.* anaerobic.

Biofilm: matrix-enclosed bacterial populations adherent to each other and/or to surfaces or interfaces.

Calculogenesis (kăl″kū-lō-jen′ĕ-sis): formation of calculus.

Calculogenic: adjective applied to bacterial plaque that is conducive to the formation of calculus.

Cariogenesis (kăr″ē-ō-jĕn′ĕ-sis): development of dental caries.

Cariogenic (kăr″ē-ō-jĕn′ik): adjective to indicate a conduciveness to the initiation of dental caries, such as a cariogenic plaque or a cariogenic food.

Facultative (fak′ul-tā″tĭv): able to live under more than one specific set of environmental conditions; contrast with **obligate.**

Flora (flo′rah): the collective organisms of a given locale.

Oral flora: the various bacteria and other microscopic organisms that inhabit the oral cavity. The mouth has an indigenous flora, meaning those organisms that are native to that area of the body. Certain organisms specifically reside in certain parts, for example, on the tongue, on the mucosa, or in the gingival sulcus.

Heterotrophic (het″er-ō-trōf′ik): not self-sustaining; feeding on others.

Intermicrobial matrix: material present between bacteria in dental plaque; derived from saliva, gingival exudate, and microorganisms.

Infection (in-fek′-shun): invasion and multiplication of a microorganism in body tissues.

Leukocyte (loo′kō-sīt): white blood corpuscle capable of ameboid movement; functions to protect the body against infection and disease. (For a description of the various white blood cells, see page 869, and Figure 59-1, page 867.)

Materia alba (mah-ter′ē-ah al′bah): white or cream-colored cheesy mass that can collect over bacterial plaque on unclean, neglected teeth; it is composed of food debris, mucin, bacteria (see text page 274).

Maturation (mach″u-ra′shun): stage or process of attaining maximal development; become mature.

Microbiota (mī″krō-bī-ō′tah): the microscopic living organisms of a region.

Microorganism (mī″krō-or′gan-izm): minute living organisms, usually microscopic; includes bacteria, rickettsiae, viruses, fungi, and protozoa.

Mycoplasma (mī″kō-plaz′mah): pleomorphic, gram-negative bacteria that lack cell walls; many are regular oral cavity residents; some are pathogenic.

Obligate (ob′lĭ-gāt): ability to survive only in a particular environment; opposite of **facultative.**

Parasite (par′ah-sīt): plant or animal that lives upon or within another living organism and draws its nourishment therefrom; may be obligate or facultative; *adj.* parasitic.

Pathogen (path′ō-jen): disease-producing agent or microorganism; *adj.* pathogenic.

Pleomorphism (plē″ō-mor′fism): assumption of various distinct forms by a single organism or within a species; *adj.* pleomorphic.

Saprophyte (sap′rō-fīt): any organism, such as bacteria, that lives upon dead or decaying organic matter.

---

primarily of glycoproteins from the saliva that are selectively adsorbed by the hydroxyapatite of the tooth surface. The adsorbed material becomes a highly insoluble coating over the teeth, calculus deposits, restorations, and complete and partial dentures.

II. TYPES OF PELLICLES[2]

A. Surface Pellicle, Unstained

The unstained pellicle is clear, translucent, in-

soluble, and not readily visible until a disclosing agent has been applied. When stained with a disclosing agent, it appears thin, with a pale staining that contrasts with the thicker, darker staining of bacterial plaque.

B. Surface Pellicle, Stained

Unstained pellicle can take on extrinsic stain and become brown, grayish, or other colors as described on page 288.

C. Subsurface Pellicle

Surface pellicle is continuous with subsurface pellicle that is embedded in tooth structure, particularly where the tooth surface is partially demineralized.[3]

III. SIGNIFICANCE OF PELLICLE

A. Protective

Pellicle appears to provide a barrier against acids; thus it may aid in reducing dental caries attack.[3]

B. Lubrication

Keeps surfaces moist; prevents drying.

C. Nidus for Bacteria

Pellicle participates in plaque formation by aiding the adherence of microorganisms.

D. Attachment of Calculus

One mode of calculus attachment is by the acquired pellicle (page 281).

BACTERIAL PLAQUE

Microbial dental plaque, commonly referred to as bacterial plaque, is a dense, nonmineralized, complex mass of colonies in a gel-like intermicrobial matrix. It adheres firmly to the acquired pellicle and hence to the teeth, calculus, and fixed and removable restorations.

The term *microbial dental plaque* is more accurate than "bacterial plaque" because microorganisms other than bacteria can be found. The organisms may include mycoplasmas, yeasts, protozoa, and viruses. Characteristics of supragingival and subgingival plaques are shown in Table 16-2.

I. STAGES IN THE FORMATION OF PLAQUE

Plaque is formed in three basic steps, namely, pellicle formation, bacterial colonization, and plaque maturation (Figure 16-2). Plaque formation does not occur randomly but involves a series of complex interactions.

A. Formation of a Pellicle

The pellicle forms on the tooth surface by selective adsorption of protein components from the saliva.

B. Bacteria Attach to the Pellicle

Initial attachment of bacteria to the pellicle is by selective adherence of specific bacteria from the oral environment. Innate characteristics of the bacteria and the pellicle determine the adhesive interactions that cause a particular organism to adhere to a particular pellicle.

C. Bacterial Multiplication and Colonization

1. Microcolonies form in layers as the bacteria multiply and grow.
2. With increased size, colonies meet and coalesce to form a continuous bacterial mass.

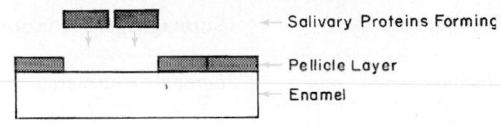

STAGE I Salivary glycoproteins are adsorbed onto dental enamel to form pellicle.

— Salivary Proteins Forming
— Pellicle Layer
— Enamel

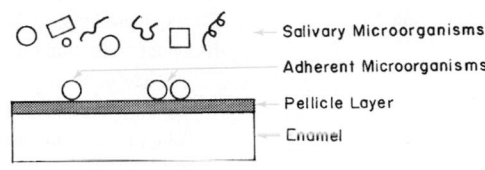

STAGE 2 Selective colonization of the pellicle by microorganisms.

— Salivary Microorganisms
— Adherent Microorganisms
— Pellicle Layer
— Enamel

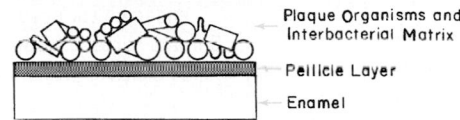

STAGE 3 Growth and maturation of plaque.

— Plaque Organisms and Interbacterial Matrix
— Pellicle Layer
— Enamel

■ FIGURE 16-2 Stages of Plaque Formation. Diagrammatic representation of the three stages of bacterial plaque formation. (Redrawn from Katz, S., McDonald, J.L., and Stookey, G.K.: *Preventive Dentistry,* Upper Montclair, NJ, DCP Publishing, 1977.)

3. Organisms of the first few hours are gram-positive cocci and rods.

D. Plaque Growth and Maturation

The increase in the mass and thickness of plaque results from
1. Continued bacterial multiplication.
2. Continuous adherence of bacteria to the plaque surface.

E. Matrix Formation

The intermicrobial substance is derived mainly from saliva for supragingival plaque, and from gingival sulcus fluid and exudate for subgingival plaque. Other components of the intermicrobial substance are the polysaccharides, glucans, and fructans or levans produced by certain bacteria from dietary sucrose. The polysaccharides are sticky and contribute to the adhesion of the plaque to the teeth.

II. CHANGES IN PLAQUE MICROORGANISMS

Bacterial plaque consists of a complex mixture of microorganisms that occur primarily as microcolonies. The population density is very high and increases as plaque ages. The probability of the development of dental caries and/or gingivitis increases as the number of microorganisms increases.

Changes in the types of organisms occur within plaque as the plaque matures. When oral hygiene practices are discontinued, the numbers of bacteria increase rapidly. The changes in oral flora follow a

TABLE 16-2 Characterisitics of Supragingival and Subgingival Plaque

Characteristic	Supragingival Plaque	Subgingival Plaque
Location	Coronal to the margin of the free gingiva	Apical to the margin of the free gingiva
Origin	Salivary glycoprotein forms pellicle Microorganisms from saliva are selectively attracted to pellicle	Downgrowth of bacteria from supragingival plaque

Distribution	Starts on proximal surfaces and other protected areas
	Heaviest collection on
	    Areas not cleaned daily by patient
	    Cervical third, especially facial
	    Lingual mandibular molars
	    Proximal surfaces
	Pit and fissure plaque
		Shallow pocket: similar to supragingival plaque
		Undisturbed; held by pocket wall
		Attached plaque covers calculus
		Unattached plaque extends to the periodontal attachment

Adhesion	Firmly attached to acquired pellicle, other bacteria, and tooth surfaces Surface bacteria (unattached): loose; washed away by saliva or swallowed	Adheres to tooth surface, subgingival pellicle, and calculus Subgingival flora: loose, floating, motile organisms in deep pocket do not adhere; they are between adherent plaque on tooth and the pocket epithelium
Retention	Rough surfaces of teeth or restorations Malpositioned teeth Carious lesions	Pocket holds plaque against tooth Overhanging margins of fillings that extend into pockets hold plaque

Shape and size	Friction of tongue, cheeks, lips, limits shape and size
	Thickness: thicker at the cervical third and on proximal surfaces
	    Healthy gingiva: thin plaque, 15 to 20 cells thick
	    Chronic gingivitis: thick plaque, 100 to 300 cells thick
		Molded by pocket wall to shape of the tooth surface
		Follows form created by subgingival calculus
		May become thicker as the diseased pocket wall becomes less tight

Structure	Adherent, densely packed microbial layer over pellicle on tooth surface Intermicrobial matrix Onset: small isolated colonies 2 to 5 days; colonies merge to form a covering of plaque	Three layers (see Figure 16–4) 1. Tooth-surface-attached plaque: many gram-positive rods and cocci 2. Unattached plaque in middle: many gram-negative, motile forms; spirochetes; leukocytes 3. Epithelium-attached plaque: gram-negative, motile forms predominate; many leukocytes migrate through epithelium
Microorganisms	Early plaque: primarily gram-positive cocci Older plaque (3 to 4 days): increased numbers of filaments and fusiforms 4 to 9 days undisturbed: more complex flora with rods, filamentous forms 7 to 14 days: vibrios, spirochetes, more gram-negative organisms	Environment conducive to growth of anaerobic population Diseased pocket: primarily gram-negative, motile, spirochetes, rods See Table 16–3
Sources of nutrients for bacterial proliferation	Saliva Ingested food	Tissue fluid (gingival sulcus fluid) Exudate Leukocytes

Significance	Etiology of
	    Gingivitis
	    Supragingival calculus
	    Dental caries (Figure 16–6)
		Etiology of
		    Gingivitis
		    Periodontal infections
		    Subgingival calculus

pattern such as that shown in Figure 16-3. The changes can be described as follows:[4]

A. Days 1 to 2

Early plaque consists primarily of gram-positive cocci. Streptococci, which dominate the bacterial population, include *Streptococcus mutans* and *Streptococcus sanguis.*

B. Days 2 to 4

The cocci still dominate, and increasing num-

bers of gram-positive filamentous forms and slender rods may be seen on the surface of the cocci colonies. Gradually, the filamentous forms grow into the cocci layer and replace many of the cocci. Slow plaque formers continue to form plaque comprised primarily of cocci for a longer time than do fast plaque formers.

C. Days 4 to 7

Filaments increase in numbers, and a more

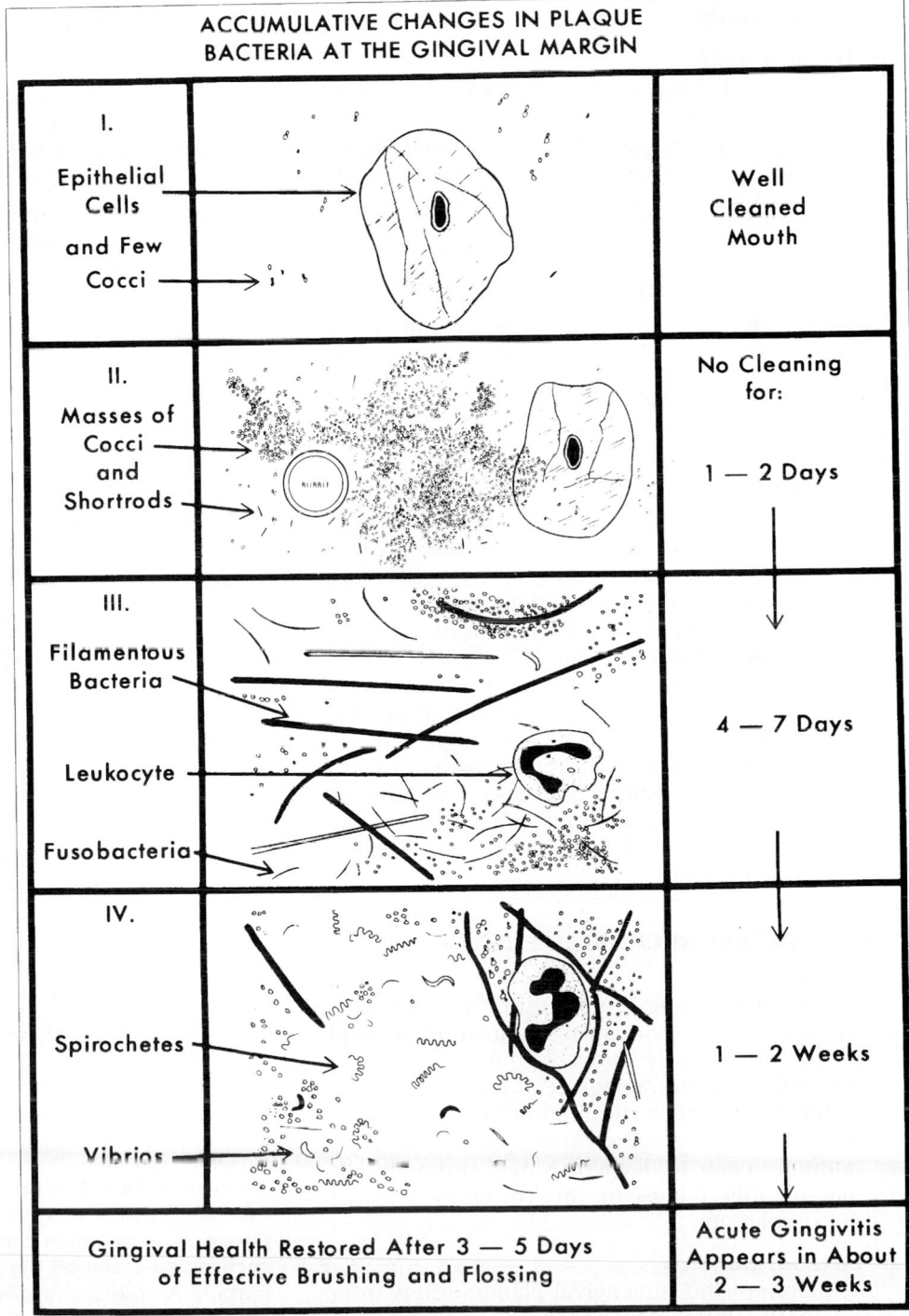

■FIGURE 16-3 **Plaque Microorganisms.** On the right are the time intervals from 1 day to 3 weeks. On the left are the changes in the plaque content that take place as plaque ages. As the numbers of microorganisms increase, the numbers of defense cells (leukocytes) also increase. (From Crawford, J.J.: Microbiology, in Barton, R.E., Matteson, S.R., and Richardson, R.E.: *The Dental Assistant,* 6th ed. Philadelphia, Lea & Febiger, 1988.)

mixed flora begins to appear with rods, filamentous forms, and fusobacteria. Plaque near the gingival margin thickens and develops a more mature flora, with gram-negative spirochetes and vibrios. As plaque spreads coronally, the new plaque has the characteristic coccal forms.

D. Days 7 to 14

Vibrios and spirochetes appear, and the number of white blood cells increases. As plaque matures and thickens, more gram-negative and anaerobic organisms appear. During this period, signs of inflammation are beginning to be observable in the gingiva.

E. Days 14 to 21

Vibrios and spirochetes are prevalent in older plaque, along with cocci and filamentous forms. The densely packed filamentous microorganisms arrange themselves perpendicular to the tooth surface in a palisade. Gingivitis is evident clinically.

III. EXPERIMENTAL GINGIVITIS[4]

Gingivitis develops in 2 to 3 weeks when plaque is left undisturbed on the tooth surfaces. Most gingivitis is reversible, and when the gingiva is treated by plaque removal procedures, the gingiva can return to health within a few days.

An experimental gingivitis program to demonstrate the effect of plaque can be conducted as follows:

A. Observe and record characteristics of the healthy gingiva at the outset. Record a gingival index, a plaque index, and a bleeding index (pages 307, 298, and 305).

B. Withhold all plaque control procedures for a period of 3 weeks.

C. Repeat clinical observations of tissues and record indices at least weekly during the test period. Note initial evidence of gingivitis.

D. Reinstate plaque removal measures after 3 weeks. Make daily observations relative to gingival bleeding and indications that healing is taking place. In 1 week, repeat gingival and plaque indices.

IV. SUBGINGIVAL MICROBIAL PLAQUE

A. Source

Subgingival plaque results from the apical proliferation of microorganisms from supragingival plaque. In the early stages of gingivitis and periodontitis, the supragingival plaque is a strong influence on the accumulation and pathogenic features of the subgingival plaque. As the periodontal pocket deepens, the supragingival plaque only relates to the coronally situated pocket plaque.

B. Microorganisms

The flora of the subgingival plaque differs from that of the supragingival plaque. The subgingival

plaque includes more anaerobic and motile organisms, and they are predominantly gram negative.

C. Organization of Subgingival Plaque (Figure 16-4)

1. *Tooth-Surface-Attached Plaque.* Over the pellicle, which covers the tooth surface, is a layer of densely packed microorganisms. Next to the tooth, on the innermost side of this layer, are many gram-positive rods and cocci. The plaque of this area is associated with calculus formation, root caries, and root resorption.

2. *Unattached Plaque.* Between the two layers of attached plaque are many motile, gram-negative organisms. The "fluid" plaque contains many white blood cells.

3. *Epithelium-Associated Plaque.* Loosely attached to the pocket epithelium are many gram-negative microorganisms and numerous white blood cells. Many virulent pathogenic

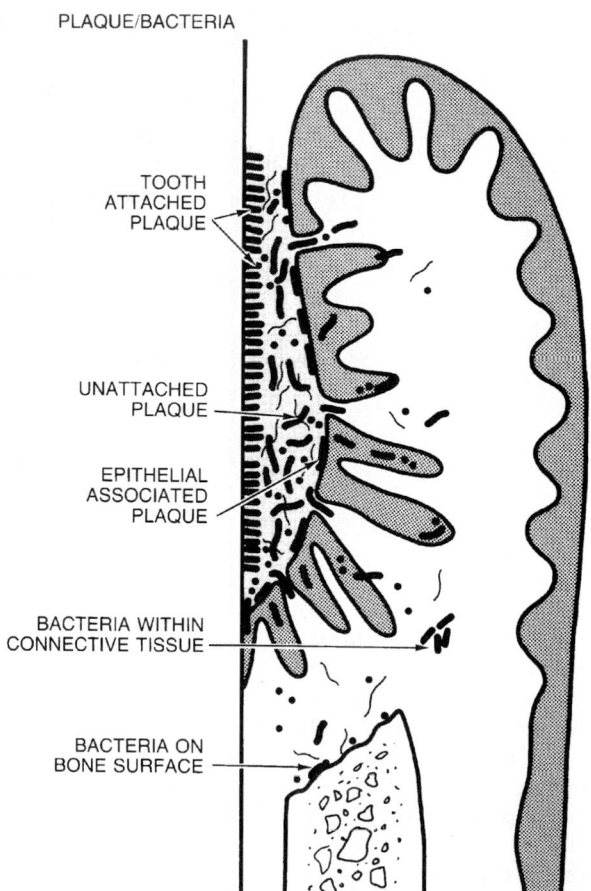

PLAQUE/BACTERIA

TOOTH ATTACHED PLAQUE

UNATTACHED PLAQUE

EPITHELIAL ASSOCIATED PLAQUE

BACTERIA WITHIN CONNECTIVE TISSUE

BACTERIA ON BONE SURFACE

■ **FIGURE 16-4 Bacterial Invasion.** Diagram of a periodontal pocket shows bacteria of attached and unattached plaque bacteria within the pocket epithelium, in the connective tissue, and on the surface of the bone. (From Carranza, F.A.: *Glickman's Clinical Periodontology*, 6th ed. Philadelphia, W.B. Saunders Co., 1984, p. 368.)

organisms in this layer may be considered a focus for the advancement of periodontal infection. From this layer, microorganisms invade the underlying connective tissue. Figure 16-4 shows bacteria within the connective tissue and on the bone surface.

D. Invasion of Microorganisms

Electron microscopy has made possible the detection of microorganisms within tissues.[5] Bacterial invasion provides a significant pathogenic mechanism for progress of periodontal infections. For example, bacteria that invade exposed dentinal tubules provide a source for recolonization within a pocket after treatment, which leads to the recurrence of the infection after a period of time.

V. COMPOSITION OF BACTERIAL PLAQUE

Plaque is composed of microorganisms and intermicrobial matrix. Organic and inorganic solids constitute approximately 20%, and water accounts for 80%. Microorganisms make up at least 70% to 80% of the solid matter, which is higher in subgingival plaque than in the supragingival form.

Composition differs between individuals and between different tooth surfaces of an individual. As plaque ages, it changes.

A. Inorganic Elements[6,7]

1. *Calcium and Phosphorus.* The concentration of calcium, phosphorus, magnesium, and fluoride is higher in plaque than in saliva, thus illustrating the ability of plaque to concentrate inorganic elements.

   Plaque on the lingual surfaces of the mandibular anterior teeth contains a higher concentration of calcium and phosphate than does plaque on the other teeth, and the amount is even higher on those same surfaces in heavy calculus formers.

2. *Fluoride.* The concentration of fluoride in plaque is higher when fluoridated water is used, and it increases following professional topical applications of fluoride and the use of fluoride-containing dentifrices and mouthrinses.

B. Organic Components

The organic intermicrobial substance surrounds the microorganisms of plaque and contains primarily carbohydrates and proteins, with small amounts of lipids.

1. *Carbohydrates.* Carbohydrates, which are produced by several types of bacteria, include glucans and fructans or levans made from dietary sucrose. Dextran is a type of glucan. These carbohydrates contribute to the following:

   a. Adherence of the microorganisms to each other and the tooth. An example is *Strep-*

tococcus mutans, which may be linked to glucans.

   b. Energy storage of carbohydrate for reserve use by plaque bacteria.

2. *Proteins*

   a. Supragingival plaque contains proteins derived from saliva.

   b. Subgingival plaque contains proteins from gingival exudate and sulcus fluid.

3. *Lipids.* The lipid content may include lipopolysaccharide endotoxins from gram-negative bacteria.

CLINICAL ASPECTS

I. DISTRIBUTION

A. Location

1. *Supragingival Plaque.* Plaque is coronal to the gingival margin.

2. *Gingival Plaque.* Plaque forms on the external surfaces of the oral epithelium and attached gingiva.

3. *Subgingival Plaque.* Plaque is located between the periodontal attachment and the gingival margin, within the sulcus or pocket.

4. *Fissure Plaque.* Plaque also develops in pits and fissures and is referred to as *fissure* plaque.

B. By Surfaces

1. *During Formation.* Supragingival plaque formation begins at the gingival margin, particularly on proximal surfaces, and increases rapidly when left undisturbed. It spreads over the gingival third and on toward the middle third of the crown.

2. *Tooth Surfaces Involved*

   a. Plaque occurs most frequently on proximal surfaces and around the gingival third, associated with protected areas (Figure 16-5).

   b. The least amounts occur on the palatal surfaces of maxillary teeth because of the activity of the tongue.

C. Factors Influencing Plaque Accumulation

In Chapter 13 (pages 231 to 233), many factors that influence deposit accumulation and disease development were outlined. A review of those factors can be helpful in conjunction with the material in this section.

1. *Crowded Teeth.* Figure 16-5 illustrates the accumulation of bacterial plaque around crowded mandibular anterior teeth. Research has shown that, when personal plaque removal efforts are made conscientiously, plaque accumulation around crowded teeth is not greater than that around teeth in good alignment.[8]

2. *Rough Surfaces.* More rapid collection occurs

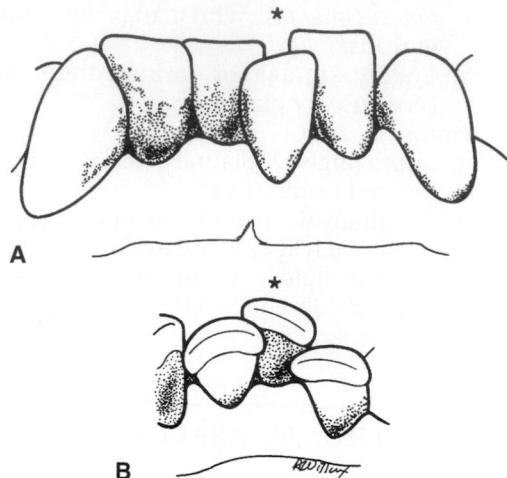

FIGURE 16-5 Plaque Accumulation in Protected Areas. Crowded mandibular anterior teeth demonstrate bacterial plaque after use of a disclosing agent. The thickest plaque is on the proximal surfaces and at the cervical thirds of the teeth. Note the central incisors in facial view **(A)** and lingual view **(B),** with thick extensive plaque on the less accessible protected surfaces.

on rough surfaces of teeth, restorations, and calculus.

3. *Difficult to Clean.* Thick, dense deposits usually collect in difficult-to-clean areas, such as under overhanging margins of crowns or fillings, under ledges of calculus, and in areas associated with carious lesions.

4. *Out of Occlusion.* Deposits may extend over an entire crown of a tooth that is unopposed, out of occlusion, or not used during mastication.

5. *Bacterial Multiplication.* The thickness of plaque results from constant cell division of the bacteria within the plaque.

II. DETECTION

A. Direct Vision
1. *Thin Plaque.* May be translucent and therefore not visible.
2. *Stained Plaque.* May acquire extrinsic stains that make it visible, for example, yellow, green, tobacco, as described on pages 286 to 289.
3. *Thick Plaque.* The tooth may appear dull, dingy, with a matted fur-like surface. Materia alba or food debris may collect over the plaque.

B. Use of Explorer or Probe
1. *Tactile Examination.* When calcification has started, plaque may feel slightly rough; otherwise the surface may feel only somewhat slippery because of the coating of soft, slimy plaque.

2. *Removal of Plaque.* When no plaque is visible, it can be detected and removed by an explorer passed over the tooth surface. When present, plaque adheres to the explorer tip.

C. Use of Disclosing Agent
When a disclosing agent is applied, plaque takes on the color and becomes readily visible (Figure 16-5). Disclosing agent should not be applied until the evaluation of the oral mucosa and gingival color has been recorded.

D. Clinical Record
1. Record plaque by location and extent (slight, moderate, or heavy). An index or plaque score is recommended (pages 298 to 302).
2. Plaque recordings and indices are kept for comparison in conjunction with the instructional plan for plaque control by the patient, for both current and maintenance appointments.
3. Plaque evaluation records are included with the complete charting and oral examination.

SIGNIFICANCE OF BACTERIAL PLAQUE

Microbial plaque plays a major role in the initiation and progression of both dental caries and periodontal diseases. Periodontal diseases and dental caries are infectious diseases caused by pathogenic microorganisms found in microbial plaques. Particular groups of microorganisms are present in association with certain infections.

Plaque is significant in the formation of dental calculus. Calculus is essentially mineralized microbial plaque (pages 280 to 281).

General oral cleanliness depends on the daily removal of bacterial plaque deposits. The accumulation of bacterial plaque on the teeth and tongue contributes to an unpleasant personal esthetic appearance as well as to halitosis.

DENTAL CARIES

Dental caries is a disease of the dental calcified structures (enamel, dentin, and cementum) that is characterized by demineralization of the mineral components and dissolution of the organic matrix. Clinical characteristics and types of cavities were described in Chapter 14.

I. ESSENTIALS FOR DENTAL CARIES
The sequence of events leading to demineralization and dental caries is shown in Figure 16-6. A diet high in cariogenic foods, along with specific microorganisms and a susceptible tooth surface, are essential (see Figure 28-1, page 443).

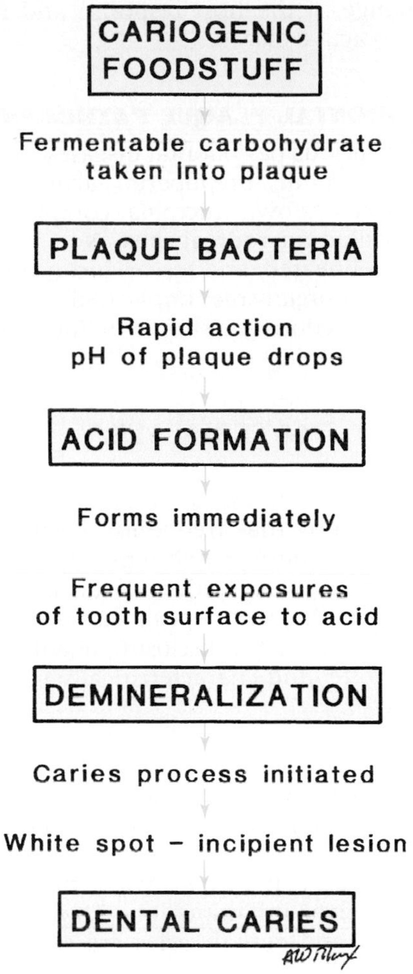

CARIOGENIC
FOODSTUFF

Fermentable carbohydrate
taken into plaque

PLAQUE BACTERIA

Rapid action
pH of plaque drops

ACID FORMATION

Forms immediately

Frequent exposures
of tooth surface to acid

DEMINERALIZATION

Caries process initiated

White spot – incipient lesion

DENTAL CARIES

FIGURE 16-6 Development of Dental Caries.
Flowchart shows the step-by-step action within the microbial plaque on the tooth surface.

A. Susceptible Tooth Surface

A tooth with optimum fluoride content resists the process of dental caries.

B. Microorganisms[9]

Mutans streptococci (*Streptococcus mutans* and *Streptococcus sobrinus*, predominantly) play a major role in caries development and progression. They appear in large numbers in carious lesions.

Historically, acidogenic lactobacilli also have been implicated. The lactobacilli may have a more important role in the progression of a carious lesion and may be less significant in its origin.

Bacterial plaque contains many acidogenic microorganisms. In addition to mutans streptococci and lactobacilli, other predominant groups of microorganisms with acidogenic potential include nonmutans streptococci and actinomyces.

C. Cariogenic Foodstuff Source

1. Cariogenic foodstuff, particularly sucrose, enters the microbial plaque.
2. Acid-forming bacteria break down the sugar to an acid.
3. Acid on the tooth surface causes subsurface demineralization.
4. Decreased salivary flow (xerostomia) and increased dietary carbohydrate promote the growth of mutans streptococci and lactobacilli in bacterial plaque.

II. CONTRIBUTING FACTORS

A. Time

Acid formation begins *immediately* when the cariogenic substance is taken into the plaque.

B. The pH of the Plaque

The pH of the plaque is lowered promptly, and 1 to 2 hours are required for the pH to return to a normal level, assuming the plaque is left undisturbed.

1. Plaque pH before eating ranges from 6.2 to 7.0; it is lower in the caries-susceptible person and higher in the caries-resistant person.
2. Immediately following sucrose intake into plaque, a rapid drop in the pH of the plaque occurs.[10,11]
3. Critical pH for enamel demineralization averages between 4.5 to 5.5, below which the enamel demineralizes. The critical pH for root surface demineralization is approximately 6.0 to 6.7.[12]
4. The amount of demineralization depends on the length of time and the frequency with which the acid with a pH below the critical pH is in contact with the tooth surface.

C. Frequency of Carbohydrate Intake

With each meal or snack that contains sucrose, the pH of the plaque is lowered (see Figure 28-6, page 451). Large amounts of sucrose eaten at mealtimes can be expected to be less cariogenic than small amounts eaten at frequent intervals during the day.[13] These and other related facts can be presented to the patient when the diet is discussed as a part of the basic instruction or as part of a total dental caries control program with dietary assessment (pages 450 to 452).

III. THE CARIOUS LESION

The incipient carious lesion begins as subsurface demineralization. Acid from bacterial action on the tooth surface passes through microchannels in the enamel, demineralization occurs, and eventually a white spot can be seen clinically. Early and continuous use of fluoride for remineralization is necessary. Dental caries formation is described on pages 238 to 242, and the use of fluoride in remineralization is covered on page 459.

EFFECT OF DIET ON PLAQUE

I. CARIOGENIC FOODS

A. Dental Caries

The relationship of the cariogenic food content of the diet and its frequency of use to the development of dental caries is well defined in research and clinical application. Dental caries initiation is outlined in Figure 16-6.

B. Effect of Sucrose on Amount and pH of Plaque

When a cariogenic diet is used, plaque forms and grows more profusely.[14] Patients fed sucrose by stomach tube had a less acidogenic plaque than did patients who were fed sucrose by mouth.[15]

II. FOOD INTAKE

Food particles are not needed in the mouth for plaque to form. In one study, neither varying the number of meals nor feeding by stomach tube affected the development of plaque.[16] In another study, less plaque developed in a group of stomach-fed patients when compared with those fed by mouth.[15]

III. TEXTURE OF DIET

The friction of mastication has been shown to affect only the occlusal and incisal thirds of the crowns of teeth. Plaque on the gingival third collected in spite of a normal diet that included coarse bread and fresh fruit[4] or chewing raw carrots three times daily as the only methods for personal care.[17] Chewing apples did not affect moderate amounts of plaque, but it did tend to remove food debris in a group of 12-year-olds.[18]

PERIODONTAL INFECTIONS

The microorganisms of bacterial plaque cause the periodontal infections. The variations in clinical manifestations in different individuals can be accounted for by the differences in the bacterial activity within the plaque, as well as by the tissue response and resistance to the microorganisms and their products.

More than 400 different species of bacteria have been known to colonize the human oral cavity. An individual may have as many as 150 at a given time.

I. BACTERIA OF HEALTHY GINGIVA

The microbiota of the healthy gingival sulcus differs from the bacteria of the diseased pocket. In health, there is a majority if aerobic, gram-positive streptococci and actinomyces. The total number of organisms and white blood cells is low, compared with a diseased pocket.

Gram-negative, pathogenic forms may be found in apparently healthy gingiva. They may be an indication of change in the host response and future susceptibility to active disease.

II. PERIODONTAL PLAQUE PATHOGENS

Each of the various periodontal diseases (for example, early onset, juvenile, prepubertal, acute, adult, peri-implantitis) has its own microbial complex of subgingival pathogenic microorganisms. Not all have been specifically delineated, and research continues.[19,20]

Major microorganisms implicated in destructive periodontal infections are shown in Table 16-3.

MATERIA ALBA

Materia alba is a loosely adherent mass of bacteria and cellular debris that frequently occurs on top of bacterial plaque where plaque removal is neglected.

Materia alba ("white material") distinguishes itself clinically as a bulky, soft deposit that is clearly visible without application of a disclosing agent. It is white, or grayish-white, and characteristically may resemble cottage cheese.

Materia alba forms over bacterial plaque. It is a product of informal accumulation of living and dead bacteria, desquamated epithelial cells, disintegrating leukocytes, salivary proteins, and particles of food debris.

Surface bacteria in contact with the gingiva contribute to gingival inflammation. Tooth surface demineralization and dental caries are seen frequently under materia alba.

Clinical distinction between materia alba, food debris, and bacterial plaque is necessary, but patient instruction for the removal of all three involves the same basic plaque control procedures. Materia alba can be removed with a water spray or oral irrigator, whereas bacterial plaque cannot.

TABLE 16-3 Pathogens in Destructive Periodontal Diseases

STRONG EVIDENCE FOR ETIOLOGY

Actinobacillus actinomycetemcomitans
Porphyromonas gingivalis
Bacteroides forsythus

MODERATE EVIDENCE FOR ETIOLOGY

Campylobacter rectus
Eubacterium nodatum
Fusobacterium nucleatum
Prevotella intermedia
Peptostreptococcus micros
Streptococcus intermedius-complex
Treponema denticola

From: *Annals of Periodontology, 1, 928,* November, 1996.

FOOD DEBRIS

Loose food particles collect about the cervical third and proximal embrasures of the teeth.

When there are open contact areas; mobility of teeth; or irregularities of occlusion, such as plunger cusps, food may be forced between the teeth during mastication, and vertical food impaction results. Horizontal or lateral food impaction occurs in facial and lingual embrasures, particularly when the interdental papillae are reduced or missing.

Food debris adds to a general unsanitary condition of the mouth. Cariogenic foods contribute to dental caries because liquefied carbohydrate diffuses rapidly into the plaque and hence to the acid-forming bacteria.

Some self-cleansing through the action of the tongue, lips, saliva, and related factors takes place (page 233). Debris removal by toothbrushing, flossing, and other aids constitutes a total plaque control program. Cleansing of debris from about fixed prostheses and orthodontic appliances is important to the plan for oral sanitation.

TECHNICAL HINTS

I. Check all surfaces of restorations and prostheses and remove rough areas and overhanging margins. Soft deposits accumulate on rough or irregular surfaces more rapidly and in greater quantity than on smooth surfaces.

II. Withhold the use of a disclosing agent until the intraoral mucosal and gingival examinations have been made. Coloring agents can disguise soft tissue changes and deviations from normal.

FACTORS TO TEACH THE PATIENT

I. Location, composition, and properties of bacterial plaque with emphasis on its role in dental caries and periodontal infections.

II. The cause and prevention of dental caries.

III. Effects of personal oral care procedures in the prevention of bacterial plaque.

IV. Plaque control procedures with special adaptations for individual needs.

V. Sources of cariogenic foodstuff in the diet with suggestions for control.

VI. Relationship of frequency of eating cariogenic foods to dental caries.

REFERENCES

1. **Schroeder,** H.E.: *Formation and Inhibition of Dental Calculus,* Vienna, Hans Huber Publishers, 1969, pp. 14–15.
2. **Meckel,** A.H.: Formation and Properties of Organic Films on Teeth, *Arch. Oral Biol., 10,* 585, July–August, 1965.
3. **Meckel,** A.H.: The Nature and Importance of Organic Deposits on Dental Enamel, *Caries Res., 2,* 104, No. 2, 1968.
4. **Löe,** H., Theilade, E., and Jensen, S.B.: Experimental Gingivitis in Man, *J. Periodontol., 36,* 177, May–June, 1965.
5. **Saglie,** R., Newman, M.G., Carranza, F.A., and Pattison, G.L.: Bacterial Invasion of Gingiva in Advanced Periodontitis in Humans, *J. Periodontol., 53,* 217, April, 1982.
6. **Mandel,** I.D.: Relation of Saliva and Plaque to Caries, *J. Dent. Res., 53,* 246, March–April, Supplement, 1974.
7. **Grøn,** P., Yao, K., and Spinelli, M.: A Study of Inorganic Constituents in Dental Plaque, *J. Dent. Res., 48,* 799, September–October, Supplement, 1969.
8. **Årtun,** J. and Osterberg, S.K.: Periodontal Status of Secondary Crowded Mandibular Incisors. Long-term Results After Orthodontic Treatment, *J. Clin. Periodontol., 14,* 261, May, 1987.
9. **Van Houte,** J., Sansone, C., Joshipura, K., and Kent, R.: Mutans Streptococci and Non-mutans Streptococci Acidogenic at Low pH, and *in vitro* Acidogenic Potential of Dental Plaque in Two Different Areas of the Human Dentition, *J. Dent. Res., 70,* 1503, December, 1991.
10. **Stephan,** R.M.: Intra-oral Hydrogen-ion Concentrations Associated with Dental Caries Activity, *J. Dent. Res., 23,* 257, August, 1944.
11. **Rosen,** S. and Weisenstein, P.R.: The Effect of Sugar Solutions on pH of Dental Plaques from Caries-susceptible and Caries-free Individuals, *J. Dent. Res., 44,* 845, September–October, 1965.
12. **Hoppenbrouwers,** P.M.M., Driessens, F.C.M., and Borggreven, J.M.P.M.: The Mineral Solubility of Human Tooth Roots, *Arch. Oral Biol., 32,* 319, No. 5, 1987.
13. **Gustafsson,** B.E., Quensel, C.-E., Lanke, L.S., Lundquist, C., Grahnén, H., Bonow, B.E., and Krasse, B.: The Vipeholm Dental Caries Study. The Effect of Different Levels of Carbohydrate Intake on Caries Activity in 436 Individuals Observed for Five Years, *Acta Odontol. Scand., 11,* 232, Nos. 3–4, 1954.
14. **Carlsson,** J. and Egelberg, J.: Effect of Diet on Early Plaque Formation in Man, *Odont. Revy, 16,* 112, No. 1, 1965.
15. **Littleton,** N.W., Carter, C.H., and Kelley, R.T.: Studies of Oral Health in Persons Nourished by Stomach Tube. I. Changes in pH of Plaque Material after the Addition of Sucrose, *J. Am. Dent. Assoc., 74,* 119, January, 1967.
16. **Egelberg,** J.: Local Effect of Diet on Plaque Formation and Development of Gingivitis in Dogs. III. Effect of Frequency of Meals and Tube Feeding, *Odont. Revy, 16,* 50, No. 1, 1965.
17. **Lindhe,** J. and Wicén, P.-O.: The Effects on the Gingivae of Chewing Fibrous Foods, *J. Periodont. Res., 4,* 193, No. 3, 1969.
18. **Birkeland,** J.M. and Jorkjend, L.: The Effect of Chewing Apples on Dental Plaque and Food Debris, *Community Dent. Oral Epidemiol., 2,* 161, No. 4, 1974.
19. **Socransky,** S.S., Haffajee, A.D., Cugini, M.A., Smith, C., and Kent, R.L.: Microbial Complexes in Subgingival Plaque, *J. Clin. Periodontol., 25,* 134, February, 1998.
20. **Haffajee,** A.D. and Socransky, S.S.: Microbial Etiological Agents of Destructive Periodontal Diseases, *Periodontology 2000, 5,* 78, 1994.

SUGGESTED READINGS

Alaluusua, S. and Maimivirta, R.: Early Plaque Accumulation—A Sign for Caries Risk in Young Children, *Community Dent. Oral Epidemiol., 22,* 273, October, 1994.

Corbet, E.F. and Davies, W.I.R.: The Role of Supragingival Plaque in the Control of Progressive Periodontal Disease, A Review, *J. Clin. Periodontol., 20,* 307, May, 1993.

Frisken, K.W.: The Incidence of Periodontopathic Microorganisms in Young Children, *Oral Microbiol. Immunol., 5,* 43, February, 1990.

Haffajee, A.D., Socransky, S.S., Smith, C., and Dibart, S.: Microbial Risk Indicators for Periodontal Attachment Loss, *J. Periodont. Res., 26,* 293, May, (Part 2), 1991.

Hellström, M.-K., Ramberg, P., Krok, L., and Lindhe, J.: The Effect of Supragingival Plaque Control on the Subgingival Microflora in Human Periodontitis, *J. Clin. Periodontol.*, *23*, 934, October, 1996.

Lang, N.P., Mombelli, A., and Attström, R.: Dental Plaque and Calculus, in Lindhe, J., Karring, T., and Lang, N.P., eds.: *Clinical Periodontology and Implant Dentistry*, 3rd ed. Copenhagen, Munksgaard, 1997, pp. 102–137.

Ramberg, P.W., Lindhe, J., and Gaffar, A.: Plaque and Gingivitis in the Deciduous and Permanent Dentition, *J. Clin. Periodontol.*, *21*, 490, August, 1994.

Sansone, C., Van Houte, J., Joshipura, K., Kent, R., and Margolis, H.C.: The Association of Mutans Streptococci and Nonmutans Streptococci Capable of Acidogenesis at a Low pH with Dental Caries on Enamel and Root Surfaces, *J. Dent. Res.*, *72*, 508, February, 1993.

Scannapieco, F.A., Stewart, E.M., and Mylotte, J.M.: Colonization of Dental Plaque by Respiratory Pathogens in Medical Intensive Care Patients, *Crit. Care Med.*, *20*, 740, June, 1992.

Socransky, S.S. and Haffajee, A.D.: Evidence of Bacterial Etiology: A Historical Perspective, *Periodontology 2000*, *5*, 7, 1994.

van Houte, J.: Role of Micro-organisms in Caries Etiology, *J. Dent. Res.*, *73*, 672, March, 1994.

Microbiology

Christersson, L.A., Fransson, C.L., Dunford, R.G., and Zambon, J.J.: Subgingival Distribution of Periodontal Pathogenic Microorganisms in Adult Periodontitis, *J. Periodontol.*, *63*, 418, May, 1992.

Columbo, A.P., Haffajee, A.D., Dewhirst, F.E., Paster, B.J., Smith, C.M., Cugini, M.A., and Socransky, S.S.: Clinical and Microbiological Features of Refractory Periodontitis Subjects, *J. Clin. Periodontol.*, *25*, 169, February, 1998.

Darveau, R.P., Tanner, A., and Page, R.C.: The Microbial Challenge in Periodontitis, *Periodontology, 2000*, *14*, 12, 1997.

Liljenberg, B., Gualini, F., Berglundh, T., Tonetti, M., and Lindhe, J.: Composition of Plaque-associated Lesions in the Gingiva and the Peri-implant Mucosa in Partially Edentulous Subjects, *J. Clin. Periodontol.*, *24*, 119, February, 1997.

Listgarten, M.A.: Electron Microscopic Observations on the Bacterial Flora of Acute Necrotizing Ulcerative Gingivitis, *J. Periodontol.*, *36*, 328, July–August, 1965.

Listgarten, M.A., Lai, C.-H., and Young, V.: Microbial Composition and Pattern of Antibiotic Resistance in Subgingival Microbial Samples From Patients with Refractory Periodontitis, *J. Periodontol.*, *64*, 155, March, 1993.

Mombelli, A., Marxer, M., Gaberthüel, T., Grunder, U., and Lang, N.P.: The Microbiota of Osseointegrated Implants in Patients with a History of Periodontal Disease, *J. Clin. Periodontol.*, *22*, 124, February, 1995.

Moore, W.E.C., Moore, L.H., Ranney, R.R., Smibert, R.M., Burmeister, J.A., and Schenkein, H.A.: The Microflora of Periodontal Sites Showing Active Destructive Progression, *J. Clin. Periodontol.*, *18*, 729, November, 1991.

Moore, W.E.C. and Moore, L.V.H.: The Bacteria of Periodontal Diseases, *Periodontology 2000*, *5*, 66, 1994.

Preber, H., Bergström, J., and Linder, L.E.: Occurrence of Periopathogens in Smoker and Non-smoker Patients, *J. Clin. Periodontol.*, *19*, 667, October, 1992.

Riviere, G.R., Smith, K.S., Carranza, N., Tzagaroulaki, E., Kay, S.L., and Dock, M.: Subgingival Distribution of *Treponema denticola*, *Treponema socranskii*, and Pathogen-related Oral Spirochetes: Prevalence and Relationship to Periodontal Status of Sampled Sites, *J. Periodontol.*, *66*, 829, October, 1995.

Russell, R.R.B.: Bacteriology of Periodontal Disease, *Curr. Opinion Dent.*, *2*, 66, September, 1992.

Shordone, L., Barone, A., Ramaglia, L., Ciaglia, R.N., and Iacono, V.J.: Antimicrobial Susceptibility of Periodontopathic Bacteria Associated with Failing Implants, *J. Periodontol.*, *66*, 69, January, 1995.

Socransky, S.S. and Haffajee, A.D.: The Bacterial Etiology of Destructive Periodontal Disease: Current Concepts, *J. Periodontol.*, *63*, 322, April, 1992 (Supplement).

Tanner, A., Maiden, M.F.J., Macuch, P.J., Murray, L.L., and Kent, R.L.: Microbiota of Health, Gingivitis, and Initial Periodontitis, *J. Clin. Periodontol.*, *25*, 85, February, 1998.

Zambon, J.J.: Periodontal Diseases: Microbial Factors, *Annals Periodont.*, *1*, 879, November, 1996.

Dental Plaque Structure and Formation

Dahlén, G., Lindhe, J., Sato, K., Hanamura, H., and Okamoto, H.: The Effect of Supragingival Plaque Control on the Subgingival Microbiota in Subjects With Periodontal Disease, *J. Clin. Periodontol.*, *19*, 802, November, 1992.

Gibbons, R.J. and van Houte, J.: On the Formation of Dental Plaques, *J. Periodontol.*, *44*, 347, June, 1973.

Katsanoulas, T., Reneé, I., and Allström, R.: The Effect of Supragingival Plaque Control on the Composition of the Subgingival Flora in Periodontal Pockets, *J. Clin. Periodontol.*, *19*, 760, November, 1992.

Listgarten, M.A.: The Structure of Dental Plaque, *Periodontology 2000*, *5*, 52, 1994.

Newman, H.N.: The Development of Dental Plaque: From Preeruptive Primary Cuticle to Acquired Pellicle to Dental Plaque to Calculus Formation, in Harris, N.O. and Christen, A.G.: *Primary Preventive Dentistry*, 4th ed. Norwalk, Connecticut, Appleton & Lange, 1995, pp. 19–38.

Quirynen, M., Dekeyser, C., and van Steenberghe, D.: The Influence of Gingival Inflammation, Tooth Type, and Timing on the Rate of Plaque Formation, *J. Periodontol.*, *62*, 219, March, 1991.

Ramberg, P., Axelsson, P., and Lindhe, J.: Plaque Formation at Healthy and Inflamed Gingival Sites in Young Individuals, *J. Clin. Periodontol.*, *22*, 85, January, 1995.

Ramberg, P., Lindhe, J., Dahlen, G., and Volpe, A.R.: The Influence of Gingival Inflammation on de novo Plaque Formation, *J. Clin. Periodontol.*, *21*, 51, January, 1994.

Scheie, A.A.: Mechanisms of Dental Plaque Formation, *Adv. Dent. Res.*, *8*, 246, July, 1994.

Transmission

Alaluusua, S., Asikainen, S., and Lai, C.-H.: Intrafamilial Transmission of *Actinobacillus actinomycetemcomitans*, *J. Periodontol.*, *62*, 207, March, 1991.

Greenstein, G. and Lamster, I.: Bacterial Transmission in Periodontal Diseases: A Critical Review, *J. Periodontol.*, *68*, 421, May, 1997.

Preus, H.R., Zambon, J.J., Dunford, R.G., and Genco, R.J.: The Distribution and Transmission of *Actinobacillus actinomycetemcomitans* in Families With Established Adult Periodontitis, *J. Periodontol.*, *65*, 2, January, 1994.

Van der Velden, U., Van Winkelhoff, A.J., Abbas, F., Arief, E.M., Timmerman, M.F., van der Weijden, G.A., and Winkel, E.G.: Longitudinal Evaluation of the Development of Periodontal Destruction in Spouses, *J. Clin. Periodontol.*, *23*, 1014, November, 1996.

Van Steenbergen, T.J.M., Petit, M.D.A., Scholte, L.H.M., van der Velden, U., and deGraaff, J.: Transmission of *Porphyromonas gingivalis* Between Spouses, *J. Clin. Periodontol.*, *20*, 340, May, 1993.

Von Troil-Linden, B., Torkko, H., Alaluusua, S., Wolf, J., Jousimies-Somer, H., and Asikainen, S.: Periodontal Findings in Spouses. A Clinical, Radiographic and Microbiological Study, *J. Clin. Periodontol.*, *22*, 93, February, 1995.

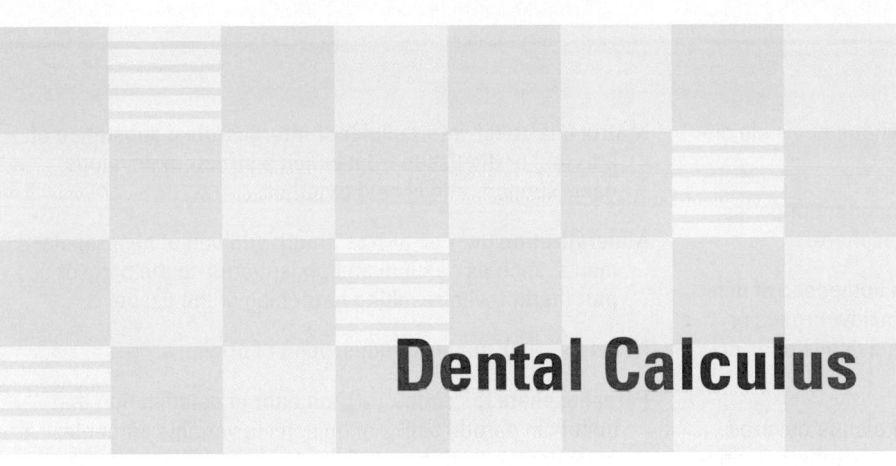

Dental Calculus

Dental calculus, which is mineralized bacterial plaque, is a hard, tenacious mass that forms on the clinical crowns of the natural teeth and on dentures and other dental prostheses. Terms and key words associated with calculus are defined in Box 17-1.

Calculus is significant in the progression of inflammatory periodontal disease. The rough surface of the subgingival calculus holds the disease-producing bacteria of the dental plaque close to the gingival tissue and perpetuates the inflamed state.

The control of plaque deposits by the patient, supplemented by complete professional calculus removal, can reduce or eliminate gingival inflammation. A major objective in nonsurgical periodontal therapy is to prepare the teeth, through calculus removal, to have biologically acceptable smooth surfaces.

Comprehensive understanding of the characteristics, origin, development, and methods of prevention of calculus is essential to patient examination, assessment, treatment, and instruction. For successful treatment and prevention, the patient needs to know the interrelationship between plaque, calculus, and oral health; the need for complete removal of calculus;

and the reasons for the painstaking manner in which scaling procedures must be carried out.

CLASSIFICATION AND DISTRIBUTION

Dental calculus is classified by its location on a tooth surface as related to the adjacent free gingival margin, that is, supragingival and subgingival (Figure 17-1).

I. SUPRAGINGIVAL CALCULUS

A. Location
On the clinical crown coronal to the margin of the gingiva.

B. Distribution
1. Most frequent sites are on the lingual surfaces of mandibular anterior teeth and the facial surfaces of maxillary first and second molars, opposite the openings of the ducts of the salivary glands.
2. Crowns of teeth out of occlusion; nonfunctioning teeth; or teeth that are neglected

BOX 17-1 KEY WORDS: Calculus

Amorphous (ah-mor'fus): without definite shape or visible differentiation in structure.

Apatite (ap'ah-tīt): crystalline mineral component of bones and teeth that contains calcium and phosphate.

Calculus (kal'kū-lus): abnormal concretion composed of mineral salts, usually occurring within the hollow organs or their passages; also called stones, such as gallstones or kidney stones.

> **Denture calculus:** mineralized bacterial plaque covered on the external surface with vital, tightly adherent, non-mineralized bacterial plaque.

Ectopic (ek-tŏp'ik): out of place; arising or produced at an abnormal site or in a tissue where it is not normally found.

> **Ectopic oral calcification:** examples are pulp stones, denticles, and salivary calculi.

Germ-free: free of microorganisms; a germ-free animal in research is reared under completely sterile conditions.

Matrix (mā'triks): intercellular or intermicrobial substance of a tissue, or the tissue from which a structure develops, gains support, and is held together.

Mineralization (min"er-al-ĭ-zā'shun): addition of mineral elements, such as calcium and phosphorus, to the body or a part thereof with resulting hardening of the tissue.

Nidus (nī'dus): nucleus; focus; point of origin.

Pyrophosphate (pī"rō-fos'fāt): inhibitor of calcification that occurs in parotid saliva of humans in variable amounts; anticalculus component of "tarter-control" dentifrices.

Saturated (sach'ĕr-āt-ed): holding all of a substance (solute) that can be dissolved in the solution.

> **Supersaturated** (soo-per-sach'ĕr-āt-ed): a solution containing more of an ingredient than can be held in solution permanently.

---

during daily plaque removal (toothbrushing, flossing, or other personal care).
3. Surfaces of dentures and dental prostheses.

C. Other Names for Supragingival Calculus
1. Supramarginal.*
2. Extragingival.

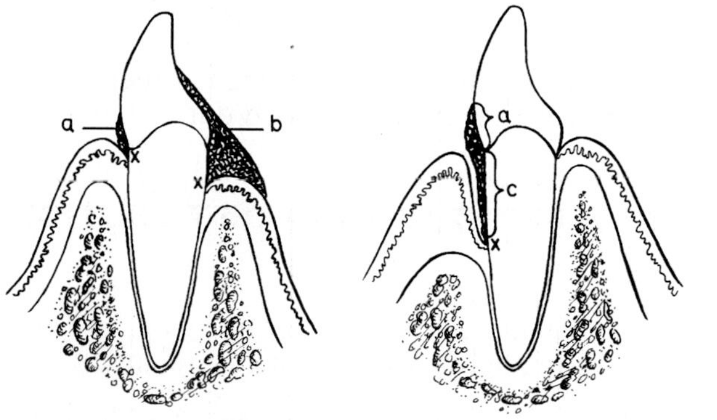

FIGURE 17-1 Dental Calculus. (a) Supragingival calculus on cervical third of a mandibular anterior tooth extends slightly subgingivally. **(b)** Supragingival calculus over crown, exposed root surface, and the margin of the gingiva. **(c)** Subgingival calculus along root to the bottom of a periodontal pocket. **(x)** Bottom of pocket.

*The terms *supra-* and *subgingival* are at present probably the most widely used. Supra- and submarginal are more specific in their definition because the margin of the free gingiva is the dividing line between the two categories. The gingiva includes free and attached.

3. Coronal, indicating that the calculus is on the anatomic crown.
4. Salivary, a term that indicates that the source of the minerals is the saliva.

II. SUBGINGIVAL CALCULUS

A. Location
On the clinical crown apical to the margin of the gingiva. It extends nearly to the bottom of the pocket. As the pocket is deepened by disease, calculus forms on the exposed root surface.

B. Distribution
1. May be generalized or localized on single teeth or a group of teeth.
2. Proximal surfaces have heaviest deposits.

C. Other Names for Subgingival Calculus
1. Submarginal.
2. Serumal; term indicates that the source of the minerals is the blood serum.

III. OCCURRENCE

Calculus occurs at any age and on both permanent and primary teeth. Incidence increases with age, and in some populations, 100% of the people older than 30 years have calculus. The increase is because of continuing accumulation, not necessarily an increased tendency to form new deposits as age advances.

CLINICAL CHARACTERISTICS

I. APPEARANCE AND CONSISTENCY

Identification of calculus prior to removal depends on knowledge of its appearance, consistency, and distribution. Appointment planning, selection of instruments, and techniques depend on understanding the texture, morphology, and mode of attachment of calculus. Table 17-1 provides a summary of clinical characteristics.

II. SUPRAGINGIVAL EXAMINATION

A. Direct Examination

Supragingival deposits may be seen directly or indirectly, using a mouth mirror.

TABLE 17-1 Clinical Characteristics of Dental Calculus

Characteristic	Supragingival Calculus	Subgingival Calculus
Color	White, creamy yellow, or gray May be stained by tobacco, food, or other pigments Slight deposits may be invisible until dried with compressed air	Light to dark brown, dark green, or black Stains derived from blood pigments from diseased pocket
Shape	Amorphous, bulky Gross deposits may (1) Form interproximal bridge between adjacent teeth (2) Extend over the margin of the gingiva (Figure 17-1b) Shape of calculus mass is determined by the anatomy of the teeth, contour of gingival margin, and pressure of the tongue, lips, cheeks	Flattened to conform with pressure from the pocket wall Combination of the following calculus formations occur* (1) Crusty, spiny, or nodular (2) Ledge or ringlike (3) Thin, smooth veneers (4) Finger- and fernlike (5) Individual calculus islands
Consistency and texture	Moderately hard Newer deposits less dense and hard Porous Surface covered with nonmineralized plaque	Brittle, flintlike Harder and more dense than supragingival calculus Newest deposits near bottom of pocket are less dense and hard Surface covered with bacterial plaque
Size and quantity	Quantity has direct relationship to (1) Personal oral care procedures and plaque control measures (2) Physical character of diet (3) Individual tendencies (4) Function and use Increased amount in tobacco smokers	Related to pocket depth Increased amount with age because of accumulation Quantity is related to personal care, diet, and individual tendency as it is with supragingival. Subgingival is primarily related to the development and progression of periodontal disease
Distribution on individual tooth	Coronal to margin of gingiva May cover a large portion of the visible clinical crown, or may form fine thin line near gingival margin	Apical to margin of gingiva Extends to bottom of the pocket and follows contour of soft tissue attachment With gingival recession, subgingival calculus may become supragingival and become covered with typical supragingival calculus
Distribution on teeth	Symmetrical arrangement on teeth except when influenced by (1) Malpositioned teeth (2) Unilateral hypofunction (3) Inconsistent personal care (4) Abrasion from food Occurs with or without associated subgingival deposits Location related to openings of the salivary gland ducts: (1) Facial surface of maxillary molars (2) Lingual surface of mandibular anterior teeth	Heaviest on proximal surfaces, lightest on facial surfaces Occurs with or without associated supragingival deposits

*Everett, F.G. and Potter, G.R.: Morphology of Submarginal Calculus, *J. Periodontol., 30,* 27, January, 1959.

B. Use of Compressed Air

Small amounts of calculus that have not been stained are frequently invisible when they are wet with saliva. With a combination of retraction, light, and drying with air, small deposits usually can be seen. An explorer may be used when visual examination is not definite (page 216).

III. SUBGINGIVAL EXAMINATION

A. Visual Examination

1. Dark edge of calculus may be seen at or just beneath the gingival margin.
2. Diseased gingival margin does not adapt closely to a tooth surface, thus permitting a view into the pocket where calculus can be seen.
3. Gentle air blast can deflect the margin from the tooth for observation into the pocket.
4. When light shines through anterior teeth during transillumination, a dark, opaque, shadowlike area seen on a proximal tooth surface could be subgingival calculus. Supragingival calculus may also be found by this method. Without calculus, stain, or thick soft deposit, the enamel is translucent.

B. Gingival Tissue Color Change

Dark calculus may reflect through a thin margin and suggest the presence of subgingival calculus.

C. Tactile Examination

1. *Probe.* While probing for sulcus/pocket characteristics, a rough subgingival tooth surface can be felt when calculus is present. Although there are other causes of roughness, subgingival calculus is the most common (pages 229 to 230).
2. *Explorer.* A fine subgingival explorer is needed that can be adapted close to the root surface all the way to the bottom of a pocket. Each subgingival area must be examined carefully to the bottom of the pocket, completely around each tooth.

IV. CLINICAL RECORD

Calculus deposits are described in the examination record. The location of supra- and subgingival deposits and their extent (slight, moderate, or heavy) must be designated.

The calculus record is included with the complete charting and oral examination (page 318).

CALCULUS FORMATION[1]

Subgingival calculus does not develop by direct extension from supragingival calculus. First, subgingival bacterial plaque forms by extension of supragingival plaque. Each plaque mineralizes separately.

Calculus results from the deposition of minerals into a plaque organic matrix. Calculus formation occurs in three basic steps: *pellicle formation, plaque formation,* and *mineralization.* Mineralization of supra- and subgingival calculus is essentially the same, although the source of the elements for mineralization is not the same.

I. PELLICLE FORMATION

The formation and characteristics of pellicle were described on pages 264 and 266. The pellicle, or cuticle, is composed of mucoproteins from the saliva and is an acellular material. Its thickness and contour vary on the tooth surface. It begins to form within minutes after all deposits have been removed from the tooth surface.

II. PLAQUE MATURATION

A. Microorganisms settle in the pellicle layer.
B. Colonies are formed. Originally, the colonies consist primarily of cocci and rod-shaped organisms. By the fifth day, the plaque is mostly made up of filamentous organisms.
C. The colonies grow together to form a cohesive plaque layer.

III. MINERALIZATION

A. Mineralization Foci (Centers) Form

Within 24 to 72 hours, more and more mineralization centers develop close to the underlying tooth surface. Eventually, the centers grow large enough to touch and unite.

B. Organic Matrix

Mineralization first occurs within the intermicrobial matrix. The filamentous microorganisms provide the matrix for the deposition of minerals.

A calculus-like deposit has been observed on the teeth of germ-free animals that have no bacterial plaque.[2-4] It may indicate that other organic substances, such as the pellicle, may mineralize. The pellicle is between the dental plaque and the tooth surface. Since the attachment of calculus is very strong, it is expected that the pellicle must mineralize to create such a firm bond.

C. Sources of Minerals

1. *Supragingival Calculus.* The source of elements for supragingival calculus is the saliva.
2. *Subgingival Calculus.* The gingival sulcus fluid and the inflammatory exudate supply the minerals for the subgingival deposits. Gingival sulcus fluid was described on page 190. Because the amount of sulcus fluid and exudate increases with increases in inflammation, more minerals are available for mineralization of subgingival plaque.

D. Crystal Formation

Mineralization consists of crystal formation,

namely, hydroxyapatite, octocalcium phosphate, whitlockite, and brushite, each with a characteristic developmental pattern. The crystals form in the intercellular matrix and on the surface of bacteria, and finally within the bacteria.[5,6]

E. Mechanism of Mineralization[7]

The mineralization process is considered the same for both supra- and subgingival calculus. Heavy calculus formers have higher salivary levels of calcium and phosphorus than do light calculus formers.[8] Light calculus formers have higher levels of parotid pyrophosphate.[9] Pyrophosphate is an inhibitor of calcification and is used in anticalculus dentifrices (page 283).

The process by which minerals, mainly calcium and phosphate, become incorporated from the saliva or gingival sulcus fluid into the plaque matrix is still not completely understood.

Current research studies point to the probability that calcification of calculus may involve the same phenomena as those of other ectopic calcifications (such as urinary or renal calculi) and may be similar to normal calcification of bone, cartilage, enamel, or dentin.

IV. FORMATION TIME

Formation time means the average number of days required for the primary soft deposit to change to the mature mineralized stage. The average time is about 12 days, within a range from 10 days for rapid calculus formers to 20 days for slow calculus formers.[8] Mineralization can begin as early as 24 to 48 hours.

Formation time depends on individual tendency, but it is strongly influenced by the roughness of the tooth surface and the care and character of personal plaque control measures. Determination of the approximate formation time for an individual is important to instruction and counseling, as well as to treatment planning for professional care and frequency of maintenance appointments.

V. STRUCTURE OF CALCULUS

A. Layers

Calculus forms in layers that are more or less parallel with the tooth surface. The layers are separated by a line that appears to be a pellicle that was deposited over the previously formed calculus, and as mineralization progressed, the pellicle became imbedded.

The lines between the layers of calculus can be called incremental lines. They form around the tooth in supragingival calculus, but form irregularly from crown to apex on the root surface in subgingival calculus. The lines are evidence that calculus grows or increases by apposition of new layers.

B. Surface

The surface of a calculus mass is rough and can be detected by use of an explorer. As observed by electron microscope, the surface roughness appears as peaks, valleys, and pits.

C. Outer Layer

The outer layer of subgingival calculus is partly calcified. On the surface is a thick, matlike, soft layer of bacterial plaque. The outer surface of the plaque on the subgingival calculus is in contact with the diseased pocket epithelium. The contents of the three layers of subgingival plaque are outlined in Table 16-2, page 268, and Figure 16-4 (page 270).

ATTACHMENT OF CALCULUS

Calculus is more readily removed from some tooth surfaces than from others. The ease or difficulty of removal can be related to the manner of attachment of the calculus to the tooth surface.

Several modes of attachment have been observed by conventional histologic techniques and by electron microscopy. On any one tooth and in any one area, more than one mode of attachment may be found.

When studying the attachment types, the character of the hard, smooth enamel surface and that of the rough, porous, cemental surface should be considered. Three general modes of attachment can be identified.[10]

I. ATTACHMENT BY MEANS OF AN ACQUIRED PELLICLE OR CUTICLE

A. The pellicle is a thin, acellular, homogeneous layer positioned between the calculus and the tooth surface.
B. Calculus attachment is superficial because no interlocking or penetration occurs.
C. Pellicle attachment occurs most frequently on enamel and newly scaled and planed root surfaces.
D. Calculus may be removed readily because of the smooth attachment.

II. ATTACHMENT TO MINUTE IRREGULARITIES IN THE TOOTH SURFACE BY MECHANICAL LOCKING INTO UNDERCUTS

A. Enamel irregularities include cracks, lamellae, and carious defects.
B. Cemental irregularities include tiny spaces left at previous locations of Sharpey's fibers, resorption lacunae, scaling grooves, cemental tears.
C. Difficult to be certain all calculus is removed when it is attached by this method.

III. ATTACHMENT BY DIRECT CONTACT BETWEEN CALCIFIED INTERCELLULAR MATRIX AND THE TOOTH SURFACE

A. Interlocking of inorganic crystals of the tooth with the mineralizing bacterial plaque.

B. Distinction between calculus and cementum is difficult during root planing.

COMPOSITION

Calculus is made up of inorganic and organic components and water. Although the percentage varies depending on the age and hardness of a deposit and the location from which the sample for analysis is taken, mature calculus usually contains between 75% and 85% inorganic components; the rest is organic components and water. The chemical content of supra- and subgingival calculus is similar.[11–13]

I. INORGANIC

A. Inorganic Components
The components are mainly calcium (Ca), phosphorus (P), carbonate (CO_3), sodium (Na), magnesium (Mg), and potassium (K).

B. Trace Elements
Various trace elements have been identified, including chlorine (Cl), zinc (Zn), strontium (Sr), bromine (Br), copper (Cu), manganese (Mn), tungsten (W), gold (Au), aluminum (Al), silicon (Si), iron (Fe), and fluorine (Fl).

C. Fluoride in Calculus
1. *Concentration.* The concentration of fluoride in calculus varies and is influenced by the amount of fluoride received from fluoride in the drinking water, topical application,[14] dentifrices,[15,16] or any form that is received by contact with the external surface of the calculus.
2. *Uptake.* The surface of the cementum, which is more permeable, has a content of fluoride higher than that of the enamel surface.

D. Crystals
At least two-thirds of the inorganic matter of calculus is crystalline, principally apatite. Predominating is hydroxyapatite, which is the same crystal present in enamel, dentin, cementum, and bone. Calculus also contains varying amounts of brushite, whitlockite, and octocalcium phosphate.[17]

E. Calculus Compared With Teeth and Bone
Dental enamel is the most highly calcified tissue in the body and contains 96% inorganic salts; dentin contains 65%, and cementum and bone contain 45% to 50%.[18] Mature calculus has approximately 75% to 85% inorganic content. A comparison of calculus with the tooth parts provides insight into the effects of instrumentation, the difficulty of distinguishing calculus from cementum or dentin when scaling subgingivally, and the modes of attachment of calculus to the tooth surface.

II. ORGANIC

The organic proportion of calculus consists of various types of nonvital microorganisms, desquamated epithelial cells, leukocytes, and mucin from the saliva. Substances identified in the organic matrix include cholesterol, cholesterol esters, phospholipids, and fatty acids in the lipid fraction; reducing sugars and carbohydrate–protein complexes in the carbohydrate fraction; and keratins, nucleoproteins, and amino acids in the protein portion.[19,20]

The microorganisms are predominantly filamentous. In early calculus, during the first 5 days, cocci are found with some rods.[19,21] Most of the organisms within calculus are considered nonviable. The plaque on the calculus surface contains viable organisms.

SIGNIFICANCE OF DENTAL CALCULUS

Calculus has long been considered to have an important role in the development, promotion, and recurrence of gingival and periodontal infections.

Significant to the rationale for calculus removal and the production of a smooth tooth surface are the points summarized here concerning the relationship of calculus to periodontal and gingival diseases.

I. RELATION TO BACTERIAL PLAQUE
A. Subgingival plaque develops as a result of downgrowth of supragingival plaque bacteria.
B. Subgingival plaque contains pathogenic bacteria that cause inflammation and destruction in the gingival tissue and lead to loss of attachment to the tooth surface and development and deepening of the pocket.

II. RELATION TO ATTACHMENT LOSS AND POCKET FORMATION
A. With increased pocket depth, greater amounts of plaque can accumulate with increased numbers of pathogenic organisms. Irritation to the pocket lining stimulates greater flow of gingival sulcus fluid, which contains minerals for subgingival calculus formation.
B. Calculus is mineralized bacterial plaque. The plaque bacteria next to the tooth surface are mineralized first.
C. Subgingival calculus is always covered by masses of active plaque bacteria. The bacterial mass is in contact with the diseased pocket epithelium and promotes gingivitis and periodontitis.
D. With its rough surface, permeable structure, and porosity, calculus can act as a reservoir

for endotoxins and tissue breakdown products.

E. Calculus is a predisposing factor in pocket development in that it provides a haven for the collection of bacterial masses on the rough surface of the calculus deposit.

PREVENTION OF CALCULUS

Dental calculus can be a cosmetic problem or a periodontal health problem (or both) for many patients. Patients at risk for calculus formation need individualized counseling. Risk factors related to calculus formation are the same as those for bacterial plaque formation. The contributing factors in disease development described in Chapter 13 (pages 231 to 234) apply to calculus and plaque and their formation and reformation.

There are several methods for coping with the problem of calculus. The patient must understand the importance of individual daily bacterial plaque removal and how professional maintenance appointments on a regular basis can supplement the personal care.

I. PROFESSIONAL REMOVAL OF CALCULUS

A. Removal of calculus provides a smooth tooth surface in an environment conducive to gingival healing.

B. The smooth surfaces can be easier for the patient to maintain.

C. With emphasis on good oral hygiene and routine professional removal, low levels of supra- and subgingival calculus have been demonstrated on a long-term basis.[22]

II. PERSONAL BACTERIAL PLAQUE CONTROL

Removal of bacterial plaque by appropriately selected brushing, flossing, and supplementary methods is a major factor in the control of dental calculus reformation.

III. ANTICALCULUS DENTIFRICE

Calculus-control dentifrices currently available contain either a pyrophosphate system or a zinc system. Their aim is to inhibit calculus crystal growth, which in turn should lessen the amount of calculus deposited on the teeth. The dentifrices do not have an effect on existing calculus deposits and are offered as a preventive measure against the formation of new calculus.

For a patient who cannot control supragingival calculus, and hence cannot achieve optimum gingival tissue health, an anticalculus dentifrice may provide motivation, as well as a supplement to mechanical plaque removal efforts.[23]

FACTORS TO TEACH THE PATIENT

I. Good oral hygiene and frequent professional care for complete scaling are consistent with low levels of supra- and subgingival calculus.

II. What calculus is and how it forms from bacterial plaque.

III. The effect of calculus on the health of the periodontal tissues and, therefore, on the general health of the oral cavity.

IV. Properties of calculus that explain the need for detailed, meticulous scaling procedures.

V. Reasons for producing a calculus-free smooth tooth surface during scaling.

VI. Plaque control measures that the patient may carry out to minimize calculus deposits.

VII. What to expect from use of an anticalculus dentifrice.

VIII. Only selecting products with an ADA Seal of Acceptance (see Figure 24-15, page 389).

REFERENCES

1. **Mandel,** I.D.: Calculus Update: Prevalence, Pathogenicity and Prevention, *J. Am. Dent. Assoc., 126,* 573, May, 1995.
2. **Fitzgerald,** R.J. and McDaniel, E.G.: Dental Calculus in the Germ-free Rat, *Arch. Oral Biol., 2,* 239, August, 1960.
3. **Gustafsson,** B.E. and Krasse, B.: Dental Calculus in Germfree Rats, *Acta Odontol. Scand., 20,* 135, Number 2, 1962.
4. **Theilade,** J., Fitzgerald, R.J., Scott, D.B., and Nylen, M.U.: Electron Microscopic Observations of Dental Calculus in Germfree and Conventional Rats, *Arch. Oral Biol., 9,* 97, January–February, 1964.
5. **Gonzales,** F. and Sognnaes, R.F.: Electronmicroscopy of Dental Calculus, *Science, 131,* 156, January 15, 1960.
6. **Zander,** H.A., Hazen, S.P., and Scott, D.B.: Mineralization of Dental Calculus, *Proc. Soc. Exp. Biol. Med., 103,* 257, February, 1960.
7. **Ingram,** G.S. and Edgar, W.M.: Calcium Salt Precipitation and Mechanisms of Inhibition Under Oral Conditions, *Adv. Dent. Res., 9,* 427, December, 1995.
8. **Schroeder,** H.E.: *Formation and Inhibition of Dental Calculus.* Vienna, Hans Huber Publishers, 1969, pp. 73–74.
9. **Vogel,** J.J. and Amdur, B.H.: Inorganic Pyrophosphate in Parotid Saliva and Its Relation to Calculus Formation, *Arch. Oral Biol., 12,* 159, January, 1967.
10. **Canis,** M.F., Kramer, G.M., and Pameijer, C.M.: Calculus Attachment. Review of the Literature and New Findings, *J. Periodontol., 50,* 406, August, 1979.
11. **Mandel,** I.D.: Biochemical Aspects of Calculus Formation, *J. Periodont. Res., 9,* 10, No. 1, 1974.
12. **Glock,** G.E. and Murray, M.M.: Chemical Investigation of Salivary Calculus, *J. Dent. Res., 17,* 257, August, 1938.
13. **Mandel,** I.D. and Levy, B.M.: Studies on Salivary Calculus. I. Histochemical and Chemical Investigations of Supra- and Subgingival Calculus, *Oral Surg., 10,* 874, August, 1957.
14. **Schait,** A. and Mühlemann, H.R.: Fluoride Uptake by Calculus Following Topical Application of Fluorides, *Helv. Odont. Acta, 15,* 132, October, 1971.
15. **Kinoshita,** S., Schait, A., Schroeder, H.E., and Mühlemann, H.R.: Origin of Fluoride in Early Dental Calculus, *Helv. Odont. Acta, 9,* 141, October, 1965.
16. **Mühlemann,** H.R., Schait, A., and Schroeder, H.E.: Salivary Origin of Fluorine in Calcified Dental Plaques, *Helv. Odont. Acta, 8,* 128, October, 1964.
17. **Grøn,** P., van Campen, G.J., and Lindstrom, I.: Human Dental

Calculus. Inorganic Chemical and Crystallographic Composition, *Arch. Oral Biol., 12,* 829, July, 1967.

18. **Melfi,** R.C.: *Permar's Oral Embryology and Microscopic Anatomy,* 9th ed. Philadelphia, Lea & Febiger, 1994, p. 85.

19. **Mandel,** I.D., Levy, B.M., and Wasserman, B.H.: Histochemistry of Calculus Formation, *J. Periodontol., 28,* 132, April, 1957.

20. **Mandel,** I.D.: Histochemical and Biochemical Aspects of Calculus Formation, *Periodontics, 1,* 43, March–April, 1963.

21. **Turesky,** S., Renstrup, G., and Glickman, I.: Histologic and Histochemical Observations Regarding Early Calculus Formation in Children and Adults, *J. Periodontol., 32,* 7, January, 1961.

22. **Anerud,** A., Löe, H., and Boysen, H.: The Natural History and Clinical Course of Calculus Formation in Man, *J. Clin. Periodontol., 18,* 160, March, 1991.

23. **Tilliss,** T.S.I.: A Closer Look at Tartar Control Dentifrices, *J. Dent. Hyg., 63,* 364, October, 1989.

SUGGESTED READINGS

Breuer, M.M., Mboya, S.A., Moroi, H., and Turesky, S.S.: Effect of Selected Beta-blockers on Supragingival Calculus Formation, *J. Periodontol., 67,* 428, April, 1996.

Brown, C.M., Hancock, E.B., O'Leary, T.J., Miller, C.H., and Sheldrake, M.A.: A Microbiological Comparison of Young Adults Based on Relative Amounts of Subgingival Calculus, *J. Periodontol., 62,* 591, October, 1991.

Carranza, F.A.: Dental Calculus, in Carranza, F.A. and Newman, M.G.: *Clinical Periodontology,* 8th ed. Philadelphia, W.B. Saunders Co., 1996, pp. 150–160.

Christersson, L.A., Grossi, S.G., Dunford, R.G., Machtei, E.E., and Genco, R.J.: Dental Plaque and Calculus: Risk Indicators for Their Formation, *J. Dent. Res., 71,* 1425, July, 1992.

Gaare, D., Rølla, G., Aryadi, F.J., and Van der Ouderaa, F.: Improvement of Gingival Health by Toothbrushing in Individuals with Large Amounts of Calculus, *J. Clin. Periodontol., 17,* 38, January, 1990.

Gaffar, A., LeGcros, R.Z., Gambogi, R.J., and Afflitto, J.: Recent Advances in Plaque, Gingivitis, Tartar and Caries Prevention Technology, *Int. Dent. J., 44,* 63, February, Supplement 1, 1994.

Galgut, P.N.: Supragingival Calculus Formation in a Group of Young Adults, *Quintessence Int., 27,* 817, December, 1996.

Hazen, S.P.: Supragingival Dental Calculus, *Periodontology 2000,* 8, 125, 1995.

MacPherson, L.M.D., Girardin, D.C., Hughes, N.J., Stephen, K.W., and Dawes, C.: The Site-specificity of Supragingival Calculus Deposition on the Lingual Surfaces of the Six Permanent Lower Anterior Teeth in Humans and the Effects of Age, Sex, Gum-chewing Habits and the Time Since Last Prophylaxis on Calculus Scores, *J. Dent. Res., 74,* 1715, October, 1995.

Mandel, I.D.: Calculus Formation and Prevention: An Overview, *Compend. Cont. Educ. Dent.,* Special Issue No. 1, pp. S1–3, 1991.

Mandel, I.D. and Gaffar, A.: Calculus Revisited. A Review, *J. Clin. Periodontol., 13,* 249, April, 1986.

Nancollas, G.H. and Johnsson, M.A.S.: Calculus Formation and Inhibition, *Adv. Dent. Res., 8,* 307, July, 1994.

Okumura, H., Nakagaki, H., Kato, K., Ito, F., Weatherall, J.A., and Robinson, C.: Distribution of Fluoride in Human Dental Calculus, *Caries Res., 27,* 271, July–August, 1993.

Rolla, G., Rykke, M., and Gaare, D.: The Role of the Acquired Enamel Pellicle in Calculus Formation, *Adv. Dent. Sci., 9,* 403, December, 1995.

Turesky, S., Breuer, M., and Coffman, G.: The Effect of Certain Systemic Medications on Oral Calculus Formation, *J. Periodontol., 63,* 871, November, 1992.

Walsh, T.F., Figures, K.H., and Lamb, D.J.: *Clinical Dental Hygiene. A Handbook for the Dental Team.* Oxford, England, Wright, 1992, pp. 56–57, 88–89, 121–122.

Anticalculus Dentifrice

Adams, D.: Calculus-inhibition Agents: A Review of Recent Clinical Trials, *Adv. Dent. Res., 9,* 410, December, 1995.

Beacham, B.E., Kurgansky, D., and Gould, W.M.: Circumoral Dermatitis and Cheilitis Caused by Tartar Control Dentifrices, *J. Am. Acad. Dermatol., 22,* 1029, June, 1990.

Chikte, U.M.E., Rudolph, M.J., and Reinach, S.G.: Anti-calculus Effects of Dentifrice Containing Pyrophosphate Compared with Control, *Clin. Prev. Dent., 14,* 29, July–August, 1992.

Disney, J.A., Graves, R.C., Cancro, L., Payonk, G., and Stewart, P.: An Evaluation of 6 Dentifrice Formulations for Supragingival Anticalculus and Antiplaque Activity, *J. Clin. Periodontol., 16,* 525, September, 1989.

Drake, D.R., Chung, J., Grigsby, W., and Wu-Yuan, C.: Synergistic Effect of Pyrophosphate and Sodium Dodecyl Sulfate on Periodontal Pathogens, *J. Periodontol., 63,* 696, August, 1992.

Gaengler, P., Kurbad, A., and Weinert, W.: Evaluation of Anticalculus Efficacy. An SEM Method of Evaluating the Effectiveness of Pyrophosphate Dentifrice on Calculus Formation, *J. Clin. Periodontol., 20,* 144, February, 1993.

Hall, R.C., Embery, G., and Shellis, R.P.: Fluoride Modulates the Inhibition of *in vitro* Hydroxyapatite Crystal Growth by Small Dentin Proteoglycan: Relevance to Dental Calculus, *Adv. Dent. Res., 9,* 433, December, 1995.

Kazmierczak, M., Mather, M., Ciancio, S., Fischman, S., and Cancro, L.: A Clinical Evaluation of Anticalculus Dentifrices, *Clin. Prev. Dent., 12,* 13, April–May, 1990.

Kowitz, G., Jacobson, J., Meng, Z., and Lucatorto, F.: The Effects of Tartar-control Toothpaste on the Oral Soft Tissues, *Oral Surg. Oral Med. Oral Pathol., 70,* 529, October, 1990.

Mellberg, J.R., Petrou, I.D., Fletcher, R., and Grote, N.: Evaluation of the Effects of a Pyrophosphate-Fluoride Anticalculus Dentifrice on Remineralization and Fluoride Uptake *in situ, Caries Res., 25,* 65, January–February, 1991.

Petrone, M., Lobene, R.R., Harrison, L.B., Volpe, A., and Petrone, D.M.: Clinical Comparison of the Anticalculus Efficacy of Three Commercially Available Dentifrices, *Clin. Prev. Dent., 13,* 18, July–August, 1991.

Scruggs, R.R., Stewart, P.W., Samuels, M.S., and Stamm, J.W.: Clinical Evaluation of Seven Anticalculus Dentifrice Formulations, *Clin. Prev. Dent., 13,* 23, January, 1991.

Segreto, V.A., Collins, E.M., D'Agostino, R., Cancro, L.P., Pfeifer, J., and Gilbert, R.J.: Anticalculus Effect of a Dentifrice Containing 0.5% Zinc Citrate Trihydrate, *Community Dent. Oral Epidemiol., 19,* 29, February, 1991.

Stephan, K.W., Saxton, C.A., Jones, C.L., Ritchie, J.A., and Morrison, T.: Control of Gingivitis and Calculus by a Dentifrice Containing a Zinc Salt and Triclosan, *J. Periodontol., 61,* 674, November, 1990.

Dental Stains and Discolorations

Discolorations of the teeth and restorations occur in three general ways: (1) stain adheres directly to the surfaces, (2) stain contained within calculus and soft deposits, and (3) stain incorporated within the tooth structure or the restorative material. Instructional and clinical procedures apply to all three. The first two types may be removed by scaling or polishing. Certain stains may be prevented by the patient's routine personal care.

The significance of stains is primarily the appearance or cosmetic effect. In general, any detrimental effect on the teeth or gingival tissues is related to the bacterial plaque or calculus in which the stain occurs. Thick deposits of stain conceivably can provide a rough surface on which bacterial plaque can collect and irritate the adjacent gingiva. Certain stains provide a means of evaluating oral cleanliness and the patient's habits of personal care. Key words that relate to dental stains and discolorations are defined in Box 18-1.

I. CLASSIFICATION OF STAINS

A. Classified by Location
1. *Extrinsic.* Extrinsic stains occur on the external surface of the tooth and may be removed by procedures of toothbrushing, scaling, and/or polishing.
2. *Intrinsic.* Intrinsic stains occur within the tooth substance and cannot be removed by techniques of scaling or polishing.

B. Classified by Source
1. *Exogenous.* Exogenous stains develop or originate from sources outside the tooth. Exogenous stains may be extrinsic and stay on the outer surface of the tooth or intrinsic and become incorporated within the tooth structure.
2. *Endogenous.* Endogenous stains develop or originate from within the tooth. Endogenous stains are always intrinsic and usually are discolorations of the dentin reflected through the enamel.

II. RECOGNITION AND IDENTIFICATION

More than one type of stain may occur and more than one etiologic factor may cause the stains of an individual's dentition. A differential diagnosis may be needed.

BOX 18-1 KEY WORDS: Dental Stains and Discolorations

Amelogenesis imperfecta (am"ĕ-lo-jen'ĕ-sis im-per-fec'tah): imperfect formation of enamel; hereditary condition in which the ameloblasts fail to lay down the enamel matrix properly or at all.

Chlorophyll (klor'ō-fĭl): green plant pigment essential to photosynthesis.

Chromogenic (krō"mō-jen'ik): producing color or pigment.

Chronologic (kron"ĕl-oj'ic): arranged in order of time.

Dentinogenesis imperfecta (den"ti-nō-jen'ĕ-sis): hereditary disorder of dentin formation in which the odontoblasts lay down an abnormal matrix; can occur in both primary and permanent dentitions.

Endogenous (en-doj'ĕ-nus): produced within or caused by factors within.

Exogenous (eks-oj'ĕ-nus): originating outside or caused by factors outside.

Extrinsic (eks-trin'sĭk): derived from or situated on the outside; external.

Hypoplasia (hī"pō-plā'zhah): incomplete development or underdevelopment of an organ or a tissue.

Intrinsic (in-trin'sik): situated entirely within.

A. Medical and Dental History

Developmental complications, medications, use of tobacco, and fluoride histories all contribute necessary information.

Accurately prepared medical and dental histories can provide information to supplement clinical observations.

B. Food Record

Assessment of a food record may aid in identifying certain contributing factors.

C. Oral Hygiene Habits

The history of personal plaque removal with the type and frequency of use of toothbrush, floss, and other supplemental materials and devices may help to explain the presence of certain stains. The state of oral hygiene and oral cleanliness is significant to the occurrence of dental stains.

III. APPLICATION OF PROCEDURES FOR STAIN REMOVAL

A. Stains Occurring Directly on the Tooth Surface

1. Stains that are directly associated with the plaque or pellicle on the surface of the enamel or exposed cementum are removed as much as possible during toothbrushing by the patient. Certain stains can be removed by scaling, whereas others require polishing.
2. When stains are tenacious, excessive polishing should be avoided. As mild an abrasive agent as possible should be used. Precautions should be taken to prevent (1) abrasion of the tooth surface or gingival margin, (2) removal of a layer of fluoride-rich tooth surface, or (3) overheating with a power-driven polisher.

B. Stains Incorporated Within Tooth Deposits

When stain is included within the substance of a soft deposit or calculus, it is removed with the deposit.

EXTRINSIC STAINS

The most frequently observed stains, yellow, green, black line, and tobacco, are described first; descriptions of the less common orange, red, and metallic stains follow.

I. YELLOW STAIN

A. Clinical Appearance

Dull, yellowish discoloration of bacterial plaque appears.

B. Distribution on Tooth Surfaces

Yellow stain is associated with presence of bacterial plaque. Note distribution of bacterial plaque, Table 16-2, page 268.

C. Occurrence

1. Common to all ages.
2. More evident when personal oral care procedures are neglected.

D. Etiology

Usually food pigments.

II. GREEN STAIN

A. Clinical Appearance

1. Light or yellowish green to very dark green.
2. Embedded in bacterial plaque.
3. Occurs in three general forms:
   a. Small curved line following contour of facial gingival crest.
   b. Smeared irregularly, may even cover entire facial surface.
   c. Streaked, following grooves or lines in enamel.

4. The stain is frequently superimposed by soft yellow or gray debris (materia alba and food debris).
5. Dark green may become embedded in surface enamel and be observed as an exogenous intrinsic stain when superficial layers of deposit are removed.
6. Enamel under stain is sometimes demineralized as a result of cariogenic plaque. The rough demineralized surface encourages plaque retention, demineralization, and recurrence of green stain.

B. Distribution on Tooth Surfaces
1. Primarily facial; may extend to proximal.
2. Most frequently facial cervical third of maxillary anterior teeth.

C. Composition
1. Chromogenic bacteria and fungi.
2. Decomposed hemoglobin.
3. Inorganic elements include calcium, potassium, sodium, silicon, magnesium, phosphorus, and other elements in small amounts.[1]

D. Occurrence
1. May occur at any age; primarily found in childhood.
2. Collects on both permanent and primary teeth.

E. Recurrence
Recurrence depends on fastidiousness of personal care procedures.

F. Etiology
Green stain results from oral uncleanliness, chromogenic bacteria, and gingival hemorrhage.
1. Chromogenic bacteria or fungi are retained and nourished in bacterial plaque where the green stain is produced.
2. Blood pigments from hemoglobin are decomposed by bacteria.
3. Predisposing factors are the presence of means for retention and proliferation of chromogenic bacteria, such as bacterial plaque, and food debris.

G. Clinical Approach
1. Do not scale the area. Often, an area of demineralized tooth structure underlies the stain and soft deposits.
2. Ask the patient to remove the soft deposits during a bacterial plaque control lesson. Initiate a daily fluoride remineralization program.

H. Other Green Stains
In addition to the clinical entity known as "green stain" that was just described, bacterial plaque and acquired pellicle may become stained a green color by a variety of substances. Differential distinction may be determined by questioning the patient or from items in the medical or dental histories. Green discoloration may result from the following:
1. Chlorophyll preparations.
2. Metallic dusts of industry.
3. Certain drugs. The stain from smoking marijuana may appear grayish green.

III. BLACK LINE STAIN

Black line stain is a highly retentive black or dark brown calculus-like stain that forms along the gingival third near the gingival margin. It may occur on primary or permanent teeth.

A. Other Names
Pigmented dental plaque, brown stain, black stain.

B. Clinical Features
1. Continuous or interrupted fine line, 1 mm wide (average), no appreciable thickness.
2. May be a wider band or even occupy entire gingival third in severe cases (rare).
3. Follows contour of gingival crest about 1 mm above crest.
4. Usually demarcated from gingival crest by clear white line of unstained enamel.
5. Appears black at bases of pits and fissures.
6. Heavy deposits slightly elevated from the tooth surface may be detected with an explorer.
7. Gingiva is firm, with little or no tendency to bleed.
8. Teeth are frequently clean and shiny, with a tendency to lower incidence of dental caries.

C. Distribution on Tooth Surfaces
1. Facial and lingual surfaces; follows contour of gingival crest onto proximal surfaces.
2. Rarely on facial surface of maxillary anterior teeth.
3. Most frequently: lingual and proximal surfaces of maxillary posterior teeth.

D. Composition and Formation[2,3]
1. Black line stain, like calculus, is composed of microorganisms embedded in an intermicrobial substance.
2. The microorganisms are primarily gram-positive rods, with other bacteria, including cocci, in smaller percentages.

   The composition of black line stain is different from the composition of supragingival calculus, in which cocci predominate. Attachment to the tooth of black line stain is by a pellicle-like structure.[4]

   Oral disease does not result from the presence of black line stain. In contrast, gingivitis is related to the formation of supragingival plaque, and in the presence of a cariogenic substrate, dental caries develops.

3. Mineralization in black line stain is similar to the formation of calculus.

E. Occurrence
1. All ages; more common in childhood.
2. More common in female patients.
3. Frequently found in clean mouths.

F. Recurrence
Black line stain tends to form again despite regular personal care, but quantity may be less when plaque control procedures are meticulous.

G. Predisposing Factors
None apparent, except a natural tendency.

IV. TOBACCO STAIN

A. Clinical Appearance
1. Light brown to dark leathery brown or black.
2. Shape
   a. Diffuse staining of bacterial plaque.
   b. Narrow band that follows contour of gingival crest, slightly above the crest.
   c. Wide, firm, tarlike band may cover cervical third and extend to central third of crown.
3. Incorporated in calculus deposit.
4. Heavy deposits (particularly from smokeless tobacco) may penetrate the enamel and become exogenous intrinsic.

B. Distribution on Tooth Surfaces
1. Cervical third, primarily.
2. Any surface, as well as pits and fissures.
3. Most frequently on lingual surfaces.

C. Composition
1. Tar and products of combustion.
2. Brown pigment from smokeless tobacco.

D. Predisposing Factors
1. Natural tendencies. The quantity of stain is not necessarily proportional to the amount of tobacco used.
2. Personal oral care procedures: increased deposits occur with neglect.
3. Extent of bacterial plaque and calculus available for adherence.

V. OTHER BROWN STAINS

A. Brown Pellicle
The acquired pellicle is smooth and structureless and recurs readily after removal.[5] The pellicle can take on stains of various colors that result from chemical alteration of the pellicle.[6]

B. Stannous Fluoride[7–9]
Light brown, sometimes yellowish, stain forms on the teeth in the pellicle after repeated use of a stannous fluoride gel or other product, or after having a topical fluoride application. The brown stain results from the formation of stannous sulfide or brown tin oxide from the reaction of the tin ion in the fluoride compound.

C. Foodstuffs
Tea, coffee, and soy sauce are often implicated in the formation of a brownish-stained pellicle. As with other brown pellicle stains, less stain occurs when the personal oral hygiene and plaque control are excellent.

D. Anti-Plaque Agents[10,11]
Chlorhexidine and alexidine are used in mouthrinses and are effective against plaque formation (page 386). A brownish stain of the tooth surfaces results, usually more pronounced on proximal and other surfaces less accessible to routine plaque control procedures. The stain also tends to form more rapidly on exposed roots than on enamel. Tooth staining has been considered a significant side effect.

E. Betel Leaf[12]
Betel leaf chewing is common among people of all ages in eastern countries. Betel has a caries-inhibiting effect.

The discoloration imparted to the teeth is a dark mahogany brown, sometimes almost black. It may become thick and hard, with partly smooth and partly rough surfaces.

Microscopically, the black deposit consists of microorganisms and mineralized material with a laminated pattern characteristic of subgingival calculus. It should be removed by scaling.

VI. ORANGE AND RED STAINS

A. Clinical Appearance
Orange or red stains appear at the cervical third.

B. Distribution on Tooth Surfaces
1. More frequently on anterior than on posterior teeth.
2. Both facial and lingual surfaces of anterior teeth.

C. Occurrence
Rare (red more rare than orange).

D. Etiology
Chromogenic bacteria.

VII. METALLIC STAINS

A. Metals or Metallic Salts From Metal-Containing Dust of Industry
1. *Clinical Appearance.* Examples of colors on teeth:
   a. Copper or brass: green or bluish-green.
   b. Iron: brown to greenish-brown.
   c. Nickel: green.
   d. Cadmium: yellow or golden brown.
2. *Distribution on Tooth Surfaces*

a. Primarily anterior; may occur on any teeth.

b. Cervical third more commonly affected.

3. *Manner of Formation*

a. Industrial worker inhales dust through mouth, bringing metallic substance in contact with teeth.

b. Metal imparts color to bacterial plaque.

c. Occasionally, stain may penetrate tooth substance and become exogenous intrinsic stain.

B. Metallic Substances Contained in Drugs

1. *Clinical Appearance.* Examples of colors on teeth:

a. Iron: black (iron sulfide) or brown.

b. Manganese (from potassium permanganate): black.

2. *Distribution on Tooth Surfaces.* Generalized, may occur on all.

3. *Manner of Formation*

a. Drug enters plaque substance, imparts color to plaque and calculus.

b. Pigment from drug may attach directly to tooth substance.

4. *Prevention.* Use a medication through a straw or in tablet or capsule form to prevent direct contact with the teeth.

ENDOGENOUS INTRINSIC STAINS

Stains incorporated within the tooth structure may be related to the period of tooth development.

I. PULPLESS TEETH

Not all pulpless teeth discolor. Improved endodontic procedures have contributed to the prevention of many discolorations formerly associated with that cause.

A. Clinical Appearance

A wide range of colors exists; stains may be light yellow-brown, slate gray, reddish-brown, dark brown, bluish-black, or black. Others have an orange or greenish tinge.

B. Manner of Formation

1. Blood and other pulp tissue elements may be made available for breakdown as a result of hemorrhages in the pulp chamber, root canal treatment, or necrosis and decomposition of the pulp tissue.

2. Pigments from the decomposed hemoglobin and pulp tissue penetrate the dentinal tubules.

II. TETRACYCLINES

A. Tetracycline antibiotics, used widely for combating many types of infections, have an affinity for mineralized tissues and are absorbed by the bones and teeth. They can be transferred through the placenta and enter fetal circulation.

B. Discoloration of the teeth of a child can result when the drug is administered to the mother during the third trimester of pregnancy or to the child in infancy and early childhood.

C. Color of teeth may be light green to dark yellow, or a gray-brown. The discoloration depends on the dosage, length of time the drug was used, and the type of tetracycline. After eruption, the teeth may fluoresce under ultraviolet light, but that property is lost with age and exposure.[14]

D. Discoloration may be generalized or limited to specific parts of individual teeth that were developing at the time of administration of the antibiotic. Reference to the Table of Tooth Development can assist in determining the patient's age at the time the drug was administered, and the patient's medical history at that age may reveal the illness for which the antibiotic was prescribed (see Tables 14-1 and 14-2, pages 238 and 239).

III. IMPERFECT TOOTH DEVELOPMENT

Defective tooth development may result from factors of genetic abnormality or environmental influences during tooth development.

A. Hereditary: Genetic[15]

1. *Amelogenesis Imperfecta:* The enamel is partially or completely missing because of a generalized disturbance of the ameloblasts. Teeth are yellowish-brown or gray-brown.

2. *Dentinogenesis Imperfecta ("Opalescent Dentin"):* The dentin is abnormal as a result of disturbances in the odontoblastic layer during development. The teeth appear translucent or opalescent and vary in color from gray to bluish-brown.

B. Enamel Hypoplasia

1. *Systemic Hypoplasia* (chronologic hypoplasia resulting from ameloblastic disturbance of short duration). Teeth erupt with white spots or with pits. Over a long period of time, the white spots may become discolored from food pigments or other substances taken into the mouth. Figure 14-5 (page 243) shows an example of chronologic hypoplasia.

2. *Local Hypoplasia* (affects single tooth). White spots may become stained as in systemic hypoplasia.

C. Dental Fluorosis

Dental fluorosis was originally called "brown stain." Later, Dr. Frederick S. McKay, who studied the condition and described it in the dental literature, named it "mottled enamel" (pages 460 and 461).

1. *Manner of Formation*
   a. Enamel hypomineralization results from ingestion of excessive fluoride ion in drinking water (more than 2 parts per million) during the period of mineralization. The enamel alterations are a result of toxic damage to the ameloblasts.
   b. When the teeth erupt, they have white spots or areas that later become discolored from oral pigments and appear light or dark brown.
   c. Severe effects of excess fluoride during development may produce cracks or pitting; the discoloration concentrates in these. This condition and appearance led to the name mottled enamel.
2. *Classification*
   Dean provided the original definitions for five grades of fluorosis. They ranged from "questionable" (a few white flecks or spots) to "severe" (marked brown staining and pitting of the enamel surfaces).[16]

   More specific classifications have been developed for clinical and research purposes.[17,18] The Tooth Surface Index of Fluorosis (TSIF) is shown in Table 29-2, page 461.

IV. OTHER SYSTEMIC CAUSES

Several types of tooth discolorations may result from blood-borne pigments.

Pigments circulating in the blood are transmitted to the dentin from the capillaries of the pulp. For example, prolonged jaundice early in life can impart a yellow or greenish discoloration to the teeth.

Erythroblastosis fetalis (Rh incompatibility) may leave a green, brown, or blue hue to the teeth.

EXOGENOUS INTRINSIC STAINS

When intrinsic stains come from an outside source, not from within the tooth, the stain is called exogenous intrinsic. Extrinsic stains, such as tobacco and green stains, can provide stain that becomes intrinsic.

Restorative materials cause staining of teeth, as described in the section that follows. Tooth-color restorations may become stained from the various extrinsic staining substances mentioned in this chapter. A few references are included in "Suggested Readings" at the end of the chapter.

I. RESTORATIVE MATERIALS

A. Silver Amalgam
1. Silver amalgam can impart a gray to black discoloration to the tooth structure around a restoration.
2. Metallic ions migrate from the amalgam restoration into the enamel and dentin.
3. Silver, tin, and mercury ions eventually contact debris at the junction of the tooth and the restoration and form sulfides, which are products of corrosion.

B. Copper Amalgam
Copper amalgam used for filling primary teeth may impart a bluish-green color.

II. ENDODONTIC THERAPY AND RESTORATIVE MATERIALS

A. Silver nitrate: bluish-black.
B. Volatile oils: yellowish-brown.
C. Strong iodine: brown.
D. Aureomycin: yellow.
E. Silver-containing root canal sealer: black.

III. DRUGS

A. Stannous Fluoride Topical Application[7]
1. Light to dark brown staining from the formation of tin sulfide.
2. Located most frequently in occlusal pits and grooves of posterior teeth and cervical third facial surfaces of anterior teeth; in carious and precarious lesions; and in margins of tooth color and amalgam restorations.
3. Staining may accompany dental caries arrestment.

B. Ammoniacal Silver Nitrate
Used in treatment of such sensitive areas as exposed cementum or for inhibition of demineralization in dental caries prevention; imparts a dark brown to black discoloration.

IV. STAIN IN DENTIN

Discoloration resulting from a carious lesion is an example.

TECHNICAL HINTS

I. Record color, type, extent, and location of stains with the patient's examination and assessment.
II. Make additions to the dental history as information is gained concerning the origin of stains such as those related to tooth development, systemic disease, occupations, or medications.
III. Avoid making patient feel self-conscious by overemphasizing the appearance of stains, particularly those that may occur in spite of conscientious bacterial plaque removal habits.
IV. Use tact when questioning patients with brown stain, because nonsmokers do not appreciate having an assumption made concerning the cause of a brown stain on the teeth.

FACTORS TO TEACH THE PATIENT

I. Predisposing factors that contribute to stain accumulation.

II. Personal care procedures that can aid in the prevention or reduction of stains.

III. Advantages of starting a smoking cessation program.

IV. Reasons for not using an abrasive dentifrice with vigorous brushing strokes to lessen or remove stain accumulation.

V. The need to avoid tobacco, coffee, tea, and other beverages or foodstuffs that can stain, to prevent discoloration of new restorations.

VI. Reasons for the difficulty of removing certain extrinsic stains during scaling and polishing.

VII. Effect of tetracyclines on developing teeth. Need to avoid use during pregnancy and by children to age 12.

REFERENCES

1. **Shay,** D.E., Haddox, J.H., and Richmond, J.L.: An Inorganic Qualitative and Quantitative Analysis of Green Stain, *J. Am. Dent. Assoc., 50,* 156, February, 1955.

2. **Theilade,** J., Slots, J., and Fejerskov, O.: The Ultrastructure of Black Stain on Human Primary Teeth, *Scand. J. Dent. Res., 81,* 528, No. 7, 1973.

3. **Slots,** J.: The Microflora of Black Stain on Human Primary Teeth, *Scand. J. Dent. Res., 82,* 484, No. 7, 1974.

4. **Theilade,** J.: Development of Bacterial Plaque in the Oral Cavity, *J. Clin. Periodontol., 4,* 1, December, 1977.

5. **Meckel,** A.H.: The Formation and Properties of Organic Films on Teeth, *Arch. Oral Biol., 10,* 585, July–August, 1965.

6. **Eriksen,** H.M. and Nordbø, H.: Extrinsic Discoloration of Teeth, *J. Clin. Periodontol., 5,* 229, November, 1978.

7. **Horowitz,** H.S. and Chamberlin, S.R.: Pigmentation of Teeth Following Topical Applications of Stannous Fluoride in a Non-fluoridated Area, *J. Public Health Dent., 31,* 32, Winter, 1971.

8. **Shannon,** I.L.: Stannous Fluoride: Does It Stain Teeth? How Does It React with Tooth Surfaces? A Review, *Gen. Dent., 26,* 64, September–October, 1978.

9. **Leverett,** D.H., McHugh, W.D., and Jensen, Ø.E.: Dental Caries and Staining After Twenty-eight Months of Rinsing with Stannous Fluoride or Sodium Fluoride, *J. Dent. Res., 65,* 424, March, 1986.

10. **Flötra,** L., Gjermo, P., Rölla, G., and Waerhaug, J.: Side Effects of Chlorhexidine Mouthwashes, *Scand. J. Dent. Res., 79,* 119, April, 1971.

11. **Formicola,** A.J., Deasy, M.J., Johnson, D.H., and Howe, E.E.: Tooth Staining Effects of an Alexidine Mouthwash, *J. Periodontol., 50,* 207, April, 1979.

12. **Reichart,** P.A., Lenz, H., König, H., Becker, J., and Mohr, U.: The Black Layer on the Teeth of Betel Chewers: a Light Microscopic, Microradiographic, and Electronmicroscopic Study, *J. Oral Pathol., 14,* 466, July, 1985.

13. **Ehrlich,** A. and Torres, H.O.: *Essentials of Dental Assisting.* Philadelphia, W.B. Saunders Co., 1992, pp. 389–393.

14. **Robinson,** H.B.G. and Miller, A.S.: *Color Atlas of Oral Pathology,* 5th ed. Philadelphia, J.B. Lippincott Co., 1990, p. 55.

15. **Ibid.,** p. 41.

16. **Dean,** H.T.: Investigation of Physiological Effects by Epidemiological Method, in Moulton, F.R., ed.: *Fluorine and Dental Health.* Washington, D.C., American Association for the Advancement of Science, No. 19, 1942.

17. **Thylstrup,** A. and Fejerskov, O.: Clinical Appearance of Dental Fluorosis in Permanent Teeth in Relation to Histologic Changes, *Community Dent. Oral Epidemiol., 6,* 315, December, 1978.

18. **Horowitz,** H.S., Driscoll, W.S., Meyers, R.J., Heifetz, S.B., and Kingman, A.: A New Method for Assessing the Prevalence of Dental Fluorosis—The Tooth Surface Index of Fluorosis, *J. Am. Dent. Assoc., 109,* 37, July 1984.

SUGGESTED READINGS

Addy, M. and Moran, J.: Mechanisms of Stain Formation on Teeth, in Particular Associated with Metal Ions and Antiseptics, *Adv. Dent. Sci., 9,* 450, December, 1995.

Barta, J.E., King, D.L., and Jorgensen, R.L.: ABO Blood Group Incompatibility and Primary Tooth Discoloration, *Pediatr. Dent., 11,* 316, December, 1989.

Cuff, M.J.A., McQuade, M.J., Scheidt, M.J., Sutherland, D.E., and Van Dyke, T.E.: The Presence of Nicotine on Root Surfaces of Periodontally Diseased Teeth in Smokers, *J. Periodontol., 60,* 564, October, 1989.

Holan, G. and Fuks, A.B.: The Diagnostic Value of Coronal Dark-gray Discoloration in Primary Teeth Following Traumatic Injuries, *Pediatr. Dent., 18,* 224, May–June, 1996.

Joiner, A., Jones, N.M., and Raven, S.J.: Investigation of Factors Influencing Stain Formation Utilizing an *in situ* Model, *Adv. Dent. Sci., 9,* 471, December, 1995.

Massler, M. and Schour, I.: *Atlas of the Mouth.* Chicago, American Dental Association, Plate 12.

Nathoo, S.A.: The Chemistry and Mechanisms of Extrinsic and Intrinsic Discoloration, *J. Am. Dent. Assoc., 128,* 6S, April, Supplement, 1997.

Nathoo, S.A. and Gaffar, A.: Studies on Dental Stains Induced by Antibacterial Agents and Rational Approaches for Bleaching Dental Stains, *Adv. Dent. Res., 9,* 462, December, 1995.

Tilliss, T.: Dental Stains and Chemotherapeutics: A Closer Look, *DentalHygienistNews, 2,* 12, January/February/March, 1989.

Chlorhexidine and Antibiotics

Addy, M., Moran, J., Griffiths, A.A., and Wills-Wood, N.J.: Extrinsic Tooth Discoloration by Metals and Chlorhexidine I. Surface Protein Denaturation or Dietary Precipitation?, *Br. Dent. J., 159,* 281, November 9, 1985.

Addy, M. and Moran, J.: Extrinsic Tooth Discoloration by Metals and Chlorhexidine. II. Clinical Staining Produced by Chlorhexidine, Iron and Tea, *Br. Dent. J., 159,* 331, November 23, 1985.

Addy, M., Al-Arrayed, F., and Moran, J.: The Use of an Oxidizing Mouthwash to Reduce Staining Associated with Chlorhexidine. Studies *in vitro* and *in vivo, J. Clin. Periodontol., 18,* 267, April, 1991.

Addy, M., Mahdavi, S.A., and Loyn, T.: Dietary Staining *in vitro* by Mouthrinses as a Comparative Measure of Antiseptic Activity and Predictor of Staining *in vivo, J. Dent., 23,* 95, April, 1995.

Beiswanger, B.B., Mallatt, M.E., Mau, M.S., Jackson, R.D., and Hennon, D.K.: The Clinical Effects of a Mouthrinse Containing 0.1% Octenidine, *J. Dent. Res., 69,* 454, February, 1990.

Berger, R.S., Mandel, E.B., Hayes, T.J., and Grimwood, R.R.: Minocycline Staining of the Oral Cavity, *J. Am. Acad. Dermatol., 21,* 1300, December, 1989.

Leard, A. and Addy, M.: The Propensity of Different Brands of Tea and Coffee to Cause Staining Associated with Chlorhexidine, *J. Clin. Periodontol., 24,* 115, February, 1997.

Parkins, F.M., Furnish, G., and Bernstein, M.: Minocycline Use Discolors Teeth, *J. Am. Dent. Assoc., 123,* 87, October, 1992.

Sanz, M., Vallcorba, N., Fabregues, S., Müller, I., and Herkströter, F.: The Effect of a Dentifrice Containing Chlorhexidine and Zinc on Plaque, Gingivitis, Calculus and Tooth Staining, *J. Clin. Periodontol., 21,* 431, July, 1994.

Wade, W., Addy, M., Hughes, J., Milsom, S., and Doherty, F.: Studies on Stannous Fluoride Toothpaste and Gel (1). Antimicrobial Properties and Staining Potential in Vitro, *J. Clin Periodontol., 24,* 81, February, 1997.

Discoloration of Restorations

Chan, K.C., Fuller, J.L., and Hormati, A.A.: The Ability of Foods to Stain Two Composite Resins, *J. Prosthet. Dent., 43,* 542, May, 1980.

Kidd, E.A.M.: The Caries Status of Tooth-coloured Restorations with Marginal Stain, *Br. Dent. J., 171,* 241, October 19, 1991.

Luce, M.S. and Campbell, C.E.: Stain Potential of Four Micro-filled Composites, *J. Prosthet. Dent., 60,* 151, August, 1988.

Nordbö, H., Attramadal, A., and Eriksen, H.M.: Iron Discoloration of Acrylic Resin Exposed to Chlorhexidine or Tannic Acid: A Model Study, *J. Prosthet. Dent., 49,* 126, January, 1983.

Um, C.M. and Ruyter, I.E.: Staining of Resin-based Veneering Materials with Coffee and Tea, *Quintessence Int., 22,* 377, May, 1981.

Indices and Scoring Methods

19

Indices and scoring methods are used in clinical practice and community programs to determine and record the state of health of individuals and groups. Several well-known and widely used indices and scoring methods are described in this chapter. In addition, an index for scoring enamel fluorosis is included on page 461 with the chapter on fluorides. "Suggested Readings" at the end of the chapter contains references to other indices. Box 19-1 defines related terminology.

Familiarity with the various types of indices may prove helpful when different evaluation criteria are needed. A distinction must be made between an individual oral health assessment score, a clinical trial, and a community health epidemiologic survey.

I. INDIVIDUAL ASSESSMENT SCORE

A. Purpose

In clinical practice, an index, plaque record, or scoring system for an individual patient can be used for education, motivation, and evaluation. The effects of personal disease control efforts, the progress of healing between professional treatments, and the maintenance of health over time can be monitored. An example is the plaque-free score described on pages 299 to 302 in which a patient is able to measure the effects of personal daily care efforts by the changes in the scores. This system may prove to be a valuable motivating device.

B. Uses

1. Provides individual assessment to help a patient recognize an oral problem.

2. Reveals the degree of effectiveness of present oral hygiene practices.
3. Motivates the person in preventive and professional care for the elimination and control of oral disease.
4. Evaluates the success of individual and professional treatment over a period of time by comparing index scores.

II. CLINICAL TRIAL

A. Purpose

A clinical trial is planned for the determination of the effect of an agent or procedure on the prevention, progression, or control of a disease. The trial is conducted by comparing an experimental group with a control group that is similar to the experimental group in every way except for the variable being studied.

Examples of indices used for clinical trials are the Plaque Index (Pl I) of Silness and Löe[1] and the Patient Hygiene Performance (PHP) of Podshadley and Haley.[2] These and other indices are described in this chapter.

B. Uses

1. Determines baseline data before experimental factors are introduced.
2. Measures the effectiveness of specific agents for the prevention, control, or treatment of oral conditions.
3. Measures the effectiveness of mechanical devices for personal care, such as toothbrushes, interdental cleaning devices, or irrigators.

BOX 19-1 KEY WORDS: Indices and Scoring Methods

Calibration (kal″ĭ-bra′shun): determination of accuracy and consistency between examiners to standardize procedures and gain reliability of recorded findings; instrument calibration is defined in Box 12-1.

Epidemiology (ep′ĭ-dē″mē-ol′o-jē): the study of the relationships of various factors that determine the frequency and distribution of diseases in the human community; study of health and disease in populations.

Incidence (in′sĭ-dens): the rate at which a certain event occurs, as the number of new cases of a specific disease occurring during a certain period of time.

Index (in′deks): a graduated, numeric scale with upper and lower limits; scores on the scale correspond to a specific criterion for individuals or populations; *pl.* indices (in′dĭ-sēz) or indexes (in-dek′sĕz).

Pilot study: a trial run of a planned study using a small sample to pretest an instrument, survey, or questionnaire.

Placebo (plah-sē′bō): an inactive substance or preparation with no intrinsic therapeutic value given to satisfy a patient's symbolic need for drug therapy; used in controlled research studies in a form identical in appearance to the material being tested.

Prevalence (prev′ah-lens): the total number of cases of a specific disease or condition in existence in a given population at a certain time.

Ramfjord Index Teeth: teeth used for epidemiologic studies of periodontal diseases: the maxillary right and mandibular left first molars, maxillary left and mandibular right first premolars, and maxillary left and mandibular right central incisors.

Reliability: ability of an index or test procedure to measure consistently at different times and under a variety of conditions; reproducibility; consistency.

Screening of a *population:* assessment of many individuals to disclose certain characteristics or a certain disease entity; *individual* screening: brief assessment for initial evaluation and classification of needs for additional examination and treatment planning.

Validity: ability of an index or test procedure to measure what it is intended to measure.

III. EPIDEMIOLOGIC SURVEY

A. Purpose
The word *epidemiology* denotes the study of disease characteristics of populations. An example of an index designed for a survey of population groups is the DMFT (Decayed, Missing, and Filled Teeth) Index.[3] It has been used with populations around the world to determine the extent of dental caries. Such a survey was not designed for evaluation of an individual patient.

B. Uses
1. Shows the prevalence and incidence of a particular condition occurring within a given population.
2. Provides baseline data to show existing dental health practices.
3. Assesses the needs of a community.
4. Compares the effects of a community program and evaluates the results.

IV. INDEX

An index is an expression of clinical observations in numeric values. It is used to describe the status of the individual or group with respect to a condition being measured. The use of a numeric scale and a standardized method for interpreting observations of a condition results in an index score that is more consistent and less subjective than a word description of that condition.

A. Descriptive Categories of Indices
1. *General Categories*
   a. Simple index: One that measures the presence or absence of a condition. An example is an index that measures the presence of bacterial plaque without evaluating its effect on the gingiva.
   b. Cumulative index: One that measures all the evidence of a condition, past and present. An example is the DMFT Index for dental caries.
2. *Types of Simple and Cumulative Indices*
   a. Irreversible: One that measures conditions that will not change. An example is an index that measures dental caries.
   b. Reversible: One that measures conditions that can be changed. Examples are indices that measure bacterial plaque.

B. Selection Criteria
A useful and effective index
1. Is simple to use and calculate.
2. Requires minimal equipment and expense.
3. Uses a minimal amount of time to complete.
4. Does not cause patient discomfort nor is otherwise unacceptable to a patient.
5. Has clear-cut criteria that are readily understandable.
6. Is as free as possible from subjective interpretation.
7. Is reproducible by the same examiner or different examiners.
8. Is amenable to statistical analysis; has validity and reliability.

V. SYSTEMS DESCRIBED IN THIS CHAPTER

A. Screening for Periodontal Health (PSR) (page 295)

B. Bacterial Plaque
1. Plaque Index (Pl I) (page 298).
2. Plaque Control Record (page 298).
3. Plaque-Free Score (page 299).

C. Plaque, Debris, Calculus
1. Patient Hygiene Performance (PHP) (page 302).
2. Simplified Oral Hygiene Index (OHI-S) (page 303).

D. Gingival Bleeding
1. Sulcus Bleeding Index (SBI) (page 305).
2. Gingival Bleeding Index (GBI) (page 305).
3. Eastman Interdental Bleeding Index (EIBI) (page 306).

E. Gingival/Periodontal
1. Gingival Index (GI) (page 307).
2. Community Periodontal Index of Treatment Needs (CPITN) (page 308).

F. Dental Caries
1. Decayed, Missing, and Filled Permanent Teeth (DMFT) (page 309).
2. Decayed, Missing, and Filled Permanent Tooth Surfaces (DMFS) (page 310).
3. Primary teeth indices (page 311).

PERIODONTAL SCREENING & RECORDING (PSR)
(American Academy of Periodontology and American Dental Association[4])

I. PURPOSE

To assess the state of periodontal health in a rapid and effective manner and to motivate the patient to seek necessary complete periodontal assessment and treatment.

II. SELECTION OF TEETH

The dentition is divided into sextants. Each tooth is examined. Posterior sextants begin distal to the canines.

III. PROCEDURE

A. Instrument
Specially designed probe used by World Health Organization for the CPITN (page 308).
1. *Markings.* At intervals from tip: 3.5, 2.0, 3.0, and 3.0 mm (total 11.5 mm) (Figure 19-1).
2. *Working Tip.* A ball 0.5 mm in diameter. The functions of the ball are

a. To aid in the detection of calculus, rough overhanging margins of restorations, and other tooth surface irregularities.

b. To facilitate assessment at the probing depth and reduce risk of overmeasurement.

3. *Color Coding.* Color-coded between 3.5 and 5.5 mm.

B. Probe Application

1. Insert probe gently into a sulcus until resistance is felt.

2. Apply a circumferential walking step to probe systematically about each tooth through each sextant.

3. Observe color-coded area of the probe for prompt identification of probing depths.

4. Remember that each sextant receives one code number corresponding to the deepest position of the color-coded portion of the probe.

C. Criteria

1. Five codes and an asterisk are used. Table 19-1 shows the clinical findings, code significance, and patient management guidelines.

2. Each code may include conditions identified with the preceding codes; for example, Code

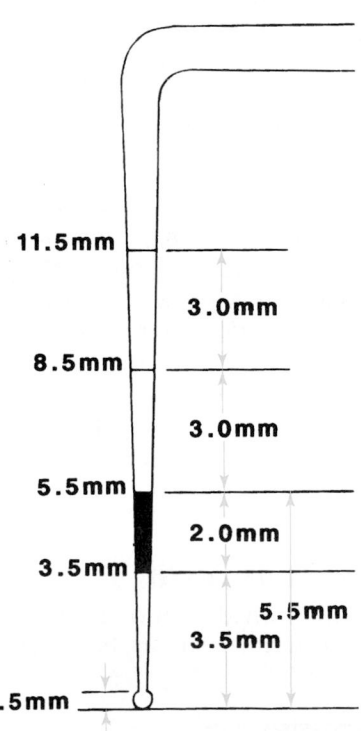

FIGURE 19-1 Periodontal Probe. The probe, with markings as shown, is used to make determinations for the PSR and the Community Periodontal Index of Treatment Needs (CPITN). (From FDI: *A Simplified Periodontal Examination for Dental Practices.* Fédération Dentaire Internationale, 64 Wimpole Street, London WIM 8AL.)

3 with probing depth from 3.5 to 5.5 mm also may include calculus, an overhanging restoration, and bleeding on probing.

3. One need not probe the remaining teeth in a sextant when a Code 4 is found. For Codes 0, 1, 2, and 3, the sextant is completely probed.

D. Recording

1. Use a simple six-box form to provide a space for each sextant. The form can be made into peel-off stickers or a rubber stamp to facilitate recording in the patient's permanent record.

2. One score is marked for each sextant; the highest code observed is recorded. When indicated, an asterisk is added to the score in the individual space with the sextant code number.

IV. SCORING

A. Follow-up Patient Management

Patients are classified into assessment and treatment planning needs by the highest coded score of their PSR (Table 19-1, right column).

B. Calculation Examples

EXAMPLE I.

4*	2	3
3	2*	4*

PSR Sextant Score

Interpretation: With Codes 3 and 4, a comprehensive periodontal examination is indicated. Asterisks mean furcation involvement in two quadrants, and a possible mucogingival involvement in the mandibular anterior sextant. When the patient has not been aware of the presence of periodontal involvement, counseling is important if cooperation and compliance are to be obtained.

EXAMPLE 2.

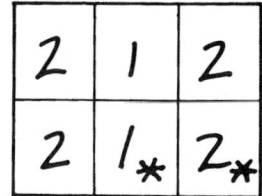

PSR Sextant Score

Interpretation: An overall Code 2 can indicate calculus and overhanging restorations that must be removed. All restorations must be checked for recurrent dental caries. Appointments for instruction in bacterial plaque control

TABLE 19-1 Periodontal Screening and Recording (PSR)[†]

Clinical Findings	Code Description	Management Guidelines
Code 0	**Code 0** • Colored area of probe is completely visible in the deepest probing depth of the sextant • No calculus, no defective margins, no bleeding	**Code 0** • Bacterial plaque control • Preventive care
Code 1	**Code 1** • Colored area of probe is completely visible in the deepest probing depth of the sextant • Smooth surfaces, no calculus, no defective margins • There is bleeding after gentle probing	**Code 1** • Bacterial plaque control • Preventive care
Code 2	**Code 2** • Colored area of probe is completely visible in the deepest probing depth • Rough surface felt may be supra- and/or sub-gingival calculus • Defective margins of restorations	**Code 2** • Bacterial plaque control instruction • Complete preventive care • Calculus removal • Correction of irregular margins of restorations
Code 3	**Code 3** • Colored area of probe is only partly visible in the deepest probing depth • Requirements for Codes 1 and 2 may be present	**Code 3** • Comprehensive periodontal assessment is indicated[‡] • Patient is counseled concerning appropriate treatment plan
Code 4	**Code 4** • Colored area of probe completely disappears • Probing depth greater than 5.5 mm	**Code 4** • Comprehensive periodontal assessment is indicated[†] • Patient is counseled concerning appropriate treatment plan
★ Clinical Abnormality	**Code ★** • Any notable feature such as furcation involvement • mobility • mucogingival problem • marked recession area	**Code ★** • Abnormality in Codes 0, 1, or 2: specific treatment is planned • In Codes 3 or 4: included in comprehensive assessment and treatment plan

[†]American Dental Association and American Academy of Periodontology, 1992.
[‡]Comprehensive periodontal assessment includes but is not limited to radiographic and clinical examination (complete soft tissue record, identification of probing depths, mobility, gingival recession, mucogingival problems, and furcation involvements).

are of primary concern. The asterisks in two quadrants may indicate minimal attached gingiva.

PLAQUE INDEX (Pl I)
(Silness and Löe[1,5])

I. PURPOSE
To assess the thickness of plaque at the gingival area.

II. SELECTION OF TEETH
The entire dentition or selected teeth can be evaluated.

A. Areas Examined
Examine four gingival areas (distal, facial, mesial, lingual) systematically for each tooth.

B. Modified Procedures
Examine only the facial, mesial, and lingual areas. Assign double score to the mesial reading, and divide the total by 4.

III. PROCEDURE
A. Dry the teeth and examine visually using adequate light, mouth mirror, and probe or explorer.
B. Evaluate bacterial plaque on the cervical third; pay no attention to plaque that has extended to the middle or incisal thirds.
C. Use probe to test the surface when no plaque is visible. Pass the probe or explorer across the tooth surface in the cervical third and near the entrance to the sulcus. When no plaque adheres to the probe tip, the area is scored 0. When plaque adheres, a score of 1 is assigned.
D. Use a disclosing agent, if necessary, to assist evaluation for the 0 to 1 scores. When the Pl I is used in conjunction with the Gingival Index (GI, page 307), the GI must be completed first because the disclosing agent masks the gingival characteristics.
E. Include plaque on the surface of calculus and on dental restorations in the cervical third in the evaluation.
F. Criteria
   0 = No plaque.
   1 = a film of plaque adhering to the free gingival margin and adjacent area of the tooth. The plaque may be recognized only after application of disclosing agent or by running the explorer across the tooth surface.
   2 = Moderate accumulation of soft deposits within the gingival pocket that can be seen with the naked eye or on the tooth and gingival margin.
   3 = Abundance of soft matter within the gingival pocket and/or on the tooth and gingival margin.

IV. SCORING

A. Pl I for Area
Each area (distal, facial, mesial, lingual or palatal) is assigned a score from 0 to 3.

B. Pl I for a Tooth
Scores for each area are totaled and divided by 4.

C. Pl I for Groups of Teeth
Scores for individual teeth may be grouped and totaled and divided by the number of teeth. For instance, a Pl I may be determined for specific teeth or groups of teeth. The right side may be compared with the left.

D. Pl I for the Individual
Add the scores for each tooth and divide by the number of teeth examined. The Pl I ranges from 0 to 3.

E. Suggested Range of Scores for Patient Reference

Rating	Scores
Excellent	0
Good	0.1–0.9
Fair	1.0–1.9
Poor	2.0–3.0

F. Pl I for a Group
Add the scores for each member of a group and divide by the number of individuals.

PLAQUE CONTROL RECORD
(O'Leary, Drake, and Naylor[6])

I. PURPOSE
To record the presence of bacterial plaque on individual tooth surfaces to permit the patient to visualize progress while learning plaque control.

II. SELECTION OF TEETH AND SURFACES
A. All teeth are included. Missing teeth are identified on the record form by a single thick horizontal line.
B. Four surfaces are recorded: facial, lingual, mesial, and distal.
C. Six areas may be recorded. The mesial and distal segments of the diagram may be divided to provide space to record proximal surfaces from the facial separately from the lingual or palatal surfaces (Figure 19-2).[7]

III. PROCEDURE
A. Apply disclosing agent or give a chewable tablet. Instruct patient to swish and rub the solution over the tooth surfaces with the tongue before rinsing.
B. Examine each tooth surface for bacterial

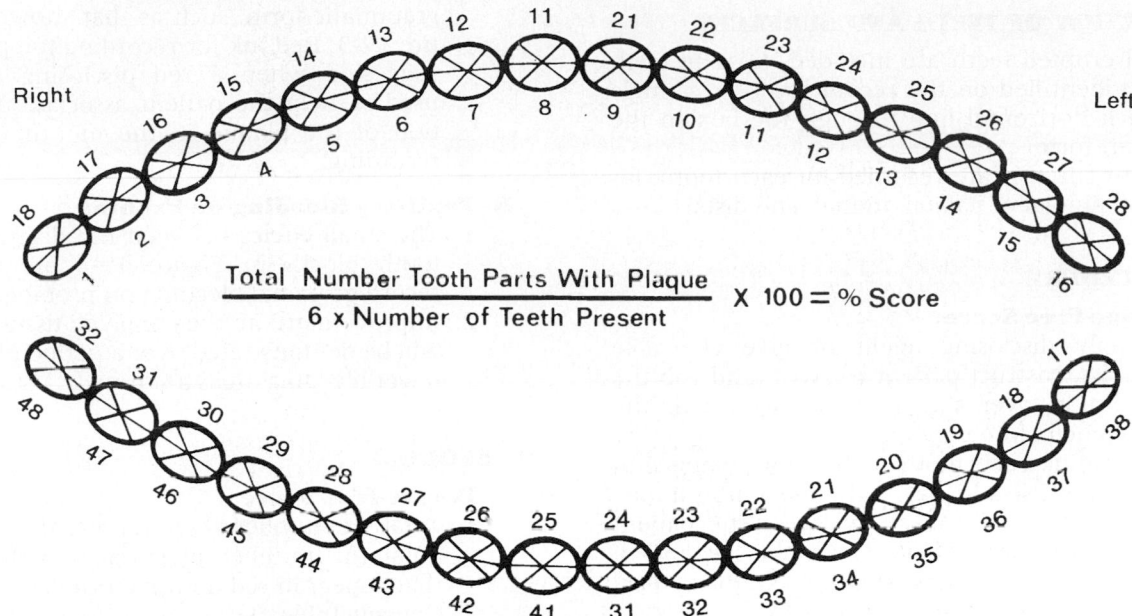

Total Number Tooth Parts With Plaque / **6 x Number of Teeth Present** X 100 = % Score

■ **FIGURE 19-2 Plaque Control Record.** Diagrammatic representation of the teeth includes spaces to record plaque on six areas of each tooth. The facial surfaces are on the outer and the lingual and palatal surfaces on the inner portion of the arches. Teeth are numbered by the ADA System on the inside and by the FDI System on the outside. (Modified from Ramfjord, S.P. and Ash, M.M.: *Periodontology and Periodontics.* Philadelphia, W.B. Saunders Co., 1979, p. 273 and from O'Leary, T.J., Drake, R.B., and Naylor, J.E.: *J. Periodontol.,* 43, 38, 1972.)

plaque at the gingival margin. No attempt is made to differentiate quantity of plaque.

C. Record by making a dash or coloring in the appropriate spaces on the diagram (Figure 19-2) to indicate plaque on facial, lingual, palatal, mesial, and/or distal surfaces.

IV. SCORING

A. Total the number of teeth present; multiply by four (or six if modification is used) to obtain the number of available surfaces. Count the number of surfaces with plaque.

B. Multiply the number of plaque-stained surfaces by 100 and divide by the total number of available surfaces to derive the percentage of surfaces with plaque.

C. Compare over subsequent appointments as the patient learns and practices plaque control. Ten percent or fewer plaque-stained surfaces can be considered a good goal, but if the plaque is regularly left in the same areas, special instruction is indicated to prevent pocket formation.

D. Calculation example for plaque control record:

Individual findings: 26 teeth scored
                                  8 surfaces with plaque

1. Multiply the number of teeth by 4:

26 × 4 = 104 surfaces

2. Percent with plaque –

$$\frac{\text{Number of surfaces with plaque} \times 100}{\text{Number of available tooth surfaces}}$$

$$= \frac{8 \times 100}{104} = \frac{800}{104} = 7.6$$

Interpretation: Although 0% is ideal, fewer than 10% plaque-stained surfaces has been suggested as a guideline in periodontal therapy. After initial therapy and when the patient has reached a 10% level of plaque control or better, necessary additional periodontal and restorative procedures may be initiated.[6] In comparison, a similar evaluation using a plaque-free score would mean that a goal of 90% or better plaque-free surfaces would have to be reached before the surgical phase of treatment could be undertaken.

PLAQUE-FREE SCORE
(Grant, Stern, Everett[8])

I. PURPOSE

To determine the location, number, and percentage of plaque-free surfaces for individual motivation and instruction. Interdental bleeding can also be documented.

II. SELECTION OF TEETH AND SURFACES

A. All erupted teeth are included. Missing teeth are identified on the record form by a single thick horizontal line through the box in the chart form.

B. Four surfaces are recorded for each tooth: facial, lingual or palatal, mesial, and distal.

III. PROCEDURE

A. Plaque-Free Score

1. Apply disclosing agent or give chewable tablet. Instruct patient to swish and rub the solution over the tooth surfaces with the tongue before rinsing.

2. Examine each tooth surface for evidence of plaque. Use adequate light and a mouth mirror for visualizing all surfaces. The patient needs a hand mirror to see the location of the plaque that has been missed during personal hygiene procedures.

3. Record in red the surfaces showing plaque. Use an appropriate tooth chart form or a dia-

grammatic form, such as that shown in Figure 19-3. Red ink for recording the plaque is suggested when a red disclosing agent is used to help the patient associate the location of the plaque in the mouth with the recording.

B. Papillary Bleeding on Probing

1. The small circles between the diagrammatic tooth blocks in Figure 19-3 are used to record proximal bleeding on probing.

2. Improvement in the gingival tissue health will be demonstrated over a period of time as fewer bleeding areas are noted.

IV. SCORING

A. Plaque-Free Score

1. Total the number of teeth present.

2. Total the number of surfaces with plaque that appear in red on the tooth diagram.

3. Consult Table 19-2:
   a. Read across the top or bottom to locate the number of teeth and total surfaces.

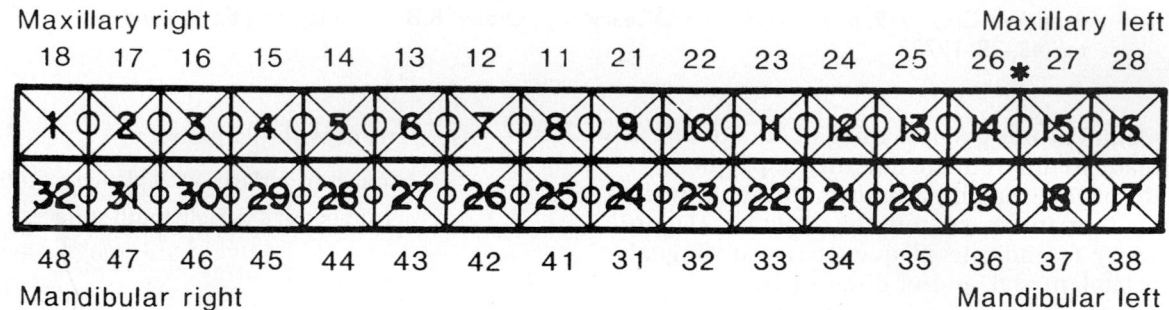

Maxillary right | Maxillary left

18 17 16 15 14 13 12 11 21 22 23 24 25 26 * 27 28

1 2 3 4 5 6 7 8 9 10 11 12 13 14 15 16

32 31 30 29 28 27 26 25 24 23 22 21 20 19 18 17

48 47 46 45 44 43 42 41 31 32 33 34 35 36 37 38

Mandibular right | Mandibular left

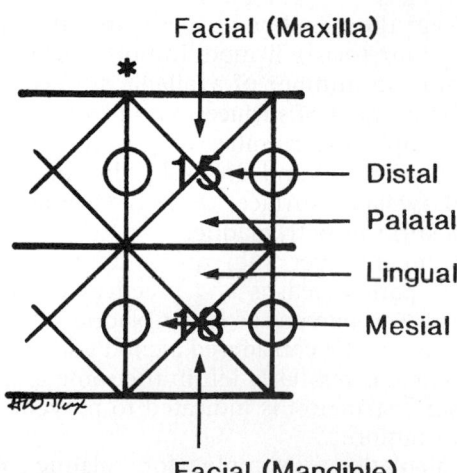

Facial (Maxilla)

Distal
Palatal
Lingual
Mesial

Facial (Mandible)

FIGURE 19-3 Plaque-free Score. Diagrammatic representation of the teeth used to record plaque and papillary bleeding. Enlargement of teeth (*) shows tooth surfaces. Teeth are numbered by the ADA System inside each block and by the FDI System outside each block. (Adapted from Grant, D.A., Stern, I.B., and Listgarten, M.A.: *Periodontics,* 6th ed. St. Louis, Mosby, 1988, p. 613.)

TABLE 19-2 Plaque-Free Score

Number of Tooth Surfaces

Number of Tooth Surfaces With Plaque	32–128	31–124	30–120	29–116	28–112	27–108	26–104	25–100	24–96	23–92	22–88	21–84	
1	99.2	99.2	99.2	99.2	99.2	99.1	99.1	99.0	99.0	99.0	98.9	98.9	
4	96.9	96.8	96.7	97.6	96.5	96.3	96.2	96.0	95.9	95.7	95.5	95.3	
7	94.6	95.4	94.2	94.0	93.8	93.6	93.3	93.0	92.8	92.4	92.1	91.7	
10	92.2	92.0	91.7	91.4	91.1	90.8	90.4	90.0	89.6	89.2	88.7	88.1	
13	89.9	89.6	89.2	88.8	88.4	88.0	87.5	87.0	86.5	85.9	85.3	84.5	
16	87.5	87.1	86.7	86.3	85.8	85.2	84.7	84.0	83.4	82.7	81.9	81.0	
19	85.2	84.7	84.2	83.7	83.1	82.5	81.8	81.0	80.3	79.4	78.5	77.4	
22	83.9	82.3	81.7	81.1	80.4	79.7	78.9	78.0	77.1	76.1	75.0	73.9	
25	80.4	79.9	79.2	78.5	77.7	76.9	76.0	75.0	74.0	72.9	71.6	70.3	
28	78.2	77.5	76.7	75.9	75.0	74.1	73.1	72.0	70.9	69.6	68.2	66.4	
31	75.8	75.0	74.2	73.3	72.4	71.3	70.2	69.0	67.8	66.4	64.8	63.1	
34	73.5	72.6	71.7	70.7	69.7	68.6	67.4	66.0	64.6	63.1	61.4	59.6	
37	71.1	70.2	69.2	68.2	67.0	65.8	64.5	63.0	61.5	59.8	58.0	56.0	
40	68.8	67.8	66.7	65.6	64.3	63.0	61.6	60.0	58.4	56.6	54.6	52.4	
43	66.5	65.4	64.2	63.0	61.7	60.2	58.7	57.0	55.3	53.3	51.2	48.9	
46	64.1	63.0	61.7	60.4	59.0	57.5	55.8	54.0	52.1	50.0	47.8	45.3	
49	61.8	60.5	59.2	57.8	56.3	54.7	52.9	51.0	49.0	46.8	44.4	41.7	
52	59.4	58.1	56.7	55.2	53.6	51.9	50.0	48.0	45.9	43.5	41.0	38.1	
55	57.1	55.7	54.2	52.6	50.9	49.1	47.2	45.0	42.8	40.3	37.5	34.6	
58	54.7	53.3	51.7	50.0	48.3	46.3	44.3	42.0	39.6	37.0	34.1	31.0	
61	52.4	50.9	49.2	47.5	45.6	43.6	41.4	39.0	36.4	33.7	30.7	27.4	
64	50.0	48.4	46.7	44.9	42.9	40.8	38.5	36.0	33.4	30.5	27.3	23.9	
67	47.7	46.0	44.2	42.3	40.2	38.0	35.6	33.0	30.3	27.2	23.9	20.3	
70	45.4	43.6	41.7	39.7	37.5	35.2	32.7	30.0	27.1	24.0	20.5	16.7	
73	43.0	41.2	39.2	37.1	34.9	32.5	29.9	27.0	24.0	20.7	17.1	13.1	
76	40.7	38.8	36.7	34.5	32.2	29.7	27.0	24.0	20.9	17.4	13.7	9.6	
79	38.3	36.3	34.2	31.9	29.5	26.9	24.1	21.0	17.8	14.2	10.3	6.0	
82	36.0	33.9	31.7	29.4	26.8	24.1	21.2	18.0	14.6	10.9	6.9	2.4	
85	33.6	31.5	29.2	26.8	24.2	21.3	18.3	15.0	11.5	7.7	3.3	—	
88	31.3	29.1	26.7	24.2	21.5	18.6	15.4	12.0	8.4	4.4	0.0	—	
91	29.0	26.7	24.2	21.6	18.8	15.8	12.5	9.0	5.3	1.1	—	1.3	79
94	27.6	24.2	21.7	19.0	16.1	13.0	9.7	6.0	2.1	—	0.0	5.0	78
97	24.3	21.8	19.2	16.4	13.4	10.2	6.8	3.0	—	—	4.0	8.8	73
100	21.9	19.4	16.7	13.8	10.8	7.5	3.9	0.0	—	2.8	7.9	12.5	70
103	19.9	17.0	14.2	11.3	8.1	4.7	1.0	—	1.5	7.0	11.9	16.3	67
106	17.2	14.6	11.7	8.7	5.4	1.9	—	0.0	5.9	11.2	15.8	20.0	64
109	14.9	12.1	9.2	6.1	2.7	—	—	4.7	10.3	15.3	19.8	23.8	61
112	12.5	9.7	6.7	3.5	0.0	—	3.4	9.4	14.8	19.5	23.7	27.5	58
115	11.2	7.3	4.2	.9	—	1.8	8.4	14.1	19.2	23.7	27.7	31.3	55
118	7.9	4.9	1.7	—	0.0	7.2	13.4	18.8	23.6	27.8	31.6	35.0	52
121	5.5	2.5	—	—	5.8	12.5	18.4	23.5	28.0	32.0	35.6	38.8	49
124	3.2	0.0	—	4.2	11.6	17.9	23.4	28.2	32.4	36.2	39.5	42.5	46
128	0.0	—	2.3	10.5	17.4	23.3	28.4	32.9	36.8	40.3	43.5	46.3	43
	—	0.0	9.1	16.7	23.1	28.6	33.4	37.5	41.2	44.5	47.4	50.0	40
	—	7.5	16.0	23.0	28.9	34.0	38.4	42.2	45.6	48.7	51.4	53.8	37
	5.6	15.0	22.8	29.2	34.7	39.3	43.4	46.9	50.0	52.8	55.3	57.5	34
	13.9	22.5	29.6	35.5	40.4	44.7	48.4	51.6	54.5	57.0	59.3	61.3	31
	22.3	30.0	36.4	41.7	46.2	50.0	53.4	56.3	58.9	61.2	63.2	65.0	28
	30.6	37.5	43.2	48.0	52.0	55.4	58.4	61.0	63.3	65.3	67.2	68.8	25
	38.9	45.0	50.0	54.2	57.7	60.8	63.4	65.7	67.7	69.5	71.1	72.5	22
	47.3	52.5	56.9	60.5	63.5	66.1	68.4	70.4	72.1	73.7	75.0	76.3	19
	55.6	60.0	63.7	66.7	69.3	71.5	73.4	75.0	76.5	78.8	79.0	80.0	16
	63.9	67.5	70.5	73.0	75.0	76.8	78.4	79.7	80.9	82.0	82.9	87.5	13
	72.3	75.0	77.3	79.2	80.8	82.2	83.4	84.4	85.3	86.2	86.9	87.5	10
	80.6	82.5	84.1	85.5	86.6	87.5	88.4	89.1	89.8	90.3	90.8	91.3	7
	88.9	90.0	91.0	91.7	92.4	92.9	93.4	93.8	94.2	94.5	94.8	95.0	4
	97.3	97.5	97.8	98.0	98.1	98.3	98.4	98.5	98.6	98.7	98.7	98.8	1
	9–36	10–40	11–44	12–48	13–52	14–56	15–60	16–64	17–68	18–72	19–76	20–80	

(From Grant, D.A., Stern, I.B., and Everett, F.G.: *Periodontics*, 5th ed. St. Louis, Mosby, 1979.)

b. Read down the side to locate the number of surfaces with plaque.

c. Find the intersection of the top and side numbers; this number is the plaque-free score, listed as a percentage.

4. To calculate without Table 19-2 for reference

a. Multiply the number of teeth by four to determine the number of available surfaces.

b. Subtract the number of surfaces with plaque from the total available surfaces to find the number of plaque-free surfaces.

c. Plaque-free score =

$$\frac{\text{Number of plaque-free surfaces} \times 100}{\text{Number of available surfaces}}$$

= Percent plaque-free surfaces

5. Evaluate plaque-free score. Ideally, 100% is the goal. When a patient maintains a percentage under 85%, check individual surfaces to determine whether plaque is usually left in the same areas. To prevent the development of specific areas of periodontal infection, remedial instruction in the areas usually missed is indicated.

B. Papillary Bleeding on Probing

1. Total the number of small circles marked for bleeding. A person with 32 teeth has 30 interdental areas. The mesial or distal surface of a tooth adjacent to an edentulous area is probed and counted.

2. Evaluate total interdental bleeding. In health, bleeding on probing does not occur.

C. Calculation Example for Plaque-Free Score

Individual findings: 24 teeth scored
37 surfaces with plaque

1. With Table 19-2

a. Locate the number of teeth across the top of Table 19-2 (24–96); the second number indicates the number of surfaces, which in this case total 96.

b. Locate the number of surfaces with plaque down the side (37); find the intersection.

c. The percentage of plaque-free surfaces is 61.5%.

2. Without reference to Table 19-2

a. Multiply the number of teeth by 4:

$24 \times 4 = 96$ available surfaces

b. Subtract the number of surfaces with plaque from total available surfaces:

$96 - 37 = 59$ plaque-free surfaces

c. Percentage of plaque-free surfaces:

$$\frac{59 \times 100}{96} = 61.5\%$$

Interpretation: On the basis of the ideal 100%, 61.5% is poor. More instruction is indicated.

PATIENT HYGIENE PERFORMANCE (PHP)
(Podshadley and Haley[2])

I. PURPOSE

To assess the extent of plaque and debris over a tooth surface. Debris is defined for the PHP as the soft foreign material consisting of bacterial plaque, materia alba, and food debris that is loosely attached to tooth surfaces.

II. SELECTION OF TEETH AND SURFACES

A. Teeth Examined
(F.D.I. system tooth numbers are in parentheses.)

Maxillary	Mandibular
No. 3 (16) Right first molar	No. 19 (36) Left first molar
No. 8 (11) Right central incisor	No. 24 (31) Left central incisor
No. 14 (26) Left first molar	No. 30 (46) Right first molar

B. Substitutions
When a first molar is missing, is less than three-fourths erupted, has a full crown, or is broken down, the second molar is used. The third molar is used when the second is missing. The adjacent central incisor is used for a missing incisor.

C. Surfaces
The facial surfaces of incisors and maxillary molars and the lingual surfaces of mandibular molars are examined. These surfaces are the same as those used for the Simplified Oral Hygiene Index (see Figure 19-5, page 303).

III. PROCEDURE

A. Apply disclosing agent. Instruct the patient to swish for 30 seconds and expectorate, but not rinse.

B. Examination is made using a mouth mirror.

C. Each tooth surface to be evaluated is subdivided (mentally) into five sections (Figure 19-4A) as follows:

1. *Vertically.* Three divisions—mesial, middle, and distal.

2. *Horizontally.* The middle third is subdivided into gingival, middle, and occlusal or incisal thirds.

D. Each of the five subdivisions is scored for the presence of stained debris as follows:

0 = No debris (or questionable).
1 = Debris definitely present.
Identify by *M* when all three molars or both incisors are missing.
Identify by *S* when a substitute tooth is used.

IV. SCORING

A. Debris Score for Individual Tooth
Add the scores for each of the five subdivisions. The scores range from 0 to 5.

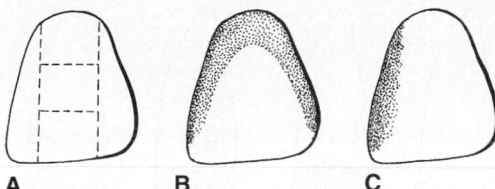

FIGURE 19-4 Patient Hygiene Performance (PHP). **(A)** Oral debris is assessed by dividing a tooth into 5 subdivisions, each of which is scored 1 when debris is shown to be present after use of a disclosing agent. **(B)** Example of debris score of 3. Shaded portion represents debris stained by disclosing agent. **(C)** Example of debris score of 1. (From Podshadley, A.G. and Haley, J.V.: A Method for Evaluating Oral Hygiene Performance, *Public Health Rep., 83,* 259, 1968.)

B. PHP for the Individual

Total the scores for the individual teeth and divide by the number of teeth examined. The PHP ranges from 0 to 5.

C. Suggested Range of Scores for Evaluation

Rating	Scores
Excellent	0–(no debris)
Good	0.1–1.7
Fair	1.8–3.4
Poor	3.5–5.0

D. Calculation Example for an Individual

Tooth	Debris Score
No. 3 (16)	5
No. 8 (11)	3
No. 14 (26)	4
No. 19 (36)	5
No. 24 (31)	2
No. 30 (46)	3
Total	22

$$PHP = \frac{\text{Total debris score}}{\text{Number of teeth scored}} = \frac{22}{6} = 3.66$$

Interpretation: According to the suggested range of scores, this person with a PHP of 3.66 would be classified as exhibiting poor hygiene performance.

E. PHP for a Group

To obtain the average PHP score for a group or population, total the individual scores and divide by the number of people examined.

SIMPLIFIED ORAL HYGIENE INDEX (OHI-S)
(Greene and Vermillion[9] and Greene[10])

I. PURPOSE

To assess oral cleanliness by estimating the tooth surface covered with debris and/or calculus.

II. COMPONENTS

The OHI-S has two components, the Simplified Debris Index (DI-S) and the Simplified Calculus Index (CI-S). The two scores may be used separately or may be combined for the OHI-S.

III. SELECTION OF TEETH AND SURFACES

A. Identify the Six Specific Teeth (Figure 19-5)

1. *Posterior.* The first fully erupted tooth distal to each second premolar is examined. The facial surfaces of the maxillary molars and the lingual surfaces of the mandibular molars are used. Although usually the first molars are used, the second or third molars also may be used.
2. *Anterior.* The facial surfaces of the maxillary right and the mandibular left central incisors are used. When either is missing, the adjacent central incisor is scored.

B. Extent

A score represents half the circumference of the selected tooth; it includes proximal surfaces to the contact areas.

IV. PROCEDURE

A. Qualification

At least two of the six possible surfaces must

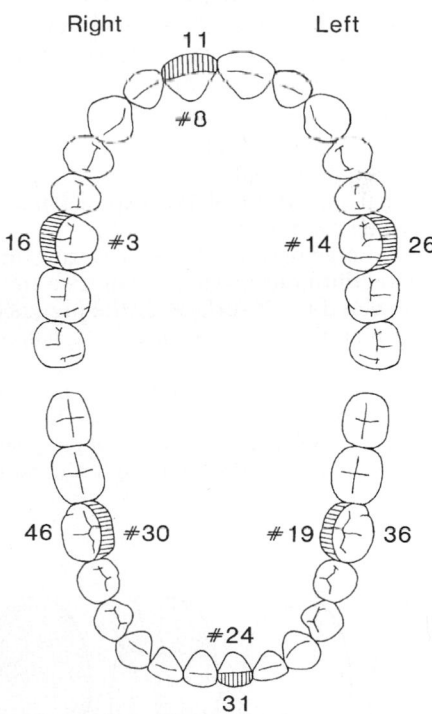

FIGURE 19-5 Simplified Oral Hygiene Index (OHI-S). Six tooth surfaces are scored as follows: facial surfaces of maxillary molars and of the maxillary right and mandibular left central incisors, and the lingual surfaces of mandibular molars. Teeth are numbered by the ADA System on the lingual surface and by the FDI System on the facial surface.

have been examined for an individual score to be calculated.

B. Record Six Debris Scores

1. *Definition of Oral Debris.* Oral debris is the soft foreign matter on the surfaces of the teeth that consists of bacterial plaque, materia alba, and food debris.
2. *Examination.* Run the side of the tip of a probe or explorer across the tooth surface to estimate the surface area covered by debris.
3. *Criteria* (Figure 19-6)

   0 = No debris or stain present.

   1 = Soft debris covering not more than one third of the tooth surface being examined, or the presence of extrinsic stains without debris, regardless of surface area covered.

   2 = Soft debris covering more than one third but not more than two-thirds of the exposed tooth surface.

   3 = Soft debris covering more than two thirds of the exposed tooth surface.

C. Record Six Calculus Scores

1. *Definition of Calculus.* Dental calculus is a hard deposit of inorganic salts composed primarily of calcium carbonate and phosphate mixed with debris, microorganisms, and desquamated epithelial cells.
2. *Examination.* Use an explorer to estimate surface area covered by supragingival calculus deposits. Identify subgingival deposits by exploring and/or probing. Record only definite deposits of hard calculus.
3. *Criteria* (Figure 19-7)

   0 = No calculus present.

   1 = Supragingival calculus covering not more than one third of the exposed tooth surface being examined.

   2 = Supragingival calculus covering more than one third but not more than two thirds of the exposed tooth surface, or the presence of individual flecks of subgingival calculus around the cervical portion of the tooth.

   3 = Supragingival calculus covering more than two thirds of the exposed tooth surface or a continuous heavy band of subgingival calculus around the cervical portion of the tooth.

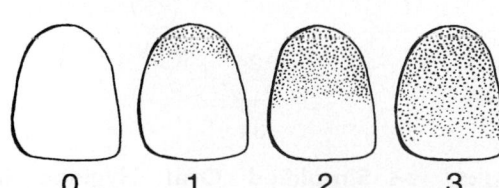

FIGURE 19-6 Simplified Oral Hygiene Index. For the Debris Index, 6 teeth (Figure 19-5) are scored. Scoring of 0 to 3 is based on tooth surfaces covered by debris as shown.

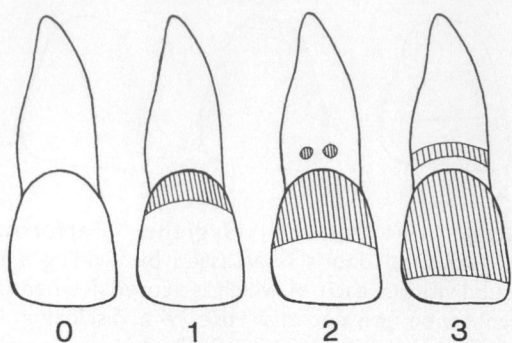

FIGURE 19-7 Simplified Oral Hygiene Index. For the Calculus Index, 6 teeth (Figure 19-5) are scored. Scoring of 0 to 3 is based on location and tooth surface area with calculus as shown. Note slight subgingival calculus recorded as 2 and more extensive subgingival calculus by 3.

V. SCORING

A. OHI-S for an Individual

1. *Determine Simplified Debris Index (DI-S) and Simplified Calculus Index (CI-S)*
   a. Divide total scores by number of sextants.
   b. DI-S and CI-S values range from 0 to 3.
2. *Simplified Oral Hygiene Index (OHI-S)*
   a. Combine the DI-S and CI-S.
   b. OHI-S value ranges from 0 to 6.

B. Suggested Range of Scores for Evaluation[10]
DI-S and CI-S

Rating	Scores
Excellent	0
Good	0.1–0.6
Fair	0.7–1.8
Poor	1.9–3.0

OHI-S

Rating	Scores
Excellent	0
Good	0.1–1.2
Fair	1.3–3.0
Poor	3.1–6.0

C. Calculation Example for an Individual

Tooth	DI-S	CI-S *Score*
Nu. 3 (16)	2	2
No. 8 (11)	1	0
No. 14 (26)	3	2
No. 19 (36)	3	2
No. 24 (31)	2	1
No. 30 (46)	2	2
Total	13	9

$$DI\text{-}S = \frac{\text{Total debris scores}}{\text{Number of teeth scored}} = \frac{13}{6} = 2.17$$

$$CI\text{-}S = \frac{\text{Total calculus scores}}{\text{Number of teeth scored}} = \frac{9}{6} = 1.50$$

$$OHI\text{-}S = DI\text{-}S + CI\text{-}S = 2.17 + 1.50 = 3.67$$

Interpretation: According to the suggested range of scores, the score for this individual (3.67) indicates a poor oral hygiene status.

D. OHI-S Group Score

Compute the average of the individual scores by totaling the scores and dividing by the number of individuals.

BLEEDING INDICES

Bleeding on gentle probing or flossing is an early sign of gingival inflammation and precedes color changes and enlargement of the gingival tissues.[11,12] Based on the principle that healthy tissue does not bleed, testing for bleeding has become a significant procedure for evaluation prior to treatment planning, after therapy to show the effects of treatment, and at maintenance appointments to determine continued control of gingival inflammation.

For patient instruction and motivation, a variety of bleeding indices and scoring methods has been developed. The Gingival Index (GI) described on page 307 includes an estimate of bleeding on probing, along with other clinical observations to score the severity of gingivitis. The GI has been used extensively in research, as well as for patient instruction and motivation.

Another example is a plaque-free score as described on pages 299 to 302. The form illustrated in Figure 19-3 has small circles that can be colored to illustrate interproximal bleeding. A series of diagrams made over several weeks can show the patient's progress toward health, as less and less bleeding is charted.

Bleeding indices described here are the Sulcus Bleeding Index developed by Mühlemann, the Gingival Bleeding Index of Carter and Barnes, and the Eastman Interdental Bleeding Index.

SULCUS BLEEDING INDEX (SBI)
(Mühlemann and Son[11])

I. PURPOSE

To locate areas of gingival sulcus bleeding upon gentle probing and thus recognize and record the presence of early (initial) inflammatory gingival disease.

II. AREAS EXAMINED

Four gingival units are scored systematically for each tooth: the labial and lingual marginal gingivae (M units), and the mesial and distal papillary gingivae (P units).

III. PROCEDURE

A. Use standardized lighting while probing each of the four areas.

B. Hold the probe parallel with the long axis of the tooth for M units, and direct the probe toward the col area for P units.

C. Wait 30 seconds after probing before scoring apparently healthy gingival units.

D. Dry the gingivae gently if necessary to observe color changes clearly.

E. Criteria

0 = Healthy appearance of P and M, no bleeding on sulcus probing.

1 = Apparently healthy P and M showing no change in color and no swelling, but bleeding from sulcus on probing.

2 = Bleeding on probing *and* change of color caused by inflammation. No swelling or macroscopic edema.

3 = Bleeding on probing *and* change in color and slight edematous swelling.

4 = (1) Bleeding on probing *and* change in color *and* obvious swelling.
(2) Bleeding on probing and obvious swelling.

5 = Bleeding on probing and spontaneous bleeding *and* change in color, marked swelling with or without ulceration.

IV. SCORING

A. SBI for Area

Each of the four gingival units (M and P) is scored 0 to 5.

B. SBI for Tooth

Scores for the four units are totaled and divided by four.

C. SBI for Individual

By totaling scores for individual teeth and dividing by the number of teeth, the SBI is determined. Indices range from 0 to 5.

GINGIVAL BLEEDING INDEX (GBI)
(Carter and Barnes[13])

I. PURPOSE

To record the presence or absence of gingival inflammation as determined by bleeding from interproximal gingival sulci.

II. AREAS EXAMINED

Each interproximal area has two sulci, which either are scored as one interdental unit or may be scored individually. Certain areas may be excluded from scoring because of accessibility, tooth position, diastemata, or other factors, and if exclusions are made, a consistent procedure should be followed for an individual and for a group if a study is to be made.

A full complement of teeth has 30 proximal areas.

In the original studies, third molars were excluded, and 26 interdental units were recorded.[13]

III. PROCEDURE

A. Instrument
Unwaxed dental floss is used. Floss has the advantages of being readily available, disposable, and usable by the instructed patient.

B. Steps
1. Pass the floss interproximally first on one side of the papilla and then on the other.
2. Curve the floss around the adjacent tooth (Figure 24-1E and F, page 374), and bring the floss below the gingival margin.
3. Move the floss up and down for one stroke, with care not to lacerate the gingiva. Adapt finger rests to provide controlled, consistent pressure.
4. Use a new length of clean floss for each area.
5. Retract for visibility of bleeding from both facial and lingual aspects.
6. Allow 30 seconds for reinspection of an area that does not show blood immediately either in the area or on the floss.

C. Criteria
Bleeding indicates the presence of disease. No attempt is made to quantify the severity of bleeding because no bleeding represents health.

IV. SCORING

The numbers of bleeding areas and scorable units are recorded. Patient participation in observing and recording over a series of appointments can increase motivation.

EASTMAN INTERDENTAL BLEEDING INDEX (EIBI)
(Abrams, Caton, and Polson[14] and Caton and Polson[15])

I. PURPOSE

To assess the presence of inflammation in the interdental area by the presence or absence of bleeding.

II. AREAS EXAMINED

Each interdental area around the entire dentition.

III. PROCEDURE

A. Instrument
Triangular wooden interdental cleaner (page 380).

B. Steps
1. Insert gently, then immediately remove, a wooden cleaner into each interdental area in such a way as to depress the papilla 1 to 2 mm (Figure 19-8).

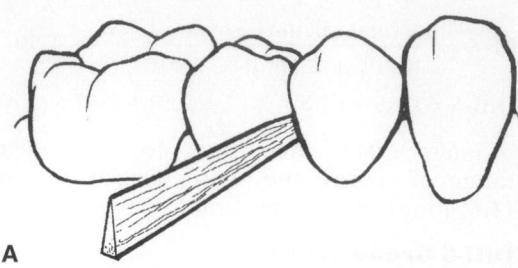

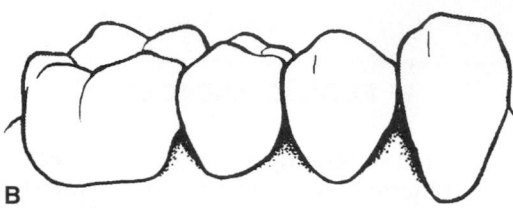

■ **FIGURE 19-8 Eastman Interdental Bleeding Index.** The test for interdental bleeding is made by inserting a wooden interdental cleaner into each interdental space. **(A)** Wooden interdental cleaner inserted in a horizontal path, parallel with the occlusal surfaces. **(B)** The presence or absence of bleeding is noted within a quadrant 15 seconds after final insertion. Bleeding indicates the presence of inflammation.

2. Make the path of insertion horizontal (parallel to the occlusal surface), taking care not to angle the point in an apical direction.
3. Insert and remove four times; move to next interproximal area.
4. Record the presence or absence of bleeding within 15 seconds for each area.

C. Scoring
1. *Number of bleeding sites.* The number may be totaled for an individual score for comparison with scores over a series of appointments.
2. *Percentage scores.* Index is expressed as a percentage of the total number of sites evaluated. Calculations can be made for total mouth, quadrants, or maxillary versus mandibular.
3. *Calculation example:*
   An adult with a complete dentition has 15 maxillary and 15 mandibular interproximal areas. The EIBI revealed 13 areas of bleeding. To calculate percentage:

$$\frac{\text{Number of bleeding areas}}{\text{Total number of areas}} \times 100$$

$$= \text{Percent bleeding area}$$

$$\frac{13}{30} \times 100 = 43\% \text{ (EIBI expressed by \%)}$$

GINGIVAL/PERIODONTAL INDICES

Measurements for gingival and periodontal indices have varied over the years. Historically, the P-M-A (Papillary-Marginal-Attached) index is attributed to Schour and Massler,[16,17] two outstanding teacher-researchers. They developed the P-M-A to assess the extent of gingival changes in large groups for epidemiologic studies.

The Periodontal Index (PI) of Russell[18] was another acclaimed contribution to the study of disease incidence. As a complex index that accounted for both gingival and periodontal changes, its aim was to survey large populations.

For screening, the PSR has been included on pages 295 to 297 and illustrated in Table 19-1. In this section the Gingival Index (GI) of Löe and Silness[19] and the Community Periodontal Index of Treatment Needs (CPITN)[20,21] will be described.

GINGIVAL INDEX (GI)
(Löe and Silness[5,19])

I. PURPOSE

To assess the severity of gingivitis based on color, consistency, and bleeding on probing.

II. SELECTION OF TEETH AND GINGIVAL AREAS

A gingival index may be determined for selected teeth or for the entire dentition.

A. Areas Examined

Four gingival areas (distal, facial, mesial, lingual) are examined systematically for each tooth.

B. Modified Procedure

The distal examination for each tooth can be omitted. The score for the mesial area is doubled, and the total score for each tooth is divided by four.

III. PROCEDURE

A. Dry the teeth and gingivae; under adequate light, use a mouth mirror and probe.
B. Use the probe to press on the gingivae to determine the degree of firmness.
C. Use the probe to run along the soft tissue wall near the entrance to the gingival sulcus to evaluate bleeding (Figure 19-9).
D. Criteria
   0 = Normal gingivae.
   1 = Mild inflammation—slight change in color, slight edema. *No bleeding on probing.*
   2 = Moderate inflammation—redness, edema, and glazing. *Bleeding on probing.*
   3 = Severe inflammation—marked redness and

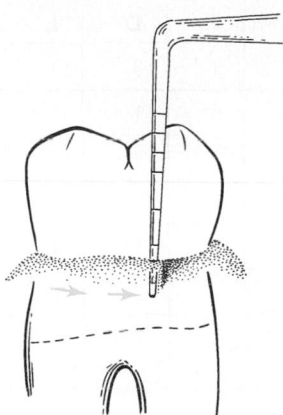

FIGURE 19-9 Gingival Index (GI). Probe stroke for bleeding evaluation. The broken line represents the level of attachment of the periodontal tissues. The probe is inserted a few millimeters and moved along the soft tissue pocket wall with light pressure in a circumferential direction. The stroke shown here is in contrast with the walking stroke used for probing depth evaluation and measurement as described on pages 208 and 209 (Figure 12-6).

edema. Ulceration. *Tendency to spontaneous bleeding.*

IV. SCORING

A. GI for Area

Each of the four gingival surfaces (distal, facial, mesial, lingual) is given a score of 0 to 3.

B. GI for a Tooth

Scores for each area are totaled and divided by four.

C. GI for Groups of Teeth

Scores for individual teeth may be grouped and totaled, and divided by the number of teeth. A GI may be determined for specific teeth, group of teeth, quadrant, or side of mouth.

D. GI for the Individual

By totaling scores and dividing by the number of teeth examined, the GI is determined. Indices range from 0 to 3.

E. Suggested Range of Scores for Patient Reference

Rating	Scores
Excellent (healthy tissue)	0
Good	0.1–1.0
Fair	1.1–2.0
Poor	2.1–3.0

F. Calculation Example for an Individual

(Using six teeth for an example of screening; teeth selected are known as the Ramfjord Index Teeth.[22])

	M	F	D	L	
3 (16)	3	1	3	1	
9 (21)	1	0	1	1	
12 (24)	2	1	2	0	
19 (36)	3	1	3	3	
25 (41)	1	1	1	1	
28 (44)	2	1	2	0	
Total	12	5	12	6	= 35

$$\text{Gingival index} = \frac{\text{Total score}}{\text{Number of surfaces}}$$

$$= \frac{35}{24} = 1.45 \text{ GI}$$

Interpretation: According to the suggested range of scores, the score for this individual (1.45) indicates only fair gingival health (moderate inflammation). The ratings for each gingival area or surface can be used to help the patient compare gingival changes and improve oral hygiene procedures.

G. GI for a Group

Add the individual GI scores and divide by the number of individuals examined.

COMMUNITY PERIODONTAL INDEX OF TREATMENT NEEDS (CPITN)

(Fédération Dentaire Internationale[20] and Ainamo et al[21])

I. PURPOSE

To screen and monitor individual or group periodontal treatment needs.

II. SELECTION OF TEETH

A. Adults (20 years and older)

1. Divide the dentition into sextants. Evaluate all teeth.
   a. Posterior sextants begin distal to canines.
   b. A sextant must have two or more functional teeth. A functional tooth is not indicated for extraction. When only one functional tooth is present, it is assessed with the adjacent sextant. The sextant with no teeth or one tooth is recorded as missing and marked X on the record form.
2. Third molars are included only when they function in place of second molars.

B. Children and Adolescents (7 to 19 years of age)

1. Divide the dentition into sextants.
2. Evaluate one tooth per sextant: all first mo-

lars, maxillary right central incisor, and mandibular left central incisor.[20]
3. When a designated tooth is missing, the sextant is recorded as missing and marked with an X.

III. PROCEDURE

A. Instrument: Specially Designed Probe for CPITN and PSR (Figure 19-1, page 296)

1. *Markings.* At intervals from tip: 3.5, 2.0, 3.0, and 3.0 mm (total 11.5 mm).
2. *Working Tip.* A ball 0.5 mm in diameter. The functions of the ball tip are
   a. To aid in detection of calculus and other tooth surface roughness.
   b. To facilitate assessment of the base of the pocket and reduce the risk of overmeasurement.
3. *Color-Coding.* Color-coded between 3.5 and 5.5 mm.

B. Probe Application

1. Objectives are to determine probing depth, bleeding response, and presence of calculus.
2. Insert probe into sulcus/pocket gently. Keep light contact with tooth surface to detect calculus; use a pressure no greater than 15 to 25 grams to reveal disease without causing patient discomfort.
3. Observe color-coded area for prompt identification of probing depth below 3.5 mm, between 3.5 and 5.5 mm (within the color-coded zone), and above the 5.5-mm level to facilitate classification.

C. Criteria

Five codes are used. Each includes conditions identified with the preceding codes; for example, Code 3 with 4- or 5-mm pockets includes calculus and bleeding, typical of Codes 1 and 2.

Code 0 = Healthy periodontal tissues.
Code 1 = Bleeding after gentle probing.
Code 2 = Supra- or subgingival calculus or defective margin of filling or crown.
Code 3 = 4- or 5-mm pocket.
Code 4 = 6-mm or deeper pathologic pocket.

D. Recording

1. Use a simple box chart for recording. The chart can be made into stick-on labels or a rubber stamp to facilitate the recording procedure on any examination form or individual patient record.
2. Place X for missing sextant.
3. Mark one score to represent each sextant. Record only the highest code that corresponds with the most severe condition.
4. Do not examine remaining teeth in a sextant after a Code 4 has been recorded.
5. The use of only Codes 0, 1, and 2 for patients aged 7 to 11 years may be advisable because of frequent occurrence of gingival ("false")

pockets without attachment loss. The possibility of periodontal disease with attachment loss, however, should not be overlooked in young patients, nor should the need to treat deep gingival pockets.

IV. SCORING

A. Periodontal Treatment Needs

Patients are classified (0, I, II, III) into treatment needs according to the highest coded score recorded during the examination.

0 = No need for treatment (Code 0).

I = Oral hygiene instruction (Code 1).

II = Oral hygiene instruction plus scaling and root planing, including elimination of plaque-retentive margins of fillings and crowns (Codes 2 and 3).

III = I + II + complex periodontal therapy that may include surgical intervention and/or deep scaling and root planing with local anesthesia (Code 4).

B. CPITN for an Individual

1. EXAMPLE 1.

⊠	2	3
4	2	⊠

Interpretation: Two sextants are marked as missing (X). Codes 2, 3, and 4 indicate need for thorough periodontal examination, charting, and detailed treatment plan.

2. EXAMPLE 2.

3	0	3
3	1	3

Interpretation: Code 1 indicates need for improved oral hygiene. Code 3 indicates need for scaling and root planing after a complete periodontal examination and charting.

C. CPITN for Groups

The recordings for a group may be presented in a variety of ways, such as the following:[21]

1. Treatment needs can be reported as the number or percentage of subjects in each treatment need category.
2. Mean number of sextants with bleeding, calculus, and moderate or deep pockets for each age group can be shown.
3. To identify high and low priorities for treatment in a community, calculations of the number and percentage of individuals with the following can be made:
   a. No sextant scoring each code.
   b. 1 to 2 sextants scoring Code 1, 2, 3, or 4.
   c. 3 to 4 sextants scoring Code 1, 2, 3, or 4.
   d. 5 to 6 sextants scoring Code 1, 2, 3, or 4.

DENTAL CARIES INDICES

The most widely used indices are the DMFT (Decayed, Missing, Filled Teeth) and DMFS (Decayed, Missing, Filled surfaces) for permanent teeth.[3] Their counterparts deft (decayed, extracted, filled teeth) and defs (decayed, extracted, filled surfaces) are used for the primary teeth.[23] For a mixed dentition, two separate indices are indicated, one for the permanent teeth and another for the primary teeth.

The indices show the number of persons affected by dental caries, the number of teeth that need treatment, and the proportion of teeth that have been treated.

DECAYED, MISSING, AND FILLED PERMANENT TEETH (DMFT)
(Klein, Palmer, and Knutson[3])

I. PURPOSE

To determine total dental caries experience, past and present.

II. SELECTION OF TEETH

A. DMFT Is Based on 28 Teeth

B. Teeth Not Counted

1. Third molars.
2. Uncrupted teeth. A tooth is considered erupted when any part projects through the gingiva. Certain types of research may require differentiation between clinical emergence, partial eruption, and full eruption.
3. Congenitally missing and supernumerary teeth.
4. Teeth removed for reasons other than dental caries, such as an impaction or during orthodontic treatment.
5. Teeth restored for reasons other than dental caries, such as trauma (fracture), cosmetic purposes, or use as a bridge abutment.
6. Primary tooth retained with the permanent successor erupted. The permanent tooth is evaluated because a primary tooth is never included in this index.

III. PROCEDURES

A. Instruments

Each tooth is examined in a systematic sequence, using a mouth mirror and adequate light. Explorers with standardized dimensions of the working ends are needed for consistency.

B. Examination

1. *Use of Explorer.* Teeth should be observed by

visual means as much as possible. Unnecessary discomfort for the patient can be avoided by exploring only questionable small lesions.

2. *Criteria for Identification of Dental Caries.* A detailed description for clinical recognition of dental caries appears on page 248, and a review of that material is suggested. In brief, for a dental caries index, a tooth can be considered carious when

   a. The lesion is clinically visible and obvious.

   b. The explorer tip can penetrate into soft yielding material.

   c. Discoloration or loss of translucency typical of undermined or demineralized enamel is apparent.

   d. The explorer tip in a pit or fissure resists removal after moderate to firm pressure on insertion.

C. Criteria for Recording

1. *Each Tooth Is Recorded Once.*
2. *"D" Recordings*
   a. When both dental caries and a restoration are present, the tooth is listed as D.
   b. When a crown is broken down as a result of dental caries, it may be recorded as D.
3. *"M" Recordings.* A tooth is considered missing
   a. When it has been extracted because of dental caries.
   b. When it is carious, nonrestorable, and indicated for extraction.
4. *"F" Recordings*
   a. Permanent and temporary fillings are recorded as F.
   b. A tooth with a defective filling but without evidence of dental caries is recorded as F.

IV. SCORING

A. Individual DMFT

1. Total each component separately.
2. Total D + M + F = DMF
Example:
   a. D = 3, M = 2, F = 5
      DMF = 3 + 2 + 5 = 10
   b. A DMF of 10 may have different derivations. An individual who had regular dental care may have a distribution: $D = 0$, $M = 0$, $F = 10$.

B. Group Average

1. Total the DMFs for each individual examined.
2. Divide the total DMFs by the number of individuals in the group.
Example: 30 individuals with a total DMF of 210.

$$\frac{210}{30} = 7.0 = \text{average DMF for the group}$$

3. This DMF average represents accumulated

dental caries experience. It can be presented by age groups.

C. Specific Treatment Needs of a Group

1. To calculate the percentage of DMF teeth needing restorations, divide the total D component by the total DMFT.
Example: D = 175, M = 55, F = 18
Total DMFT = 248

$$\frac{D}{DMF} = \frac{175}{248} = 0.70 \text{ or } 70\% \text{ of the teeth need restorations}$$

2. To calculate the percent of *all* teeth lost by extraction because of dental caries: 20 individuals have 28 × 20 = 560 permanent teeth.

$$\frac{M}{\text{Total teeth}} = \frac{55}{560} = 0.09 \text{ or } 9\% \text{ of all their teeth lost because of dental caries}$$

3. The same type of calculation can be used to determine the percentage of filled teeth.

DECAYED, MISSING, AND FILLED PERMANENT TOOTH SURFACES (DMFS)
(Klein, Palmer, and Knutson[3])

I. PURPOSE

To determine total dental caries experience, past and present, by recording tooth surfaces involved instead of teeth, as in the DMFT previously described.

II. SELECTION OF TEETH AND SURFACES

A. Teeth Not Counted
The same as listed for the DMFT (page 309).

B. Surfaces

1. *Posterior Teeth.* Each tooth has five surfaces examined and recorded: facial, lingual, mesial, distal, and occlusal.
2. *Anterior Teeth.* Each tooth has four surfaces for evaluation: facial, lingual, mesial, and distal.
3. *Total Surface Count for a DMFS.* 128 surfaces. Of 28 teeth, 16 are posterior (16 × 5 = 80) and 12 are anterior (12 × 4 = 48).
4. *Missing Posterior Teeth.* Recorded as five surfaces. The number of surfaces that were carious before extraction usually cannot be determined.

III. PROCEDURES

The same criteria for instruments and examination apply as listed previously for DMFT. In all surveys, specific criteria must be predetermined.

IV. SCORING

A. Individual DMFS

Teeth present = 24 (4 teeth have not yet erupted)
D (surfaces) = 3, M = 0, F (surfaces) = 8
DMFS = D + M + F = 3 + 0 + 8 = 11

B. Group DMFS

A group of 20 individuals 15 to 18 years old

lives in a community with fluoridated water. All have lived there continuously except three who moved there from a nonfluoridated town after reaching 12 years of age. The following data show the distribution of DMFS:

10 individuals (each with 0 DMFS)	0
7 individuals (DMFS = 2,2,3,3,3,3,4)	20
3 individuals who had not lived continuously in the area (DMFS = 9,12,12)	33
Total DMFS	53

$$\text{Average DMFS for the group} = \frac{53}{20} = 2.65$$

Interpretation: The differences between those who had not lived with fluoridation are notable. The two groups should be presented separately because of the wide difference. The group average DMFS is 2.65, whereas the DMFS for those who lived in the fluoridated area all their lives is 1.18, and the DMFS for the other three is 11.0.

DECAYED, INDICATED FOR EXTRACTION, AND FILLED TEETH OR SURFACES (dft and dfs) (deft and defs)[23]
(Gruebbel[23])

I. PURPOSE

To determine the dental caries experience as shown for the primary teeth present in the oral cavity by evaluating teeth or surfaces.

II. SELECTION OF TEETH OR SURFACES

A. deft or dft
20 teeth evaluated.

B. defs or dfs
88 surfaces evaluated.
1. *Posterior Teeth.* Each has five surfaces: facial, lingual or palatal, mesial, distal, and occlusal. (8 teeth × 5 surfaces = 40 surfaces.)
2. *Anterior Teeth.* Each has four surfaces: facial, lingual or palatal, mesial, and distal. (12 teeth × 4 surfaces = 48 surfaces.)

C. Teeth Not Counted
1. Missing teeth, including unerupted and congenitally missing.
2. Supernumerary teeth.
3. Teeth restored for reasons other than dental caries are not counted as f.

III. PROCEDURE

A. Instruments and Examination
Same as for DMFT (page 309).

B. Criteria for Identification of Dental Caries
Same as for DMFT.

C. Criteria for def
d = number of primary teeth or surfaces with dental caries but not restored.

e = number of teeth indicated for extraction because of dental caries.

f = number of filled primary teeth on surfaces that do not have dental caries (each surface is scored once only, "d" has first score).

D. Difference Between deft/defs and dft/dfs
In the deft and defs, both "d" and "e" are used to describe teeth with dental caries. Thus, d and e are sometimes combined, and the index becomes the "dft" or "dfs."

IV. SCORING

A. Individual dft
A 2½-year-old child with nursing caries (page 240) has 18 teeth. Teeth A (55) and J (65) are unerupted. There is no sign of dental caries in teeth M (73), N (72), O (71), P (81), Q (82), and R (83). All other teeth have two carious surfaces each, except B (54), which is broken down to the gum line.

Summary:	
Total teeth =	18
Caries-free =	6
"d" teeth =	12
"f" teeth =	0

dft = d + f = 12 + 0 = 12

Interpretation: 12 of 18 teeth with carious lesions indicates a serious need for dental treatment and a prevention program for the child.

B. Individual dfs
Using the same 2½-year-old child to calculate dfs:

Total number of carious surfaces:	11 × 2 = 22
Tooth B:	1 × 5 = 5
Total dfs	27

Interpretation: The child has 48 anterior surfaces (12 teeth × 4 surfaces) and 30 posterior surfaces (6 teeth × 5 surfaces) to total 78 surfaces.

$$\frac{dfs}{\text{Number of surfaces}} = \frac{27}{78}$$

$$= 0.34 \text{ or } 34\% \text{ of the surface in need of dental treatment}$$

C. Mixed Dentition
A DMFT or DMFS and a deft or defs are never added together. Each child is given a separate index for permanent teeth and another for primary teeth. The index for the permanent teeth is usually determined first, and then the index for the primary teeth is prepared separately.

DECAYED, MISSING, AND FILLED (dmft or dmfs)
(Gruebbel[23])

I. PURPOSE

To determine dental caries experience past and present for children older than 7 and up to 11 or 12 years of age.

II. SELECTION OF TEETH OR SURFACES

A. dmft: 12 teeth evaluated (8 primary molars; 4 primary canines).

B. dmfs: 56 surfaces evaluated.
   1. Primary molars: 8×5 surfaces each = 40.
   2. Primary canines: 4×4 surfaces each = 16.

C. A primary molar or canine is presumed missing because of dental caries when it has been lost before the normal exfoliation time.

D. Each tooth is counted only once. When both dental caries and a restoration are present, the tooth or surface is listed as *d*, dental caries.

III. PROCEDURE

A. Instruments and examination are the same as for DMFT or DMFS (page 309).

B. Criteria for dmft or dmfs

d = number of primary molars and canines or number of surfaces that are carious (**decayed**).

m = number of primary molars and canines **miss**ing.

f = number of **f**illed primary molars and canines without caries (teeth or surfaces).

IV. SCORING

A. Individual dmf

A 5-year-old boy has all primary molars and canines present.

Examination reveals d = 2, m = 0, f = 1

dmf = d + m + f = 2 + 0 + 1 = 3 dmf

B. Mixed Dentition

Permanent and primary teeth are evaluated separately. A DMFT or DMFS and a dmft and a dmfs are never added together.

TECHNICAL HINTS

I. Select an index or scoring method that best fits the needs of the situation or patient.

II. Calibrate criteria for each index used.

III. Implement an index at the beginning of an appointment series.

IV. Permit the patient to graph or chart the plaque or gingival index used and correlate the numeric values with the oral findings that may be seen.

V. Keep a continuing record, graph, or chart for index recording in the patient's permanent file for observation and review at each maintenance appointment.

FACTORS TO TEACH THE PATIENT

I. How an index is used and calculated, and what the scores mean.

II. Correlation of index scores with current oral health practices and procedures.

III. Procedures to follow to improve index scores and bring the oral tissues to health.

REFERENCES

1. **Silness,** J. and Löe, H.: Periodontal Disease in Pregnancy. II. Correlation Between Oral Hygiene and Periodontal Condition, *Acta Odontol. Scand., 22,* 121, No. 1, 1964.

2. **Podshadley,** A.G. and Haley, J.V.: A Method for Evaluating Oral Hygiene Performance, *Public Health Rep., 83,* 259, March, 1968.

3. **Klein,** H., Palmer, C.E., and Knutson, J.W.: Studies on Dental Caries. I. Dental Status and Dental Needs of Elementary School Children, *Public Health Rep., 53,* 751, May 13, 1938.

4. **American Academy of Periodontology and American Dental Association:** *Periodontal Screening & Recording.* Sponsored by Procter & Gamble, June, 1992.

5. **Löe,** H.: The Gingival Index, the Plaque Index and the Retention Index Systems, *J. Periodontol., 38,* 610, November–December, 1967 (Part II).

6. **O'Leary,** T.J., Drake, R.B., and Naylor, J.E.: The Plaque Control Record, *J. Periodontol., 43,* 38, January, 1972.

7. **Ramfjord,** S.P. and Ash, M.M.: *Periodontology and Periodontics.* Philadelphia, W.B. Saunders Co., 1979, p. 273.

8. **Grant,** D.A., Stern, I.B., and Everett, F.G.: *Periodontics,* 5th ed. St. Louis, Mosby, 1979, pp. 529–531.

9. **Greene,** J.C. and Vermillion, J.R.: The Simplified Oral Hygiene Index, *J. Am. Dent. Assoc., 68,* 7, January, 1964.

10. **Greene,** J.C.: The Oral Hygiene Index—Development and Uses, *J. Periodontol., 38,* 625, November–December, 1967 (Part II).

11. **Mühlemann,** H.R. and Son, S.: Gingival Sulcus Bleeding—A Leading Symptom in Initial Gingivitis, *Helv. Odontol. Acta, 15,* 107, October, 1971.

12. **Meitner,** S.W., Zander, H.A., Iker, H.P., and Polson, A.M.: Identification of Inflamed Gingival Surfaces, *J. Clin. Periodontol., 6,* 93, April, 1979.

13. **Carter,** H.G. and Barnes, G.P.: The Gingival Bleeding Index, *J. Periodontol., 45,* 801, November, 1974.

14. **Abrams,** K., Caton, J., and Polson, A.: Histologic Comparisons of Interproximal Gingival Tissues Related to the Presence or Absence of Bleeding, *J. Periodontol., 55,* 629, November, 1984.

15. **Caton,** J.G. and Polson, A.M.: The Interdental Bleeding Index: A Simplified Procedure for Monitoring Gingival Health, *Compend. Cont. Educ. Dent., 6,* 88, February, 1985.

16. **Schour,** I. and Massler, M.: Prevalence of Gingivitis in Young Adults, *J. Dent. Res., 27,* 733, Abstract No. 33, December, 1948.

17. **Massler,** M.: The P-M-A Index for the Assessment of Gingivitis, *J. Periodontol., 38,* 592, November–December, 1967 (Part II).

18. **Russell,** A.L.: A System of Classification and Scoring for Prevalence Surveys of Periodontal Disease, *J. Dent. Res., 35,* 350, June, 1956.

19. **Löe,** H. and Silness, J.: Periodontal Disease in Pregnancy. I. Prevalence and Severity, *Acta Odontol. Scand., 21,* 533, No. 6, 1963.

20. **Fédération Dentaire Internationale:** A Simplified Periodontal Examination for Dental Practices, FDI WG6 and Joint FDI/WHO WG1, Fédération Dentaire Internationale, 64 Wimpole Street, London, WIM 8AL.

21. **Ainamo,** J., Barmes, D., Beagrie, G., Cutress, T., Martin, J., and Sardo-Infirri, J.: Development of the World Health Organization (WHO) Community Periodontal Index of Treatment Needs (CPITN), *Int. Dent. J., 32,* 281, September, 1982.

22. **Ramfjord,** S.P.: Indices for Prevalence and Incidence of Periodontal Disease, *J. Periodontol., 30,* 51, January, 1959.

23. **Gruebbel,** A.O.: A Measurement of Dental Caries Prevalence and Treatment Service for Deciduous Teeth, *J. Dent. Res., 23,* 163, June, 1944.

SUGGESTED READINGS

Ainamo, J., Etemadzadeh, H., and Kallio, P.: Comparability and Discriminating Power of 4 Plaque Quantifications, *J. Clin. Periodontol., 20, 244,* April, 1993.

Burt, B.A. and Eklund, S.A.: *Dentistry, Dental Practice, and the Community,* 4th ed. Philadelphia, W.B. Saunders Co., 1992, pp. 57–77.

Lobene, R.R., Mankodi, S.M., Ciancio, S.G., Lamm, R.A., Charles, C.H., and Ross, N.M.: Correlations Among Gingival Indices: A Methodology Study, *J. Periodontol., 60,* 159, March, 1989.

Marks, R.G., Magnusson, I., Taylor, M., Clouser, B., Maruniak, J., and Clark, W.B.: Evaluation of Reliability and Reproducibility of Dental Indices, *J. Clin. Periodontol., 20,* 54, January, 1993.

Palat, M., Gomez, C., Scherer, W., Hittelman, E., and LoPresti, J.: Indicators of Gingival Inflammation: The Gingival Index vs Sulcular Temperature Measurements, *J. Practical Hyg., 2,* 25, January/ February, 1993.

Quirynen, M., Dekeyser, C., and van Steenberghe, D.: Discriminating Power of Five Plaque Indices, *J. Periodontol, 62,* 100, February, 1991.

Silness, J. and Røynstrand, T.: Partial Mouth Recording of Plaque, Gingivitis and Probing Depth in Adolescents, *J. Clin. Periodontol., 15,* 189, March, 1988.

Summers, C.J., Gooch, B.F., Marianos, D.W., Malvitz, D.M., and Bond, W.W.: Practical Infection Control in Oral Health Surveys and Screenings, *J. Am. Dent. Assoc., 125,* 1213, September, 1994.

Tal, H. and Rosenberg, M.: Estimation of Dental Plaque Levels and Gingival Inflammation Using a Simple Oral Rinse Technique, *J. Periodontol., 61,* 339, June, 1990.

Toevs, S.E. and Lukken, K.M.: Assessing Interproximal Gingival Health, *J. Dent. Hyg., 63,* 228, June, 1989.

Toevs, S.E. and Lukken, K.M.: Bleeding As An Indicator of Health or Disease. Clinical Application of this Parameter, *J. Dent. Hyg., 64,* 256, July–August, 1990.

Periodontal Disease Indices

Almas, K., Bulman, J.S., and Newman, H.N.: Assessment of Periodontal Status with CPITN and Conventional Periodontal Indices, *J. Clin. Periodontol., 18,* 654, October, 1991.

Barnett, M.L.: Suitability of Gingival Indices for Use in Therapeutic Trials: Is Bleeding a sine qua non? *J. Clin. Periodontol., 23,* 582, June, 1996.

Bentley, C.D. and Disney, J.A.: A Comparison of Partial and Full Mouth Scoring of Plaque and Gingivitis in Oral Hygiene Studies, *J. Clin. Periodontol., 22,* 131, February, 1995.

Blieden, T.M., Caton, J.G., Proskin, H.M., Stein, S.H., and Wagener, C.J.: Examiner Reliability for an Invasive Gingival Bleeding Index, *J. Clin. Periodontol., 19,* 262, April, 1992.

Butler, B.L., Morejon, O., and Low, S.B.: An Accurate Time-efficient Method to Assess Plaque Accumulation, *J. Am. Dent. Assoc., 127,* 1763, December, 1996.

Khocht, A., Zohn, H., Deasy, M., and Chang, K.-M.: Screening for Periodontal Disease: Radiographs vs. PSR, *J. Am. Dent. Assoc., 127,* 749, June, 1996.

Mojon, P., Chung, J.-P., Favre, P., and Budtz-Jorgensen, E.: Examiner Agreement on Periodontal Indices During Dental Surveys of Elders, *J. Clin. Periodontol., 23,* 56, January, 1996.

Newbrun, E.: Indices to Measure Gingival Bleeding, *J. Periodontol., 67,* 555, June, 1996.

Spolsky, V.W. and Gornbein, J.A.: Comparing Measures of Reliability for Indices of Gingivitis and Plaque, *J. Periodontol., 67,* 853, September, 1996.

Sterrett, J.D., Hawkins, C.H., Pelletier, L., and Murphy, H.J.: The Use of Accurate Gingival Indices in Current Periodontal Literature, *Can. Dent. Hyg./Probe, 24,* 85, Summer, 1990.

Other Indices

Addy, M., Renton-Harper, P., and Myatt, G.: A Plaque Index for Occlusal Surfaces and Fissures: Measurement of Repeatability and Plaque Removal, *J. Clin. Periodontol., 25,* 164, February, 1998.

Aherne, C.A., O'Mullane, D., and Barrett, B.E.: Indices of Root Surface Caries, *J. Dent. Res., 69,* 1222, May, 1990.

Donachie, M.A. and Walls, A.W.G.: Assessment of Tooth Wear in an Aging Population, *J. Dent., 23,* 157, June, 1995.

Katz, R.V.: Development of an Index for the Prevalence of Root Caries, *J. Dent. Res., 63,* 814, Special Issue, May, 1984.

Koch, A.L., Gershen, J.A., and Marcus, M.: A Children's Oral Health Status Index Based on Dentists' Judgment, *J. Am. Dent. Assoc., 110,* 36, January, 1985.

Lobene, R.R., Weatherford, T., Ross, N.M., Lamn, R.A., and Menaker, L.: A Modified Gingival Index for Use in Clinical Trials, *Clin. Prev. Dent., 8,* 3, January–February, 1986.

Massler, M. and Schour, I.: The P-M-A Index of Gingivitis, *J. Dent. Res., 28,* 634, Abstract Number 7, December, 1949.

Quigley, G.A. and Hein, J.W.: Comparative Cleansing Efficiency of Manual and Power Brushing, *J. Am. Dent. Assoc., 65,* 26, July, 1962.

Silberman, S.L., Trubman, A., Duncan, W.K., and Meydrech, E.F.: A Simplified Hypoplasia Index, *J. Public Health Dent., 50,* 282, Summer, 1990.

Records and Charting

Patient health records provide a means of communication between the members of the health team themselves, as well as with their patients. Coordinated planning and continuity of care can be facilitated. The records serve as a basis for the evaluation of the quality of care and aid when a review is made of the effectiveness of patient care practices. Data from health records are utilized in research and education.

Comprehensive health histories, informed consent forms, and accurate documentation are essential to a safe, thorough, and caring practice. They are both business and legal documents for protection of health-care workers.

Complete and accurate examinations with proper documentation by records and chartings are basic to all patient care. All findings from the comprehensive assessment are recorded. Some systems of recording involve the completion of forms with topics and spaces to check or fill in the information, whereas others call for a prose-style summary.

Radiographs, study casts, photographs, and all other materials collected during the initial examination and during continuing patient appointments are official parts of the permanent records. Each part must be dated.

A filing system is needed that has accessibility to the health records by authorized personnel only. The privacy of records must be maintained.

Computerized systems have many advantages for integration of the records into the total practice. Appointment schedules, medical alerts, and financial aspects all can be part of the data management by the computer.

I. PURPOSES FOR CHARTING

The purpose of each type of charting is defined by its title: the dental charting includes diagrammatic representation of existing conditions of the teeth, whereas the periodontal charting indicates clinical features of the periodontium. Separate types of chart forms may be used to record the special features of each, or the two may be combined on one chart. Neatness in the markings of symbols, drawings, and labels goes hand in hand with the accuracy of the examination itself.

An accurate, detailed, and carefully recorded charting is used as follows:

A. For Care Planning
The charting is a graphic representation of the existing condition of the patient's teeth and periodontium from which needed treatment procedures can be organized into a treatment plan.

B. For Counseling Treatment
During dental and dental hygiene appoint-

ments, the charting is useful for guiding specific procedures.

C. For Evaluation
The outcome and degree of lasting effects of treatment are determined by comparing the findings of the initially recorded examination with periodic follow-up examinations.

D. For Protection
In the event of misunderstanding by a patient, or if legal questions should arise, the records and chartings are realistic evidence.

E. For Identification
In the event of emergency, accident, or disaster, a patient may be identified by the teeth for which a record has been maintained.

II. MATERIALS FOR CHARTING

A. Instruments
1. Probe.
2. Sharp explorers.
3. Clear and unscratched mouth mirror.
4. Dental floss.
5. Gauze sponges.
6. Air tip and saliva ejector.
7. Topical anesthetic if probing proves discomforting to the patient.

B. Study Casts

C. Radiographs
1. Advanced preparation of the radiographic survey facilitates coordination between clinical and radiographic examinations. The completely processed and mounted radiographs provide greater assurance of a thorough analysis.
2. A bitewing survey may be sufficient for the charting of dental caries, but a periapical survey is essential for periodontal evaluation.

D. Form for Manual Charting
Many variations of chart forms are in current use, some available commercially, some designed by the individual practitioner to meet particular needs. Specifications for an adequate form include ample space to chart neatly, accurately, and completely; to label as needed for clarity; and to record in a manner that can be interpreted by all who use it. Three types of forms are described here.
1. *Anatomic Tooth Drawings of the Complete Teeth.* Such a chart form lends itself to combined dental and periodontal charting. Figure 20-2 is an example of this type of chart form (page 317).
2. *Anatomic Drawings of the Crowns of Teeth Only.* Difficult to chart adequately the periodontal findings; designed primarily for charting dental caries.
3. *Geometric.* A diagrammatic representation for each tooth with space for each surface; generally does not include the roots. Without roots, the diagram would not be useful for periodontal charting.

Each tooth in the geometric chart shown in Figure 20-1 includes two circles. The inner circle represents the occlusal surface, and the outer circle, divided into four parts, represents the mesial, facial, distal, and lingual. The individual tooth diagrams may be arranged in a linear format (Figure 20-1*A*) or in arches to simulate the oral cavity (Figure 20-1*B*).

E. Computerized Systems
Voice-operated or mouse-controlled computer systems aid greatly in saving time and solving the problem of cross-contamination by way of chart forms and utensils.

CLINIC PROCEDURES

I. PATIENT PREPARATION

A. Patient Position
Position for optimum visibility and accessibility.

B. Illumination
Maximum illumination is important. Use direct or indirect (mirror) light or transillumination.

II. SEQUENCE FOR CHARTING

A. Basic Entries
1. *Name, Birth Date*
2. *Date.* Every entry must be dated.
3. *Missing Teeth.* When radiographs are available in advance, missing teeth can be charted before the clinic appointment. Whether dental or periodontal charting is completed first, marking the missing teeth will be necessary.

B. Systematic Procedure
The use of a set routine is prerequisite to accomplishing a complete and accurate charting, not only for the tooth surface-to-surface pattern, but also for the parts of the charting itself.

Charting of all of one kind of item for the entire mouth, rather than complete chartings of one tooth, helps to obtain accuracy because only one train of thought is required at a time. For example, in the dental charting, record all the restorations first. Then start again at the first tooth and chart all the deviations from normal. Charting all restorations and deviations for each tooth separately is a less efficient method.

DENTAL RECORDS AND CHARTING

The patient's permanent records include the itemized findings of the clinical and radiographic examinations along with subjective symptoms reported by the patient. Material for the dental records has been in-

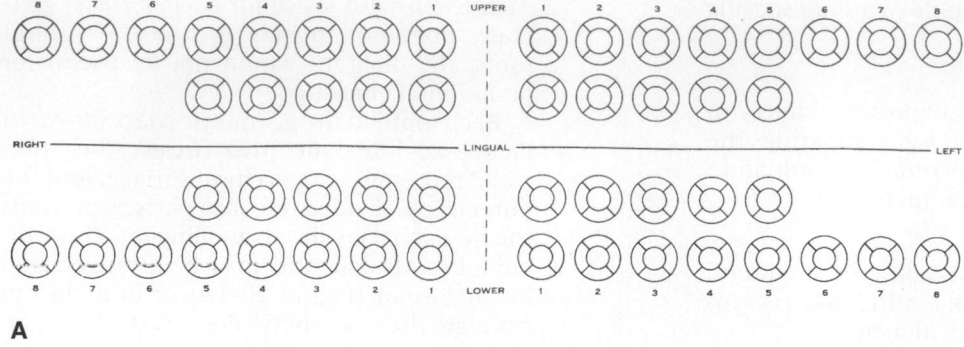

A

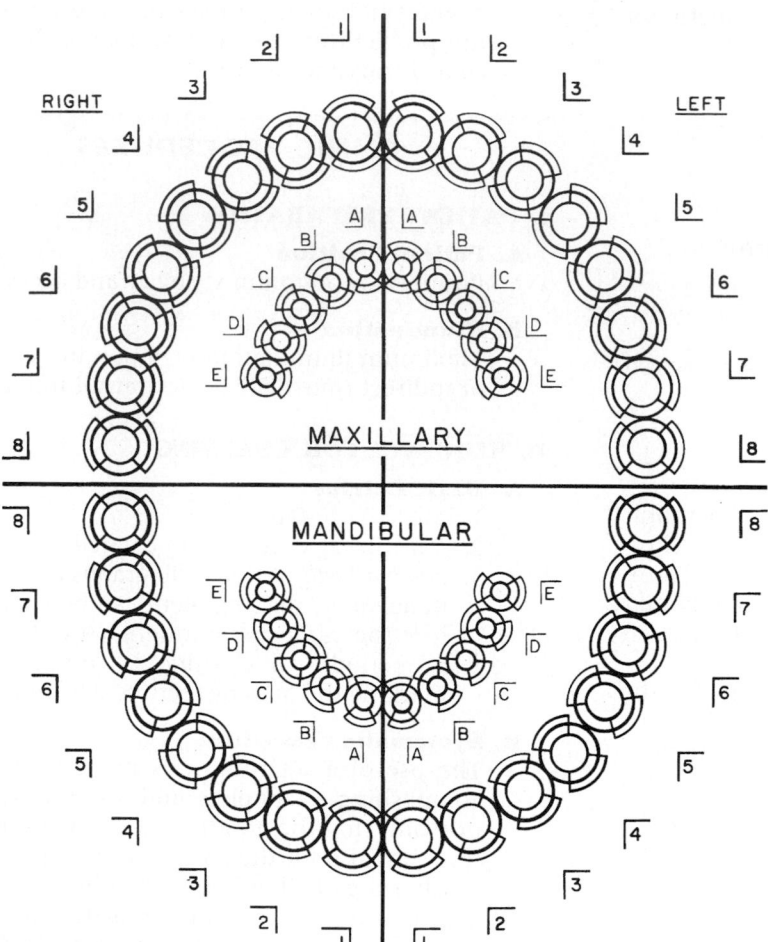

B

FIGURE 20-1 Geometric Charting Form. Type A. Linear format with primary teeth between the permanent teeth. **Type B.** Permanent teeth in arch form with primary teeth inside. Teeth are numbered by quadrant numbers 1 through 8.

cluded in Chapter 14 and for occlusion in Chapter 15. Mobility of teeth has been included with the periodontal examination because the causes of mobility are periodontally oriented.

After initial entries are recorded, additions are made to show the progress of treatment. At each periodic maintenance visit, new and comparative records and chartings must be prepared.

The need for meticulous examination and recording cannot be overemphasized. Finding and recording a carious lesion may mean saving a tooth for the pa-

tient's lifetime; inadvertent neglect of a tooth may lead eventually to a need for endodontic therapy or even extraction.

I. BEFORE PATIENT APPOINTMENT

Radiographs and study casts prepared at an initial appointment before clinical examination for charting help to conserve patient chair time.

A. Radiographic Charting

The following may be charted without the presence of the patient: missing, unerupted, impacted teeth; endodontic restorations; overhanging margins of existing restorations; proximal surface carious lesions; and any other deviation from normal evident from the radiographs.

Supplemental and confirmational observations and checks are made during the clinical examination with the patient. For example, when an overhanging restoration is noted but dental caries is not visible in the radiograph, examination by exploration is required because the restoration may be superimposed over the carious lesion.

B. Study Casts

Record the classification of occlusion (pages 258 to 259).

II. PATIENT APPOINTMENT

Figure 20-2 is an example of a quadrant of dental charting using anatomic tooth drawings. Dental findings can also be charted on a geometric form, such as that shown in Figure 20-1.

A. Chart missing teeth.

B. Chart existing restorations, including fixed and removable prostheses.

C. Chart sealants.

D. Chart apparent carious lesions and other deviations from normal.

E. Coordinate clinical and radiographic findings.

F. Use dental floss. Chart inadequate contact areas and observe proximal surface roughness. Fraying of dental floss as it is passed over a rough proximal surface may mean the de-

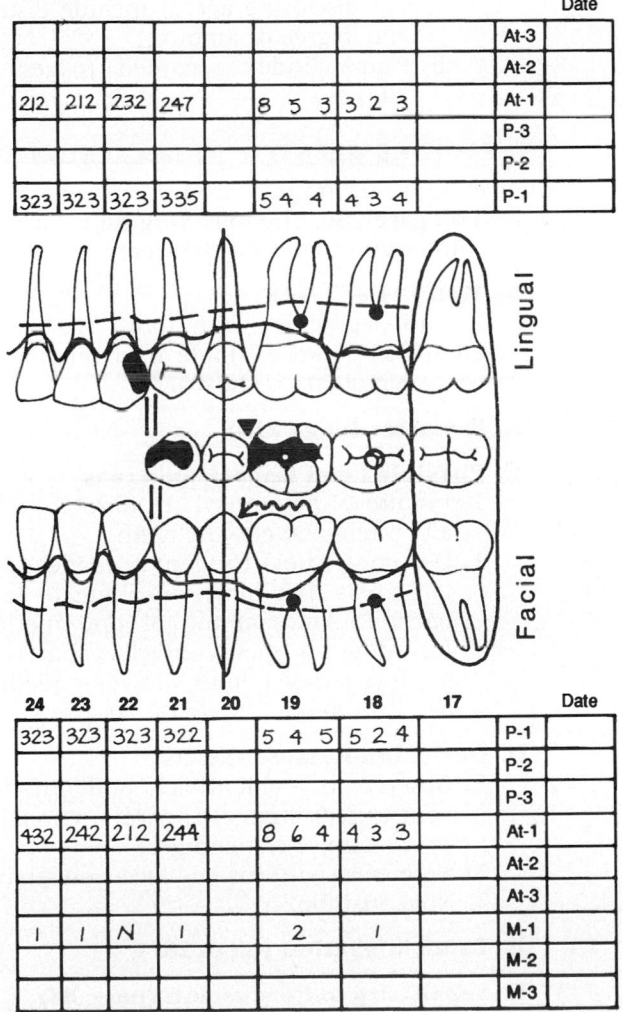

Key

Missing Tooth: | or X
Unerupted or impacted: Encircle tooth
Drift and Migration: ∿∿∿
Open Contact: ||
Food Impaction: ↓ (at occlusal)

Periodontal Chart

Gingival Margin: Black line
Mucogingival Junction: Dashed line
Furca involved: ● (in furcation)
Probing depths: (mm) P-1, P-2, P-3
Clinical attachment level: (mm) At-1, At-2, At-3

Dental Chart

Dental Caries: red
Restorations: blue
Defective Restoration: circle with red
Overhang: ▼ (at occlusal)
Mobility: (+, N, 1, 2, 3) M-1, M-2, M-3
Fremitus: F-1 (recorded on maxillary only)

■ **FIGURE 20-2 Periodontal and Dental Charting.** Section of a charting (mandibular left quadrant) shows combined dental and periodontal charting. Dental caries and restorations are usually marked with colored pencils, such as blue for restorations and red for dental caries, on the anatomic crowns or roots. The gingival margin is clearly drawn to show areas of recession. Boxes at the apices of each tooth provide spaces for probing depths and clinical attachment level recordings, as well as for mobility notations.

fective margin of a restoration, a sharp cavity margin, or dental calculus.

G. Chart pulp vitality. Record numbers in the permanent record. Chart forms sometimes include a specific place for the recording of such data. Procedures were described on page 250.

H. Chart tooth sensitivity. The patient may report hypersensitive areas, or they may be discovered during instrumentation. Record the tooth number and surface for reference during the treatment phase.

PERIODONTAL RECORDS AND CHARTING

The patient's permanent records include the itemized findings of all the clinical and radiographic examinations. Material for the periodontal charting has been described on pages 212 to 213. Entries should be clear and easily understood by all who read them and use them in continuing treatment.

Additions to the records are made to show the progress of treatment and comparative observations throughout the series of treatment appointments. After the mouth has been brought to a state of health, a maintenance plan is outlined. At each succeeding appointment, new and comparative records and chartings are made.

Basic periodontal recordings are listed here.

I. CLINICAL OBSERVATIONS OF THE GINGIVA

A. Describe Gingiva
Color, size, position, shape, consistency, and surface texture; extent of bleeding when probed; and areas where exudate can be pressed from the pockets (pages 193 to 199 and Table 11-1, pages 194 and 195).

B. Describe Distribution of Gingival Changes
Localized or generalized; specify the areas of severest disease involvement. Use tooth numbers to identify adjacent gingival tissue. Tooth numbering systems are described on pages 84 to 85.

C. Describe Degree of Severity of Disease
Slight, moderate, severe.

II. ITEMS TO BE CHARTED

A. Missing teeth.
B. Gingival line (margin) and mucogingival lines (junctions).
C. Probing depths.
D. Areas of suspected mucogingival involvement.
E. Furcation involvement.
F. Abnormal frenal attachments.
G. Mobility and fremitus of teeth.

III. DEPOSITS

A. Stains
1. *Extrinsic.* Record type of stain, color, distribution; specific location by tooth number; whether slight, moderate, or heavy.
2. *Intrinsic.* Record separately from extrinsic and identify by type when known.

B. Calculus
Record distribution and amount of supragingival and subgingival calculus separately for treatment planning purposes.

C. Soft Deposits
1. *Food Debris.* Distribution and amount. Record location by teeth when the plaque control instruction requires special emphasis on a particular area.
2. *Bacterial Plaque*
   a. Record direct observations with or without disclosing agent; include distribution and degree or amount.
   b. Plaque index recorded (pages 298 to 302).

IV. FACTORS RELATED TO OCCLUSION

Clinical signs of trauma from occlusion were described on page 262. The following list is for consideration with other records for the treatment planning.

A. Mobility of Teeth
Record degree for each tooth (page 218). In Figure 20-2, an example of a method for recording mobility is shown.

B. Fremitus (page 219)

C. Possible Food Impaction Areas
1. Inquire of patient where fibrous foods usually catch between the teeth.
2. Use dental floss to identify inadequate contact areas that may contribute to food impaction. An example of one method for recording an open contact is shown by the vertical parallel lines between teeth numbered 21 and 22 in Figure 20-2.

D. Occlusion-Related Habits
1. Observe for evidence of, and question patient concerning, such parafunctional habits as bruxism or clenching.
2. Note wear patterns and facets on study cast.
3. Note attrition.

E. Tooth Migration (page 261)

F. Sensitivity to Percussion (page 84)

G. Radiographic Evidences
Related to trauma from occlusion (page 262).

V. RADIOGRAPHIC FINDINGS

Specific notes should be made to correlate the radiographic findings with the clinical observations just listed. Details of radiographic findings in periodontal disease were described on pages 219 to 222. The following should be noted in particular:

A. Height of bone as related to the cemento-enamel junction.
B. Horizontal or angular shape of remaining bone.
C. Intact, broken, or missing crestal lamina dura.
D. Furcation involvement.
E. Widening of periodontal ligament space.
F. Overhanging fillings, large carious lesions, and other bacterial plaque–retention factors.

TECHNICAL HINTS

I. Use a record form with adequate space for recording details.
II. Prepare permanent records in ink.
III. Use abbreviations and symbols only if their meaning is clear to all who read them.
IV. Check that all records are complete, accurate, clearly stated, readable, and neat.
V. Plan appointments, when possible, in order that radiographs and study casts will be available prior to and at the time of clinical charting. When the medical and dental history and the extraoral and intraoral examinations can be completed in advance, time can be saved. Necessary consultations with a patient's physician, preparation with premedication when indicated for the patient susceptible to bacteremia, or other special adaptation can be made.

FACTORS TO TEACH THE PATIENT

I. Interpretation of all recordings; meaning of all numbers used, such as for probing depths.
II. The importance of making a complete study of the patient's oral problems before beginning treatment.
III. Advantages of cooperation and patience in furnishing information that will help dental personnel to interpret observations accurately so that the correct diagnosis and appropriate treatment plan can be made.
IV. Assurance that all information received is completely confidential, and that the records are locked when the office is closed.

SUGGESTED READINGS

Ekstein, E.C.: Dental Office Record Keeping and Its Impact on Anticipated Litigation, *Compend. Cont. Educ. Dent., 14,* 590, May, 1993.

Eubanks, S.: The Dental Assistant's Role in Risk Management. Patient Records, *Dent. Assist., 61,* 18, Second Quarter, 1992.

Keselyak, N. and Maschak, L.: The Problem-oriented Dental Record: A Key to Dental Hygiene Treatment Planning and the Problem-Solving Model for Dental Hygiene Practice, *Can. Dent. Hyg./Probe, 27,* 15, January/February, 1993.

McCullough, C.: Clinical Applications of Voice Chart Computer Technology in the Practice of Dental Hygiene, *J. Pract. Hyg., 4,* 29, November/December, 1995.

Nunn, P.: SOAP for Whiter, Brighter Notes! *Access, 8,* 26, February, 1994.

Schutte, D.W. and Sansome, K.C.: Defensible Dental Records, Walk-in Patients, *DentalHygienistNews, 9,* 10, Number 3, 1996.

Sfikas, P.M.: Guarding the Files. Your Role in Maintaining the Confidentiality of Patient Records, *J. Am. Dent. Assoc., 127,* 1248, August, 1996.

Stach, D.J.: The Complete Dental Record, in Woodall, I.R.: *Comprehensive Dental Hygiene Care,* 4th ed. St. Louis, Mosby, 1993, pp. 70–77.

Summers, C.J., Gooch, B.F., Marianos, D.W., Malvitz, D.M., and Bond, W.W.: Practical Infection Control in Oral Health Surveys and Screenings, *J. Am. Dent. Assoc., 125,* 1213, September, 1994.

Williams, V.: Getting the Required Information in 10 Minutes, *Access, 8,* 38, January, 1994.

Woodward, B.: Sounding Board. The Computer-based Patient Record and Confidentiality, *N. Engl. J. Med., 333,* 1419, November 23, 1995.

Forensic Identification

Beale, D.R.: The Importance of Dental Records for Identification, *N.Z. Dent. J., 87,* 84, July, 1991.

Clark, D.H., ed.: *Practical Forensic Odontology.* Oxford, Wright, 1992, pp. 101–109 (Dental Record Interpretation).

O'Reilly, P.: An Overview of Forensic Dentistry, *Clin. Prev. Dent., 8,* 16, January–February, 1986.

Parker, L.S.: Dental Detectives, *RDH, 10,* 14, February, 1990.

Planning Dental Hygiene Care

CHAPTER OUTLINE

In the dental hygiene process of care described in Chapter 1 and illustrated in Figure 21-1, assessment data are used to formulate the dental hygiene diagnosis. Then, taking into consideration the dental hygiene prognosis, a dental hygiene care plan and appointment sequence can be formalized. Terms and key words used in conjunction with these steps are defined in Box 21-1.

I. ASSESSMENT

Assessment includes the gathering of details of the health status of the patient, and analysis and synthesis of that data. The application of clinical judgment and critical thinking skills are necessary to arrive at a dental hygiene diagnosis. Assessment procedures are described in detail in Chapters 6 through 20.

II. DENTAL HYGIENE DIAGNOSIS

A. Basis for Diagnosis
1. Data collected during the patient interview, including the patient's chief complaint and comprehensive personal/social, medical, and dental health histories.
2. Data collected during a thorough physical assessment of vital signs, extraoral and intraoral tissue examination, and dental and periodontal chartings may reveal symptoms that have not previously been apparent to the patient.
3. Identification of the individual patient's oral problems.
4. Identification of corresponding treatment or education needs that may be addressed by providing oral care services that are within the dental hygienist's legal scope of practice.
5. Identification of treatment needs that may be addressed by consultation with another licensed health-care professional.

B. Diagnostic Statements
1. Provide the basis for planning interventions that achieve oral health outcomes for which the dental hygienist is considered responsible.
2. Reflect expected treatment outcomes and identify patient responses that are changeable by dental hygiene interventions.

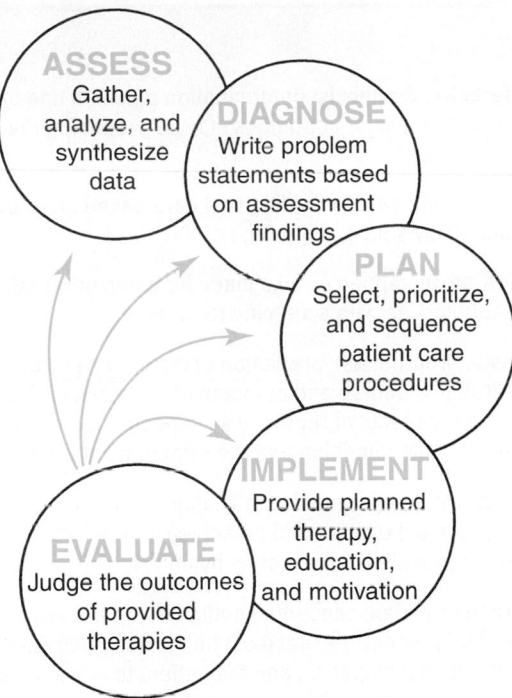

FIGURE 21-1 The Five Components of the Dental Hygiene Process of Care. Planning for dental hygiene care depends upon all of the interrelated components.

3. Exclude those diagnoses requiring surgery, prescriptive medication, or other modes of treatment intervention that are legally defined as dental practice.

C. Diagnostic Models

Medical and dental models of diagnosis evaluate assessment data and classify diagnostic statements according to disease processes. Most nursing models encompass a broader focus that addresses the health functioning of individuals and describe actual or potential health problems that nurses are able and licensed to treat.

In recent years, several proposed dental hygiene models have been developed that incorporate components from a variety of existing health-care models. The models, many of which are still being tested, are meant to give direction and a scientific basis from which to make diagnostic decisions and formulate patient care plans.

1. *Dental Hygiene Diagnostic Model*[1]
   a. Diagnostic statements are developed by following a series of six steps that form the process of diagnostic decision-making: (1) initial review, (2) hypothesis formation, (3) inquiry strategy, (4) problem synthesis, (5) diagnostic decision-making, and (6) learning from the process.
   b. Recorded in patient treatment records using the notation "DHDx" and accompa-

nied by a treatment plan or treatment goal statement.[2]

2. *Human Needs Model*[3]
   a. Diagnostic statements are based on whether the specific criteria defining eight human needs are met or unmet by the patient's current oral health status.
   b. Written by outlining goals to be obtained for resolving each observed deficit.[4,5]

3. *Dental Hygiene Process Model*[6]
   a. Diagnostic statements identify the patient's problem in terms of response rather than need and state the possible etiology. Statements are classified into several categories, which include general systemic, soft tissue, periodontal, oral hygiene, and dental categories.
   b. Written by stating the problem and the etiological factor joined by the phrase "related to."

4. *Oral Health–Related Quality of Life (OHRQL) Model*[7]
   a. Diagnostic statements for individuals/populations are based on the assessment of domains related to health/preclinical disease; biological/physiological disease; and the broad-based sequelae to disease such as symptom status, functional status, health perceptions, and overall quality of life.
   b. Dental hygiene actions are formulated for each domain, incorporating a multidisciplinary approach to care.

III. DENTAL HYGIENE PROGNOSIS

A. Outcome Expected

The dental hygiene prognosis is a look ahead to an anticipated outcome. In other words it is a statement of results (outcomes) that are expected to be achieved by the dental hygiene intervention.

B. Use of Risk Factors and Assessments

By using information from the assessment and by determining probable outcomes, the dental hygienist and the patient together may select interventions with the potential to reverse a patient's oral problem or at least, with time and continued care, result in a state of optimal oral health for the patient. The prognosis might be based on the treatment alternatives selected and on patient commitment to personal care and preventive regimens.

IV. DENTAL HYGIENE CARE PLAN

The dental hygiene care plan is an essential part of the integrated components in the dental hygiene process of care illustrated in Figure 21-1. The written care plan is a prioritized sequence of evidence-based dental hygiene interventions predicated on the dental hygiene diagnosis of the patient's oral problems.

BOX 21-1 KEY WORDS: Dental Hygiene Care Plan

Assessment (ah-ses'ment): the critical analysis and valuation or judgment of a particular condition, situation, or other subject of appraisal.

Chief complaint: the patient's concern as stated during the initial health history preparation; may be the reason for seeking professional care; the complaint such as pain or discomfort may require emergency dental diagnosis.

Consent: voluntary agreement with an action proposed by another.

Informed consent: a patient's voluntary agreement to a treatment plan after details of the proposed treatment have been presented and comprehended by the patient.

Informed refusal: a patient's decision to refuse recommended treatment after all options, potential risks, and potential benefits have been thoroughly explained.

Definitive care: complete care; end point at which all treatment required at the time has been completed.

Diagnose (di'ag-nōs): to identify or recognize a disease or problem.

Diagnosis (di"ag-no'sis): a concise technical description of the cause, nature, or manifestations of a condition, situation, or problem. Identification of a disease or deviation from normal condition by recognition of characteristic signs and symptoms.

Dental hygiene diagnosis: identification of an existing or potential oral health problem that a dental hygienist is qualified and licensed to treat.

Differential diagnosis: determination of which one of several diseases or conditions may be producing the symptoms.

Evidence-based care: providing oral care based on relevant, scientifically sound, research.

Intervention: to happen or take place between other events; to intervene, as with a specific treatment.

Prognosis (prog-no'sis): prediction of outcome; a forecast of the probable course and outcome of an attack of disease and the prospects of recovery as expected by the nature of the specific condition and the symptoms of the case.

Dental hygiene prognosis: an evaluation of the results (outcomes) expected to be achieved from oral treatment provided by the dental hygienist.

Total treatment plan: sequential outline of the essential services and procedures that must be carried out by the dentist, the dental hygienist, and the patient to eliminate disease and restore the oral cavity to health and normal function.

Dental hygiene care plan: the services within the framework of the total treatment plan to be carried out by the dental hygienist.

Planned treatment and educational procedures are carried out within the patient's total oral treatment plan. The parts of a master treatment plan, including the components of the dental and dental hygiene care plan, are listed in Table 21-1. The dental hygiene care plan outlines actions within the scope of dental hygiene practice as defined by each state's practice act.

Except for emergency treatment, dental hygiene care and education logically precede other phases of treatment. The success of restorative, prosthetic, orthodontic, and other special dentistry depends on soft tissue health. One primary objective of dental hygiene therapy is to restore and maintain health of the gingival tissues. Thus, the dental hygiene care plan has a major influence on the future oral health of the patient.

PLANNING FOR DENTAL HYGIENE CARE

The objective is to prepare a flexible, realistic dental hygiene care plan and sequence of procedures based on the patient's needs. Planned care is determined by assessment data collected and/or diagnostic statements that identify problems in the patient's oral health status. Care recommendations should be evidence-based treatment modalities supported by current research findings.

The dental hygiene care plan is integrated with the patient's total treatment plan, which encompasses the patient's restorative and surgical needs. Consideration is given to the following factors that may require specific adaptation in treatment or education in the care plan.

I. RISK FACTORS

Whether or not the patient presents for dental hygiene care with current oral disease, several risk factors can be noted that increase the patient's potential for diminished oral health status. When a patient presents for dental hygiene care exhibiting one or more of these risk factors, it is essential to develop a care plan that addresses the need for preventive education and counseling.

TABLE 21-1 Components of a Master Treatment Plan

Phase	Procedures	Included in the Dental Hygiene Care Plan
Preliminary Phase	• Assessment data collection • Emergency care (pain, biopsy) • Removal of hopeless teeth • Provisional replacement to restore function	✓
Phase I Therapy	• Bacterial plaque control • Introduction of additional preventive measures (diet changes, fluorides, mouthguard) • Calculus removal • Correction of restorative and prosthetic irritants (plaque traps, overhangs) • Restorative caries control (excavation and restoration) • Occlusal therapy • Minor orthodontic movement	✓ ✓ ✓
Outcomes Evaluation of Phase I	• Probing depths • Clinical signs of inflammation • Bacterial plaque control • Patient's participation	✓ ✓ ✓ ✓
Phase II Surgical	• Periodontal • Endodontic • Implant placement	
Phase III Restorative	• Final restorations • Fixed/removable prostheses	
Evaluation of Overall Outcomes	• Final polish for restorations • Periodontal response to restorations/implants • Other response to restorations	✓ ✓
Phase IV Maintenance	• Appointments for continuing care and supervision • Refining plaque control techniques	✓ ✓

Adapted from: Carranza, F.A.: The Treatment Plan, in: Carranza, F.A. and Newman, M.G.: *Clinical Periodontology*, 8th ed. Philadelphia, W.B. Saunders, 1996, p. 400.

A. Risk Factors for Periodontal Infections or Poor Response to Periodontal Therapy
1. Behavioral Factors (tobacco use, oral hygiene neglect)
2. Systemic Diseases (diabetes, HIV infection)
3. Other Systemic Conditions (osteoporosis, osteopenia)
4. Hormonal Considerations (pregnancy, menopause)
5. Nutritional Status
6. Iatrogenic Factors (overhangs, open contacts, and residual calculus)

B. Risk Factors for Caries
1. Behavioral Factors (inadequate oral hygiene, frequent use of cariogenic foods)
2. Low Fluoride
3. Exposed Root Surfaces
4. Xerostomia
5. History of Dental Caries/Restorative Dentistry

C. Periodontal Disease as a Risk Factor for Systemic Conditions
1. Preterm Low Birth Weight[8]
2. Bacterial Pneumonia[9]
3. Cardiovascular Disease[10]

II. PATIENT'S OVERALL HEALTH RISK

A. Physical Status
The extent of the patient's medical risk determines modifications necessary during treatment. Patient positioning, sequence and timing of treatments, and prevention of medical complications need consideration.

B. ASA Classification[11]
A classification system adopted by the American Society of Anesthesiologists is outlined in Table 21-2 with examples of physical manifestations and suggested treatment modification levels.

TABLE 21-2 ASA Physical Status Classification System

	ASA Classification	Examples of Physical Manifestations	Treatment (Tx) Considerations
ASA* I	Without systemic disease; a normal, healthy, patient with little or no dental anxiety	Able to walk one flight of stairs with no distress	No Tx modifications necessary
ASA II	Mild systemic disease or extreme dental anxiety	Must stop after walking one flight of stairs because of distress Well-controlled chronic conditions Upper respiratory infections Healthy pregnant woman Allergies	Minimal risk; minor Tx modifications may be necessary
ASA III	Systemic disease that limits activity but is not incapacitating	Must stop en route walking one flight of stairs Chronic cardiovascular conditions Controlled insulin-dependent diabetes Chronic pulmonary diseases Elevated blood pressure	Elective Tx not contraindicated; but serious consideration of Tx modifications may be necessary
ASA IV	Incapacitating disease that is a constant threat to life	Unable to walk up one flight of stairs Unstable cardiovascular conditions Extremely elevated blood pressure Uncontrolled epilepsy Insulin-dependent diabetes	Conservative, non-invasive management of emergency dental conditions; more complex intervention may require hospitalization during Tx
ASA V	Patient is moribund and not expected to survive	End-stage renal, hepatic, infectious disease or terminal cancer	Only palliative Tx delivered

*American Society of Anesthesiologists: New Classification of Physical Status, *Anesthesiology*, 24, 111, January–February, 1963.

　Reference: Malamed, S.F.: *Medical Emergencies in the Dental Office*, 4th ed. St. Louis, Mosby, 1993, pp. 41–43.

III. ORAL HEALTH-CARE KNOWLEDGE LEVEL OF THE PATIENT

Before planning individualized patient care, an attempt is made to assess the patient's oral health knowledge level. From that baseline, planned educational interventions build on current knowledge rather than provide information too far above or below the patient's current understanding.

IV. ROLE OF THE PATIENT

Planning for oral hygiene instruction and use of oral hygiene aids is based on understanding of the patient's role in attaining and maintaining oral health. A patient must participate when the goals are determined for oral health outcomes. The willingness and/or ability to participate in planned oral health behaviors will be the key to reaching goals set during planning.

V. TISSUE CONDITIONING

Preparation or conditioning of the gingival tissue for scaling can be of particular significance when there is spongy, soft tissue that bleeds on slight provocation, and when the area is generally septic from plaque and debris accumulation.

Tissue conditioning is accomplished by initiating pretreatment plaque control measures and prescribing a concentrated daily program of plaque removal and warm saltwater rinsing. A quadrant that needs tissue conditioning is not selected for scaling until gingival healing and patient cooperation have been demonstrated.

Anticipated outcomes of such a program include:

A. Gingival Healing
The tissue becomes less edematous, bleeding is minimized, and scaling procedures are facilitated.

B. General Oral Cleanliness With Lowered Bacterial Accumulation
There is less likelihood that bacteremias will be produced during scaling, and there is less contamination in the aerosols produced.

C. Learning by the Patient
The patient can practice and see benefits of plaque removal.

VI. THE PERIODONTAL DIAGNOSIS

Planning for number and length of appointments in a

treatment sequence will be affected by the patient's periodontal diagnosis.

A. Current Periodontal Status
Criteria for determining a patient's current periodontal status include:
1. Current and past periodontal condition
2. Location of past or current periodontal disease
3. Severity of the individual patient's disease patterns
4. Modifiers that affect the progress of the disease

B. Case Type
For purposes of determining the sequence and number of appointments required for initial nonsurgical periodontal therapy, division of the periodontal diagnosis into case types is useful. However, this designation does not differentiate between patients with gingival tissue that is healthy at the present time or is in a currently active disease state.
1. Case Type I: gingivitis
2. Case Type II: slight periodontitis
3. Case Type III: moderate periodontitis
4. Case Type IV: advanced periodontitis

VII. PATIENT COMFORT

A. Quadrant Selection
When the patient indicates an area of discomfort, that area may be treated first. To make the first scaling less complicated and help orient an anxious patient to procedures to be followed, either the quadrant with the fewest teeth or the least severe periodontal infection may be selected.

B. Anesthesia
The need for anesthesia is determined by severity of the periodontal infection, depth of pockets, consistency and distribution of calculus, potential patient discomfort during scaling, and the sensitivity of the patient's tissues. When two quadrants are to be treated at the same appointment, it will minimize patient post-treatment discomfort to select a maxillary and mandibular quadrant of the same side.

VIII. PREPROCEDURAL ANTIMICROBIAL RINSING

A. Purposes
Preprocedural removal of bacterial plaque will lower the bacterial count in aerosols and decrease potential for bacteremia.
1. The first choice for bacterial removal is patient brushing and flossing.
2. Rinsing with an antibacterial mouthwash has been shown to be beneficial in lowering bacterial counts and contributing to less bacteremia.[12]

B. Procedure
1. Vigorous rinsing, forcing the fluid between the teeth, for 1 to 2 minutes can remove loose debris and surface bacteria approximately 1 mm below the gingival margin.[13]
2. Even rinsing with water will have some effect on bacteria, however chlorhexidine rinses have the most substantivity.[14]

IX. MAINTENANCE DURING THERAPY
When restorative, prosthetic, or orthodontic treatment extends over a period of time, periodic appointments are needed for monitoring the continued success of the patient's self-care. A gingival tissue assessment, checks with the probe to determine bleeding, plaque checks with disclosing agents, additional instruction for the care of new prostheses or implants, and motivational encouragement are essential.

X. FOUR-HANDED DENTAL HYGIENE
Planning patient care while working with a dental assistant allows for the use of flexible scheduling.[15] If there are two treatment chairs available, patients are seated in an overlapping time frame. A well-trained dental hygiene assistant can be delegated such tasks as patient reception and seating, medical history update, radiographs, oral hygiene instruction, and clean-up/disinfection of the unit in preparation for the next patient.

SEQUENCING AND PRIORITIZING PATIENT CARE

I. OBJECTIVES
The expected outcomes of preparing a well-sequenced dental hygiene care plan are:

A. Provide Evidence-Based, Individualized Patient Care
In addition to planning care to address the individual patient's needs as determined in the collection of assessment data, patient care is based on documented scientific evidence of success. Health-care providers must be able to assess the value of information available in product advertising and in the scientific literature.

B. Eliminate and Control Etiologic and Predisposing Disease Factors
The principal etiologic agents in both dental caries and periodontal and gingival diseases are the microorganisms of bacterial plaque. The overall goal of the dental hygiene care plan is to control the etiologic agent and, thus, to prevent future recurrence of the same conditions.

C. Eliminate the Signs and Symptoms of Disease
Measures to eliminate signs of disease such as

gingival bleeding and probing depths are included in the care plan. Elimination of disease symptoms of conditions outside the dental hygiene scope of practice, such as carious lesions, would be part of the patient's total treatment plan. Planning for dental interventions would include occlusal adjustment, restoration of teeth, replacement of missing teeth, orthodontic tooth movement, and periodontal surgery.

D. Promote Oral Health and Prevent Recurrence of Disease

Methods used to achieve optimum oral health are education, counseling, and the supervision of the patient in daily self-care. Encouragement of maintenance and provision of regular follow-up, supervision, and dental hygiene care are necessary if the patient is to meet the goals.

II. CRITERIA FOR DETERMINING TREATMENT SEQUENCE

Sequence planning involves first the identification of overall treatment and education patterns appropriate for an individual patient's needs. Then an outline of a series of dental hygiene appointments with specific services, treatment procedures, and educational interventions is included. The success of restorative, prosthetic, orthodontic, and other specialty dentistry depends on obtaining and maintaining soft tissue health.

Treatment sequence defines the order in which the parts of an individual appointment are to be carried out. The sequence is determined by numerous factors, including urgency of treatment, need for treating etiologic factors first, the severity and extent of conditions, and certain patient requirements.

A. Urgency

When discomfort or pain is present, the area involved requires first attention. In the dental hygiene care plan, this could apply to an area of the gingiva that is particularly difficult to clean because of inaccessibility. Immediate treatment is indicated in an area with a periodontal abscess or with necrotizing ulcerative gingivitis (NUG). Specially adapted plaque control instruction and/or scaling may be needed.

B. Existing Etiologic Factors

In patients with gingival or periodontal infection, success of the treatment depends on thorough, daily plaque removal to prevent recurrence of the infection. Dental caries may also develop unless continued attention is devoted to preventive measures.

Factors that caused or contributed to the existing condition must be arrested or controlled. Therefore plaque control measures must be introduced and success evaluated in the care plan before scaling will be effective.

C. Severity and Extent of the Condition

Findings that indicate the severity of gingival or periodontal infection include changes in color, size, shape, consistency, and bleeding of the gingiva; probing depths; mobility of the teeth; and radiographic signs. To determine length of appointments and sequencing of procedures, consideration must be given to probing depths in relation to the distribution of dental calculus. Number and length of appointments planned can increase with severity of the condition.

Planning considerations graded by the severity of infection might include the following:

1. *Moderate to Advanced Periodontal Disease.* For the patient who requires complicated periodontal, restorative, and prosthetic treatment, the dental hygiene care plan includes preventive and preparatory procedures, as well as maintenance during therapy, post-surgical care, and re-evaluation follow-up.

2. *Moderate or Slight Periodontal Disease.* The dental hygiene care plan includes the preventive phase and complete periodontal debridement, and it may include root planing. This treatment may be definitive, or the follow-up evaluation may show the need for surgical or other additional treatment.

3. *Gingivitis With Supra- and Subgingival Calculus.* The preventive phase and complete periodontal debridement are indicated. Tissue re-evaluation is necessary, especially for patients who began the treatment sequence with poor oral hygiene and require further motivation in order to attain oral health goals. The treatment may be definitive.

4. *Gingivitis With Slight Supragingival Calculus or No Calculus.* Dental hygiene services usually constitute the definitive treatment. To eliminate gingival inflammation, bacterial (plaque) debridement, and plaque control education may be the total treatment, which is supplemented by scaling when calculus is present.

D. Individual Patient Requirements

Items from the patient history that may require adaptation in appointment length, spacing, or sequencing when planning dental hygiene care include:

1. *Antibiotic Premedication.* Current recommended standard prophylactic regimens and a list of conditions that require antibiotic premedication appear on pages 101 to 104. For patients who need antibiotics, all instrumentation, including the examination procedures that require the use of instruments (probing, exploring), as well as tooth movement for mobility determination, are done under antibiotic coverage.

Bacteremias have been demonstrated during brushing, flossing, and other disease control measures. For patients with poor oral hygiene, early introduction of plaque control measures in the care plan is imperative. Initial instruction and practice of plaque-removing procedures are carried out while the patient is premedicated.

Efficient use of appointment time and/or spacing of appointment dates will avoid prolonged antibiotic coverage.

2. *Systemic Diseases.* Chronic disease will influence the content and length of appointments.
3. *Physical Disability.* Physical limitations will require adaptation of appointment plan.

PREPARATION OF A CARE PLAN

When writing the actual plan, each patient is considered individually. Figure 21-2 shows one suggested format for an individualized, sequenced appointment plan for multiple appointments. The format includes space to write dental hygiene diagnostic statements. In addition, treatment procedures and specific areas or quadrants to be treated at each appointment can be designated. Educational strategies or individualized

Dental Hygiene Appointment Plan

Patient Name: _____   Date: _____

Initial Therapy: _____
or
Maintenance: _____

Dental Hygiene Diagnosis:

Periodontal Diagnosis:

Appt #	Plan for Treatment and Services	Plan for Education and Counseling
1	Procedures: 1. 2. 3.	1. 2. 3. 4.
2	Procedures: 1. 2. 3.	1. 2. 3. 4.
3	Procedures: 1. 2. 3.	1. 2. 3. 4.
4	Procedures: 1. 2. 3.	1. 2. 3. 4.

FIGURE 21-2 Appointment Plan Format. The written appointment plan should include the dental hygiene diagnosis as well as sequenced treatment procedures and planned educational intervention for each appointment.

oral hygiene instruction are prioritized and listed for each appointment.

Examples of treatment sequences and plans are found in special areas of this book. An outline for maintenance appointments can be found on page 644, and a treatment sequence for a patient with necrotizing ulcerative gingivitis is found on pages 580 to 582. A suggested outline for conducting a plaque control program using a series of lessons is found on pages 337 to 339.

INFORMED CONSENT

It is every patient's right to possess knowledge that will allow shared decision-making with the oral care provider while treatment is being planned. Informed consent is a legal concept that can exist even without a written document. Informed consent can be lacking, even when a document has been signed, if the patient has not had the opportunity to comprehend and evaluate the risks and benefits of the suggested treatment.

I. INFORMED CONSENT

Table 21-3 provides criteria necessary for obtaining informed consent. Before being asked to sign the care plan, the patient must be informed of all of the treatment options available and consent to follow the recommendations in the agreed-upon care plan.

"Expressed consent" is given either orally or in writing. "Implied consent" granted by the patient's presence in the dental chair only applies to data collection procedures, data analysis, and treatment planning.[16]

II. INFORMED REFUSAL

The patient's right to autonomy in making decisions regarding oral treatment requires that practitioners respect a patient's decision to refuse treatment.[17] Refusal of care as well as any recommended treatment options are documented in the patient's permanent record.

TECHNICAL HINTS

I. Complete, accurate records are essential. Misunderstandings can lead to legal involvement.
II. Standardized, triplicate format consent forms that are printed with the care provider's official name and address will provide a copy to be given to the patient, a copy for the patient's file, and a copy for any necessary specialists.
III. While there are exceptions for emergency treatment, all care plans or informed consent forms should be signed by the patient whenever possible. Plans for minors or mentally disabled patients should be discussed with and signed by a parent or guardian, particularly when anesthesia must be used or prescriptions issued.
IV. When practice acts require that the dentist administer the anesthesia for the dental hygiene patient, the dental hygienist may maximize efficiency by recording the time of the patient's appointment on the dentist's daily schedule.

FACTORS TO TEACH THE PATIENT

I. Why a dental hygiene care plan is made.
II. Why patient input into the final care plan is important. Which parts of the plan are to be carried out by the patient. How the roles of patient and members of the dental team are interrelated in eliminating the patient's oral problems.
III. A clear explanation of how the dental hygiene care plan is an integral part of a total treatment plan, providing continued tissue maintenance during long-term dental, orthodontic, or surgical periodontal treatment.
IV. The long-term effects of comprehensive continuing care.
V. Why disease control measures must be learned before, and in conjunction with, scaling.
VI. Significance of the indices as guides for evaluating the health of the gingiva and the outcomes of the dental hygiene interventions.
VII. What presurgical preparation means, what it consists of, and what its expected advantages are.

TABLE 21-3 Informed Consent

INFORMATION TO DISCLOSE

- *Diagnosis:* description of patient's problem(s).
- *Treatment:* nature and rationale for the proposed treatment(s).
- *Alternatives:* viable alternatives to the proposed treatment(s).
- *Consequences:* risks and benefits of all proposed treatment alternatives including physical and psychologic effects, costs, and potential resulting problems.
- *Prognosis:* expected outcome with treatment(s), with alternative treatments, and without treatment.

PRINCIPLES OF INFORMING

- Assess the patient's ability to give informed consent.
- Simplify the terminology so that the patient can understand.
- Encourage the patient and family to ask questions.
- Continue to assess the patient's understanding and reeducate as often as necessary.
- Document all relevant factors and include signed form in patient record.

Adapted from Stuart, G.W. and Sundeen, S.J.: *Principles and Practice of Psychiatric Nursing.* St. Louis, Mosby–Year Book, 1995, p. 183.

VIII. The potential detrimental effects to the oral cavity if the patient chooses not to accept the treatment alternatives outlined by the clinician in the care plan.

REFERENCES

1. **Gurenlian**, J.R.: Diagnostic Decision Making, in: Woodall, I.R., ed.: *Comprehensive Dental Hygiene Care*, 4th ed. St. Louis, Mosby, 1993, pp. 361–370.
2. **Gurenlian**, J.R.: Recording the Dental Hygiene Diagnosis, *Access, 8*, 16, November, 1994.
3. **Darby**, M.L. and Walsh, M.M.: *Dental Hygiene Theory and Practice*. Philadelphia, W.B. Saunders, 1994, pp. 29–34, 401–415.
4. **UCSF Research Team**, National Center for Dental Hygiene Research, Philadelphia. Modified Client Assessment Tool Based on Human Needs Theory, *DHChat List Serv Archives*, http://jcffline.tju.edu/DIINet/research/dhchat/humanneedsbg.hmtl, February, 1997.
5. **Devore**, L.R. and Dean, M.-C.: Strategies for Oral Health Promotion and Disease Prevention and Control, in: Darby M.L., ed.: *Mosby's Comprehensive Review of Dental Hygiene*, 4th ed. St Louis, Mosby, 1998, pp. 494–495.
6. **Mueller-Joseph**, L. and Petersen, M.: *Dental Hygiene Process: Diagnosis and Care Planning*. Albany, Delmar, 1995, pp. 46–63.
7. **Williams**, K.-B., Gadbury-Amyot, C.C., Krust Bray, K., Manne, D., and Collins, P.: Oral Health–related Quality of Life: A Model for Dental Hygiene, *J. Dent. Hyg., 72*, 19, Spring, 1998.
8. **Offenbacher**, S., Katz, V., Fertik, G., Collins, J., Boyd, D., Maynor, G., McKaig, R., and Beck, J.: Periodontal Infection as a Possible Risk Factor for Preterm Low Birth Weight, *J. Periodontol., 67*, 1103, October, Supplement, 1996.
9. **Scannapieco**, F.A. and Mylotte, J.M.: Relationships Between Periodontal Disease and Bacterial Pneumonia, *J. Periodontol., 67*, 1114, October, Supplement, 1996.
10. **Beck**, J., Garcia, R., Heiss, G., Vokonas, P.S., and Offenbacher, S.: Periodontal Disease and Cardiovascular Disease, *J. Periodontol., 67*, 1123, October, Supplement, 1996.
11. **American Society of Anesthesiologists**: New Classification of Physical Status, *Anesthesiology, 24*, 111, January–February, 1963.
12. **Fine**, D.H., Korik, I., Furgang, D., Myers, R., Olshan, A., Barnett, M.L., and Vincent, J.: Assessing Pre-procedural Subgingival Irrigation and Rinsing with an Antiseptic Mouthrinse to Reduce Bacteremia, *J. Am. Dent. Assoc., 127*, 641, May, 1996.
13. **Wunderlich**, R.C., Singleton, M., O'Brien, W.J., and Caffesse, R.G.: Subgingival Penetration of an Applied Solution, *Int. J. Periodontics Restorative Dent., 4*, 64, Number 5, 1984.
14. **Veksler**, A.E., Kayrouz, G.A., and Newman, M.G.: Reduction of Salivary Bacteria by Pre-procedural Rinses with Chlorhexidine 0.12%, *J. Periodontol., 62*, 649, November, 1991.
15. **Blitz**, P. and Wright, V.: It Takes Two, *RDH, 14*, 18, September, 1994.
16. **Schoen**, D.H. and Dean, M.-C.: *Contemporary Periodontal Instrumentation*. Philadelphia, W.B. Saunders, 1996, p. 208.
17. **Odom**, J.G. and Bowers, D.F.: Informed Consent and Refusal, in: Weinstein, B.D.: *Dental Ethics*. Philadelphia, Lea & Febiger, 1993, pp. 65–80.

SUGGESTED READINGS

Coleman, G.C.: Dental Treatment Planning, in Coleman, G.C. and Nelson, J.: *Principles of Oral Diagnosis*. St. Louis, Mosby, 1993, pp. 210–248.

Fisher, E.T.: General Dentist and Periodontist Working Together. *Compend. Cont. Dent. Educ., 11*, 454, July, 1990.
Levine, R. A.: A Patient Centered Periodontal Program for the 1990s, Part I, *Compend. Cont. Dent. Educ.,11*, 222, April, 1990; Part II, p. 274, May , 1990.
McCullough, C.: Diagnosis and Treatment Planning, *Access, 7*, 26, April, 1993.
Miller, S.S.: Dental Hygiene Diagnosis, *RDH, 2*, 46, July–August, 1982.
Page, R.C. and Beck, J.D.: Risk Assessment for Periodontal Diseases, *Int. Dent. J., 47*, 61, April, 1997.
Pattison, A.M. and Pattison, G.L.: *Periodontal Instrumentation*, 2nd ed. Norwalk, CT, Appleton & Lange, 1992, pp. 329–335.
Taptich, B.J., Iyer, P.W., and Bernocchi-Losey, D.: *Nursing Diagnosis and Care Planning*, 2nd ed. Philadelphia, W.B. Saunders, 1994, pp. 3–33.

Evidence-based Care

Evidence-based Medicine Working Group: Evidence-based Health Care: A New Approach to Teaching the Practice of Health Care, *J. Dent. Educ.,58*, 648, August, 1994.
Leake, J.L., Main, P.A., and Woodward, G.L.: Developing Evidence Based Guidelines for Children's Dental Care in a Dental Public Health Unit in Ontario, Canada, *Community Dent Health.,14*, 11, March, 1997.
McCulloch, C.A.G.: Can Evidence-Based Dental Health Care Assure Quality?, *J. Dent. Educ., 58*, 654, August, 1994.
Raphael, K. and Marbach, J.J.: Evidence-based Care of Musculoskeletal Facial Pain: Implications for the Clinical Science of Dentistry, *J. Am. Dent. Assoc., 128*, 73, January, 1997.

Informed Consent

American Academy of Periodontology: *Informed Consent for Surgical Periodontics*. Chicago, American Academy of Periodontology, 1997.
Chiodo, G.T. and Tolle, S.W.: Informed Consent Across Cultures, *Gen. Dent., 45*, 421, September–October, 1997.
Litch, C.S. and Liggett, M.L.: Consent for Dental Therapy in Severely Ill Patients, *J. Dent. Educ., 56*, 298, May, 1992.
Odom, J.G., Odom, S.S., and Jolly, D.E.: Informed Consent and the Geriatric Dental Patient, *Spec. Care Dentist., 12*, 202, September/October, 1992.
Robbins, K.S.: Medical-legal Considerations, in Malamed, S.F.: *Handbook of Medical Emergencies in the Dental Office*, 4th ed. St. Louis, Mosby, 1993, pp. 91–101.
Woodman, R.C. and Malz, V.L.: Informed Consent and the Elderly Patient, *Spec. Care Dentist., 14*, 65, March/April, 1994.

Prognosis

McGuire, M.K.: Prognosis Versus Actual Outcome: A Long-term Survey of 100 Treated Periodontal Patients Under Maintenance Care, *J. Periodontol., 62*, 51, January, 1991.
McGuire, M.K. and Nunn, M.E.: Prognosis Versus Actual Outcome. II. The Effectiveness of Clinical Parameters in Developing an Accurate Prognosis, *J. Periodontol., 67*, 658, July, 1996.
McGuire, M.K. and Nunn, M.E.: Prognosis Versus Actual Outcome. III. The Effectiveness of Clinical Parameters in Accurately Predicting Tooth Survival, *J. Periodontol., 67*, 666, July, 1996.

IV

PREVENTION

Health Promotion and Disease Prevention

22

The dental hygienist is a primary care provider of preventive services. As a specialist in oral health care, the dental hygienist is involved at all levels of prevention, primary, secondary, and tertiary (page 3).

In Part IV of this book, Prevention, for which this chapter is an introduction, objectives, information, and procedures for primary prevention are described. Box 22-1 defines key terms related to health promotion and disease prevention for the individual patient.

Within the process of dental hygiene care, the needs of a patient are assessed from the histories and clinical findings, a dental hygiene diagnosis is made, and the care plan is outlined. When planning the sequence of treatment for the patient, initiation of preventive measures precedes clinical services except in an emergency. One important reason is that the patient must learn and practice procedures of daily self-care if oral health is to be attained and maintained.

STEPS IN A PREVENTIVE PROGRAM

Each patient needs a preventive care plan. To plan and carry out a preventive program takes a cooperative effort by the patient and members of the dental team. Details of the basic steps listed below were described either in previous chapters or will be parts of the chapters to follow.

I. ASSESS THE PATIENT'S NEEDS

A. Review all information from the histories, radiographic and clinical examinations, and chartings.

B. Identify the presence and severity of infection and the risk factors for oral health.

C. Utilize indices to rate the extent of the needs

BOX 22-I KEY WORDS: Health Promotion and Disease Prevention

Behavior: manner in which an individual acts or performs.

Behavior modification: approach to correct undesirable behavior through systematic manipulation of environmental and behavioral variables; treatment procedure for certain mental and physical disorders.

Communication: verbal or nonverbal interaction or interchange; nonverbal, without spoken words, may be accomplished through pictures, gestures, facial expressions, or posture.

Compliance: extent to which a person's health behaviors coincide with dental/medical health advice.

Dental health education: the provision of oral health information to people in such a way that they can apply it in everyday living.

Dysphagia (dis-fā′je-ah): difficulty in swallowing.

Evaluation: appraisal of changes in a patient's behavior or oral health status that have resulted from interventions by the professional health-care worker.

Halitophobia: imaginary halitosis; constant fear of having bad breath; somtimes related to underlying psychiatric condition.

Health education: combination of learning opportunities planned to facilitate and reinforce voluntary behavior conducive to the health of the individual or group.

Health promotion: planned combination of educational, economic, organizational, or environmental support for actions conducive to health of individuals or groups.

Learning: acquiring knowledge or skills through study, instruction, or experience; true learning means that knowledge acquired is applied in everyday living.

Affective domain: the domain of learning concerned with attitudes, interests, and appreciations.

Cognitive domain: the domain of learning concerned with knowledge outcomes and intellectual abilities.

Psychomotor domain: the domain of learning concerned with levels of motor skills.

Marketing: the task of establishing, maintaining, and enhancing patient relationships so that the goals of the patient, the group, or the community can be achieved.

Motivation: inner driving force that prompts an individual to act to satisfy a need or desire or to accomplish a particular goal.

Noncompliance: failure to carry out a prescribed health-care plan, for example, failure to take medications as prescribed.

Organoleptic (or″gă-no-lep′tik): stimulating any of the organs of sensation; susceptible to a sensory stimulus.

Preventive dental hygiene: sum total of the efforts to promote, restore, and maintain the oral health of the individual.

Putrefaction (pu″trĕ-fak′shun): enzymatic decomposition, especially of proteins with the production of foul-smelling compounds such as hydrogen sulfide, ammonia, and mercaptans.

Volatile sulfur compounds (VSCs): hydrogen sulfide; methyl mercaptan; and to a lesser extent, dimethyl sulfide and dimethyl disulfide produced by microbial metabolism and which create oral malodor.

Xerogenic (ze″ro-gen′ik): producing or causing dry mouth.

---

and provide a baseline for continuing comparisons. For most patients a bacterial plaque score can be helpful for showing the patient the extent of the gingival problem, and a dietary record along with the charting of carious lesions help show the dental problem.

D. Does the patient show willingness and readiness to learn? How may cultural values and beliefs promote or block the patient's response and compliance?

II. PLAN FOR INTERVENTION

A. Apply information about the patient, such as educational level, occupation, socioeconomic background, and attitudes toward oral health and oral care.

B. Determine the current personal oral care procedures carried out by the patient and the frequency.

C. Note factors that may affect the patient's dexterity when using oral cleaning devices such as an occupation that requires manual or digital skill.

D. Recognize the influence of age and physical and mental disabilities. Will another person (parent or other caregiver) be needed to carry out the necessary procedures?

E. Outline the procedures needed and work out goals with the patient.

F. Explain what can occur if the patient does not follow the care plan.

III. IMPLEMENTATION

A. How can the patient best be helped to be

aware of personal oral health problems and to learn and practice more effective health behaviors?

B. Provide motivating demonstration and supervision for daily self-care, bacterial plaque removal, self-applied fluoride, and other applicable preventive measures.

C. Introduce tobacco use cessation when indicated.

D. Show methods for self-evaluation.

E. Spread instruction over several appointments while clinical procedures are being completed. Learning takes time and reinforcement.

IV. PERFORM CLINICAL PREVENTIVE SERVICES

A. Complete scaling and bacterial debridement.

B. Apply caries-preventive agents: fluoride, sealants.

V. EVALUATE PROGRESSIVE CHANGES

A. Can the patient demonstrate the procedures for self-care? Do the teeth and gingiva show the benefits of learning?

B. Record a bacterial plaque score at each appointment and compare previous recordings with the patient.

C. At appropriate intervals, probe to note improvement in tissue quality, bleeding on probing, and probing depths.

D. Provide preventive counseling for corrective action when goals are not met.

VI. PLAN SHORT- AND LONG-TERM MAINTENANCE

A. Determine appropriate maintenance intervals.

B. Reevaluate to monitor continuance of preventive practices.

C. Provide supplemental care for the patient who does not respond to basic therapy.

PATIENT COUNSELING

Personalized patient counseling contributes first to the knowledge, attitudes, and practices of the individual and then, through the individual, to the family and the community. Periodontal infections and dental caries can be prevented or controlled, and therefore, teeth can be preserved throughout the lifetime of the individual.

For most patients major attention must be placed on control of dental caries and/or periodontal infection with emphasis on microbial plaque control and tobacco use cessation. Attention also should be paid to prevention of oral accidents such as those related to mouth protectors for contact sports, safety belts for automobiles, and children's accidents that lead to fractured anterior teeth.

Knowledge of and belief in health facts are not enough. Benefits result only when knowledge is put into action. Learning occurs when an individual changes behavior and when beneficial changes are incorporated into everyday living.

MOTIVATION

An individual is motivated to practice behavior that leads to achievement of goals that are valued. Instruction can be effective if the patient considers oral health a valuable asset.

Stimulation of behavior, or motivation, stems from basic physiologic or social needs. Peer group approval and the need to conform to group standards, as well as the fear of disapproval or rejection when, for example, appearance of the teeth or odor of the breath is unacceptable, are frequently much stronger motivating factors than is a health reason, such as freedom from infection or the ability to chew food.

THE LEARNING PROCESS

I. PRINCIPLES OF LEARNING

A. Learning is more effective when an individual is physiologically and psychologically ready to learn.

B. Individual differences must be considered if effective learning is to take place.

C. Motivation is essential for learning.

D. What an individual learns in a given situation depends on what is recognized and understood.

E. Transfer of learning is facilitated by recognition of similarities and dissimilarities between past experiences and the present situation.

F. An individual learns what is actually used.

G. Learning takes place more effectively in situations from which the individual derives feelings of satisfaction.

H. Evaluation of the results of instruction is essential to determine whether learning is taking place.

II. THE LEARNING LADDER[1]

Figure 22-1 illustrates the six steps from learner unawareness to habit formation. When beginning to help a patient learn about oral health and what the individual's needs are, one must determine where the patient stands on the ladder and start from there. Briefly, the ladder steps are as follows:

A. Unawareness

Many patients have little concept of the new information about dental and periodontal infections and how they are prevented or controlled.

B. Awareness

Patients may have a good knowledge of the sci-

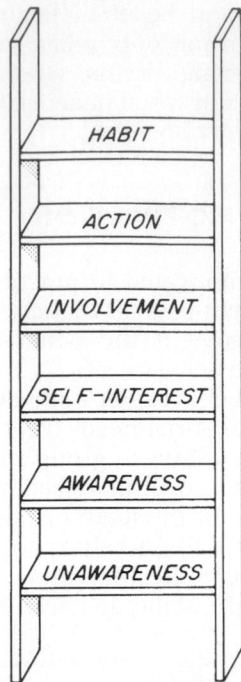

FIGURE 22-1 The Learning Ladder. Learning takes place in a series of steps from unawareness through interest and involvement to habit formation. See the text for the description of each step on the ladder. (From Harris, N.O. and Christen, A.G.: *Primary Preventive Dentistry*, 4th ed. Norwalk, CT, Appleton & Lange, 1995.)

entific facts, but do not apply the facts to personal action.

C. Self-Interest

Realization of the application of facts/knowledge to the well-being of the individual is an initial motivation.

D. Involvement

With awareness and application to self, the response to action is forthcoming when attitude is influenced.

E. Action

Testing new knowledge and beginning of change in behavior may lead to an increased awareness that a real health goal is possible to attain.

F. Habit

Self-satisfaction in the comfort and value of sound teeth and healthy periodontal tissues helps to make certain practices become part of a daily routine. Ultimate motivation is finally reached.

INDIVIDUAL PATIENT PLANNING

Initial instruction for most new patients will be personal plaque removal procedures. Each patient will have individual requirements.

All of the factors that apply to an individual patient are matched with the available bacterial plaque removal procedures. These include the selection of a toothbrush, toothbrushing method, interdental care devices and methods, dentifrice, and applied techniques for implants and fixed and removable dental prostheses.

With a clear definition of the needs of a patient, a recommended regimen or program can be outlined. The patient is shown the oral condition, changes and benefits that can be expected are explained, and cooperation is solicited. In this framework, the patient helps to formulate the goals that must be accomplished.

I. WHEN TO TEACH

The initial instruction is best given *first,* before any clinical treatment. Reasons related to the educational aspects are as follows:

A. Emphasis on Importance of Self-Care

Clinical professional services have only short-term effectiveness if the patient does not maintain tissue health through daily plaque removal. If considered first, and first in succeeding appointments, the degree of importance placed on self-care procedures by the dental team will become apparent to the patient.

B. Teaching Is More Effective

If instruction is delayed until after the clinical procedures in an appointment,
1. Time may be limited.
2. The gingival margin may be sensitive from instrumentation.
3. Blood clots forming after scaling and root planing must not be disturbed so healing can progress favorably.
4. Patient may be tired, anxious to leave, and less receptive to instruction.

C. Plaque on Patient's Teeth

1. *Plaque Is the Lesson.* With removal of tooth deposits during scaling, the opportunity to utilize the patient's existing plaque for demonstration is lost.
2. *Use a Disclosing Agent (pages 342 to 344).* With the use of a disclosing agent, a method of instruction is available that clearly and dramatically can show the patient what is to be accomplished. Bacterial plaque is not visible on most teeth without staining. Words fail to impress upon the patient that bacterial colonies exist on the teeth and that these multitudes of microorganisms are the responsible agents for dental and periodontal infections.

II. THE SETTING

A. Teaching Facility

A specific area may be set aside and furnished

for plaque control instruction in a dental office or clinic. Such an area should be planned with mirrors for the patient to use to observe the stained plaque on posterior teeth and distal surfaces. The patient also should be able to see placement of the toothbrush and floss in all areas of the mouth. Requirements for such a facility for a patient in a wheelchair are described on pages 742 to 743 and in Figure 50-2.

B. At the Dental Unit

Because of the need for the light and rinsing facilities during the demonstration, instruction may be given best at the dental chair. Without an extensive display of instruments and other equipment to distract the patient, and with the clinician seated beside the dental chair at the patient's eye level, an atmosphere conducive to learning can be created.

PRESENTATION, DEMONSTRATION, PRACTICE

A suggested outline for conducting the bacterial plaque control program follows. Various adaptations will be needed to tailor the plan to individual patients.

Equipment and methods for oral care are described in Chapters 23, 24, 25, 26; dietary analysis in Chapter 28; and fluorides in Chapter 29. For the patient who uses tobacco, suggested procedures to introduce tobacco use cessation are presented in Chapter 27. Control of bacterial plaque is basic to all patient preventive programs.

Each of the "lessons" described in the following outline is meant to represent the opening few minutes of each appointment before instrumentation for scaling. A plaque index or score (pages 298 to 302) and/or a bleeding index (pages 305 to 306) is made at the start. The index or score is understood by the patient, and new and review instructions are provided as indicated.

I. FIRST LESSON

A. Objective
Orientation to bacterial plaque removal.

B. Description
Describe the formation and composition of bacterial plaque, its relationship to oral disease (dental caries and periodontal infection), and specifically the relationship to the patient's present condition. Present an overview of the plaque control program, what it can accomplish, and its purposes in relation to professional treatment.

C. Illustration
Sketch on a pad of paper or use prepared materials. Show a tooth and gingiva and point out

where the bacterial masses collect to form plaque. Explain briefly how inflammation develops in the gingiva. Divide the material over more than one instruction period. Too long a "lecture" with too many facts and details at one time may mean the patient cannot absorb any of them.

1. *Patient With Gingivitis.* Show and explain the formation of dental calculus and how periodontal disease can develop if gingivitis is left untreated.
2. *Patient With Periodontitis.* Introduce pocket formation and the reasons for pocket elimination.
3. *Patient Whose Most Severe Problem Is Dental Caries.* When a food record for assessment is to be prepared, orientation to the preparation of the food record precludes discussion of plaque, cariogenic foods, and dental caries until the dietary record is obtained (pages 444 to 448).

D. Demonstration
1. While the patient observes in a mirror, a healthy area of gingiva and an inflamed area can be compared.
2. A probe is used to show a gingival sulcus and/or increased pocket depth related to periodontal involvement. Bleeding on probing is an important indicator of disease and should be recorded.
3. Remove a sample of plaque with a curet to demonstrate the thickness and consistency of plaque and to use for a phase microscope demonstration when available.

E. Application of a Disclosing Agent
1. *Explain Its Purpose.* Discoloration of plaque shows where the masses of bacteria accumulate.
2. *Apply Disclosing Agent.* Use a topical application and provide diluted concentrate for a rinse; or request the patient to chew a tablet, swish for approximately 1 minute, and rinse (page 344).
3. *Examine the Teeth With the Patient.* Point out the stained plaque and explain how the bacteria must be removed to control inflammation.
4. *Record Plaque Score or Index* (pages 298 to 302). Explain the score to the patient and use it to compare at future evaluations.
5. *Observe Location.* Observation of the location of disclosed plaque guides the instruction for plaque removal.

F. Instruction
1. *Keep Instruction Simple.* It may be better not to teach both flossing and brushing during the first control lesson, depending on the patient's background and experience.
2. *Floss First*

a. Review objective.

b. Show manner of holding the floss, inserting proximally, pressing around the tooth, and activating for plaque removal (Figure 24-1, page 374).

c. Examine in mirror to observe proximal areas where plaque has been removed.

3. *Brush.* Select a soft brush and ask the patient to remove the stained plaque. No specific brushing instructions should be given at this time so that the patient can concentrate on the single objective related to plaque removal.

4. *After Brushing, Examine the Teeth With the Patient.* The patient will see where accessible plaque was removed.

5. *Explain.* The use of a toothbrush is the most effective means of plaque removal for facial and lingual surfaces. Dental floss and other interdental devices are needed for the proximal tooth surfaces.

6. *Additional Devices: Care of Fixed Prostheses and Implants.* Instruction for care of a new prosthesis must be provided at the same appointment as its placement. The use of floss threaders is described on page 401. Dental implants need special attention (pages 420 to 422).

G. Summary of Lesson I

1. Review the basic objectives of learning about plaque composition, occurrence, and relationship to oral disease, and learning about the use of a disclosing agent to aid in plaque detection and removal.

2. At the first lesson, a specific toothbrushing method is not necessarily presented. The basic objectives should not be obscured by inclusion of excess information or diversion of the patient's thinking by concentration on details of brush position. The exceptions are:

a. The patient who demonstrates an acceptable brushing technique and whose mouth has been kept reasonably clean and shows no signs of detrimental brushing may only need to be shown a few special adaptations for the difficult-to-reach areas or other improvements.

b. The patient who demonstrates a brushing method that is detrimental, such as a vigorous horizontal stroke or a haphazard scrub-brush method, and whose teeth and/or gingiva show the effects of harmful brushing needs an introduction to a less destructive method.

H. Instruction at End of Appointment

1. Encourage use of disclosing agent at home; provide patient with tablets or instructions for purchasing. Suggest using a tablet for daily plaque checks.

2. Emphasize the need for cleaning regularly for complete daily bacterial plaque removal. Discuss carrying a toothbrush and dental floss for use when not at home.

3. When extra brushes cannot be supplied, explain that the toothbrush that has been used that day will be kept in the office for use during future appointments. Write down the specific name (number) of the brush for the patient to purchase for home use.

I. Patient Records

Methods, procedures, and patient progress and problems should be recorded following each appointment. The documented record can be reviewed before each appointment as a guide to continuing instruction.

II. SECOND LESSON

A. Objectives

To evaluate patient's success to date and to review and expand the knowledge content of the previous lesson.

B. Evaluation

1. *Examine the Gingival Tissue With the Patient.* Evaluate and compare with notes recorded from previous examination. Changes in color, size, and bleeding on probing should be noted and recorded.

2. *Apply the Disclosing Agent.* Evaluate the plaque as the patient self-evaluates, using a hand mirror. Chart plaque index or other record and compare, with the patient, with previous scores or indices.

C. Review and Extension of Knowledge

1. Invite questions from patient concerning plaque formation and gingival and periodontal infections to determine how clearly information from the previous lesson was understood and retained.

2. Always commend and compliment the patient for successes and improvements.

3. Discuss dentifrice recommendation when information from the dental history and the oral examination indicates the need for a change.

4. Explain why the patient needs a more scientific brushing method (or how a few alterations in the previous method can improve the oral condition).

5. Relate brushing to the treatment phase of oral care.

D. Demonstration

When not done previously, demonstrate the brushing technique of choice for this particular patient.

1. Show the basic stroke on the anterior teeth where the patient can observe brush position and activation. Explain each step.

Demonstrate brush position for each quadrant.

2. Instruction is divided appropriately to permit the patient to learn at a comfortable pace. When a patient has a power-assisted brush, initial instruction should be given with the manual brush so that proficiency can be attained with both. The patient should be asked to bring the power-assisted brush to the next appointment for demonstration and instruction.

E. Practice

1. Each position around each arch must be practiced because of the variations in grasp of brush and hand positions; the difficulty of access; and the individual tooth positions, particularly malpositions.

2. A recommended sequence for plaque removal that includes all areas and the tongue is discussed with the patient.

F. Instructions for Home Procedures

Use disclosing agent after flossing and brushing to test completeness of plaque removal. A mouth mirror for the patient to use at home can be helpful. Inexpensive plastic mirrors are available specifically for this purpose.

III. CONTINUOUS INSTRUCTION

A. Number of Lessons

It is not possible to predict in advance the number of specific teaching sessions a patient will need to demonstrate mastery of the recommended procedures and to show by the appearance of the teeth and health of the gingiva that the practices have been carried out daily. When additional supervision is indicated after professional treatment has been completed, short appointments may be scheduled in conjunction with dental appointments.

One learning experience is rarely adequate. When a patient has been able to maintain relatively clean teeth and clinically healthy gingiva and can demonstrate an acceptable toothbrushing method, a review of difficult-to-reach areas can be made and re-evaluated at a follow-up appointment.

B. Relationship to Gingival Health

When areas of gingival marginal redness and sponginess persist, tooth surfaces are checked carefully for residual calculus, and scaling and planing are completed as indicated. When the patient consistently fails to remove dental plaque in certain areas, a re-evaluation of the program is made. Perhaps the selected procedures are too difficult for the patient to accomplish or perhaps supplementary measures are needed.

C. Maintenance

After the initial instruction series, a follow-up is scheduled after a short interval for the first maintenance appointment. One must evaluate the patient's ability to continue adequate self-care and determine whether true learning has resulted and new habits have been adopted. *Learning means that a change in behavior has occurred.*

At each maintenance appointment, a plaque score or index is recorded, and the patient can evaluate the progress made. The complete procedures for the maintenance appointment are described on pages 644 to 645.

IV. INSTRUCTION ADAPTABILITY

The methods for presentation, demonstration, practice, and evaluation described in the previous pages can be adapted readily to various age levels. Awareness of the changing motivation and interests of the young to the elderly, and adaptations of terminology with respect for the patient's level of understanding, ease the transition from patient to patient.

Others for whom instruction is provided are the caregivers who attend patients who are unable to care for themselves. In Part VI, the various chapters that pertain to patients with disabilities include suggestions for patient care. Aids and devices are described on pages 749 to 754.

THE PRESCHOOL CHILD

The establishment of positive health habits and attitudes in the adult has its beginnings in childhood. Even before birth and during the first year after birth, the parent's education for prevention of dental caries and gingival infection should begin.

After birth, regular daily systemic fluoride in the absence of fluoridation, as well as attention to the control of cariogenic foods, can mean a great deal to the future oral health of the child. Nursing caries was described on page 240. Infant and toddler care and instruction are included on pages 660 to 662.

I. EARLY PLAQUE CONTROL

Conditioning a child to associate cleaning of the oral cavity with total body cleanliness should begin before the first teeth erupt. A small, soft toothbrush is advised. Other information relative to a child's oral care is included on page 660 and Table 43-3.

As time goes on, the child will want to use the brush, particularly if given the opportunity to watch the parents brush their teeth. At first, a tiny child may only chew on the brush, but eventually he or she may try to imitate the parents. Gradually, an actual brushing procedure can be encouraged.

For several years the parents will have the responsibility for brushing the child's teeth after meals and flossing and brushing before the child retires. The age varies with the individual child relative to when the child can take on the responsibility. It has been suggested that when a child attends to bathing, personal toothbrushing may also be done. Parental supervision and encouragement must continue for a few more years for most children.

II. PROFESSIONAL INSTRUCTION

A. The First Dental Appointment

Early visits to the dental office for orientation and getting acquainted are to be encouraged. If the infant has not had a dental emergency and therefore has not yet visited the dental office, oral examination and preventive health education are indicated within 6 months of the eruption of the first primary tooth and no later than 12 months of age.[2] Instruction in plaque control for child and parent should be introduced at the first appointment along with other preventive measures.

B. Instruction for the Child

1. *Toothbrush Selection.* A child-sized, soft nylon brush is recommended. When possible, let the child select the brush from assorted colors.
2. *Method.* Control of bacterial plaque at the gingival margin and on proximal tooth surfaces requires the same emphasis for the very young as for patients of other ages. Although the very young child has a short interest span for specific instruction, the parent can be coached to assist with supplementary home instruction.

III. INSTRUCTION FOR THE PARENT

The parent who is a patient in the same dental practice may be familiar already with the teaching methods used and well oriented to the importance of bacterial plaque control. Transfer of knowledge and skills to care of the child can be relatively easy. When the child is a patient in a pedodontic specialty practice or the parent is a patient elsewhere, orientation is needed in accord with the parent's present knowledge.

A. Disclosing Agent

1. The use of tablets is preferable for older preschool children who will chew them, so that tablets can be used at home for the parent to evaluate plaque control. One-half tablet is sufficient. When a young child cannot understand about chewing the tablet, disclosing solution can be applied.
2. Examination is accomplished by giving the child a mirror to "watch" the teeth. The plaque deposits are pointed out and discussed with the parent, and a little plaque is removed with a probe or curet to illustrate.

B. Demonstration

The brushing method of choice is shown to the parent while the child is in the dental chair under the light.

C. Procedure and Practice

1. *Provide Natural Setting.* Procedures are demonstrated to both the child and parent to simulate the home setting. Several positions for parent and child are effective and are shown in Figure 50-11 on page 754.
2. *Demonstrate Head Support.* Show the parent how, if the child's teeth are brushed from the front, the child's head falls back, unsupported, and seeing into the mouth is difficult.
3. *Suggested Standing Position.* Child stands in front of parent and leans back against the parent. Parent cradles the child's head with the nondominant arm and brings the hand around to hold the chin in the palm of the hand and to retract the lips and cheek with the fingers.
4. *Brush Mandibular Teeth.* Retract lip for anterior teeth and cheek for posterior teeth. The back of the brush head retracts the tongue.
5. *Brush Maxillary Teeth.* Child is asked to tip the head back so that the parent can look in the mouth while fingers retract the upper lip for anterior teeth and the cheek for posterior teeth.
6. *Apply Dental Floss.* With the child's head supported as described for brushing, the parent can be shown how finger and hand rests (fulcrums) can be maintained while floss is applied. When primary teeth are widely spaced, brushing may be adapted to remove plaque from all surfaces without a need for flossing. The parent can use nylon yarn, if more efficient, for proximal surfaces.
7. *Recommend Dentifrice.* A fluoride dentifrice is essential, even when fluoride is in the drinking water. The amount of fluoride dentifrice used should be no greater than the size of a small pea as illustrated in Figure 29-8 (page 472).

   When a child has a dental caries problem, additional measures may be recommended. As the child matures and develops the ability to rinse, a daily fluoride rinse can be used.

D. Summary

Instructions include brushing after each meal and using the disclosing test before one of the brushings. In a nonfluoridated area, the most beneficial procedure is to use a fluoride supplement (mouthrinse and swallow, or chewable tablet, pages 463 to 464) at bedtime after thorough plaque removal by toothbrushing and flossing.

E. Second Appointment

Procedure follows that for an adult. The gingiva are examined, and bleeding on probing is evaluated; plaque is disclosed and neglected areas are discovered; the child and then the parent demonstrate brushing. Suggestions for improvement are offered.

As needed, calculus and dental stain are removed professionally. Brushing demonstration precedes each succeeding restorative appointment until proficiency is demonstrated.

IV. MAINTENANCE

Instruction continues with each 3- to 4-month maintenance appointment.

THE TEACHING SYSTEM

A simple, direct approach, such as has been described, with specific content and unembellished material focuses the attention of the patient on the central theme: control of oral bacteria. The more practical, realistic, and goal centered the components of instruction can be, the more effective the outcomes will be in terms of treatment and prevention of recurrence of infection. An *informed,* knowledgeable patient will have reasons for *practicing* appropriate, scientifically based, self-care measures.

A teaching system must be re-evaluated from time to time, particularly as new research reveals new aspects of prevention and treatment. New devices for plaque removal and gingival care may become available, and these must be studied before recommendations to patients can be made.

The teaching system presented in this chapter has a built-in evaluation of patient learning. The outcomes of learning are shown by examination and demonstration: examination for the gingival characteristics consistent with health; demonstration of disclosable plaque; and demonstration of the patient's ability to use floss and brush for plaque removal without harm to the oral tissues.

Because the ultimate objective of plaque control is to prevent dental caries and periodontal infections, the oral health history of the patient over several years can be used to document a true evaluation. The teaching system must involve development of the patient's attitudes relative to continuing professional supervision and regular appointments for examination and treatment.

EVALUATION OF TEACHING AIDS

I. GENERAL CHARACTERISTICS

Evaluation of teaching aids involves consideration of the following:

A. Simplicity
Ease of management, ready obtainability, ease of understanding by the patient.

B. Content
Practical, scientifically sound, meaningful.

C. Level of Orientation
Appropriate for the individual patient.

D. Durability
If reusable, the teaching aids must maintain their cleanliness and freshness. Washable materials can be selected when available.

E. Cost
Reasonable. Cost relates to their essential value in reaching goals.

F. Objectives
1. Objective of a teaching aid must be clear and readily understood by the patient.
2. In teaching, activities should be reality centered, not fantasy centered. A well-intentioned visual aid may provide entertainment rather than education and have no transfer value, in terms of the actual oral health lesson, to the behavioral pattern of the patient.

II. READING MATERIAL FOR THE PATIENT

Effectively presented informational books and leaflets can supplement and reinforce individually presented instruction. Selected with a purpose, a booklet or other printed material may be presented to the patient to read while at the dental office, or it may be given for "homework." The booklet's contents must be reviewed with the patient; particular sections may be marked to personalize the instruction and encourage reading. Indiscriminate distribution of printed materials is pointless.

Obtaining copies of and reviewing newly available materials are essential parts of a dental hygienist's work, even as a teacher reviews new textbooks and materials for possible use in a classroom.

Instruction sheets and leaflets can be custom-made with the cooperation and recommendations of the dentist. It is especially helpful to have postcare instructions and plaque control procedures outlined so that the patient can have a reference for home use. Materials can be personalized by writing on them the patient's name and special procedures or reminders.

III. USE OF MODELS

A. Patient's Study Cast
The cast can be useful to explain oral conditions or restorations, such as the need to replace missing teeth. With certain patients, aspects of bacterial plaque control can be demonstrated, provided the patient is properly oriented to associate the cast with the teeth in the mouth.

B. Commercially Available Models
Although plastic models (dentoforms) have been used extensively for teaching toothbrushing methods, their meaningfulness to the patient has not been demonstrated. When a toothbrush is available for demonstration directly in the mouth and for a patient to use to practice brushing under supervision, the need for taking the time to demonstrate on a model first may be questioned.

When teaching is by means of the model and brush only, and particularly when the oversized model is used, the patient's learning should be carefully evaluated. All three of the patient evaluation methods described in this chapter (gingival status, disclosed plaque, and ability of patient to brush) should be utilized.

The model and the large toothbrush probably do not represent a problem to the patient, and most patients can imitate the motions of the toothbrush on the model accurately when asked. The difficulty comes in transferring the motions to the mouth and relating such motions to the bacterial collections on the teeth. The more complex the technique, the greater the difficulty of transfer.

USE OF DISCLOSING AGENTS

A disclosing agent is a preparation in liquid, tablet, or lozenge form that contains a dye or other coloring agent. In dental hygiene, a disclosing agent is used to identify bacterial plaque deposits for instruction, evaluation, and research. Key words related to disclosing agents are defined in Box 22-2.

Bacterial plaque is nearly colorless unless stained by foods, beverages, or tobacco. After use of a disclosing agent, the soft deposits pick up and hold the color of the agent. On the other hand, the dye can be rinsed off readily from plaque-free surfaces (Figure 22-2). After staining, the deposits that can be seen distinctly provide a valuable visual aid in patient instruction. Such a procedure can demonstrate dramatically to the patient the presence of deposits and the areas that need special attention during personal oral care.

I. PURPOSES

A disclosing agent clearly demarcates soft deposits that might otherwise be invisible and therefore facilitates the following:

A. Personalized patient instruction in the location of soft deposits and the techniques for removal.

B. Self-assessment by the patient on a daily basis during initial instruction and periodic checks thereafter.

C. Continuing evaluation of the effectiveness of the instruction for the patient.
   1. Determining the need for revisions of the plaque control procedures.
   2. Studying the long-term effects over successive maintenance appointments.

D. Preparation of plaque indices (pages 298 to 302).

E. Conducting research studies to gain new information about the incidence and formation of deposits on the teeth, the effectiveness of specific devices for bacterial plaque control and antiplaque agents, and to evaluate clinical and instructional group health programs.

II. PROPERTIES OF AN ACCEPTABLE DISCLOSING AGENT

A. Intensity of Color

A distinct staining of deposits should be evident. The color should contrast with normal colors of the oral cavity.

B. Duration of Intensity

The color should not rinse off immediately with ordinary rinsing methods, nor should it be removable by the saliva for the period of time required to complete the instruction or clinical service. The color should be removed from the gingival tissue and lips by the completion of the appointment, however, as the patient may have a personal reaction to color retained for a long period of time.

BOX 22-2 KEY WORDS AND ABBREVIATIONS: Disclosing Agents

Diffusion (dĭ-fu′zhun): process of being widely spread.

Diffusibility: refers to the ability of a disclosing agent to spread readily over a tooth surface and flow into the interproximal areas.

Disclosing agent (dis-klo′zing): selective dye in solution, tablet, or lozenge form used to visualize and identify bacterial plaque on the surfaces of the teeth.

Eosin (e′o-sin): rose-colored dye used for preparing histologic specimens for microscopic study; companion dye with **hematoxylin** for the well-known "H & E" that stains nuclei blue and the cytoplasm pink.

Erythrosin (ĕ-rith′ro-sin): red-colored dye used in solution or tablet form for a disclosing agent in the identification of bacterial plaque on teeth.

F.D.&C. (Food Drug & Cosmetic): United States Food, Drug, and Cosmetic Act regulates the packaging, labeling, importing, and exporting of such products as disclosing agents.

Fluorescein (floo-res′e-in): bright yellow fluorescing dye effective for disclosing bacterial plaque on teeth; used in ophthalmology to reveal corneal lesions of the eye.

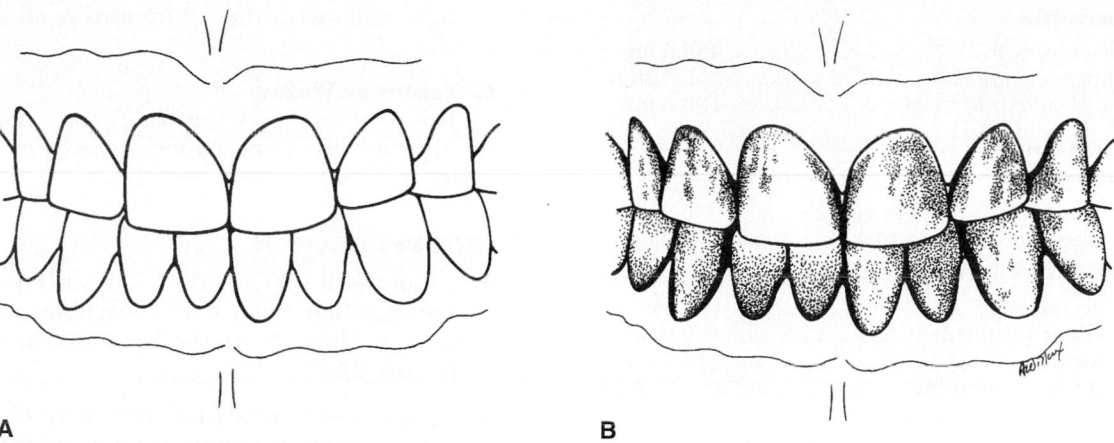

A   B

■ **FIGURE 22-2 Use of Disclosing Agent. (A)** Appearance of the teeth before application of a disclosing agent. Bacterial plaque and pellicle are usually invisible. **(B)** After use of a disclosing agent on the same teeth as those shown in **A.** Bacterial plaque and pellicle take on the color of the dye used in the disclosing agent. As noted, soft deposits are extensive, and are especially thick on the proximal surfaces.

C. Taste

The patient should not be made uncomfortable by an unpleasant or highly flavored substance. The main reason for using the disclosant is to motivate the patient; therefore, the use of the agent should be pleasant and encourage cooperation.

D. Irritation to the Mucous Membrane

The patient should be questioned concerning the possibility of an idiosyncrasy to an ingredient. When this information is obtained, it should be entered on the patient's permanent history record. Because of the possibility of allergy, more than one type of disclosing agent should be available for use.

E. Diffusibility

A solution should be thin enough so it can be applied readily to the exposed surfaces of the teeth, yet thick enough to impart an intense color to bacterial plaque.

F. Astringent and Antiseptic Properties

These properties may be highly desirable in that the disclosing agent may contribute other factors to the treatment procedures. The application of an antiseptic before scaling is frequently recommended, and if an antiseptic disclosing agent is used, one solution can serve a dual purpose.

A disclosant may inhibit the growth of microorganisms. In quantitative plaque research studies, therefore, disclosing agents without antibacterial properties should be used.

III. FORMULAE

A variety of disclosing agents has been used. Skinner's iodine solution was formerly the most classic

and widely used. In general, iodine solutions are less desirable because of their unpleasant flavor.

Aniline dyes have been shown to have carcinogenic potential. Therefore, the use of basic fuchsin and beta rose (flavored basic fuchsin) has been discouraged.

The formulae of a few disclosing agents are included in this chapter. Other well-known agents are Buckley's, Berwick's, Talbot's iodo-glycerol, and Metaphen solutions.

A. Iodine Preparations

1. Skinner's Solution

Iodine crystals	3.3 g
Potassium iodide	1.0 g
Zinc iodide	1.0 g
Water (distilled)	16.0 mL
Glycerin	16.0 mL

2. Diluted Tincture of Iodine

Tincture of iodine	21.0 mL
Water (distilled)	15.0 mL

B. Mercurochrome Preparations

1. Mercurochrome Solution (5%)

Mercurochrome	1.5 g
Water (distilled) to make	30.0 mL

2. Flavored Mercurochrome Disclosing Solution

Mercurochrome	13.5 g
Water (distilled)	3.0 L
Oil of peppermint	3 drops
Artificial noncariogenic sweetener	

C. Bismarck Brown (Easlick's Disclosing Solution)

Bismarck Brown	3.0 g
Ethyl alcohol	10.0 mL
Glycerin	120.0 mL
Anise (flavoring)	1 drop

D. Merbromin

Merbromin, N.F........................... 450.0 mg
Oil of peppermint .... 1 drop
Water (distilled) to make...................... 100.0 mL

E. Erythrosin

1. Concentrate for Application by Rinsing

   F.D.&C. Red No. 3 or No. 28 .... 6.0 g
   Water (distilled) to make............... 100.0 mL

2. For Direct Topical Application

   Erythrosin................................... 0.8 g
   Water (distilled)........................... 100.0 mL
   Alcohol (95%) .... 10.0 mL
   Oil of peppermint .... 2 drops

3. Tablet[3]

   F.D.&C. Red No. 3 .... 15.0 mg
   Sodium chloride 0.747%
   Sodium sucaryl 0.747%
   Calcium stearate 0.995%
   Soluble saccharin......................... 0.186%
   White oil 0.124%
   Flavoring...................................... 2.239%
   Sorbitol to make a 7-grain tablet

F. Fast Green

F.D.&C. Green No. 3 5% or 2.5%

G. Fluorescein[4]

F.D.&C. Yellow No. 8 (used with a special ultra-violet light source to make the agent visible)

H. Two-Tone[5]

F.D.&C. Green No. 3
F.D.&C. Red No. 3
Thicker (older) plaque stains blue; thinner (newer) plaque stains red.

IV. METHODS FOR APPLICATION

Make gingival tissue evaluation before application because disclosing agent masks tissue colors.

A. Solution for Direct Application (Painting)

1. Have patient rinse to remove food particles and heavy saliva.
2. Apply water-based lubricant generously to prevent staining of the lips.
3. Dry the teeth with compressed air, retracting cheek or tongue.
4. Use swab or small cotton pellet to carry the solution to the teeth.
5. Apply solution generously to the crowns of the teeth only.
6. Direct the patient to spread the agent over all surfaces of the teeth with the tongue.
7. Examine the distribution of agent and request the patient to rinse if indicated.

B. Rinsing

A few drops of a concentrated preparation are placed in a paper cup and water is added for the appropriate dilution. Instruct the patient to rinse and swish the solution over all tooth surfaces.

C. Tablet or Wafer

The patient chews the wafer (one half may be sufficient for some patients), swishes it around for 30 to 60 seconds, and rinses.

V. INTERPRETATION

A. Clean tooth surfaces do not absorb the coloring agent; when pellicle and bacterial plaque are present, they absorb the agent and are disclosed (Figure 22-2).

B. Pellicle stains as a thin, relatively clear covering, whereas bacterial plaque appears darker, thicker, and more opaque.

C. Two-Tone

1. *Red Plaque.* Newly formed, thin, usually supragingival.
2. *Blue Plaque.* Thicker, older, more tenacious; usually it is seen at and just below gingival margin, especially on proximal surfaces and where brush or floss is not easily applied; may be associated with calculus deposits.

VI. PATIENT INSTRUCTION

Because plaque and pellicle are frequently invisible to a patient, a disclosing agent can provide a visual method for patient instruction.

A. Explain Bacterial Plaque

The patient needs to be informed about the composition and effect of plaque in the production of gingival and periodontal infections, with particular reference to the individual mouth.

B. Show Location and Distribution of Plaque

With a mirror, the patient can observe the teeth and the disclosed bacterial plaque. A small mouth mirror is needed to show the lingual surfaces and posterior facial areas.

Show the special areas of concern. Relate the tinted areas to the health of the gingiva.

C. Demonstrate Methods for Daily Plaque Removal

A plan for instruction is outlined on pages 337 to 339. The techniques for toothbrushing and interdental care are described in Chapters 23 and 24.

TECHNICAL HINTS FOR DISCLOSING AGENTS

I. Avoid using disclosing or antiseptic solutions on teeth that have tooth-color restorations because these materials may be stained by coloring agents.

II. Do not apply a disclosing agent before a sealant is to be placed.

III. Purchase solutions in small quantities. Do not keep solutions containing alcohol longer than 2 or 3 months because the alcohol will evaporate and render the solution too highly concentrated.

IV. Use small bottles with dropper caps for solutions. Transfer solution to a dappen dish for use. Do not contaminate the solution by dipping cotton pliers with pellet directly into the container bottle.

V. Request local druggist to stock disclosing tablets for patients to purchase. Advise patients of the stores where the agents may be purchased.

VI. Source for two-tone disclosing agent:

RHODES TO HEALTH
Marilyn Rhodes, R.D.H.
4335 Bermuda Avenue
Oakland, CA 94619-3020
Phone 510-531-0348
1-800-530-0348
www.rhodestohealth.com

XEROSTOMIA

Saliva has many functions in the oral cavity relating to the maintenance of health of the teeth and soft tissues. It is protective in its functions of lubrication and cleansing. It contains immunoglobulins, electrolytes, and other substances that aid in resistance to disease (Table 22-1).

Xerostomia means dryness of the mouth. It is caused by absence or diminished quantity of saliva. Lack of saliva and the resulting dry mouth are important contributing factors to oral discomfort and disease, particularly dental caries. Xerostomia is a symptom, not a disease entity.

TABLE 22-1 Functions of Saliva

Lubrication of membranes, gingiva, teeth
Cleansing in self-cleansing mechanism
Tasting
Digestion: Food breakdown: chewing
               Food bolus formation
               Swallowing
Protection against diseases
    Antibacterial
    Antifungal
    Antiviral
Buffering: pH control
Remineralization
    Protection against demineralization
Speech
Carrier of antibodies, hormones, enzymes
    Provide data for diagnostic testing

I. CAUSES OF XEROSTOMIA

Xerostomia may be permanent or temporary. Temporary dry mouth occurs in diseases accompanied by high fever with dehydration or fluid loss; with control of certain diseases, such as diabetes or hyperthyroidism, salivary flow returns to normal. Major causes of permanent xerostomia are as follows:

A. Radiation to Head and Neck for Cancer Therapy
Permanent damage to the salivary glands can result (pages 727 to 728).

B. Surgical Removal of Glands
The glands may be removed because of neoplasm.

C. Sjögren's Syndrome[6]
The syndrome is an autoimmune disorder of the salivary and lacrimal glands with symptoms of polyarthritis, enlarged parotid glands, marked xerostomia, and dryness of the eyes.

D. Pharmacologically Induced Xerostomia
Many drugs that are common prescription items produce dry mouth as a side effect.[7] Table 22-2 shows a partial list of the classes of drugs that decrease salivary function.

II. EFFECTS OF XEROSTOMIA

During patient examination and history preparation, questions and clinical observations can point to the existence of dry mouth even when a patient does not complain of the symptoms.

A. Clinical Symptoms
1. Feeling of oral dryness; tongue sticks to palate.
2. Difficulty with mastication, swallowing, or speech.
3. Impaired taste.
4. Thirst, with resultant increased use of fluids; licking of lips.
5. Smarting, burning, and soreness of mucosa and tongue.

TABLE 22-2 Partial List of Classes of Drugs That Decrease Salivary Function

Anticholinergics
Antihistamines
Antihypertensives
Antianxiety
Anticonvulsants
Diuretics
Narcotics
Antidepressants (tricyclic)

B. Oral Effects

1. Heavy bacterial plaque, materia alba, and debris accumulation can lead to increased severity of periodontal infection and dental caries.
2. Predisposition to dental caries, particularly root caries.
3. Problems of denture wearing.
4. Dietary changes because of discomfort during eating; may use large quantities of liquid to soften food for swallowing.

III. MANAGEMENT OF XEROSTOMIA[8,9]

A. Pilocarpine Therapy[9,10]

Pilocarpine acts to increase salivary output. Patients with Sjögren's syndrome or other causes of xerostomia can get relief.

B. Prevention of Dental Caries

Severe, rampant dental caries related to any cause needs prompt counseling and treatment. One example is radiation therapy described on pages 728 to 729. Even before the radiation treatments are started, oral hygiene and caries prevention instruction must start, and a fluoride program must be initiated.

C. Personal Care Program

1. Rigorous plaque control effort by the patient for bacterial plaque removal.
2. Multiple fluorides may be recommended; use of dentifrice, rinse, and brush-on gel (or tray).
3. Advise patient to void tobacco and alcohol, and to use foods that are noncariogenic.

D. Environmental Factors

Patient may need to adjust air humidification in living quarters.

E. Use of a Saliva Substitute[10]

A saliva substitute is a preparation with physical and chemical properties similar to those of real saliva. The ideal substitute should be able to coat the mucosa and teeth to keep them moist, reduce enamel solubility, and remineralize the surface, as well as to help prevent accumulation of bacterial plaque.

Saliva substitutes contain carboxymethylcellulose (CMC) and the minerals calcium and phosphorous, fluoride, and other ions typical of normal human saliva. A small amount is sprayed into the mouth and distributed over all surfaces with the tongue. Patients can use the preparation at will, as needed for comfort.

F. Early Recognition

Dental hygienists are often the first to observe dry mouth (during the intraoral examination) and the first to hear the complaints of the patient of the discomforts caused. Early diagnosis and early treatment of Sjögren's syndrome or other causes of xerostomia can provide a major contribution to the general and oral health of the patient.

HALITOSIS

Halitosis, an unpleasant odor of exhaled air, is a symptom of importance in the complete consideration of health promotion and disease prevention. The sources or causes may be local or systemic. Bad breath can and should be a health concern.

The effects on the individual may be to create a sensitivity leading to a social handicap that can impair general daily living and personal relationships. When a patient asks about the breath, the request for help must be taken seriously.

Halitosis is also known as oral malodor, fetor ex ore, or just bad breath. It is sometimes called by names related to the cause such as "hunger breath," "menstrual breath," "tobacco breath," or "garlic breath."

I. ETIOLOGY

At least 90% of all malodor originates in the oral cavity, whereas the remaining 10% has systemic or nonoral causes.

A. Oral Causes and Contributing Factors

1. Periodontal Infections: odor from subgingival bacterial plaque
2. Tongue coating harbors microorganisms
3. Xerostomia
4. Faulty restorations retaining food and bacteria
5. Unclean dentures
6. Oral pathologic lesions: carcinomas
7. Throat infection
8. Cleft palate

B. Systemic and Non-Oral Factors[11]

1. Renal or hepatic failure
2. Carcinomas
3. Diabetes
4. Upper respiratory; nasal passages
5. Cirrhosis of the liver

II. ASSESSMENT

The normal breath of a healthy person with healthy oral tissues is nonodiferous or mildly sweet smelling. Suggestions for the assessment are included here. The list of predisposing and etiologic factors should provide a guide to specific areas of concern.

A. Medical, Dental, and Personal History[12]

1. Systemic influences: relate to list of causes
2. Medications history: side effects of dry mouth
3. Tobacco use
4. Diet, eating habits

B. Extraoral Examination

1. *Organoleptic.* Smelling of the exhaled air is

the simplest and most common method for identification.

2. *Detection Oral Source.* When the odor is detected from the open mouth, but not from the nose when the mouth is closed, it can be assumed that the odor has an oral origin.

C. Intraoral Examination
1. Tongue coating
2. Evidence of mouth breathing
3. Xerostomia: dry mucosa
4. Other: see "Oral Causes and Contributing Factors"

D. Complete Periodontal Examination
1. General personal care : state of oral hygiene
2. Probing for attachment levels, probing depths; periodontal status
3. Evidence of neglect; past history of dental hygiene care.

E. Measurement of Oral Malodor[13]
1. *Composition.* The majority of malodor arises in the mouth from microbial metabolism. Volatile sulphur compounds (VSCs) are produced consisting of hydrogen sulfide, methyl mercaptan, and lesser amounts of dimethyl sulfide and dimethyl disulfide. The VSCs are much higher in patients with periodontal diseases.[14]
2. *Instrumental Examination.* A VSC monitor has been developed especially for use in research to test the effects of mouthrinses and other products on oral malodors. A portable sulfide monitor (halimeter) is available for obtaining either or both oral or nasal readings to differentiate the sources of malodor.[15]

III. INTERVENTIONS

A. Dental Hygiene Care Plan
Objectives are based on achieving optimum gingival and periodontal health. Daily microbial plaque control and cleaning of all fixed and removable prostheses and implants are mandatory. All potential sources of plaque retention must be removed and carious lesions restored.

B. Plan for Instruction
The plan for instruction is outlined on pages 337 to 339. For patients who want to use a mouthrinse to help produce pleasant oral odors, they should be advised that mouthrinses have only temporary effects on malodor. Rinses with alcohol, glycerin, or strong oxidizing agents that can have detrimental effects on the oral tissues when used extensively must be avoided.

C. Tongue Cleaning
Brushing and scraping of the dorsal surface of the tongue is a daily requirement. A tongue scraper is shown in Figure 23-13, page 365. The tongue is a major source of the organisms producing VSCs.[16]

FACTORS TO TEACH THE PATIENT

I. The relationship between preventive measures and clinical services.

II. Why particular preventive measures were selected for the particular patient.

III. Self-assessment and methods for determining health of gingiva; assessment of bacterial plaque after use of a disclosing agent.

IV. Objectives for bacterial plaque infection control.

V. Treatment measures for xerostomia, such as diet, personal care, and where to obtain and how to use a saliva substitute.

VI. Purposes for use of disclosing agents; the appearance of stained bacterial plaque and the methods of daily care necessary to keep plaque controlled.

VII. For the parent, method of application of a disclosing agent to a small child's teeth to evaluate the presence of plaque.

REFERENCES

1. **Christen,** A.G. and Katz, C.A.: Understanding Human Motivation, in Harris, N.O. and Christen, A.G.: *Primary Preventive Dentistry,* 4th ed. Norwalk, CT, Appleton & Lange, 1995, pp. 393–396.

2. **American Academy of Pediatric Dentistry:** A.A.P.D. Oral Health Policies, *Pediatr. Dent., 20,* 72, Special Issue, Number 6, November, 1998.

3. **Arnim,** S.S.: Use of Disclosing Agents for Measuring Tooth Cleanliness, *J. Periodontol., 34,* 227, May, 1963.

4. **Lang,** N.P., Ostergaard, E., and Löe, H.: A Fluorescent Plaque Disclosing Agent, *J. Periodont. Res., 7,* 59, Number 1, 1972.

5. **Block,** P.L., Lobene, R.R., and Derdivanis, J.P.: A Two-tone Dye Test for Dental Plaque, *J. Periodontol., 43,* 423, July, 1972.

6. **Fox,** P.C., Brennan, M., Pillemer, S., Radfar, L., Yamano, S., and Baum, B.J.: Sjögren's Syndrome: A Model for Dental Care in the 21st Century, *J. Am. Dent. Assoc., 129,* 719, June, 1998.

7. **Felder,** R.S., Millar, S.B., and Henry, R.H.: Oral Manifestations of Drug Therapy, *Spec. Care Dentist., 8,* 119, May–June, 1988.

8. **Fox,** P.C.: Management of Dry Mouth, *Dent. Clin. North Am., 41,* 863, October, 1997.

9. **Lockhart,** P.B., Fox, P.C., Gentry, A.C., Acharya, R., and Norton, J.: Pilot Study of Controlled-release Pilocarpine in Normal Subjects, *Oral Surg. Oral Med. Oral Pathol. Oral Radiol. Endod., 82,* 517, November, 1996.

10. **Yagiela,** J.: Agents Affecting Salivation, in American Dental Association, Council on Scientific Affairs: *ADA Guide to Dental Therapeutics.* Chicago, ADA Publishing Co., 1998, pp. 186–198.

11. **Preti,** G., Clark, L., Cowart, B.J., Feldman, R.S., Lowry, L.D., Weber, E., and Young, I.M.: Non-oral Etiologies of Oral Malodor and Altered Chemosensation, *J. Periodontol., 63,* 790, September, 1992.

12. **Bosy,** A.: Oral Malodor: Philosophical and Practical Aspects, *J. Can. Dent. Assoc., 63,* 196, March, 1997.

13. **Rosenberg,** M. and McCulloch, C.A.G.: Measurement of Oral Malodor: Current Methods and Future Prospects, *J. Periodontol., 63,* 776, September, 1992.

14. **Yaegaki,** K. and Sanada, K.: Biochemical and Clinical Factors Influencing Oral Malodor in Periodontal Patients, *J. Periodontol., 63,* 783, September, 1992.

15. **Ratcliff**, R.: Current Concepts in the Causes and Treatment of Halitosis, *J. Pract. Hyg., 6*, 47, July/August, 1997.

16. **DeBoever**, E.H. and Loesche, W.J.: Assessing the Contribution of Anaerobic Microflora of the Tongue to Oral Malodor, *J. Am. Dent. Assoc., 126*, 1385, October, 1995.

SUGGESTED READINGS

Albandar, J.M., Buischi, Y.A.P., Mayer, M.P.A., and Axelsson, P.: Long-term Effect of Two Preventive Programs on the Incidence of Plaque and Gingivitis in Adolescents, *J. Periodontol., 65*, 605, June, 1994.

Al-Yahfoufi, Z., Mombelli, A., Wicki, A., and Lang, N.P.: The Effect of Plaque Control in Subjects with Shallow Pockets and High Prevalence of Periodontal Pathogens, *J. Clin Periodontol., 22*, 78, January, 1995.

Bader, J.D., Rozier, R.G., McFall, W.T., and Ramsey, D.L.: Association of Dental Health Knowledge with Periodontal Conditions among Regular Patients, *Community Dent. Oral Epidemiol., 18, 32*, February, 1990.

Baker, K.A.: The Role of Dental Professionals and the Patient in Plaque Control, *Periodontology 2000, 8*, 108, 1995.

Bruerd, B.: Focus Group. Evaluating Oral Health Education Materials, *DentalHygienistNews, 8*, 21, Spring, 1996.

Chopoorian, K.: How Adults Learn: The Dental Hygienist as an Educator, *DentalHygienistNews, 9*, 3, Number 2, 1996.

Christensen, G.J.: Educating Patients About Dental Procedures, *J. Am. Dent. Assoc., 126*, 371, March, 1995.

Chu, R. and Craig, B.: Understanding the Determinants of Preventive Oral Health Behaviours, *Can. Dent. Hyg. Assoc./Probe, 30*, 12, January/February, 1996.

Gluch-Scranton, J. and Tedesco, A.-M.: Individualizing Dental Hygiene Patient Management Throughout the Life Span, *Sem. Dent. Hyg., 4*, 1, January, 1994.

Ivanovic, M. and Lekic, P.: Transient Effect of a Short-term Educational Programme without Prophylaxis on Control of Plaque and Gingival Inflammation in School Children, *J. Clin. Periodontol., 23*, 750, August, 1996.

Kiyak, H.A.: Behavioural Techniques in Oral Health Promotion, *Can. Dent. Hyg. Assoc./Probe, 26*, 112, Autumn, 1992.

Lachapelle, D., Desaulniers, G., and Bujold, N.: Dental Health Education for Adolescents: Assessing Attitude and Knowledge Following Two Educational Approaches, *Can. J. Public Health, 80*, 339, September–October, 1989.

Lang, W.P., Farghaly, M.M., and Ronis, D.L.: The Relation of Preventive Dental Behaviors to Periodontal Health Status, *J. Clin. Periodontol., 21*, 194, March, 1994.

Liebman, J.: Dental Hygienists as Adult Educators, *Access, 9*, 47, September–October, 1995.

Lim, L.P., Davies, W.I.R., Yuen, K.W., and Ma, M.H.: Comparison of Modes of Oral Hygiene Instruction in Improving Gingival Health, *J. Clin. Periodontol., 23*, 693, July, 1996.

McConaughy, F.L., Lukken, K.M., and Toevs, S.E.: Health Promotion Behaviors of Private Practice Dental Hygienists, *J. Dent. Hyg., 65*, 222, June, 1991.

McConaughy, F.L., Toevs, S.E., and Lukken, K.M.: Adult Clients' Recall of Oral Health Education Services Received in Private Practice, *J. Dent. Hyg., 69*, 202, September–October, 1995.

McCullough, C.: Personal Oral Hygiene: The Most Important Component in Managing Periodontal Health, *Access, 7*, 33, December, 1993.

Stabholz, A. and Mann, J.: Periodontal Health and the Role of the Dental Hygienist, *Int. Dent. J., 48*, 50, February, 1998.

Testa, M.A. and Simonson, D.C.: Assessment of Quality-of-Life Outcomes, *N. Engl. J. Med., 334*, 835, March 28, 1996.

Motivation, Compliance, Communication

Albrecht, G. and Hoogstraten, J.: Satisfaction as a Determinant of Compliance, *Community Dent. Oral Epidemiol., 26*, 139, April, 1998.

Bagley, J.G. and Low, K.G.: Enhancing Flossing Compliance in College Freshmen, *Clin. Prev. Dent., 14*, 25, November/December, 1992.

Brown, J.: Creating Agreement: Understanding the Resistant Patient, *DentalHygienistNews, 3*, 14, Summer, 1990.

DeVore, C.H., Beck, F.M., and Horton, J.E.: Plaque Score Changes Based Primarily on Patient Performance at Specific Time Intervals, *J. Periodontol., 61*, 343, June, 1990.

Feinstein, J.A.: Choosing Educational Materials Patients Understand, *DentalHygienistNews, 5*, 4, Winter, 1992.

Gluch-Scranton, J.: Motivational Strategies in Dental Hygiene Care, *Seminars in Dental Hygiene, 3*, 1, July, 1991.

Hellstadius, K., Åsman, B., and Gustafsson, A.: Improved Maintenance of Plaque Control by Electrical Toothbrushing in Periodontitis Patients with Low Compliance, *J. Clin. Periodontol., 20*, 235, April, 1993.

Levine, R.A. and Wilson, T.G.: Compliance as a Major Risk Factor in Periodontal Disease Progression, *Compend. Cont. Educ. Dent., 13*, 1072, December, 1992.

Stewart, J.E., Jacobs-Schoen, M., Padilla, M.R., Maeder, L.A., Wolfe, G.R., and Hartz, G.W.: The Effect of a Cognitive Behavioral Intervention on Oral Hygiene, *J. Clin. Periodontol., 18*, 219, April, 1991.

Tedesco, L.A., Keffer, M.A., Davis, E.L., and Christersson, L.A.: Effect of a Social Cognitive Intervention on Oral Health Status, Behavior Reports, and Cognitions, *J. Periodontol., 63*, 567, July, 1992.

Weinstein, P., Getz, T., and Milgrom, P.: Helping Patients Change Their Oral Self-care, *DentalHygienistNews, 6*, 11, Spring, 1993.

Weinstein, R., Tosolin, F., Ghilardi, L., and Zanardelli, E.: Psychological Intervention in Patients with Poor Compliance, *J. Clin. Periodontol., 23*, 283, March, 1996.

Weiss, B.D. and Coyne, C.: Communicating with Patients Who Cannot Read, *N. Engl. J. Med., 337*, 272, July 24, 1997.

Children

Hamilton, M.E. and Coulby, W.M.: Oral Health Knowledge and Habits of Senior Elementary School Students, *J. Public Health Dent., 51*, 212, Fall, 1991.

Macgregor, I.D.M. and Balding, J.W.: Self-esteem as a Predictor of Toothbrushing Behaviour in Young Adolescents, *J. Clin. Periodontol., 18*, 312, May, 1991.

Ogasawara, T., Watanabe, T., and Kasahara, H.: Readiness for Toothbrushing of Young Children, *ASDC J. Dent. Child., 59*, 353, September–October, 1992.

Raynor, J.A.: A Dental Health Education Programme, Including Home Visits, for Nursery School Children, *Br. Dent. J., 172*, 57, January 25, 1992.

Rise, J., Wold, B., and Aarö, L.E.: Determinants of Dental Health Behaviors in Nordic Schoolchildren, *Community Dent. Oral Epidemiol., 19*, 14, February, 1991.

Schneider, H.S.: Parental Education Leads to Preventive Dental Treatment for Patients under the Age of Four, *ASDC J. Dent. Child., 60*, 33, January–February, 1993.

Schou, L., Currie, C., and McQueen, D.: Using a "Lifestyle" Perspective to Understand Toothbrushing Behavior in Scottish Schoolchildren, *Community Dent. Oral Epidemiol., 18*, 230, October, 1990.

Disclosing Agents

Baab, D.A., Broadwell, A.H., and Williams, B.L.: A Comparison of Antimicrobial Activity of Four Disclosant Dyes, *J. Dent. Res., 62*, 837, July, 1983.

Kipioti, A., Tsamis, A., and Mitsis, F.: Disclosing Agents in Plaque Control. Evaluation of Their Role During Periodontal Treatment, *Clin. Prev. Dent., 6*, 9, November–December, 1984.

Leknes, K.N. and Lie, T.: Erythrosin Staining in Clinical Disclosure of Plaque, *Quintessence Int., 19*, 199, March, 1988.

Lim, L.P., Tay, F.B.K., Waite, I.M., and Cornick, D.E.R.: A Comparison of 4 Techniques for Clinical Detection of Early Plaque Formed During Different Dietary Regimes, *J. Clin. Periodontol., 13*, 658, August, 1986.

Pitcher, G.R., Newman, H.N., and Strahan, J.D.: Access to Subgingival Plaque by Disclosing Agents Using Mouthrinsing and Direct Irrigation, *J. Clin. Periodontol., 7*, 300, August, 1980.

Rapley, J.W. and Brunsvold, M.A.: The Effects of Erythrosine on Alveolar Bone and Gingival Connective Tissue in Dogs, *J. Periodontol., 62*, 132, February, 1991.

Tan, A.E.S.: Disclosing Agents in Plaque Control: A Review, *J. West. Soc. Periodont. Periodont. Abstr., 29*, 81, Number 3, 1981.

Tan, A.E.S. and Wade, A.B.: The Role of Visual Feedback by a Disclosing Agent in Plaque Control, *J. Clin. Periodontol., 7*, 140, April, 1980.

Saliva

Edgar, W.M.: Saliva: Its Secretion, Composition and Functions, *Br. Dent. J., 172*, 305, April 25, 1992.

Epstein, J.B.: The Role of Saliva in Oral Health and the Causes and Effects of Xerostomia, *J. Can. Dent. Assoc., 58*, 217, March, 1992.

Hall, H.D.: Protective and Maintenance Functions of Human Saliva, *Quintessence Int., 24*, 813, November, 1993.

Mandel, I.D.: The Role of Saliva in Maintaining Oral Homeostasis, *J. Am. Dent. Assoc., 119*, 298, August, 1989.

Mandel, I.D.: The Diagnostic Uses of Saliva, *J. Oral Pathol. Med., 19*, 119, March, 1990.

NIDR, Public Information and Reports: Saliva: A Promising Diagnostic and Monitoring Tool, *J. Am. Dent. Assoc., 125*, 867, July, 1994.

Ship, J.A., Fox, P.C., and Baum, B.J.: How Much Saliva Is Enough? "Normal" Function Defined, *J. Am. Dent. Assoc., 122*, 63, March, 1991.

Shugars, D.C. and Wahl, S.M.: The Role of the Oral Environment in HIV-1 Transmission, *J. Am. Dent. Assoc., 129*, 851, July, 1998.

Xerostomia

Al-Hashimi, I.: Management of Xerostomia, *DentalHygienistNews, 7*, 17, Fall, 1994.

Butt, G.M.: Drug-induced Xerostomia, *J. Can. Dent. Assoc., 57*, 391, May, 1991.

Ettinger, R.L.: Review: Xerostomia: A Symptom Which Acts Like a Disease, *Age Ageing, 25*, 409, September, 1996.

Garg, A.K. and Kirsch, E.R.: Xerostomia: Recognition and Management of Hypofunction of the Salivary Glands, *Compend. Cont. Educ. Dent., 16*, 574, June, 1995.

Kindelan, S.A., Yeoman, C.M., Douglas, C.W.I., and Franklin, C.: A Comparison of Intraoral *Candida* Carriage in Sjögren's Syndrome Patients with Healthy Xerostomic Controls, *Oral Surg. Oral Med. Oral Pathol. Oral Radiol. Endod., 85*, 162, February, 1998.

McDonald, E. and Marino, C.: Dry Mouth: Diagnosing and Treating Its Multiple Causes, *Geriatrics, 46*, 61, March, 1991.

Najera, M.P., Al-Hashimi, I., Plemons, J.M., Rivera-Hidalgo, F., Rees, T.D., Haghighat, N., and Wright, J.M.: Prevalence of Periodontal Disease in Patients with Sjögren's Syndrome, *Oral Surg. Oral Med. Oral Pathol. Oral Radiol. Endod., 83*, 453, April, 1997.

Sciubba, J.J.: Sjögren's Syndrome: Pathology, Oral Presentation, and Dental Management, *Compend. Cont. Educ. Dent., 15*, 1084, September, 1994.

Sreebny, L.M.: Dry Mouth and Salivary Gland Hypofunction,

Part I: Diagnosis, *Compend. Cont. Educ. Dent., 9*, 569, July/August, 1988.

Sreebny, L.M.: Dry Mouth and Salivary Gland Hypofunction. Part II: Etiology and Patient Evaluation, *Compend. Cont. Educ. Dent., 9*, 630, September, 1988.

Sreebny, L.M.: Dry Mouth and Salivary Gland Hypofunction. Part III: Treatment, *Compend. Cont. Educ. Dent., 9*, 716, October, 1988.

Oral Lubricants

Furumoto, E.K., Barker, G.J., Carter-Hanson, C., and Barker, B.F.: Subjective and Clinical Evaluation of Oral Lubricants in Xerostomic Patients, *Spec. Care Dentist., 18*, 113, May/June, 1998.

Olsson, H. and Axéll, T.: Objective and Subjective Efficacy of Saliva Substitutes Containing Mucin and Carboxymethylcellulose, *Scand. J. Dent. Res., 99*, 316, August, 1991.

Olsson, H., Spak, C.-J., and Axéll, T.: The Effect of a Chewing Gum on Salivary Secretion, Oral Mucosal Friction, and the Feeling of Dry Mouth in Xerostomic Patients, *Acta Odontol. Scand., 49*, 273, October, 1991.

van der Reijden, W.A., Buijs, M.J., Damen, J.J.M., Veerman, E.C.I., ten Cate, J.M., and Amerongen, A.V.N.: Influence of Polymers for Use in Saliva Substitutes on De- and Remineralization of Enamel in vitro, *Caries Res., 31*, 216, May–June, 1997.

Halitosis

Bosy, A., Kulkarni, G.V., Rosenberg, M., and McCulloch, C.A.G.: Relationship of Oral Malodor to Periodontitis: Evidence of Independence in Discrete Subpopulations, *J. Periodontol., 65*, 37, January, 1994.

Carlson-Mann, L.: The Use of Tongue Cleaners in the Treatment of Halitosis, *Can. Dent. Hyg. Assoc./Probe, 32*, 114, May/June, 1998.

Kleinberg, I. and Westbay, G.: Salivary and Metabolic Factors Involved in Oral Malodor Formation, *J. Periodontol., 63*, 768, September, 1992.

Kozlovsky, A., Gordon, D., Gelernter, I., Loesche, W.J., and Rosenberg, M.: Correlation Between the BANA Test and Oral Malodor Parameters, *J. Dent. Res., 73*, 1036, May, 1994.

McDowell, J.D. and Kassebaum, D.K.: Diagnosing and Treating Halitosis, *J. Am. Dent. Assoc., 124*, 55, July, 1993.

Richter, J.L.: Diagnosis and Treatment of Halitosis, *Compend. Cont. Educ. Dent., 17*, 370, April, 1996.

Rosenberg, M.: Clinical Assessment of Bad Breath, *J. Am. Dent. Assoc., 127*, 475, April, 1996.

Rosenberg, M.: First International Workshop on Oral Malodor, *J. Dent. Res., 73*, 586, March, 1994.

Rosenberg, M., Kulkarni, G.V., Bosy, A., and McCulloch, C.A.G.: Reproducibility and Sensitivity of Oral Malodor Measurements with a Portable Sulphide Monitor, *J. Dent. Res., 70*, 1436, November, 1991.

Shimura, M., Watanabe, S., Iwakura, M., Oshikiri, Y., Kusumoto, M., Ikawa, K., and Sakamoto, S.: Correlation Between Measurements Using a New Halitosis Monitor and Organoleptic Assessment, *J. Periodontol., 68*, 1182, December, 1997.

23

Oral Infection Control: Toothbrushes and Toothbrushing

The toothbrush is the principal instrument in general use for accomplishing bacterial plaque removal as a necessary part of oral disease control. Many different designs of toothbrushes and supplementary devices have been manufactured and promoted.

Patients who have not previously received professional advice concerning the best brush for their particular oral conditions probably have used brushes selected on the basis of cost, availability, advertising claims, family tradition, or habit. Because of the variety in shapes, sizes, textures, and other characteristics, dental professionals must become familiar with the many available products to advise patients appropriately.

BOX 23-1 KEY WORDS: Toothbrushes

Abrasion (ah-brā′zhun) **(gingiva):** lesion of the gingiva that results from mechanical removal of the surface epithelium.

Abrasion (tooth): loss of tooth structure produced by a mechanical cause (such as a hard-bristled toothbrush used with excessive pressure and an abrasive dentifrice); abrasion contrasts with erosion, which involves a chemical process.

Bristle (bris′l): individual short, stiff, natural hair of an animal; historically, toothbrush bristles were taken from a hog or wild boar, but current toothbrush bristles are made of nylon and are called filaments.

End rounded: characteristic shape of each toothbrush filament; a special manufacturing process removes all sharp edges and provides smooth, rounded ends to prevent injury to gingiva or tooth structure during use.

Filament (fĭl′ah-ment): individual synthetic fiber; a single element of a **tuft** fixed into a toothbrush head.

  Curved filament: a nylon filament curved to follow the curvature of the tooth and enter the sulcus at about a 45° angle.

Mechanical plaque control: oral hygiene methods for removal of bacterial plaque from tooth surfaces using a toothbrush and selected devices for interdental cleaning; contrasts with chemotherapeutic plaque control in which an antimicrobial agent is used.

Power-assisted toothbrush: a brush driven by electricity or battery; also called automatic, electric, or mechanical (in contrast with manual).

Stiffness: the reaction force exerted per unit area of the brush during deflection; the term stiffness is used interchangeably with **firmness** of toothbrush bristles or filaments; the stiffness depends primarily on the length and diameter of the filaments.

Sulcular (sŭl′kū-lar) **brushing:** a method in which the end-rounded filament tips are activated at and just below the gingival margin for the purpose of loosening and removing bacterial plaque from the gingival sulcus.

Toothbrush head: the part of the toothbrush composed of the tufts and the **stock** (extension of the handle where the tufts are attached).

Tuft: a cluster of bristles or filaments secured together in one hole in the head of a toothbrush.

Key words relating to toothbrushes are listed in Box 23-1 with their definitions.

DEVELOPMENT OF TOOTHBRUSHES[1-4]

Crudely contrived toothpicks, presumably used for relief from food impaction, are believed to be the earliest implements devised for the care of the teeth. Excavations in Mesopotamia uncovered elaborate gold toothpicks used by the Sumerians about 3000 B.C.

The earliest record of the "chewstick," which has been considered the primitive toothbrush, dates back in the Chinese literature to about 1600 B.C. The care of the mouth was associated with religious training and ritual: the Buddhists had a "toothstick," and the Mohammedans used the "miswak" or "siwak." Chewsticks, made from various types of tasty woods by crushing an end and spreading the fibers in a brush-like manner, are still used by many Asiatic and African people.

The Ebers Papyrus, compiled about 1500 B.C. and dating probably at about 4000 B.C., contained reference to conditions similar to periodontal diseases and to preparations used as mouthwashes and dentifrices. The writings of Hippocrates (about 300 B.C.) include descriptions of diseased gums related to calculus and of complex preparations for the treatment of unhealthy mouths.

I. EARLY TOOTHBRUSHES

It is believed that the first brush made of hog's bristles was mentioned in the early Chinese literature. Pierre Fauchard in 1728 in *Le Chirurgien Dentiste* described many aspects of oral health. He condemned the toothbrush made of horse's hair because it was rough and destructive to the teeth and advised the use of sponges or herb roots. Fauchard recommended scaling of teeth and developed instruments and splints for loose teeth, as well as dentifrices and mouthwashes.

One of the earlier toothbrushes made in England was produced by William Addis about 1780. By the early 19th century, craftsmen in various European countries constructed handles of gold, ivory, or ebony in which replaceable brush heads could be fitted. The first patent for a toothbrush in the United States was issued to H. N. Wadsworth in the middle of the 19th century.

Many new varieties of toothbrushes were developed around 1900, when celluloid was available for the manufacture of toothbrush handles. In 1919, the American Academy of Periodontology defined specifications for toothbrush design and brushing methods in an attempt to standardize professional recommendations.[5]

Nylon came into use in toothbrush construction in 1938. World War II complications prevented Chinese export of wild boar bristles, and synthetic materials were substituted for natural bristles. Since then, synthetic materials have been improved and manufacturer's specifications standardized. Nearly all current toothbrushes are made exclusively of synthetic materials. Powered toothbrushes, although developed earlier, were not actively promoted until about 1960.

II. BRUSHING METHODS

Historically, the purpose of brushing was to provide *massage* to increase the resistance of the gingival tissue. Massage or friction from a hard-bristled brush was believed to *increase keratinization,* which, in turn, resulted in the resistance to bacterial invasion.[6]

Koecker, in 1842,[7] wrote that, after the dentist has scaled off the tartar, the patient must clean the teeth every morning and after every meal with a hard brush and an astringent powder. For the inner surfaces he recommended a conical-shaped brush of fine hog's bristles. For the outer surfaces, he believed the brush should be oblong of the "best white horsehair." He instructed the patient to press hard against the gums so the bristles go between the teeth and "between the edges of the gums and the roots of the teeth. The pressure of the brush is to be applied in the direction from the crowns of the teeth towards the roots, so the mucus, which adheres to the roots under the edges of the gums, may be completely detached, and after that, removed by the friction in a direction towards the grinding surfaces."

MANUAL TOOTHBRUSHES

I. CHARACTERISTICS OF AN EFFECTIVE TOOTHBRUSH[8]

A. Conforms to individual patient requirements in size, shape, and texture.
B. Is easily and efficiently manipulated.
C. Is readily cleaned and aerated; impervious to moisture.
D. Is durable and inexpensive.
E. Has prime functional properties of flexibility, softness, and diameter of the bristles or filaments, and of strength, rigidity, and lightness of the handle.
F. Has end-rounded filaments or bristles.
G. Is designed for utility, efficiency, and cleanliness.

II. GENERAL DESCRIPTION

A. Parts (Figure 23-1)
1. *Handle:* The part grasped in the hand during toothbrushing.
2. *Head:* The working end; consists of tufts of bristles or filaments and the stock where the tufts are secured.
3. *Shank:* The section that connects the head and the handle.

B. Dimensions
1. *Total Brush Length:* About 15 to 19 cm (6 to 7.5 inches); junior and child sizes may be shorter.
2. *Head:* Should be only large enough to accommodate the tufts.
   a. Length of brushing plane, 25.4 to 31.8 mm (1 to 1¼ inches); width, 7.9 to 9.5 mm (5⁄16 to 3⁄8 inch).
   b. Bristle or filament height, 11 mm (7⁄16 inch).

III. HANDLE

A. Composition
Nearly all current brush handles are plastics, which combine durability, imperviousness to moisture, pleasing appearance, low cost, sufficient rigidity, and smooth texture.

B. Shape
1. *Preferred Characteristics*
   a. Easy to grasp.
   b. Does not slip or rotate during use.
   c. No sharp corners or projections.
   d. Light weight, consistent with strength.
2. *Variations.* A twist, curve, offset, or angle in the shank with or without thumb rests may assist the patient in the adaptation of the brush to difficult-to-reach areas. Slight devi-

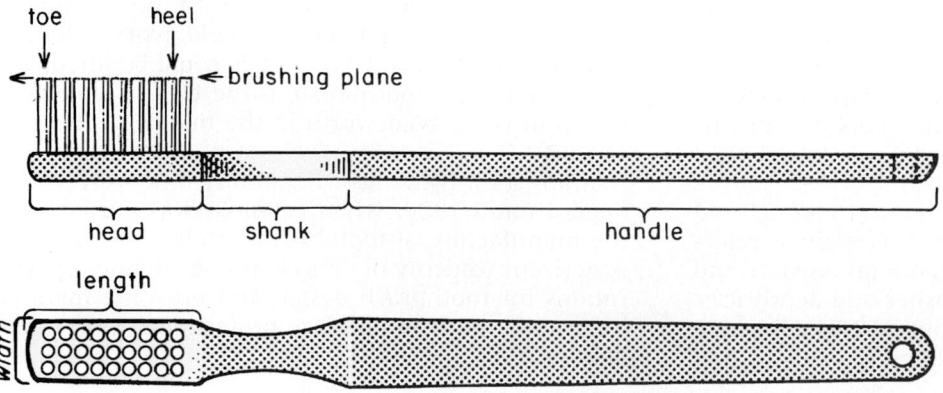

■ **FIGURE 23-1 Parts of a Toothbrush.**

ations may not complicate manipulation or affect control of the brush placement and pressure.

Bent or thickened handles can be helpful for use by patients with certain types of disability (pages 749 to 751).

IV. HEAD

A. Design

1. *Tufted:* Is 5 to 11 tufts long and 2 to 4 rows wide, spaced for easy cleaning of the brush.
2. *Multitufted:* Is 10 or 12 tufts long and 3 or 4 rows wide, spaced closely to provide a smooth brushing plane and to allow the filaments to support each other.

B. Brushing Plane (profile)

Brushes are available with variously shaped filament profiles. The brushing plane is also referred to as the trim, which is the characteristic arrangement of the tips of the filaments at the brushing surface.

The trim may range from filaments of equal lengths (flat planes) to those with variable lengths, such as dome-shaped, rippled, bi-level (Figure 23-2), or curved shape (see Figure 23-6, page 358). When used properly, all can reduce plaque and gingivitis.

All filaments should be soft and end-rounded for safety to oral soft tissues and tooth structure. Efficiency for cleaning the hard-to-reach areas, such as extension onto proximal surfaces, malpositioned teeth, or exposed root surfaces, depends on individual patient abilities and understanding.

V. BRISTLES AND FILAMENTS

Most current toothbrushes have nylon filaments. Natural bristles are relatively unsanitary, and their physical qualifications cannot be standardized.

The stiffness depends on the diameter and length of the filament. Brushes designated as soft, medium, or hard are not comparatively consistent between manufacturers.

A. Factors Influencing Stiffness

1. *Diameter.* Thinner filaments are softer and more resilient.
2. *Length.* Shorter filaments are stiffer and have less flexibility.
3. *Number of Filaments in a Tuft.* Each filament gives support to the adjacent filaments; each tuft gives support to adjacent tufts.
4. *Curvature of Filaments.* Curved filaments may be more flexible and less stiff than straight filaments of equal length and diameter; there is no straight end-line force applied as with the straight filament.

B. Natural Bristles

1. *Source.* Historically, bristles were obtained from the hair of the hog or wild boar.

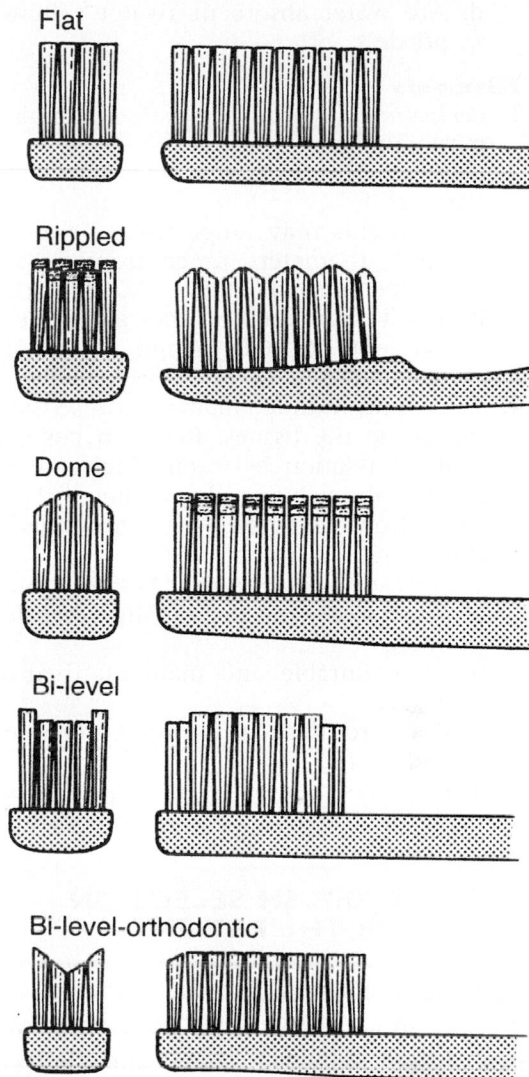

FIGURE 23-2 Brush Trim Profiles. A variety of filament profiles are available. In addition to the classic flat planed brush, other trims include the rippled, dome, and bilevel. Brushes for use over orthodontic appliances are made with various bilevel shapes.

2. *Uniformity.* Bristles are not consistent in texture or wearing properties. Their inherent resiliency varies with the breed of animal, as well as with the geographic location and season when the bristles were taken.
3. *Diameter.* They vary in size from 0.087 mm (0.0035 inch) to 0.475 mm (0.019 inch), depending on the portion of the bristle and the age and life of the animal.
4. *Shape.* Bristles have deficient, irregular, frequently open ends.
5. *Disadvantages.*[9] Toothbrushes with natural bristles are not recommended because the bristles
   a. Cannot be standardized.
   b. Wear more rapidly and irregularly.
   c. Are hollow, thereby allowing microorganisms and debris to collect inside.

d. Are water absorbent (water softens the bristle).

C. Filaments

1. *Composition.* Synthetic, plastic materials, primarily nylon.
2. *Uniformity.* Controlled.
3. *Diameter*
   a. Filaments may range from extra soft to hard. Diameters range from 0.15 mm (0.006 inch) to 0.3 mm (0.012 inch).
   b. Small interdental brushes are made with filaments of 0.075 mm (0.003 inch) (pages 376 to 377).
4. *Shape.* End-rounded filaments cause the least trauma to the tissues. Research has shown a direct relation between gingival damage and the absence of end-rounding.[10,11] Figure 23-3 shows examples of nonrounded and end-rounded filaments.[11]
5. *Advantages of Filaments Over Natural Bristles*
   a. Rinse clean and dry rapidly when left in open.
   b. More durable and maintain their form longer.
   c. Ends, rounded and closed, repel water and debris.
   d. More resistant to accumulation of bacteria and fungi than are natural bristles.

TOOTHBRUSH SELECTION FOR THE PATIENT

I. INFLUENCING FACTORS

Factors that influence the selection of the proper toothbrush for an individual patient include the following:

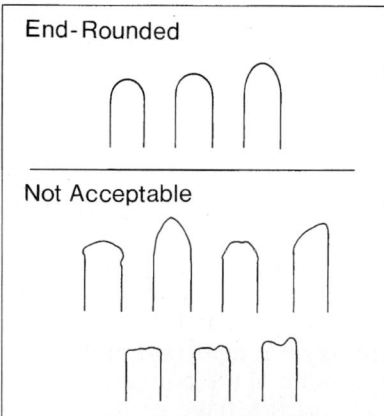

■ FIGURE 23-3 End-Rounded Filaments. Examples of the shape of acceptable end-rounding and of those that are not acceptable are shown. (From Silverstone, L.M. and Featherstone, M.J.: A Scanning Electron Microscope Study of the End Rounding of Bristles in Eight Toothbrush Types, *Quintessence Int.,* 19, 3, February, 1988.)

A. Patient

1. Ability of the patient to use the brush and remove plaque from all tooth surfaces without damage to the soft tissue or tooth structure.
2. Manual dexterity of patient.
3. Motivation, ability, and willingness to follow the prescribed procedures.

B. Gingiva

1. Status of gingival or periodontal health.
2. Anatomic configurations of the gingiva.

C. Position of Teeth

Displaced teeth require variations in brush placement.

1. Crowded teeth (Figure 16-5, page 272).
2. Open contacts (Figure 13-4, page 232).

D. Shape of Teeth and Exposed Roots

E. Personal Preferences

1. Professional personnel may prefer to instruct patients in certain methods and with certain brushes.
2. Patient may have preferences and may resist change.

F. Method Selected

Method of brushing to be recommended and instructed.

II. TOOTHBRUSH SIZE AND SHAPE

The brush selected must be able to be adapted to all facial, lingual, palatal, and occlusal surfaces for bacterial plaque removal.

III. SOFT NYLON BRUSH

The following are suggested as advantages for the use of a soft end-rounded brush that is applied appropriately.

A. More effective in cleaning the cervical areas, both proximal and marginal.
B. Less traumatic to the gingival tissue; therefore, patients can brush at the cervical areas without fear of discomfort or soft tissue laceration.
C. Can be directed into the sulcus for sulcular brushing and into interproximal areas for cleaning the proximal surfaces.
D. Applicable around fixed orthodontic appliances or fixation appliances used to treat a fractured jaw.
E. Tooth abrasion and/or gingival recession can be prevented or may be less severe in an overvigorous brusher.
F. More effective use for sensitive gingiva in such conditions as necrotizing ulcerative gingivitis or severe gingivitis, or during healing stages following scaling and root planing or periodontal surgery.

G. Small size is ideal for a young child as a first brush on primary teeth.

GUIDELINES FOR TOOTHBRUSHING

Complete toothbrushing instruction for a patient involves teaching what, when, where, and how. In addition to descriptions of specific toothbrushing methods, the succeeding sections consider the grasp of the brush, the sequence and amount of brushing, the areas of limited access, and supplementary brushing for the occlusal surfaces and the tongue. The possible detrimental effects from improper toothbrushing and variations for special conditions are described. The care of toothbrushes is outlined.

I. GRASP OF BRUSH

A. Objectives

Manipulation of the brush for successful removal of bacterial plaque can be related to the manner in which the brush is held. Patients may need specific instruction in how to hold and place the brush. When they start to brush to remove the bacterial plaque that has been colored with a disclosing agent, the tenaciousness of the plaque and the need for controlled pressure can be realized. With a light, comfortable grasp, the following can be expected:

1. Control of the brush during all movements.
2. Effective positioning at the beginning of each brushing stroke, follow through during the complete stroke, and repositioning for the next stroke.
3. Sensitivity to the amount of pressure applied.

B. Procedure

1. Grasp toothbrush handle in the palm of the hand with thumb against the shank.
   a. Near enough to the head of the brush so that it can be controlled effectively.
   b. Not so close to the head of the brush that manipulation of the brush is hindered or that fingers can touch the anterior teeth when reaching the brush head to molar regions.
2. Direct filaments in the direction needed for placement on the teeth; direction depends on the brushing method to be used.
3. Adapt grasp for the various positions of the brush head on the teeth throughout the procedure; adjust to permit unrestricted movement of the wrist and arm.
4. Apply appropriate pressure for removal of the bacterial plaque. Too much pressure, however, bends the filaments and curves them away from the area where brushing is needed.

II. SEQUENCE

A. The procedure in brushing, for any method used, should ensure complete coverage for each tooth surface.
B. Start brushing from a molar region of one arch around to the opposite side, then back around the lingual or facial. Repeat in the opposing arch.
C. Each brush placement must overlap the previous one for thorough coverage (Figure 23-4).
D. Encourage the patient to begin by brushing one of the areas of greatest individual need as shown by disclosing agent.
   1. Areas that are most frequently missed.
   2. Areas that are most difficult for brush placement and/or manipulation, such as the right side for the right-handed brusher or the left side for the left-handed brusher.
E. Suggest that the sequence be varied at least once each day so that the same areas are not always brushed last when time may be limited and plaque removal may be less complete.

III. AMOUNT OF BRUSHING

The main consideration is the removal of the bacterial plaque. All surfaces of all teeth need to be brushed clean. The number of strokes and length of time spent depends on the patient's ability and efficiency in accomplishing the task.

A. The Count System

To ensure thorough coverage with an even distribution of amount of brushing and to help the patient concentrate on the performance, a system of counting can be useful.

1. Count 6 strokes in each area (or 5 or 10, whichever is most appropriate for the partic-

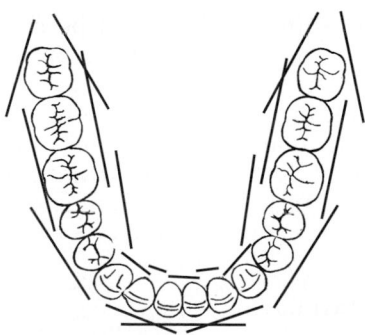

■ FIGURE 23-4 Brushing Positions. Each brush position, as represented by a black line, should overlap the previous position. Note placement at canines, where the distal aspect of the canine is brushed with the premolars and the mesial aspect is brushed with the incisors. Short lines on the lingual anterior aspect indicate brush placed vertically (Figure 23-10). The maxillary teeth require a similar number of brushing positions.

ular patient) for modified Stillman or other method in which a stroke is used.

   2. Count slowly to 10 for each brush position while brush is vibrated and filament ends are held in position for the Bass, Charters, or other vibratory method.

B. The Clock System

Some patients brush thoroughly while watching a clock or an egg timer for 3 or 4 minutes. Timed procedures cannot guarantee thorough coverage, because single areas that are most accessible may get more brushing time.

C. Combination

For many patients, use of the "count" system in combination with the "clock" system produces the most complete removal of bacterial plaque.

IV. FREQUENCY OF BRUSHING

Because of individual variations, one set rule for frequency cannot be applied. The emphasis in patient education should be placed on complete plaque control rather than on number of brushings.

For the control of bacterial plaque, and for oral sanitation and halitosis prevention, at least two brushings, accompanied by appropriate interdental care, are recommended for each day. *The longer the bacteria remain undisturbed, the greater the pathogenic potential of the plaque.*

A clean mouth before going to sleep should be encouraged. Bacteria thrive in the dark, warm, moist climate of the oral environment. Patients who use a chewable fluoride tablet, mouthrinse, or gel application before going to bed should complete their plaque removal before fluoride application.

METHODS FOR TOOTHBRUSHING

Most toothbrushing methods can be classified based on the position and motion of the brush. Noted beside certain categories that follow are names of methods that utilize the designated motion as part or all of their particular procedure. Some of these methods are recorded for descriptive, comparative, or historic purposes only, and are not currently recommended. A few even may have been shown to be detrimental.

   A. Sulcular: Bass.

   B. Simultaneous Sulcular: Collis.

   C. Roll: Rolling stroke, modified Stillman.

   D. Vibratory: Stillman, Charters, Bass.

   E. Circular: Fones.

   F. Vertical: Leonard.

   G. Horizontal.

   H. Physiologic: Smith.

   I. Scrub-brush.

THE BASS METHOD: SULCULAR BRUSHING

The Bass method is widely accepted as an effective method for bacterial plaque removal adjacent to and directly beneath the gingival margin. The area at the gingival margin is the most significant in the control of gingival and periodontal infections.

I. PURPOSES AND INDICATIONS

   A. For all patients for bacterial plaque removal adjacent to and directly beneath the gingival margin.
   B. For open interproximal areas, cervical areas beneath the height of contour of the enamel, and exposed root surfaces.
   C. For the patient who has had periodontal surgery.
   D. For adaptation to abutment teeth, under the gingival border of a fixed partial denture, and orthodontic appliances (Figure 25-2, page 397).

II. PROCEDURE[12]

A. Position the Brush

   1. *Filaments.* Direct the filaments apically (up for maxillary, down for mandibular teeth). Even though the brush placement calls for directing the filaments at a 45° angle, it is usually easier and safer for the patient to first place the sides of the filaments parallel with the long axis of the tooth. From that position the brush can be turned slightly and brought to the gingival margin to the 45° angle (Figure 23-5).
   2. *Gingival Sulcus.* Place the brush with the filament tips directed straight into the gingival sulcus. The filaments will be directed at approximately 45° to the long axis of the tooth, as shown in Figure 23-5A.

B. Strokes

   1. *Press Lightly Without Flexing.* Press lightly so the filament tips enter the gingival sulci and embrasures and cover the gingival margin. Do not bend the filaments with excess pressure.
   2. *Vibrate the Brush.* Vibrate the brush back and forth with very short strokes without disengaging the tips of the filaments from the sulci. Count at least 10 vibrations.

C. Reposition the Brush

Apply the brush to the next group of two or three teeth. Take care to overlap placement, as shown in Figure 23-4.

D. Repeat Stroke

The entire stroke (steps A through C) is re-

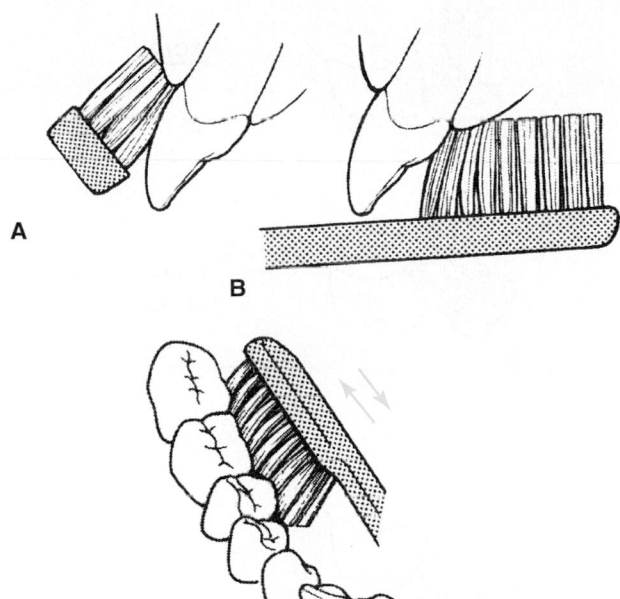

FIGURE 23-5 Sulcular Brushing. (A) Filament tips are directed into the gingival sulcus at approximately 45° to the long axis of the tooth. **(B)** Position for palatal surface of maxillary anterior teeth. **(C)** Brush in position for lingual surfaces of mandibular posterior teeth.

peated at each position around the maxillary and mandibular arches, both facially and lingually.

E. Position Brush for Lingual and Palatal Anterior Surfaces (Figure 23-5B)

Hold the brush the long narrow way for the anterior components. The filaments are kept straight and directed into the sulci.

III. PROBLEMS

A. An overeager brusher may convert the previously mentioned "very short strokes" into a vigorous scrub that causes injury to the gingival margin.

B. Dexterity requirement may be too high for certain patients. Because a 45° angle can be difficult to visualize, emphasis should be on placing the tips of the filaments into the sulcus.

C. Rolling stroke procedure may precede the sulcular brushing when a patient believes it helps to clean the teeth. The two methods should be performed separately rather than trying to combine them in what has been referred to as a "modified Bass."

The procedure of rolling the brush down over the crown after the vibratory part of the sulcular brush stroke has several disadvantages: (1) too often the brush is hastily and carelessly replaced into the sulcus position, or the opposite is true, and considerable time is consumed in the attempt to replace the brush carefully; (2) gingival margin injury by the constant replacement of the brush can result; and (3) patient may tend to roll the brush down over the crown prematurely, thereby accomplishing very little sulcular brushing.

THE COLLIS METHOD: SIMULTANEOUS SULCULAR

An adaptation of the sulcular brushing method is made when a Collis curved brush is used. The ability to brush three surfaces at the same time can provide added advantages.

I. PURPOSES AND INDICATIONS

All of the purposes and indications previously listed for sulcular brushing apply when a Collis curved brush is used. In addition, the following are special applications:

A. For patients with limited range of motion when a conventional sulcular technique may be difficult for the patient to master.

B. For aides and caretakers who provide oral care for disabled patients.

C. For parents or other caretakers responsible for children's care and supervision.

II. PROCEDURE

A. Position the Brush

1. *Filaments.* Direct the curved filaments apically (up for maxillary and down for mandibular teeth). Tilt the toe of the brush head and slide it over the teeth in the canine area.

2. *Gingival Sulcus.* The outer filaments enter the sulcus at a 45° angle automatically.

3. *For Gingival Recession.* Tilt the brush toward the facial or lingual to reach into the sulcus and adapt to cervical areas below the height of contour of the crown and to the exposed root surfaces (Figure 23-6A).

B. Strokes

Once the brush has straddled the teeth, apply short back-and-forth strokes typical of sulcular brushing.

C. Reposition the Brush

Apply the brush to the next group of two or three teeth. Take care to overlap placement as shown in Figure 23-4.

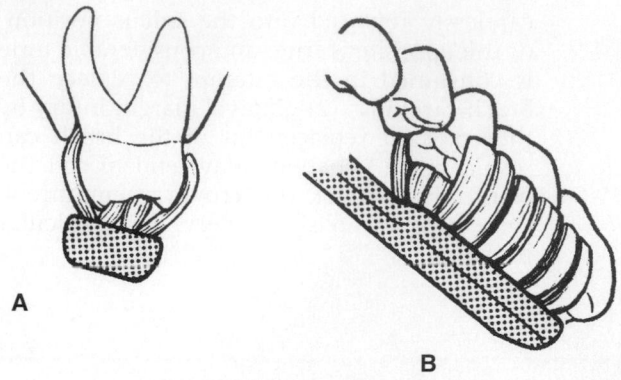

FIGURE 23-6 Use of Collis Simultaneous Sulcular Brush. (A) Curved filaments are placed over the crown and tipped to facial or palatal (lingual) to reach under the gingiva for sulcular brushing. **(B)** Shows position of curved filaments for posterior teeth.

THE ROLL OR ROLLING STROKE METHOD

I. PURPOSES AND INDICATIONS

A. Cleaning gingiva and removing plaque, materia alba, and food debris from the teeth without emphasis on gingival sulcus.
   1. Meant for children with relatively healthy gingiva and normal tissue contour when a sulcular technique may seem difficult for the patient to master.
   2. Meant for general cleaning in conjunction with the use of a vibratory technique (Bass, Charters, Stillman).
B. Useful for preparatory instruction (first lesson) for modified Stillman method because the initial brush placement is the same. This can be particularly helpful when there is a question as to how complicated a technique the patient can master and practice.

II. PROCEDURE[5,13]

A. Position the Brush
1. *Filaments.* Direct filaments apically (up for maxillary, down for mandibular teeth).
2. *Place Side of Brush on the Attached Gingiva.* The filaments are directed apically. When the plastic portion of the brush head is level with the occlusal or incisal plane, generally the brush is at the proper height, as shown in Figure 23-7*A*.

B. Strokes
1. *Press to Flex the Filaments.* The sides of the filaments are pressed lightly against the gingiva. The gingiva will blanch.
2. *Roll the Brush Slowly Over the Teeth.* As the brush is rolled, the wrist is turned slightly.

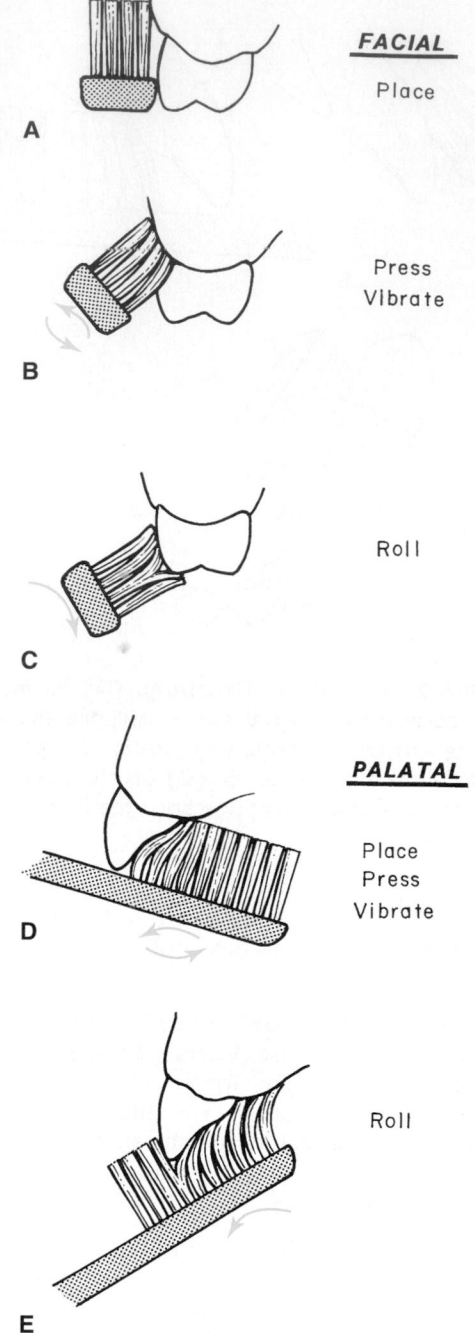

FIGURE 23-7 Modified Stillman Method of Brushing. (A) Initial brush placement with sides of bristles or filaments against the attached gingiva. **(B)** The brush is pressed and angled, then vibrated. **(C)** Vibrating is continued as the brush is rolled slowly over the crown. **(D)** Maxillary anterior lingual placement with the brush applied the long way. **(E)** Vibrating continues as the brush is rolled over the crown and interdental areas. Placement is similar for the lingual surfaces of the mandibular anterior teeth. The roll or rolling stroke brushing method has the same brush positions.

The filaments remain flexed and follow the contours of the teeth, thereby permitting cleaning of the cervical areas. Some filaments may reach interdentally.

C. Replace and Repeat Five Times or More

The entire stroke (steps A and B) is repeated at least five times for each tooth or group of teeth. When the brush is removed and repositioned, the wrist is rotated, the brush is moved away from the teeth, and the cheek is stretched facially with the back of the brush head. Care must be taken not to drag the filament tips over the gingival margin when the brush is returned to the initial position (Figure 23-7A).

D. Overlap Strokes

When moving the brush to an adjacent position, overlap the brush position, as shown in Figure 23-4.

E. Position Brush for Anterior Lingual or Palatal Surfaces

1. Use the brush the long, narrow way.
2. Hook the heel of the brush on the incisal edge (Figure 23-7D).
3. Press (down for maxillary, up for mandibular) until the filaments lie flat against the teeth and gingiva.
4. Press and roll (curve up for mandibular, down for maxillary teeth).
5. Replace and repeat five times for each brush width.

III. PROBLEMS

A. Brushing too high during initial placement can lacerate the alveolar mucosa.
B. Tendency to use quick, sweeping strokes results in no brushing for the cervical third of the tooth because the brush tips pass over rather than into the area; likewise for the interproximal areas.
C. Replacing brush with filament tips directed into the gingiva can produce punctate lesions (page 366).

THE STILLMAN METHOD

As originally described by Stillman,[14] the method was designed for massage and stimulation, as well as for cleaning the cervical areas. The brush ends were placed partly on the gingiva and partly on the cervical areas of the tooth and were directed slightly apically. Pressure was applied to effect a blanching. The handle was given a slight rotary motion, and the brush ends were maintained in position on the tooth surface. After several applications, the brush was moved to the adjacent tooth.

THE MODIFIED STILLMAN METHOD

A modified Stillman, which incorporates a rolling stroke after the vibratory (rotary) phase, frequently is used. The modifications minimize the possibility of gingival trauma and increase the plaque removal effects.[15]

I. PURPOSES AND INDICATIONS

A. Bacterial plaque removal from cervical areas below the height of contour of the crown and from exposed proximal surfaces.
B. General application for cleaning tooth surfaces and massage of the gingiva.

II. PROCEDURE (FIGURE 23-7)

A. Position the Brush

1. *Filaments.* Direct filaments apically (up for maxillary, down for mandibular teeth).
2. *Place Side of Brush on the Attached Gingiva.* The filaments are directed apically. When the plastic portion of the brush head is level with the occlusal or incisal plane, generally the brush is at the proper height, as shown in Figure 23-7A.

B. Strokes

1. *Press to Flex the Filaments.* The sides of the filaments are pressed lightly against the gingiva. The gingiva will blanch.
2. *Angle the Filaments.* Turn the handle by rotating the wrist so that the filaments are directed at an angle of approximately 45° with the long axis of the tooth.
3. *Activate the Brush.* Use a slight rotary motion. Maintain light pressure on the filaments, and keep the tips of the filaments in position with constant contact. Count to 10 slowly as the brush is vibrated by a rotary motion of the handle.
4. *Roll and Vibrate the Brush.* Turn the wrist and work the vibrating brush slowly down over the gingiva and tooth. Make some of the filaments reach interdentally.

C. Replace Brush for Repeat Stroke

Reposition the brush by rotating the wrist. Avoid dragging the filaments back over the free gingival margin by holding the brush out, slightly away from the tooth.

D. Repeat Stroke Five Times or More

The entire stroke (steps A through C) is repeated at least five times for each tooth or group of teeth. When moving the brush to an adjacent position, overlap the brush position, as shown in Figure 23-4.

E. Position Brush for Anterior Lingual and Palatal Surfaces

1. Position the brush the long, narrow way for

the anterior components, as described for the rolling stroke technique and shown in Figure 23-7*D* and *E*.

2. Press and vibrate, roll, and repeat.

III. PROBLEMS

A. Without careful placement and using a brush with end-rounded filaments, tissue laceration can result. Light pressure is needed.

B. Patient may try to move the brush into the rolling stroke too quickly, and the vibratory aspect may be ineffective for plaque removal at the gingival margin.

THE CHARTERS METHOD

During his long productive dental career, Dr. W. J. Charters emphasized the importance of prevention. The interproximal toothbrushing method that he taught had as its objectives cleanliness through removal of the "film and mucin" from the proximal surfaces and gingival massage through mechanical stimulation.

Among his many published papers, Charters described two brush positions, one at a right angle to the long axis of the tooth[16] and another at a 45° angle with the tips of the bristles toward the occlusal plane.[17] The right-angle position might have been intended primarily for patients with interdental periodontal tissue loss, where access permitted the bristles to enter the embrasure.

For either brush position, the instructions were to force the tips into the interproximal area. "With the bristles between the teeth, as much pressure as possible is exerted, giving the brush several slight rotary or vibratory movements. This causes the sides of the bristles to come in contact with the gum margin, producing an ideal massage."[17]

The classic periodontal textbooks[18] have described the Charters method with the bristles directed toward the occlusal plane at a 45° angle with the long axis. This method is described as follows.

I. PURPOSES AND INDICATIONS

A. Loosen debris and bacterial plaque.

B. Massage and stimulate marginal and interdental gingiva.

C. Aid in plaque removal from proximal tooth surfaces when interproximal tissue is missing, for example, following periodontal surgery.

D. Adapt to cervical areas below the height of contour of the crown and to exposed root surfaces.

E. Remove bacterial plaque from abutment teeth and under the gingival border of a fixed partial denture (bridge) or from the undersurface of a sanitary bridge.

F. Cleansing orthodontic appliances (Figure 25-2*C*, page 397).

II. PROCEDURE[17]

A. Apply Rolling Stroke Procedure
Instruct in a basic rolling stroke for general cleaning to be accomplished first.

B. Position the Brush

1. *Filaments.* Hold brush (outside the oral cavity) with filaments directed toward the occlusal or incisal plane of the teeth that will be brushed. The tips are pointed down for application to the maxillary and pointed up for application to the mandibular arch. Insert the brush held in the direction it will be used.

2. *Place the Brush.* Place the sides of the filaments against the enamel with the brush tips toward the occlusal or incisal plane.

3. *Angle the Filaments.* Angle at approximately 45° to the occlusal or incisal plane. Slide the brush to a position at the junction of the free gingival margin and the tooth surface (Figure 23-8*B*). Note contrast with position for the Stillman method (Figure 23-8*A*).

C. Strokes

1. *Press Lightly.* Press lightly to flex the filaments and force the tips between the teeth. The sides of the filaments are pressed against the gingival margin.

2. *Vibrate the Brush.* Vibrate gently but firmly, keeping the tips of the filaments in contact. Count to 10 slowly as the brush is vibrated by a rotary motion of the handle.

D. Reposition the Brush and Repeat
Repeat steps B and C, as described, several times in each position around the dental arches.

E. Overlap Strokes
When moving the brush to an adjacent position, overlap the brush position, as shown in Figure 23-4.

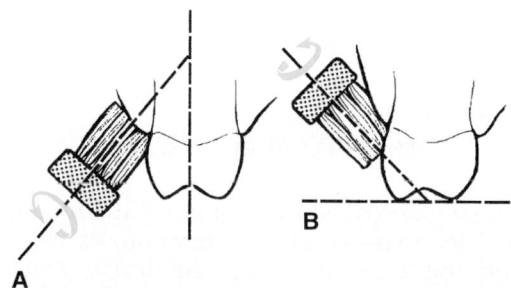

■ **FIGURE 23-8 Charters and Stillman Methods Compared. (A)** Stillman. The brush is angled at approximately 45° to the long axis of the tooth. **(B)** Charters. The brush is angled at approximately 45° to the occlusal plane, with brush tips directed toward the occlusal or incisal surfaces.

F. Position Brush for Anterior Lingual and Palatal Surfaces

Because the Charters brush position is difficult to accomplish on the lingual surfaces, a modified Stillman technique is frequently advised. When the Charters method is preferred, the positions are as follows:

1. *Posterior*
   a. With brush tips pointed toward the occlusal surfaces, extend the brush handle across the incisal edge of the canine of the side opposite that to be brushed.
   b. Place the sides of the toe-end filaments against the distal surface of the most posterior tooth and subsequently at each embrasure.
   c. Press and vibrate.
2. *Anterior*
   a. With brush handle parallel with the long axis of the tooth, place the sides of the toe-end filaments over the interproximal embrasure.
   b. Press and vibrate.

G. Application of Brush for Fixed Partial Denture

When placing the brush, check that the filament tips are directed under the gingival border of the pontic.

III. PROBLEMS

A. Brush ends do not engage the gingival sulcus to remove subgingival bacterial accumulations.
B. In some areas, the correct brush placement is limited or impossible; therefore, modifications become necessary, consequently adding to the complexity of the procedure.
C. Requirements in digital dexterity are high.

OTHER TOOTHBRUSHING METHODS

The rolling stroke, modified Stillman, and Bass are probably the methods most used for patient instruction either directly or as guidelines with variations. Other methods that have been used are included here. The technique and intent of some of the methods overlap. Assessment prior to special instruction may reveal that a mixture of techniques may be in use by a patient.

I. CIRCULAR: THE FONES METHOD

Many patients, especially schoolchildren, probably received instruction in this method because it was advocated by Fones, who founded the first course for dental hygienists. He described the technique in the first dental hygiene text, which was used for many years by dental hygiene students throughout the United States.

Although now considered possibly detrimental for adults, particularly when used by a vigorous brusher, this method may be recommended as an easy-to-learn first technique for young children. A soft brush with 0.006- to 0.008-inch filament diameter is selected. In abbreviated form, the technique described by Dr. Fones includes the following:[19]

A. With the teeth closed, place the brush inside the cheek with the brush tips lightly contacting the gingiva over the last maxillary molar.
B. Use a fast, wide, circular motion that sweeps from the maxillary gingiva to the mandibular gingiva with very little pressure (Figure 23-9).
C. Bring anterior teeth in edge-to-edge contact, and hold lip out when necessary to make the continuous circular strokes.
D. Lingual and palatal tooth surfaces require an in-and-out stroke. Brush sweeps across palate on the maxillary arch and back and forth to the molars on the mandibular arch.

II. VERTICAL: LEONARD METHOD

As described by Hirschfeld,[20] the up-and-down stroke was employed when teeth were cleaned with a primitive crude twig toothbrush. The true vertical stroke passes from the gingiva over the maxillary teeth to the gingiva over the mandibular teeth, with a vigorous sweeping motion.

Leonard described and advocated a vertical stroke in which maxillary and mandibular teeth were brushed separately. Paraphrased, his method is described as follows:[21]

A. With the teeth edge-to-edge, place the brush with the filaments against the teeth at right angles to the long axes of the teeth.
B. Brush vigorously, without great pressure, with a stroke that is mostly up and down on the tooth surfaces, with just a slight rotation

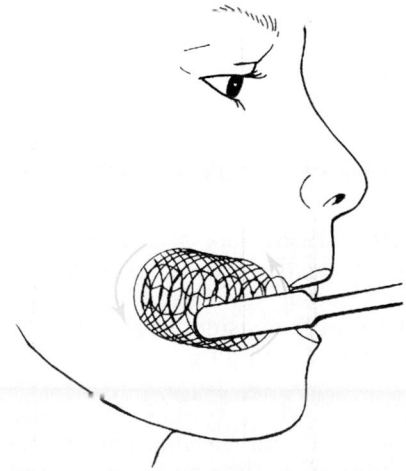

☐ **FIGURE 23-9 Fones Method of Brushing.** With the teeth closed, a circular motion extends from the maxillary gingiva to the mandibular gingiva using a light pressure.

or circular movement after striking the gingival margin with force.

C. Use enough pressure to force the filaments into the embrasures, but not enough to damage the brush.

D. The upper and lower teeth are not brushed in the same series of strokes. The teeth are placed edge-to-edge to keep the brush from slipping over the occlusal or incisal surfaces.

III. HORIZONTAL

Horizontal or crosswise brushing is generally recognized as detrimental. An unlimited sweep with a horizontal scrubbing motion bears pressure on teeth that are most facially inclined or prominent. With the use of an abrasive dentifrice, such brushing may produce tooth abrasion. Because the interdental areas are not touched by this method, bacterial plaque can remain undisturbed on proximal surfaces.

IV. PHYSIOLOGIC: SMITH'S METHOD

The physiologic method was described by Smith[22] and advocated later by Bell.[23] It was based on the principle that the toothbrush should follow the same physiologic pathway that food follows when it traverses over the tissues in a "natural" masticating act.

A soft brush with "small tufts of fine bristles arranged in four parallel rows and trimmed to an even length" was used in a brushing stroke directed down over the lower teeth onto the gingiva and upward over the teeth for the maxillary. Smith also suggested a few gentle horizontal strokes to clean the portion of the sulci directly over the bifurcations of the roots.

V. SCRUB-BRUSH

A scrub-brush procedure consists of vigorously combined horizontal, vertical, and circular strokes, with some vibratory motions for certain areas. Without caution, vigorous scrubbing can encourage gingival recession and, with a dentifrice of sufficient abrasiveness, can create areas of tooth abrasion.

POWER-ASSISTED TOOTHBRUSHES

Power-assisted brushes are also known as automatic, mechanical, or electric brushes. The American Dental Association Council on Scientific Affairs evaluates and classifies power-assisted brushes for the reduction of bacterial plaque and gingivitis (Figure 24-15, page 389).[24]

Comparisons have been made in research between the power-assisted and the manual brushes to determine the ability of each type to remove plaque, prevent calculus development, and reduce the incidence of gingivitis. Both types have been shown effective when used correctly.

I. DESCRIPTION

A. Motion

The action on different models may be one of the following:

1. Rotational.
2. Counter-rotational.
3. Oscillating counter-rotational.

B. Power Source

1. *Direct.* Cord from electrical outlet connects directly to the toothbrush handle.
2. *Replaceable Batteries.* Disadvantage in the nuisance and cost of repeatedly replacing or recharging batteries; also, as the batteries lose their power, the brush is slowed. Corrosion may be a problem if water gets into the case.
3. *Rechargeable.* The instrument is placed into a stand that contains the recharger and is connected to the electrical outlet. A few models have a recharger built into the handle.
4. *Switches.* A few models require that the push button be held down during operation. This requirement may present difficulties for some patients, such as small children or persons with certain types of disabilities.

C. Speeds

Speeds vary from low to high among the different models. Some have the speed coordinated with the filament texture. The number of strokes per minute varies from, for example, as low as 1000 cycles per minute for a replaceable battery type to about 3600 oscillations per minute for an arcuate model. The rechargeable battery types operate at approximately 2000 complete strokes per minute.

II. PURPOSES AND INDICATIONS

A. General Application

Power-assisted brushes have been developed to facilitate mechanical removal of bacterial plaque and food debris from the teeth and the gingiva.

All the general objectives that apply to the use of manual brushes can be applied to power-assisted brushes. They may be especially helpful for people who lack the manual dexterity needed to handle a manual brush successfully.

B. Special Dental Treatment

With instruction and supervision, a power-assisted brush recommended by a dental professional may be of special benefit for a patient with plaque-retentive areas or devices.

1. Those who wear orthodontic appliances (pages 395 to 397).
2. Those undergoing complex restorative and prosthodontic treatment (pages 411 to 415).
3. Those with dental implants (pages 419 to 422).

C. Patients With Disabilities

The thick handles of power-assisted brushes have been shown to be easily handled and manipulated by patients with certain disabilities, especially when grasping is difficult to accomplish (pages 749 to 751).

D. Patients Unable to Brush

A power-assisted brush may be readily handled by a parent or caregiver.

III. INSTRUCTION

With a manual brush, an individual must learn to apply the brush tips in certain ways so that each surface of each tooth can be reached, slight pressure can be applied for a thorough brushing effect, and the stroke can be repeated a number of times. With a power-assisted brush, the action is built-in. The only muscle training required is turning the handle to apply the brush to each surface of each tooth and holding it on each surface for a reasonable length of time in a correct position.

IV. METHODS FOR USE

The general suggestions presented here are basic and, as with all brushing techniques, need adaptations for an individual mouth. Familiarity with the instructions provided by the manufacturers of the various power-assisted brushes is a prerequisite.

A. Select brush with soft end-rounded filaments.
B. Select dentifrice with minimum abrasivity. The extra strokes made by a power-assisted brush can increase the effects of abrasion to the tooth surface.
C. Place a small amount of dentifrice on the brush and spread the dentifrice over the teeth to prevent splashing when the power is turned on.
D. Any of the brushing methods previously described in this chapter can be applied for use with a power-assisted brush.
E. Vary the brush position for each tooth surface. Brush each tooth and surrounding gingiva separately.
   1. Apply the brush for sulcular brushing to the distal, facial, and mesial surfaces of each tooth as the brush is moved from the most posterior teeth toward the anterior, quadrant by quadrant.
   2. Turn the brush to reach proximal areas.
   3. Angulate for access to surfaces of rotated, crowded, or otherwise displaced teeth.
   4. Retract lip with fingers of other hand to give access to and visibility of anterior facial surfaces, particularly including prominent canines.
   5. Modify brush positions for application to proximal surfaces when interdental papillae are missing. Brush head may be positioned parallel with the long axis and inserted vertically.
F. Make strokes slowly, with a slight steady pressure. Pressure should not be great enough at any time to bend the filaments.
G. Precautions
   1. Synthetic restorations should be avoided or treated without pressure because they can wear down under repeated application of the fast-moving filaments with dentifrice.
   2. Avoid pressure with abrasive dentifrice over exposed cementum or dentin.

SUPPLEMENTAL BRUSHING

I. PROBLEM AREAS

Each surface of each tooth must be brushed. Initial instruction necessarily may be limited to a basic procedure, particularly when it varies from the patient's present procedures.

At succeeding lessons, the special hard-to-get areas are shown to the patient. Suggestions are made and demonstrated for brush adaptation for areas that were missed. Methods for cleaning the interdental areas and fixed and removable prostheses are described in Chapters 24 and 25.

Attention in teaching should be given to the following:

A. Facially displaced teeth, especially canines and premolars, where the zone of attached gingiva on the facial may be minimal and where toothbrush abrasion frequently occurs.
B. Inclined teeth, for example, lingual surfaces of mandibular molars that are inclined lingually.
C. Exposed root surfaces; cemental and dentinal surfaces.
D. Overlapped teeth or wide embrasures, which require use of vertical brush position (Figure 23-10).
E. Surfaces of teeth next to edentulous areas (Figure 24-6, page 377).
F. Exposed furcation areas (Figure 24-10, page 379).
G. Right canine and lateral incisor, both maxillary and mandibular, which are commonly missed by right-handed brushers; the opposite is true for left-handed brushers.
H. Distal surfaces of most posterior teeth (Figure 23-11). At best, the brush may reach only the distal line angles. Supplementation with dental floss, yarn, or tufted dental floss is needed for the distal surface (page 374 [Figure 24-1G] and page 376 [Figure 24-4C]).

II. OCCLUSAL BRUSHING

A. Objectives

1. Loosen plaque microorganisms packed in pits and fissures.

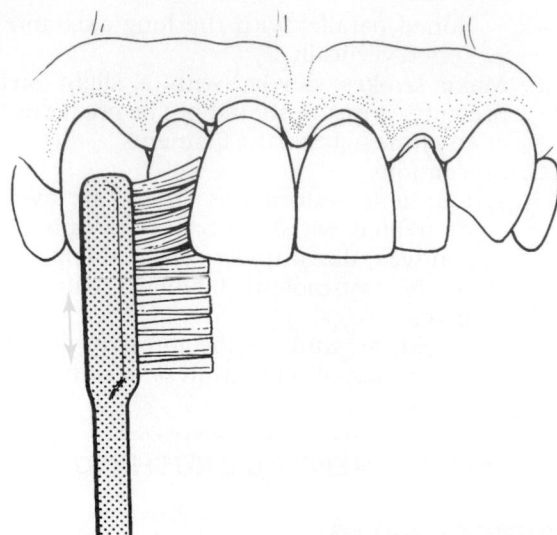

FIGURE 23-10 Brush in Vertical Position. For overlapped teeth, open interproximal areas, and selected areas of recession, the bacterial plaque on proximal tooth surfaces can be conveniently removed with the brush held in a vertical position.

2. Remove plaque deposits from occlusal surfaces of teeth out of occlusion or not used during mastication.
3. Remove plaque from the margins of restorations.
4. Clean pits and fissures to prepare for sealants.

B. Procedure

1. Place brush on occlusal surfaces of molar teeth with filament tips pointed into the occlusal pits at a right angle. The handle should be parallel with the occlusal surface. The toe of the brush should cover the distal grooves of the most posterior tooth (Figure 23-12A).
2. Two acceptable strokes are suggested.
   a. Vibrate the brush in a slight circular movement while maintaining the fila-

ment tips on the occlusal surface throughout a count of 10. Press moderately so filaments do not bend but go straight into the pits and fissures (Figure 23-12C).
   b. Force the filaments against the occlusal surface with sharp, quick strokes; lift the brush off each time to dislodge debris; repeat about 10 times.
3. Move brush to premolar area, overlapping previous brush position.

C. Precaution

Long scrubbing strokes from anterior to posterior on an occlusal surface may contact only the prominent parts of the cusps (Figure 23-12B and C).

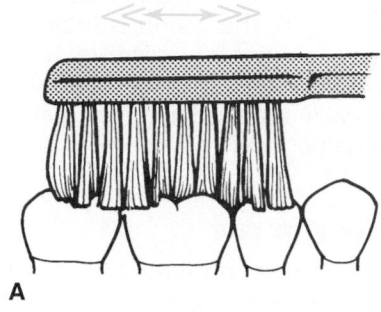

A

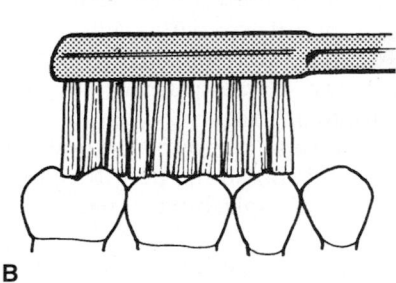

B

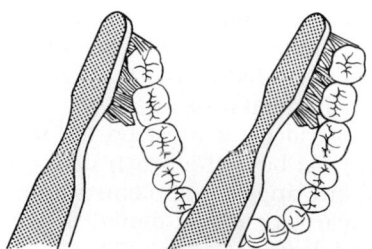

FIGURE 23-11 Brushing Problems. Brush placement to remove plaque from the distal surfaces of the most posterior teeth. The distobuccal surface is approached by stretching the cheek; the distolingual surface is approached by directing the brush across from the canine of the opposite side.

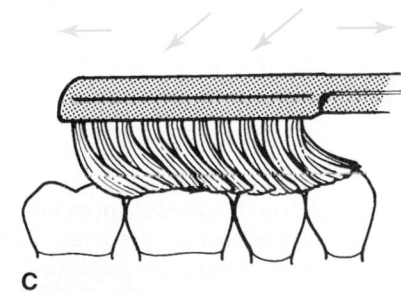

C

FIGURE 23-12 Occlusal Brushing. (A) Vibrating brush with light pressure while maintaining filament tips on the occlusal surface permits tips to work their way into pits and fissures. **(B)** Long horizontal strokes contact only the cusp tips. **(C)** Excess pressure curves the filaments so that tips cannot get into the pits and fissures.

III. TONGUE CLEANING

Total mouth cleanliness includes tongue care.

A. Microorganisms of the Tongue

1. Main foci for oral microorganisms are
   a. Dorsum of tongue.
   b. Gingival sulci and pockets.
   c. Bacterial plaque on all teeth.
2. Microorganisms in saliva are principally from the tongue.
3. The microflora of the tongue is not constant, but changes frequently.[25]

B. Effects of Cleaning the Tongue

1. Retards bacterial plaque formation and total plaque accumulation.
2. Reduces number of microorganisms.
3. Reduces potential for halitosis (pages 346 to 347).
4. Contributes to overall cleanliness.

C. Anatomic Features of Tongue Conducive to Debris Retention

1. *Surface Papillae.* Numerous filiform papillae extend as minute projections, whereas fungiform papillae are not as high and create elevations and depressions that entrap debris and microorganisms (Figure 11-2, page 188).
2. *Fissured Tongue.* Fissures may be several millimeters deep and retain debris.

D. Brushing Procedure

1. Hold the brush handle at a right angle to the midline of the tongue and direct the brush tips toward the throat.
2. With the tongue extruded, the sides of the filaments are placed on the posterior part of the tongue surface.
3. With light pressure, draw the brush forward and over the tip of the tongue. Repeat three or four times. Do not scrub the papillae.

E. Tongue Scraper

Tongue cleaners or scrapers may be made of plastic, stainless steel, or other flexible metal. They are curved and wide enough to fit over the tongue surface without hitting the teeth. Some are made with a single handle, whereas others have two ends to hold, as shown in Figure 23-13.

1. *Purpose.* By removing debris and microorganisms, the patient can expect tongue scraping to contribute to overall mouth cleanliness, reduce the numbers of bacteria available for plaque formation, and lessen mouth odors. The procedure can be especially helpful for the patient who has xerostomia, a coated tongue, deep fissures, or who smokes.
2. *Procedure.* Place the arch toward the posterior of the dorsal surface (Figure 23-13). Press with a light but firm stroke, and pull for-

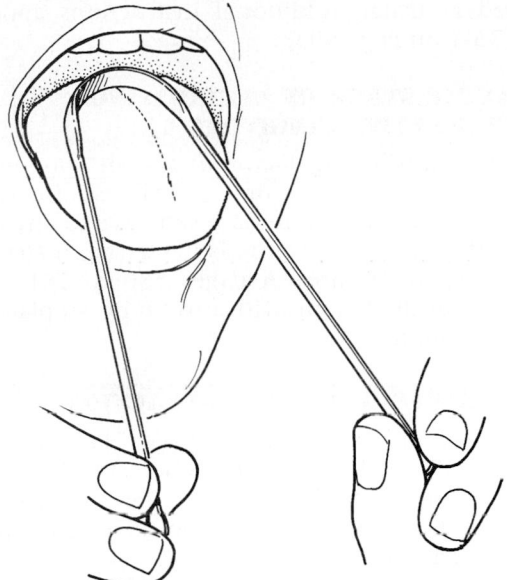

FIGURE 23-13 Tongue Scraper. A variety of plastic or flexible metal scrapers are available to clean the dorsal surface of the tongue. The scraper is pressed over the tongue with a light but firm stroke.

ward. Repeat several times, covering the entire surface of the tongue. Wash the tongue scraper under running water.

TOOTHBRUSHING FOR SPECIAL CONDITIONS

Even when an unusual oral condition develops, a patient must be encouraged to brush wherever possible to reduce the possibility of infection and promote healing. Prolonged omission of techniques of plaque removal is never indicated. Examples of conditions that may require a temporary departure from personal care routines follow.

I. ACUTE ORAL INFLAMMATORY OR TRAUMATIC LESIONS

When an acute oral condition precludes normal brushing, the patient should be instructed to brush all areas of the mouth that are not affected and to resume regular plaque control measures on the affected area as soon as possible. Rinsing with a warm, mild saline solution can encourage healing and debris removal.

II. FOLLOWING PERIODONTAL SURGERY

Patients must receive specific instructions concerning brushing while sutures and/or a dressing are in place. Because direct, vigorous brushing of a periodontal dressing could cause its displacement, brushing of the occlusal surfaces and light strokes over the dressing may be advised. Other teeth and gingiva should be brushed as usual. Additional instructions appear in Table 36-1 on page 593.

III. ACUTE STAGE OF NECROTIZING ULCERATIVE GINGIVITIS

A major contributing factor in the development of this disease is a lack of oral cleanliness. During the acute stage, the oral tissues are sensitive to any touch, and toothbrushing therefore is neglected. Instructions for these patients are on pages 580 to 581. A soft brush is indicated along with careful brush placement to avoid trauma.

IV. FOLLOWING DENTAL EXTRACTION

Instructions may be found on page 711 and include brushing all teeth and gingiva except the surgical wound area. Teeth adjacent to the extraction site need cleaning as soon as possible to reduce bacterial collections and to promote healing.

V. FOLLOWING DENTAL RESTORATIONS

Patients tend to avoid brushing a new crown, newly placed fixed partial denture, or other prosthesis. Specific instructions should be given at the time of insertion.

TOOTHBRUSH TRAUMA: THE GINGIVA

Trauma to the gingiva occurs most frequently on the facial surfaces over teeth prominent in the dental arch. The lesions frequently are found over canines and premolars.

Lesions are especially apt to occur after initial instruction in use of a new method of brushing. The patient may be overzealous or may have misunderstood correct brush placement. Examination of a patient's gingiva within a few days to a week after instruction can be important.

I. ACUTE ALTERATIONS

Acute lesions are usually lacerations or ulcerations. The severity of the lesion may depend on the frequency and extent of brushing, as well as on the stiffness of the filaments and the force applied.

A. Appearance
1. Scuffed epithelial surface with denuded underlying connective tissue.
2. Punctate lesions that appear as red pinpoint spots.
3. Diffuse redness and denuded attached gingiva.

B. Precipitating Factors
1. Horizontal or vertical scrub toothbrushing method.
2. Excess pressure applied using firm palm grasp of handle.[26]
3. Use of abrasive dentifrice.[27]

4. Overvigorous placement and application of the toothbrush.
5. Penetration of gingiva by filament ends.
6. Use of toothbrush with frayed, broken bristles or filaments.
7. Application of filaments beyond attached gingiva.

II. CHRONIC ALTERATIONS

A. Changes in Gingival Contour
1. *Appearance*
   a. Rolled, bulbous, hard, firm marginal gingiva, in "piled up" or festoon shape ("McCall's festoon," Figure 11-10*D*, page 196).
   b. Gingival cleft, which is a narrow groove or slit that extends from the crest of the gingiva to the attached gingiva ("Stillman's cleft," Figure 11-11, page 197).
2. *Location*
   a. Usually appear only on the facial gingiva, because of the vigor with which toothbrush is used.
   b. Frequently inversely related to the right- or left-handedness of the patient.
   c. Areas most often involved are around canines or teeth in labioversion or buccoversion.

B. Gingival Recession
1. *Appearance.* Margin has moved apically and cementum is exposed.
2. *Predisposing Factors*
   a. Anatomic: Narrow band of attached gingiva and thin facial bone over teeth malposed in labioversion.
   b. Toothbrushing habits: Vigorous pressured brushing with abrasive dentifrice and worn brush.

C. Suggested Corrective Measures
1. Recommend use of a soft toothbrush with end-rounded filaments.
2. Correct the patient's toothbrushing method; demonstrate a toothbrushing method better suited to the oral condition.
3. Temporary cessation of brushing the traumatized area may be needed. An antimicrobial rinse may assist in the healing process.

TOOTHBRUSH TRAUMA: DENTAL ABRASION

I. APPEARANCE

Wedge-shaped indentations with smooth, shiny surfaces (Figure 14-8, page 245).

Abrasion is the loss of tooth substance produced by mechanical wear other than that caused by mastication. Abrasion also may be defined as the pathologic wearing away of tooth substance through some abnormal mechanical process, in contrast with erosion that generally involves a chemical process.

II. LOCATION OF ABRADED AREAS

A. Primarily on facial surfaces, especially of canines, premolars, and sometimes first molars, or, on any tooth in buccoversion or labioversion, those most available to the pressure of the toothbrush. The canines are susceptible because of their prominence on the curvature of the dental arches.
B. Most abraded areas are on the cervical areas of exposed root surfaces, but occasionally they may occur on the enamel. When adjacent teeth are involved, the lesions appear in line with each other.

III. CONTRIBUTING FACTORS

A. Hard toothbrush with abrasive agent in the dentifrice.
B. Horizontal brushing with excessive pressure.
C. Form of filament ends: Abrasion is less frequent when filaments are end-rounded.
D. Prominence of the tooth surface labially or buccally.

IV. CORRECTIVE MEASURES

A. Explain the problem to the patient to ensure full cooperation.
B. Advise use of a specific brush with end-rounded filaments.
C. Change or correct the toothbrushing procedure.
D. Recommend a less abrasive dentifrice.
E. Use a smaller amount of dentifrice.
   1. Start brushing in the area of the dentition where the most plaque and calculus are noted at a maintenance appointment.
   2. Avoid applying the dentifrice vigorously to the same tooth surfaces.

CARE OF TOOTHBRUSHES

When discussing the type and features of the brush selected for an individual patient, the number of brushes needed and the frequency of replacement should be included. Perhaps an ideal time to teach cleaning and daily care of brushes would be after a practice session when the brush has to be washed and cleaned for storage at the dental office.

The condition of a brush depends on many factors, including the amount and manner of use, the type of care, and the quality of the brush at the start.

I. SUPPLY OF BRUSHES

A. Advise at least two brushes for home use and a third in a portable container for use at work, school, or travel.

B. Purchase of brushes should be staggered so that all brushes are not new at the same time and, more important, so that they are all not old at the same time, thereby resulting in less than optimum maintenance of the gingival condition.

II. BRUSH REPLACEMENT

A. Frequent replacement recommended; at least every 2 to 3 months.
B. Brushes should be replaced before filaments become splayed, frayed, or lose resiliency. Duration of a brush is influenced by many factors, including frequency and method of use.
C. Brush contamination occurs with use.[28,29] Contamination has the potential for causing systemic or localized infection.
D. Patients who are debilitated, immunosuppressed, have a known infection, or are about to undergo surgery for any reason can be advised to disinfect their brushes or use disposable brushes.[28]

III. CLEANING TOOTHBRUSHES

A. Clean thoroughly after each use.
B. Hold brush head under strong stream of warm water from faucet to force particles, dentifrice, and bacteria from between the filaments.
C. Tap the handle on edge of sink to remove remaining particles.
D. Use one toothbrush to clean another brush; filaments can be worked between those of the other brush to remove resistant debris.
E. Rinse completely and tap out excess water.

IV. BRUSH STORAGE

A. Brushes should be kept in open air with head in an upright position, apart from contact with other brushes, particularly those of another person.
B. Portable brush container should have sufficient holes to give air temporarily until the brush can be completely exposed for drying. A closed container encourages bacterial growth.

REFERENCES

1. **Hirschfeld,** I.: *The Toothbrush: Its Use and Abuse.* Brooklyn, NY, Dental Items of Interest, 1939, pp. 1–27.
2. **Kimery,** M.J. and Stallard, R.E.: The Evolutionary Development and Contemporary Utilization of Various Oral Hygiene Procedures, *Periodont Abstr, 16,* 90, September, 1968.
3. **McCauley,** H.B.: Toothbrushes, Toothbrush Materials and Design, *J. Am. Dent. Assoc., 33,* 283, March 1, 1946.
4. **Weinberger,** B.W.: *An Introduction to the History of Dentistry.* St. Louis, Mosby, 1948, pp. 43, 140–144.
5. **American Academy of Periodontology,** Committee Report: The Tooth Brush and Methods of Cleaning the Teeth, *Dent. Items Interest, 42,* 193, March, 1920.

6. **Alexander,** J.F.: Toothbrushes and Toothbrushing, in Menaker, L., ed.: *The Biologic Basis of Dental Caries.* Hagerstown, MD, Harper & Row, 1980, pp. 482–496.
7. **Koecker,** L.: *Principles of Dental Surgery, Exhibiting a New Method of Treating the Diseases of the Teeth and Gums.* Baltimore, MD, American Society of Dental Surgeons, 1842, Chapter III, pp. 155–156.
8. **American Dental Association,** Council on Dental Therapeutics: *Accepted Dental Therapeutics,* 40th ed. Chicago, American Dental Association, 1984, pp. 386–387.
9. **Massassati,** A. and Frank, R.M.: Scanning Electron Microscopy of Unused and Used Manual Toothbrushes, *J. Clin. Periodontol., 9,* 148, March, 1982.
10. **Breitenmoser,** J., Mörmann, W., and Mühlemann, H.R.: Damaging Effects of Toothbrush Bristle End Form on Gingiva, *J. Periodontol., 50,* 212, April, 1979.
11. **Silverstone,** L.M. and Featherstone, M.J.: A Scanning Electron Microscope Study of the End Rounding of Bristles in Eight Toothbrush Types, *Quintessence Int., 19,* 3, February, 1988.
12. **Bass,** C.C.: An Effective Method of Personal Oral Hygiene, *J. Louisiana State Med. Soc., 106,* 100, March, 1954.
13. **Hard,** D.: Oral Prophylaxis, in Bunting, R.W.: *Oral Hygiene,* 3rd ed. Philadelphia, Lea & Febiger, 1957, pp. 280–283.
14. **Stillman,** P.R.: A Philosophy of the Treatment of Periodontal Disease, *Dent. Digest, 38,* 315, September, 1932.
15. **Hirschfeld:** op. cit., p. 380.
16. **Charters,** W.J.: Home Care of the Mouth. I. Proper Home Care of the Mouth, *J. Periodontol., 19,* 136, October, 1948.
17. **Charters,** W.J.: Eliminating Mouth Infections with the Toothbrush and Other Stimulating Instruments, *Dent. Digest, 38,* 130, April, 1932.
18. **Miller,** S.C.: *Textbook of Periodontia,* 3rd ed. Philadelphia, The Blakiston Co., 1950, pp. 327–328.
19. **Fones,** A.C., ed.: *Mouth Hygiene,* 4th ed. Philadelphia, Lea & Febiger, 1934, pp. 299–306.
20. **Hirschfeld:** op. cit., pp. 369–371.
21. **Leonard,** H.J.: Conservative Treatment of Periodontoclasia, *J. Am. Dent. Assoc., 26,* 1308, August, 1939.
22. **Smith,** T.S.: Anatomic and Physiologic Conditions Governing the Use of the Toothbrush, *J. Am. Dent. Assoc., 27,* 874, June, 1940.
23. **Bell,** D.G.: Home Care of the Mouth. III. Teaching Home Care to the Patient, *J. Periodontol., 19,* 140, October, 1948.
24. **American Dental Association,** Council on Scientific Affairs: *Products of Excellence. ADA Seal Program.* Chicago, American Dental Association, Revised annually.
25. **Van der Weijden,** G.A. and Van der Velden, U.: Fluctuation of the Microbiota of the Tongue in Humans, *J. Clin. Periodontol., 18,* 26, January, 1991.
26. **Niemi,** M.-L., Ainamo, J., and Etemadzadeh, H.: The Effect of Toothbrush Grip on Gingival Abrasion and Plaque Removal During Toothbrushing, *J. Clin. Periodontol., 14,* 19, January, 1987.
27. **Niemi,** M.-L., Sandholm, L., and Ainamo, J.: Frequency of Gingival Lesions After Standardized Brushing as Related to Stiffness of Toothbrush and Abrasiveness of Dentifrice, *J. Clin. Periodontol., 11,* 254, April, 1984.
28. **Glass,** R.T.: The Infected Toothbrush, the Infected Denture, and Transmission of Disease: A Review, *Compend. Cont. Educ. Dent., 13,* 592, July, 1992.
29. **Müller,** H.-P., Lange, D.E., and Müller, R.F.: Actinobacillus actinomycetemcomitans Contamination of Toothbrushes from Patients Harbouring the Organism, *J. Clin. Periodontol., 16,* 388, July, 1989.

Dean, D.H., Beeson, L.D., Cannon, D.F., and Plunkett, C.B.: Condition of Toothbrushes in Use: Correlation with Behavioral and Socio-economic Factors, *Clin. Prev. Dent., 14,* 14, January/February, 1992.
Kieser, J. and Groeneveld, H.: A Clinical Evaluation of a Novel Toothbrush Design, *J. Clin. Periodontol., 24,* 419, June, 1997.
Menon, M.V. and Coykendall, A.L.: Effect of Tongue Scraping, *J. Dent. Res., 73,* 1492, September, 1994.
Raitio, M., Möttönen, M., and Uhari, M.: Toothbrushing and the Occurrence of Salivary Mutans streptococci in Children at Day Care Centers, *Caries Res., 29,* 280, July–August, 1995.
Salman, R.A.: Roentgeno-oddities. Toothbrush Ingestion, *Oral Surg. Oral Med. Oral Pathol., 66,* 386, September, 1988.
Van der Weijden, G.A., Timmerman, M.F., Reijerse, E., Snoek, C.M., and van der Velden, U.: Toothbrushing Force in Relation to Plaque Removal, *J. Clin. Periodontol., 23,* 724, August, 1996.
Waerhaug, J: Effect of Toothbrushing on Subgingival Plaque Formation, *J. Periodontol., 52,* 30, January, 1981.

Toothbrush Trials

Agerholm, D.M.: A Clinical Trial to Evaluate Plaque Removal with a Double-headed Toothbrush, *Br. Dent. J., 170,* 411, June 8, 1991.
Beatty, C.F., Fallon, P.A., and Marshall, D.D.: Comparative Analysis of the Plaque Removal Ability of .007 and .008 Toothbrush Bristles, *Clin. Prev. Dent., 12,* 22, December, 1990.
Davies, A.L., Rooney, J.C., Constable, G.M., and Lamb, D.J.: The Effect of Variations in Toothbrush Design on Dental Plaque Scores, *Clin. Prev. Dent., 10,* 3, May–June, 1988.
Dean, D.H.: Toothbrushes with Graduated Wear: Correlation With *In Vitro* Cleansing Performance, *Clin. Prev. Dent., 13,* 25, July–August, 1991.
Gibson, M.T., Joyston-Bechal, S., and Smales, F.C.: Clinical Evaluation of Plaque Removal with a Double-headed Toothbrush, *J. Clin. Periodontol., 15,* 94, February, 1988.
Mandel, I.D.: The Plaque Fighters: Choosing a Weapon, *J. Am. Dent. Assoc., 124,* 71, April, 1993.
Park, K.K., Matis, B.A., and Christen, A.G.: Choosing an Effective Toothbrush, *Clin. Prev. Dent., 7,* 5, July–August, 1985.
Stabbe, K.A., Tishk, M.N., Overman, P.R., and Love, J.W.: A Comparison of Plaque Reaccumulation and Patient Acceptance Using a Conventional Toothbrush and a Newly Designed Toothbrush, *Clin. Prev. Dent., 10,* 10, September–October, 1988.
Thevissen, E., Quirynen, M., and van Steenberghe, D.: Plaque Removing Effect of a Convex-shaped Brush Compared with a Conventional Flat Brush, *J. Periodontol., 58,* 861, December, 1987.
Volpe, A.R., Emling, R.C., and Yankell, S.L.: The Toothbrush: A New Dimension in Design, Engineering, and Clinical Evaluation, *J. Clin. Dent., 3,* C1–C33, Supplement C, 1992.

Power-Assisted Brushes

Ainamo, J., Xie, Q., Ainamo, A., and Kallio, P.: Assessment of the Effect of an Oscillating/Rotating Electric Toothbrush on Oral Health. A 12-month Longitudinal Study, *J. Clin. Periodontol., 24,* 28, January, 1997.
Bader, H.I.: Review of Currently Available Battery-operated Toothbrushes, *Compend. Cont. Educ. Dent., 13,* 1162, December, 1992.
Barnes, C.M.: Powered Toothbrushes: Evidence Warrants Wider Recommendations, *Access, 12,* 56, May–June, 1998.
Boyd, R.L.: Clinical and Laboratory Evaluation of Powered Electric Toothbrushes: Review of the Literature, *J. Clin. Dent., 8,* 67, Number 3, 1997.
Khambay, B.S. and Walmsley, A.D.: An *in vitro* Evaluation of Electric Toothbrushes, *Quintessence Int., 26,* 841, December, 1995.
Khocht, A., Spindel, L., and Person, P.: A Comparative Clinical Study of the Safety and Efficacy of Three Toothbrushes, *J. Periodontol., 63,* 603, July, 1992.
O'Beirne, G., Johnson, R.H., Persson, G.R., and Spektor, M.D.: Efficacy of a Sonic Toothbrush on Inflammation and Probing Depth in Adult Periodontitis, *J. Periodontol., 67,* 900, September, 1996.
Shibly, O., Schifferle, R.E., Ciancio, S.G., Tarakji, M., and

SUGGESTED READINGS

Claydon, N. and Addy, M.: Comparative Single-use Plaque Removal by Toothbrushes of Different Designs, *J. Clin. Periodontol., 23,* 1112, December, 1996.
Daly, C.G., Chapple, C.C., and Cameron, A.C.: Effect of Toothbrush Wear on Plaque Control, *J. Clin. Periodontol., 23,* 45, January, 1996.

Mather, M.L.: A Clinical Comparison of 2 Electric Toothbrush Designs, *J. Clin. Periodontol., 24*, 260, April, 1997.

Shultz, P.H., Killoy, W.J., Rapley, J.W., and Shultz, R.E.: A Clinical Comparison of Subgingival and Interproximal Plaque Removal Effectiveness: Electric vs. Manual Toothbrushing, *J. Pract. Hyg., 4*, 31, March/April, 1995.

Silverstone, L.M., Tilliss, T.S.I., Cross-Poline, G.N., Van der Linden, E., Stach, D.J., and Featherstone, M.J.: A Six-week Study Comparing Efficacy of a Rotary Electric Toothbrush with a Conventional Toothbrush, *Clin. Prev. Dent., 14*, 29, March–April, 1992.

Taylor, J.Y., Wood, C.L., Garnick, J.J., and Thompson, W.O.: Removal of Interproximal Subgingival Plaque by Hand and Automatic Toothbrushes, *J. Periodontol., 66*, 191, March, 1995.

Tritten, C.B. and Armitage, G.C.: Comparison of a Sonic and a Manual Toothbrush for Efficacy in Supragingival Plaque Removal and Reduction of Gingivitis, *J. Clin. Periodontol., 23*, 641, July, 1996.

Chewing Sticks

Eid, M.A., Selim, H.A., and Al-Shammery, A.R.: The Relationship Between Chewing Sticks (Miswak) and Periodontal Health. Part I. Review of the Literature and Profile of the Subjects, *Quintessence Int., 21*, 913, November, 1990.

Eid, M.A., Al-Shammery, A.R., and Selim, H.A.: The Relationship Between Chewing Sticks (Miswak) and Periodontal Health. II. Relationship to Plaque, Gingivitis, Pocket Depth, and Attachment Loss, *Quintessence Int., 21*, 1019, December, 1990.

Gazi, M., Saini, T., Ashri, N., and Lambourne, A.: Miswak Chewing Stick Versus Conventional Toothbrush as an Oral Hygiene Aid, *Clin. Prev. Dent., 12*, 19, October–November, 1990.

van Palenstein Helderman, W.H., Munck, L., Mushendwa, S., and Mrema, F.G.: Cleaning Effectiveness of Chewing Sticks Among Tanzanian Schoolchildren, *J. Clin. Periodontol., 19*, 460, August, 1992.

Trauma From Toothbrushing

Khocht, A., Simon, G., Person, P., and Denepitiya, J.L.: Gingival Recession in Relation to History of Hard Toothbrush Use, *J. Periodontol., 64*, 900, September, 1993.

Nemcovsky, C.E. and Artzi, Z.: Erosion-Abrasion Lesions Revisited, *Compend. Cont. Educ. Dent., 17*, 416, April, 1996.

Pearlman, B.A.: A Mistaken Health Belief Resulting in Gingival Injury: A Case Report, *J. Periodontol., 65*, 284, March, 1994.

Schemehorn, B.R. and Zwart, A.C.: The Dentin Abrasivity Potential of a New Electric Toothbrush, *Am. J. Dent., 9*, S19, Special Issue, July, 1996.

Spieler, E.L.: The Softer Touch, *RDH, 16*, 38, January, 1996.

Toothbrush Contamination

Caudry, S.D., Klitorinos, A., and Chan, E.C.S.: Contaminated Toothbrushes and Their Disinfection, *J. Can. Dent. Assoc., 61*, 511, June, 1995.

Denny, F.W.: Risk of Toothbrushes in the Transmission of Respiratory Infections, *Pediatr. Infect. Dis. J., 10*, 710, September, 1991.

Meier, S., Collier, C., Scaletta, M.G., Stephens, J., Kimbrough, R., and Kettering, J.D.: An *in vitro* Investigation of the Efficacy of CPC for Use in Toothbrush Decontamination, *J. Dent. Hyg., 70*, 161, July–August, 1996.

Interdental Care and Chemotherapy

Traditionally, toothbrushing has been considered to be first in line as the method for cleaning the teeth and removing bacterial plaque for the prevention of gingival and periodontal infections. Toothbrushing cannot accomplish plaque removal for the proximal tooth surfaces and adjacent gingiva to the same degree that it does for the facial, lingual, and palatal aspects. Interdental plaque control, therefore, is essential to complete the patient's self-care program.

Objectives and procedures for devices for proximal bacterial plaque removal are included in this chapter. Key words are defined in Box 24-1. Particular applications are given for care of teeth and soft tissues related to dental prostheses in Chapter 25. In Chapter 26, the necessary adaptations for a mouth with complete rehabilitation and dental implants are described.

When the preventive treatment plan is outlined for an individual, assessment is made of the oral condition, the problem areas, and the overall prognosis for health improvement or maintenance. Measures for interdental plaque control are selected to complement plaque control by toothbrushing.

At first, the simplest procedures are selected for the patient's convenience and ease of learning. The daily oral care regimen also must be kept at a realistic level with respect to the time the patient is able or willing to spend. As the values the patient places on oral health increase over time, and as the preventive maintenance program becomes a priority in the patient's lifelong self-care health goals, a more refined program can be introduced.

THE INTERDENTAL AREA

Normally, the interdental gingiva fills the gingival embrasure and the area beneath the contact area. The removal of bacterial plaque from a normal shallow

---

BOX 24-1 KEY WORDS: Interdental Care and Chemotherapy

Antimicrobial agent: chemical that has a bacteriostatic or bactericidal effect on microbial plaque.

Astringent (ah-strin'jent): a substance that causes contraction or shrinkage and arrests discharges.

Cannula (kan'ū-lah): a tubular instrument placed into a cavity to introduce or drain fluid.

Chemotherapy: treatment of disease by means of chemical substances or pharmaceutical agents.

Col (kawl): the depression in the gingival tissue under a contact area between the lingual (palatal) papilla and the facial papilla.

Embrasure (em-brā-zhur): V-shaped spillway space next to the contact area of adjacent teeth, narrowest at the contact and widening toward the facial, lingual (palatal), and occlusal contacts.

Humectant (hū-mek'tant): substance contained in a product (such as in a dentifrice) to retain moisture and prevent hardening upon exposure to air.

Hydrokinetic activity (hī"drō-kǐ-net'ik): activity relating to motions of fluids or the forces that produce or affect such motions: opposite of hydrostatic.

Hydrostatic (hī"drō-stat'ik): relating to the equilibrium of a liquid and the pressure exerted by the liquid at rest.

Hydrotherapy (hī"drō-ther'ah-pē): the use of forced intermittent or steady stream of water for cleansing or therapeutic purposes.

Interproximal space: the triangular region bounded by the proximal surfaces of contacting teeth and the alveolar bone between the teeth, which forms the base of the triangle; the space is normally filled with the interdental papilla.

Irrigant: substance used for irrigation.

Irrigation (ir"i-gā'shun): flushing of a specific site or area with a stream of fluid; application of a continuous or pulsated stream of fluid to a part of the body for a cleansing or therapeutic purpose.

    Oral irrigation: targeted delivery of water or solution to specific locations within the mouth.

    Supragingival irrigation: the point of delivery of the irrigation is at or coronal to the free gingival margin.

    Subgingival irrigation: intentional irrigation of a gingival crevice or periodontal pocket when the point of delivery is directed under the gingival margin.

Irrigator: a device usually consisting of a reservoir with a flexible delivery tube that uses pressure to flush an area.

Isotonic (ī"sō-ton'ik): having a uniform tonicity or tension; denoting solutions with the same osmotic pressure.

Lavage (lah-vahzh'): a flushing action using large quantities of water or other liquid; also called irrigation.

Substantivity: the ability of an agent to be bound to the pellicle and tooth surface and to be released over an extended period of time with the retention of its potency.

Synergism (sin'er-jizm): process whereby the joint action of separate agents is greater than the sum of their effects taken separately.

Synergistic effect: coordinated action; acting jointly; for example, one drug might enhance the effect of another drug.

sulcus and from the enamel under the proximal gingival tissue usually can be accomplished with dental floss without adding more complicated procedures.

When the interdental papilla is missing or reduced in height, the tooth surfaces are exposed, the shape of the interdental gingiva is changed, and the embrasures are open. A review of the gingival and dental anatomy of the interdental area can give meaning to and clarify the role and purpose of the various devices available for interdental care.

I. GINGIVAL ANATOMY

A. Posterior Teeth

Between adjacent posterior teeth are two papillae, one facial and one lingual or palatal. They are connected by a col, a depressed concave area that follows the shape of the apical border of the contact area (Figure 11-8A, page 192).

B. Anterior Teeth

Between anterior teeth in contact is a single papilla with a pyramidal shape. As shown in Figure 11-8B (page 192), the tip of the papilla may form a small col under the contact area.

C. Epithelium

The epithelium covering a col is usually thin and not keratinized. It is less resistant to bacterial infection than are keratinized surfaces. When inflammation is present in the interdental tissue, the papillae become enlarged with inflammatory cells and fluids, and the col becomes deeper.

The col is in a protected area when the teeth are in alignment and the contact area is normal. The col is generally inaccessible to ordinary toothbrushing. Because of its concave center, the col can harbor microorganisms. Most gingival disease starts in the col areas, and the incidence of gingivitis is greatest in the interdental tissues.[1]

II. PROXIMAL TOOTH SURFACES

With bacterial infection and loss of gingival attachment, the interdental papillae are reduced in height, and the proximal tooth surfaces become exposed. Bacterial plaque can accumulate.

Irregularities of tooth position, such as rotation or overlapping, and deviations related to malocclusion or tooth loss may be present. Such complications prevent easy access for removal of bacterial deposits by the individual. Figure 16-5 on page 272 illustrates this problem.

The root surface morphology of the proximal surfaces is typical for each tooth type. Concavities and grooves are predisposed to bacterial accumulations.[2,3] With advanced periodontitis, furcation areas of maxillary first premolars and maxillary molars open onto the proximal surfaces.

III. SELECTIVE INTERDENTAL PLAQUE REMOVAL

Vibratory and sulcular toothbrushing, such as that performed with the Charters, Stillman, and Bass methods, can be successful to some degree in removing bacterial plaque near the line angles of the facial and lingual or palatal embrasures. The brush may be adapted in a vertical position, as shown in Figure 23-10 on page 364, for additional access. More than a toothbrush is needed, however, for complete plaque and debris removal from the proximal tooth surfaces. With judicious selection and use of the various methods for interdental care, disease control can be accomplished by the motivated patient.

DENTAL FLOSS AND TAPE

The effective use of dental floss contributes to gingival health by removing bacterial plaque[4-7] and reducing interproximal bleeding.[8] Dental floss is most effective when interdental papillae are present and there has not been loss of attachment with root surface exposure.[9] As recession occurs, dental floss may still be used, but greater time, effort, and dexterity are required for complete removal of bacterial plaque from the exposed proximal tooth surfaces.

I. TYPES OF FLOSS

Research has shown no difference in the effectiveness of waxed or unwaxed floss for plaque removal.[4,6,10-12] Plaque removal depends on how floss is applied. For optimal patient compliance, the patient may use a preferred type.[4,13]

A. Materials

1. *Silk.* Historically floss was made of silk fibers loosely twisted together to form a strand and waxed for interproximal cleaning.
2. *Nylon.* Nylon multifilaments, waxed or unwaxed, have been widely used in circular (floss) or flat (tape) form for bacterial plaque removal from proximal tooth surfaces.
3. *Expanded PTFE.* Plastic monofilament polytetrafluoroethylene with wax is used for proximal tooth surface plaque removal.

B. Features of Waxed or Expanded PTFE

1. Smooth surface provided by the wax covering helps to prevent trauma to soft tissue.
2. Slides through contact area with ease.
3. Monofilament type resists breakage or shredding when passed over irregular tooth surface, restoration, or calculus deposit.
4. Wax gives strength and durability during application; shredding or breakage is rare.

C. Unwaxed

1. Thinner floss may be helpful when contact areas are tight; however, forcing the floss through may break the floss.

2. Pressure against a tooth surface spreads the nylon fibers and gives wider surface for plaque removal.
3. Sharper thin edge requires special attention to prevent injury to the gingival tissue when guiding floss through a tight contact area or when moving the floss on the tooth surface in an apical direction.
4. Squeaking sound effect when floss moves over a clean tooth surface may provide a motivation for patient thoroughness.
5. Unwaxed floss, which frays when rubbed over an irregular tooth surface, rough surface of a restoration, or a calculus deposit, might cause the patient to become aggravated and discouraged, thereby resulting in lost motivation to floss regularly.
6. Floss that is tightly wound around fingers tends to cut, hurt, and cause discomfort. This problem is not usually as evident with wide dental tape or with waxed floss or tape.

II. PROCEDURE

When dental floss is applied with firm pressure to a flat or convex proximal tooth surface, bacterial plaque can be removed. Older plaque is tenacious and may require several strokes for removal. When floss is placed over a concave surface, contact is not possible (Figure 24-8A, page 378), and supplementary devices are needed to completely remove a bacterial deposit.

A. When to Floss
For most patients, dental floss should be used before toothbrushing. The following reasons may apply:
1. When proximal tooth surfaces are deplaqued, the fluoride from a dentifrice used while brushing reaches the proximal surfaces for prevention of dental caries.
2. When brushing is accomplished first, flossing may not be carried out.
   a. The mouth feels clean; the need for flossing may not be appreciated.
   b. Time may be short and flossing can be postponed.

B. Floss Preparation
1. Hold a 12- to 15-inch length of floss with the thumb and index finger of each hand; grasp firmly with only ½ inch of floss between the finger tips. The ends of the floss may be tucked into the palm and held by the ring and little finger, or the floss may be wrapped around the middle fingers (Figure 24-1A, B, and C).
2. A circle of floss may be made by tying the ends together; the circle may be rotated as the floss is used (Figure 24-2).[14]

C. Application
1. *Maxillary Teeth.* Direct the floss up by holding the floss over two thumbs or a thumb and an index finger as shown in Figure 24-1A and B. Rest a side of a finger on teeth of opposite side of the maxillary arch to provide balance and a fulcrum.
2. *Mandibular Teeth.* Direct the floss down by holding the two index fingers on top of the strand. One index finger holds the floss on the lingual aspect and the other on the facial aspect (Figure 24-1C). The side of the finger on the lingual side is held on the teeth of the opposite side of the mouth to serve as a fulcrum or rest.

D. Insertion
1. Hold floss firmly in a diagonal or oblique position (Figure 24-3).
2. Guide the floss past each contact area with a gentle sawing motion (Figure 24-1D).
3. Control floss to prevent snapping through the contact area onto the gingival tissue.

E. Cleaning Stroke
1. Clean adjacent teeth separately; for the distal aspect, curve the floss mesially, and for the mesial aspect, curve the floss distally, around the tooth (Figure 24-1E and F).
2. Pass the floss below the gingival margin, curve to adapt the floss around the tooth, press, and slide up and down over the tooth surface. Repeat.
3. Loop the floss over the distal surfaces of the most posterior teeth in each quadrant and the teeth next to edentulous areas (Figure 24-1G). Hold firmly against the tooth and move the floss in both an up-and-down motion and a "shoeshine" stroke.

F. Additional Suggestions
1. Slide the floss to a new, unused portion for succeeding proximal tooth surfaces.
2. Floss may be doubled to provide a wider rubbing surface.
3. When a dentifrice is used with the floss, dental tape may be better than floss in retaining the dentifrice against the tooth.

III. PRECAUTIONS

A. Pressure in Col Area
The col area is not keratinized and is vulnerable to bacterial invasion. Plaque control of the area is of great importance because most gingival and periodontal infection begins in the col area.

Too great a pressure with floss one or more times daily, particularly very fine floss that tends to cut more easily than thicker floss, can be destructive to the attachment. Excess pressure of the floss against the attachment is particularly significant in children in whom teeth are in the process of eruption and the junctional epithelium is less firmly attached.

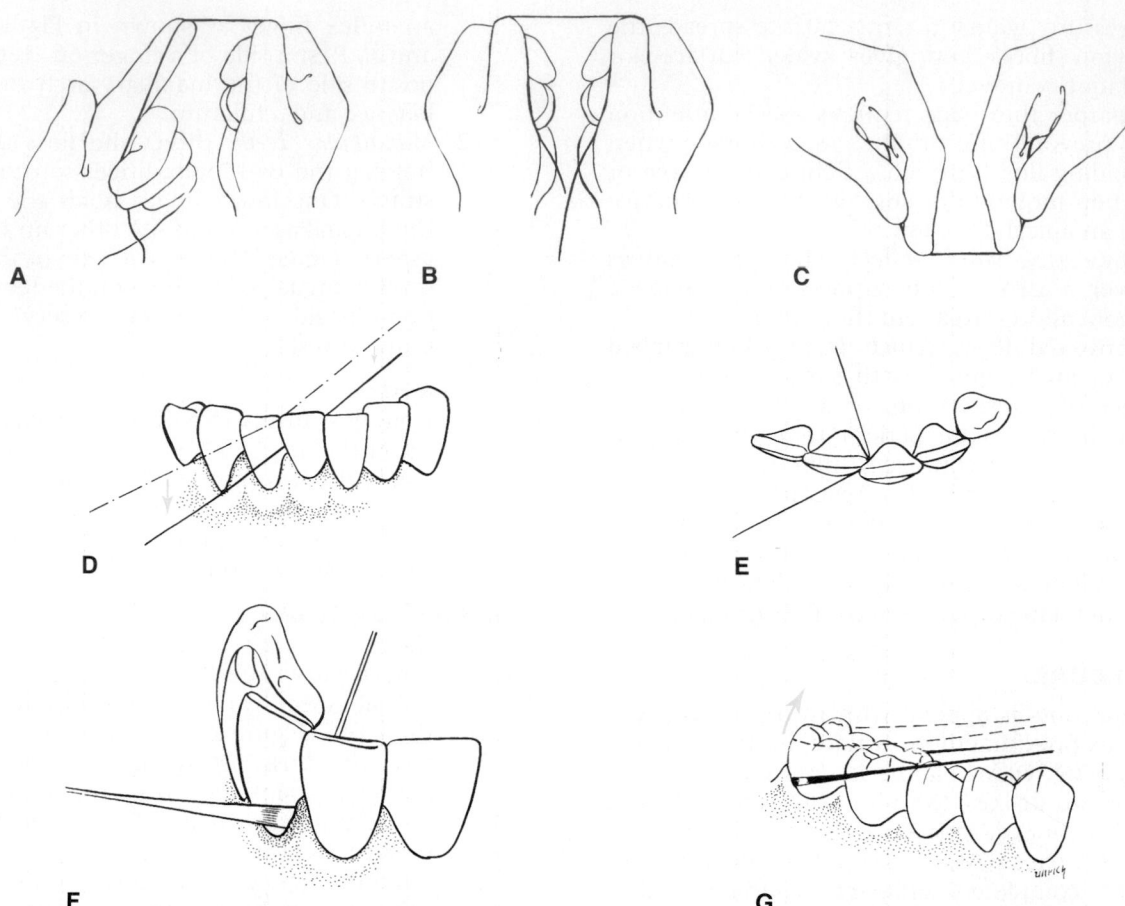

■ **FIGURE 24-1 Use of Dental Floss.** For maxillary insertion, hold the floss between the thumb and index finger **(A)** or between thumbs **(B).** Grasp the floss firmly. Allow only 1/2-inch length between fingers. **(C)** For the mandibular teeth, direct the floss down, guided by the index fingers. **(D)** Work the floss slowly between the teeth in a short sawing motion. Avoid snapping through the contact area. **(E)** Curve the floss around the tooth in a C-shape. Hold the floss toward the mesial for cleaning the distal surfaces and toward the distal for cleaning the mesial surfaces. **(F)** Press the floss firmly against the tooth. Move gently beneath the gingiva until tissue resistance is felt. Slide the floss horizontally and vertically with pressure to remove bacterial plaque. **(G)** Begin flossing with the distal surface of the most posterior tooth, and work systematically around the arch.

B. Prevention of Floss Cuts and Floss Clefts

1. *Location.* Floss cuts or clefts occur primarily on facial and lingual or palatal surfaces directly beside or in the middle of an interdental papilla. They appear as straight-line cuts from the gingival margin and may result in a floss cleft (page 196).

2. *Causes*
   a. Using too long a piece of floss between the fingers when held for insertion.
   b. Snapping the floss through the contact area.
   c. Not curving the floss about the teeth; holding floss straight across the papilla.
   d. Not using a rest to prevent undue pressure.

C. Aid for Flossing

A floss holder can be helpful for a person with a disability or for a parent or caregiver serving a child or patient. Floss holders are described on pages 751 and 752.

TUFTED DENTAL FLOSS

I. DESCRIPTION

Tufted dental floss is also called a floss/yarn combination. Regular dental floss is alternated with a thickened tufted portion. Two variations are available commercially.

A. Single, Precut Lengths

"Super Floss"[15] is available in a 2-foot length composed of a 5-inch tufted portion adjacent to a 3-inch stiffened end for inserting under a

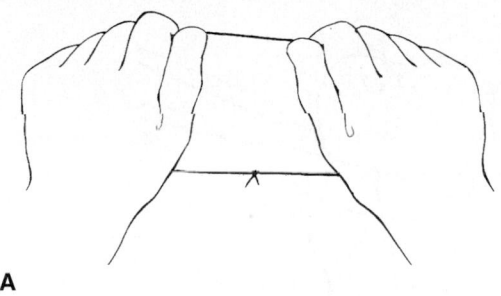

A

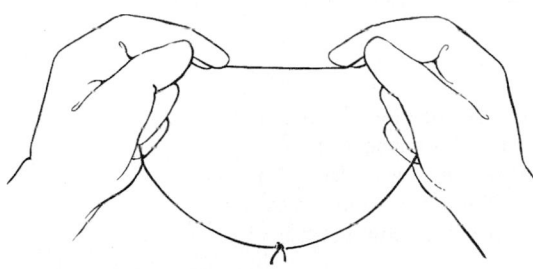

B

▪ **FIGURE 24-2 Circle of Floss.** The ends of the floss are tied together for convenient holding. A child may be able to manage floss better with this technique. **(A)** Floss held for maxillary teeth. **(B)** Floss held for mandibular teeth.

fixed appliance or orthodontic attachment (Figure 24-4*A*).

B. Roll
"NUFloss"[16] is available in a roll that is similar to that of regular floss and has a cutting device to allow selection of a preferred length. The tufted portions (about 1 inch long) alternate with the plain floss (about 1½ inches long) (Figure 24-4*B*).

II. INDICATIONS FOR USE
A. Plaque removal from tooth surfaces adjacent to wide embrasures where interdental papillae have been lost.
B. Plaque removal from mesial and distal abut-

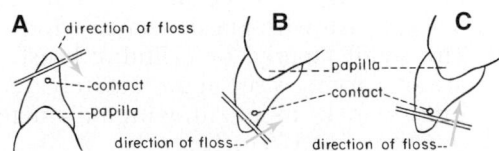

▪ **FIGURE 24-3 Insertion of Floss.** Hold floss in a diagonal or oblique position over the teeth where the floss will be inserted. Arrows indicate the direction of movement of the floss. **(A)** Floss held for mandibular insertion. **(B)** Floss held for maxillary insertion. **(C)** Floss held incorrectly. When floss is held horizontally, the possibility for damage to the papilla is greater.

ments and under pontic of a fixed partial denture or orthodontic appliance. The stiff end of "Super Floss" is inserted; "NUFloss" is threaded using a floss threader (see Figures 25-9 and 25-10, page 401).

III. PROCEDURE
A. Individual Surface of Tooth or Implant
Curve floss and/or tufted portion around the tooth or implant in a "C" to remove bacterial plaque. Move floss vertically and horizontally (Figure 24-4*C*).

B. Fixed Partial Denture
Thread tufted floss over pontic and apply to distal surface of the mesial abutment and mesial surface of the distal abutment (Figure 25-10, page 401).

KNITTING YARN

I. INDICATIONS FOR USE
A. For tooth surfaces adjacent to wide proximal spaces, dental floss is too narrow and does not remove plaque efficiently.
B. For mesial and distal abutments of fixed partial dentures and under pontics, use a floss threader (page 401).
C. For isolated teeth, teeth separated by a diastema, and distal surfaces of most posterior teeth.

II. PROCEDURE
A. Fold yarn double. Use about 8 inches of 3- or 4-ply smooth synthetic yarn. Loop through about 8 inches of dental floss; tie floss with one overhand knot.
B. Insert floss through the contact area. Draw the yarn into the embrasure (Figure 24-5).
C. Clean adjacent teeth separately with a facial–lingual, back-and-forth stroke. Hold the ends of the yarn distally and then around mesially.
D. For specific areas where a papilla may be high or access is not otherwise sufficient for the wide yarn, use the dental floss end of the combination.
E. Apply dentifrice.
F. For closed contacts, use a floss threader (see Figure 25-10, page 401).

GAUZE STRIP

I. INDICATIONS FOR USE
A. For proximal surfaces of widely spaced teeth. Gauze is too thick to pass through contact areas.
B. For surfaces of teeth next to edentulous areas.

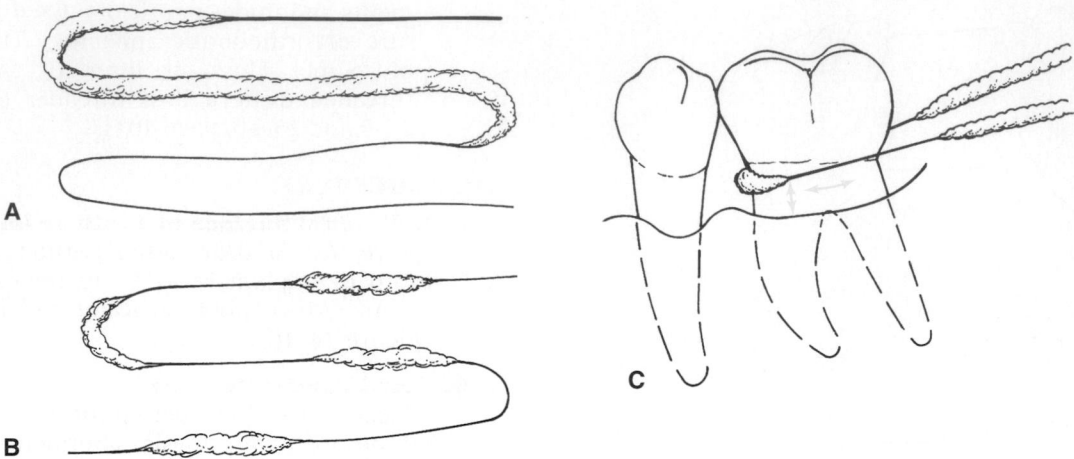

FIGURE 24-4 Tufted Dental Floss. The floss/yarn combination may be "Super Floss" **(A)** in a precut length with a tufted portion and a 3-inch stiffened end for insertion under a fixed prosthesis, or "NUFloss." **(B)** With tufted portions alternated with plain floss. A preferred length of "NUFloss" is obtained from the container. **(C)** "NUFloss" applied to the proximal surface of a molar. It may be used in an up-and-down and a shoe-shine stroke.

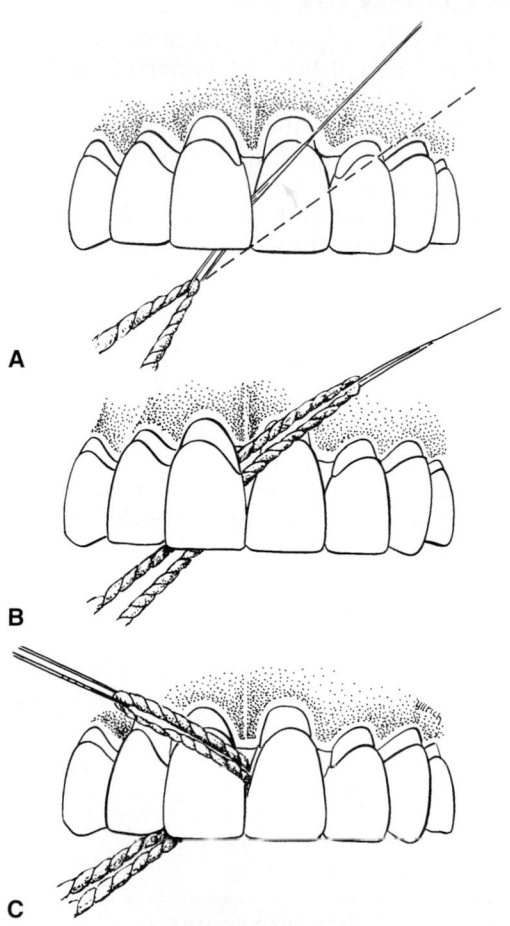

FIGURE 24-5 Knitting Yarn. (A) Yarn is looped through dental floss, and the floss is drawn through the contact area in the usual manner, shown by the arrow. **(B)** Yarn is drawn through the embrasure. **(C)** Yarn is positioned against the surface of the tooth for plaque removal. When tooth contact is missing and space permits, the yarn is used without floss.

C. For distal and mesial surfaces of abutment teeth.

D. For areas under posterior cantilevered section of a fixed appliance, such as the distal portion of a denture supported by implants.

II. PROCEDURE

A. Cut 1-inch gauze bandage into a 6- to 8-inch length, and fold in thirds or down the center.

B. Position the fold of the gauze on the cervical area next to the gingival crest and work back and forth several times; hold ends in a distal direction to clean a mesial surface, and in a mesial direction to clean a distal surface (Figure 24-6).

INTERDENTAL BRUSHES

I. TYPES

A. Small Insert Brushes With Reusable Handle

1. Soft nylon filaments are twisted into a fine stainless steel wire for insertion into a handle with an angulated shank (Figure 24-7D). Select brush with plastic-coated wire.

2. The small tapered or cylindric brush heads are of varying sizes approximately 12 to 15 mm (½ inch) in length, with a diameter of 3 to 5 mm (⅛ to ¼ inch).

B. Brush With Wire Handle

1. Soft nylon filaments are twisted into a fine stainless steel wire. The wire is continuous with the handle, which is approximately 35 to 45 mm (1½ to 1¾ inches) in length (Figure 24-7C).

2. The filaments form a narrow brush approxi-

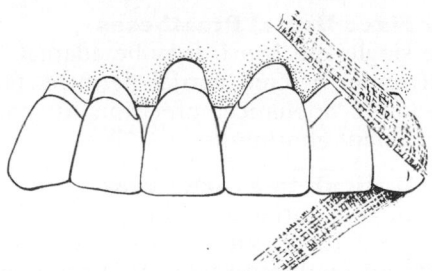

FIGURE 24-6 Gauze Strip. A 6- or 8-inch length of 1-inch bandage is folded in thirds and placed around a tooth adjacent to an edentulous area, a tooth with interdental spacing, or the distal surface of the most posterior tooth. A shoe-shine stroke is used to clean the bacterial plaque from the surface.

mately 30 to 35 mm (1¼ to 1½ inches) in length and 5 to 8 mm (¼ to ⁵⁄₁₆ inches) in diameter.

II. INDICATIONS FOR USE

When sufficient space is available for the insertion of an interdental brush without excess force, the following applications are indicated:

A. For Removal of Bacterial Plaque and Debris

1. Proximal tooth surfaces adjacent to open embrasures, orthodontic appliances, fixed prostheses, dental implants, periodontal splints, and space maintainers, and other areas that are hard to reach with a regular toothbrush.
2. Concave proximal surfaces where dental floss and other interdental aids cannot reach (Figure 24-8A). Floss bridges over a concave surface, whereas the interproximal brush can reach and cleanse (Figure 24-8B).[1,17]
3. Exposed Class IV furcations (Figure 13-3, page 230).

B. For Application of Chemotherapeutic Agents

1. Fluoride dentifrice, gel, and/or mouthrinse for prevention of dental caries, particularly root surface caries and for surfaces adjacent to any prosthesis.
2. Antibacterial agents for control of bacterial plaque and the prevention of gingivitis.
3. Desensitizing agents.

III. PROCEDURE

A. Select brush of appropriate diameter.
B. Moisten the brush and insert at an angle in keeping with gingival form; brush in and out.

IV. CARE OF BRUSHES

A. Clean brush during use to remove debris and plaque by holding under actively running water.
B. Clean thoroughly after use and dry in open air.
C. Discard when filaments become loose or deformed.

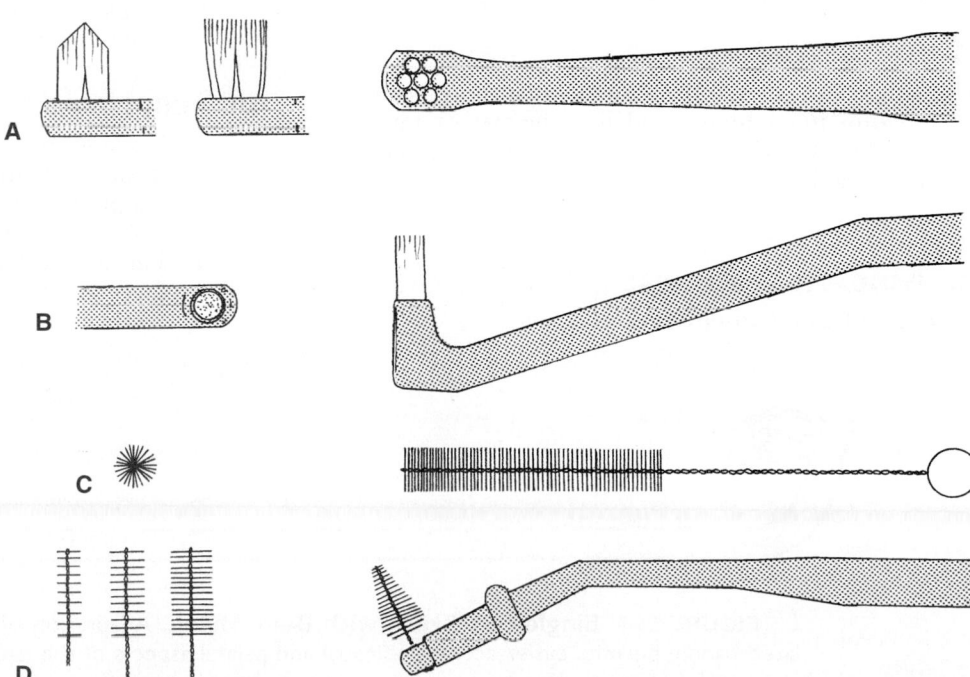

FIGURE 24-7 Single-tuft and Interdental Brushes. **(A)** Single-tuft brush with tapered and flat groups of filaments. **(B)** Single-tuft brush on handle with angulated shank. **(C)** Interdental brush with filaments twisted into a fine wire that ends in a handle. **(D)** Insert brushes for a reusable handle with an angulated shank.

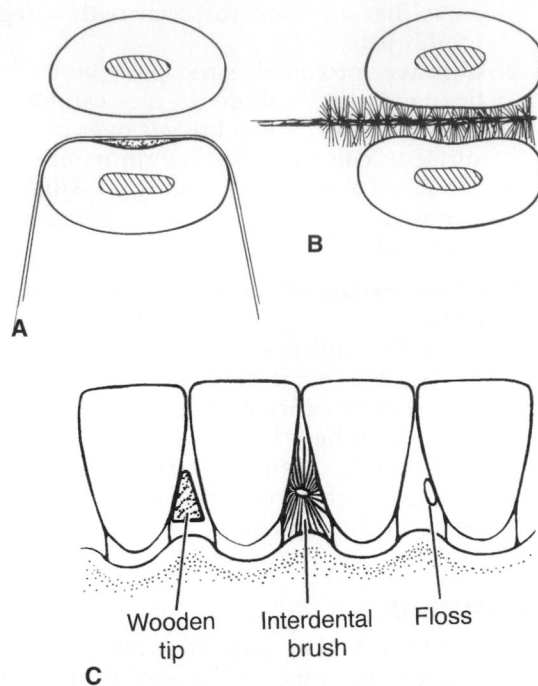

FIGURE 24-8 Interdental Care. (A) Floss positioned on the mesial surface of a maxillary first premolar shows the inability of the floss to remove bacterial plaque on a concave proximal tooth surface. **(B)** Use of an interdental brush in the same interproximal area to show how the proximal surfaces can be cleaned free of bacterial plaque. **(C)** Comparison of the access of a wooden tip, an interdental brush, and a piece of dental floss to an open interdental area.

SINGLE-TUFT BRUSH (END-TUFT, UNITUFT)

I. DESCRIPTION

The single tuft, or group of small tufts, may be from 3 to 6 mm in diameter and may be flat or tapered (Figure 24-7*A* and *B*). The handle may be straight or contra-angled.

II. INDICATIONS FOR USE

A. For Open Interproximal Areas

B. For Fixed Dental Prostheses
The single-tuft brush may be adaptable around and under a fixed partial denture, pontic, orthodontic appliance, precision attachment, or an implant abutment.

C. For Difficult-to-Reach Areas
The lingual surfaces of the mandibular molars, abutment teeth, the distal surfaces of the most posterior teeth, and teeth that are crowded are examples of areas where an end-tuft brush may prove of value. The shank may be bent for easy adaptation (Figure 24-9).

III. PROCEDURE

A. Direct the end of the tuft into the interproximal area and along the gingival margin.
B. Combine a rotating motion with intermittent pressure.
C. Use a sulcular brushing stroke.

INTERDENTAL TIP

I. COMPOSITION AND DESIGN

Conical or pyramidal flexible rubber or plastic tip is attached to the end of the handle of a toothbrush or is on a special plastic handle. The soft, pliable rubber tip is preferred because it can be adapted to the interdental area and below the gingival margin more easily than can the hard, more rigid plastic tip.

II. INDICATIONS FOR USE

A. For cleaning debris from the interdental area and for removal of bacterial plaque by rubbing the exposed tooth surfaces.
B. For plaque removal at and just below the gingival margin.

III. PROCEDURE

A. Trace along the gingival margin with the tip positioned just beneath the margin. The adaptation is similar to the toothpick in holder (see Figure 24-11).
B. For additional cleaning of the proximal surfaces of the teeth, rub the tip against the teeth as it is moved in and out of an embra-

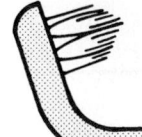

FIGURE 24-9 Single-tuft Brush with Bent Shank. Adaptation of brush with angulated handle permits easier access to lingual and palatal aspects of the natural teeth, as well as to orthodontic appliances, prostheses, and implant abutments.

sure and under a contact area. Position tip with the gingival form; take care not to flatten the interdental tissue.

C. Rinse the tip as indicated during use to remove debris, and wash thoroughly at the finish.

PIPE CLEANER

I. INDICATIONS FOR USE

A. For proximal surfaces when interdental gingiva is missing.
B. For open furcation areas.

II. PROCEDURE

A. Use one-third of a regular-length pipe cleaner at a time. Check wire end to prevent damage to the gingiva or scratching of the cemental surface.
B. Carefully work the end of the cleaner through the space. Take care not to press wire end into the gingiva.
C. Work back and forth pressing toward one surface and then the other.
D. Slide pipe cleaner between exposed roots of a furcation. Work back and forth (Figure 24-10).

TOOTHPICK IN HOLDER

I. DESCRIPTION

A round toothpick is inserted into a plastic handle with contra-angled ends for adaptation to the tooth surface at the gingival margin for plaque removal.

II. INDICATIONS FOR USE

A. Patient With Periodontitis

For plaque removal at and just under the gin-

gival margin, for interdental cleaning, particularly for concave proximal tooth surfaces, and for exposed furcation area.

B. Orthodontic Patient

For plaque removal at gingival margin above appliance and for cleaning around fixed appliances (see Figure 25-3, page 397).

III. PROCEDURE

A. Prepare Instrument

1. Insert round tapered toothpick into the end of the holder. One type of holder has angulated ends for use in various positions.
2. Twist the toothpick firmly into place. Break off the long end cleanly so that sharp edges cannot scratch the inner cheek or the tongue during use.

B. Application

1. Apply toothpick at the gingival margin. At a right-angle application, with moderate pressure, trace the gingival margin around each tooth.
2. To remove plaque just below the gingival margin, apply the end at less than 45°, maintain the tip on the tooth surface, and follow around the sulcus or pocket (Figure 24-11).
3. Use a tip that has become frayed from use as a small cleaning "brush" to rub on tooth surfaces where plaque has collected. Check for and remove loose bits of wood that could become deposited in the sulcus or gingiva.
4. For hypersensitive spots, usually at the cervical third of a tooth, the patient can use the tip daily to massage dentifrice for desensitization.
5. When a contact is inadequate and the patient indicates that floss or toothpicks are required to relieve pressure from impacted food, dental attention may be needed. The area should be charted or otherwise brought to the attention of the dentist.

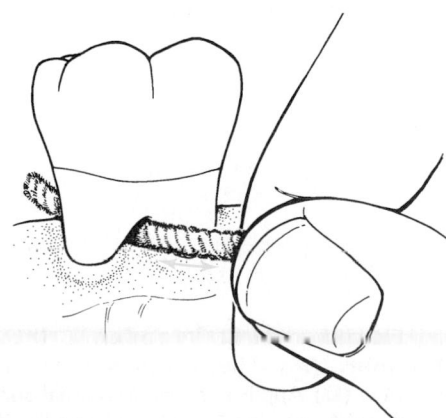
FIGURE 24-10 Pipe Cleaner. An exposed furcation area may be cleaned by inserting a pipe cleaner and moving it back and forth.

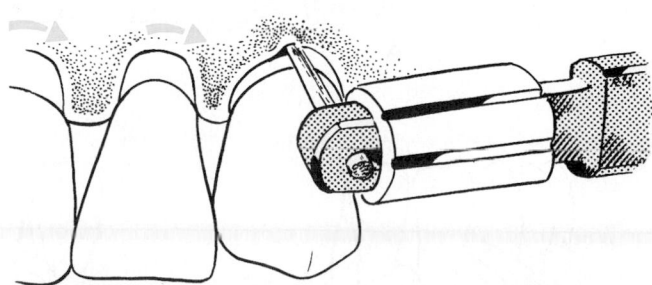
FIGURE 24-11 Toothpick in Holder for Bacterial Plaque at Gingival Margin. The tip is placed at or just below the gingival margin. Trace the margin around each tooth.

WOODEN INTERDENTAL CLEANER

I. DESCRIPTION

The wooden cleaner is a 2-inch-long device made of bass wood or birchwood. It is triangular in cross section as shown in Figure 24-12.

II. INDICATIONS FOR USE

A. Application

For cleaning proximal tooth surfaces where the tooth surfaces are exposed and interdental gingiva missing. Space must be adequate; otherwise the gingival tissue can be traumatized.

B. Limitation

As with most interdental devices, the wooden cleaner is advised only for the patient who follows instructions carefully. A fresh cleaner may be advised for each arch or quadrant because the wood may become splayed.

III. PROCEDURE

A. Fulcrum (Rest)

First teach the patient to use a rest by placing the hand on the cheek or chin, or by placing a finger on the gingiva convenient to the place where the tip will be applied. This precaution helps to prevent insertion of the wedge with too much pressure.

B. Preparation

Soften the wood by placing the pointed end in the mouth and moistening with saliva.

C. Directions

1. Hold the base of the triangular wedge toward the gingival border of the interdental area and insert with the tip pointed slightly toward the occlusal or incisal surfaces to follow the contour of the embrasure (Figure 24-12*B* and *C*). When the wedge is held horizontally, the interdental tissue can be flattened.

2. Clean the tooth surfaces by moving the wedge in and out while applying a burnishing stroke with moderate pressure first to one side of the embrasure and then to the other, about four strokes each.

3. Discard the cleaner as soon as the first signs of splaying are evident.

CHEMOTHERAPY

Chapter 23 and the first part of this chapter described various methods for mechanical bacterial plaque control. The objective in mechanical removal of plaque deposits is the physical clearing away of microorganisms and their pathogenic products to prevent or treat dental and periodontal infections.

The mechanical devices also are used to apply agents for chemotherapy. For example, the toothbrush is used to apply a dentifrice that contains fluoride for dental caries control. The irrigator, described in the next section, is a mechanical device that has a cleansing role when plain water is used as the irrigant, but it can also be used to deliver an antimicrobial agent for treatment of gingival infection.

Chemotherapy for preventive or therapeutic oral disease control can be applied by either systemic or local methods (page 568). Systemic chemotherapy can be the prescription of an antibiotic specific for periodontal pathogenic microorganisms, such as tetracycline to control *Actinobacillus actinomycetemcomitans* in the treatment of juvenile periodontitis.

The four general local methods for chemotherapy are (1) irrigation, (2) use of a mouthrinse, (3) use of a dentifrice, and (4) local delivery of a slow-release agent to a periodontal pocket.

Treatment using a local method may be performed by the patient as recommended and demonstrated by the dentist and dental hygienist. An example is patient-applied supragingival and/or subgingival irrigation described in the following section.

Other local treatment is performed as part of the professional care during appointments. One example

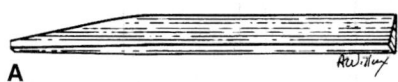

A

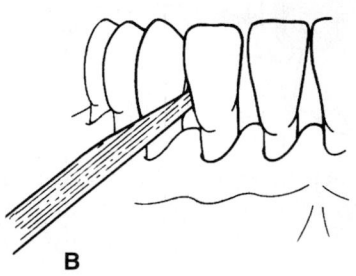

B

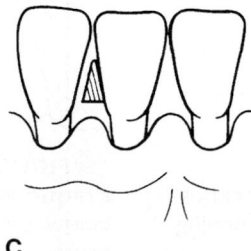

C

■ FIGURE 24-12 **Wooden Interdental Cleaner. (A)** The 2-inch wooden triangular cleaner. **(B)** Application on proximal surface of a tooth with missing interdental papilla. The base of the triangle is on the gingival side. **(C)** The side of the triangle is rubbed in and out against the proximal surface to remove bacterial plaque.

is professionally administered subgingival irrigation; another example is the application of an antibiotic or other antimicrobial agent placed into a pocket for slow release. Professionally applied chemotherapy is described in Chapter 34, pages 568 to 573.

ORAL IRRIGATION

Irrigation is the targeted application of a pulsated or steady stream of water or other irrigant for cleansing and/or therapeutic purposes. Oral irrigation can be applied by the patient or the clinician. For the patient, irrigation can be a part of the routine personal bacterial plaque control program and used as instructed. Professionally administered irrigation may be indicated prior to and/or following initial therapy appointments for scaling and root planing and during supportive periodontal treatment.

Oral irrigation is an adjunctive method for the arrest and control of gingival infection. The control of gingival and periodontal infections requires the control of risk factors including the microbial challenge. Oral irrigation helps to keep the subgingival bacterial challenge at levels compatible with health. Since lipopolysaccharides are instrumental in initiating the inflammatory response, and because the subgingival area is a haven for the microflora, irrigation may prove to be a necessary link in maintaining periodontal health. Irrigation disrupts microbial colonization.

Mechanical devices, including toothbrushes and interdental implements, can accomplish bacterial plaque removal supragingivally and slightly below the gingival margin for the motivated patient. For selected patients in need of enhanced subgingival access, irrigation can supplement other efforts. Instruction and supervision are provided by the oral health professional.

Oral irrigation devices are evaluated by the American Dental Association, Council on Scientific Affairs. The Seal of Acceptance signifies the safety and effectiveness of the product (see Figure 24-15, page 389).

DESCRIPTION OF IRRIGATORS

I. POWER-DRIVEN DEVICE

    A. Generates an intermittent or pulsating jet of fluid with an adjustable dial for regulation of pressure.

    B. Delivers through a hand-held interchangeable tip that rotates 360° for application at the gingival margin.

    C. Maintains steady flow or pulsation of irrigant from a reservoir.

    D. Provides reservoir container for convenient measurement of antimicrobial or other agent. Some reservoirs are calibrated for easy instruction and documentation.

II. NON-POWER-DRIVEN DEVICE

    A. Attaches to a household water supply: faucet or shower.

    B. Delivers through a hand-held interchangeable tip that can be turned for application at the gingival margin.

    C. Cannot definitively control water pressure.

    D. Non-pulsating flow of irrigant.

DELIVERY METHODS

The target of oral irrigation is the loosely attached subgingival bacterial plaque. When the *pulsated* irrigant is directed perpendicularly to the long axis of the tooth, two zones of hydrokinetic activity are created. The first is the impact zone where the irrigant makes initial contact, and the second is the flushing zone where the irrigant is deflected from the tooth surface.[18]

The lavage action of irrigation produces quantitative and qualitative changes in the subgingival microflora.[19]

I. STANDARD JET TIP

A. Delivery Tips

    1. Monojet (single stream) (Figure 24-13*B*).

    2. Fractionated microjet (Figure 24-13*A*).

    3. Pulsating and non-pulsating.

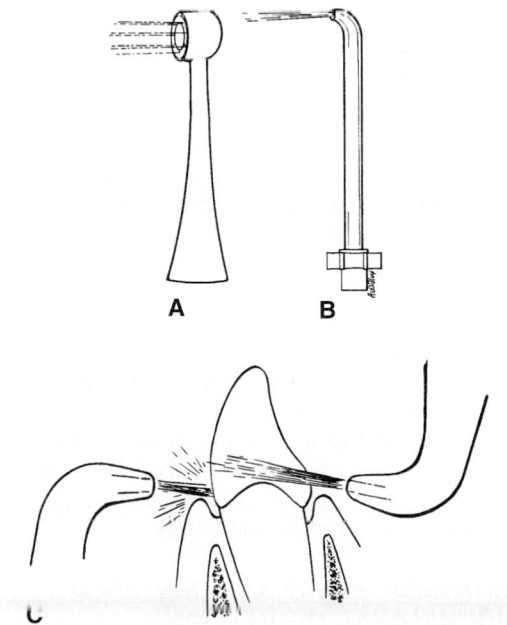

A   B

C

FIGURE 24-13 Supragingival Irrigation. (A) Fractionated microjet tip (multiple streams) for home irrigator. **(B)** Monojet tip (single stream). **(C)** Monojet delivery tip used in horizontal direction through interproximal area. Only low pressures are recommended.

B. Procedure
1. Direct the jet tip toward the interdental area until almost touching the tooth surfaces; hold tip at a right angle to the long axis of the tooth (Figure 24-13*C*).
2. Start on the lowest pressure setting; increase slightly over time depending on the condition of the gingiva and tissue comfort. Lean over the sink.
3. Follow a definite pattern around the mouth, maxillary arch first, then the mandibular; apply 5 to 6 seconds at each interdental area.

C. Special Instructions
1. Keep irrigator at a low pressure; keep tip directed at the gingival margin.
2. Irrigation imparts a clean feeling to the mouth; the patient must understand that irrigation is an adjunct and not a substitute for regular toothbrushing and interdental care.

II. SPECIALIZED TIPS
A. Delivery Tips
1. *Angulation.* For application at or below the gingival margin for targeted delivery of water or antimicrobial agent.
2. *Types*
   a. Soft rubber tip designed to be placed 2 mm below the gingival margin (Figure 24-14*A*).
   b. Tapered plastic tip designed to be placed at the gingival margin (Figure 24-14*B*).
   c. Metal or plastic cannula tip for placement below the gingival margin, possibly to the base of pocket.

B. Procedure
1. Identify appropriate areas for use (for example, specific pocket, furca, or implant).[20]
2. Set unit pressure on lowest setting or follow the manufacturer's instructions.
3. Direct the tip at or below the gingival margin according to the manufacturer's directions and as demonstrated by the dental professional (Figure 24-14*C*).
4. Activate flow of solution for 5 to 6 seconds into designated area; stop flow and move to next designated area.
5. When using a metal or plastic cannula, care must be taken to ensure the patient can place the tip subgingivally and deliver the agent accurately and safely.

III. PROFESSIONALLY ADMINISTERED SUBGINGIVAL IRRIGATION
Supplementary irrigation may be indicated as an adjunct to nonsurgical periodontal therapy. The procedure for professionally administered irrigation is described on page 568.

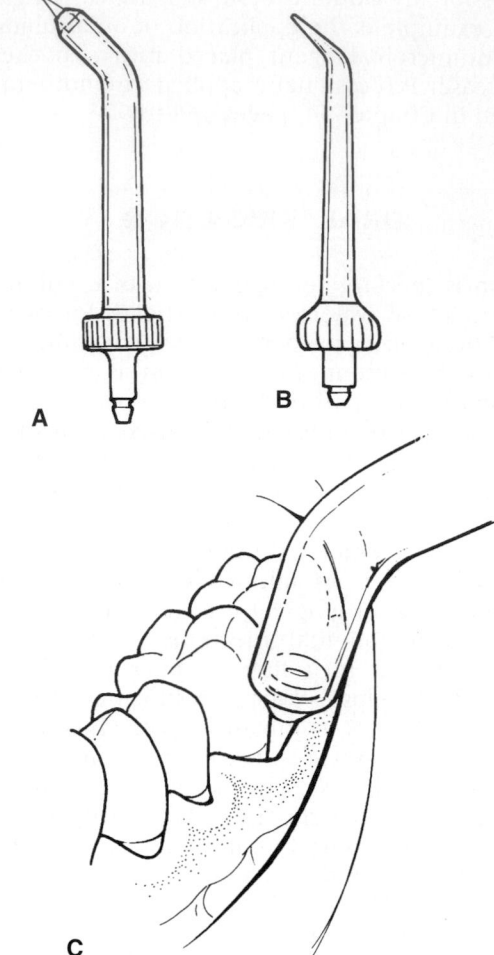

FIGURE 24-14 Patient-Applied Subgingival Irrigation. (A) and **(B)** Special tips for use by the patient. **(C)** Soft rubber tip, designed to be placed 2 mm below gingival margin, in position for irrigation.

BENEFICIAL EFFECTS FROM IRRIGATION

Benefits that have been shown from the use of an oral irrigator include the reduction of bacterial plaque and gingivitis, reduction or alteration of microbial flora, subgingival access to pathogenic microorganisms, delivery of antimicrobial agents, and removal of bacteria and debris for oral cleanliness and sanitation.

I. REDUCTION OF GINGIVITIS
Supragingival irrigation is effective for removing loosely attached bacterial plaque and reducing gingivitis. When an antimicrobial agent is used in the irrigator, reduction of supragingival plaque and gingivitis is enhanced.[21–23]

II. REDUCTION OR ALTERATION OF MICROBIAL FLORA
Both supra- and subgingival irrigation reduce micro-

bial counts and disrupt microbial colonization.[19,23,24] The duration of bacterial suppression varies with frequency of irrigation and therefore is related to patient motivation and compliance.

III. PENETRATION INTO POCKET: SUBGINGIVAL ACCESS

The standard jet tip placed at the gingival margin can penetrate below the gingival margin a few millimeters or beyond.[25–27] When a specialized tip (Figure 24-14) is used to dispense the fluid, penetration has been shown up to 70% and 90% of the pocket depth and beyond.[27,28]

IV. DELIVERY OF ANTIMICROBIAL AGENTS

The effectiveness of an antimicrobial agent is enhanced when delivered by an oral irrigator. When used as a mouthrinse, an agent does not usually penetrate subgingivally sufficiently to influence the subgingival microflora to a significant degree.

Agents that have been researched for use in an irrigator include chlorhexidine gluconate,[22,23,29,30] stannous fluoride,[29,31–33] phenolic compounds (essential oils),[21,34] and sanguinaria.[35,36]

V. PERIODONTAL MAINTENANCE

Oral irrigation has been shown to improve the following clinical parameters for periodontal maintenance patients: gingival index, bleeding on probing, and probing depths.[37–40]

APPLICATIONS FOR PRACTICE

A patient without gingival or periodontal infection who has achieved adequate skills for daily plaque removal and who conscientiously keeps regular maintenance appointments for professional supervision may not see additional clinical benefits from the use of home irrigation. However, since the inflammatory response is subclinical in the early stages, the patient may benefit from the addition of irrigation if there are other risk factors to be considered.

I. ADVANTAGES OF HOME IRRIGATION

A. Patient Participation in Therapy
The patient is a cotherapist through daily irrigation with an antimicrobial agent and can contribute to a more positive response to professional treatments for gingivitis with or without coexisting periodontitis.

B. Removal of Loose Bacterial Plaque From Problem Areas
Areas that are difficult to access, such as open interdental areas, malpositioned teeth, exposed furcas, and postperiodontal surgery problem areas, can benefit from home irrigation.

C. Care for Special Needs Areas
1. Prosthetic replacements, fixed partial dentures, prostheses.
2. Orthodontic appliances.
3. Intermaxillary fixation appliances for orthognathic surgery[41] and fractured jaw (page 718).
4. Complex restorations and other extensive rehabilitation.
5. Implant maintenance with soft rubber specialized tip.

D. Postponement of Surgery
The patient who is unable to proceed with essential periodontal surgical therapy and is being maintained by frequent professional appointments may benefit from irrigation with an effective antimicrobial agent that aids in the control of subgingival microorganisms.

II. CONTRAINDICATION

The health history of a patient who requires antibiotic premedication for dental and dental hygiene treatment should be reviewed before introducing the use of an oral irrigator or other mechanical device. The American Heart Association recommendations state that although oral irrigating devices have been implicated in producing bacteremia, the relation to infective endocarditis is not known.[42]

The incidence of bacteremia from irrigation ranges from a low of 6% in patients with gingivitis to a high of 50% in patients with periodontitis.[43,44] The patient's physician can be contacted for advice when a question arises about the use of adjunctive oral hygiene aids that can create bacteremia.

MOUTHRINSES

Mouthrinsing is a supragingival procedure. Even vigorous rinsing does not force the fluid into a sulcus or pocket more than a few millimeters.[25,45]

Mouthrinses may be classified as cosmetic or therapeutic. When claims for therapeutic value have not been scientifically substantiated, the repeated use of a product may be harmful.

Mouthrinses that claim no therapeutic or disease preventive value are not included in the acceptance program of the American Dental Association, Council on Scientific Affairs. At present, the routine unsupervised use of medicated mouthrinses by the public cannot be considered appropriate.

When recording information about the oral health practices of a patient as part of the medical and dental history, it can be determined whether a particular mouthrinse is used, the frequency of its use, and what the patient believes to be the benefit from its use. If any detrimental effects are suspected after the oral examination, or if adverse effects are known to be possible, the patient can be informed and alternate procedures for rinsing can be recommended.

I. PURPOSES AND USES

A. Dental Office or Clinic

1. Pretreatment rinse to reduce microorganisms, thereby providing a more aseptic working field.[46,47]
2. Pretreatment rinse to reduce aerosol contamination during use of handpiece and ultrasonic scaler[48] (page 558).
3. To facilitate impression procedures (page 173).
4. To rinse and refresh the mouth during film placement for radiography and following a dental or dental hygiene procedure.
5. Fluoride rinse after scaling, after coronal polishing, after polishing restorations, to replace surface fluoride removed during the treatment.
6. Fluoride rinse as part of the caries prevention program, particularly after scaling to prevent root caries.

B. Patient at Home

1. *Mouth Cleaning.* Vigorous rinsing to dislodge food debris contributes to general oral cleanliness. Rinsing with clear water after meals and after snacks, particularly sweet snacks, has been suggested when toothbrushing and interdental cleaning are not possible.

   The limitations of rinsing for cleansing should be understood. Although rinsing aids in the removal of gross debris and unattached surface microorganisms, attached plaque is not disturbed.
2. *Postsurgical Care*
   a. After oral surgery as directed (page 711).
   b. After periodontal surgery (see Table 36-1, page 593).
   c. Antiplaque rinse to promote healing when tissues are not ready for routine brushing. Chlorhexidine use is described on page 386.
3. *After Nonsurgical Periodontal Therapy* (pages 560 to 561). A saline rinse can promote healing of the gingival tissues, and a fluoride rinse can benefit the exposed root planed surfaces for dental caries prevention.
4. *Treatment.* During pathologic conditions, such as necrotizing ulcerative gingivitis, rinsing is used to remove debris, encourage healing, and soothe tender gingiva (pages 580 to 581).
5. *Dental Caries Prevention.* The use of fluoride mouthrinses for dental caries control is included in the chapter on fluoride application (pages 470 to 471).
6. *Cosmetic Purposes.* Advertising claims can be misleading, and patients need assistance in interpreting what they read and hear. With-

out advice, people may select a mouthrinse on the basis of advertising promises or flavor. Purposes and effects that may be expected from the use of a cosmetic mouthrinse are the following:
   a. Removes loose debris when rinsing is vigorous.
   b. Gives temporary benefit through mechanical reduction in numbers of oral microorganisms.
   c. Imparts a pleasant taste, odor, and refreshing sensation to the oral cavity.
   d. Contributes to a temporary suppression of halitosis when causes are local (page 347).

II. PROCEDURE FOR RINSING

Many patients, particularly children, must be shown specifically how to rinse. The method can be practiced under supervision.

Uninstructed patients may hold fluid in their mouths and bow the head from side to side, or perform some other action that cannot force the water about and between the teeth. Table 24-1 suggests steps for teaching a patient how to rinse.

III. CHARACTERISTICS OF AN EFFECTIVE MOUTHRINSE

Suggested requirements for an effective chemotherapeutic agent include at least the following:[49]

A. Nontoxic
The agent should not damage oral tissues or create systemic disturbances.

B. No or Limited Absorption
The agent should not be absorbed through the membranes of the gastrointestinal tract. The action should be confined to bacterial plaque.

C. Substantivity
Substantivity means the ability of an agent to be bound to the pellicle and tooth surface and to be released over an extended period of time with retention of potency. With time, the bac-

---

TABLE 24-1 How to Rinse

1. Take a small amount of the fluid into the mouth.
2. Close lips; hold teeth slightly apart.
3. Force the fluid through the interdental areas with pressure.
4. Use the lips, cheeks, and tongue action to force the fluid back and forth between the teeth.
5. Balloon the cheeks, then suck them in, alternately several times.
6. Divide the mouth into three parts—front, right, and left.
7. Concentrate the rinsing first on the front, then on the right, and then on the left side.
8. Expectorate or swallow according to directions.

terial succession and, ultimately, disease are altered.

D. Bacterial Specificity

The agent may have a broad antimicrobial spectrum, but it should have specificity for the organisms most pathogenic for a given infection. The agent may act directly on the organism, may interfere with bacterial attachment, may act on the plaque matrix, or may alter the tooth surface.

E. Low Induced Drug Resistance

Long-range effectiveness is lost when a drug induces resistance of microorganisms.

SELF-PREPARED MOUTHRINSES

Plain water, saline solutions, or solutions of bicarbonate of soda may be considered the most practical mouthrinses from the point of view of availability, cost, and effectiveness for debris removal and general oral cleanliness. Frequently prescribed or recommended, they may be helpful in postoperative care following dental and dental hygiene procedures.

When a salt solution is of greater strength than the physiologic salt solution concentration of body cells, fluid is drawn out of the cells by osmosis to balance the concentration. This action may produce a reduction of edema and related benefits. The patient history must be checked, as a patient on a low-salt or sodium-free diet should not use a saline rinse.

I. WATER

II. ISOTONIC SODIUM CHLORIDE SOLUTION

A. Isotonic is normal or physiologic salt solution, which is 0.9% aqueous solution; same concentration as cellular fluids.
B. Preparation (household measurements): level ½ teaspoonful salt added to 1 cup (8 ounces) of warm water.

III. HYPERTONIC SODIUM CHLORIDE SOLUTION

A. A salt solution that has an osmotic pressure greater than that of physiologic salt solution is hypertonic.
B. Preparation (household measurements): ½ teaspoonful salt added to ½ cup (4 ounces) of warm water.

IV. SODIUM BICARBONATE SOLUTION

Level ½ teaspoonful soda added to 1 cup (8 ounces) of warm water.

V. SODIUM CHLORIDE—SODIUM BICARBONATE SOLUTION (FLAVORED)

Sodium chloride	2.0 g (½ teaspoonful)
Sodium bicarbonate	1.0 g (¼ teaspoonful)
Amaranth solution	2.0 mL (½ teaspoonful)
Peppermint water to make	240.0 mL (8-ounce glass)

COMMERCIAL MOUTHRINSE INGREDIENTS[50]

Basic ingredients for both cosmetic and therapeutic oral rinses include water, alcohol, flavoring oils, and coloring materials.

I. WATER

Makes up the largest percentage by volume.

II. ALCOHOL

Ethyl alcohol is used to increase the solubility of the essential oils. The concentration may be as much as 15% to 30%. Alcohol lowers surface tension and is mildly astringent.

III. FLAVORING

Essential oils and their derivatives (eucalyptus oil, oil of wintergreen) or aromatic waters (peppermint, spearmint, wintergreen, or others) are used.

IV. COLORING

Must not discolor oral tissues.

V. SWEETENING AGENT

Artificial noncariogenic sweetener.

VI. ACTIVE INGREDIENTS

Commercial mouthrinses generally contain more than one active ingredient and, therefore, may advertise more than one claim for usefulness. Several factors influence how effective an agent may be, including the dilution by the saliva, the length of time the agent may be in contact with the tissue or bacteria, and the effect that contact with the organic matter of the mouth may have in changing the action. The following agents and products are for information only and should not be considered recommendations.

A. **Oxygenating Agents**[51]
1. *Purposes*
a. Cleansing. The effervescence makes these agents effective in debridement.
b. Antimicrobial. Action is limited; the agent is effective only as long as oxygen is being released.
2. *Active Ingredients*
Hydrogen peroxide (hydrogen peroxide USP diluted with water)
Sodium perborate
Urea peroxide
3. *Precaution.* Continued use of hydrogen peroxide solution, as well as of most other oxygen-liberating drugs after the treatment of a

disease, can lead to sponginess of the gingiva; formation of black hairy tongue; hypersensitivity of exposed root surfaces; and, because an acid is produced when water is added, demineralization of tooth surfaces.[52,53]

B. Astringents
1. *Purpose:* Shrink tissues.
2. *Use:* During impression making.
3. *Active Ingredients*

   Zinc chloride
   Zinc acetate
   Alum
   Tannic, acetic, and citric acids
4. *Precaution:* The agents are acid in water solution and can cause tooth demineralization and tissue irritation with repeated use.

C. Anodynes
1. *Purposes:* Alleviate pain, soothe sore spots.
2. *Uses:* Temporary pain relief for lesions of mucous membranes; during radiographic film exposure; as aid in impression making.
3. *Active Ingredients*

   Phenol derivatives
   Essential oils

D. Buffering Agents
1. *Purpose and Uses:* Reduce oral acidity created by the fermentation of food debris; dissolve mucinous films; give relief for soreness of soft tissues.
2. *Active Ingredients*

   Sodium borate solution NF
   Sodium perborate NF
   Sodium bicarbonate USP

E. Deodorizing Agents
1. *Purpose:* Neutralize odors from decomposed oral debris.
2. *Use:* Lessen possibility of halitosis from local causes.
3. *Active Ingredients:* Chlorophyll and other deodorizing agents.

F. Antimicrobial Agents
1. *Purposes*
   a. Reduce the oral microbacterial count.
   b. Inhibit bacterial activity.
2. *Active Ingredients*

Bisbiguanides	Chlorhexidine
	Alexidine
Bispyridines	Octenidine
Pyrimidines	Hexetidine
Halogens	Iodine
	Iodophores
	Fluorides
Phenolic compounds	Phenol; thymol
	Hexylresorcinol
	Listerine (thymol, eucalyptol, menthol; methylsalicylate)
Quaternary ammonium compounds	Cetylpyridinium chloride
	Benzethonium chloride
Herbal extract	Sanguinarine

CHLORHEXIDINE

Chlorhexidine has been tested extensively and has been shown to be the most effective antiplaque and antigingivitis chemotherapeutic agent available.

I. PREPARATIONS

A. 0.2% Chlorhexidine Gluconate
Early studies showed that twice-daily use of 0.2% rinse prevented bacterial plaque accumulation and gingivitis.[54] The 0.2% solution has been used extensively throughout the world except in the United States.

B. 0.12% Chlorhexidine Gluconate
The 0.12% solution has approval in the United States. Research has shown that the clinical effects of 0.12% mouthrinse compare favorably with those of the 0.2% mouthrinse.[55]

II. MECHANISM OF ACTION

A. Bactericidal
Chlorhexidine is active against a wide range of gram-positive and gram-negative microorganisms and fungi. It alters the bacterial cell wall so that lysis occurs, and the cell is destroyed.

B. Substantivity
Chlorhexidine is rapidly adsorbed to teeth and pellicle and is released slowly, thus prolonging the bactericidal effect.

III. CLINICAL USES
No chemotherapeutic agent is intended to substitute for mechanical plaque removal on a daily basis.
A. As a preprocedural rinse to lower the oral bacterial count and hence lower the contamination of aerosols produced during treatment procedures.
B. Decreases supragingival bacterial plaque formation and inhibits development of gingivitis.
C. Used for short-term adjunctive therapy following surgical treatment that limits the amount of mechanical plaque removal because of healing tissue, dressings, or accessibility.
D. Used for selected patients to control inflammation in necrotizing ulcerative gingivitis and to encourage and motivate patients when oral hygiene has been neglected for a period of time.
E. Suppresses *Streptococcus mutans;* prevents smooth surface dental caries.[56]

IV. SIDE EFFECTS

Brown staining of teeth has been the most generalized side effect. Certain patients, however, also develop one or more of the following conditions:

A. Temporary loss of taste.

B. Discomfort from the bitter taste of the mouthrinse. Masking with a flavoring agent has been customary with more recent commercial products.

C. Burning sensations of the mucosa.

D. Dryness and soreness of the mucosa.

E. Epithelial desquamation.

F. Discoloration of the teeth, tongue, and restorations.

G. Slight increase in supragingival calculus formation related to the dead bacteria that remain as a result of the bactericidal action of the chlorhexidine. The dead bacteria are trapped in the usual calculus formation process.

DENTIFRICES

A dentifrice is a substance used with a toothbrush or other applicator to remove bacterial plaque, materia alba, and debris from the gingiva and teeth for *cosmetic* and *sanitary* purposes, and for applying specific agents to the tooth surfaces for *preventive* and/or *therapeutic* purposes. As a result of research, current knowledge can be applied to aid the patient in the selection of an appropriate dentifrice that will benefit the teeth and gingiva and help to maintain them in a healthy state.

BASIC COMPONENTS[50]

Powder dentifrices contain abrasives, detergents, flavoring, and sweetener. Paste and gel dentifrices contain the same ingredients plus binders, humectants, preservative, and water. Either may have a coloring agent. The range of content of the various ingredients in commercially available dentifrices is as follows:

Detergent	1% to 2%
Cleaning and polishing agents	20% to 40%
Binder (thickener)	1% to 2%
Humectant	20% to 40%
Flavoring	1% to 1.5%
Water	20% to 40%
Therapeutic agent	1% to 2%
Preservative, sweetener, and coloring agent	2% to 3%

A therapeutic dentifrice has a drug or chemical agent added for a specific preventive or treatment action. In manufacturing products, a major problem is to combine agents that are compatible with each other.

I. DETERGENTS (FOAMING AGENTS OR SURFACTANTS)

A. Purposes

To lower surface tension; penetrate and loosen surface deposits and stains; emulsify debris for easy removal by the toothbrush; and contribute to the foaming action, which many people like.

B. Criteria for Use

Nontoxic, neutral in reaction, active in acid or alkaline media, stable, compatible with other dentifrice ingredients, no distinctive flavor, and foaming characteristics.

C. Substances Used

Sodium lauryl sulfate USP
Sodium n-lauryl sarcosinate

II. CLEANING AND POLISHING AGENTS

A dentifrice may have a combination of agents in an *abrasive system* to accommodate both cleaning and polishing objectives.

A. Purposes

An abrasive is used to clean, and a polishing agent is used to produce a smooth, shiny tooth surface that resists discoloration and bacterial accumulation and retention.

B. Criteria for Use

The ideal abrasive cleans well with no damage to the tooth surface and provides a high polish that can prevent or delay the reaccumulation of stains and deposits.

C. Abrasives Used

Calcium carbonate
Calcium pyrophosphate
Dicalcium phosphate, dihydrate
Dicalcium phosphate, anhydrous
Insoluble sodium metaphosphate (IMP)
Hydrated aluminum oxide
Silica, silicates, and dehydrated silica gels
For gel dentifrices:[50]
    Synthetic amorphous silica zerogel
    Synthetic amorphous complex aluminosilicate salt

III. BINDERS (THICKENERS)

A. Purpose

To prevent separation of the solid and liquid ingredients during storage.

B. Criteria

Stable, nontoxic, compatible with other ingredients.

C. Types Used

Organic hydrophilic colloids
Alginates
Synthetic derivatives of cellulose

Organic colloids require a preservative to prevent microbial growth.

IV. HUMECTANTS

A. Purposes

To retain moisture and prevent hardening on exposure to air; to stabilize the preparation.

B. Criteria

Stable, nontoxic.

C. Substances Used

Glycerin
Sorbitol
Propylene glycol

These agents require a preservative to prevent microbial growth.

V. PRESERVATIVES

A. Purpose

To prevent bacterial growth; to prolong shelf life.

B. Criterion

Compatible with other ingredients.

C. Substances Used

Alcohols
Benzoates
Formaldehyde
Dichlorinated phenols

VI. SWEETENING AGENTS

A. Purpose

To impart a pleasant flavor for patient acceptance.

B. Criterion

Must be noncariogenic.

C. Substances Used

Artificial noncariogenic sweetener
Sorbitol and glycerin, used as humectants, contribute to sweet flavor

VII. FLAVORING AGENTS

A. Purposes

To make the dentifrice desirable; to mask other ingredients that may have a less pleasant flavor.

B. Criteria

Remain unchanged during manufacturing and storage; compatible with other ingredients.

C. Substances Used

Essential oils (peppermint, cinnamon, wintergreen, clove)
Menthol
Artificial noncariogenic sweetener

VIII. COLORING AGENTS

A. Purpose

Attractiveness.

B. Criteria

Does not stain teeth or discolor other oral tissues.

C. Types

Vegetable dyes.

PROPHYLACTIC OR THERAPEUTIC DENTIFRICES

The American Dental Association, Council on Scientific Affairs evaluates dentifrices that claim therapeutic value.

I. ACTION OF THERAPEUTIC AGENTS[51]

A. Dental caries prevention
B. Tooth sensitivity reduction
C. Calculus formation reduction
D. Bacterial plaque formation reduction
E. Gingivitis reduction
F. Tooth-whitening cosmetic effect

II. DENTIFRICE SELECTION

The dentifrice that has been used by a patient should be recorded with other information about self-care habits when the dental history is prepared. Later the dentifrice must be evaluated and a change recommended when necessary in accord with the individual oral condition and treatment objectives.

There are specific reasons for recommending the use of particular dentifrices and for discouraging the use of others. The patient expects professional advice in keeping with current research. In addition to having ADA acceptance, the factors described in the following sections should be considered in dentifrice selection.

A. Dental Caries Control and Remineralization

Over the years, research on chlorophyll dentifrices; ammoniated dentifrices; dentifrices containing such enzyme inhibitors as sodium n-lauryl sarcosinate and sodium dehydroacetate; and antibiotics, such as penicillin and tyrothricin, contributed to the search for a major break into dental caries prevention. Research has shown that fluoride dentifrices contribute the greatest benefits at present.

Problems with dentifrice formulation have been related to finding compatible constituents to combine with the active ingredient in the dentifrice formula.

The use of a fluoride-containing dentifrice is generally recommended for all age groups and is mandatory for children. Fluoride for prevention of root caries is necessary after gingival recession and root exposure after periodontal therapy.

Fluoride dentifrices are described on page 471.

B. Gingival Health: Control of Bacterial Plaque

The health of the gingival tissue and the prevention of periodontal infections are prime objectives when using a toothbrush and interdental aids for bacterial plaque removal from proximal tooth surfaces. With the addition of a chemotherapeutic agent, the dentifrice can provide the medium for application of the agent to the teeth and gingiva.

C. Calculus-Prevention Agents

Ingredients and the properties and limitations of such agents are described with calculus, page 283. The "tartar-control" dentifrices also contain fluoride for dental caries prevention.

D. Desensitization

Fluorides and potassium nitrate are the principle agents shown to be effective. They are included with other methods of desensitization on page 600. Because most tooth sensitivity is related to areas of exposed dentin and cementum, attention must be paid to the abrasiveness of a dentifrice to avoid products that may uncover the dentinal tubules and cause additional sensitivity.

III. FACTORS AFFECTING ABRASIVENESS

A. Stiffness of the toothbrush used: the harder the brush, the more abrasive.

B. Force or pressure used during brushing: the greater the force, the more abrasive.

C. Concentration of the dentifrice: the greater the dilution, the less abrasive.

D. Exposure of cementum and/or dentin: patient needs instruction in the use of a brush with end-rounded filaments.

AMERICAN DENTAL ASSOCIATION ACCEPTANCE PROGRAM

Approval of a product is shown by use of the *ADA Seal of Acceptance* (Figure 24-15). The council publishes a list of all accepted items. The depth and importance of the seal program is recognized internationally.

I. PURPOSES

A. To determine the safety and effectiveness of a product.

B. To review advertising claims.

C. To inform the profession and the public about the safety and efficacy of the product.

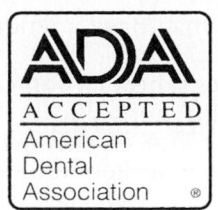

■ **FIGURE 24-15 Seal of Acceptance, The American Dental Association, Council on Scientific Affairs.** Seal may be used for therapeutics, materials, instruments, and equipment that meet ADA guidelines for safety and effectiveness.

II. PRODUCTS CONSIDERED

A. Drugs and chemicals used in the diagnosis, treatment, or prevention of oral diseases.

B. Chemicals that may affect the health of dentists, dental hygienists, other team members, and the public.

C. Dental materials, instruments, and equipment.

III. REQUIREMENTS

A. Information to Be Provided

1. Composition: properties and quantities of all ingredients and vehicles.

2. Objective data from clinical and laboratory studies.
   a. To support the product's safety and efficacy.
   b. ADA guidelines and protocol to be followed.

3. Advertising, promotional claims, and patient education materials.

B. Reapplication

1. Every 3 years.

2. Changes in the composition of any product require a new application at any time.

TECHNICAL HINTS

I. While preparing the patient's dental history, inquire about and record specific devices, dentifrices, mouthrinses, or other auxiliary aids used, in anticipation of evaluation for professional advice needed.

II. Request that a patient bring for demonstration a plaque control device being used to ensure that, although not producing symptoms currently, no harm is being done that could cause problems after long-term use.

III. Take care that preparations containing alcohol are not recommended for use by alcoholic patients, recovering alcoholic patients, or young people that may have a tendency toward alcoholism.

IV. Check patient history for risk of bacteremia and need for antibiotic premedication while teaching the use of new plaque removal devices. Those who floss only every 2 to 3 days are subject to bacteremia.[57]

FACTORS TO TEACH THE PATIENT

I. Significance of American Dental Association product acceptance stamp. How to select approved products.

II. Ask dental hygienist and dentist about new products and whether they are appropriate to use.

III. How to use each supplementary aid for bacterial plaque removal. Bring implements to the office for approval of how each is being used.

IV. Avoid prolonged use of commercial mouthrinses.

V. How to prepare saline rinse for use after a scaling appointment.

REFERENCES

1. **Smukler,** H., Nager, M.C., and Tolmie, P.C.: Interproximal Tooth Morphology and Its Effect on Plaque Removal, *Quintessence Int., 20,* 249, April, 1989.
2. **Gher,** M.E. and Vernino, A.R.: Root Morphology—Clinical Significance in Pathogenesis and Treatment of Periodontal Disease, *J. Am. Dent. Assoc., 101,* 627, October, 1980.
3. **Fox,** S.C. and Bosworth, B.L.: A Morphological Survey of Proximal Root Concavities: A Consideration in Periodontal Therapy, *J. Am. Dent. Assoc., 114,* 811, June, 1987.
4. **Ciancio,** S.G., Shibly, O., and Farber, G.A.: Clinical Evaluation of the Effect of Two Types of Dental Floss on Plaque and Gingival Health, *Clin. Prev. Dent., 14,* 14, May/June, 1992.
5. **Abelson,** D.C., Barton, J.E., Maietti, G.M., and Cowherd, M.G.: Evaluation of Interproximal Cleaning by Two Types of Dental Floss, *Clin. Prev. Dent., 3,* 19, July–August, 1981.
6. **Lobene,** R.R., Soparkar, P.M., and Newman, M.B.: Use of Dental Floss. Effect on Plaque and Gingivitis, *Clin. Prev. Dent., 4,* 5, January–February, 1982.
7. **Hanes,** P.J., O'Dell, N.L., Baker, M.R., Keagle, J.G., and Davis, H.C.: The Effect of Tensile Strength on the Clinical Effectiveness and Patient Acceptance of Dental Floss, *J. Clin. Periodontol., 19,* 30, January, 1992.
8. **Graves,** R.C., Disney, J.A., and Stamm, J.W.: Comparative Effectiveness of Flossing and Brushing in Reducing Interproximal Bleeding, *J. Periodontol., 60,* 243, May, 1989.
9. **Killoy,** W.J., Chairman, Discussion Section II, Consensus Report: *Proceedings of the World Workshop in Clinical Periodontics.* American Academy of Periodontology, Princeton, NJ, 1989, pp. 11–15.
10. **Hill,** H.C., Levi, P.A., and Glickman, I.: The Effects of Waxed and Unwaxed Dental Floss on Interdental Plaque Accumulation and Interdental Gingival Health, *J. Periodontol., 44,* 411, July, 1973.
11. **Lamberts,** D.M., Wunderlich, R.C., and Caffesse, R.G.: The Effect of Waxed and Unwaxed Dental Floss on Gingival Health. Part I. Plaque Removal and Gingival Response, *J. Periodontol., 53,* 393, June, 1982.
12. **Wunderlich,** R.C., Lamberts, D.M., and Caffesse, R.G.: The Effect of Waxed and Unwaxed Dental Floss on Gingival Health. Part II. Crevicular Fluid Flow and Gingival Bleeding, *J. Periodontol., 53,* 397, June, 1982.
13. **Beaumont,** R.H.: Patient Preference for Waxed or Unwaxed Dental Floss, *J. Periodontol., 61,* 123, February, 1990.
14. **Masters,** D.H.: Oral Hygiene Procedure for the Periodontal Patient, *Dent. Clin. North Am., 13,* 3, January, 1969.
15. **SUPER-FLOSS,** Oral-B Laboratories, Inc., 600 Clipper Drive, Belmont, CA 94002-4199.
16. **NU-FLOSS,** 1311 W. Webster Ave., Winter Park, FL 32789.
17. **Kiger,** R.D., Nylund, K., and Feller, R.P.: A Comparison of Proximal Plaque Removal Using Floss and Interdental Brushes, *J. Clin. Periodontol., 18,* 681, October, 1991.
18. **Lugassy,** A.A., Lautenschlager, E.P., and Katrana, D.: Characterization of Water Spray Devices, *J. Dent. Res., 50,* 466, March–April, 1971.
19. **Cobb,** C.M., Rodgers, R.L., and Killoy, W.J.: Ultrastructural Examination of Human Periodontal Pockets Following the Use of an Oral Irrigation Device *in vivo, J. Periodontol., 59,* 155, March, 1988.
20. **Felo,** A., Shibly, O., Ciancio, S.G., Lauciello, F.R., and Ho, A.: Effects of Subgingival Chlorhexidine Irrigation on Peri-implant Maintenance, *Am. J. Dent., 10,* 107, April, 1997.
21. **Ciancio,** S.G., Mather, M.L., Zambon, J.J., and Reynolds, H.S.: Effect of a Chemotherapeutic Agent Delivered by an Oral Irrigation Device on Plaque, Gingivitis, and Subgingival Microflora, *J. Periodontol., 60,* 310, June, 1989.
22. **Flemmig,** T.F., Newman, M.G., Doherty, F.M., Grossman, E., Meckel, A.H., and Bakdash, M.B.: Supragingival Irrigation with 0.06% Chlorhexidine in Naturally Occurring Gingivitis. I. 6 Month Clinical Observations, *J. Periodontol., 61,* 112, February, 1990.
23. **Brownstein,** C.N., Briggs, S.D., Schweitzer, K.L., Briner, W.W., and Kornman, K.S.: Irrigation with Chlorhexidine to Resolve Naturally Occurring Gingivitis, *J. Clin. Periodontol., 17,* 588, September, 1990.
24. **Newman,** M.G., Flemmig, T.F., Nachnani, S., Rodrigues, A., Calsina, G., Lee, Y.-S., deCamargo, P., Doherty, F.M., and Bakdash, B.: Irrigation with 0.06% Chlorhexidine in Naturally Occurring Gingivitis. II. 6 Months Microbiological Observations, *J. Periodontol., 61,* 427, July, 1990.
25. **Wunderlich,** R.C., Singleton, M., O'Brien, W.J., and Caffesse, R.G.: Subgingival Penetration of an Applied Solution, *Int. J. Periodontics Restorative Dent., 4,* 64, Number 5, 1984.
26. **Eakle,** W.S., Ford, C., and Boyd, R.L.: Depth of Penetration in Periodontal Pockets with Oral Irrigation, *J. Clin. Periodontol., 13,* 39, January, 1986.
27. **Boyd,** R.L., Hollander, B.N., and Eakle, W.S.: Comparison of a Subgingivally Placed Cannula Oral Irrigator Tip with a Supragingivally Placed Standard Irrigator Tip, *J. Clin. Periodontol., 19,* 340, May, 1992.
28. **Braun,** R.E. and Ciancio, S.G.: Subgingival Delivery by an Oral Irrigation Device, *J. Periodontol., 63,* 469, May, 1992.
29. **Krust,** K.S., Drisko, C.L., Gross, K., Overman, P., and Tira, D.E.: The Effects of Subgingival Irrigation with Chlorhexidine and Stannous Fluoride. A Preliminary Investigation, *J. Dent. Hyg., 65,* 289, July–August, 1991.
30. **Walsh,** T.F., Glenwright, H.D., and Hull, P.S.: Clinical Effects of Pulsed Oral Irrigation with 0.2% Chlorhexidine Digluconate in Patients with Adult Periodontitis, *J. Clin. Periodontol., 19,* 245, April, 1992.
31. **Mazza,** J.E., Newman, M.G., and Sims, T.N.: Clinical and Antimicrobial Effect of Stannous Fluoride on Periodontitis, *J. Clin. Periodontol., 8,* 203, June, 1981.
32. **Boyd,** R.L., Leggott, P., Quinn, R., Buchanan, S., Eakle, W., and Chambers, D.: Effect of Self-administered Daily Irrigation with 0.02% SnF_2 on Periodontal Disease Activity, *J. Clin. Periodontol., 12,* 420, July, 1985.
33. **Schmid,** E., Kornman, K.S., and Tinanoff, N.: Changes of Subgingival Total Colony Forming Units and Black Pigmented Bacteroides After a Single Irrigation of Periodontal Pockets with 1.64% SnF_2, *J. Periodontol., 56,* 330, June, 1985.
34. **Harper,** D.S., Gordon, J., Fine, J., and Hovliaras, C.: Effect of

Subgingival Irrigation with an Antiseptic Mouthrinse on Periodontal Pocket Microflora, *J. Dent. Res., 70,* 324, Abstract No. 474, Special Issue, April, 1991.

35. **Southard,** G.L., Parsons, L.G., Thomas, L.G., Woodall, I.R., and Jones, B.J.B.: Effect of Sanguinaria Extract on Development of Plaque and Gingivitis when Supragingivally Delivered as a Manual Rinse or Under Pressure in an Oral Irrigator, *J. Clin. Periodontol., 14,* 377, August, 1987.
36. **Parsons,** L.G., Thomas, L.G., Southard, G.L., Woodall, I.R., and Jones, B.J.B.: Effect of Sanguinaria Extract on Established Plaque and Gingivitis when Supragingivally Delivered as a Manual Rinse or Under Pressure in an Oral Irrigator, *J. Clin. Periodontol., 14,* 381, August, 1987.
37. **Fine,** J.B., Harper, D.S., Gordon, J.M., Hovliaras, C.A., and Charles, C.H.: Short-term Microbiological and Clinical Effects of Subgingival Irrigation with an Antimicrobial Mouthrinse, *J. Periodontol., 65,* 30, January, 1994.
38. **Newman,** M.G., Cattabriga, M., Etienne, D., Flemmig, T., Sanz, M., Kornman, K.S., Doherty, F., Moore, D.J., and Ross, C.: Effectiveness of Adjunctive Irrigation in Early Periodontitis: Multi-center Evaluation, *J. Periodontol., 65,* 224, March, 1994.
39. **Chaves,** E.S., Kornman, K.S., Manwell, M.A., Jones, A.A., Newbold, D.A., and Wood, R.C.: Mechanism of Irrigation Effects on Gingivitis, *J. Periodontol., 65,* 1016, November, 1994.
40. **Flemmig,** T.F., Epp, B., Funkenhauser, Z., Newman, M.G., Kornman, K.S., Haubitz, I., and Klaiber, B.: Adjunctive Supragingival Irrigation with Acetylsalicyclic Acid in Periodontal Supportive Therapy, *J. Clin. Periodontol., 22,* 427, June, 1995.
41. **Phelps-Sandall,** B.A. and Oxford, S.J.: Effectiveness of Oral Hygiene Techniques on Plaque and Gingivitis in Patients Placed in Intermaxillary Fixation, *Oral Surg. Oral Med. Oral Pathol., 56,* 487, November, 1983.
42. **Dajani,** A.S., Taubert, K.A., Wilson, W., Bolger, A.F., Bayer, A., Ferrieri, P., Gewitz, M.H., Shulman, S.T., Nouri, S., Newburger, J.W., Hutto, C., Pallasch, T.J., Gage, T.W., Levison, M.E., Peter, G., and Zuccaro, G.: Prevention of Bacterial Endocarditis. Recommendations by the American Heart Association, *JAMA, 277,* 1794, June 11, 1997.
43. **Romans,** A.R. and App, G.R.: Bacteremia, a Result from Oral Irrigation in Subjects with Gingivitis, *J. Periodontol., 42,* 757, December, 1971.
44. **Felix,** J.E., Rosen, S., and App, G.R.: Detection of Bacteremia after the Use of an Oral Irrigation Device in Subjects with Periodontitis, *J. Periodontol., 42,* 785, December, 1971.
45. **Pitcher,** G.R., Newman, H.N., and Strahan, J.D.: Access to Subgingival Plaque by Disclosing Agents Using Mouthrinsing and Direct Irrigation, *J. Clin. Periodontol., 7,* 300, August, 1980.
46. **Scopp,** I.W. and Orvieto, L.D.: Gingival Degerming by Povidone-iodine Irrigation: Bacteremia Reduction in Extraction Procedures, *J. Am. Dent. Assoc., 83,* 1294, December, 1971.
47. **Veksler,** A.E., Kayrouz, G.A., and Newman, M.G.: Reduction of Salivary Bacteria by Pre-procedural Rinses with Chlorhexidine 0.12%, *J. Periodontol., 62,* 649, November, 1991.
48. **Fine,** D.H., Mendieta, C., Barnett, M.L., Furgang, D., Meyers, R., Olshan, A., and Vincent, J.: Efficacy of Preprocedural Rinsing with an Antiseptic in Reducing Viable Bacteria in Dental Aerosols, *J. Periodontol., 63,* 821, October, 1992.
49. **Newbrun,** E.: Chemical and Mechanical Removal of Plaque, *Compend. Cont. Educ. Dent., 6,* S110, Supplement No. 6, 1985.
50. **Volpe,** A.R.: Dentifrices and Mouth Rinses, in Stallard, R.E., ed.: *A Textbook of Preventive Dentistry,* 2nd ed. Philadelphia, W.B. Saunders Co., 1982, pp. 170–216.
51. **Mariotti,** A.J.: Mouthrinses and Dentifrices, in American Dental Association, Council on Scientific Affairs: *ADA Guide to Dental Therapeutics.* Chicago, ADA Publishing Co., 1998, pp. 199–213.
52. **Ciancio,** S.G.: Non-surgical Periodontal Treatment, in *Proceedings of the World Workshop in Clinical Periodontics.* American Academy of Periodontology, Princeton, NJ, 1989, p. II-2.
53. **Rees,** T.D. and Orth, C.F.: Oral Ulcerations with Use of Hydrogen Peroxide, *J. Periodontol., 57,* 689, November, 1986.
54. **Löe,** H. and Schiøtt, C.R.: The Effect of Mouthrinses and Topical Application of Chlorhexidine on the Development of Dental Plaque and Gingivitis in Man, *J. Periodont. Res., 5,* 79, Number 2, 1970.
55. **Segreto,** V.A., Collins, E.M., Beiswanger, B.B., de la Rosa, M., Isaacs, R.L., Lang, N.P., Mallatt, M.E., and Meckel, A.H.: A Comparison of Mouthrinses Containing Two Concentrations of Chlorhexidine, *J. Periodont. Res., 21,* 23, Supplement Number 16, 1986.
56. **van Rijkom,** H.M., Truin, G.J., and van't Hof, M.A.: A Meta-analysis of Clinical Studies on the Caries-inhibiting Effect of Chlorhexidine Treatment, *J. Dent. Res., 75,* 790, February, 1996.
57. **Carroll,** G.C. and Sebor, R.J.: Dental Flossing and Its Relationship to Transient Bacteremia, *J. Periodontol., 51,* 691, December, 1980.

SUGGESTED READINGS

Addy, M. and Moran, J.M.: Evaluation of Oral Hygiene Products: Science is True; Don't Be Misled by the Facts, *Periodontology 2000, 15,* 40, 1997.

Seymour, R.A. and Heasman, P.A.: Pharmacological Control of Periodontal Disease. II. Antimicrobial Agents, *J. Dent., 23,* 5, February, 1995.

Tipton, D.A., Braxton, S.D., and Dabbous, M.K.: Effects of a Bleaching Agent on Human Gingival Fibroblasts, *J. Periodontol., 66,* 7, January, 1995.

Whall, C.W.: The How and Why of the ADA's Evaluation Program for Dental Therapeutic Products, *J. Public Health Dent., 52,* 338, Number 6, Special Issue, 1992.

Interdental Care

Beatty, C.F., Fallon, P.A., and Marshall, D.D.: A Comparison of the Effectiveness of Two Wooden Interdental Cleaners, *Contact Internat, 12,* 6, June, 1998.

Carter-Hanson, C., Gadbury-Amyot, C., and Killoy, W.: Comparison of the Plaque Removal Efficacy of a New Flossing Aid (Quik Floss®) to Finger Flossing, *J. Clin. Periodontol., 23,* 873, September, 1996.

Caton, J.G., Blieden, T.M., Lowenguth, R.A., Frantz, B.J., Wagener, C.J., Doblin, J.M., Stein, S.H., and Proskin, H.M.: Comparison Between Mechanical Cleaning and an Antimicrobial Rinse for the Treatment and Prevention of Interdental Gingivitis, *J. Clin. Periodontol., 20,* 172, March, 1993.

Checchi, L., Biagini, G., Zucchini, C., and DeLuca, M.: Clinical and Morphologic Response to Interdental Brushing Therapy, *Quintessence Int., 22,* 483, June, 1991.

Kleisner, J. and Imfeld, T.: Evaluation of the Efficacy of Interdental Cleaning Devices. How to Design a Clinical Study, *J. Clin. Periodontol., 20,* 707, November, 1993.

Latcham, N.: The Effect of Overhang Removal on Increasing Patients' Flossing Frequency, *Clin. Prev. Dent., 12,* 22, April–May, 1990.

Rodrigues, C.R., Ando, T., Singer, J.M., and Issáo, M.: The Effect of Training on the Ability of Children to Use Dental Floss, *ASDC J. Dent. Child., 63,* 39, January–February, 1996.

Irrigation

Asari, A.M., Newman, H.N., Wilson, M., and Bulman, J.S.: 0.1%/0.2% Commercial Chlorhexidine Solutions as Subgingival Irrigants in Chronic Periodontitis, *J. Clin. Periodontol., 23,* 320, April, 1996.

Cline, N.V.: Subgingival Irrigation: Efficacy in Nonsurgical Periodontal Therapy, *Access, 11,* 14, February, 1997.

Greenstein, G.: Subgingival Irrigation—An Adjunct to Periodontal Therapy. Current Status and Future Directions, *J. Dent. Hyg., 64,* 389, October, 1990.

Greenstein, G.: Supragingival and Subgingival Irrigation: Practical Application in the Treatment of Periodontal Diseases, *Compend. Cont. Educ. Dent., 13,* 1098, December, 1992.

Linden, G.J. and Newman, H.N.: The Effects of Subgingival Irrigation with Low Dosage Metronidazole on Periodontal Inflammation, *J. Clin. Periodontol., 18,* 177, March, 1991.

Shiloah, J. and Hovious, L.A.: The Role of Subgingival Irrigations in the Treatment of Periodontitis, *J. Periodontol., 64,* 835, September, 1993.

Stein, M.: A Literature Review. Oral Irrigation Therapy. The Adjunctive Roles for Home and Professional Use, *Can. Dent. Hyg. Assoc./Probe, 27,* 18, January/February, 1993.

Mouthrinses

Binney, A., Addy, M., and Newcombe, R.G.: The Effect of a Number of Commercial Mouthrinses Compared with Toothpaste on Plaque Regrowth, *J. Periodontol., 63,* 839, October, 1992.

Brecx, M., Brownstone, E., MacDonald, L., Gelskey, S., and Cheang, M.: Efficacy of Listerine®, Meridol®, and Chlorhexidine Mouthrinses as Supplements to Regular Toothcleaning Measures, *J. Periodontol., 19,* 202, March, 1992.

Fine, D.: Evaluation of Antimicrobial Mouthrinses and Their Bactericidal Effectiveness, *J. Am. Dent. Assoc., 125,* 11-S, Supplement, August, 1994.

Jenkins, S., Addy, M., and Newcombe, R.: Evaluation of a Mouthrinse Containing Chlorhexidine and Fluoride as an Adjunct to Oral Hygiene, *J. Clin. Periodontol., 20,* 20, January, 1993.

Jenkins, S., Addy, M., and Newcombe, R.G.: A Comparison of Cetylpyridinium Chloride, Triclosan and Chlorhexidine Mouthrinse Formulations for Effects on Plaque Regrowth, *J. Clin. Periodontol., 21,* 441, July, 1994.

Mandel, I.D.: Antimicrobial Mouthrinses: Overview and Update, *J. Am. Dent. Assoc., 125,* 2S, Supplement, August, 1994.

Ramberg, P., Furuichi, Y., Volpe, A.R., Gaffar, A., and Lindhe, J.: The Effects of Antimicrobial Mouthrinses on de novo Plaque Formation at Sites with Healthy and Inflamed Gingivae, *J. Clin. Periodontol., 23,* 7, January, 1996.

Renton-Harper, P., Addy, M., Moran, J., Doherty, F.M., and Newcombe, R.G.: A Comparison of Chlorhexidine, Cetylpyridinium Chloride, Triclosan, and C31G Mouthrinse Products for Plaque Inhibition, *J. Periodontol., 67,* 486, May, 1996.

Rethman, J.: A Clinical Overview of Oral Rinses, *J. Pract. Hyg., 6,* 17, January/February, 1997.

Settembrini, L., Penugonda, B., Scherer, W., Strassler, H., and Hittelman, E.: Alcohol-containing Mouthwashes: Effect on Composite Color, *Operative Dent., 20,* 14, January–February, 1995.

Dentifrices

Addy, M., Greenman, J., Renton-Harper, P., Newcombe, R., and Doherty, F.: Studies on Stannous Fluoride Toothpaste and Gel.(Part 2). Effects on Salivary Bacterial Counts and Plaque Regrowth *in vivo, J. Clin. Periodontol., 24,* 86, February, 1997.

Binney, A., Addy, M., McKeown, S., and Everett, L.: The Choice of Controls in Toothpaste Studies. The Effect of a Number of Commercially Available Toothpastes Compared to Water on 4-day Plaque Regrowth, *J. Clin. Periodontol., 23,* 456, May, 1996.

Cutress, T., Howell, P.T., Finidori, C., and Abdullah, F.: Caries Preventive Effect of High Fluoride and Xylitol Containing Dentifrices, *ASDC J. Dent. Child., 59,* 313, July–August, 1992.

Hill, M. and Moore, R.L.: Advances in Home Therapy for Gingivitis—Revolution or Evolution? *J. Pract. Hyg., 6,* 2, Supplement, November–December, 1997.

Jenkins, S., Addy, M., and Newcombe, R.: The Effects of a Chlorhexidine Toothpaste on the Development of Plaque, Gingivitis and Tooth Staining, *J. Clin. Periodontol., 20,* 59, January, 1993.

Levy, S.M., Maurice, T.J., and Jakobsen, J.R.: Dentifrice Use Among Preschool Children, *J. Am. Dent. Assoc., 124,* 57, September, 1993.

Owens, J., Addy, M., and Faulkner, J.: An 18-week Home-use Study Comparing the Oral Hygiene and Gingival Health Benefits of Triclosan and Fluoride Toothpastes, *J. Clin. Periodontol., 24,* 626, September, 1997.

Wade, W., Addy, M., Hughes, J., Milsom, S., and Doherty, F.: Studies on Stannous Fluoride Toothpaste and Gel. (Part 1). Antimicrobial Properties and Staining Potential *in vitro, J. Clin. Periodontol., 24,* 81, February, 1997.

Walker, C., Borden, L.C., Zambon, J.J., Bonta, C.Y., DeVizio, W., and Volpe, A.R.: The Effects of a 0.3% Triclosan-containing Dentifrice on the Microbial Composition of Supragingival Plaque, *J. Clin. Periodontol., 21,* 334, May, 1994.

Chlorhexidine

Al-Tannir, M.A. and Goodman, H.S.: A Review of Chlorhexidine and Its Use in Special Populations, *Spec. Care Dentist., 14,* 116, May/June, 1994.

Christie, P., Claffey, N., and Renvert, S.: The Use of 0.2% Chlorhexidine in the Absence of a Structured Mechanical Regimen of Oral Hygiene Following the Non-surgical Treatment of Periodontitis, *J. Clin. Periodontol., 25,* 15, January, 1998.

Emilson, C.G.: Potential Efficacy of Chlorhexidine Against *Mutans streptococci* and Human Dental Caries, *J. Dent. Res., 73,* 682, March, 1994.

Johnson, B.T.: Uses of Chlorhexidine in Dentistry, *Gen. Dent., 43,* 126, March–April, 1995.

Kidd, E.A.M.: Role of Chlorhexidine in the Management of Dental Caries, *Int. Dent. J., 41,* 279, October, 1991.

Lee, Y.C., Charles, S.L., and Holborow, D.W.: The Effect of Local Application of Chlorhexidine on Plaque and Gingivitis, *New Zeal. Dent. J., 92,* 13, March, 1996.

McKenzie, W.T., Forgas, L., Vernino, A.R., Parker, D., and Limestall, J.D.: Comparison of a 0.12% Chlorhexidine Mouthrinse and an Essential Oil Mouthrinse on Oral Health in Institutionalized, Mentally Handicapped Adults: One-year Results, *J. Periodontol., 63,* 187, March, 1992.

Mendieta, C., Vallcorba, N., Binney, A., and Addy, M.: Comparison of 2 Chlorhexidine Mouthwashes on Plaque Regrowth *in vivo* and Dietary Staining *in vitro, J. Clin. Periodontol., 21,* 296, April, 1994.

Owens, J., Addy, M., Faulkner, J., Lockwood, C., and Adair, R.: A Short-term Clinical Study Design to Investigate the Chemical Plaque Inhibitory Properties of Mouthrinses When Used as Adjuncts to Toothpastes: Applied to Chlorhexidine, *J. Clin. Periodontol., 24,* 732, October, 1997.

Persson, R.E., Truelove, E.L., LeResche, L., and Robinovitch, M.R.: Therapeutic Effects of Daily or Weekly Chlorhexidine Rinsing on Oral Health of a Geriatric Population, *Oral Surg. Oral Med. Oral Pathol., 72,* 184, August, 1991.

Pilatti, G.L. and Sampaio, J.E.C.: The Influence of Chlorhexidine on the Severity of Cyclosporin A–induced Gingival Overgrowth, *J. Periodontol., 68,* 900, September, 1997.

Sanz, M., Vallcorba, N., Fabreques, S., Muller, I., and Herkströter, F.: The Effect of a Dentifrice Containing Chlorhexidine and Zinc on Plaque, Gingivitis, Calculus and Tooth Staining, *J. Clin. Periodontol., 21,* 431, July, 1994.

Smith, R.G., Moran, J., Addy, M., Doherty, F., and Newcombe, R.G.: Comparative Staining *in vitro* and Plaque Inhibitory Properties *in vivo* of 0.12% and 0.2% Chlorhexidine Mouthrinses, *J. Clin. Periodontol., 22,* 613, August, 1995.

Tellefsen, G., Larsen, G., Kaligithi, R., Zimmerman, G.J., and Wikesjo, U.M.E.: Use of Chlorhexidine Chewing Gum Significantly Reduces Dental Plaque Formation Compared to Use of Similar Xylitol and Sorbitol Products, *J. Periodontol., 67,* 181, March, 1996.

Peroxide

American Dental Association, Council on Dental Therapeutics: Guidelines for the Acceptance of Peroxide-containing Oral Hygiene Products, *J. Am. Dent. Assoc., 125,* 1140, August, 1994.

Harfst, S.: Baking Soda Revisited, *DentalHygienistNews, 4,* 7, Fall, 1991.

Lewinstein, I., Hirschfeld, Z., Stabbolz, A., and Rotstein, I.: Effect of Hydrogen Peroxide and Sodium Perborate on the Microhardness of Human Enamel and Dentin, *J. Endodont., 20,* 61, February, 1994.

Marshall, M.V., Cancro, L.P., and Fischman, S.L.: Hydrogen Peroxide: A Review of Its Use in Dentistry, *J. Periodontol., 66,* 786, September, 1995.

Triclosan

Furuichi, Y., Ramberg, P., Krok, L., and Lindhe, J.: Short-term Effects of Triclosan on Healing Following Subgingival Scaling, *J. Clin. Periodontol., 24*, 777, October, 1997.

Gaffar, A., Scherl, D., Afflitto, J., and Coleman, E.J.: The Effect of Triclosan on Mediators of Gingival Inflammation, *J. Clin. Periodontol., 22*, 480, June, 1995.

Lindhe, J., Rosling, B., Socransky, S.S., and Volpe, A.R.: The Effect of a Triclosan-containing Dentifrice on Established Plaque and Gingivitis, *J. Clin. Periodontol., 20*, 327, May, 1993.

Mankodi, S., Walker, C., Conforti, N., DeVizio, W., McCool, J.J., and Volpe, A.R.: Clinical Effect of a Triclosan-containing Dentifrice on Plaque and Gingivitis: A Six-month Study, *Clin. Prev. Dent., 14*, 4, November–December, 1992.

Moran, J., Addy, M., and Newcombe, R.: A 4-day Plaque Regrowth Study Comparing an Essential Oil Mouthrinse with a Triclosan Mouthrinse, *J. Clin. Periodontol., 24*, 636, September, 1997.

Ramberg, P., Furuichi, Y., Sherl, D., Volpe, A.R., Nabi, N., Gaffar, A., and Lindhe, J.: The Effect of Triclosan on Developing Gingivitis, *J. Clin. Periodontol., 22*, 442, June, 1995.

Rosling, B., Wannfors, B., Volpe, A.R., Furuichi, Y., Ramberg, P., and Lindhe, J.: The Use of Triclosan/copolymer Dentifrice May Retard the Progression of Periodontitis, *J. Clin. Periodontol., 24*, 873, December, 1997.

Rosling, B., Dahlen, G., Volpe, A., Furuichi, Y., Ramberg, P., and Lindhe, J.: Effect of Triclosan on the Subgingival Microbiota of Periodontitis-susceptible Subjects, *J. Clin. Periodontol., 24*, 881, December, 1997.

Wade, W.G. and Addy, M.: Antibacterial Activity of Some Triclosan-containing Toothpastes and Their Ingredients, *J. Periodontol., 63*, 280, April, 1992.

25

Care of Dental Prostheses

Total cleanliness of the oral cavity for the health of the teeth and supporting structures involves specific procedures for the care of the natural teeth and all replacements, both fixed and removable. A *prosthesis* is an artificial replacement of a missing part of the body, and a dental prosthesis replaces one or more teeth. Other definitions may be studied in Box 25-1. Additional definitions pertaining to orthodontic appliances are included in Box 41-1 (see page 637).

The fit and function of a dental prosthesis depend to a large degree on the cooperation of the patient in daily cleaning of the prosthesis and bacterial plaque control for the remaining natural teeth. Likewise, orthodontic appliances must be kept clean and peri-odontal health maintained if the treatment is to have long-term success.

The patient's cooperation depends to a degree on the motivation, information, and sense of appreciation and concern imparted by the members of the dental team. For the natural teeth involved, instruction begins early, before construction of the partial denture or placement of orthodontic appliances. Instruction is supplemented when an appliance is inserted to demonstrate specific techniques for daily care. Continuing supervision and review of procedures at succeeding appointments and maintenance appointments are required.

A patient may have more than one prosthesis. For

BOX 25-1 KEY WORDS: Dental Prostheses*

Abutment (ah-but'ment): a tooth or implant used for the support or retention of a fixed or removable prosthesis.

Denture (den'chur): artificial substitute for missing natural teeth and adjacent tissues.

Complete denture: dental prosthesis that replaces the entire dentition and associated structures; may be a complete maxillary denture or a complete mandibular, or both.

Immediate denture: a complete or removable partial denture fabricated in advance for placement immediately following the removal of natural teeth.

Fixed partial denture: a replacement for one or more missing teeth that is securely retained to natural teeth, tooth roots, and/or dental implant abutments that furnish the primary support for the prosthesis; also called a fixed prosthesis.

Removable partial denture: a dental prosthesis that supplies teeth and/or associated structures in a partially edentulous jaw and can be removed and replaced at will.

Denture adhesive: a soft material used to adhere a denture to the underlying mucosa; also referred to as an adherent.

Hawley retainer: a removable plastic and wire appliance used to stabilize teeth; may be modified for special applications during or after orthodontic therapy.

Obturator (ob'tŭ-rā'tor): a prosthesis used to close a congenital or acquired opening, such as for a cleft palate, an area lost because of trauma, or after surgery for removal of a diseased area.

Pontic (pon'tik): an artificial tooth on a partial denture that replaces a missing natural tooth, restores its function, and usually occupies the space previously filled by the natural crown.

Precision attachment: a type of connector that consists of a metal receptacle and a close-fitting part; the metal receptacle usually is included within the restoration of an abutment tooth, and the close-fitting part is attached to a pontic or removable partial denture framework.

Preventive orthodontics: dental services intended to prevent the development of a malocclusion by maintaining the integrity of an otherwise normally developing dentition.

Prosthesis (pros-thē'sĭs): artificial replacement of an absent part of the body; may be a therapeutic device to improve or alter function; may be a device employed to aid in accomplishing a desired surgical result.

Rest: a rigid, stabilizing extension of a fixed or removable partial denture that contacts a remaining tooth or teeth; prevents movement toward the mucosa and transmits functional forces to the teeth.

Space maintainer: prosthetic replacement for prematurely lost primary teeth to prevent closure of the space before eruption of the permanent successors.

*Definitions in this chapter that pertain to prosthodontics are taken or adapted from and are in accord with the *Glossary of Prosthodontic Terms*, 6th ed., 1993, of the Academy of Prosthodontics Foundation.
   Definitions pertaining to orthodontic appliances are taken or adapted from the Orthodontic Glossary of the American Society of Orthodontists.

---

example, a complete maxillary denture may be accompanied by both fixed and removable partial dentures in the mandibular arch. For this patient, the regimen for personal care involves the natural teeth as well as the fixed and removable dentures. A program of instruction must be worked out for each patient, depending on individual needs. Examples of fixed and removable prostheses and appliances are listed in Table 25-1.

ORTHODONTIC APPLIANCES

Without a strong and persistent preventive care program before, during, and following completion of orthodontic treatment, a high dental caries rate has been associated with orthodontic treatment. Gingival and periodontal infections during and following treatment are not unusual. An individualized preventive

program that includes a specific plan of instruction, motivation, and supervision is essential for the patient with orthodontic appliances. The patient must understand that much more effort is required while in treatment than was required before the appliances were placed.

The patient may be under care with regular appointments for a long period, frequently over a few years. Periodic communication between the patient's referring dentist and dental hygienist is necessary to coordinate instruction along with other necessary dental and dental hygiene care.

I. COMPLICATING FACTORS

A. Age Group

Many orthodontic patients are in the preteen and teenage years, periods when the incidence of gingivitis is high. The incidence of periodon-

TABLE 25-1   Types of Oral Prostheses and Appliances

FIXED

Orthodontic appliance
Space maintainer
Fixed partial denture
Periodontal splint
Implant-supported complete denture

REMOVABLE

Removable orthodontic appliance
Removable space maintainer
Hawley appliance
Removable partial denture
   Natural teeth supported
   Implant supported
Complete denture
Overdenture
Obturator

tal infection increases from early childhood to late teenage years.

B. Gingivitis

Bacterial plaque retention by orthodontic appliances leads to gingivitis. The degree can vary from slight to severe with gingival enlargement, particularly of the interdental papillae. The tissue may greatly enlarge and cover the fixed appliance. The enlarged tissue with pockets provides additional plaque-retentive areas.

C. Position of Teeth

Teeth that are irregularly positioned are naturally more susceptible to the retention of bacterial deposits and are more difficult to clean. With the severe malocclusions presented by orthodontic patients at the outset, this factor becomes even more significant.

D. Problems With Appliances

1. Orthodontic appliances retain plaque and debris.
2. Accidents may cause wires to bend adversely and become embedded in the gingiva. A loosened band may be forced under the gingiva.
3. Removable appliances or their clasps may press excessively against the gingiva.
4. Rubber bands used during therapy may slip under the gingiva and detach the junctional epithelium.

E. Self-Care Is Difficult

Even the patient who tries to maintain oral cleanliness has difficulty because the appliances are in the way and interfere with the application of the toothbrush and other devices used for plaque control.

II. DISEASE CONTROL

A rigid program for dental caries and periodontal disease control is needed. The selection of plaque control procedures for an individual patient is determined by the anatomic features of the gingiva, the position of the teeth, and the type and position of the orthodontic appliance.

Many types of appliances are utilized for orthodontic treatment. Fixed orthodontic appliances may consist of brackets bonded directly to the tooth surfaces after an acid etch procedure, as shown in Figure 41-1 (page 637). Other appliances are bands cemented around each tooth with brackets attached to the bands to support an arch wire. Figures 25-2 and 25-3 show teeth with complete bands.

A. General Instructions

1. Give instructions before appliances are placed. Every attempt must be made to have the oral tissues in health and the patient motivated to perform thorough daily plaque removal.
2. Perform brushing before a mirror so that brush application is accurate and brushing is thorough.
3. Use a disclosing solution rinse to assist in self-evaluation. Orthodontic patients may experience difficulty in chewing disclosing wafers without discomfort or pain.
4. Recommend an approved fluoride dentifrice to aid in dental caries control.
5. Place emphasis in brushing on sulcular brushing and cleaning the area between the orthodontic bands and brackets and the gingiva.

B. Toothbrushing: Brush Selection

1. *Soft brush.* A soft brush with end-rounded filaments generally is recommended.
2. *Bi-level.* A special bi-level orthodontic brush designed with spaced rows of soft nylon filaments and with a middle row that is shorter can be applied directly over the fixed appliance. It is used with a short horizontal stroke (Figure 25-1).
3. *Power-assisted.* Used with soft filaments, a light stroke, and at a low speed, power-assisted brushes have been shown very effective for gingival health and cleaning around appliances.

C. Brushing Procedure

1. *Sulcular brushing.* A sulcular method is needed by most patients for cleaning the appliances and maintaining the gingiva.
2. *Adapt for appliance.* Special adaptation is required for facial surfaces. Place the brush with filament ends directed toward the occlusal surface (Charters position, see Figure 23-8) to clean over the wire and bracket (or under for mandibular arch); place in Still-

man position for the opposite side (Figure 25-2).

3. *Clean all surfaces.* To ensure cleanliness, one should brush the appliances in any way that the filaments can be manipulated. Insert the brush from below, over, and above the arch wire; rotate and vibrate to remove plaque and debris.

4. *Lingual and palatal.* Approach to brushing is similar to the basic strokes used on the facial surfaces.

D. Additional Measures

1. *Interdental Aids.* The previously described applications for the interdental tip and toothpick in holder (pages 378 and 379) also apply for care of the orthodontic patient (Figure 25-3).

   A floss threader is needed for plaque removal from proximal tooth surfaces when the appliance prevents passage of floss from the occlusal aspect. Tufted dental floss or yarn used in the floss threader can remove plaque more efficiently than can regular dental floss.

   An interdental brush and a single-tuft brush can be particularly beneficial around individual teeth. The entire system should be kept as simple as possible.

2. *Oral Irrigation.*[1] Most orthodontic patients can benefit from the regular use of an irrigator for removal of loose bacterial plaque and food debris and prevention of gingival inflammation.

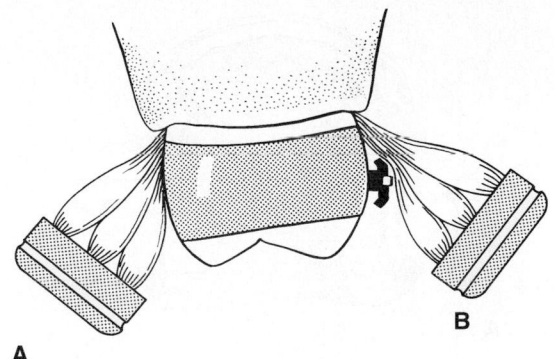

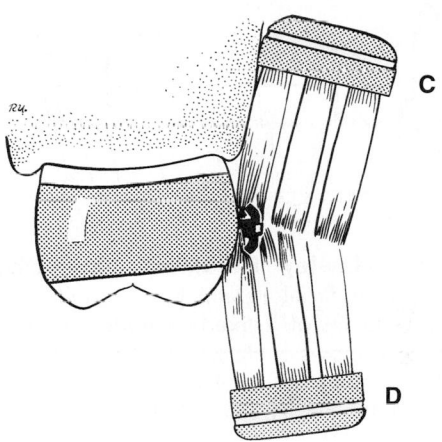

■FIGURE 25-2 **Toothbrushing for Orthodontic Appliance. (A)** Sulcular brushing for periodontal tissues. **(B)** Facial surface over bracket. **(C)** Cleaning the bracket using brush in Charters brushing position for the gingival side. **(D)** Brush in Stillman position for occlusal side of the bracket and arch wire.

III. CARE OF REMOVABLE APPLIANCE OR HAWLEY RETAINER (FIGURE 25-4)

After fixed appliances have been removed, a retainer is worn to give support to the teeth while the bone and other supporting tissues are stabilizing.

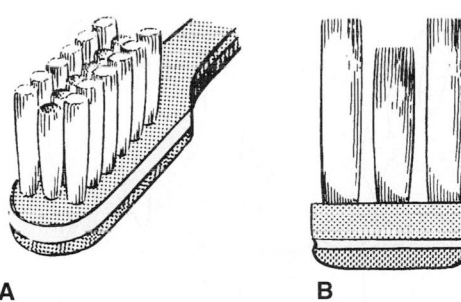

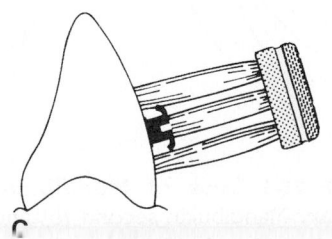

■FIGURE 25-1 **Orthodontic Bi-level Toothbrush. (A)** Middle row of filaments trimmed shorter to fit over a fixed appliance. **(B)** Cross section. **(C)** Brush held over a bracket. Another bi-level shape is shown in Figure 23-2, page 353.

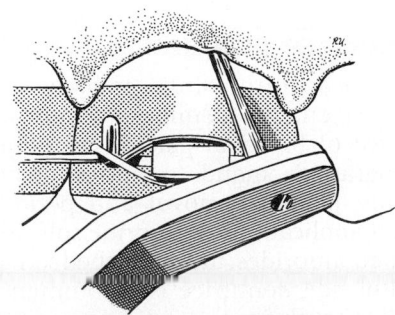

■FIGURE 25-3 **Toothpick Holder for Orthodontic Patient.** Moistened toothpick in holder can be applied for cleaning about appliances and in the subgingival area of the sulcus. Directions for use of the device are on page 379.

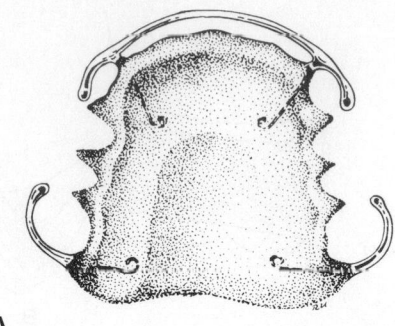

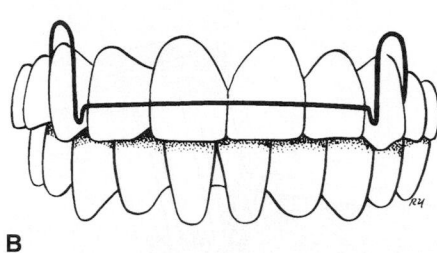

FIGURE 25-4 Hawley Retainer. (A) Removable acrylic retainer with facial retaining wire and clasps to be worn after removal of a fixed orthodontic appliance. **(B)** Anterior view shows a Hawley appliance in position. The method for cleaning the appliance is similar to that for cleaning a removable denture (page 402).

   A. Clean the appliance after each meal and before retiring. Instructions for cleaning procedures and agents for removable appliances are described with the care of the removable denture (pages 402 to 403).

   B. Brush and rinse teeth and gingival tissue under the appliance each time the appliance is removed. Unless necessary as directed by the orthodontist, the health of the underlying tissues is best maintained when the appliance is not kept in the mouth continuously.

   C. Brush the mucosa under the appliance. Methods are described on page 407.

   D. Keep appliance in a container with water when it is out of the mouth.

IV. SELF-APPLIED FLUORIDE

A patient with an orthodontic appliance has an increased risk of enamel demineralization and dental caries because of bacterial plaque retention. A daily fluoride program is mandatory to supplement mechanical daily plaque removal and periodic professional topical applications of fluoride solution or gel.

   Self-applied fluorides are described on pages 469 to 472. A fluoride dentifrice is recommended, along with a daily mouthrinse, gel tray, or brush-on gel. Encouragement, repetition, reinforcement, and motivation are needed to achieve continuing interest and cooperation of an orthodontic patient in both the plaque control and the self-applied fluoride programs.

SPACE MAINTAINERS

When teeth are lost, the surrounding teeth tend to move toward the space. The loss of a permanent tooth is illustrated in Figure 25-5. After the extraction of the mandibular first molar, the second and third molars inclined mesially and the maxillary first molar supererupted into the space. Prevention of such disruption of occlusion and function is a primary reason for the use of fixed or removable dental prostheses described in the next sections of this chapter.

   The premature loss of one or more primary molars disrupts the eruption pattern of the developing permanent teeth. The loss of a second primary molar creates a serious situation because the permanent molars begin to migrate mesially. The permanent premolars may be closed in and prevented from eruption, as shown in Figure 25-6.

   Many malocclusions result from early loss or prolonged retention of primary teeth. When a primary tooth cannot be saved through treatment and restoration, the space then must be held. The use of a space maintainer is a form of preventive orthodontics.

I. TYPES OF SPACE MAINTAINERS

The two general types of space maintainers are *fixed* and *removable*. An advantage of a fixed maintainer is that the patient cannot lose or forget to wear it. Some

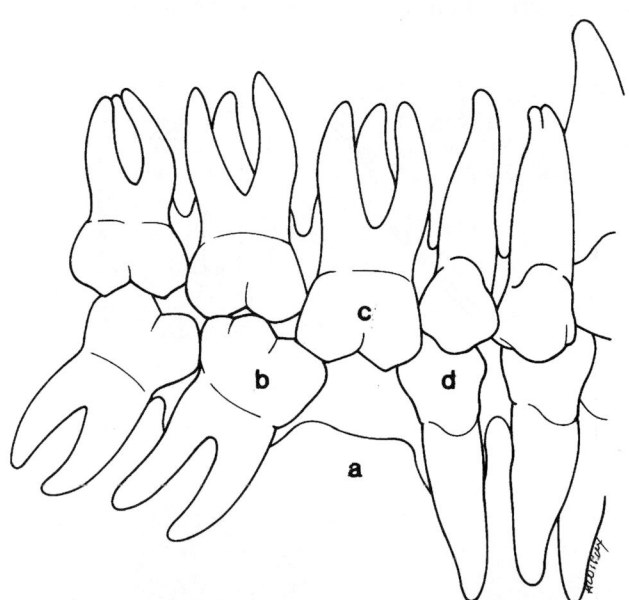

FIGURE 25-5 Loss of Mandibular First Permanent Molar. Mandibular second *(b)* and third molars incline into the space from which the first molar was removed *(a)*. Second premolar *(d)* drifts distally. Maxillary first molar *(c)* supererupts into the space. Occlusion and mastication are disabled, and predisposition to periodontal involvement around the irregularly positioned teeth is greatly increased.

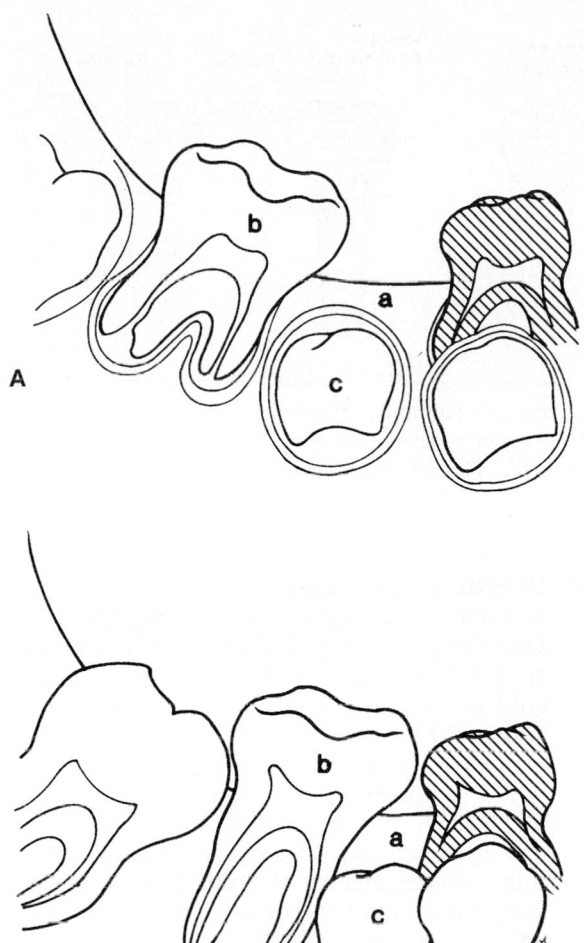

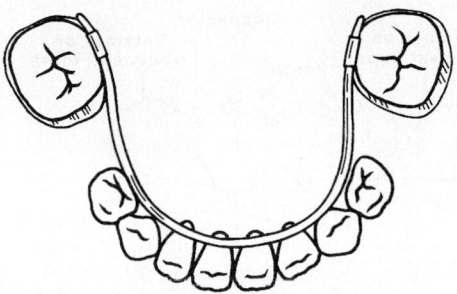

FIGURE 25-7 Space Maintainer. Bilateral lingual mandibular space maintainer with orthodontic bands cemented around the permanent molars to hold the lingual arch wire. Space from which primary molar was removed is being maintained for eruption of the permanent premolar.

Adaptation of methods is needed for cleaning the lingual arch wire and the lingual aspect of the molar bands for an appliance such as that shown in Figure 25-7. A single-tuft brush with a bent shank may prove helpful (see Figure 24-9, page 378). Prevention of dental caries and gingivitis can be especially important during the ages of mixed dentition.

III. REMOVABLE SPACE MAINTAINER

A. Description
The removable appliance is constructed with an acrylic base and stainless steel wire formed into clasps. A lingual bar of stainless steel may be used for a mandibular appliance.

B. Personal Care Procedures
The removable space maintainer is similar to a removable partial denture, and the methods for denture hygiene described on pages 402 to 403 apply. Care of natural teeth, the abutments, and clasped teeth requires continuing demonstration and motivation for the young patient.

FIGURE 25-6 Premature Loss of Second Primary Molar. (A) Developing first permanent molar *(b)* inclines and drifts mesially into the space *(a)* from which the second primary molar was removed. Developing second premolar *(c)* is crowded. **(B)** Space from which molar was removed *(a)* is nearly closed by the mesial drift and eruption of the first permanent molar *(b)*. Developing second premolar *(c)* is closed in and prevented from eruption. Note that the second permanent molar has impacted against the first molar.

space maintainers may be designed for function during mastication, and others may have orthodontic attachments to move teeth.

II. FIXED SPACE MAINTAINER

A. Description
A fixed appliance is made of orthodontic arch wire soldered to a band or bands placed around natural teeth, usually around molars. A bilateral lingual appliance is shown in Figure 25-7.

B. Personal Care Procedures
Bacterial plaque control can be accomplished by using many of the methods described for orthodontic appliances (pages 396 to 397).

FIXED PARTIAL DENTURES

I. DESCRIPTION
Fixed partial dentures, formerly called dental "bridges," are composed of abutments, connectors, and pontics as defined in Box 25-1 and shown in Figure 25-8.

II. CHARACTERISTICS

A. Types of Fixed Partial Dentures
1. *Natural Teeth Supported*
   a. Bilateral: Supported by one or more natural teeth at each end (Figure 25-8*A*).
   b. Cantilever: Supported by one or more teeth at one end only (Figure 25-8*B*).
   c. Resin-bonded cast metal bridge: Uses resin-bonded retainer attached to etched

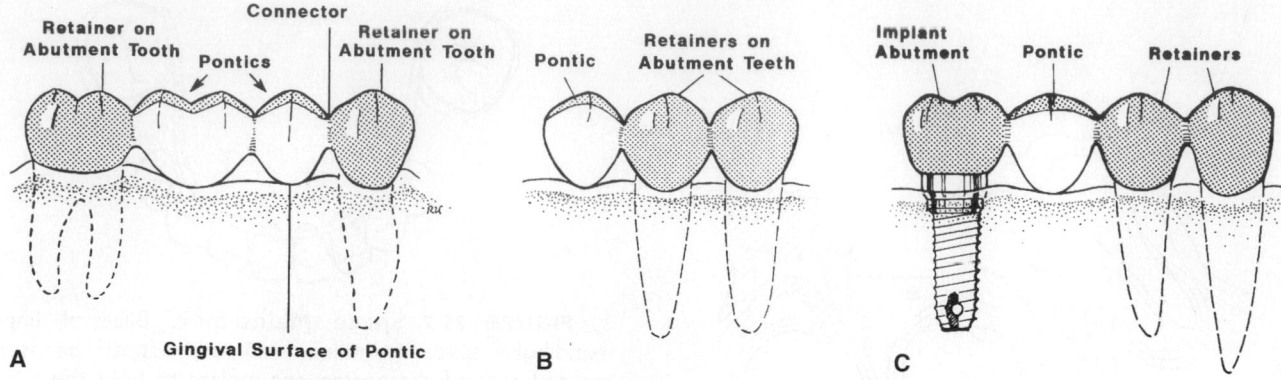

FIGURE 25-8 **Fixed Partial Dentures. (A)** Characteristic parts of mandibular four-unit fixed partial denture. Cast gold crowns on the abutment teeth serve as the retainers for this bridge. **(B)** Cantilever bridge supported by double abutment. **(C)** Fixed partial denture with natural teeth and implant abutments.

enamel; characterized by little or no removal of tooth structure.
2. *Implant Supported* (Figure 25-8*C*): Blade, cylinder, and screw types of implants used for abutments are shown in Figure 26-5 (page 417).

B. Criteria for Fixed Partial Denture[2]
1. Harmonious with the teeth and surrounding periodontium.
2. All parts accessible for cleaning by the patient and the professional person.
3. Must not interfere with the cleaning regimen for the remaining natural dentition.
4. Must not traumatize oral tissues.

CARE PROCEDURES

I. DEBRIS REMOVAL

When suggesting a procedure to follow for cleaning the oral cavity when a fixed partial denture is present, debris removal with an oral irrigator may be recommended as a first step. By removing food and debris, access of the toothbrush and other aids for plaque removal is facilitated. Procedure for use of an oral irrigator is described on pages 331 to 382.

II. PLAQUE REMOVAL FROM ABUTMENT TEETH

Nearly all the methods proposed for bacterial plaque control in the two previous chapters may be applicable to abutment teeth. The proximal surface and gingiva of an abutment tooth adjacent to a pontic require special attention.

A. Toothbrushing
Sulcular brushing is generally indicated. The area of the tooth surface adjacent to and beneath the gingival margin must be kept meticulously free of bacterial plaque.

B. Dentifrice Selection
A nonabrasive dentifrice is indicated to prevent the possibility of abrasion when pontic or crown facings are made of acrylic, when the gold of the partial denture is highly polished and could be scratched, and when areas of root exposure are on abutment teeth.

A fluoride-containing dentifrice is important for protection of remaining tooth surfaces, particularly exposed cementum. Acidulated fluoride preparations are contraindicated for porcelain and composite restorations (pages 631 to 633).[3]

C. Additional Interdental Care
An interdental plaque removal method is indicated. The method is selected on the basis of the individual patient or the prosthesis. The interdental cleaning device is adapted specifically to the distal surface of the mesial abutment and the mesial surface of the distal abutment, and from both facial and lingual aspects.

The same interdental cleaning procedure can usually be applied to the gingival surface of the fixed partial denture. Interdental cleaning methods and devices are described on pages 373 to 380.

III. THE PROSTHESIS

A. Areas Requiring Emphasis
The gingival surfaces of the pontics and beneath the connectors are particularly prone to plaque retention.

B. Toothbrushing
A toothbrush in the Charters position may be helpful for cleaning the gingival surface of the pontic from the facial aspect. The filaments can be directed under the pontic to clean the gingival surface. Charters brush position is described on page 360.

C. Dental Floss

1. Thread a 12- to 15-inch length into a floss threader. Several types are available (Figure 25-9).
2. Apply threader between an abutment and pontic.
3. Draw the floss through, and using single or double thickness, remove loose debris (Figure 25-10).
4. Apply dentifrice and a new section of the floss with moderate pressure to the undersurface (gingival surface) of the pontic and then to the proximal surfaces of each abutment tooth to remove bacterial plaque. Remove floss.

D. Knitting Yarn

Put length of yarn or tufted floss in floss threader and pull through under the prosthesis for a cleaning device that is thicker than floss alone (Figure 24-5, page 376).

E. Other Interdental Devices

A pipe cleaner, an interdental brush, a single-tuft brush, or an interdental tip should be recommended and demonstrated as indicated by the requirements of the individual prosthesis. These devices usually fit mesial and distal to the

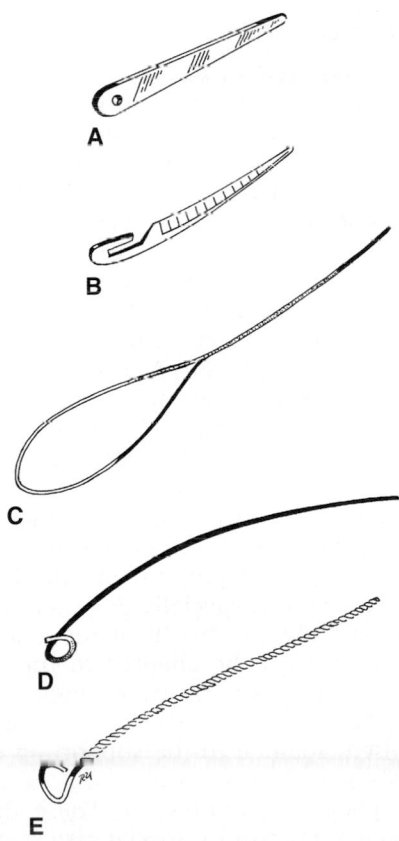

FIGURE 25-9 Floss Threaders. (A) Clear plastic with closed eye. **(B)** Tinted plastic with open eye. **(C)** Soft plastic loop. **(D)** Flexible wire. **(E)** Twisted wire.

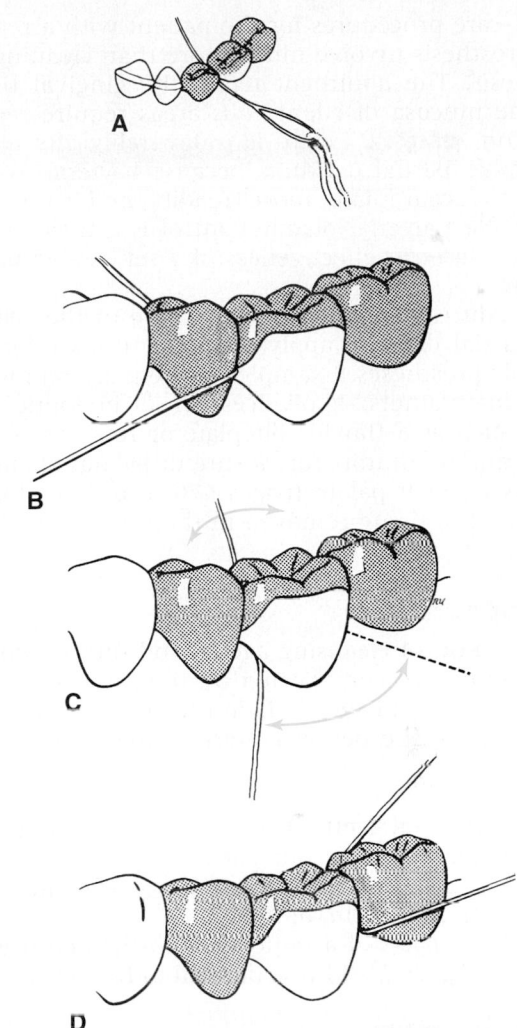

FIGURE 25-10 Use of Floss Threader. (A) Use floss threader to draw the floss (or yarn or tufted floss) between abutment and a pontic. **(B)** Apply floss to the distal surface of the mesial abutment; pull through 1 or 2 inches. **(C)** Slide floss under pontic. Move back and forth several times, as shown by the arrows, to remove bacterial plaque from the gingival surface of the pontic. **(D)** Apply new section of floss to the mesial surface of the distal abutment.

pontic, but not over the gingival surface of the pontic. Yarn or tufted floss with threader is essential.

REMOVABLE PARTIAL DENTURES

The removable partial denture replaces one or more, but less than all, of the natural teeth and associated structures, and it can be removed from the mouth and replaced at will. Depending on the location and number of remaining natural teeth, a partial denture may receive all its support from the teeth, or it may be partly tooth borne and partly tissue borne.

Self-care procedures for the patient with a removable prosthesis involve much more than cleaning the prosthesis. The abutment teeth, the gingival tissue, and the mucosa of edentulous areas require regular attention. Gingival health is unfavorably affected by removable partial dentures because bacterial plaque tends to accumulate more readily and in greater quantities. Bacterial plaque control is a major factor in the long-term effectiveness of a removable partial denture.

Procedures suggested here for care of the removable partial denture apply also to various other removable prostheses. Examples of these are removable space maintainers; appliances for orthodontic purposes, such as a Hawley biteplate or retainer (Figure 25-4); and obturators for closure of palatal openings, such as for cleft palate (pages 670 to 671) or for replacement of tissue removed in the treatment of oral cancer.

I. DESCRIPTION

The selection of cleansing agents and the procedures for cleaning are complicated by the intricacy of the metallic parts and their relation to the natural teeth, as well as by the dental materials used in construction.

The denture base rests on the oral mucosa and carries the artificial teeth. The base is most frequently made of plastic resin, but alloys of gold or chrome have also been used. The teeth may be made of porcelain, plastic resin, or metal.

The basic parts of a removable partial denture are shown in Figure 25-11 and defined in Box 25-1.

II. OBJECTIVES

A. The Prosthesis

Because natural teeth are adjacent to the prosthesis, objectives for cleaning the prosthesis take on added significance. The basic objectives are to remove irritants to the oral tissues (primarily bacterial plaque), prevent mouth odors, and improve appearance.

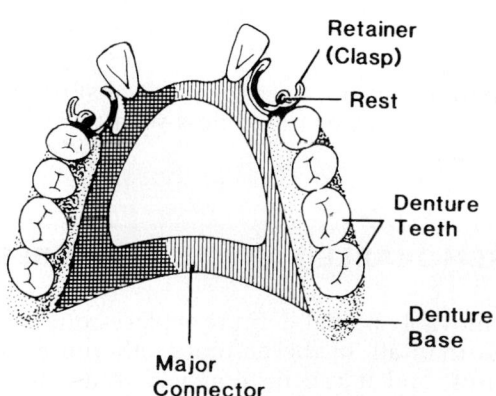

FIGURE 25-11 Removable Partial Denture. Components of a removable partial denture shown for a maxillary prosthesis.

Labels: Retainer (Clasp); Rest; Denture Teeth; Denture Base; Major Connector

B. The Natural Teeth

The objective is to control plaque for the prevention of dental caries and periodontal infection.

CLEANING A REMOVABLE PROSTHESIS

Rinsing, immersion, and brushing methods, as well as the cleansing agents described for the complete denture on pages 404 to 405, apply alike to the partial prosthesis, with the few additions noted as follows.

I. RINSING

After each meal, the denture and the natural teeth should be brushed. When regular cleaning facilities are not available, rinsing is important for both the natural teeth and the removable prosthesis. While the appliance is out, the tongue can be used to rub the sides of abutment teeth.

II. IMMERSION

Before immersion, the denture must be cleaned by rinsing and brushing to remove all bacterial plaque and debris. An agent known to discolor metal can be avoided. Procedures for immersion cleaning are described on pages 405 to 406.

III. BRUSHING

A. Recommended Brushes

1. *Toothbrush.* One or more should be reserved for the natural teeth. The use of a regular toothbrush for care of a removable prosthesis is not recommended. When a patient chooses to do so, however, a separate brush is definitely indicated. Brushing the clasps and other metal parts can deform the filaments and make the brush ineffective for use on the natural teeth.

2. *Power-Assisted Brush.* A power-assisted toothbrush is sometimes appropriate for the natural teeth of the patient with a partial denture. The power-assisted brush, however, should not be used in and about the intricate clasps and other parts of a removable prosthesis because of the danger of catching the brush and damaging the prosthesis.

3. *Clasp Brush.* A specially designed narrow, tapered, cylindric brush about 2 to 3 inches long that can be adapted to the inner surfaces of clasps is recommended (Figure 25-12). Clasps and their connectors are closely adapted to the supporting teeth, and the protected internal surfaces are prone to plaque accumulation. These difficult-to-clean areas require special care.

4. *Denture Brush.* A denture brush is shown in Figure 25-14 and described on page 406. It is an excellent brush for cleaning all the

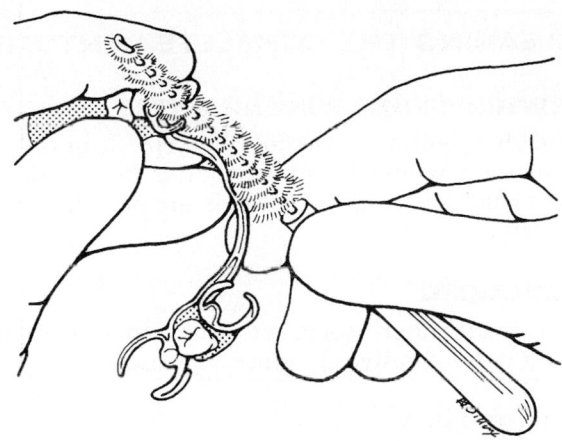

FIGURE 25-12 Clasp Brush. A brush specially designed to remove bacterial plaque from the inside surfaces of clasps is available. The denture must be held carefully to avoid accidents.

smooth surfaces and the metal bars of the partial denture.

B. Precautions During Brushing

Too tight a grasp of a partial prosthesis can result in bending or fracture of clasps or bars. Filaments of a brush can inadvertently catch the prosthesis and cause it to drop. Partial filling of the sink with water or lining of the sink with a face cloth or towel is necessary to prevent accidents that cause breakage (page 407).

THE NATURAL TEETH

I. PLAQUE CONTROL

Toothbrushing and interdental cleaning methods selected for the particular needs of the patient must be followed meticulously. The longevity of the removable appliance depends on the health of the supporting teeth, and in turn, the health of the natural teeth depends on the cleanliness of the prosthesis.

II. DENTAL CARIES CONTROL

The topical application of fluoride; the use of a fluoride dentifrice and other self-applied fluoride measures, such as a daily mouthrinse or application of a gel; and the control of refined sugars in the diet must be definite parts of the complete program of oral care for the patient with a removable prosthesis.

The patient must be constantly alert to the control of plaque retention by the prosthesis and to the need for rinsing immediately after eating when brushing is not possible. For the patient who has been caries-susceptible and whose teeth are missing because of dental caries, a dietary assessment and specific dental caries control program may increase a patient's motivation.

COMPLETE DENTURES

One should not assume that the patient who is new to the dental office and is wearing dentures or a denture knows the proper methods for caring for the prostheses. During questioning for the patient history, information about the method and frequency of denture care is recorded. Later, the dentures are examined and the current method of care is reviewed. Alternate cleansing agents, devices, or procedures are recommended and demonstrated as needed.

Instruction may be given to the patient receiving a maxillary and mandibular denture for the first time, to the patient whose dentures have been remade or relined, or to the patient with a single denture that opposes natural teeth. Another patient may be receiving an immediate denture. Types of dentures and characteristics of the edentulous mouth are described on pages 698 to 701.

I. COMPONENTS OF A COMPLETE DENTURE (FIGURE 25-13)

In an effort to understand the effects of various cleansing agents and devices, information about the structure and material of the parts of a denture is pertinent.

A. Denture Base

The part of a denture that rests on the oral mucosa and to which the teeth are attached is the denture base. Most denture bases are made of plastic resin. Others may be metal, for example, chrome-cobalt or gold, in combination with a plastic resin.

B. Surfaces

1. *Impression Surface.* Also called the tissue or inner surface, the impression surface is the part that lies adjacent to the mucous membrane of the alveolar ridge and immediately

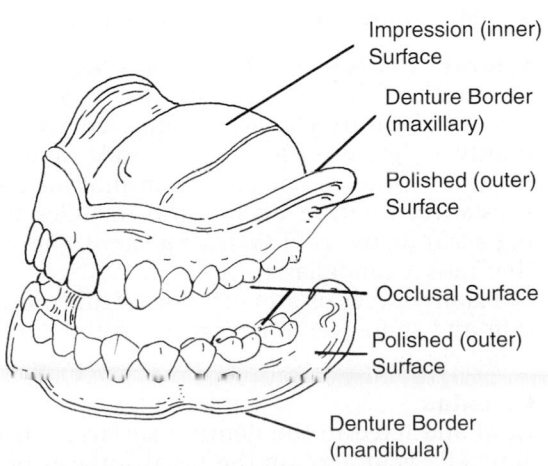

Impression (inner) Surface

Denture Border (maxillary)

Polished (outer) Surface

Occlusal Surface

Polished (outer) Surface

Denture Border (mandibular)

FIGURE 25-13 Complete Denture. The surfaces and borders of maxillary and mandibular dentures.

associated parts; in the maxillary, the tissue surface is adjacent to the hard palate.

2. *Polished Surface.* The external or outer surface is highly polished. The occlusal and impression surfaces are not polished.

3. *Occlusal Surface.* The portion of the surface of a denture that makes contact or near contact with the corresponding surface of the opposing denture or natural teeth is the occlusal surface.

C. Teeth

The denture teeth may be made of plastic resin or porcelain. Some posterior teeth have metal occlusal inserts. Anterior porcelain teeth have metal pins for retention.

II. PURPOSES FOR CLEANING

Inadequate oral tissue care and denture hygiene practices are major causes of oral lesions under dentures.

A. Prevent Irritation to the Oral Tissues

1. *Mechanical Irritants.* Rough deposits of plaque, calculus, thick stains.

2. *Chemical Irritants.* Products of putrefaction of food debris and bacterial metabolic products.

B. Control Infection

Reactions to bacterial denture plaque and/or secondary infections by way of traumatic lesions may occur.

C. Prevent Mouth Odors

D. Maintain Appearance

III. DENTURE DEPOSITS

Accumulation of stains and deposits on dentures varies between individuals in a manner similar to that on natural teeth. The phases of deposit formation may be divided as follows:

A. Mucin and Food Debris on the Denture Surface

Readily removed by rinsing and brushing.

B. Denture Pellicle and Bacterial Plaque

Denture pellicle forms readily after a denture is cleaned. Denture plaque is composed predominantly of gram-positive cocci, rods, and filamentous forms of bacteria in an intermicrobial substance. Denture plaque also includes varying accumulations of *Candida albicans,* the yeast that causes candidiasis.

Plaque serves as a matrix for calculus formation and stain accumulation when the denture is not cleaned.

C. Calculus

Hard and fixed to the denture surface, calculus generally is located on the facial surfaces of the maxillary molars and the lingual surfaces of the mandibular anterior region.

CLEANING THE COMPLETE DENTURE

I. RINSING UNDER RUNNING WATER

Although a denture that could be kept clean only by this method would be unusual, the use of rinsing after meals when other methods are not possible is necessary.

II. BRUSHING

Brush with water, soap, or other mild cleansing agent. Coarse abrasives produce scratches.

III. IMMERSION

The denture is soaked in a solvent or detergent in which chemical action removes or loosens stains and deposits that can then be rinsed or brushed away.

IV. MECHANICAL DENTURE CLEANSERS

Commercially available devices include ultrasonic, sonic, magnetic, and agitating mechanisms that can be combined with an immersion agent. The action of the mechanical cleansing device seems to make the solution more efficient than a solution used alone. Ultrasonic cleaning during a professional appointment is described on pages 615 to 616.

V. DENTURE CLEANSERS[4-7]

A. Requirements for a Denture Cleanser[4]

1. Easy for a patient to use.
2. Reasonably priced.
3. Effective removal of denture deposits (organic and inorganic) without abrasion of the denture surface.
4. Bactericidal and fungicidal action.
5. Nontoxic.
6. Harmless to the dental materials used for partial or complete dentures.

B. Chemical Solution Cleansers (Immersion)

1. *Alkaline Hypochlorite*
   a. Active ingredient: Dilute sodium hypochlorite with bleaching properties.
   b. Action: Loosens debris and light stains; bleaching; dissolves mucin; dissolves plaque matrix.
   c. Example: Household bleach.
   d. Disadvantage: Odor; tarnish; surface pitting; bleaching effect on soft lining materials and denture materials containing fibers.
2. *Alkaline Peroxide*
   a. Active ingredient: Alkaline detergent with an oxygen-liberating agent (sodium perborate or percarbonate).
   b. Action: Loosens debris and light stains by an oxygen-liberating mechanism. A preventive cleanser should be used regularly from the day a denture has been cleaned

professionally to prevent accumulation of heavy deposits.

   c. Examples: Most proprietary cleansers are in the form of a powder or tablet that is dropped into water to create the alkaline solution of hydrogen peroxide.

   d. Disadvantage: Does not remove heavy stains or calculus.

3. *Dilute Acids*

   a. Active ingredient: Inorganic acids.

   b. Action: Dissolves inorganic components of denture deposits.

   c. Examples: 3% to 5% hydrochloric acid alone or with phosphoric acid; commercially prepared ultrasonic solutions. The strong acids (although in dilute forms) are not recommended for home use by the patient. Acetic acid (vinegar) has been used with some success when deposits were not old and hard.

   d. Disadvantage: Corrosion of metal parts of a denture.

4. *Enzymes.* The enzymes act to break down plaque proteins and polysaccharides. Enzyme agents have been incorporated into various immersion-type cleansers.

5. *Disinfectants.* A sanitary denture is necessary for the prevention of inflammation in the oral mucosa under the denture. Types of denture-induced lesions are described on pages 701 to 702. Regular daily maintenance procedures must be carried out.

     Patient instruction in disinfection of a denture is recommended. Disinfection can be accomplished by several EPA-registered products.[8]

     Full-strength, commercially available sodium hypochlorite (household bleach) has been shown to be an antimicrobial agent. Before disinfection, preclean the denture under running water taking care not to splash and thus contaminate the area. To disinfect, immerse the denture for 5 minutes in full-strength bleach.[9] Because bleach can fade the color of a denture, immersion should be timed at 5 minutes, and the denture should be rinsed completely.

C. Abrasive Cleansers (Brushing)

1. *Denture Pastes and Powders, Toothpastes and Powders*

   a. Active ingredient: An abrasive, such as calcium carbonate (see Dentifrices, page 387).

   b. Action: Mechanical removal of bacterial plaque and stains by brushing.

   c. Examples: Various commercial products.

   d. Disadvantages: Can abrade the plastic resin denture base and acrylic teeth. A paste with low abrasiveness should be selected.

2. *Household Agents*

   a. Active ingredient: Detergent and/or abrasive agent.

   b. Examples: Salt and bicarbonate of soda are mildly abrasive; hand soap is cleansing and not particularly abrasive. Scouring powders or other excessively abrasive cleansers should not be used.

GENERAL CLEANING PROCEDURES

I. WHEN TO CLEAN

  A. Regularly after each meal and before retiring.

  B. Chemical immersion daily or twice weekly, depending on the rate of formation of calculus and stain and the type of solution used.

    1. May be at one of the daily cleanings.

    2. Suggested while bathing.

    3. Overnight when denture is removed as instructed by the dentist.

II. SELECTION OF PROCEDURE FOR CLEANING

Immersion, followed by brushing, is recommended. When unable to clean, rinsing after eating is advised.

III. PREPARATION FOR CLEANING

  A. Rinse the denture thoroughly when it is taken from the mouth to remove saliva and loose debris.*

  B. Remove denture-adhesive material.

    1. *Definition.* A denture adhesive is a commercially available paste or powder preparation. A patient may use it under the direction of the dentist for temporary stabilization. An occasional patient may use an adhesive indefinitely in an attempt to get along with ill-fitting dentures that should be adjusted or rebased.

    2. *Method.* Use a brush with light pressure to remove the adhesive.

  C. Denture-bearing mucosa. Rinse and clean with a brush twice or more times daily (pages 407 to 408).

IV. CLEANING BY IMMERSION

  A. Advantages

    1. The solution reaches all areas of the denture for a complete cleaning.

    2. Minimizes the danger of dropping the appliance. Prevents need for handling, which is required during brushing.

    3. Offers safe storage when dentures are out of the mouth.

---

*Procedure for removal of a denture for a patient is described on page 615. It may be necessary to instruct a caregiver for a disabled patient.

4. Aids persons with limited ability to manage a brush.
5. When cleaning is distasteful, immersion involves the least handling and observation. This advantage is particularly attractive to a caregiver who must clean the denture of a helpless patient.

B. Procedure
1. Place denture in a plastic container with fitted cover that is maintained specifically for this purpose.
2. Use only warm water for rinsing and for mixing the solution. Warm water promotes the action of the cleanser. Hot water should never be used because it can distort plastic resin.
3. Follow manufacturer's specifications to ensure correct dilution of cleanser.
4. Check that the denture is completely submerged in the solution; cover the container.
5. When the denture is removed, rinse under running water and remove loosened debris and chemicals before proceeding to clean by brushing.
6. Empty and clean container daily. Mix fresh solution to prevent contamination and growth of microorganisms.[10]

C. Solutions
1. *Proprietary:* Available in powder or tablet form.
   a. Preparation: Add measured warm water as directed by the manufacturer.
   b. Length of immersion: Usually 10 to 15 minutes or as suggested by the manufacturer. Because the action depends on the mechanical bubbling effect of released oxygen, the solution has little value after the available oxygen has been released.
   c. Effect: The solutions are only effective against loose debris; denture cleanliness depends on regular daily immersion supplemented by brushing.
2. *Hypochlorite Solution:* Household bleach (5% sodium hypochlorite) and Calgone. Calgone acts to improve the penetrating and detaching power of the bleach.
   a. Proportions
      1 tablespoon (15 mL) sodium hypochlorite (household bleach)
      2 teaspoons (8 mL) Calgone
      4 ounces (114 mL) water
   b. Length of immersion: Usually 10 to 15 minutes. When stains or calculus form, the patient should be instructed to soak the denture overnight provided there are no metal parts that can become corroded.

V. CLEANING BY BRUSHING
A. Type of Brush
1. *Denture Brush.* A good-quality denture brush with end-rounded filaments is recommended. The styles of denture brushes vary. One type shown in Figure 25-14 is designed with two arrangements of filaments. One group in a large round arrangement of tufts permits access to the inner, curved impression surface of the denture. The second group of tufts is arranged to form a rectangular brush for convenient adaptation to the polished and occlusal denture surfaces. Another design is shown in Figure 50-10, page 753.
2. *Other Brushes.* A few patients prefer not to have a denture brush for personal reasons. A hand brush can be used, provided the filaments are long enough to reach into the deeper portions of the impression surfaces. Prerequisite is that each area of each surface of the denture must be reached by the brush if bacterial plaque formation is to be controlled.

If a patient prefers to use an ordinary toothbrush, a multitufted soft nylon brush with end-rounded filaments should be acceptable if access to all the inner curvatures is possible without applying undue pressure on certain parts in the attempt to clean others. The patient who wears a single denture should keep separate brushes for the natural teeth and the denture to maintain the brush for the natural teeth in the best condition possible.

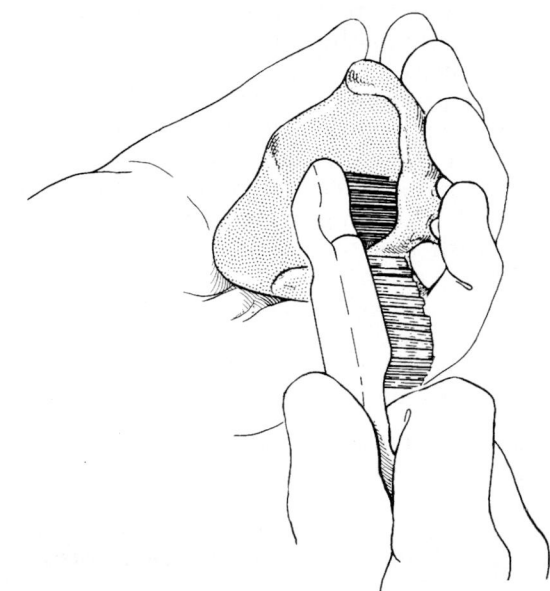

■ **FIGURE 25-14 Denture Brush.** The denture is held securely, but without squeezing, in the palm of the nonworking hand. Place a face cloth in the bottom of the sink and partially fill with water. The specially designed brush is preferred because one group of tufts is arranged to provide access to the inner impression surface of the denture, as shown.

B. Procedure
1. Grasp denture in palm of hand securely, but without a squeezing pressure because dentures can be broken (Figure 25-14).
2. Hold the denture low in a sink in which a towel, wash cloth, or rubber mat has been spread over the bottom to serve as a cushion should the denture be dropped. The sink should be partially filled with water.
3. Apply warm water, nonabrasive cleanser, and brush to all areas of the denture. Particular attention should be paid to the impression surfaces where configurations of the surface correspond with those of the oral topography. The anterior areas of the inner surfaces of both the maxillary and mandibular dentures require special adaptations of the brush.
4. Rinse denture and brush under running water. Use the brush to remove denture cleanser that may be retained in the grooves.
5. Visually check each area carefully for bacterial plaque. Teach the patient to run a finger over the surfaces to find "slippery" plaque areas.

C. Precautions Related to Brushing
1. Overzealous brushing with an abrasive cleansing agent on the impression surface could alter the fit of the denture.
2. Plastic resin can be abraded. Scratches make a rough surface; the denture may become more subject to the collection of debris and calculus.
3. Possibility of incomplete coverage during cleaning, particularly in the more inaccessible areas.
4. Possibility of cleaning with uneven pressure when the brush is applied more vigorously to accessible areas.
5. Danger of dropping and breaking the denture is increased when it is wet and, therefore, slippery.
6. Patient who requires eyeglasses should be advised to wear them when brushing to watch the procedure and to observe the cleanliness of the denture after brushing.

VI. ADDITIONAL INSTRUCTIONS

A. Care of Plastic Resin
An appliance made with plastic resin should be immersed in water or cleansing solution when it is not in the mouth.

B. Prevention of Denture Deposits
When the denture is kept clean by regular procedures from the time of insertion, accumulation of heavy stains and calculus can be prevented.

C. Professional Maintenance
A denture should never be scraped by the patient with a sharp instrument in the attempt to remove calculus deposits. When the cleaning methods recommended in this chapter do not remove deposits, the denture should be taken to the dental hygienist and dentist for professional cleaning. A regular maintenance plan is arranged.

D. Paste Cleaners
Paste cleansers (dentifrices or denture pastes) may cling and be difficult to rinse from the denture. Residual chemical agents, such as essential oils, may cause inflammatory or allergic reactions of the oral mucosa, and phenolic agents can have deleterious effects on plastic resin.

E. Soft Lining Materials
Temporary soft conditioning lining material may be sensitive to proprietary cleansers. Washing with cold water and a soft cloth, cotton, or soft brush (gently) can be suggested. The denture plaque should be removed several times each day. Outer, polished surfaces should be thoroughly brushed in the usual manner. When the denture is placed in water overnight, the teeth should be placed down so that the soft material at the denture border cannot become deformed.

THE UNDERLYING MUCOSA

I. RINSING

Each time the denture is removed, the mouth should be rinsed thoroughly with warm water or a mild salt solution (page 385). The patient can learn to clean the mucosa by rubbing over the edentulous areas with the tongue.

II. CLEANING

The edentulous mucosa should be brushed at least once daily. A soft brush with end-rounded filaments is applied in long, straight strokes from posterior to anterior.

Concurrently, the tongue is cleaned. Use a tongue scraper as described on page 365.

III. MASSAGE

For stimulation of circulation and increased resistance to trauma, frequent massage is recommended. Methods for massage that may be suggested to the patient are the following:

A. Digital
Place thumb and index finger over the ridge and apply massage with a press-and-release stroke. The palate may be rubbed with the ball of the thumb.

B. Soft Toothbrush
Apply sides of filaments and vibratory motion

to each area. Prevent trauma to the tissue by placing the brush carefully and avoiding scrubbing with undue pressure.

C. Power-Assisted Brush
Apply to each area with smooth, even strokes.

COMPLETE OVERDENTURE

An overdenture is a complete denture supported by both retained natural teeth or implants and the soft tissue of the residual alveolar ridge. It also has been known as an overlay denture, coping denture, and tooth-mucosa-supported denture.

I. PURPOSES
The advantages of an overdenture when compared with a denture in a completely edentulous mouth are that the natural teeth
- A. Help to preserve bone.
- B. Allow the remaining teeth to bear occlusal pressures, thereby reducing the pressures placed on edentulous areas.
- C. Improve stability and retention of the denture.
- D. Improve the patient's tactile and proprioceptive senses by having the periodontal ligament present.
- E. Increase the patient's psychologic acceptance of the denture. The patient does not feel that all natural teeth have been lost.

II. CRITERIA
The overdenture should be considered for any patient whose treatment plan calls for extraction of all teeth. Teeth to be preserved must meet certain standards of health.

A. Periodontal Condition
Because wearing the overdenture brings stress to the periodontium, the tissues must have, or be treatable to obtain, the following:
1. Healthy gingiva. There must be no bleeding or other signs of inflammation; minimal probing depth; and all requirements of health (Table 11-1, pages 194 to 195).
2. A band of attached gingiva (pages 211 to 212).

B. Bone Support
The bone level following tooth preparation must be adequate to withstand occlusal forces.

C. Teeth
Teeth must have minimal mobility. Teeth selected are frequently the mandibular canines and premolars and the maxillary canines.

III. PREPARATION OF THE TEETH

A. Endodontics
Most preserved teeth need endodontic therapy because the crown will be reduced.

B. Periodontics
Treatment procedures depend on clinical findings, but they may include measures to eliminate inflammation and pockets, to increase the zone of attached gingiva, or to reshape the architecture of the bone or gingival tissue.

C. Restorative
1. Tooth crowns are reduced to short rounded preparations or, for some patients, to the level and contour of the gingival margin.
2. An amalgam or composite restoration may cover the root canals, or the teeth may be protected by a gold coping (Figure 25-15*B*). A coping is a cast thin metal covering or cap.
3. The gold coping may be used as a retainer for a retentive attachment.

DENTAL HYGIENE CARE AND INSTRUCTION

The patient must be well informed concerning the problems of care of the retained teeth and gingiva. A high degree of motivation to want to save the remaining teeth is the primary concern.

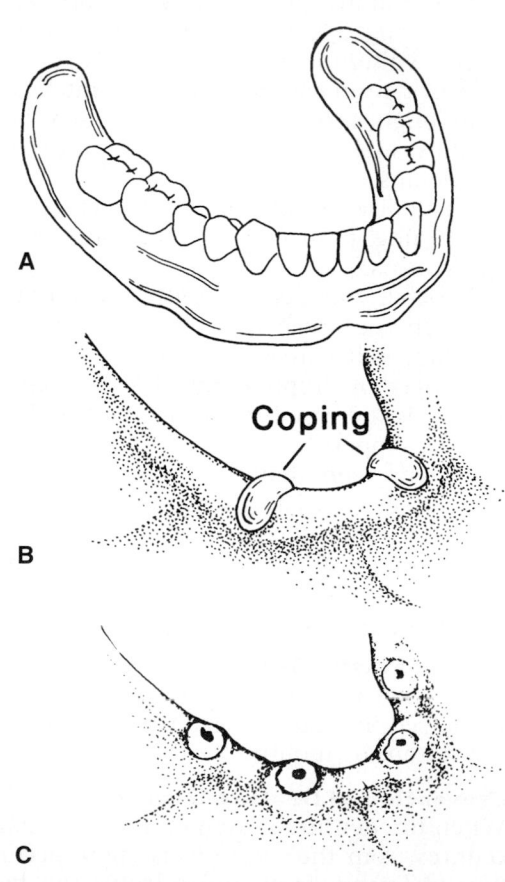

FIGURE 25-15 Overdenture. (A) Mandibular complete denture. **(B)** Support provided by gold cap copings. **(C)** Natural teeth with amalgam restoration in the coronal portion of the root canal opening.

I. DENTURE CARE

The impression surface of the denture must be kept meticulously free from plaque accumulation. Denture care is outlined on pages 404 to 407. Implant care is described on pages 419 to 422.

II. GINGIVAL TISSUE AND NATURAL TEETH

A. Complete daily bacterial plaque removal using a soft brush with end-rounded filaments or a power-assisted toothbrush is needed.

B. Interdental tip or a toothpick in holder should be used daily to trace around each natural tooth to clean subgingivally (pages 378 to 379).

C. Massage of the edentulous mucosa contributes to complete oral health (page 407).

III. FLUORIDE

A specific fluoride application plan must be included. The requirements depend partly on the past history of dental caries. When the teeth have been extracted because of dental caries, caries control measures take on special significance, particularly if dietary habits remain the same. Current dietary habits must be checked by asking the patient to keep a daily food record (pages 444 to 449). Limitations on cariogenic foods intake can be recommended accordingly.

A. Fluoride Self-Application

All patients must use a fluoride dentifrice. In addition, a mouthrinse and/or a gel tray can be recommended. After cleaning, the patient's denture can be used for a custom tray, and the gel drops can be placed inside at the locations of the natural teeth. Pressure of the denture as it is seated forces the gel about the teeth. Higher concentrations of sodium fluoride (5000 ppm) have been shown to be more protective for overdenture abutments.[11]

B. Professional Topical Applications

When daily mouthrinse or gel tray is not carried out regularly by the patient or when additional fluoride is indicated, professional topical applications are made. Because frequent maintenance appointments are needed to check the health of the gingival tissues, an application can be made at each such appointment. Benefit is derived from fluoride in direct proportion to the frequency of application: the more frequent the application of fluoride, the greater the benefit derived.

IV. SEALANTS

Application of sealants to overdenture abutment teeth has been shown effective in the prevention of dental caries.[12]

V. MAINTENANCE APPOINTMENTS

Supervision by frequent maintenance appointments for scaling and bacterial debridement, topical fluoride applications, and motivation and instruction for plaque control are essential. Check for integrity of each sealant and replace as necessary.

TECHNICAL HINTS

I. Review instructions for each patient with a fixed or removable prosthesis. Do not assume that, because a denture has been in use for a long time, the patient knows how to clean it properly or how to care for the adjacent soft tissue.

II. Wearing an overdenture day and night can be a major risk factor for periodontal infection and dental caries in the natural abutment teeth.[13]

III. Prevent cross-contamination when receiving a removable prosthesis from a patient by:
   A. Wearing protective gloves.
   B. Offering a container or disposable napkin in which the patient can place the denture.
   C. Rinsing the prosthesis under running water, taking care not to splash.
   D. Wearing gloves and a mask while cleaning the appliance, and directing scrub strokes away from oneself and into the sink to prevent contamination.

IV. Acrylic restorations, crowns, and pontics are subject to toothbrush dentifrice abrasion. Select soft brush and nonabrasive cleansing material.

V. Provide printed instructions for each patient. Personalize the instructions with notations related to particular problem areas of the patient.

VI. Source of educational materials:

American Dental Association
Department of Salable Materials
211 East Chicago Avenue
Chicago, IL 60611

Request current catalog. Samples of booklets are available on request.

REFERENCES

1. **Attarzadeh,** F.: Water Irrigating Devices for the Orthodontic Patient, *Int. J. Orthod., 24,* 15, Spring, 1986.
2. **Obreschkow,** C.: Oral Hygiene and Periodontal Considerations in Restorative Treatment with Prefabricated Attachments and Precision-milled Prosthetic Devices, *Int. J. Periodontics Restorative Dent., 4,* 73, No. 1, 1985.
3. **American Dental Association,** Council on Dental Materials, Instruments and Equipment and Council on Dental Therapeutics: Status Report: Effect of Acidulated Phosphate Fluoride on Porcelain and Composite Restorations, *J. Am. Dent. Assoc., 116,* 115, January, 1988.
4. **Abelson,** D.C.: Denture Plaque and Denture Cleansers: Review of the Literature, *Gerodontics, 1,* 202, October, 1985.
5. **Budtz-Jörgensen,** E.: Materials and Methods for Cleaning Dentures, *J. Prosthet. Dent., 42,* 619, December, 1979.

6. **Gallagher,** J.B., Jr.: *Handbook For Complete Dentures.* Boston, Tufts University School of Dental Medicine, 1981.

7. **American Dental Association,** Council on Dental Materials, Instruments, and Equipment: Denture Cleansers, *J. Am. Dent. Assoc., 106,* 77, January, 1983.

8. **Cottone,** J.A., Terezhalmy, G.T., and Molinari, J.A.: *Practical Infection Control in Dentistry,* 2nd ed. Baltimore, Williams & Wilkins, 1996, pp. 241–244.

9. **Rudd,** R.W., Senia, E.S., McCleskey, F.K., and Adams, E.D.: Sterilization of Complete Dentures with Sodium Hypochlorite, *J. Prosthet Dent., 51,* 318, March, 1984.

10. **DePaola,** L.G. and Minah, G.E.: Isolation of Pathogenic Microorganisms from Dentures and Denture-soaking Containers of Myelosuppressed Cancer Patients, *J. Prosthet. Dent., 49,* 20, January, 1983.

11. **Ettinger,** R.L., Olson, R.J., Wefel, J.S., and Asmussen, C.: In Vitro Evaluation of Topical Fluorides for Overdenture Abutments, *J. Prosthet. Dent., 78,* 309, September, 1997.

12. **Kurtz,** K.S.: Adjunctive Caries Control in Overdenture Abutment Teeth: A New Modality, *J. Am. Dent. Assoc., 126,* 213, February, 1995.

13. **Budtz-Jörgensen,** E.: Effects of Denture-wearing Habits on Periodontal Health of Abutment Teeth in Patients with Overdentures, *J. Clin. Periodontol., 21,* 265, April, 1994.

SUGGESTED READINGS

Asad, T., Watkinson, A.C., and Huggett, R.: The Effect of Disinfection Procedures on Flexural Properties of Denture Base Acrylic Resins, *J. Prosthet. Dent., 68,* 191, July, 1992.

Assery, M., Sugrue, P.C., Graser, G.N., and Eisenberg, A.D.: Control of Microbial Contamination with Commercially Available Cleaning Solutions, *J. Prosthet. Dent., 67,* 275, February, 1992.

Chan, E.C., Iugovaz, I., Siboo, R., Bilyk, M., Barolet, R., Amsel, R., Wooley, C., and Klitorimos, A.: Comparison of Two Popular Methods for Removal and Killing of Bacteria from Dentures, *J. Can. Dent. Assoc., 57,* 937, December, 1991.

Cook, R.J.: Response of the Oral Mucosa to Denture Wearing, *J. Dent., 19,* 135, June, 1991.

Glass, R.T.: The Infected Toothbrush, the Infected Denture, and Transmission of Disease: A Review, *Compend. Cont. Educ. Dent., 13,* 592, July, 1992.

Jagger, D.C. and Harrison, A.: Denture Cleansing—The Best Approach, *Br. Dent. J., 178,* 413, June 10, 1995.

Ma, T., Johnson, G.H., and Gordon, G.E.: Effects of Chemical Disinfectants on the Surface Characteristics and Color of Denture Resins, *J. Prosthet. Dent., 77,* 197, February, 1997.

McNeme, S.J., vonGonten, A.S., and Woolsey, G.D.: Effects of Laboratory Disinfecting Agents on Color Stability of Denture Acrylic Resins, *J. Prosthet Dent., 66,* 132, July, 1991.

Merchant, V. and Molinari, J.A.: Infection Control in Prosthodontics: A Choice No Longer, *Gen. Dent., 37,* 29, January–February, 1989.

Nakamoto, K., Tamamoto, M., and Hamada, T.: Evaluation of Denture Cleansers With and Without Enzymes Against *Candida albicans, J. Prosthet. Dent., 66,* 792, December, 1991.

Obatake, R.M., Collard, S.M., Martin, J., and Ladd, G.D.: The Effects of Sodium Fluoride and Stannous Fluoride on the Surface Roughness of Intraoral Magnet Systems, *J. Prosthet. Dent., 66,* 553, October, 1991.

Orthodontics

Alexander, S.A.: Effects of Orthodontic Attachments on the Gingival Health of Permanent Second Molars, *Am. J. Orthod. Dentofacial Orthop., 100,* 337, October, 1991.

Atack, N.E., Sandy, J.R., and Addy, M.: Periodontal and Microbiological Changes Associated with the Placement of Orthodontic Appliances. A Review, *J. Periodontol., 67,* 78, February, 1996.

Berglund, L.J. and Small, C.L.: Effective Oral Hygiene for Orthodontic Patients, *J. Clin. Orthod., 24,* 315, May, 1990.

Brightman, L.J., Terezhalmy, G.T., Greenwell, H., Jacobs, M., and Enlow, D.H.: The Effects of a 0.12% Chlorhexidine Gluconate Mouthrinse on Orthodontic Patients Aged 11 Through 17 with Established Gingivitis, *Am. J. Orthod. Dentofacial Orthop., 100,* 324, October, 1991.

Casey, G.R.: Maintenance of Oral Hygiene and Dental Health During Orthodontic Therapy, *Clin. Prev. Dent., 10,* 11, January–February, 1988.

Cooney, B.M.: The Periodontally Compromised Adult Orthodontic Patient, *DentalHygienistNews, 5,* 7, Summer, 1992.

Geiger, A.M., Gorelick, L., Gwinnett, A.J., and Benson, B.J.: Reducing White Spot Lesions in Orthodontic Populations with Fluoride Rinsing, *Am. J. Orthod. Dentofacial Orthop., 101,* 403, May, 1992.

Huser, M.C., Baehni, P.C., and Lang, R.: Effects of Orthodontic Bands on Microbiologic and Clinical Parameters, *Am. J. Orthod. Dentofacial Orthop., 97,* 213, March, 1990.

Jackson, C.L.: Comparison Between Electric Toothbrushing and Manual Toothbrushing, With and Without Oral Irrigation, for Oral Hygiene of Orthodontic Patients, *Am. J. Orthod. Dentofacial Orthop., 99,* 15, January, 1991.

Kilicoglu, H., Yildirim, M., and Polater, H.: Comparison of the Effectiveness of Two Types of Toothbrushes on the Oral Hygiene of Patients Undergoing Orthodontic Treatment with Fixed Appliances, *Am. J. Orthod. Dentofacial Orthop., 111,* 591, June, 1997.

Morris, C.: Dental Hygiene and Orthodontics: An Advantageous Partnership, *Compend. Oral Hyg., 4,* 3, Number 1, 1997.

Riordan, D.J.: Effects of Orthodontic Treatment on Nutrient Intake, *Am. J. Orthod. Dentofacial Orthop., 111,* 554, May, 1997.

Schlein, R.A., Kudlick, E.M., Reindorf, C.A., Gregory, J., and Royal, G.C.: Toothbrushing and Transient Bacteremia in Patients Undergoing Orthodontic Treatment, *Am. J. Orthod. Dentofacial Orthop., 99,* 466, May, 1991.

Trimpeneers, L.M., Wijgaerts, I.A., Grognard, N.A., Dermaut, L.R., and Adriaens, P.A.: Effect of Electric Toothbrushes Versus Manual Toothbrushes on Removal of Plaque and Periodontal Status During Orthodontic Treatment, *Am. J. Orthod. Dentofacial Orthop., 111,* 492, May, 1997.

Trombeli, L., Scabbia, A., Griselli, A., Zangari, F., and Calura, G.: Clinical Evaluation of Plaque Removal by Counterrotational Electric Toothbrush in Orthodontic Patients, *Quintessence Int., 26,* 199, March, 1995.

Overdentures

Ettinger, R.L. and Jakobsen, J.: Caries: A Problem in an Overdenture Population, *Community Dent. Oral Epidemiol., 18,* 42, February, 1990.

Figures, K.H., Ellis, B., and Lamb, D.J.: Fluoride Penetration into Dentine Abutments *in vitro, Caries Res., 24,* 301, September–October, 1990.

Gomes, B.C. and Renner, R.P.: Periodontal Considerations of the Removable Partial Overdenture, *Dent. Clin. North Am., 34,* 653, October, 1990.

Keltjens, H.M.A.M., Schaeken, M.J.M., van der Hoeven, J.S., and Hendriks, J.C.M.: Caries Control in Overdenture Patients: 18-month Evaluation on Fluoride and Chlorhexidine Therapies, *Caries Res., 24,* 371, September–October, 1990.

McDermott, I.G. and Samant, A.: An Overview of Removable Partial Overdentures, *Compend. Cont. Educ. Dent., 11,* 106, February, 1990.

Walters, R.A.: Design, Preparation, and Maintenance of Overdenture Abutments, *Dent. Clin. North Am., 34,* 631, October, 1990.

Yamaga, T. and Nokubi, T.: Clinical Observations of Noncoping Overdenture Abutments Protected by Tannin-fluoride Preparation, *J. Prosthet. Dent., 78,* 315, September, 1997.

26

The Patient With Oral Rehabilitation and Implants

Complete oral rehabilitation refers to the combined treatment of the teeth and periodontium to restore health, function, and physical form. As generally used, *oral rehabilitation* applies to involved extensive restorative procedures in a mouth that cannot be treated with routine dental care. It is also known as *mouth rehabilitation, occlusal rehabilitation, occluso-rehabilitation, complete reconstruction,* or *periodontal prosthesis.* Key words are defined in Box 26-1. Other terms used in this chapter were defined in Box 25-1, page 395, particularly the types and parts of dental prostheses.

The term *periodontal prosthesis* is used to designate restorative and prosthodontic treatment that is necessary for the treatment of advanced periodontal disease. The prosthesis used may be a splint for immobilization or stabilization of a group of teeth or an entire arch, maxillary or mandibular.

Periodontal, restorative, and prosthodontic treatments are interdependent. The function and duration of all restorative and prosthodontic treatments depend directly on the health of the periodontium, which provides the attachment and support necessary for the restored teeth. Periodontal health, in turn, is influenced by restorative and prosthodontic treatment. Many predisposing factors that contribute to the initiation, development, and progress of periodontal infections are a direct result of untreated dental caries, incomplete or inadequate restorations, unreplaced missing teeth, and inadequate occlusal relationships built into restorations or prostheses.

I. OBJECTIVES OF COMPLETE REHABILITATION

Objectives for complete rehabilitation involve the same principles as for all oral care and include the need to

BOX 26-1 KEY WORDS: Rehabilitation and Implants*

Crown: an artificial replacement that restores missing tooth structure by surrounding part or all of the remaining structure with a material, such as cast metal or porcelain, or a combination of materials, such as metal and porcelain fused (veneer crown).

Embrasure (em-brā'zhur): the space defined by proximal surfaces of adjacent teeth where those surfaces diverge apically, facially, lingually, or occlusally from an area of contact.

Furcation (fur-kā'shun) **invasion:** pathologic resorption of bone within a furcation; a periodontal bony defect.

Hydroxyapatite ceramic: a composition of calcium and phosphate to provide a dense, nonresorbable, biocompatible ceramic used for dental implants; metal implants may be coated with tricalcium phosphate or hydroxyapatite.

Implant: an alloplastic (inert metal or plastic) material or device grafted or inserted surgically into intact tissues for diagnostic, prosthetic, therapeutic, or experimental purposes.

Inlay: a fixed restoration placed within tooth structure, prepared outside the mouth, and subsequently cemented into the tooth to restore intracoronal tooth structure; may be made of porcelain, composite resin, or cast gold.

Occlusal adjustment: treatment in which the occluding surfaces of teeth are reshaped by grinding to create harmonious contact relationships between maxillary and mandibular teeth; also known as occlusal equilibration or selective grinding.

Odontoplasty (ō-don"tō-plas'tē): the reshaping of a portion of a tooth; may be performed for therapeutic or esthetic purposes.

Onlay: a fixed restoration that is prepared outside the mouth and is subsequently cemented onto the tooth; it restores the occlusal surface, the mesial-distal or lingual-facial margins, and covers or replaces one or more cusps.

Osseous (os'ē-us) **integration:** the apparent direct attachment or connection of osseous tissue to an inert, alloplastic material without intervening connective tissue. Also called **osseointegration.**

Peri-implantitis (per"ē-ĭm-plan-tī'tĭs): inflammation of the tissue around a dental implant and/or its abutment.

Splint: an apparatus, appliance, or device used to prevent motion or displacement of fractured or movable parts.

Dental splint: designed to immobilize and stabilize teeth in the same dental arch.

Supportive periodontal treatment: an extension of periodontal therapy; includes procedures performed at selected time intervals to review the general health history, reassess the status of periodontal health, and provide preventive oral hygiene care; also called **periodontal maintenance** or **preventive maintenance.**

Titanium: a uniquely biocompatible metal used for implants either in the commercially pure form or as an alloy.

Titanium alloy: the most common titanium alloy (Ti-6A1-4V) used for dental implants contains 6% aluminum to increase strength and decrease weight, and 4% vanadium to prevent corrosion.

Tomography: a radiographic technique that provides a distinct image of a selected plane through the body; the images of structures that lie above and below that plane are blurred.

Veneer: a layer of tooth-color material (composite or porcelain) that is bonded or cemented to a prepared tooth surface.

*Definitions in this chapter that pertain to prosthodontics are taken or adapted from and are in accord with the *Glossary of Prosthodontic Terms,* 6th ed., 1993, of the Academy of Prosthodontics Foundation.

Definitions that relate to periodontics are taken or adapted from the *Glossary of Periodontal Terms,* 3rd ed., 1992, of the American Academy of Periodontology.

A. Restore optimal functional occlusion.
B. Maintain the health of the periodontium.
C. Produce biologically contoured restorations in harmony with normal oral physiology.
D. Replace missing teeth.
E. Provide support to teeth with advanced bone loss and marked mobility.
F. Provide desirable esthetics.
G. Establish acceptable phonetics.

II. COMPONENTS OF TREATMENT

Complete oral reconstruction means total mouth involvement, which brings in many phases of dentistry, often accomplished by individual specialists. The overall treatment plan may include some or all of the following:

A. Extensive periodontal therapy involving various surgical procedures.
B. Occlusal adjustment.
C. Endodontic therapy.
D. Correction of oral habits.
E. Orthodontic tooth movement.
F. Splinting of teeth temporarily or permanently.
G. Dental implants.
H. Restorations involving individual teeth: crowns, inlays, onlays.
I. Replacement of teeth by fixed and/or removable prostheses.

III. ACCOMPLISHMENT OF TREATMENT

Treatment may be long and involved for the patient who undergoes complete oral rehabilitation. It requires patience, persistence, and dedication of the patient, the dental hygienist, and the dentist.

The dental hygiene treatment plan overlaps every phase of the total treatment, beginning with the initial preparation of the patient's mouth. Maintenance and supervision of the patient's self care program are essential throughout restorative and prosthodontic therapy and continuing into the maintenance phase.

Specific measures for self-care in terms of plaque removal and dental caries prevention must be selected and supervised. The patient is shown how to self-evaluate, so that minor deviations from normal can be recognized and called to the attention of the clinician.

CHARACTERISTICS OF THE REHABILITATED MOUTH

To select the appropriate methods for bacterial plaque control and dental caries prevention, one must assess existing conditions, such as contour and position of the gingiva, contour of restorations, and problem areas adjacent to fixed prostheses. When these are known, the variety of possible techniques and devices for plaque removal can be reviewed and a plan for care outlined.

A patient who has undergone extensive periodontal therapy and restorative and prosthodontic rehabilitation may have some or all of the characteristics listed here. Each condition may require specially selected or adapted self-care measures for bacterial plaque control. Fixed and removable appliances can provide many areas for bacterial plaque and debris retention.

I. PERIODONTAL FINDINGS

A. Gingival recession.
B. Exposed root surfaces.
C. Exposed furcation areas.
D. Alterations of gingival contour; the gingival margins may be rolled or rounded.
E. Changes in size and shape of the gingival embrasures.
　1. Missing interdental papillae; wide embrasures with gingival recession and increased root exposure (Figure 26-1).
　2. Narrowed embrasures created by overcontoured restorations or variously shaped pontics (Figure 26-2).

II. SINGLE TOOTH RESTORATIONS

A. The gingival margin around a crown restoration may appear bluish or bluish-red when the crown margin is below the gingival margin.
B. Various restorations may require selective cleaning agents.

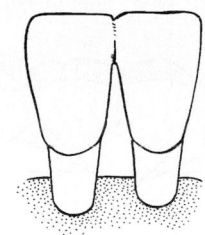

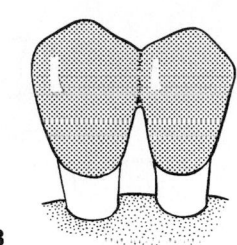

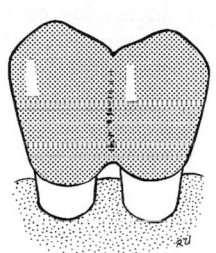

FIGURE 26-1 Gingival Embrasures. (A) Wide embrasure between two central incisors with missing interdental papilla and gingival recession. **(B)** Double abutment with closed contact area with open embrasure provides access for plaque removal. **(C)** Overcontoured crowns of a double abutment with a narrowed embrasure that provides limited access for bacterial plaque and debris removal.

III. FIXED PROSTHESES

The parts of a fixed prosthesis are shown on page 400 in Figure 25-8.
　A patient may have
　　A. Fixed splinting around long segments of, or an entire, arch (Figure 26-3).
　　B. Natural abutment teeth with difficult access areas adjacent to a pontic.
　　C. Implant abutment surfaces.
　　D. Closed contacts between teeth involved in a multitooth prosthesis.
　　E. Gingival surfaces of pontics.
　　F. Wide and triangular embrasures created by pontics or narrow, unnatural, non-self-cleansing areas created by improperly shaped pontics (Figure 26-2B).

IV. REMOVABLE PROSTHESES

A. Complete denture may be used in one dental arch opposing natural teeth and partial dentures, fixed or removable.

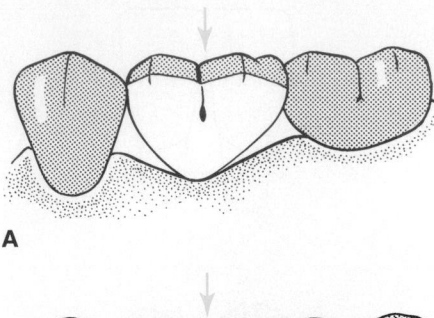

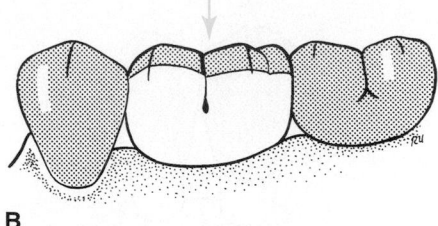

FIGURE 26-2 Shape of Pontics. Mandibular three-unit fixed partial denture. **(A)** "Bullet"-shaped pontic with wide embrasures for access for bacterial plaque removal. **(B)** Improperly shaped pontic with closed embrasures and wide gingival surface for plaque retention. Arrows indicate pontics.

B. Partial denture
1. Creation of potential areas of bacterial plaque and debris retention.
   a. Alteration of tooth form by clasp, rest, or precision attachment (defined in Box 25-1, page 395).
   b. Improperly contoured edge of the partial denture at the junction of the partial denture and the abutment tooth.

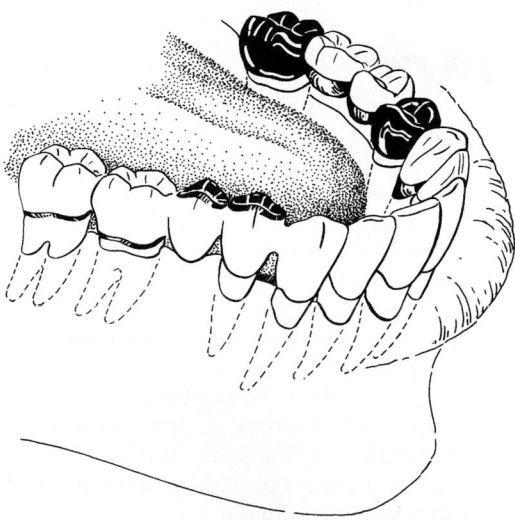

FIGURE 26-3 Complete-Arch Fixed Splint. A continuous therapeutic fixed appliance stabilizes periodontally involved teeth and replaces missing components to provide appropriate occlusal relationships. Numerous problem areas for bacterial plaque removal exist.

2. Partial denture may impinge on the gingiva surrounding the abutment tooth.
3. Double abutment (two natural teeth with crowns that are soldered or cast together) has a closed contact requiring lateral (from facial or lingual aspects) access to the gingival embrasure (Figure 26-1*B* and *C*).
4. The mucosa under the partial denture needs special care.

SELF-CARE FOR THE REHABILITATED MOUTH

These special patients require greater than average attention, patience, and teaching skill to obtain a favorable result that will ensure continuing health of the patient's periodontal tissues. Total commitment on the part of the patient is necessary if the selected plan is to meet the requirements for daily care.

I. PLANNING THE DISEASE CONTROL PROGRAM

The control program should be planned as a concentrated effort to maintain the gingival tissue, the exposed tooth structure, and, hence, the underlying supporting periodontium, as well as the restorations and prostheses. The instructions have three parts: first, before the surgical, restorative, and prosthodontic treatment; second, during therapy; and third, after reconstruction.

A. Part 1
Basic plaque control measures are learned and practiced by the patient during the preparatory phase. During these lessons, principles for self-evaluation can be presented.

B. Part 2
During therapy, adaptations are needed for applying techniques to temporary restorations. When the treatment extends over a long period, regular dental hygiene appointments for careful monitoring of the gingival health are essential.

C. Part 3
After therapy is completed, another set of self-care procedures is required to meet the needs of the rehabilitated mouth. Special devices and techniques are selected and tried until the most efficient and thorough procedures are determined.

II. PLAQUE CONTROL: SELECTION OF METHODS[1]

Any of the methods and procedures described in Chapters 23, 24, and 25 may be needed in the care of the oral soft tissues, tooth surfaces, restorations, and fixed and removable prostheses. After assessment, methods selected must allow the patient to accomplish complete daily plaque removal from each area around every tooth or replacement. A summary of devices and methods is provided in Table 26-1.

Most patients need a method for each of the following:

A. Debris removal, particularly from interproximal areas and around fixed implants and prostheses.
B. Sulcular brushing procedure adapted for complete coverage for anatomic variations.
C. Interdental plaque removal
　1. Proximal surfaces of natural and restored teeth, including exposed roots where access exists from the incisal or occlusal surfaces.
　2. Proximal surfaces of abutment teeth under closed contact areas (Figure 26-4).
　3. Mesial and/or distal surfaces of teeth without proximal contact.
D. Removal of bacterial plaque around a fixed partial denture must include the gingival and proximal surfaces of pontics.
E. Cleaning a removable prosthesis and care of the supporting tissues.

III. FLUORIDES

A. Selection of Fluorides

For the patient with porcelain or composite

TABLE 26-1 Care of the Rehabilitated Mouth

Problem	Device/Method	Special Adaptations
Debris removal	Water irrigation Toothbrush	Wide embrasures Under fixed partial dentures
Sulcular brushing	Toothbrush with soft, end-rounded filaments	Facial and lingual surfaces Distal surfaces of most-posterior teeth, particularly terminal abutment
Proximal surfaces, plaque removal	Floss Floss with threader Yarn with floss and/or threader Toothpick holder Pipe cleaner Interdental brush Single-tuft brush	Abutment teeth Proximal root surfaces Pontic surfaces Narrowed embrasures
Proximal surfaces, open contacts	Gauze strip Yarn	Terminal abutment of removable partial denture Distal surfaces of most-posterior teeth in the dental arch
Exposed furcation, molars	Pipe cleaner Floss/yarn in threader Interdental brush Interdental rubber tip	Rotated tooth
Exposed furcation, maxillary first premolar	Interdental brush Interdental rubber tip	Fused root with groove
Exposed root surfaces	Fluoride dentifrice Dentifrice containing desensitizing agent	Desensitization Prevent abrasion of cementum or dentin
Fixed partial denture	Toothbrush (soft, end-rounded) Floss threader with floss/yarn Any other proximal surface procedures as applicable	Gingival surfaces of pontics Proximal surfaces of pontics and retainers
Edentulous gingiva under removable denture	Toothbrush (soft nylon) (manual or power-assisted) Digital massage	Stimulation and plaque removal
Tongue cleaning	Toothbrush (soft nylon) Tongue scraper	Deep fissures
Removable denture	Denture brush Clasp brush Chemical cleanser for immersion	Clasps

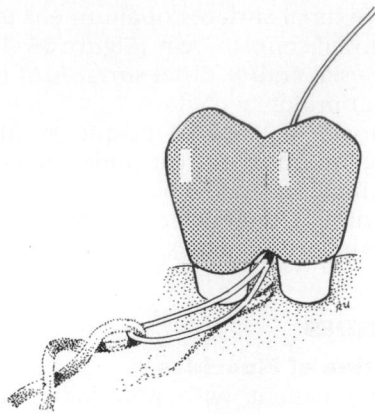

■ FIGURE 26-4 Bacterial Plaque Removal from Embrasure. A floss threader is used with yarn or tufted floss to clean under a double abutment embrasure. Narrowed embrasure from overcontoured crown increases plaque and debris retention and makes cleaning difficult.

resin restorations, an acidulated fluoride preparation must be avoided. Porcelain and composite resin restorations become pitted and rough with repeated applications of a fluoride solution with an acidic pH.[2]

Neutral fluoride products with low viscosity and low fluoride concentration can be advised.

B. Personal Daily Program

Fluoride dentifrice, along with daily mouthrinse or brush-on gel, is recommended to prevent root caries. For certain patients in the root caries risk groups and those with multiple sensitive teeth, a custom-tray application should be used daily.

C. Professional Topical Applications

When the patient does not drink fluoridated water routinely or use self-treatment methods on a regular basis, additional fluoride may be deemed beneficial. Professional applications are recommended for each maintenance appointment.

IV. DIETARY ASSESSMENT

Whether the need for the rehabilitation was related to extensive dental caries or to a periodontal disease, dietary counseling is indicated. Every possible means must be taken to prevent carious lesions of the exposed root surfaces about the restorations. Overall dietary factors should be checked to ensure support from a nutritional standpoint. Procedures for obtaining the food record and conducting the counseling session are described on pages 444 to 449.

V. PROCEDURE

No fixed procedure applies to every patient. A personalized sequence must be worked out, often by trial and error.

A. Outline a possible sequence
  1. Select methods and devices that can meet the requirements of the individual oral characteristics.
  2. Demonstrate the use of the methods and have the patient practice under supervision. Avoid presenting too many procedures in one lesson, which can confuse and discourage the patient.
  3. Provide step-by-step written directions for home reference.
B. Recheck successes within a few days and at least by 1 week.
  1. Assess gingival tissue (Table 11-1, pages 194 and 195).
  2. Assess plaque. Use a disclosing agent to provide the patient with an evaluation of areas that need additional attention.
  3. Assess performance
    a. Observe patient's dexterity in managing the self-care methods for plaque removal.
    b. Note relationship of procedures used by the patient to areas where disclosing agent revealed plaque retention.
  4. Make necessary adjustments to simplify and clarify, so that all areas are completely deplaqued daily.
C. Re-evaluate weekly or as frequently as needed to maintain the patient's motivation, to follow the health of the gingival tissues, and to recognize a need for changes in the procedures used.

VI. SAMPLE PROCEDURE

The patient described in this section has a complete maxillary fixed partial denture (splint), which has several natural teeth as abutments and four areas of double pontics; a mandibular removable partial denture with double abutments connecting mandibular canines and first premolars on each side; and wide embrasures between mandibular incisors caused by previous periodontal infection, which has since been treated with periodontal surgery.

The patient might use the following procedure:

A. Morning, After Eating
  1. Completely brush with power-assisted brush (containing softest filaments available); apply the brush to proximal surfaces.
  2. Brush partial removable denture manually and rinse thoroughly.

B. Noon, After Eating (Away From Home)
  1. Rinse partial denture under running water.
  2. Use manual toothbrush, covering all surfaces as thoroughly as possible.
  3. Rinse carefully, forcing the water under fixed partial denture areas.

C. Evening, After All Eating
  1. Remove partial denture, rinse under run-

ning water, and place in cleansing solution. (Complete procedure for partial removable denture is described on pages 402 and 403).

2. Use water irrigator to remove debris from all parts of fixed splint and from all proximal surfaces of mandibular teeth.

3. Use toothbrush for facial and lingual sulcular brushing; apply the brush interdentally as much as possible. Use sodium fluoride dentifrice.

4. Brush tongue and edentulous gingiva under removable denture.

5. Use dental floss and/or yarn for accessible proximal surfaces.

6. Clean all gingival and proximal surfaces of fixed partial denture. Use floss and yarn with floss threader for all proximal and gingival surfaces not accessible from incisal or occlusal aspects. Interdental brush may be needed for certain wide embrasures.

7. Use yarn or gauze strip for distal surfaces of the abutment teeth for the mandibular removable denture (mandibular premolars).

8. Use toothpick holder with dentifrice containing a desensitizing agent to massage hypersensitive areas of exposed roots.

9. Rinse with fluoride mouthrinse; vigorously force the solution between the teeth and under fixed appliances.

10. Clean partial denture, using denture brush and clasp brush, and rinse the denture thoroughly.

VII. MAINTENANCE PLAN

Continuing supervision of the patient with oral rehabilitation is an absolute essential. The well-informed and conscientious patient who devotes up to an hour each day on personal care procedures expects a maintenance appointment that thoroughly evaluates the gingival tissue, the rehabilitation prostheses, and the completeness of plaque control efforts.

Everything listed on pages 644 and 645 for inclusion in the maintenance examination applies with special meaning and emphasis to the rehabilitated patient. What could seem like a minute area of gingival bleeding on probing, whether the pocket is shallow or has started to deepen, should be a warning signal that an area may not be covered by present self-care procedures and needs some form of treatment. *Each millimeter of gingival sulcus must be probed carefully to detect incipient changes.*

DENTAL IMPLANTS

A *dental implant* may be placed within or on mandibular or maxillary bone either to replace teeth or to provide a stable and retentive base for support of a fixed or removable prosthesis. The various plates and screws used in the treatment of fractured bones are also implants.

The success of an implant can depend on many factors, especially including patient understanding and skills for direct daily care of the prosthesis and the surrounding soft tissues. Frequent maintenance appointments for careful supervision and patient motivation are essential components for implant success.

TYPES OF DENTAL IMPLANTS

The three general categories of dental implants are described here. They are endosseous, subperiosteal, and transosteal. The endosseous implants are the most widely used.

I. ENDOSSEOUS (ENDOSTEAL)

A. Location
The implant is placed within the bone.

B. Examples
Blade, screw, and cylinder types are used (Figure 26-5).

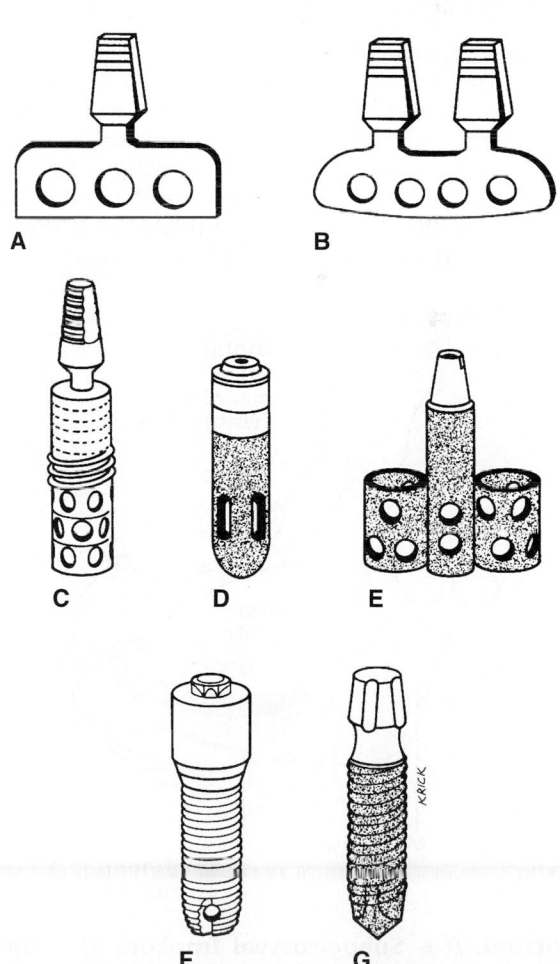

■ **FIGURE 26-5 Endosseous Implants. A** and **B.** Blade types. **C, D,** and **E.** Cylinder types. **F** and **G.** Screw types.

C. Materials

The three basic types of biomaterials are metals and alloys, ceramics and carbon, and polymers.[3]

D. Description[4]

The support, body, or fixture is placed in bone during the first surgical step and left covered by mucosal tissue for several months while implant bonds with the bone. The abutment, post, or neck is then exposed through the soft tissue at a second-stage surgical procedure. Placement of the prosthesis follows.

II. SUBPERIOSTEAL

A. Location

The implant is placed over the bone, under the periosteum.

B. Example

A custom-fabricated framework of metal rests over the bone of the mandible or maxilla; it may be the complete arch or unilateral (Figure 26-6).

C. Material

Cobalt-chromium-molybdenum (Vitallium) or titanium are used.

D. Description[5,6]

1. *Two-step.* In the first step, a surgical flap is used to reflect mucosal tissues and to expose the underlying bone. An impression is made of the bony ridge. The metallic unit is cast and then placed in a second surgical step. Usually, four posts protrude into the oral cavity to hold the complete denture.

2. *One-step.* Computer-assisted tomography design and manufacturing have been applied, using a reformatted computed tomography scan from which approximate casts of the maxilla or mandible can be made. The implant is designed on this replica and is placed in one surgical procedure.

III. TRANSOSTEAL (TRANSOSSEOUS)

A. Location

The implant is placed through the bone.

B. Example

The mandibular staple bone plate (Figure 26-7).

C. Materials

Stainless steel, ceramic-coated materials, and titanium alloy.

D. Description[7,8]

A metal plate, fitted to the inferior border of the mandible, has five to seven pins extending toward the occlusal surface. Usually, two terminal pins protrude into the oral cavity to hold the overdenture. The pins are connected by a crossbar. The transosteal implant can be used when the patient has an atrophic edentulous mandible or a congenital or traumatic deformity of the mandible.

PREPARATION AND PLACEMENT

I. PATIENT SELECTION

Careful screening is essential at the start. Generally acceptable physical health and a real desire to go through the required treatment are prerequisite. Diagnosis and treatment planning are based on a risk-benefit analysis and follow a detailed medical, dental, and behavioral history along with an oral and radio-

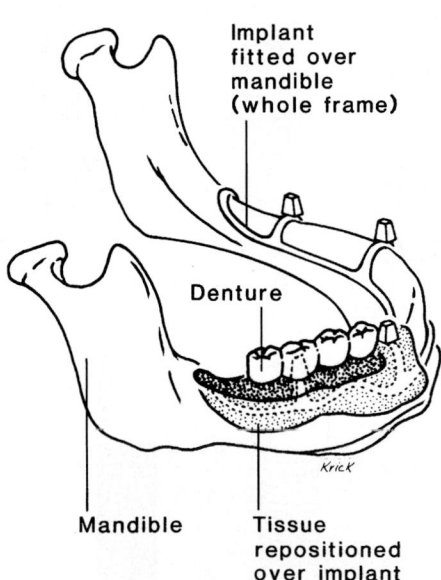

FIGURE 26-6 Subperiosteal Implant. The custom-fabricated framework is shown on the left side of the mandible; on the right side, the framework is shown by dotted lines under the denture.

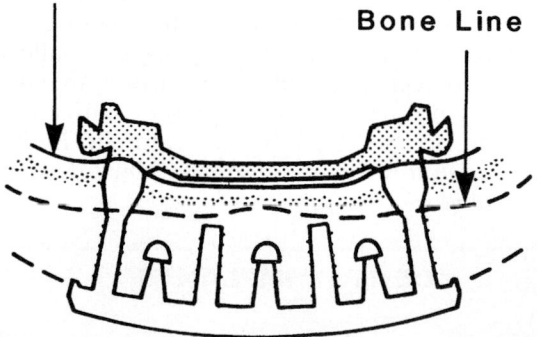

FIGURE 26-7 Transosteal Implant. Mandibular staple bone plate in the anterior region shows metal plate at the lower border of the mandible, with pins extending toward the occlusal surface. Terminal pins protrude into the oral cavity to hold the overdenture.

graphic examination. Sometimes a psychologic examination is used.

A. Systemic Health
1. *Medical History.* The patient must be free of systemic conditions that can interfere with healing or acceptance of the implant. Biocompatibility of the implant with body tissues is essential.
2. *Contraindications.* Examples of conditions that may make a patient a poor risk include recent radiation therapy to the affected part, uncontrolled diabetes mellitus, alcoholism or heavy alcohol intake, substance abuse including tobacco use, an immunosuppressive disease or medication, anticoagulant medication, psychosis, or paranoia.

B. Oral Examination
1. Radiographic evidence of adequate depth of alveolar bone is needed.
2. The presence of an active oral disease, such as periodontitis, contraindicates implant placement until the disease is treated and under control.

C. Oral Hygiene
The patient must demonstrate consistent and effective personal oral care.

II. INFORMATION FOR THE PATIENT

A. Explain procedures to be performed and the time schedule.
B. Explain possible complications.
C. Emphasize the role of personal oral care and the need for daily bacterial plaque control.
D. Obtain an informed consent statement and agreement of understanding.

III. SURGICAL STEPS

Acceptable bone integration has occurred with certain single-stage endosseous implants, but the generally accepted method is a two-stage procedure. The entire implant usually cannot be inserted in one step because forces of occlusion (chewing, biting) cause mobility and prevent bone healing. When the implant is first placed it must be stabilized. Movement of the implant may cause the formation of a fibrous tissue layer instead of osseointegration.

The surgical procedure requires atraumatic placement of the implant into the bone. Whenever microorganisms are introduced during a surgical procedure, healing can be impaired. Manufacturers prepare implants in sterile packages.

IV. PROSTHODONTIC STEPS

Attention to ideal requirements for acceptable prostheses is necessary. Margins, embrasure shapes, crown contours, contact areas, and occlusal harmony must be designed to prevent bacterial plaque collection and permit thorough disease control procedures by the patient.

IMPLANT INTERFACES

An implant has an inner interface with the *bone* and a *soft tissue* interface where the terminal pin, abutment, post, or other protruding portion of the implant is surrounded by the mucosal or gingival tissue.

I. IMPLANT/BONE INTERFACE
Osseointegration refers to direct structural and functional union between the implant and healthy living bone. No discernible connective tissue is between the bone and the implant.

II. IMPLANT/SOFT TISSUE INTERFACE
The external environment of an implant is the oral cavity, with saliva, bacterial plaque, and debris.

A. Biologic Seal (Permucosal Seal)
Between the implant or post and the soft tissue, a biologic seal must exist to prevent microorganisms and inflammation-producing agents from entering the tissues.

B. Soft Tissue Connection
Sulcular epithelium is in contact with the implant surface. The attachment appears similar to the epithelial attachment of the junctional epithelium of a natural tooth. Hemidesmosomes and basal lamina have been identified. The epithelium resembles a long junctional epithelium.

PERI-IMPLANT HYGIENE

A key requirement for implant success is the disease control program for the tissue surrounding the implant. Meticulous hygiene is a necessity for which repeated instruction may be needed.

I. CARE OF THE NATURAL TEETH
Transmission of microorganisms from the natural teeth and periodontal pockets to the peri-implant tissues can occur. The pockets around the teeth act as natural reservoirs, and periodontal pathogens from the pockets colonize in the tissue around the implants. It is therefore of utmost importance that, before placement of the implants, the periodontal condition be treated and brought to a healthy state. Then, after the placement of the implants, the maintenance program emphasizes care of the natural teeth and tissues as well as the peri-implant tissues.

II. BACTERIAL PLAQUE (IMPLANT PLAQUE)
Plaque microorganisms around implants with healthy permucosal tissue have been shown to be like the

flora around natural teeth. Gram-positive, nonmotile, coccoid, and other forms of bacteria predominate.[11,12,13]

The tissues around implant posts or abutments react to microorganisms and their toxic products in a manner similar to the gingiva surrounding natural teeth. When inflammation and pocket depths increase, the total number of microorganisms including spirochetes and motile rods increase also.[13]

III. PLANNING THE DISEASE CONTROL PROGRAM

A. Relation to Treatment
Supervision of a patient's oral hygiene must begin prior to the surgical phase for implant placement and carry on throughout the treatment phases.

B. Types of Prostheses
Implant-supported prostheses may be partial, complete, fixed, removable, or single-tooth replacements. Prostheses may be supported by natural teeth and/or implants. An individual may have a variety of areas and prostheses to care for.

IV. SELECTION OF PLAQUE-REMOVAL METHODS

Any of the methods for plaque removal described in Chapters 23, 24, and 25 may be required in various combinations. Each patient needs an individually planned program so that each type of abutment and prosthesis can be maintained in a plaque-free environment.

A. Conventional Prosthesis
Removable or fixed, partial or complete dentures made of conventional dental materials are to be cleaned by the usual methods described earlier. Suggestions provided here pertain primarily to the posts, abutments, or other protruding portions of implants.

B. Precautions
1. Prevent damage to implant materials. Care must be taken to use implements, dentifrices, or other cleaning agents that will not scratch or abrade the titanium or other material. Only smooth plastic or wooden implements should be used.
2. Each device should be checked before use. Toothbrush filaments must be smooth, soft, and end rounded to prevent damage to the peri-implant tissue. Soft, end-rounded, power-assisted brushes can be applied effectively.

C. Subperiosteal Implant
The posts and surrounding tissue need to be cleaned completely around the circumference. Yarn or gauze strip can be used with a floss threader to position the material under the crossbar.

D. Endosseus Implant
1. *Abutments or Posts.* A floss threader can be used to position yarn or a gauze bandage strip around an abutment and under a fixed prosthesis. Tufted dental floss is also highly effective. Interdental brushes and single end-tuft brushes are adaptable. The end-tuft brush bent at the neck is particularly useful on lingual and palatal surfaces (see Figure 24-9, page 378).
2. *Undersurface of Fixed Prosthesis With Cantilever.* Several endosseous implants may be placed anterior to the mental foramen, and the complete overdenture may have a cantilevered portion distal to the terminal implant. Cleaning plaque from under the cantilever may be accomplished by using gauze strips.

V. RINSING AND IRRIGATION

A. General Cleaning
Use of an irrigator can remove debris before specific cleaning with toothbrush and auxiliary aids.

B. Chemotherapy
1. Rinsing or daily irrigation with an approved antimicrobial can be recommended to help minimize bacterial accumulation and inflammation. Specific directions for preparation of the solution and use of the irrigator must be demonstrated.
2. Chlorhexidine, 0.12%, has been shown to be effective. A cotton swab or interdental brush, dipped in the solution, can be applied directly to the gingival margins to help to prevent staining of oral tissues or tooth-color restorations.[14]

VI. FLUORIDE MEASURES FOR DENTAL CARIES CONTROL

For the patient with natural teeth, daily fluoride self-application should be incorporated into the regime (pages 469 to 472). Titanium implants may be corroded by acidic fluoride preparations or preparations with a high fluoride concentration.[15,16] Low-concentration neutral sodium fluoride is recommended.

MAINTENANCE

I. BASIC CRITERIA FOR IMPLANT SUCCESS

The long-term success of an implant is assessed by routine, frequent examinations. A healthy implant shows the following:
A. No pain or discomfort reported by the patient.
B. No mobility.
C. No bleeding or increased probing depths on gentle probing.

D. No bone loss or peri-implant radiolucency in a radiograph.

E. No clinical signs of peri-implantitis (Table 11-1, pages 194 to 195).

II. FREQUENCY OF APPOINTMENTS

The patient's daily oral plaque removal and regular supervision and monitoring through maintenance appointments directly influence the long-term success of an implant. When teeth were lost originally because of lack of daily plaque control by the patient, a more intense program of education and practice may be needed. Neglect may have been caused by lack of knowledge about, or appreciation for, preventive measures.

Each patient must have a personalized appointment interval, depending on individual needs. The first series of appointments following placement of the implant(s) should start within a week and be scheduled weekly until healing is completed and the patient has demonstrated the ability to control the bacterial plaque.

Maintenance appointments during the first year may be at 1- or 2-month intervals.

III. THE MAINTENANCE APPOINTMENT

Factors outlined for a maintenance appointment (pages 644 to 645) apply to a patient with an implant.

A. Health History Review; Vital Signs; Intraoral/Extraoral Examination

Basic review questions can reveal the present state of health, recent illnesses, changes in medications, and other current information. Comparisons with previous records permit assessment of vital signs and extraoral/intraoral observations.

B. Selective Radiographs

A standard procedure must be used in order that comparisons can be made for bone level to determine status of implant stability. Special film placement devices have been developed.[17,18]

C. Periodontal Assessment

1. *Peri-Implant Tissue.* Visual examination should show no signs of inflammation as evidenced by the usual criteria of changes in color, size, shape, and consistency.
2. *Probing.* Probe gently to determine bleeding tendency. A plastic probe must be used.
3. *Mobility Determination.*
4. *Deposits.* Bacterial plaque can be tested with a disclosing agent. The gingival surfaces of fixed prostheses should be checked carefully.

   Calculus is usually not extensive, hard, or firmly attached to implant abutments or other protruding parts, provided the patient has been faithful with daily procedures and professional maintenance appointments.

D. Review of Personal Bacterial Plaque Control Procedures

The patient demonstrates self-care methods, and the clinician provides recommendations for improvements.

E. Instrumentation

Each type of implant requires attention to certain features. Manufacturer's instructions should be followed. Care must be taken not to scratch or alter in any way the surfaces of titanium and other materials making up the implant superstructures.

1. *Calculus Removal.* Plastic instruments are indicated for titanium. Figure 26-8 shows vari-

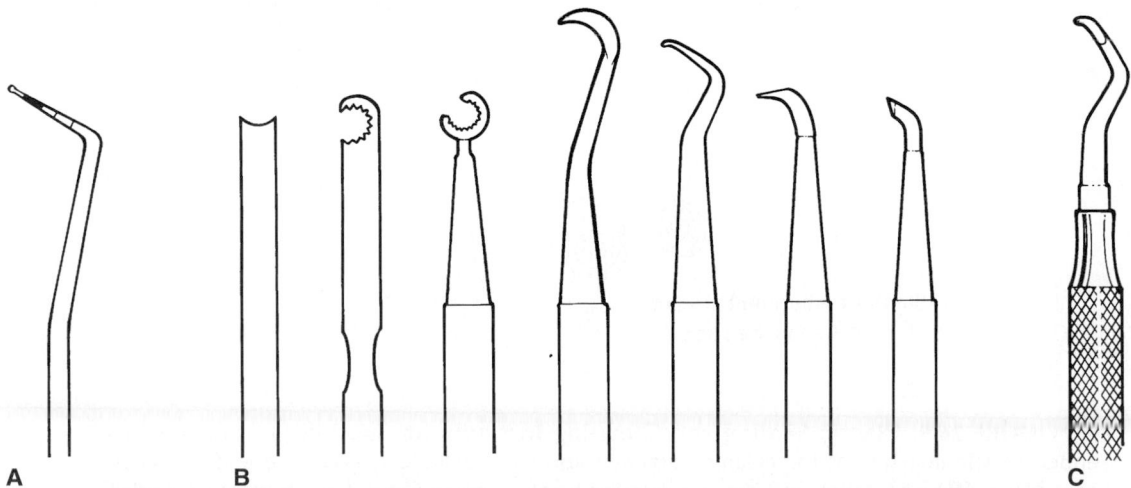

FIGURE 26-8 Plastic Instrument Designs for Implants. (A) Plastic probe with same markings as that in Figure 19-1 (page 296). **(B)** Scalers and curets. **(C)** Exchangeable plastic curet tip fitted to metal handle for convenient sterilization and replacement. (*Implacare*, HuFriedy, used with permission.)

ous plastic instruments that have been developed for use on implants. In Figure 26-9, adaptation of plastic instruments to implant abutments is illustrated.

2. *Prevention of Damage to the Implant Surface.* Severe abrasion can result from application of an ultrasonic scaler.

3. *Stain Removal.* Unless necessary for esthetics, stain removal is not included routinely. When selective stain removal with a rubber cup is indicated, only a nonabrasive agent should be used and applied gently. An air-powder polisher can be used with a light, sweeping, low-pressured application.[19–21]

4. *Professional Subgingival Irrigation.* The use of 0.12% chlorhexidine after professional instrumentation may be another treatment alternative when peri-implantitis has been present. Irrigation with chlorhexidine gluconate has been shown to be a safe procedure around implants.[22,23]

FACTORS TO TEACH THE PATIENT

I. IMPORTANCE OF DAILY CARE

The health of the periodontal tissues and the duration of the restorations and prostheses depend on daily self-care by the patient.

II. NEED FOR CONCENTRATION

More thought and concentration are required to maintain the mouth with advanced restorative dentistry, periodontal prostheses, or implants than are needed for an average mouth.

III. TIME REQUIREMENT

Cleaning a mouth with complex restorations takes longer. Time must be allotted in the daily schedule for complete cleaning and plaque removal once each day, supplemented by cleaning at least three times each day, or after each meal.

IV. DILIGENCE AND THOROUGHNESS

Do not go easy with the brush and other devices in the attempt to protect the restorations from breakage. *Protection* is for the gingival tissues and the preservation of the periodontium and is accomplished only by thorough bacterial plaque removal around every tooth.

V. IMPORTANCE OF MAINTENANCE

Frequent, regular appointments for professional supervision and cooperative care are necessary.

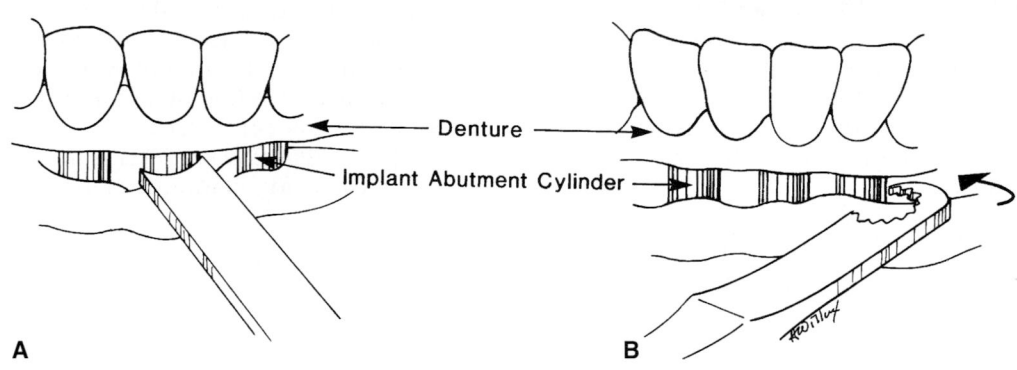

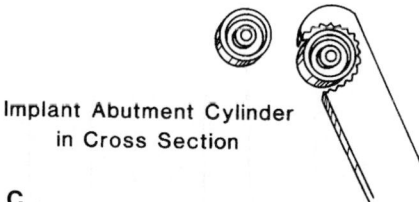

■ **FIGURE 26-9 Plastic Scaling and Cleaning Instrument.** Specially designed double-ended plastic instrument for cleaning titanium abutment cylinders. **(A)** One end is a crescent blade. **(B)** The other end is a semicircular hook to apply around an abutment cylinder, shown in **(C)**. (Adapted from Balshi, T.J.: Hygiene Maintenance Procedures for Patients Treated with the Tissue Integrated Prosthesis [Osseointegration], *Quintessence Int., 17,* 95, February, 1986).

REFERENCES

1. **Bradbury,** E., Harvard University School of Dental Medicine, Boston, personal communication.
2. **American Dental Association,** Council on Dental Materials, Instruments, and Equipment and Council on Dental Therapeutics: Status Report: Effect of Acidulated Phosphate Fluoride on Porcelain and Composite Restorations, *J. Am. Dent. Assoc., 116,* 115, January, 1988.
3. **Lemons,** J.E.: Dental Implant Biomaterials, *J. Am. Dent. Assoc., 121,* 716, December, 1990.
4. **Albrektsson,** T., Zarb, G., Worthington, P., and Eriksson, A.R.: The Long-term Efficacy of Currently Used Dental Implants: A Review and Proposed Criteria of Success, *Int. J. Oral Maxillofac. Implants, 1,* 11, No. 1, 1986.
5. **Harris,** B.W.: A New Technique for the Subperiosteal Implant, *J. Am. Dent. Assoc., 121,* 422, September, 1990.
6. **Homoly,** P.A.: The Restorative and Surgical Technique for the Full Maxillary Subperiosteal Implant, *J. Am. Dent. Assoc., 121,* 404, September, 1990.
7. **Cranin,** A.N., Sher, J., and Schilb, T.P.: The Transosteal Implant: A 17-year Review and Report, *J. Prosthet. Dent., 55,* 709, June, 1986.
8. **Small,** I.A.: The Fixed Mandibular Implant: Its Use in Reconstructive Prosthetics, *J. Am. Dent. Assoc., 121,* 369, September, 1990.
9. **Donley,** T.G. and Gillette, W.B.: Titanium Endosseous Implant-Soft Tissue Interface: A Literature Review, *J. Periodontol., 62,* 153, February, 1991.
10. **Cochran,** D.: Implant Therapy I, *Annals of Periodontol., 1,* 710, November, 1996.
11. **Mombelli,** A. and Lang, N.P.: Microbial Aspects of Implant Dentistry, *Periodontology 2000, 4,* 74, 1994.
12. **Mombelli,** A., Marxer, M., Gaberthüel, T., Grunder, U., and Lang, N.P.: The Microbiota of Osseointegrated Implants in Patients with a History of Periodontal Disease, *J. Clin. Periodontol., 22,* 124, February, 1995.
13. **Schou,** S., Holmstrup, P., Hjorting-Hansen, E., and Lang, N.P.: Plaque-induced Marginal Tissue Reactions of Osseointegrated Oral Implants: A Review of the Literature, *Clin. Oral Impl. Res., 3,* 149, December, 1992.
14. **Koutsonikos,** A., Federico, J., and Yukna, R.A.: Implant Maintenance, *J. Pract. Hyg., 5,* 11, March/April, 1996.
15. **Siirilä,** H.S. and Könönen, M.: The Effect of Oral Topical Fluorides on the Surface of Commercially Pure Titanium, *Int. J. Oral Maxillofac. Implants, 6,* 50, Number 1, 1991.
16. **Probster,** L., Lin, W., and Hüttemann, H.: Effect of Fluoride Prophylactic Agents on Titanium Surfaces, *Int. J. Oral Maxillofac. Implants, 7,* 390, Fall, 1992.
17. **Cox,** J.F. and Pharoah, M.: An Alternative Holder For Radiographic Evaluation of Tissue-integrated Prostheses, *J. Prosthet. Dent., 56,* 338, September, 1986.
18. **Meijer,** H.J.A., Steen, W.H.A., and Bosman, F.: Standardized Radiographs of the Alveolar Crest Around Implants in the Mandible, *J. Prosthet. Dent., 68,* 318, August, 1992.
19. **Barnes,** C.M., Fleming, L.S., and Mueninghoff, L.A.: An SEM Evaluation of the In-vitro Effects of an Air-abrasive System on Various Implant Surfaces, *Int. J. Oral Maxillofac. Implants, 6,* 463, Number 4, 1991.
20. **Brookshire,** F.V.G., Nagy, W.W., Dhuru, V.B., Ziebert, G.J., and Chada, S.: The Qualitative Effects of Various Types of Hygiene Instrumentation on Commercially Pure Titanium and Titanium Alloy Implant Abutments: An in vitro and Scanning Electron Microscope Study, *J. Prosthet. Dent., 78,* 286, September, 1997.
21. **Chairay,** J.-P., Boulekbache, H., Jean, A., Soyer, A., and Bouchard, P.: Scanning Electron Microscopic Evaluation of the Effects of an Air-abrasive System on Dental Implants: A Comparative in vitro Study Between Machined and Plasma-sprayed Titanium Surfaces, *J. Periodontol., 68,* 1215, December, 1997.
22. **Lavigne,** S.E., Krust-Bray, K.S., Williams, K.B., Killoy, W.J., and Theisen, F.: Effects of Subgingival Irrigation with Chlorhexidine on the Periodontal Status of Patients with HA-coated Integral Dental Implants, *Int. J. Oral Maxillofac. Implants, 9,* 156, Number 2, 1994.
23. **Felo,** A., Shibly, O., Ciancio, S.G., Lauciello, F.R., and Ho, A.: Effects of Subgingival Chlorhexidine Irrigation on Peri-implant Maintenance, *Am. J. Dent., 10,* 107, April, 1997.

SUGGESTED READINGS

Bader, J.D., Rozier, R.G., McFall, W.T., and Ramsey, D.L.: Effect of Crown Margins on Periodontal Conditions in Regularly Attending Patients, *J. Prosthet. Dent., 65,* 75, January, 1991.

Brunsvold, M.A. and Lane, J.J.: The Prevalence of Overhanging Dental Restorations and Their Relationship to Periodontal Disease, *J. Clin. Periodontol., 17,* 67, February, 1990.

Cronin, R.J. and Cagna, D.R.: An Update on Fixed Prosthodontics, *J. Am. Dent. Assoc., 128,* 425, April, 1997.

Freilich, M.A., Breeding, L.C., Keagle, J.G., and Garnick, J.J.: Fixed Partial Dentures Supported by Periodontally Compromised Teeth, *J. Prosthet. Dent., 65,* 607, May, 1991.

Kois, J.C. and Spear, F.M.: Periodontal Prosthesis: Creating Successful Restorations, *J. Am. Dent. Assoc., 123,* 108, October, 1992.

Kourkouta, S., Walsh, T.F., and Davis, L.G.: The Effect of Porcelain Laminate Veneers on Gingival Health and Bacterial Plaque Characteristics, *J. Clin. Periodontol., 21,* 638, October, 1994.

Lundgren, D.: Prosthetic Reconstruction of Dentitions Seriously Compromised by Periodontal Disease, *J. Clin. Periodontol., 18,* 390, July, 1991.

Romberg, E., Wood., M., Thompson, V.P., Morrison, G.V., and Suzuki, J.B.: 10-year Periodontal Response to Resin Bonded Bridges, *J. Periodontol., 66,* 973, November, 1995.

Van Dijken, J.W.V. and Sjöström, S.: The Effect of Glass Ionomer Cement and Composite Resin Fillings on Marginal Gingiva, *J. Clin. Periodontol., 18,* 200, March, 1991.

Wright, P.S. and Hellyer, P.H.: Gingival Recession Related to Removable Partial Dentures in Older Patients, *J. Prosthet. Dent., 74,* 602, December, 1995.

Dental Implants

Albrektsson, T. and Sennerby, L.: State of the Art in Oral Implants, *J. Clin. Periodontol., 18,* 474, July, 1991.

Balshi, T.J.: Candidates and Requirements for Single Tooth Implant Prostheses, *Int. J. Periodont. Restorative Dent., 14,* 317, August, 1994.

Berglundh, T. and Lindhe, J.: Dimension of the Periimplant Mucosa. Biological Width Revisited, *J. Clin. Periodontol., 23,* 971, October, 1996.

Eckert, S.E.: Food and Drug Administration Requirements for Dental Implants, *J. Prosthet. Dent., 74,* 162, August, 1995.

Meffert, R.M., Langer, B., and Fritz, M.E.: Dental Implants: A Review, *J. Periodontol., 63,* 859, November, 1992.

Meffert, R.M: Issues Related to Single-tooth Implants, *J. Am. Dent. Assoc., 128,* 1383, October, 1997.

Nunn, P.J.: Peri-implant Disease: The New Kid in the Chair, *Access, 11,* 12, May–June, 1997.

Schnitman, P.A.: Implant Dentistry: Where Are We Now?, *J. Am. Dent. Assoc., 124,* 39, April, 1993.

Schulte, W.: Implants and the Periodontium, *Internat. Dent. J., 45,* 16, February, 1995.

Slavkin, H.C.: Biomimicry, Dental Implants and Clinical Trials, *J. Am. Dent. Assoc., 129,* 226, February, 1998.

Implant Applications

Bain, C.A.: Smoking and Implant Failure: Benefits of a Smoking Cessation Protocol, *Int. J. Oral Maxillofac. Implants, 11,* 756, November–December, 1996.

Bida, D.F.: The Use of Dental Implants in the Treatment of Athletic Injuries, *J. Oral Implantol., 17,* 172, Number 2, 1991.

Blanchaert, R.H.: Implants in the Medically Challenged Patient, *Dent. Clin. North Am., 42,* 35, January, 1998.

Block, M.S. and Kent, J.N.: Placement of Endosseous Implants into Tooth Extraction Sites, *J. Oral Maxillofac. Surg., 49,* 1269, December, 1991.

Lemons, J.E., Laskin, D.M., Roberts, W.E., Tarnow, D.P., Shipman, C., Paczkowski, C., Lorey, R.E., and English, C.: Changes in Patient Screening for a Clinical Study of Dental Implants after Increased Awareness of Tobacco Use as a Risk Factor, *J. Oral Maxillofac. Surg., 55,* 72, Supplement 5, December, 1997.

Mengel, R., Stelzel, M., Hasse, C., and Flores-de-Jacoby, L.: Osseointegrated Implants in Patients Treated for Generalized Severe Adult Periodontitis. An Interim Report, *J. Periodontol., 67,* 782, August, 1996.

Silverstein, L.H., Koch, J.P., Lefkove, M.D., Garnick, J.J., Singh, B., and Steflik, D.E.: Nifedipine-induced Gingival Enlargement Around Dental Implants: A Clinical Report, *J. Oral Implantol., 21,* 116, Number 2, 1995.

Smith, R.A., Berger, R., and Dodson, T.B.: Risk Factors Associated with Dental Implants in Healthy and Medically Compromised Patients, *Int. J. Oral Maxillofac. Implants, 7,* 367, Number 3, 1992.

Steiner, M., Windchy, A., Gould, A.R., Kushner, G.M., and Weber, R.: Effects of Chemotherapy in Patients with Dental Implants, *J. Oral Implantol., 21,* 142, Number 2, 1995.

Peri-Implant Microbiology

Bauman, G.R., Mills, M., Rapley, J.W., and Hallmon, W.W.: Plaque-induced Inflammation Around Implants, *Int. J. Oral Maxillofac. Implants, 7,* 330, Number 3, 1992.

Ericsson, I., Persson, L.G., Berglundh, T., Marinello, C.P., Lindhe, J., and Klinge, B.: Different Types of Inflammatory Reactions in Peri-implant Soft Tissues, *J. Clin. Periodontol., 22,* 255, March, 1995.

George, K., Zafiropoulos, G.-G.K., Murat, Y., Hubertus, S., and Nisengard, R.J.: Clinical and Microbiological Status of Osseointegrated Implants, *J. Periodontol., 65,* 766, August, 1994.

Gouvoussis, J., Sindhusake, D., and Yeung, S.: Cross-infection from Periodontitis Sites to Failing Implant Sites in the Same Mouth, *Int. J. Oral Maxillofac. Implants, 12,* 666, September/October, 1997.

Lambert, P.M., Morris, H.F., and Ochi, S.: The Influence of 0.12% Chlorhexidine Digluconate Rinses on the Incidence of Infectious Complications and Implant Success, *J. Oral Maxillofac. Surg., 55,* 25, Supplement 5, December, 1997.

Nelson, S.K., Knoernschild, K.L., Robinson, F.G., and Schuster, G.S.: Lipopolysaccharide Affinity for Titanium Implant Biomaterials, *J. Prosthet. Dent., 77,* 76, January, 1997.

Ong, E.S.-M., Newman, H.N., Wilson, M., and Bulman, J.S.: The Occurrence of Periodontitis-related Microorganisms in Relation to Titanium Implants, *J. Periodontol., 63,* 200, March, 1992.

Quirynen, H.C., Van der mei, C.M.L., Bollen, A., Schotte, M., Marechal, G.I., Doornbusch, G.I., Naert, I., Busscher, H.J., and van Steenberghe, D.: An *in vivo* Study of the Influence of the Surface Roughness of Implants on the Microbiology of Supra- and Subgingival Plaque, *J. Dent. Res., 72,* 1304, September, 1993.

Quirynen, M., Papaioannou, W., and van Steenberghe, D.: Intraoral Transmission and the Colonization of Oral Hard Surfaces, *J. Periodontol., 67,* 986, October, 1996.

Rimondini, L., Fare, S., Brambilla, E., Felloni, A., Consonni, C., Brossa, F., and Carrassi, A.: The Effect of Surface Roughness on Early *in vivo* Plaque Colonization on Titanium, *J. Periodontol., 68,* 556, June, 1997.

Sbordone, L., Barone, A., Ramaglia, L., Ciaglia, R.N., and Iacono, V.J.: Antimicrobial Susceptibility of Periodontopathic Bacteria Associated with Failing Implants, *J. Periodontol., 66,* 69, January, 1995.

Instruments

Cross-Poline, G.N., Shaklee, R.L., and Stach, D.J.: Effect of Implant Curets on Titanium Implant Surfaces, *Am. J. Dent., 10,* 41, February, 1997.

Dmytryk, J.J., Fox, S.C., and Moriarty, J.D.: The Effects of Scaling Titanium Implant Surfaces With Metal and Plastic Instruments on Cell Attachment, *J. Periodontol., 61,* 491, August, 1990.

Fox, S.C., Moriarty, J.D., and Kusy, R.P.: The Effects of Scaling a Titanium Implant Surface with Metal and Plastic Instruments: An in vitro Study, *J. Periodontol., 61,* 485, August, 1990.

Hallmon, W.W., Waldrop, T.C., Meffert, R.M., and Wade, B.W.: A Comparative Study of the Effects of Metallic, Nonmetallic, and Sonic Instrumentation on Titanium Abutment Surfaces, *Int. J. Oral Maxillofac. Implants, 11,* 96, Number 1, 1996.

Kuempel, D.R., Johnson, G.K., Zaharias, R.S., and Keller, J.C.: The Effects of Scaling Procedures on Epithelial Cell Growth on Titanium Surfaces, *J. Periodontol., 66,* 228, March, 1995.

Kwan, J.Y., Zablotsky, M.H., and Meffert, R.M.: Implant Maintenance Using a Modified Ultrasonic Instrument, *J. Dent. Hyg., 64,* 422, November–December, 1990.

Parham, P.L., Cobb, C.M., French, A.A., Love, J.W., Drisko, C.L., and Killoy, W.J.: Effects of an Air-powder Abrasive System on Plasma-sprayed Titanium Implant Surfaces: An *in vitro* Evaluation, *J. Oral Implantol., 15,* 78, Number 2, 1989.

Implant Care and Maintenance

Ciancio, S.G., Lauciello, F., Shibly, O., Vitello, M., and Mather, M.: The Effect of an Antiseptic Mouthrinse on Implant Maintenance: Plaque and Peri-implant Gingival Tissues, *J. Periodontol., 66,* 962, November, 1995.

Daniels, A.H.: Home Care Parameters for the Implant Patient, *J. Pract. Hyg., 4,* 15, September/October, 1995.

DuCoin, F.J.: Dental Implant Hygiene and Maintenance: Home and Professional Care, *J. Oral Implantol., 22,* 72, Number 1, 1996.

Lang, N.P. and Nyman, S.R.: Supportive Maintenance Care for Patients with Implants and Advanced Restorative Therapy, *Periodontology 2000, 4,* 119, 1994.

LeBeau, J.: Maintaining the Long-term Health of the Dental Implant and the Implant-borne Restoration, *Compend. Oral Hyg., 3,* 3, Number 3, 1997.

Lochhead, M.A.: Osseointegrated Implants. A Part of our Future Here and Now, *Can. Dent. Hyg./Probe, 27,* 89, May/June, 1993.

McCollum, J., O'Neal, R.B., Brennan, W.A., Van Dyke, T.E., and Horner, J.A.: The Effect of Titanium Implant Abutment Surface Irregularities on Plaque Accumulation *in vivo, J. Periodontol., 63,* 802, October, 1992.

Speelman, J.A., Collaert, B., and Klinge, B.: Evaluation of Different Methods to Clean Titanium Abutments. A Scanning Electron Microscopic Study, *Clin. Oral Implants Res., 3,* 120, September, 1992.

Strong, S.S. and Strong, S.M.: The Dental Implant Maintenance Visit, *J. Pract. Hyg., 4,* 29, September/October, 1995.

Tomlinson, J.O.: Maintaining Implants at Home, *J. Pract. Hyg., 4,* 22, September/October, 1995.

Toumelin-Chemla, F., Rouelle, F., and Burdairon, G.: Corrosive Properties of Fluoride-containing Odontologic Gels Against Titanium, *J. Dent., 24,* 109, January/March, 1996.

Yukna, R.A.: Optimizing Clinical Success with Implants: Maintenance and Care, *Compend. Cont. Educ. Dent., 14,* S5554, Supplement 15, 1993.

The Patient Who Uses Tobacco

The deleterious health effects of all forms of tobacco products have been recognized for many years.[1] During patient assessment the habits of the patient are determined, and the need for developing interventions to modify risk behaviors is entered into the care plan.

It is the responsibility of all dental professionals to provide patients who use tobacco with the opportunity to enter a tobacco cessation program. Dental professionals must also play a vital role in preventing tobacco use. Key words relating to tobacco use and cessation are defined in Box 27-1. Box 27-2 defines the various forms of tobacco.

HEALTH HAZARDS

Tobacco is toxic to humans. Tobacco use is the single most preventable cause of illness and death in our society. Many children begin smoking each day. For that

---

BOX 27-1 KEY WORDS AND ABBREVIATIONS: Tobacco Use

Chemical dependency: generic term relating to psychological or physical dependency, or both, on an exogenous substance.

Cotinine (ko'tĭ-nēn): a by-product of nicotine found in body fluids; cotinine levels are used in behavioral research to determine recent use of nicotine-containing products and in clinical research to determine correlations between cotinine levels and oral disease.

Drug abuse: any use of a drug that causes physical, psychological, economic, legal, and/or social harm to the person who uses or other persons affected by the user's behavior.

Drug addiction: a chronic disorder leading to negative physical, psychological, or social consequences from compulsive use of a substance; characterized by continued use despite negative effects encountered by use.

Dysphoria (dis-for'e-ah): generalized feeling of ill-being, malaise, restlessness, and discomfort.

Nicotine (nik'o-teen): a poisonous, addictive stimulant that is the chief psychoactive ingredient in tobacco.

Nicotine gum: polacrilex lozenge or gum developed to aid in smoking cessation; available as an over-the-counter product.

Nicotine nasal spray: a nicotine withdrawal product used nasally by the patient to aid in smoking cessation.

Nicotine patch: a transdermal form of nicotine withdrawal therapy.

Nitrosamines: cancer-causing chemicals found in tobacco.

Oral cancer: in this chapter, the term "oral cancer" includes cancer of the lips, tongue, floor of the mouth, palate, gingiva, alveolar mucosa, buccal mucosa, and oropharynx.

Placenta abruptio (plah-sen'tah ab-rup'she-o): premature detachment of a normally situated placenta.

Placenta previa (plah-sen'tah prev'e-ah): placenta implanted in the lower segment of the uterus extending to the margin of the internal opening of the cervix; may obstruct opening partially or completely.

Psychoactive drug (si"ko-ak'tiv): possessing the ability to alter mood, behavior, cognitive processes, or mental tension.

Pyrolysis (pi-rol'ĭ-sis): chemical decomposition of a substance by heat.

Smoke: visible vapor and gases given off by a burning substance.

Environmental tobacco smoke (ETS) or passive smoke: tobacco smoke present in room air resulting from ignited tobacco products burning in an ashtray or exhaled by a smoker (people who are currently smoking are also exposed to other smokers' sidestream smoke).

Mainstream smoke: smoke that is inhaled directly into the user's lungs.

Sidestream smoke: the aerosol emitted directly into the surrounding air from the lit end of a smoldering tobacco product; may be inhaled by the user; is a major component of environmental smoke.

Sudden infant death syndrome (SIDS): sudden and unexpected death of an apparently healthy infant; typically occurring between the ages of 3 weeks and 5 months.

Thiocyanate (thy"o-si'ah-nāt): found in tobacco smoke, a by-product of hydrogen cyanide used to determine recent use of smoked tobacco products.

Transdermal: method of drug delivery by patch on skin; a mode for slow release over extended time.

Transmucosal: type of drug delivery by infiltration of mucosal lining.

---

age group, it will be many years before the permanent effects of tobacco use will be manifest. Evidence from tobacco addiction studies has revealed that a high percentage of today's addicted adult cigarette smokers began tobacco use in their teens. Offspring of smokers are more likely to become smokers.[2]

As years of tobacco use accumulate, so do the systemic and oral health effects of all forms of tobacco. Life expectancy is shortened. The number of years lost depends on many factors. Those who quit prior to age 50 years have one-half the risk of dying within 15 years as compared to smokers who continue.[3]

COMPONENTS OF TOBACCO PRODUCTS

Processed tobacco products contain many compounds that act solely or in concert with other components to produce tobacco's deleterious health effects. Nicotine leads to dependence while other components such as aromatic hydrocarbons, polonium-210, and N-nitrosamines are carcinogenic agents.

Once tobacco is ignited, tar, carbon monoxide, and other products produced become part of mainstream smoke and also are found in environmental tobacco smoke. Figure 27-1 illustrates the smoking process.

BOX 27-2 KEY WORDS: Tobacco Products

Smoking tobacco: any form of tobacco that is ignited and smoked by the user.

Cigar: a small, rolled form of tobacco leaf that is smoked by the user.

Cigarette: a cylindrical, paper-enclosed form of tobacco that is smoked by the user.

Pipe tobacco: ground leaf tobacco manufactured for smoking through a pipe.

Tobacco pipe: a tube with a bowl at one end used to smoke tobacco.

Smokeless (spit) tobacco: term used to define all forms of tobacco that are primarily used orally.

Chaw: a golf-ball-sized portion of chewing tobacco held in the user's mouth usually inside the cheek or between the lower lip, gingiva, and mucosa.

Chewing tobacco: tobacco available in loose-leaf, twist, and plug forms manufactured by air-drying tobacco leaves; held inside cheek and/or chewed (chaw).

Quid: a pinch of snuff held in the user's mouth for various periods of time.

Snuff: fire-cured, finely ground or powdered tobacco sold in both dry and moist forms; not chewed but a small amount ("pinch" or "quid") is placed and held between cheek and gingiva or lower lip, gingiva, and mucosa.

Spit tobacco: a synonymous term for smokeless tobacco products.

METABOLISM OF NICOTINE[4,5]

Absorption of nicotine occurs through the lungs, skin, and oral or nasal mucosa, depending on the route of administration. Absorption of tobacco that is smoked (cigarettes, pipes, and cigars) is influenced by several factors listed in Figure 27-1. Regardless of type of tobacco products used, nicotine is primarily eliminated by liver metabolism and excreted through the kidneys in acid urine.

I. NICOTINE FROM SMOKING

A. Absorption: Lungs

Nicotine enters the lungs and quickly passes into arterial circulation by way of blood vessels lining the sacs of the bronchi.

B. Distribution

1. *To the Brain*. Nicotine is delivered efficiently to the brain by the blood stream in less than 20 seconds.
2. *Changes in the Liver*. Nicotine is metabolized in the liver into cotinine. Cotinine concentrations in the blood, urine, and saliva are used to assess whether or not a person uses tobacco, what level of exposure the person has, and the level of exposure of nonsmokers to passive or environmental smoke.
3. *Peak Plasma Concentration*. Peak plasma concentration of nicotine occurs approximately 10 minutes after the onset of smoking and rapidly declines over the next 20 to 30 minutes.
4. *Dissemination*. Nicotine is spread to all body tissues.
5. *Duration*. Smallest amounts of nicotine from tobacco smoke (one puff) will remain in the body for 8 to 12 hours.

II. SMOKELESS TOBACCO[6]

Smokeless tobacco is the term applied to all forms of snuff and chewing tobacco that are not smoked but are placed in the mouth.

A. Absorption: Oral Cavity

1. Direct: through the gingiva and oral mucous membranes.
2. After placing the quid in the mouth, nicotine gradually enters the blood stream; peak concentrations are reached within 30 minutes.
3. As compared with cigarette smoking, nicotine concentration declines over 2 hours.
4. Smokeless tobacco users experience nicotine blood plasma levels similar to the nicotine blood levels of smokers.

B. Absorption: Intestinal

1. The majority of juice produced by smokeless tobacco is expectorated.
2. Juice that is intentionally and/or accidentally swallowed by the user is absorbed through the blood vessels lining the small intestine.

SYSTEMIC EFFECTS

Use of tobacco products influences every system of the body. Table 27-1 shows smoking-related conditions. The diseases that affect each system have mild to deadly consequences.

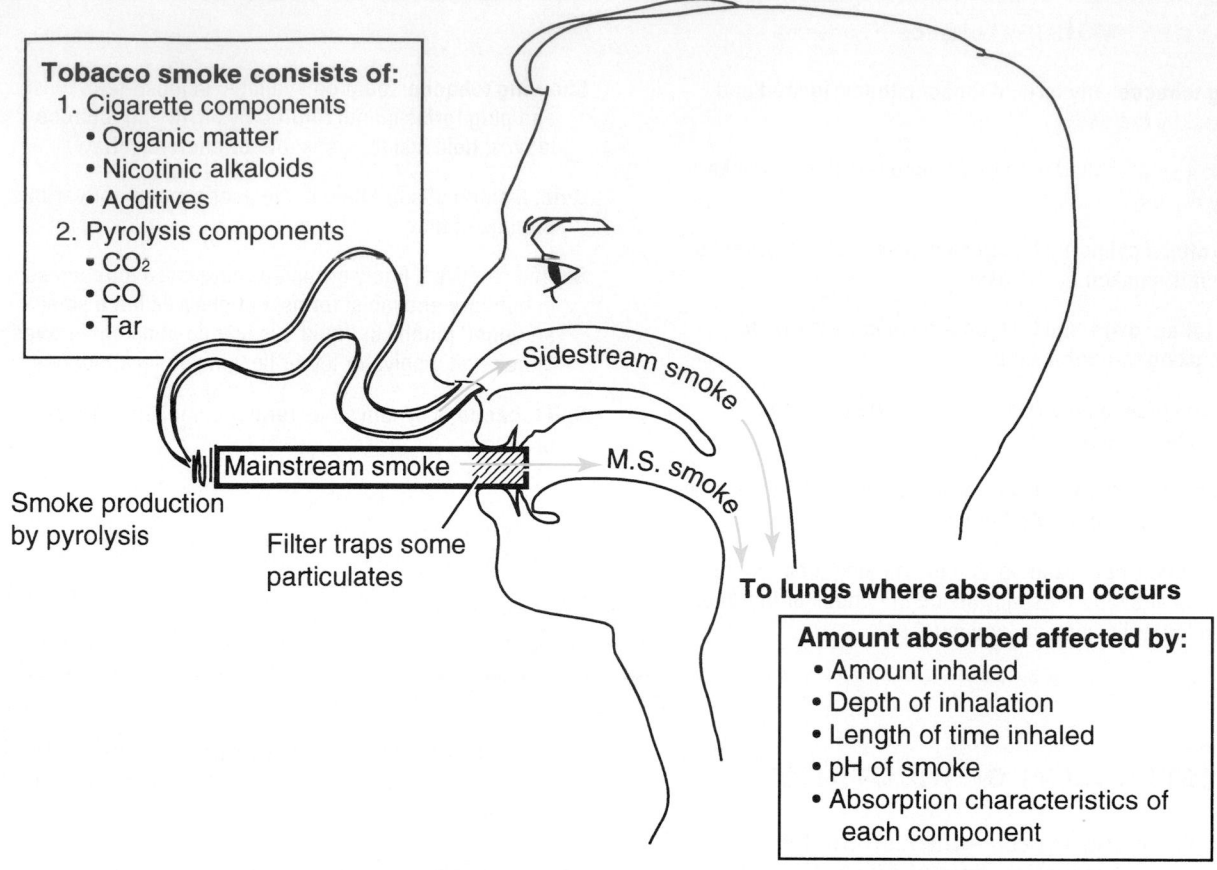

Tobacco smoke consists of:
1. Cigarette components
   - Organic matter
   - Nicotinic alkaloids
   - Additives
2. Pyrolysis components
   - CO_2
   - CO
   - Tar

Smoke production by pyrolysis

Filter traps some particulates

Sidestream smoke

Mainstream smoke

M.S. smoke

To lungs where absorption occurs

Amount absorbed affected by:
- Amount inhaled
- Depth of inhalation
- Length of time inhaled
- pH of smoke
- Absorption characteristics of each component

FIGURE 27-1 Components of mainstream smoke and factors influencing absorption by the lungs. Adapted with permission from Schmitz, J.M., Schneider, N.G., and Jarvik, M.E.: Nicotine, in Lowinson, J.H., Ruiz, P., Millman, R.B., and Langrod, J.G., eds.: *Substance Abuse. A Comprehensive Textbook,* 3rd ed., Baltimore, Williams & Wilkins, 1997, page 277. (Reproduced with permission from Henningfield, J.E.: *Behavioral Pharmacology of Cigarette Smoking.* In: Thompson, T., Dews, P.D., Barrett, J.E., eds.: Advances in Behavioral Pharmacology, vol 4. Orlando, Academic Press, 1984, page 138.)

TABLE 27-1 Disease Consequences of Tobacco Use*

Cancer	Respiratory Diseases	Cardiovascular Diseases	Pregnancy Infant Health	Other Conditions
Oral cavity*	Chronic obstructive	Atherosclerosis	Abortion	Osteoporosis
Lung	pulmonary	Coronary artery disease	Fetal neonatal death	Alzheimer's disease
Larynx	disease (COPD)	Hypertension*	Placenta abruptio	Wrinkling
Pharynx	Emphysema	Aortic aneurysm	Placenta previa	Concomitant use of
Esophagus	Bronchitis	Arterial thrombosis	Premature/prolonged	other drugs*
Stomach (peptic ulcer*)	Asthma	Stroke	membrane rupture	Early menopause
Bladder	Bacterial pneumonia		Preterm labor	
Uterine cervix	Tuberculosis		Preeclampsia	
Breast			Growth retardation	
			Sudden infant death syndrome	

*Associated with smoke and smokeless tobacco use.

I. CARDIOVASCULAR[7]

Smoking aggravates and accelerates the development of atherosclerosis and is a major risk factor for coronary heart disease. There is even greater risk with age over 50 years, use of oral contraceptives, and a familial history of coronary heart disease.

II. PULMONARY DISEASES

Smoking is the major cause of chronic obstructive pulmonary disease. Smokers have increased risk for bronchitis and emphysema, which are the major causes of chronic obstructive pulmonary diseases.

III. CANCER

One-third of all cancer deaths in the United States are directly linked to cigarette smoking. Lung cancer is the leading cause of cancer death for both black and white men and women; 80% of all lung cancers are directly related to cigarette smoking. Approximately 75% of oral cancers are related to smoking and the use of smokeless tobacco.

IV. TOBACCO AND USE OF OTHER DRUGS

Smokers are more likely to consume alcohol. The combined use of alcohol and tobacco places the patient at greater risk for oral neoplasms and other oral problems. Heavy cigarette smoking is also highly correlated with cocaine and marijuana use.[8]

ENVIRONMENTAL TOBACCO SMOKE

Environmental smoke is composed of side-stream smoke emitted into the air from burning cigarettes between puffs, exhaled mainstream smoke, and vaporized components that diffuse through cigarette paper. Environmental smoke is also called passive, secondary, involuntary, or second-hand smoke.

In indoor areas, environmental smoke can last for many hours depending on ventilation. Exposure for certain workers and families can be extensive. Fortunately, many public areas, hospitals, and commercial work areas are now mandated smoke free.

Individuals exposed to environmental tobacco smoke are at risk for the same health problems as is the active smoker. A nonsmoker may be more sensitive to the toxic effects than the habitual smoker because the system of the smoker adapts to compensate for the deleterious effects of continued smoking.

I. TOXICITY

Many chemicals are contained in passive smoke including the same carcinogenic compounds as those in mainstream smoke. Some toxic components are actually in higher concentrations in side-stream smoke than in mainstream smoke.

II. LUNG AND RESPIRATORY EFFECTS

Smoking is the primary cause of lung cancer, from both active and passive smoking.[9]

III. CARDIOVASCULAR EFFECTS[10-12]

The majority of annual deaths from exposure to environmental tobacco smoke are attributed to heart disease. The effect on the cardiovascular system of passive and active smokers is similar.

PRENATAL AND CHILDREN[13,14]

The involuntary smoke that reaches the fetus, the infant, and growing children comes from their parents who smoke, from the environment of day-care facilities, preschool, and other surroundings. The non-smoking mother who is exposed to passive smoke can also be a source. All of the smoke exposures adversely affect the physical, behavioral, and mental health of the children.

A. *In utero*
1. Transplacental passage of harmful smoke components.
2. Risks for adverse pregnancy, with outcomes of miscarriage, placenta previa, low birth weight, and increased perinatal mortality.
3. Association with cleft lip and cleft palate.[15]
4. Risk for delayed tooth formation.[16]

B. **Infancy**
1. Chemicals are passed to the baby in breast milk of mothers who smoke.
2. Increased incidence of lower respiratory tract illness.
3. Increased risk of sudden infant death syndrome.[17]

C. **Young Children**
1. Decreased lung function; increased chronic respiratory symptoms.
2. Children with asthma have additional episodes and a worsened condition.
3. Increased incidence of middle ear infections.
4. Behavior problems; less academic achievement in school, possibly related to missing school during illnesses.

ORAL MANIFESTATIONS OF TOBACCO USE

Periodontal diseases and oral cancers provide the most serious, destructive effects of tobacco use on the oral tissues. Table 27-2 lists examples of the wide variety of oral consequences of tobacco use. The long list includes life-threatening cancers, severe periodontal infections with potential tooth loss, soft mucosal and palatal tissues changes, as well as the esthetic personal influences.

Variables that determine the extent of oral tissue damage include the type of tobacco products, the length of time used in years, and the number of daily exposures. Questions in a patient's health history can provide leading information relative to the patient's

TABLE 27-2 Oral Consequences of Tobacco Use

Cancer and Pre-Cancer	Periodontal Problems	Soft Tissue Problems	Hard Tissue Problems	Esthetic Factors	Exacerbation— Oral Signs in Systemic Diseases
Squamous cell Verrucous (ST) Leukoplakia	ANUG and ANUP Relapse during maintenance Increased risk for peri-implantitis and peri-implant bone loss Localized recession and clinical attachment loss	Nicotine stomatitis (P) Smoker's melanosis Black hairy tongue Median rhomboid glossitis Chronic hyperplastic candidiasis Leukodema (P) Hyperkeratosis (ST) Dry socket Delayed wound healing	Occlusal or incisal abrasion (P), (ST) Cervical abrasion (ST) Dehiscence of bone (ST) Tooth loss	Halitosis Dental stains Prosthesis stains Orthodontic appliance stains Discoloration of restorations Impaired taste and smell	HIV/AIDS Type 1 and Type 2 diabetes

Key: mainly associated with (ST) smokeless tobacco; (P) pipe; (C) cigars; no notation = smoked tobacco.

habits. The extraoral/intraoral examination gives visual examples for use in encouraging the patient to start a tobacco cessation program.

TOBACCO AND PERIODONTAL INFECTIONS

Smoking is a major risk factor for periodontitis, and smokers are at high risk for developing more severe periodontitis than nonsmokers. The effects of smoking on the periodontal tissues are apparent upon clinical examination.

I. MECHANISMS FOR PERIODONTAL TISSUE DESTRUCTION

A. Microorganisms: Smoking increases the risk for subgingival infection.[18]

B. Immunosuppressive Effects
1. Impairment of host immune factors.
2. Peripheral neutrophil phagocytosis significantly impaired; ability of the phagocytes to kill pathogens is impaired.[19,20]
3. Reduction of serum IgG2 levels; associated with more severe periodontal destruction.[21]

C. Inhibition of Fibroblast Function: Connective tissue metabolism altered; increased collagenase activity.[22]

D. Impaired Bone Cell Function: Reduction of skeletal bone mineral content.

II. CLINICAL EFFECTS OF SMOKING

A. Clinical Characteristics
1. Gingiva: fibrotic with minimal redness relative to disease severity.
2. More severe disease (at younger adult ages) compared with same-age nonsmoker: more bone loss, greater probing depths and attachment loss.
3. Pocketing greater in anterior and maxillary lingual sites.
4. Gingival recession noted about anterior teeth.
5. Subgingival temperature above normal in smokers: indicator of disease.[23]

B. Response to Treatment
1. Resistance to conventional therapy.
2. Dental implants have greater risk for the development of peri-implantitis.[24]
3. Delayed healing after surgical and nonsurgical procedures.

NICOTINE ADDICTION

Nicotine is tobacco's psychoactive agent, and its use leads to tolerance, dependence, and addiction. With cessation of use, symptoms of withdrawal are produced. Cigarette smoking is the most widely used tobacco form that leads to addiction.

I. TOLERANCE

A. Physiologic Adaptation
The *tolerance* of a psychoactive substance means the physiologic adaptation to the effect of the

drug. When there is exposure to a constant amount, the effects on the user are lessened as time passes.

B. Amount of Use

As tolerance increases, an increased dosage is required to maintain the intensity and duration of effects.

II. DEPENDENCE

A. Characteristics of Dependence

As increased amounts are needed over time, the loss of control over the amount and frequency of tobacco use shows evidence of dependence. Some facts about dependence are included in Table 27-3. The criteria for nicotine dependency are outlined in Table 27-4.

B. Reinforcing Effect

There is a direct effect on the brain receptors that increases the compulsion to use tobacco. Positive reinforcement is produced with tobacco use, and withdrawal symptoms are produced by abrupt stopping.

III. ADDICTION

Addiction is a chronic disorder characterized by a compulsive use of a substance. The effects result in physical, psychologic, and/or social harm to the user, but there is continued use in spite of that harm. Biologic, psychologic, social, and many other factors contribute to the development and continuation of tobacco use. Factors affecting the development of addiction include the following:

TABLE 27-3 Facts About Nicotine Dependency

- Nicotine addiction is similar to that produced by other substances such as alcohol, cocaine, and heroin.
- Tolerance to nicotine is demonstrated as the user experiences less nausea and dizziness following initial use.
- Tobacco abuse: While moderate alcohol use is considered safe, any use of tobacco products is considered a health hazard. Therefore, use is not discussed since any amount is considered abuse.
- Nicotine addiction may be the most challenging of all addictions for complete recovery.
- 70% of smokers report that they would like to quit but only about ⅓ make a quit attempt each year; of these only about 2.5% are successful.
- Many tobacco users make many unsuccessful quit attempts before stopping use for indefinite or extended periods of time.
- Successfully quitting smokeless tobacco use may be equally or more difficult than stopping smoking and should not be considered a viable alternative for smokers who can quit.

Adapted from *American Psychiatric Association: Diagnostic and Statistical Manual of Mental Disorders* (DSM-IV), 4th ed. Washington, D.C., American Psychiatric Association, 1994, pp. 243–247; and Schmitz, J.M., Schneider, N.G., and Jarvik, M.E.: Nicotine, in Lowinson, J.H., Ruiz, P., Millman, R.B., and Langrod, J.G. eds.: *Substance Abuse: A Comprehensive Textbook*, 3rd ed. Baltimore, Williams & Wilkins, 1997, pp. 276–294.

TABLE 27-4 Criteria for Nicotine Dependency

- Tolerance
- Withdrawal symptoms when use discontinued
- Used in greater amounts over longer period of time than intended
- A persistent desire or unsuccessful efforts to cut down or quit
- A great deal of time spent using the substance
- Giving up important social, occupational, or recreational activities because of use of the substance
- Continued use despite knowledge of medical problems related to use and/or social and legal problems resulting from use

Adapted from *American Psychiatric Association. Diagnostic and Statistical Manual of Mental Disorders* (DSM-IV), 4th ed. Washington, D.C., American Psychiatric Association, 1994, pp. 243–247; and Schmitz, J.M., Schneider, N.G., and Jarvik, M.E.: Nicotine, in Lowinson, J.H., Ruiz, P., Millman, R.B., and Langrod, J.G. eds.: *Substance Abuse: A Comprehensive Textbook*, 3rd ed. Baltimore, Williams & Wilkins, 1997, pp. 276–294.

A. Properties of a psychoactive drug (dose)
B. Family and peer influences; social acceptability
C. Existing psychiatric disorders
D. Cost and availability of the drug
E. Influence of advertising

IV. WITHDRAWAL

Withdrawal refers to the cessation of nicotine use by an individual in whom dependence is established. When the use of products containing nicotine is stopped abruptly, within 24 hours the user will likely experience maximal physical and/or psychologic withdrawal symptoms. Table 27-5 summarizes typical symptoms related to withdrawal from nicotine.

A. Duration

Most symptoms diminish over a few weeks. Relapse is common within 1 week when the withdrawal symptoms are at a peak. Cravings for tobacco, increased appetite, and weight gain may persist for months or years.

TABLE 27-5 Criteria for Nicotine Withdrawal Syndrome

- Dysphoric or depressed mood
- Insomnia
- Irritability, frustration, and anger
- Anxiety
- Difficulty concentrating
- Restlessness
- Decreased heart rate
- Increased appetite or weight gain
- Cravings for tobacco

Adapted from *American Psychiatric Association: Diagnostic and Statistical Manual of Mental Disorders* (DSM-IV), 4th ed. Washington, D.C., American Psychiatric Association, 1994, pp. 243–247; and Schmitz, J.M., Schneider, N.G., and Jarvik, M.E.: Nicotine, in Lowinson, J.H., Ruiz, P., Millman, R.B., and Langrod, J.G. eds.: *Substance Abuse: A Comprehensive Textbook*, 3rd ed. Baltimore, Williams & Wilkins, 1997, pp. 276–294.

B. Alleviation of Symptoms

Table 27-6 suggests activities to use to overcome withdrawal of nicotine. The principle is to prevent relapse.

TREATMENT[4]

Smoking cessation methods, or treatment for nicotine addiction, can be considered in two categories: *self-help* and *assisted strategies*.

I. REASONS FOR QUITTING

Before any degree of success can be expected, the individual must make a concerted effort and must believe in the significance of the effort. Objectives will be personal. Typical reasons include the following:

A. General health awareness
B. Specific health problem related directly or indirectly to smoking
C. Effect on family
　1. Need to act as role model
　2. Awareness of effects of passive smoke
D. Pregnancy: effect on fetus
E. Cost
F. Social pressures: smoking not acceptable in many settings
G. Realization of the dangers of addiction; desire to gain control of one's life

II. SELF-HELP INTERVENTIONS

A. Cold turkey: with lifestyle changes of exercise and diet modifications.

B. Reducing number of tobacco exposures daily; using brand with lower nicotine content; budgeting the financial investment.
C. Over-the-counter nicotine patches and gum are available. Patients must be warned to follow the manufacturer's instruction carefully and seek professional help and recommendations.
D. Joining friend or family member in cessation.

III. ASSISTED STRATEGIES

A. Behavior modification: counseling, group therapy
B. Pharmacologic: Table 27-7 provides an overview of FDA-approved therapies
　1. Nicotine replacement therapy
　2. Non-nicotine medications
C. Combined behavioral and pharmacologic
　The best outcomes have been shown when combined methods are used.

PHARMACEUTICALS USED FOR TREATMENT OF NICOTINE ADDICTION[25]

I. OBJECTIVES AND RATIONALE

A. Make it easier to abstain from tobacco by partial replacement of the nicotine or by countering nicotine's action.
B. Reduce withdrawal symptoms.
C. Fulfill in part the craving for tobacco by sustaining tolerance.

TABLE 27-6 Alleviating Nicotine Withdrawal Symptoms

Symptom	Activities
Mood changes: 　anxiety, nervousness, stressed feelings	Breathe deeply; exhale through pursed lips Take a walk or other relaxation exercise Avoid caffeine Participate in self-reward activity such as purchasing new compact disk
Sleep disturbances	Avoid caffeine Avoid exercise immediately before bedtime Stay up later than usual Avoid resting or watching TV in bed; get in bed only at bedtime
Appetite increase	Eat only when you are hungry Eat low-fat, low-calorie snacks Chew sugarless gum or eat sugarless hard candy Drink additional glasses of water
Cravings	Delay smoking or dipping: Use tactics such as waiting 1 more minute; often cravings pass in 5 or 10 minutes Take deep breaths; exhale through pursed lips Exercise; take a walk Avoid places where you most commonly used tobacco

(Taken from *Enough Snuff: A Guide to Quitting Smokeless Tobacco*, 1997, Applied Behavior Science, Point Richmond, CA, with permission from Dr. H.H. Severson.)

TABLE 27-7 FDA-Approved Pharmaceutical Agents

Agent	Dosage	Comments
Nicotine Replacement Agents	Follow manufacturer's instructions	Part of comprehensive behavioral cessation program to relieve withdrawal symptoms. Do not use with other tobacco products.
Nicotine transdermal patch	5 to 22 mg/day Step-down dosing	Used 4 to 8 weeks Gradual withdrawal
Nicotine Polacrilex (gum)	Range: 2 to 4 mg/day Average 9 to 12 pieces per day	Use whenever urge to smoke arises Not to exceed 96 mg per day
Nicotine inhalation system	10 puffs through mouthpiece 6 to 16 cartridges per day	Step down dosing
Nicotine nasal spray	Range from 2 to 4 mg per dose	One spray in each nostril (not sniffed or inhaled)
Non-Nicotine Agent Bupropion HCl	150 mg/day for 3 days, then 150 mg 2 per day for 7–12 weeks	Antidepressant; decreases craving

(Data from: Dr. Robert Mecklenburg, Chair, National Dental and Tobacco Free Steering Committee, National Cancer Institute, 12304 River's Edge Drive, Potomac, MD 20854.)

D. Provide some effects (mood, cognitive changes) previously derived from nicotine.

II. CONSIDERATIONS

A. Discourage casual use of pharmaceuticals. Failure following improper use can discourage future quit attempts.
B. Inform patient of signs and symptoms of nicotine overdose. Included are nausea, vomiting, dizziness, weakness, or rapid heart beat.
C. Consult physician prior to use if under age 18 years or contraindications are present.

III. CONTRAINDICATIONS

A. Self-medication without examination.
B. Allergy or sensitivity to nicotine product (rare).
C. Pregnancy: nicotine in the blood stream, although in much lesser amount, can still reach fetus.
D. Nicotine polacrilex (gum): hypertension; using medication for asthma, depression, or diabetes; cardiovascular disease; stomach ulcers.
E. Nicotine patch: same as nicotine gum; in addition some patients may be allergic to patch adhesive.

IV. TYPES

A. Nicotine Polacrilex (Gum)

1. *Transmucosal delivery:* nicotine released in mouth during "chewing."
2. *Content:* 2-mg or 4-mg forms to be used up to 12 pieces per day.
3. *Directions:* use up to 12 pieces per day or about one per hour for 12 weeks.
4. *Requirements:* avoid tobacco and acidic foods and beverages while using gum.
5. *How to use:* chew, then park gum between the cheek and gingiva for 1 minute; repeat for 30 minutes; reposition gum in different areas of the mouth; gum should be held in place most of the time rather than chewed; carefully dispose of used gum.

B. Nicotine Patch

1. *Transdermal delivery:* nicotine released through skin.
2. *Directions:* one patch placed on rising; removed at bedtime; no tobacco use; careful disposal of used patch.
3. *Advantages:* fewer side effects than gum; single application per day.
4. *Supplementation with nicotine gum:* patch has slow, steady delivery, and gum may be used for quick relief from uncontrollable urge for cigarette; may be used with sustained release bupropion to help a smoker quit.

C. Other Preparations: nasal spray, vapor inhalation system.

NICOTINE-FREE THERAPY

Non-nicotine medications such as antidepressants have had success with selected patients. Sustained-release bupropion is a prescription drug available for smoking cessation patients not medicated for depression or seizures. Bupropion is also an aid to weight control following smoking cessation.[26]

Other antidepressants have also been successful in smoking cessation. New medications may prove helpful to patients for whom nicotine replacement therapy is unsuccessful.[27]

DENTAL HYGIENE CARE FOR THE PATIENT WHO USES TOBACCO

The patient who uses any form of tobacco presents a unique challenge to the oral health team. Specific treatment modifications are indicated. Helping the patient to quit tobacco use becomes an integral part of the care plan.

ASSESSMENT

I. PATIENT HISTORY

A. Update
Tobacco use status must be assessed at each appointment. Current information is needed for proper assessment, dental hygiene diagnosis, and care planning because tobacco use can lead to many oral and systemic problems.

B. Patient History Form
The basic history form used by all patients needs one or two questions to determine whether the patient currently uses tobacco and the type of tobacco (smoked or smokeless).

C. Special Questionnaire for Tobacco Users
The National Cancer Institute's standard tobacco use survey form is included as Figure 27-2.

D. Alert to Medical Problems
Identification of problems that result from tobacco use with concomitant use of alcohol, cocaine, or marijuana is significant. Modifications of clinic procedures may be indicated, especially for anesthesia, prognosis of outcome of treatment, and possible emergencies related to cardiovascular or respiratory difficulties.

II. VITAL SIGNS

A. Blood Pressure
Hypertension is related to all forms of tobacco use.

B. The Fifth Vital Sign
Tobacco use status is considered a vital sign along with temperature, pulse, respiratory rate, and blood pressure (Figure 7-1, page 107).[28]

III. EXTRAORAL EXAMINATION

A. Breath and Body Odor
1. *Halitosis.*
2. *Electropositive smoke.* Smoke from cigars and other smoked tobacco products clings to skin, hair, and clothes and results in body odor.
3. *Alcoholic beverages.* Tobacco users frequently consume alcoholic beverages.

B. Fingers
Smokers of nonfiltered cigarettes: yellowish-brown discoloring of the fingers and fingernails.

C. Skin
Smokers experience premature and more extensive facial wrinkling.

D. Lips
Pipe and cigar smokers are at risk for development of precancerous and cancerous lip lesions.

IV. INTRAORAL EXAMINATION
For a summary of intraoral findings see Table 27-2. Conducting a thorough extra- and intraoral examination for each patient is a routine part of practice, but the tobacco-using patient must receive an extensive examination.

A. Detection of an Intraoral Lesion or Problem
Upon detecting a tobacco-related problem or lesion, the clinician will
1. *Show the patient.* Provide a simple, but thorough, explanation related to the nature of the condition.
2. *Explain.* Make certain that the patient understands the consequences of continuing tobacco use as it relates to the progress of the problem or lesion.
3. *Record.* A well-detailed description of the lesion and information provided to the patient concerning the lesion must be noted in the patient's record.

B. Referral Indications
Should a lesion persist for more than 2 weeks, a biopsy is indicated (page 126).
1. *Refer* the patient for biopsy.
2. *Ascertain.* Check to be certain that the patient undergoes the biopsy and receives results.
3. *Consult.* Pathologist that reviews the biopsy provides the pertinent information.
4. *Document.* Results are entered in the patient's treatment record.

C. Oral Self-Examination
Oral self-examination must be taught to all patients who use tobacco. The significance of oral self-examination in this high-risk group can not

---

TOBACCO USE ASSESSMENT FORM

Name:_____ Date_____

1. Do you **use** tobacco in any form? ☐ Yes ☐ No
1A. If no, have you ever used tobacco in the past? ☐ Yes ☐ No
    How long did you use tobacco? Years___ Months___
    How long ago did you stop? Years___ Months___

If you are not currently a tobacco user, no other questions should be answered. Thank you for completing this form.

Questions 2-10 are for current tobacco users only.

2. **If you smoke,** what type (check)   How many? (Number)
    ☐ Cigarettes   Cigarettes per day___
    ☐ Cigars   Cigars per day___
    ☐ Pipes   Bowls per day___

3. **If you chew/use snuff,** what type?   How much?
    ☐ Snuff   Days a can lasts___
    ☐ Chewing   Pouches per week___
    ☐ Other (describe)   Amount_____per_____

3A. **How long** do you keep a chew in your mouth? ____minutes

4. **How many days** of the week do you use tobacco? 7 6 5 4 3 2 1

5. **How soon** after you wake do you first use tobacco?
    Within 30 minutes?___   More than 30 minutes?___

6. Does the person **closest to you** use tobacco? ☐ Yes ☐ No

7. **How interested are you** in stopping your use of tobacco?
    ☐ not at all   ☐ a little   ☐ somewhat   ☐ Yes   ☐ very much

8. Have you ever **tried to stop** using tobacco before? ☐ Yes ☐ No

9. Have you **discussed stopping** with your physician? ☐ Yes ☐ No

10. If you decided to stop using tobacco completely during the next two weeks, **how confident are you** that you would succeed?
    ☐ not at all   ☐ a little   ☐ somewhat   ☐ very confident

---

FIGURE 27-2 Tobacco Use Assessment Form. With basic information about the type of tobacco product and extent of use, a cessation program can be introduced. (From Mecklenburg, R.E., Greenspan, D., Kleinman, D.V., Manley, M.W., Niessen, L.C., Robertson, P.B., and Winn, D.E.: *Tobacco Effects in the Mouth.* U.S. Department of Health and Human Services, Public Health Service, National Cancer Institute and National Institute of Dental Research, NIH Publication No. 94-3330, Reprinted March, 1994.)

be overstated. Teach patients to perform an oral self-examination by using the same techniques and components of the professional extraoral and intraoral examination as illustrated and explained in Chapter 8 (pages 118 to 120).

D. Detect, Relate, Motivate

Lesions that are a direct consequence of use are pointed out to the patient. The presence of tobacco-related problems/lesions can serve as a powerful motivational tool to encourage a quit attempt. The demonstration of the arrest or elimination of tobacco-related problems/lesions as the patient continues a nonuse status will aid in achieving permanent cessation.

V. CONSULTATION

Patients who do not seek routine medical care need referral to a physician for evaluation. Detection of underlying medical problems is essential so that necessary dental treatment modifications may be utilized.

CLINICAL TREATMENT PROCEDURES

Patients who use tobacco have more dental stain, calculus, and periodontal problems and therefore require longer and more frequent appointments.

I. BACTERIAL PLAQUE CONTROL

Self-care for daily bacterial plaque control is first in the care plan. Immaculate oral hygiene is required by this group of high-risk patients due to susceptibility to periodontal infections, oral cancer, other soft tissue alterations, and dental caries.

II. SCALING AND ROOT PLANING

A. Inform Patient
1. Healing will be jeopardized by continued tobacco use.
2. Users can not expect the same treatment result as nonusers.[29]

B. Power-Driven Instruments

1. Precautions should be taken to avoid ingestion of bacteria, water, and other debris. Patients who smoke often have pulmonary and cardiovascular complications.
2. Patient with cardiac pacemaker: Appropriate precautions should be taken as suggested by the manufacturer and the patient's cardiologist.

III. OTHER PATIENT INSTRUCTION

A. Diet and Nutrition

1. Tobacco use decreases appetite. As a result, users may become poorly nourished.
2. Desire to control body weight by use of tobacco products may impede a patient's entry into a cessation program or result in relapse.
3. Dietary and exercise suggestions can be provided.
4. Most smokeless tobacco products are sweetened with sugar or molasses, which increases cariogenic potential. Flavorings such as mint or licorice may be added.

B. Nonalcoholic Rinses

Long-term use of alcohol-containing antibacterial agents, mouthrinses, and other oral hygiene products cannot be recommended due to the synergistic effect of alcohol and tobacco in the initiation of head and neck cancers. Tobacco users may be aware of halitosis associated with tobacco use and frequently use alcohol containing mouthrinses to mask unpleasant odors.

TOBACCO CESSATION PROGRAM[30]

A program for tobacco use cessation provides an essential service in the dental hygiene care plan. At any given time many patients admit they would like to quit, and about one-third of all patients are ready to make a serious quit attempt.

Interventions and their outcome will vary depending on the motivation and experience of the clinician and the acceptance and adherence of the individual. Even a minimal intervention conducted by a clinician may help a patient to become tobacco free.

PREPARATION: DENTAL TEAM ORGANIZATION

I. GROUP AGREEMENT

A. All personnel may not directly advise and assist patients, but agreement, support, and cooperation of all are needed.
B. Study facts: review oral manifestations.
C. Study facts: see Tables 27-3 and 27-4 to understand nicotine dependency.

D. Attend a continuing education course or other training program.

II. COORDINATOR

Suggested responsibilities for the program coordinator are as follows:

A. Contact patients for follow-up.
B. Act as coach for patients who relapse.
C. Ensure adequate documentation in patient records.
D. Order/re-order patient literature.

III. MAKE CLINIC ENVIRONMENT TOBACCO FREE

A. Remove ashtrays; post signs indicating a tobacco-free environment.
B. Reception area: avoid reading materials that advertise tobacco products.

IV. PREPARE OR OBTAIN MATERIALS

V. SET EXAMPLE

Team members who have been tobacco users must be encouraged to enter a cessation program. Provide reimbursement for pharmacologic adjunct therapy and other treatment costs.

THE FOUR As[30]

A suggested program involves the "4 As": Ask, Advise, Assist, Arrange. A cessation program flow chart to show the steps and progressive actions is presented in Figure 27-3.

I. ASK

A. Obtain Patient Confidence

Many minors use tobacco products without parental knowledge or consent. Due to increasing social unacceptance of tobacco use, patients may be hesitant to disclose their habit.

B. Present Questions Carefully

Questions related to tobacco are presented without judgment. Tobacco use is addressed as a health issue and not a moral and/or social issue. The questions are to gain facts, and the patient must not be placed on the defensive.

II. ADVISE

A. Advise to Stop

Current users must be strongly encouraged to quit. All members of the office staff must reinforce the message.

B. Motivate Patient

Clearly state the consequences of continued use and the benefits of stopping.

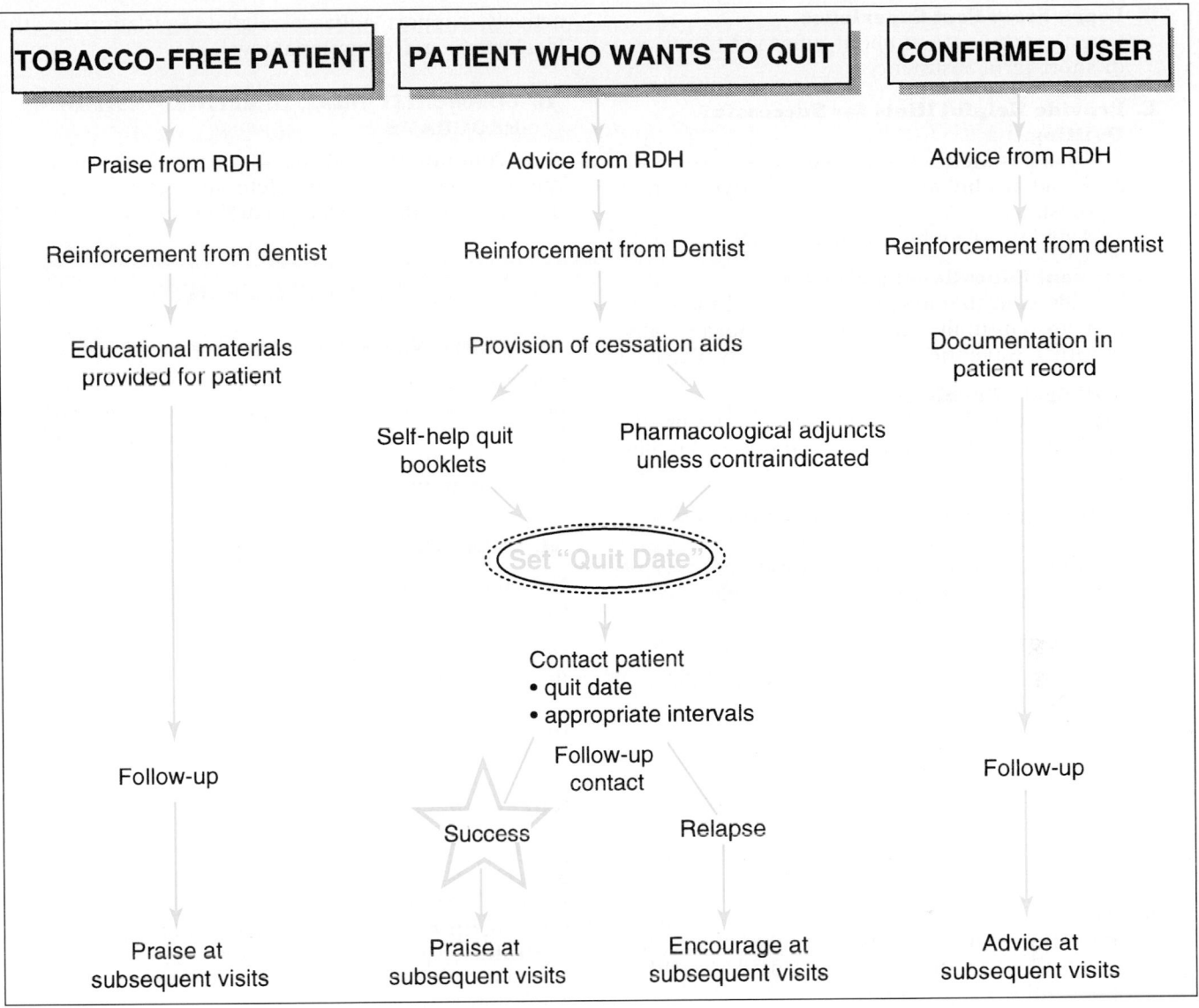

FIGURE 27-3 Tobacco Cessation. Flow chart to show how the **4 As** can be incorporated into the clinic setting.

C. Personalize the Message

Each patient will have individual reasons for quitting. A mother who smokes may be more concerned about the effect of the second-hand smoke from her cigarettes on her children than her own oral health.

D. Show Willingness to Help

E. Relate Oral Findings

When a tobacco-related problem/lesion is detected, inform and then show the patient. Explain poor prognosis for treatment if tobacco use continues.

F. Resistant Patient

For the patient not ready to stop or indifferent to suggestion, care is taken not to antagonize. Document the data obtained and record conversation for reference at future appointments.

Provide literature to help motivate. Ask and Advise at the next dental visit.

III. ASSIST

When a patient has shown interest in making an attempt to quit, assistance is given.

A. Set Quit Date

Help the patient to set a realistic quit date soon, at least within 2 weeks.

B. Alert Family and Friends

Advise the patient to spread the word that a quit date has been set; request support.

C. Remove Tobacco Products

Inform the patient that all tobacco products, paraphernalia, ashtrays, and the like must be removed from home and work site.

D. Learn From Past Experience
Question the patient about what led to relapse or short-term abstinence.

E. Provide Helpful Hints for Successful Quitting
1. Total abstinence is required.
2. Avoid alcohol and use of other psychoactive substances.
3. Avoid people who use tobacco.

F. Present Educational Materials
Provide educational and motivational materials that are culturally, racially, and educationally sensitive. Have the materials readily available.

G. Anticipate Problems
Explain withdrawal symptoms and discuss methods for alleviation of symptoms (Tables 27-5 and 27-6).

H. Encourage Use of Pharmaceutical Agents
Advise use of nicotine replacement or non-nicotine product to aid in cessation. Review manufacturer's directions for use (Table 27-7).

IV. ARRANGE
Follow-up contact with each patient is essential for success. Schedule future office appointments or make telephone contact.

A. Contact the Patient on the Quit Date
The first contact is on the quit date. The second contact should be made about 1 to 2 weeks after the quit date. Schedule subsequent contacts as needed to discuss progress.

B. Praise
The patient who has remained tobacco free deserves appreciation and congratulations. Offer opportunity for questions.

C. In Case of Relapse
1. Ask the patient to recall and record the conditions that led to re-use.
2. Encourage the patient to set another quit date, reminding the patient that each attempt is a learning experience and many quit attempts are needed by some patients before achieving success.
3. Review the use of pharmaceutical agents.
4. For the patient who requests a more intensive cessation program, provide addresses and contact numbers.

ADVOCACY

I. PUBLIC HEALTH POLICY
All members of the oral health team need to be knowledgeable about tobacco-related health promotion and public health policy activities. It is the professional responsibility of clinicians to be aware of and actively support tobacco-related legislation at the local, state, and/or national level.

II. COMMUNITY ORAL HEALTH EDUCATIONAL PROGRAMS
Any community oral health educational program cannot be considered complete unless tobacco education is included. Excellent materials are available.

TECHNICAL HINTS

I. COMPLETION OF TRAINING PROGRAM
Clinicians can be especially effective when they complete a formal training program such as the National Cancer Institute's *How to Help Your Patients Be Tobacco Free* before implementing a dental office tobacco cessation program.

II. SOURCES
National Cancer Institute
Office of Cancer Communications
Building 31, Room 4B43
National Institutes of Health
Bethesda, MD 20892

National Dental Tobacco Free Steering Committee
Dr. Robert Mecklenburg
12304 River's Edge Drive
Potomac, MD 20854

National Oral Health Information Clearinghouse (NOHIC)
1 NOHIC Way
Bethesda, MD 29892-3500
1-800-4-CANCER

Oral Health America: America's Fund for Dental Health
National Spit Tobacco Educational Program (NSTEP)
410 N Michigan Ave, Suite 352
Chicago, IL 60611
312-836-9900

Oregon Research Institute
Dr. Herbert Severson
1715 Franklin Blvd
Eugene, OR 97403
541-484-2123
Fax: 541-484-1108

FACTORS TO TEACH THE PATIENT

I. How to perform a self-examination of the oral cavity.
II. The most effective method to stop using tobacco is never to start.
III. Use of tobacco during pregnancy is related to low birth weight and other problems in newborn infants.
IV. Young children experiment or frequently use tobacco products. Parental awareness and guidance is needed.

V. Any form of social tobacco use (including cigars) can lead to addiction.

VI. Breathing environmental or second-hand smoke can lead to the same serious health problems in nonsmokers as in the smokers themselves. Children are especially susceptible.

VII. Information concerning tobacco legislation and public health policy so patients can make informed choices related to a tobacco-smoke-free society.

VIII. After attempting to quit tobacco use, relapse may occur. Should this happen, the 4-A program can be repeated. Successful quitting may require many attempts over a period of years.

IX. Oral health team members are appropriately trained to help patients become tobacco free.

REFERENCES

1. **Pindborg**, J.J.: Tobacco and Gingivitis. II. Correlation Between Consumption of Tobacco, Ulceromembranous Gingivitis and Calculus, *J. Dent. Res., 28,* 460, October, 1949.

2. **Stein**, Z.: Smoking and Reproductive Health, *J. Am. Med. Women's Assoc., 51,* 29, January/April, 1996.

3. **United States Department of Health and Human Services:** *The Health Benefits of Smoking Cessation: A Report of the Surgeon General, Executive Summary.* Public Health Service, Centers for Disease Control, Center for Chronic Disease Prevention and Health Promotion. DHHS Publication No. (CDC) 90-8416, 1990, in *MMWR, 39,* RR-12, October 5, 1990, p. vi.

4. **Schmitz**, J.M., Schneider, N.G., and Jarvik, M.E.: Nicotine, in Lowinson, J.H., Ruiz, P., Millman, R.B., and Langrod, J.G., eds.: *Substance Abuse. A Comprehensive Textbook,* 3rd ed. Baltimore, Williams & Wilkins, 1997, pp. 276–294.

5. **Benowitz**, N.L., Porchet, H., Scheiner, L., and Jacob, P.: Nicotine Absorption and Cardiovascular Effects with Smokeless Tobacco Use: Comparison with Cigarettes and Nicotine Gum, *Clin. Pharmacol. Thera., 44,* 23, July, 1988.

6. **Hatsukami**, D., Nelson, R., and Jensen, J.: Smokeless Tobacco: Current Status and Future Directions, *Brit. J. Addict., 86,* 559, May, 1991.

7. **Holbrook**, J.H., Grundy, S.M., Hennekens, C.H., Kannel, W.B., and Strong, J.P.: Cigarette Smoking and Cardiovascular Diseases. A Statement for Health Professionals by a Task Force Appointed by the Steering Committee of the American Heart Association, *Circulation, 70,* 1114A, December, 1984.

8. **Henningfield**, J.E., Clayton, R., and Pollin, W.: Involvement of Tobacco in Alcoholism and Illicit Drug Use, *Brit. J. Addict., 85,* 279, February, 1990.

9. **Fontham**, E.T.H., Correa, P., Reynolds, P., Wu-Williams, A., Buffler, P.A., Greenberg, R.S., Chen, V.W., Alterman, T., Boyd, P., Austin, D.F., and Liff, J.: Environmental Tobacco Smoke and Lung Cancer in Nonsmoking Women. A Multicenter Study, *JAMA, 271,* 1752, June 8, 1994.

10. **Taylor**, A.E., Johnson, D.C., and Kazemi, H.: Environmental Tobacco Smoke and Cardiovascular Disease. A Position Paper from the Council on Cardiopulmonary and Critical Care, American Heart Association, *Circulation, 86,* 700, August, 1992.

11. **Glantz**, S.A. and Parmley, W.W.: Passive Smoking and Heart Disease: Mechanisms and Risk, *JAMA, 273,* 1047, April 5, 1995.

12. **Wells**, A.J.: Passive Smoking as a Cause of Heart Disease, *J. Am. Coll. Cardiol., 24,* 546, August, 1994.

13. **Charlton**, A.: Children and Passive Smoking: A Review, *J. Fam. Pract., 38,* 267, March, 1994.

14. **American Heart Association,** Committee on Atherosclerosis and Hypertension in Children, Council on Cardiovascular Disease in the Young: Active and Passive Tobacco Exposure: A Serious Pediatric Health Problem, *Circulation, 90,* 2581, November, 1994.

15. **Khoury**, M. J., Gomez-Farias, M., and Mulinare, J.: Does Maternal Cigarette Smoking During Pregnancy Cause Cleft Lip and Palate in the Offspring?, *Am. J. Dis. Child., 143,* 333, March, 1989.

16. **Kieser**, J. A., Groeneveld, H. T., and da Silva, P.: Delayed Tooth Formation in Children Exposed to Tobacco Smoke, *J. Clin. Pediatr. Dent., 20,* 97, Winter, 1996.

17. **Klonoff-Cohen**, H. S., Edelstein, S. L., Lefkowitz, E.S., Srinivasan, I. P., Kaegi, D., Chang, J. C., and Wiley, K.I: The Effect of Passive Smoking and Tobacco Exposure Through Breast Milk on Sudden Infant Death Syndrome, *JAMA, 273,* 795, March 8, 1995.

18. **Zambon**, J.J., Grossi, S.G., Machtei, E.E., Ho, A.W., Dunford, R., and Genco, R.J.: Cigarette Smoking Increases the Risk for Subgingival Infection with Periodontal Pathogens, *J. Periodontol., 67,* 1050, October, 1996.

19. **MacFarlane**, G.D., Herzberg, M. C., Wolff, L. F., and Hardie, N.A.: Refractory Periodontitis Associated with Abnormal Polymorphonuclear Leukocyte Phagocytosis and Cigarette Smoking, *J. Periodontol., 63,* 908, November, 1992.

20. **Pabst**, M. J., Pabst, K. M., Collier, J. A., Coleman, T. C., Lemons-Prince, M. L., Godat, M. S., Waring, M.B., and Babu, J. P.: Inhibition of Neutrophil and Monocyte Defensive Functions by Nicotine. *J. Periodontol., 66,* 1047, December, 1995.

21. **Tew**, J.G., Zhang, J.-B., Quinn, S., Tangada, S., Nakashima, K., Gunsolley, J.C., Schenkein, H.A., and Califano, J.V.: Antibody of the IgG2 Subclass, *Actinobacillus actinomycetemcomitans,* and Early-onset Periodontitis, *J. Periodontol., 67,* 317, March, Supplement, 1996.

22. **Tipton**, D. A. and Dabbous, M.K.: Effects of Nicotine on Proliferation and Extracellular Matrix Production of Human Gingival Fibroblasts *in vitro. J. Periodontol., 66,* 1056, December, 1995.

23. **Dinsdale**, C.R.J., Rawlinson, A., and Walsh, T.F.: Subgingival Temperature in Smokers and Non-smokers with Periodontal Disease, *J. Clin. Periodontol., 24,* 761, October, 1997.

24. **Haas**, R., Haimböck, W., Mailath, G., and Watzek., G.: The Relationship of Smoking on Peri-implant Tissue: A Retrospective Study, *J. Prosthet. Dent., 76,* 592 , December, 1996.

25. **Henningfield**, J.E.: Nicotine Medications for Smoking Cessation, *N. Engl. J. Med., 333,* 1196, November 2, 1995.

26. **Hurt**, R. D., Sachs, D.P.L., Glover, E.D., Offord, K.P., Johnston, J.A., Dale, L. C., Khayrallah, M A., Schroeder, D.R., Glover, P.N., Sullivan, C. R., Croghan, I.T., and Sullivan, P.M.: A Comparison of Sustained-release Bupropion and Placebo for Smoking Cessation, *N. Engl. J. Med., 337,* 1195, October 23, 1997.

27. **Benowitz**, N.L.: Treating Tobacco Addiction: Nicotine or No Nicotine? *N. Engl. J. Med., 337,* 1230, October 23, 1997.

28. **Fiore**, M.C.: The New Vital Sign: Assessing and Documenting Smoking Status, *JAMA, 266,* 3183, December 11, 1991.

29. **Grossi**, S.G., Zambon, J., and Machtei, E., Schifferle, R., Andreana, S., Genco, R. J., Cummins, D., and Harrap, G.: Effects of Smoking and Smoking Cessation on Healing after Mechanical Periodontal Therapy. *J. Am. Dent. Assoc., 128,* 599, May, 1997.

30. **Mecklenburg**, R.E., Christen, A.G., Gerbert, B., Gift, H. C., Glynn, T.J., Jones, R.B., Lindsay, E., Manley, M.W., and Severson, H.: *How to Help Your Patients Stop Using Tobacco: A National Cancer Institute Manual for the Oral Health Team,* Smoking and Tobacco Control Program, National Cancer Institute, U.S. Department of Health and Human Services, Public Health Service, NIH Publication 91-3191, December 1990.

SUGGESTED READINGS

ADHA Committee on Tobacco Use, Prevention and Cessation: Resource List, *J. Dent. Hyg., 69,* 56, March–April, 1995.

Andrews, J.A., Severson, H.H., Lichtenstein, E., and Gordon, J.S.: Relationship Between Tobacco Use and Self-Reported Oral Hygiene Habits, *J. Am. Dent. Assoc., 129,* 313, March, 1998.

Christen, A.G. and Klein, J.A.: *Tobacco and Your Oral Health.* Carol Stream, IL, *Quintessence,* 1997, 35 pp.

Christen, A.G., McDonald, J.L., and Christen, J.A.: *The Impact of Tobacco Use and Cessation on Nonmalignant and Precancerous Oral and Dental Diseases and Conditions,* Indiana University School of Dentistry, Department of Preventive and Community Dentistry, 1121 W. Michigan St., Indianapolis, Indiana 46202-5186.

Conley, L.J., Bush, T.J., Buchbinder, S.P., Penley, K.A., Judson, F.N., and Holmberg, S.D.: The Association Between Cigarette Smoking and Selected HIV-related Medical Conditions, *AIDS, 10*, 1121, September, 1996.

Gold, D.R., Wang, X., Wypij, D., Speizer, F.E., Ware, J.H., and Dockery, D.W.: Effects of Cigarette Smoking on Lung Function in Adolescent Boys and Girls, *N. Engl. J. Med., 335*, 931, September 26, 1996.

Hovell, M.F., Slymen, D.J., Jones, J.A., Hofstetter, C.R., Burkham-Kreitner, S., Conway, T.L., Rubin, B., and Noel, D.: An Adolescent Tobacco-use Prevention Trial in Orthodontic Offices, *Am. J. Public Health, 86*, 1760, December, 1996.

Kessler, D.A., Witt, A.M., Barnett, P.S., Zeller, M.R., Natanblut, S.L., Wilkenfeld, J.P., Lorraine, C.C., Thompson, L.J., and Schultz, W.B.: The Food and Drug Administration's Regulation of Tobacco Products, *N. Engl. J. Med., 335*, 988, September 26, 1996.

Mainous, A.G. and Hueston, W.J.: The Effect of Smoking Cessation During Pregnancy on Preterm Delivery and Low Birthweight, *J. Fam. Pract., 38*, 262, March, 1994.

Mecklenburg, R.E., Greenspan, D., Kleinman, D.V., Manley, M.W., Niessen, L.C., Robertson, P. B., and Winn, D.E.: *Tobacco Effects In The Mouth*. U.S. Department of Health and Human Services, Pubic Health Service, National Institutes of Health, NIH Publication 94-3330.

Tomar, S. L., Husten, C.G., and Manley, M.W.: Do Dentists and Physicians Advise Tobacco Users to Quit? *J. Am. Dent. Assoc., 127*, 259, February, 1996.

Periodontal Diseases and Implants

American Academy of Periodontology, Research, Science and Therapy Committee: Position Paper: Tobacco Use and the Periodontal Patient, *J. Periodontol., 67*, 51, January, 1996.

Haber, J.: Cigarette Smoking: A Major Risk Factor for Periodontitis, *Compend. Cont. Educ. Dent., 15*, 1002, August, 1994.

Haber, J.: Cigarette Smoking. A Major Risk Factor for Periodontitis, *DentalHygienistNews, 8*, 3, Number 3, 1995.

Hamel, S.B. and Craig, B.J.: The Effects of Cigarette Smoking on Periodontal Disease, *Canad. Dent. Hyg. Assoc., PROBE, 31*, 204, November/December, 1997.

Kaldahl, W.B., Johnson, G.K., Patil, K.D., and Kalkwarf, K.L.: Levels of Cigarette Consumption and Response to Periodontal Therapy, *J. Periodontol., 67*, 675, July, 1996.

Kinane, D.F. and Radvar, M.: The Effect of Smoking on Mechanical and Antimicrobial Periodontal Therapy, *J. Periodontol., 68*, 467, May, 1997.

Krall, E.A., Garvey, A.J., and Garcia, R.I.: Alveolar Bone Loss and Tooth Loss in Male Cigar and Pipe Smokers, *J. Am. Dent. Assoc., 130*, 57, January, 1999.

Lindquist, L.W., Carlsson, G.E., and Jemt, T.: Association Between Marginal Bone Loss Around Osseointegrated Mandibular Implants and Smoking Habits: A 10-year Follow-up Study, *J. Dent. Res., 76*, 1667, October, 1997.

Preber, H., Linder, L., and Bergström, J.: Periodontal Healing and Periopathogenic Microflora in Smokers and Non-smokers, *J. Clin. Periodontol., 22*, 946, December, 1995.

Qandil, R., Sandhu, H.S., and Matthews, D.C.: Tobacco Smoking and Periodontal Diseases, *J. Can. Dent. Assoc., 63*, 187, March 1997.

Rosen, P.S., Marks, M.H., and Reynolds, M.A.: Influence of Smoking on Long-term Clinical Results of Intrabony Defects Treated with Regenerative Therapy, *J. Periodontol., 67*, 1159, November, 1996.

Schenkein, H.A., Gunsolley, J.C., Koertge, T.E., Schenkein, J.G., and Tew, J.G.: Smoking and Its Effects on Early-onset Periodontitis, *J. Am. Dent. Assoc., 126*, 1107, August, 1995.

Stach, D.J.: Cigarette Smoking as a Risk Factor in Periodontal Disease, *Case Studies in Periodontal Management, 1*, 1, October, 1995.

Trombelli, L. and Scabbia, A.: Healing Response of Gingival Recession Defects Following Guided Tissue Regeneration Procedures in Smokers and Non-smokers, *J. Clin. Periodontol., 24*, 529, August, 1997.

Smokeless

Connolly, G.N., Winn, D.M., Hecht, S.S., Henningfield, J.E., Walker, B., and Hoffmann, D.: The Reemergence of Smokeless Tobacco, *N. Engl. J. Med., 314*, 1020, April 17, 1986.

Fried, J.L.: The Periodontal Ramifications of Smokeless Tobacco Use, *Case Studies in Periodontal Management*, II, 1, April, 1996.

Greene, J.C. and Walsh, M.M., eds.: Smokeless (Spit) Tobacco: A Review of the State of the Science, (Symposium), *Adv. Dent. Res., 11*, 305–359, (7 articles), September, 1997.

Robertson, P.B., Derouen, T.A., Ernster, V., Grady, D., Greene, J., Mancl, L., McDonald, D., and Walsh, M.M.: Smokeless Tobacco Use: How it Affects the Performance of Major League Baseball Players, *J. Am. Dent. Assoc., 126*, 1115, August, 1995.

Stevens, V.J., Severson, H., Lichtenstein, E., Little, S.J., and Leben, J.: Making the Most of a Teachable Moment: A Smokeless-Tobacco Cessation Intervention in the Dental Office, *Am. J. Public Health, 85*, 231, February, 1995.

Tomar, S.L., Winn, D.M., Swango, P.A., Giovino, G.A., and Kleinman, D.V.: Oral Mucosal Smokeless Tobacco Lesions Among Adolescents in the United States, *J. Dent. Res., 76*, 1277, June, 1997.

Williams, N.J., Arheart, K.L., and Klesges, R.: A Smokeless Tobacco Cessation Program for Postsecondary Students, *Health Values, 19*, 33, May/June, 1995.

Winn, D.M., Blot, W.J., Shy, C.M., Pickle, L.W., Toledo, A., and Fraumeni, J.F.: Snuff Dipping and Oral Cancer Among Women in Southern United States, *N. Engl. J. Med., 304*, 745, March 26, 1981.

Tobacco Cessation

American Medical Association, Smoking Cessation Clinical Practice Guideline Panel and Staff: The Agency for Health Care Policy and Research Smoking Cessation Clinical Practice Guideline, *JAMA, 275*, 1270, April 24, 1996.

Biron, C.: Smoking Deterrents Can Help Kick the Habit, But Side Effects Need to Be Closely Monitored, *RDH, 16*, 30, June, 1996.

Christen, A.G., McDonald, J.L., Klein, J.A., Christen, J.A., and Guba, C.J.: *A Smoking Cessation Program for the Dental Office*, Department of Oral Biology, Indiana University School of Dentistry, Indianapolis, Indiana, 1994.

Dadian, T. and Pirk, S.: Tobacco Use Cessation. An Ethical Consideration, *DentalHygienistNews, 10*, 10, Number 1, 1997.

Eres, J.: Market Review, *Access, 11*, 46, July, 1997.

Fiore, M.C., Smith, S.S., Jorenby, D.E., and Baker, T.B.: The Effectiveness of the Nicotine Patch for Smoking Cessation. A Meta-analysis, *JAMA, 271*, 1940, June 22–29, 1994.

Hjalmarson, A., Nilsson, F., Sjöström, L., and Wiklund, O.: The Nicotine Inhaler in Smoking Cessation, *Arch. Intern. Med., 157*, 1721, August 11–25, 1997.

Klein, J.A.: Smoking Cessation and Avoidance: How Dental Hygienists Can Help Their Patients, *J. Pract. Hyg., 1*, 18, November/December, 1992.

Little, S.J. and Stevens, V.J.: Dental Hygiene's Role in Reducing Tobacco Use. A Literature Review and Recommendations for Action, *J. Dent. Hyg., 65*, 346, September, 1991.

Ostrowski, D.J. and DeNelsky, G.Y.: Pharmacologic Management of Patients Using Smoking Cessation Aids, *Dent. Clin. North Am., 40*, 779, July, 1996.

Severson, H.H., Andrews, J.A., Lichtenstein, E., Gordon, J.S., and Barckley, M.F.: Using the Hygiene Visit to Deliver a Tobacco Cessation Program: Results from a Randomized Clinical Trial, *J. Am. Dent. Assoc., 129*, 993, July, 1998.

Somerman, M. and Mecklenberg, R.E.: Cessation of Tobacco Use, in American Dental Association: *ADA Guide to Dental Therapeutics*. Chicago, ADA Publishing Co., 1998, pp. 505–516.

Wood, G.J., Cecchini, J.J., Nathason, N., and Hiroshige, K.: Office-based Training in Tobacco Cessation for Dental Professionals, *J. Am. Dent. Assoc., 128*, 216, February, 1997.

Diet and Dietary Assessment

Planning for a total preventive program for an individual patient involves consideration of dietary and nutritional factors. The status of oral health can be affected by nutrition, diet, and food habits. Adequate nutrition maintains general health and can contribute to a higher degree of oral health. Box 28-1 defines terminology related to nutrition, diet, and oral health.

Instruction relating to diet is coordinated with other phases of teaching. To give information about a diet conducive to oral health is a responsibility of the dental professional, and to help motivate a patient to adopt new eating patterns is a challenge. Teaching must be made practical and possible to apply if it is to have impact on such forceful influences. The overall goal is to make the recommendations and modifications as close to the original pattern of eating as possible.

Food selection by an individual is influenced by age, sex, geographic location, economic status, available foods, family traditions, religion, cultural habits, prejudices, fallacies, and advertising, as well as emotional and social factors. Consideration can be given when making recommendations for dietary changes. The complications associated with eating disorders are described on pages 830 to 833 in Chapter 56.

ORAL RELATIONSHIPS

I. PERIODONTAL TISSUES[1-3]

A. Nutritional Deficiencies

1. Protein, vitamins, and other nutrients are essential for the health of the periodontal tissues, just as they are for the health of the tissues throughout the body.

2. A nutritional deficiency has never been shown to be the specific cause of periodontal pocket formation, gingivitis, or periodontal infections. For these conditions to develop, plaque microorganisms must be present.

3. Certain nutritional deficiencies (notably protein, ascorbic acid, and vitamin B complex) may modify gingival tissue resistance so that

BOX 28-1 KEY WORDS AND ABBREVIATIONS: Diet and Dietary Analysis

A.I.: Adequate intake; the recommended nutrient intake of specific population groups, such as infants, that appears to support health; AIs have been established for calcium, vitamin D, and fluoride for all age groups.

Anticariogenic: foods that do not lower the plaque pH; encourage remineralization.

Cariogenic (kar″ē-ō-jen′ik): conducive to dental caries; the degree of cariogenicity depends on many factors, including physical form, texture, and consistency of the carbohydrate-containing food; its retention and clearance time from the oral cavity; and the frequency of use.

Cariogenic exposure: individual ingestion of a cariogenic food that exposes the tooth surface and lowers the pH in the bacterial plaque.

Clearance time: the time from the cariogenic exposure until the food is cleared from the oral cavity; influenced by consistency and quantity of saliva; by the action of the tongue, lips, and cheeks; and by the consistency of food.

Diet: customary amount and kind of food and drink taken by an individual from day to day.

Dietary assessment: separation of a dietary food record into individual components of the Food Guide Pyramid; assessment of quality, of whether the individual is using an adequate diet, and of where modifications are needed.

D.R.I.: dietary reference intakes; a comprehensive term for categories of reference values that concentrate on maintaining a healthy state for the healthy general population. The categories include the R.D.A., A.I., E.A.R., and U.L.

E.A.R.: estimated average requirement; estimates the nutrient requirements of the average individual; categorized by age and gender; foundation for the R.D.A.

Malnutrition: poor nourishment resulting from improper diet or some defect of metabolism that prevents the body from utilizing its intake of food properly.

Meal plan: a selectively planned or prescribed regimen of food to meet certain needs of the individual.

Noncariogenic food: does not support or promote bacterial growth responsible for caries formation.

Nutrient (nu′trē-ent): a chemical substance in foods that is needed by the body for building and repair; the six classes of nutrients are proteins, fats, carbohydates, minerals, vitamins, and water.

Nutrient dense: providing a higher nutrient value than calories. Particularly important for those individuals on a low-calorie meal plan to be certain to get adequate nutrients.

Nutrition: sum of processes involved in taking nutrients into the body and assimilating and utilizing them; includes ingestion, digestion, absorption, transport, utilization of nutrients, and excretion of waste products.

Nutritional deficiency: inadequacy of nutrients in the tissues; the result of inadequate dietary intake or impairment of digestion, absorption, transport, or metabolism.

R.D.A.: recommended dietary allowances; recommendations for the average amounts of nutrients that should be consumed daily by healthy people to achieve adequate nutrient intake; categorized by age and gender.

Registered dietitian: a health professional with a minimum of a bachelor's degree in nutrition or dietetics who has attended an internship program or equivalent and passed the registration exam, all under the approval of the American Dietetic Association (A.D.A.). Continuing education is required to keep credentials current.

U.L.: tolerable upper intake levels; maximum intake by an individual that is unlikely to create risks of adverse health effects in almost all healthy individuals. U.L.'s were established to avoid toxicity due to excess intake of specific nutrients from food, fortified food, water, and nutrient supplements.

U.S.D.A.: United States Department of Agriculture.

U.S.D.H.H.S.: United States Department of Health and Human Services.

---

an inflammatory condition (initiated by plaque microorganisms) may be accelerated or increased in intensity.
4. The effects of periodontal infection can alter the capacity of the tissues to utilize available nutrients; therefore, the potential for healing and repair is modified.

B. Consistency of Food
1. Soft sticky foods cling to the teeth and gingiva and encourage food and debris accumulation. Microorganisms are protected and

nourished, thus leading to increased amounts of bacterial plaque.
2. Firm fibrous foods, such as raw carrots or apples, may stimulate the tissues and improve circulation. Additionally, firm foods increase salivary flow, which acts as a buffer against plaque and aids in oral clearance.

C. Dietary Assessment
Patients with acute gingival disease or necrotizing ulcerative gingivitis, and most patients undergoing periodontal therapy, need specific in-

struction in diet selection. A dietary assessment is necessary if a true idea of the patient's diet is to be available for study. Procedures for the assessment are described later in this chapter.

II. SKIN AND MUCOUS MEMBRANE

A. Nutritional Deficiencies

Severe nutritional deficiencies are not limited to underdeveloped areas of the world but are increasing in rural and inner-city areas in the United States. Deficiencies tend to produce symptoms of mixed clinical entities, but infrequently symptoms of a severe acute disease may be seen. When certain oral symptoms suggest nutritional deficiencies, most likely the patient is suffering from multiple deficiencies.

Ordinarily, the effects of a deficiency are chronic and run a slow, gradual course. The clinical manifestations are influenced by trauma, local irritation, or systemic factors, such as a chronic disease, when tissue resistance may be lowered.

B. Oral Lesions

Types of oral lesions that suggest the possibility of an underlying nutritional deficiency are stomatitis, glossitis, hemorrhagic gingiva, chelitis, localized ulcerations, and areas of atrophic change.[4] Nutrients that are considered particularly associated with the health of the oral mucosa are protein, iron, ascorbic acid, and the B complex vitamins.

C. Extraoral Lesions

During extraoral examination, abnormalities are frequently noted. Deficiencies of various nutritional elements include dry skin, hair loss, spoon-shaped or brittle nails, or pale skin. Abnormalities related to anorexia nervosa are described on page 831.

D. Instruction

Assistance to patients through recommendations for an adequate diet for general health contribute to preserving the integrity of the oral mucosa.

III. DENTAL CARIES[5-7]

A. Prevention

Fluoride is the essential mineral for dental caries prevention. The complexity of dental caries formation is shown in Figure 28-1, which illustrates how a cariogenic diet, specific microorganisms, saliva composition, and a susceptible tooth surface together provide the environment for dental caries formation.

B. Role of Cariogenic Foods[8]

Dental caries is the result of action on the external surface of the tooth. Instead of being a deficiency disease, it can be considered the result of an excess of cariogenic foods. Fermentable car-

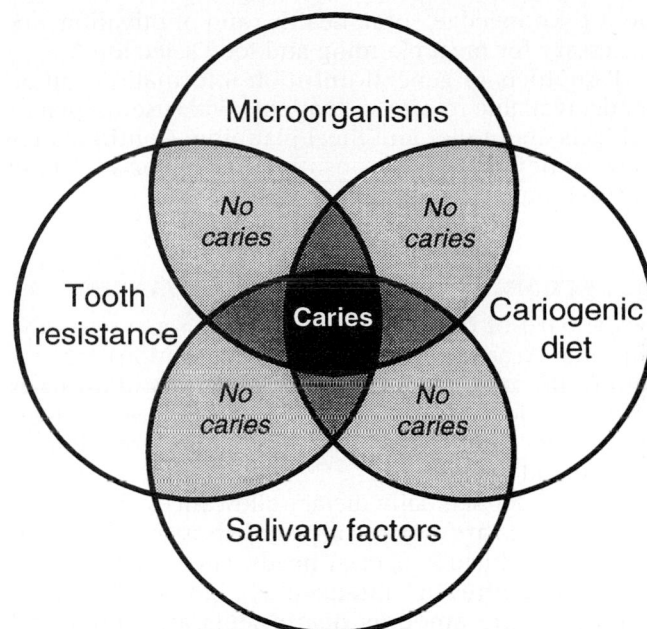

FIGURE 28-1 Dental Caries Process. Four overlapping circles illustrate the factors involved in the development of dental caries. All four act together, and as shown by the center, dental caries results. (Adapted from United States Department of Health and Human Services, Public Health Service, National Institute of Dental Research: *Broadening the Scope. Long-Range Research Plan for the 1990s*, NIH Publication No. 90-1188, Washington, D.C., United States Government Printing Office, 1990).

bohydrates produce acids when acted on by specific plaque microorganisms. These factors were reviewed in connection with bacterial plaque on pages 272 to 274.

C. Dietary Assessment and Counseling

The use of dietary assessment in the instruction of patients (or primary caregivers*) relative to dental caries control has proven to be helpful to many people. Specific personal recommendations can be made.

DAILY FOOD REQUIREMENTS

Instruction centers around helping patients learn about the foods that make up an adequate diet and improve their food selection. Poor food habits, such as missed meals, omission of essential foods, regular use of non-nutritious snacks, or illogical dieting, frequently are important considerations for recommendations related to nutritional practices for oral health. Generalities may be useful to a degree, but for daily application, specific suggestions related to the pa-

*Primary caregiver refers to the individual who has most responsibility for the patient, such as the mother of a child or a daughter of an elderly person.

tient's knowledge, oral health, and motivation are necessary for meal planning and food selection.

Pamphlets of general nutrition information can be made available to provide patients with useful, practical facts about diet and meal planning. Continued review of new materials constitutes an important phase of teaching.

I. RECOMMENDED DIETARY ALLOWANCES

A standard of dietary adequacy was prepared by the National Academy of Sciences (10th edition) for certain nutrients.[9] The recommended dietary allowances (RDAs) reflect adequate intake for healthy individuals to prevent a deficiency state. The values are adjusted for age and gender.

Recommended daily dietary allowances are not the same for all, are not recommended as an ideal diet, and do not include special needs, such as during illness. The figures are intended as a guide. The designations of the amounts of nutrients are impractical for patient instruction. To be meaningful, nutrients must be expressed in terms of the foods that contain them and how much of each of these foods must be consumed daily to meet the requirements.

For example, 60 mg of vitamin C per day is the RDA for most adults, which is the equivalent of 4 oz of orange juice. For patients who smoke, the requirement increases to 100 mg per day.

A maximum value has been established for calcium, phosphorus, magnesium, vitamin D, and fluoride and are referred to as the Dietary Reference Intakes (DRI). DRIs are categorized further for other nutrition-related values as well. Like the RDAs, the DRIs were established for the healthy general population. The purpose is to avoid overconsumption as well as to prevent disease.[10]

II. THE FOOD GUIDE PYRAMID

Fulfilling minimum requirements of nutrients for the maintenance of health and resistance to disease is not a problem when a wide variety of foods is included in the diet each day. The foods that contain the essential nutrients and whose nutrient value exceeds the calorie content are called nutrient-dense foods.

Foods have been divided into five groups: the milk group, the meat and alternative protein group, the vegetable group, the fruit group, and the grain group. The food guide pyramid is shown in Figure 28-2.

Coordinated with the food guide pyramid to explain healthy behaviors and food choices are the dietary guidelines for Americans. Both were designed to educate individuals to meet nutritional requirements, promote health, support active lives, and reduce or prevent the risk of chronic disease. The educational tool was established by the USDA and USDHHS. Table 28-1 summarizes the dietary guidelines.

TABLE 28-1   Dietary Guidelines for Americans
• Eat a variety of foods • Balance the food you eat with physical activity—maintain or improve your weight • Choose a diet with plenty of grain products, vegetables, and fruits • Choose a diet low in fat, saturated fat, and cholesterol • Choose a diet moderate in sugars • Choose a diet moderate in salt and sodium • If you drink alcoholic beverages, do so in moderation
(From U.S. Department of Agriculture and U.S. Department of Health and Human Services: Home and Garden Bulletin No. 232, 4th ed., 1995.)

III. APPLICATIONS

The size of the servings of food varies with age and physiologic states. Servings for children are smaller; for teenagers, servings are extra large or increased in number. Nutritional requirements for teenage boys are higher than at any other time in their lives, and for girls, the only time the requirements will be higher will be during pregnancy and lactation. Dietary requirements for pregnancy are summarized in the chapter on prenatal care, page 659.

With aging, total energy requirements decrease, but the components of the daily requirements remain the same or actually increase for several nutrients. Calcium requirements, for example, increase for those over the age of 51 years for the reduction of bone resorption. Therefore, food choices for the elderly should be nutrient dense. Tissue building and repair continue throughout life, and nutrients must be supplied accordingly. Problems of the diet of aging persons are summarized on pages 693 to 694.

COUNSELING FOR DENTAL CARIES CONTROL[11]

Control of bacterial plaque and of cariogenic food intake, strengthening of the tooth surface to resist caries activity, and presence of saliva are essentials in the prevention of dental caries. Figure 28-1 shows that inattention to all of these factors is necessary for dental caries to develop.

Control of dental caries by diet accompanies procedures for control of bacterial plaque. They are part of the total oral health program that also includes pit and fissure sealants, the restoration of carious teeth, and the implementation of fluoride therapy.

THE DIETARY ASSESSMENT

A dietary assessment is used as a guide for instruction of the patient. Whether the assessment is made to help a patient whose major oral health problem is

Food Guide Pyramid
A Guide to Daily Food Choices

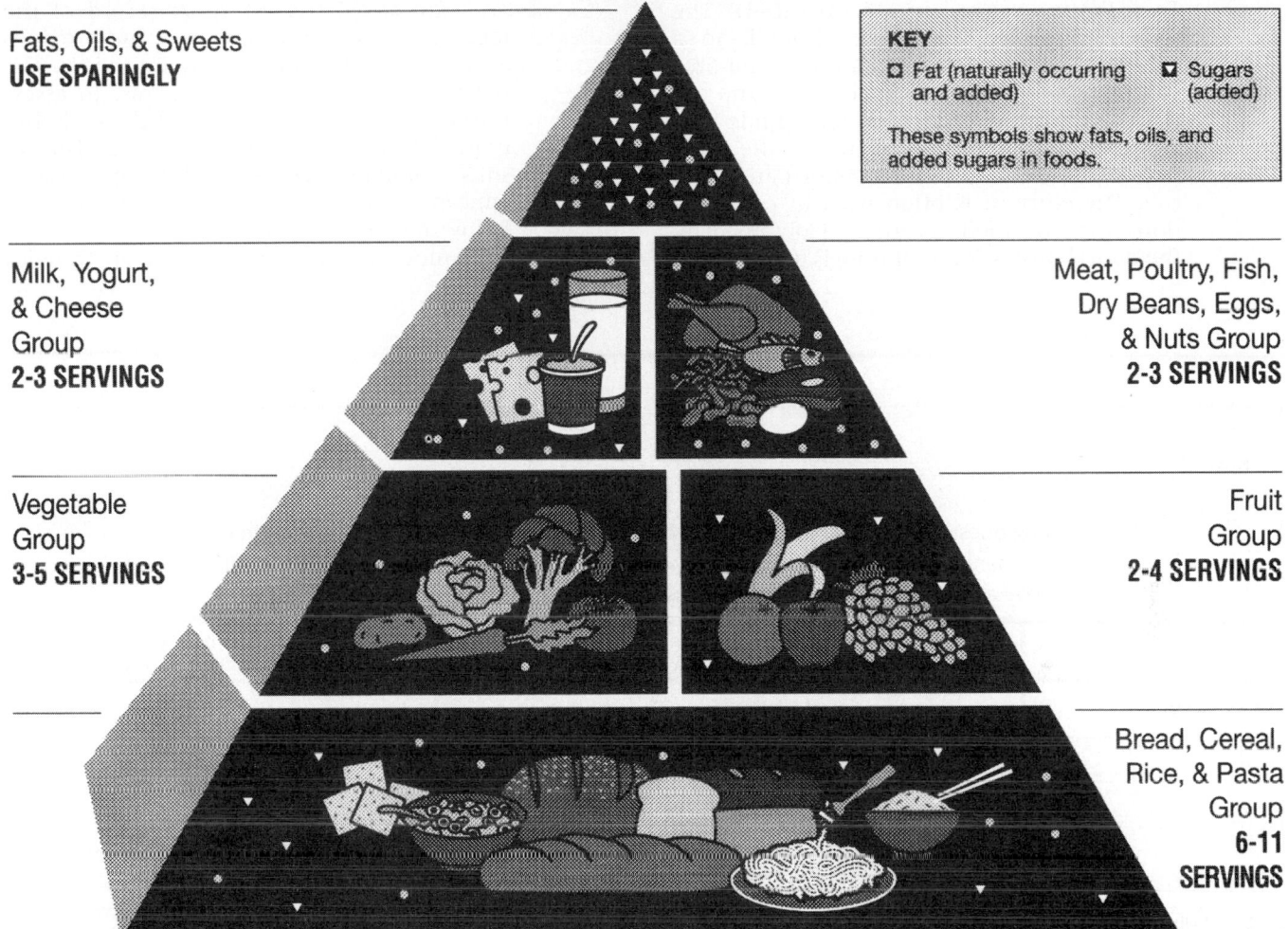

Fats, Oils, & Sweets
USE SPARINGLY

KEY
☐ Fat (naturally occurring and added)   ▼ Sugars (added)

These symbols show fats, oils, and added sugars in foods.

Milk, Yogurt, & Cheese Group
2-3 SERVINGS

Meat, Poultry, Fish, Dry Beans, Eggs, & Nuts Group
2-3 SERVINGS

Vegetable Group
3-5 SERVINGS

Fruit Group
2-4 SERVINGS

Bread, Cereal, Rice, & Pasta Group
6-11 SERVINGS

■ **FIGURE 28-2 The Food Guide Pyramid.** The purpose of the guide to daily food choices is to help the public make food choices for a healthful diet that reflect current scientific knowledge about the diet's relationship to health. (Published by the United States Department of Agriculture and the Department of Health and Human Services, 1990.)

dental caries or a periodontal infection, the same general procedures can be followed.

I. OBJECTIVES OF A DIETARY ASSESSMENT

A. To provide an opportunity for a patient to study personal dietary habits objectively.
B. To obtain an overall picture of the types of food in the patient's diet, food preferences, and quantity of food eaten.
C. To study the food habits and snacking patterns.
D. To record frequency of use and when the cariogenic food is consumed.
E. To determine the overall consistency of the diet and the fibrous foods that are regularly included.
F. To identify the nutritional status of an individual with regard to overall requirements.

G. To provide a basis for making individual recommendations for changes in the diet important to the health of the oral mucosa and the periodontium and to the prevention of dental caries.

II. COMPONENTS OF A DIETARY ASSESSMENT

A. Clinical Evaluation

Detects high-risk patients by noting factors suggestive of a nutritional problem.

1. Information obtained from a medical and social history.[11,12] Included are medications taken, disease states, disabilities, learning limitations, significant unintentional change in body weight, and factors that influence food use and food intake.
2. Observations from intra- and extraoral ex-

aminations. Examples are the physical signs and symptoms of malnutrition.

B. Forms Used for Assessment

1. *Food Frequency Checklist* (Figure 28-3). The patient indicates frequency of foods in a specified period of time. It is quick and provides enough information to assess the patient's diet compared to the food guide pyramid. A disadvantage of using the food frequency checklist alone is poor patient recall. Therefore, it is often used in combination with the food record and obtained by the dental professional. If time is a factor, the food frequency checklist can be filled out while the patient is waiting for the appointment.

2. *Food Record* (Figure 28-4). A record of the food eaten by the patient over the previous 24 hours can be obtained by interview. The record allows the dental hygienist to assess nutrients, food groups, form of the carbohydrate intake, and snacking patterns. The results should be reviewed and the appropriate education given at that appointment or a follow-up appointment.

A more accurate account of an individ-

FOOD FREQUENCY CHECKLIST

NAME _____

The following questions will help show your (your child's) normal eating behavior. This information will allow the dental health team to thoroughly evaluate your (your child's) dental status. Please mark how often you ate or drank each of these items in the past week.

Food Item	Never	1-3 Times per Month	1-3 Times per Week	5 or More Times per Week	1 - 2 Times per Day	3 - 4 Times per Day	5 or More Times per Day
Fruit and Juices							
Vegetables, other than starchy choices							
Potatoes and other starchy choices							
Milk and Yogurt							
Meat, Fish, Poultry, Eggs							
Cheese							
Cereals (Cold and Hot)							
Cookies, Cake, Pies Pastries							
Candy							
Soda							
Diet Soda							
Gum							
Sugarfree Gum							
Alcohol							

FIGURE 28-3 Food Frequency Checklist. Dietary evaluation tool to determine how often a patient consumes a specific food. It is often used in conjunction with a Food Record (Figure 28-4). The patient could fill it out while waiting for an appointment. (Adapted from Thompson, F.E. and Byers, T.B.: Dietary Assessment Resource Manual. *J. Nutrition, 124,* (II Supplement), 2297S, 1994.

ual's intake is to have the patient fill out the food intake for a specified period (3 to 7 days). This will give the patient a more active role in the assessment and a chance to observe areas that require modification. The increased time of recording intake provides a truer picture of the patient's usual diet. Provide the patient with three to seven copies of the food record.

III. PRESENTATION OF THE FOOD RECORD TO THE PATIENT[11]

Information obtained from the food record is directly proportional to the care taken in explanation of the food record and its purpose and relation to oral health.

A. Explain the Purpose

Many patients may not understand a connection between diet and oral health. Briefly describe how the diet relates to the dental situation to provide a foundation for the education to follow. The patient more likely will see the value of completing the food record as requested. Avoid mention of specific foods since the patient may not provide a true diary if what will be checked is known in advance.

B. Explain the Form

Written and oral instructions for use of the food record should be provided. Suggestions are made for listing various foods and the use of household measurements for indicating quantity (Table 28-2). Written instructions for com-

FOOD RECORD

NAME _____ DATE _____

Time	Place	Food Eaten (amount)	Number of Servings in Each Food Group							
			Grain	Fruit	Vegetable	Meat	Milk	Fat	Other CHO	Free* Foods
Example: 6:00am	Kitchen	2 slices WW toast 1 Tbsp diet marg. ½ cup Orange juice	2	1				1		
Total Servings in each group										

*A Free Food is any food that contains less than 20 calories/serving

■ **FIGURE 28-4 Food Record.** Example of a form for the patient to use to record the daily diet. A booklet of 3 to 7 forms can be assembled for a longer record.

TABLE 28-2 Food Record Instructions

- Write down everything eaten on the food record form provided.
- Record each meal as soon after eating as possible to avoid forgetting.
- Do not choose days when dieting, fasting, or ill.
- Be accurate in determining the amounts eaten, using household measurements (example, ½ cup cereal, 3 oz. fish, 1 tsp. margarine).
- Use brand names whenever possible.
- Record added sauces, gravies, condiments, and all extras (example: sugar or cream in coffee, mayonnaise, chewing gum, cough drops).
- Record food preparation methods (example: baked, fried, boiled, grilled).
- Record all fluids; include water and alcoholic beverages.

pleting the food record, along with the orally presented instructions, can encourage the patient to provide a more accurate portrayal of eating behaviors.

C. Complete the Current Day's Food Record With the Patient
This helps to illustrate how to itemize and how to list the foods in the order they are eaten.

D. General Directions
1. Emphasize importance of completing each meal's record as soon after eating as possible to avoid forgetting.
2. Encourage use of typical days, uncomplicated by illness, dieting, holidays, or other unusual events.
3. Review details of recording the component parts of a combination dish, such as a salad, sandwich, casserole, or soup.
4. Indicate need for recording nutritional supplements and all fluids.
5. Request that meals eaten other than at home be identified by writing "restaurant," "guest at friend's home," or "party."
6. Instruct to select consecutive days and at least one weekend day.

IV. RECEIVING THE COMPLETED FOOD RECORD
The appointment for receiving the food record should follow soon after its completion.

A. Obtain Supplemental Data
Question the patient to clarify presented information and obtain further information:
1. Whether the diary represents that of a typical day or week.
2. Influences on appetite.
3. Food likes and dislikes; preferences; intolerances; allergies.
4. Frequency of dining out.
5. Current diet being followed in the home.

6. Average alcohol intake.
7. Which family member is doing the cooking and food shopping.

B. Review Patient's Food Record
Review with the patient each day's recorded food list and supplement details that have been omitted.
1. Common omissions
   a. Garnishes: Frosting, whipped cream, butter or margarine on vegetables, salad dressings?
   b. Beverages: Quantity, sweetened, decaffeinated?
   c. Snacks: Kind, brand, quantity?
   d. Chewing gum or mints: Sugarless, amount?
   e. Canned fruit: Packed in water or heavy or light syrup?
   f. Fruit and vegetables: Canned, fresh, frozen?
   g. Cereal: Kind, milk, sugar, quantity?
   h. Potato: Baked, buttered, fried?
   i. Seasonings or sauces: Quantity, type?
2. Determine common food habits, such as snacking at night or fast food choices at lunch.

V. SUMMARY AND ANALYSIS
Three principal parts of the food record to analyze are the number of servings in each food group, the cariogenic foods, and the consistency of the diet.

A. Nutritional Assessment of the Diet
1. Comparison of servings with the food groups (Figure 28-2).
2. A suggested procedure is to use a check sheet to mark daily portions of each food group (Figure 28-5).
   a. Each food eaten is put into a food group, with consideration that more than one serving may have been consumed.
   b. Totals for the week may be added and the average per day calculated. The average can be compared to the recommended servings of each food group.
   c. Gross excesses and deficiencies can be identified readily.

B. Cariogenic Foods
1. Identify types of cariogenic foods included.
2. Frequency of use
   a. Daily or occasionally.
   b. Number of between-meal snacks and how many of these include cariogenic foods.
   c. Frequency is more relevant than quantity.
3. Consistency of cariogenic foods relates to probable length of time food might remain on the tooth surface.
4. Time of use: during, end of, or between meals.
5. Water taken at times when it could aid in rinsing sugars from the tooth surfaces.

Dietary Analysis

Name _____

Age _____ Date _____

FOOD GROUPS		DAY 1	2	3	4	5	6	7	Daily Average	Recommended Daily Amounts				Adequate	Inadequate
Milk Group										Child 2 - 3	Adol. 4	Adult to 50 3 - 4	51 & older 4		
Meat Group - meat, fish, poultry, eggs, dry beans										2 - 3 servings (total of 5-7 oz.)					
Vegetable Group										3 - 5 servings					
Fruit Group										2 - 4 servings					
Bread & Cereals Group										6 - 11 servings					
SWEETS									Total	NOTES AND RECOMMENDATIONS					
Liquid	With meal														
	End of meal														
	Between meals														
Soft - sticky/ retentive	With meal														
	End of meal														
	Between meals														
Hard - long-lasting	With meal														
	End of meal														
	Between meals														

FIGURE 28-5 Dietary Analysis Recording Sheet. From the food record kept by the patient (Figure 28-4), each serving is entered as a check in the space beside the appropriate food group. They are totaled, averaged, and compared with the recommended daily amounts on the right. The lower section provides space to categorize and count cariogenic foods.

6. During the counseling appointment, ask the patient to underline or circle in red the foods that are cariogenic on the food record. The experience can be impressive to the patient. People usually do not realize how many of the foods they are eating are cariogenic.

C. Consistency of Diet

1. *Types of Fibrous Foods Used.* Uncooked, crisp, raw fruits and vegetables are examples of foods that promote saliva flow.
2. *Frequency of Use.* Daily or occasionally.
3. *Time of Use*
   a. During meal, end of meal, or between meals.
   b. Relationship to providing cleansing and buffering mechanism through an increase in saliva production.

D. Assessment of the Food Record

1. The patient can identify desirable and undesirable practices.
2. Corroborate findings with clinical findings and the patient's oral health problems to prepare for the counseling session.

PREPARATION FOR ADDITIONAL COUNSELING OF PATIENT

I. DEFINE OBJECTIVES

A. To help the patient understand the individual oral problems and appreciate the need for changing habits.

B. To explain specific alterations in the diet necessary for improved general and oral health.

C. For dental caries control, to promote the modification of cariogenic foods, particularly those between meals, and to substitute noncariogenic foods.

II. PLANNING FACTORS

A. Patient Attitude
Consider patient's willingness and ability to cooperate as shown by previous conscientiousness in keeping appointments and following personal oral care procedures.

B. Problem Areas
Identify problems that arise in presenting changes in the diet as they apply to this particular patient.
1. Difficulty in change of any habit.
2. Patient may feel dissatisfied without the usual or customary foods. Many patients will not even attempt to make any modifications if the recommendations are too numerous or overwhelming.
3. Lack of appreciation of need for change because of limited knowledge concerning diet and nutrition and their relationship to oral health.
4. Common misconception that concentrated sugar is an indispensable source of energy.
5. Degree of emphasis: dental disease does not kill anyone and nothing drastic is going to happen if minor deviations from the recommended diet occur.
6. Social prejudices.
7. Cultural patterns.
8. Financial considerations.
9. Emotional disturbances that have led to or contributed to specific cravings, such as for sweets.
10. Parental attitude that removal of sweets from the diet would deprive the child of normal childhood pleasures.

III. SELECT APPROPRIATE TEACHING AIDS

A. Patient's radiographs, charting, and food record.
B. Diagrams, food models, food labels, or charts applicable to material to be presented.
C. Instructive leaflets to illustrate patient's special dietary or oral health needs.
D. An outline of a realistic diet plan with specific suggestions for food substitutes.
E. A list of snack suggestions.

COUNSELING PROCEDURES

I. SETTING
The conference must be held in a setting free from interruptions and distracting background sounds and away from the clinical treatment setting. Having participants sit comfortably also contributes to an atmosphere conducive to learning. The room can be equipped with limited educational aids, such as posters, pamphlets, food labels, and food models, but it should not be cluttered to the point of confusion.

For a younger patient, the primary caregiver should be encouraged to be present because this individual supervises the child's eating and plaque control activities. For any age, it is particularly important for the person who plans and prepares the family meals and does the grocery shopping to be present in order to educate him or her about appropriate food choices.

II. POINTERS FOR SUCCESS OF A CONFERENCE

A. Be prepared, on time.
B. Plan for only a few simple visual aids.
C. Concentrate on the factors related to the patient's diet-based dental problem.
D. Encourage parents to exclude small children (other than patient) from the conference, because they may create distractions.
E. Develop a permissive atmosphere.
F. Take care not to follow a written outline of recommendations so rigidly that the conference lacks spontaneity.
G. Include all people present in the discussion. Encourage feedback. Ask questions that require more than a "yes" or "no" response.
H. Guide the patient to develop their own behavior changes for greater compliance.
I. Use a conversational tone of voice.
J. Make certain that all questions from patient or parent are discussed adequately.
K. Avoid note taking during the conference as much as possible.

III. PRESENTATION

A. Review of Purposes of the Meeting
Provide explanation as to how diet relates to the patient's particular problem.

B. Clarification of "Cariogenic" Foods
The patient cannot be told simply to "cut out the sweets." The meaning of "sweets" must be made clear, and specific suggestions should be provided for making modifications. Many people think of sweets as candy only and do not realize the sugar content of many other foods. The meaning of cariogenic food can be illustrated by using examples from the patient's own food diary.

C. Review of Dental Caries Initiation
Discuss the principles for understanding the role of fermentable carbohydrates in dental caries initiation.
1. Cariogenic food on the tooth surface is changed to acid within 2 to 4 minutes. Use Figure 16-6 (page 273) as an illustration.
2. Acid left undisturbed is not all cleared from the mouth for 20 to 40 minutes.

D. Frequency and Time of Exposure[13,14]

1. Each exposure of the tooth surface to sucrose or other cariogenic food in a meal or snack increases the amount of acid on the tooth. The pH drops to below 5.5, which is the critical level for demineralization. Figure 28-6 illustrates how the frequent intake of sucrose lowers the pH for several hours in a day.

2. The actual amount of a cariogenic food is not as important as when and how often the tooth is exposed.

E. Retention

1. The texture of the food that is cariogenic influences the length of time the food stays in the mouth (whether sticky or combined with a sticky food).

2. Vigorous rinsing after eating a cariogenic food may help to remove part of the food, but not the plaque adhered to the tooth surface.

3. Cariogenic foods taken after brushing and flossing before retiring are not cleared readily because salivary flow decreases during sleep.

4. Cariogenic liquids are removed quickly and the enamel will be exposed to an acidic environment for a shorter period of time than retentive or solid foods.

IV. SPECIFIC DIETARY RECOMMENDATIONS

A. Examination of the Patient's Food Records

Taking the 3- to 7-day food records and consolidating them to the dietary analysis recording sheet (Figure 28-5) will assist the patient to observe the overall picture of the food intake. The patient can identify the deficiencies and excesses and suggest alternate choices.

Major changes in food habits are difficult to make for any individual. Application of the knowledge of the principles of learning (page 335) and the skills of a counselor are essential. One must attempt to retain as many as possible of the patient's present food habits and to make recommendations that can be adapted to the patient's pattern of living.

1. Discuss foods from each food group that are liked by the patient and can be added to the diet, or find acceptable substitutions for the cariogenic food choices. For example, the patient may accept light yogurt as an alternative to ice cream for a snack, but an apple may not be an appealing suggestion. The patient needs to be involved in making changes in his/her own diet.

2. Guide the patient to select those items from

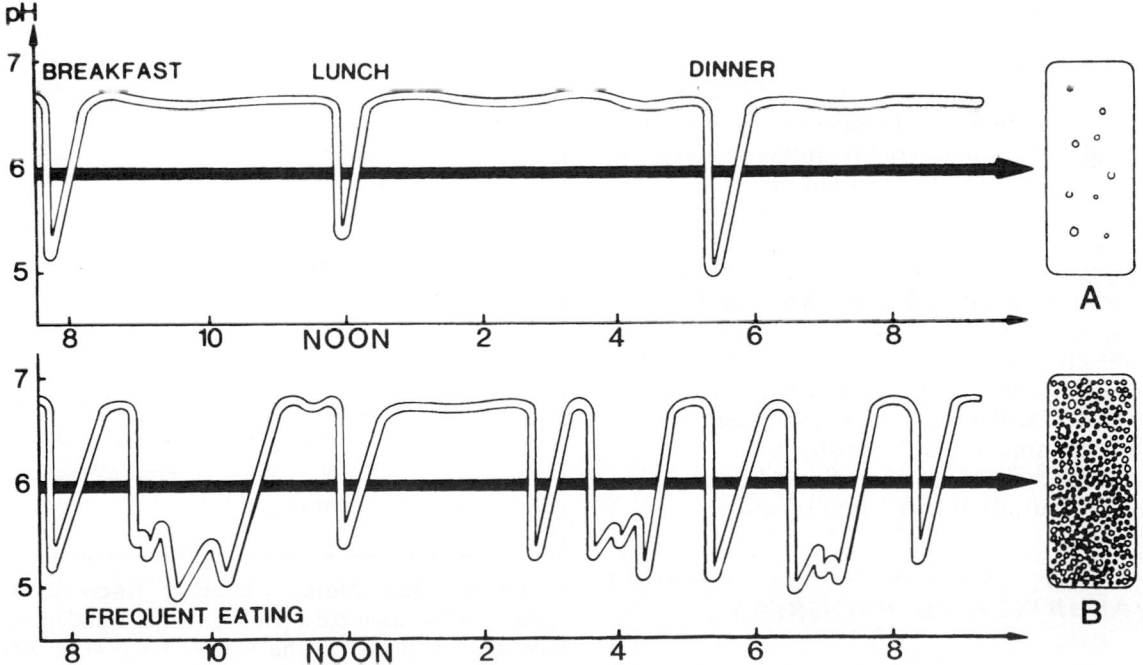

■ **FIGURE 28-6 Cariogenic Foods and Plaque pH.** The range of pH in the bacterial plaque from 5 to 7 pH is shown on the left. Time intervals are shown across the bottom of each graph. The double-line curve represents the variations in plaque pH throughout a day. Each time sugar or a cariogenic food is taken in, the pH of the plaque drops to or below the critical pH (5.2 to 5.5). As shown in the lower graph, frequent eating keeps the pH at the critical level below which enamel demineralization can occur. On the right, A shows that bacterial counts are lower, whereas in B, aciduric microorganisms are greatly increased in numbers. The critical pH for the root surfaces is 6.0 to 6.7. (Adapted from Larmas, M.: Int. Dent. J., 35, 109, June, 1985.)

the present diet that need changing and to make suggestions for appropriate substitutes.

3. To enhance compliance, allow the patient to create his/her own meal plan for 1 day (Figure 28-7).
   a. Incorporate the principles discussed in the counseling.
   b. Make modifications the patient can achieve realistically and is willing to try.
   c. Avoid too many changes that may overwhelm the patient.
   d. Determine if the patient understood the information presented and the motivation level.

B. Basic Principles for Dietary Changes

The following suggestions represent basic principles to be applied. More specific recommendations can be added as they relate to an individual family. Directions must be simple and specific, because the interpretation of many new ideas can be difficult for the patient.

1. Incorporate foods from the food groups to complete the patient's diet.
2. Limit the use of cariogenic foods to mealtimes. Pay particular attention to the final food used in the meal because it may remain on the teeth if immediate toothbrushing or rinsing is not possible.
3. Foods that require chewing are helpful by increasing salivary flow. Saliva provides additional buffering effects and removes cariogenic foods more promptly.
4. Limit between-meal snacking and select snacks from noncariogenic foods, such as plain milk, cheese and crackers, peanut butter on sliced apples, cream cheese on celery, and sugar-free gelatin or pudding.
5. Use as little concentrated sweet in the preparation of foods as possible. In baking, the amount of granulated or brown sugar can be decreased by half. Observe care in the purchase of prepared foods; for example, use unsweetened fruit juice, canned fruits with no sugar added, or diet sodas. Natural sugars are just as detrimental as refined sugars (for example, honey, maple syrup).
6. Encourage daily use of fluoride through water, foods, dentifrices, and rinses.

MENU PLANNING RECORD

Instructions: Create a realistic menu for one day.

Time	Meal
______	*Breakfast:*
______	*A.M. Snack:*
______	*Lunch:*
______	*P.M. Snack:*
______	*Dinner:*
______	*Evening Snack:*

Totals in a day: Fruits ____ Vegetables ____
Milk ____ Starch/Bread ____
Fat ____ Protein/Meat ____
Other ____

FIGURE 28-7 Menu Planning Record. An educational aid to evaluate a patient's understanding of the information discussed in the dietary counseling. Allow the patient to create a menu for 1 day, making realistic modifications as discussed during the counseling session to promote positive oral health. (Adapted from Davis, J.R. and Stegeman, C.A.: *The Dental Hygienist's Guide to Nutritional Care.* 1998, p. 420).

EVALUATION OF PROGRESS

The success of the dental caries control guidelines and meal plan depends on learning by the patient. Learning implies a change of behavior and progress toward goals that are clearly understood by the learner.

I. IMMEDIATE EVALUATION

The patient's expressed interest and demonstration of

cooperation in the caries control program indicate that at least temporarily the patient is motivated.

II. THREE-MONTH FOLLOW-UP

A. Request patient to keep a 3- to 7-day food record for assessment and evaluation.
B. Review plaque control procedures and provide suggestions as needed.
C. Recommend ideas for further modifications when indicated. Smaller goals may need to be established for greater adherence.
D. Document progress, additional material reviewed, and plan for continued change.

III. SIX-MONTH FOLLOW-UP

A. Perform examination and clinical procedures
1. Scaling as needed.
2. Topical application of fluoride, depending on self-applied fluoride program.
3. Charting of carious lesions.
B. Compare dental caries incidence with previous chartings and completed restorative dentistry.
C. Make dietary recommendations in accord with new assessment.
D. Document progress, education provided, and plan.

IV. OVERALL EVALUATION

A. Consistent reduction in dental caries rate in the years following the initial counseling shows sustained change in habits.
B. Patient's and parents' attitudes toward maintaining adequate oral health habits of personal care, diet containing minimum cariogenic foods, and routine professional dental care indicate application of learning.

FACTORS TO TEACH THE PATIENT

I. MEDICATIONS WITH SUCROSE

Medications, particularly those in liquid form or chewable, often contain sucrose or other cariogenic sugar. When chronically ill patients, especially children, have liquid or chewable medication that must be taken several times each day, the harm to the teeth can be severe. If the medication cannot be given in a less cariogenic form, the mouth should be cleared of the cariogenic sugar immediately following each dose by toothbrushing, rinsing, and flossing.[15,16]

II. MEDICATIONS WITH SIDE EFFECT OF XEROSTOMIA

Diuretics, hypertensives, and antidepressants are among several classes of medication that cause xerostomia. The elderly are a common population group to assess for xerostomia due to the possibility of multiple medications. Xerostomia increases the risk of

dental caries development since the beneficial effects of saliva in protecting against caries is limited. It also becomes difficult for the patient to chew and swallow certain foods; therefore the nutrient intake may be compromised. Further information on xerostomia can be found on pages 345 to 346.

III. CAUSE OF DENTAL CARIES

A. Explain how dental caries forms and how the acid is produced on the tooth surface by microorganisms in the plaque.
B. Use Figure 28-1 to illustrate the interaction of the sugar and other cariogenic foods with the tooth surface and the microorganisms, and show the relation of frequency of eating to acid production by using Figure 28-6.

REFERENCES

1. **Carranza**, F.A. and Newman, M.G.: *Clinical Periodontology*, 8th ed. Philadelphia, W.B. Saunders Co., 1996, pp. 185–188, 241, 254, 371–372.
2. **Genco**, R.J., Goldman, H.M., and Cohen, D.W., eds.: *Contemporary Periodontics*. St. Louis, Mosby, 1990, pp. 264–266.
3. **Enwonwu**, C.O.: Interface of Malnutrition and Periodontal Disease, *Am. J. Clin. Nutr., 61*, 430S, February, Supplement, 1995.
4. **Robinson**, H.B.G. and Miller, A.S.: *Color Atlas of Oral Pathology*, 5th ed. Philadelphia, J.B. Lippincott Co., 1990, p. 141.
5. **Newbrun**, E.: Preventing Dental Caries: Current and Prospective Strategies, *J. Am. Dent. Assoc., 123*, 68, May, 1992.
6. **Newbrun**, E.: Preventing Dental Caries: Breaking the Chain of Transmission, *J. Am. Dent. Assoc., 123*, 55, June, 1992.
7. **Dodds**, M.W.J. and Wefel, J.S.: The Developing Carious Lesion, in Harris, N.O. and Christen, A.G.: *Primary Preventive Dentistry*, 4th ed. Norwalk, CT, Appleton & Lange, 1995, pp. 39–60.
8. **Palmer**, C.A.: Nutrition, Diet, and Oral Conditions, in Harris, N.O. and Christen, A.G.: *Primary Preventive Dentistry*, 4th ed. Norwalk, CT, Appleton & Lange, 1995, pp. 369–373.
9. **National Research Council**, Committee on Dietary Allowances, Food and Nutrition Board: *Recommended Dietary Allowances*, 10th ed. Washington, D.C., National Academy of Sciences, Office of Publications, 1989.
10. **American Dairy Association and Dairy Council**: Dietary Reference Intakes: Calcium and Related Nutrients, *Dairy Council Digest, 68*, 31, November/December, 1997.
11. **Davis**, J.R. and Stegeman, C.A.: *The Dental Hygienist's Guide to Nutritional Care*. Philadelphia, W.B. Saunders Co., 1998, pp. 3–31, 363–378, 400–426.
12. **Brown**, J.P.: Indicators for Caries Management from the Patient History, *J. Dent. Educ., 61*, 855, November, 1997.
13. **Suddick**, R.P. and Dodds, M.W.J.: Caries Activity Estimates and Implications: Insights into Risk Versus Activity, *J. Dent. Educ., 61*, 876, November, 1997.
14. **McBean**, L.D.: Diet and Dental Caries: An Overview, *Dairy Council Digest, 65*, 1, January/February, 1994.
15. **Fitzsimons**, D., Dwyer, J.T., Palmer, C., and Boyd, L.D.: Nutrition and Oral Health Guidelines for Pregnant Women, Infants, and Children, *J. Am. Diet. Assoc., 98*, 182, February, 1998.
16. **Howell**, R.B. and Houpt, M.: More Than One Factor Can Influence Caries Development in HIV-positive Children, (letter), *Pediatr. Dent., 13*, 247, July/August, 1991.

SUGGESTED READINGS

American Dietetic Association: Oral Health and Nutrition, *J. Am. Diet. Assoc., 96*, 184, February, 1996.

Anusavice, K.J.: Efficacy of Nonsurgical Management of the Initial Caries Lesion, *J. Dent. Educ., 61*, 895, November, 1997.

Baker, M.: Food for Lifelong Living, *RDH, 12*, 18, November, 1992.

Eronat, N. and Eden, E.: A Comparative Study of Some Influencing Factors of Rampant or Nursing Caries in Preschool Children, *J. Clin. Pediatr. Dent., 16*, 275, Summer, 1992.

Institute of Medicine, Standing Committee on Scientific Evaluation of Dietary Reference Intakes, Food and Nutrition Board: *Dietary Reference Intakes for Calcium, Phosphorus, Magnesium, Vitamin D, and Fluoride*, Washington, D.C., National Academy Press, 1997.

Lessard, G.M.: Discussion: Nutritional Aspects of Oral Health—New Perspectives, *Am. J. Clin. Nutr., 61*, 446S, February, 1995.

Pennington, J.A.: Derivation of Daily Values Used for Nutrition Labeling, *J. Am. Diet. Assoc., 97*, 1407, December, 1997.

Popkin, B.M., Siega-Riz, A.M., and Haines, P.S.: A Comparison of Dietary Trends Among Racial and Socioeconomic Groups in the United States, *N. Engl. J. Med., 335*, 716, September 5, 1996.

Slavkin, H.C.: Nutrients and Micronutrients: Progress in Science-based Understanding, *J. Am. Dent. Assoc., 128*, 1306, September, 1997.

Souba, W.W.: Nutritional Support, *N. Engl. J. Med., 336*, 41, January 2, 1997.

Dental Caries and Diet

Gedalia, I., Ionat-Bendat, D., and Ben-Mosheh, S.: Tooth Enamel Softening with a Cola Type Drink and Rehardening with Hard Cheese or Stimulated Saliva *in situ, J. Oral Rehabil., 18*, 501, November, 1991.

Gustafsson, B.E., Quensel, C-E., Lanke, L.S., Lundquist, C., Grahnen, H., Bonow, B.E., and Krasse, B.: The Vipeholm Dental Caries Study. The Effect of Different Levels of Carbohydrate Intake on Caries Activity in 436 Individuals Observed for 5 Years, *Acta Odontol. Scand., 11*, 232, Numbers 3/4, 1954.

Hargreaves, J.A.: Discussion: Diet and Nutrition in Dental Health and Disease, *Am. J. Clin. Nutr., 61*, 447S, February, 1995.

Kashket, S., van Houte, J., Lopez, L.R., and Stocks, S.: Lack of Correlation Between Food Retention on the Human Dentition and Consumer Perception of Food Stickiness, *J. Dent. Res., 70*, 1314, October, 1991.

Moss, S.J.: Relationships Between Fluoride, Saliva, and Diet, *DentalHygienistNews, 7*, 3, Fall, 1994.

Papas, A.S., Joshi, A., Palmer, C.A., Giunta, J.L., and Dwyer, J.T.: Relationship of Diet to Root Caries, *Am. J. Clin. Nutr., 61*, 423S, February, 1995.

Riordan, D.J.: Effects of Orthodontic Treatment on Nutrient Intake, *Am. J. Orthod. Dentofac. Orthop., 111*, 554, May, 1997.

Schnuth, M.L.: You and Your Vegetarian Patients, *RDH, 14*, 12, April, 1994.

Stacey, M.A. and Wright, F.A.C.: Diet and Feeding Patterns in High Risk Pre-school Children, *Aust. Dent. J., 36*, 421, December, 1991.

Stegeman, C.A., Carroll, D.K., and Schierling, J.: The Battle of the Fermentable Carbohydrates, *Access, 12*, 38, March, 1998.

Sundin, B., Granath, L., and Birkhed, D.: Variation of Posterior Approximal Caries Incidence with Consumption of Sweets with Regard to Other Caries-related Factors in 15–18-year-olds, *Community Dent. Oral Epidemiol., 20*, 76, April, 1992.

Yiu, C.K.Y. and Wei, S.H.Y.: Management of Rampant Caries in Children, *Quintessence Int., 23*, 159, March, 1992.

Counseling: Education

Altshuler, B.D.: Nutrition Education. The Role of the Dental Hygienist, *DentalHygienistNews, 7*, 3, Summer, 1994.

Dreizen, S.: Dietary and Nutritional Counseling in the Prevention and Control of Oral Disease, *Compend. Cont. Educ. Dent., 10*, 558, October, 1989.

Freeman, R. and Sheiham, A.: Understanding Decision-making Processes for Sugar Consumption in Adolescence, *Community Dent. Oral Epidemiol., 25*, 228, June, 1997.

Kidd, E.A.M.: The Use of Diet Analysis and Advice in the Management of Dental Caries in Adult Patients, *Operative Dent., 20*, 86, May–June, 1995.

Caries Activity Tests

Arnim, S.S. and Sweet, A.P.: Acid Production by Mouth Organisms. Use of Aqueous Methyl Red for Patient Education, *Dent. Radiogr. Photogr., 29*, 1, Number 1, 1956.

Bowden, G.H.: Does Assessment of Microbial Composition of Plaque/Saliva Allow for Diagnosis of Disease Activity of Individuals? *Community Dent. Oral Epidemiol., 25*, 76, February, 1997.

Bratthall, D., Hoszek, A., and Zhao, X.: Evaluation of a Simplified Method for Site-specific Determination of Mutans Streptococci Levels, *Swed. Dent. J., 20*, 215, Number 6, 1996.

Dasanayake, A.P., Caufield, P.W., Cutter, G.R., Roseman, J.M., and Köhler, B.: Differences in the Detection and Enumeration of Mutans Streptococci Due to Differences in Methods, *Arch. Oral Biol., 40*, 345, April, 1995.

Kimmel, L. and Tinanoff, N.: A Modified Mitis Salivarius Medium for a Caries Diagnostic Test, *Oral Microbiol. Immunol., 6*, 275, October, 1991.

Koroluk, L., Hoover, J.N., and Komiyama, K.: The Sensitivity and Specificity of a Colorimetric Microbiological Caries Activity Test (Cariostat) in Preschool Children, *Pediatr. Dent., 16*, 276, July/August, 1994.

Moss, M.E. and Zero, D.T.: An Overview of Caries Risk Assessment, and its Potential Utility, *J. Dent. Educ., 59*, 932, October, 1995.

Park, K.K. and Banting, D.W.: Caries Activity Testing, in Harris, N.O. and Christen, A.G.: *Primary Preventive Dentistry*, 4th ed. Norwalk, CT, Appleton & Lange, 1995, pp. 289–315.

Powell, L.V.: Caries Risk Assessment: Relevance to the Practitioner, *J. Am. Dent. Assoc., 129*, 349, March, 1998.

Schlagenhauf, U., Pommerencke, K., and Weiger, R.: Influence of Toothbrushing, Eating and Smoking on Dentocult SM Strip Mutans Test Scores, *Oral Microbiol. Immunol., 10*, 98, April, 1995.

Snyder, M.L.: A Simple Colorimetric Method for the Estimation of Relative Numbers of Lactobacilli in the Saliva, *J. Dent. Res., 19*, 349, August, 1940.

Tanzer, J.M.: Salivary and Plaque Microbiological Tests and the Management of Dental Caries, *J. Dent. Educ., 61*, 866, November, 1997.

Fluorides

The use of fluorides provides the most effective method for dental caries prevention and control. Although historically associated primarily with dental caries, the action of fluoride on bacterial plaque also has important therapeutic and preventive effects on the control of periodontal infections and the maintenance of health.

Fluoride is important for optimum oral health at all ages. Fluoride is made available at the tooth surface by two general means: *systemically,* by way of the circulation to developing teeth, and *topically,* directly to the exposed surfaces of erupted teeth throughout life.

Fluoride as a systemic nutrient is available from the community drinking water, either naturally or by fluoridation; from prescribed dietary supplements; or in small amounts from certain foods. Key words associated with fluoride and fluoride therapy are defined in Box 29-1.

FLUORIDE METABOLISM[1]

I. FLUORIDE INTAKE

Fluoride is taken in by way of fluoridated water; supplemental tablets; and, in small amounts, foods. Foods and beverages prepared at home or processed commercially using water containing fluoride are significant sources of fluoride. In addition, varying amounts are ingested from dentifrices, mouthrinses, and other fluoride products used by the individual.

II. ABSORPTION

A. Gastrointestinal Tract
Rapid absorption; the rate and amount of absorption depends on the solubility of the fluoride compound. There is less absorption when the fluoride is taken with milk or food.

B. Blood Stream
Maximum blood levels are reached within 30 minutes of intake. The level fluctuates with intake. Normal plasma levels are very low. The fluoride concentration in the saliva ranges from 0.01 to 0.04 ppm, which is less than the plasma level.

III. DISTRIBUTION AND RETENTION
A. Fluoride is distributed by the plasma to all tissues and organs. There is a strong affinity for the calcified tissues.
B. Approximately 99% of the fluoride in the body is located in the mineralized tissues.
C. Concentrations of fluoride are at the surfaces next to the tissue fluid supplying the fluoride.
D. The fluoride ion (F) is stored as an integral part of the crystal lattice of fluorapatite. The amount stored varies with the intake, the time of exposure, and the age and stage of the development of the individual. The teeth

store small amounts, with highest levels on the tooth surface.

IV. EXCRETION
Most fluoride is excreted through the kidneys, with a small amount excreted by the sweat glands and feces. There is limited transfer from plasma to breast milk for excretion by that route.

FLUORIDE AND TOOTH DEVELOPMENT

Fluoride is a nutrient essential to the formation of sound teeth and bones, as are calcium, phosphorus, and other elements obtained from food and water.

The teeth can acquire fluoride during three periods: during the *mineralization stage* of tooth development, *after mineralization* and before eruption, and *after eruption.* At this point of study, a review of the histology of tooth development and mineralization can be a helpful supplement to the information included here.[2,3]

I. PRE-ERUPTIVE: MINERALIZATION STAGE
A. Fluoride is deposited during the formation of the enamel, starting at the dentinoenamel junction, after the enamel matrix has been laid down by the ameloblasts (Figure 29-1A).
B. Fluoride is incorporated as fluorapatite during mineralization. Table 14-1 (page 238) shows the weeks *in utero* when the hard tissue formation begins for the primary teeth. The first permanent molar begins to mineralize at birth (Table 14-2, page 239).
C. Fluoride is available to the developing teeth by way of the blood plasma to the tissues surrounding the tooth buds.
D. Sources of fluoride include drinking water and other ingested fluoride, such as that from tablets, drops, and foods.
E. During mineralization, when there is excess fluoride, the normal activity of the ameloblasts may be inhibited, and a defective enamel matrix can form. This mechanism can lead to dental fluorosis. Dental fluorosis is a form of hypomineralization that results from ingestion of an excess amount of fluoride during tooth development.

II. PRE-ERUPTIVE: MATURATION STAGE
A. After mineralization is complete and before eruption, fluoride deposition continues in the surface of the enamel (Figure 29-1B).
B. Fluoride is taken up from the nutrient tissue fluids surrounding the tooth crown. Much more fluoride is acquired by the outer surface during this period than in the underlying layers of enamel during mineralization. Children who are exposed to fluoride for the first time within the 2 years prior to eruption benefit

BOX 29-1 KEY WORDS AND ABBREVIATIONS: Fluorides

Abrasive system: substances with cleaning and polishing properties utilized in the formulation of a dentifrice; must be compatible with fluoride compounds and other ingredients and not alter the tooth structure unfavorably.

Acidogenic (as″ĭ-dō-jen′ik): producing acid or acidity.

Apatite (ap′ah-tīt): a group of minerals of the general formula $Ca_{10}(PO_4)_6X_2$ wherein the X might include hydroxyl (OH), carbonate (CO), fluoride (F), or oxygen (O); crystalline mineral component of hard tissues (bones and teeth).

> **Hydroxyapatite** (hī-drok″sē-ap′ah-tīt): $Ca_{10}(PO_4)_6(OH)_2$; the form of apatite that is the principal mineral component of teeth, bones, and calculus.

> **Fluorapatite** (floor-ap′ah-tit): the form of hydroxyapatite in which fluoride ions have replaced some of the hydroxyl ions; with fluoride, the apatite is less soluble and therefore more resistant to the acids formed by plaque bacteria from carbohydrate intake.

> **Fluorhydroxyapatite:** apatite formed when low concentrations of fluoride react with tooth mineral; at higher concentrations, calcium fluoride is formed.

Cariogenic challenge: exposure of a tooth surface to an acid attack; acid is from the action of plaque bacteria and cariogenic food ingested.

Cariostatic (kar″ē-ō-stă′tĭk): exerting an inhibitory action on the progress of dental caries.

Defluoridation: lowering the amount of fluoride in fluoridated water to an optimum level for the prevention of dental caries and dental fluorosis.

Demineralization (dē-min″er-al-ĭ-zā′shun): excessive loss of mineral or inorganic salts from body tissues.

Efficacy: with reference to a product: an efficacious product produces a statistically and clinically significant benefit under ideal testing conditions in carefully controlled clinical trials.

Enolase (ē′nō-lās): enzyme involved in glycolysis and sugar transport.

Fluoride (floo″rīd): a salt of hydrofluoric acid; occurs in many tissues and is stored primarily in bones and teeth.

Fluorosis (floo″rō′sis): form of enamel hypomineralization due to excessive ingestion of fluoride during the development and mineralization of the teeth; depending on the length of exposure and the ppm of the fluoride, the fluorosed area may appear as a small white spot or as severe brown staining with pitting.

Gel. semisolid or solid phase of a colloidal solution.

Glass ionomer (ī-on′ō-mer): dental material used for restorations and for bases under composite or amalgam restorations; ionomers adhere to dentin and enamel, release fluoride, reduce microleakage, and prevent secondary (recurrent) dental caries.

Glycolysis (glī-kol″ĭ-sis): process by which sugar is metabolized by bacteria to produce acid.

Hypocalcification (hī″pō-kal″sĭ-fĭ-kā′shun): deficient calcification.

> **Enamel hypocalcification:** defect of enamel maturation caused by hereditary or systemic irregularities.

Maturation (mach-ū-rā′shun): stage or process of becoming mature or attaining maximal development; with respect to tooth development, maturation results from the continuous dynamic exchange of ions into the surface of the enamel from pellicle, bacterial plaque, and oral fluids.

O.T.C.: over the counter.

ppm: parts per million; measure used to designate the amount of fluoride used for optimum level in fluoridated water, dentifrice, and other fluoride-containing preparations.

Remineralization (rē-min″er-al-ĭ-zā′shun): restoration of mineral elements; enhanced by presence of fluoride; remineralized lesions are more resistant to initiation of dental caries than is normal tooth structure.

Subsurface lesion: demineralized area below the surface of the enamel created by acid that has passed through micropores between enamel rods; subject to remineralization by action of fluoride.

Thixotrophic: type of gel that sets in a gel-like state but becomes fluid under stress; the fluid form permits the solution to flow into interdental areas.

"White spot": term used to describe a small area on the surface of enamel that contrasts in appearance with the rest of the surface and may be visible only when the tooth is dried; two types of white spots can be differentiated: an area of demineralization and an area of fluorosis (also referred to as an "enamel opacity").

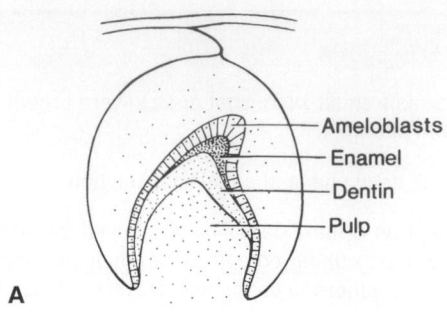

A

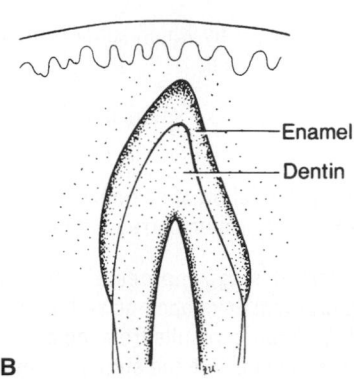

B

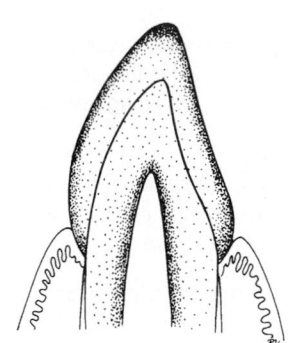

C   ▦ Fluoride

▢ **FIGURE 29-1 Systemic Fluoride.** Dots represent fluoride ions in the tissues and distributed throughout the tooth. **(A)** Developing tooth during mineralization shows fluoride from water and other systemic sources deposited in the enamel and dentin. **(B)** Maturation stage prior to eruption, when fluoride is taken up from tissue fluids around the crown. **(C)** Erupted tooth continues to take up fluoride on the surface from external sources. Note concentrated fluoride deposition on the enamel surface and on the pulpal surface of the dentin.

from fluoride acquired during this pre-eruptive stage.

III. POSTERUPTIVE

A. After eruption and throughout the life span of the teeth, fluoride from the drinking water, dentifrice, mouthrinses, and other surface ex-

posures acts to inhibit demineralization and enhance remineralization (Figure 29-2).

B. Uptake is rapid on the enamel surface during the first years after eruption. It is greater at high levels than at low levels of fluoride, especially from supplements used as chewable tablets or a swish-and-swallow liquid (page 463). Continuing intake of drinking water with fluoride provides a topical source as it washes over the teeth.

TOOTH SURFACE FLUORIDE[4]

Fluoride concentration is greatest on the surface next to the source of fluoride. For the enamel of the erupted tooth, that is the surface exposed to the oral cavity. For the dentin the highest concentration is at the pulpal surface.

I. FLUORIDE IN ENAMEL

A. Uptake

Uptake of fluoride depends on the level of fluo-

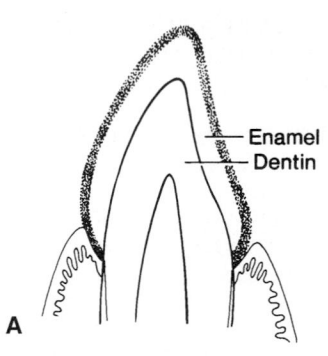

A

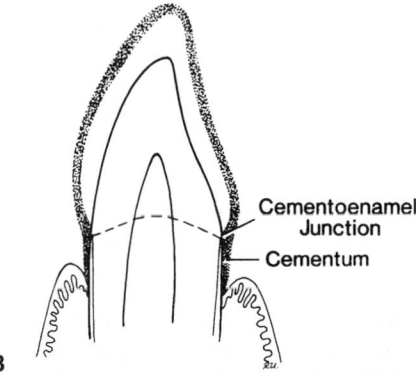

B

▢ **FIGURE 29-2 Fluoride Acquisition After Eruption. (A)** Fluoride on the enamel surface taken up from external sources, including dentifrice, rinse, topical application, and water from fluoridation passing over the tooth. **(B)** Gingival recession exposes the cementum to external sources of fluoride for the prevention of root caries and the alleviation of sensitivity.

ride taken in and the length of time of exposure.

B. Fluoride in the Enamel Surface

Fluoride is a natural constituent of enamel. The outer surface has the highest concentration, and the amount decreases toward the interior of the tooth. For example, 3000 ppm may exist at the surface, but at a depth of 50 μm, only 100 ppm may be found.

II. FLUORIDE IN DENTIN[4]

The fluoride level is greater in dentin than in enamel. The highest concentration is at the pulpal surface, where exchanges take place. Newly formed dentin (primary or secondary) absorbs fluoride rapidly.

III. FLUORIDE IN CEMENTUM[4]

The level of fluoride in cementum is high and increases with age. With recession of the clinical attachment level in periodontal infection, the root surface is exposed to the fluids of the oral cavity as shown in Figure 29-2B. Fluoride is then available to the cementum from the saliva and all the sources used by the patient, including drinking water, dentifrice, and mouthrinse.

DEMINERALIZATION— REMINERALIZATION

I. DEMINERALIZATION

Demineralization means breakdown of the tooth structure with a loss of mineral content, primarily calcium, phosphorus, and fluoride. Demineralization leads to a "white spot," the early lesion that with further demineralization breaks through the tooth surface to form the carious lesion of dental caries. The caries process was described in Chapter 16 (pages 272 to 273) and illustrated in the flowchart in Figure 16-6.

II. REMINERALIZATION

Remineralization is the process in reverse. The minerals are restored to the crystal structure, and tooth destruction is arrested. When early remineralization occurs, the white spot will "harden" and the area may be hypermineralized as compared with the enamel around it.

III. FLUORIDE IN BACTERIAL PLAQUE[5]

A. Composition and Sources

Bacterial plaque may contain from 5 to 50 ppm fluoride. The content varies greatly and is constantly changing.

The sources of plaque fluoride include saliva, gingival sulcus fluid, certain foods and liquids in the diet, topically applied agents including fluoridation, and possibly the fluoride from the demineralizing tooth surface underneath the plaque layer.

B. Exchanges With Tooth Surface

Dental plaque is in direct contact with the tooth surface. The plaque fluid transports the fluoride, other minerals, and the organic acids to the tooth surface.

There is a continuous exchange of minerals between plaque and the enamel crystals at the tooth surface, depending on the pH created by the organic acids. The presence of fluoride ions acts to control the demineralization process.

C. Microchannels to Subsurface

The acids produced in the bacterial plaque act on the enamel to form microchannels through the surface. Demineralization occurs in the subsurface layer and is visible under a microscope. Figure 29-3 shows a cross section of enamel with a subsurface demineralized area. Eventually the area can be detected on clinical examination when the spot may become chalky or discolored by food or tobacco.

IV. FLUORIDE ACTION

The effect of fluoride to prevent or reduce the incidence of dental caries is a combination of several actions. The fluoride of fluoridated drinking water and dietary supplements provides pre-eruption and posteruption benefits. Other fluoride preparations, professionally administered and/or self-applied, con-

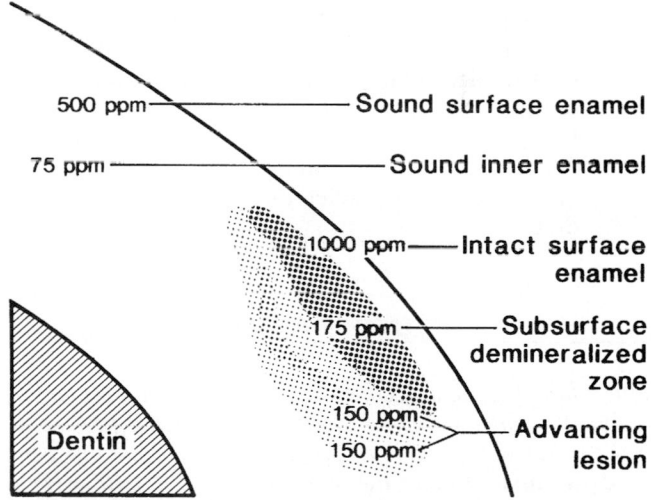

FIGURE 29-3 Examples of Enamel Fluoride Content. A demineralized area readily takes up available fluoride. As shown, the fluoride content (1000 ppm) of the relatively intact surface over a subsurface demineralized white spot is higher than that of the sound surface enamel (500 ppm). The body of the advancing lesion has a higher fluoride content (150 ppm) than does the sound inner enamel (75 ppm). (Drawn after Melberg, J.R., Ripa, L.W., and Leske, G.S.: *Fluoride in Preventive Dentistry. Theory and Clinical Applications*, Chicago, Quintessence, 1983, p. 31.)

tribute to both the enamel and the root surface of the erupted tooth.

A. Effects of Fluoride
1. Prevent demineralization.
2. Enhance remineralization of incipient lesions.
3. Alter the action of plaque bacteria.
4. Aid posteruptive maturation of the enamel surface.
5. Reduce enamel solubility and increase enamel resistance.

B. Formation of Calcium Fluoride[6]
When preparations with a high content of fluoride are applied to the teeth, calcium fluoride (CaF) precipitates out to provide free fluoride ions (F). The fluoride ions act as a reservoir of fluoride during demineralization and remineralization.

The fluoride ions remain in solution until the pH drops below 6.0 in dental plaque during a cariogenic challenge. The ions then released can prevent demineralization by entering the partially demineralized crystals to begin remineralization.

Remineralized areas often have increased mineral content over their previous state. Note in Figure 29-3 that the enamel over the demineralized area has the highest fluoride concentration. The presence of fluoride ions greatly enhances remineralization.

C. Prevention of Demineralization
Daily exposures to fluoridated drinking water, dentifrice, and mouthrinse with fluoride are basic to maintaining the balance of mineralization of the teeth. Complete oral hygiene with daily removal of bacterial plaque is also essential for coping with acid exposures from repeated cariogenic challenges, which in turn can be controlled by selection of a noncariogenic diet.

FLUORIDATION

Fluoridation is the adjustment of the fluoride ion content of a domestic water supply to the optimum physiologic concentration that will provide maximum protection against dental caries and enhance the appearance of the teeth with a minimum possibility of producing objectionable enamel fluorosis.[7] Fluoridation has been established as the most efficient, effective, reliable, and inexpensive means for improving oral health.

I. HISTORICAL ASPECTS[8]

A. Mottled Enamel and Dental Caries
Early in the 20th century, Dr. Frederick S. McKay began his extensive studies to find the cause of "brown stain," which later was called mottled enamel and now is known as *dental flu-orosis*. He observed that people with mottled enamel had significantly less dental caries.[9] He associated the condition with the drinking water, but tests were inconclusive until 1931, when H.V. Churchill, a chemist, pinpointed fluorine as the specific element related to the tooth changes.[10]

B. Background for Fluoridation
Epidemiologic studies of the 1930s sponsored by the United States Public Health Service and directed by Dr. H. Trendley Dean led to the conclusion that the level of fluoride in the water optimum for dental caries prevention averages 1 ppm. Clinically objectionable dental fluorosis is associated with levels well over 2 ppm.[11]

From this knowledge and the fact that many healthy people had lived long lives in communities where the fluoride content of the water was much greater than 1 ppm, the concept of adding fluoride to the water developed. It was still necessary, however, to show that the benefits from controlled fluoridation could parallel those of natural fluoride.

C. Fluoridation—1945
The first communities were fluoridated in 1945. Research in the communities began before fluoridation was started to obtain baseline information, and it continued over the years with detailed examinations and reports in the following communities and their scientific controls:

Fluoridation	Control City
Grand Rapids, Michigan (January, 1945)	Muskegon, Michigan
Newburgh, New York (May, 1945)	Kingston, New York
Brantford, Ontario (June, 1945)	Sarnia, Ontario
Evanston, Illinois (February, 1947)	Oak Park, Illinois

Aurora, Illinois, where the natural fluoride level is optimum (1.2 ppm), was used to compare the benefits of natural fluoride in the water supply with those of fluoridation, as well as with a fluoride-free city, Rockford, Illinois.

The research conducted in these cities, as well as other research done throughout the world, has documented the influence of fluoride on oral health. The effects and benefits itemized in a following section summarize important features of fluoridation; examples of research findings are given for illustration.

II. WATER SUPPLY ADJUSTMENT

A. Fluoride Level
The optimum fluoride level for water in temperate climates is 1 ppm. For warmer and colder climates, the amount can be adjusted

from approximately 0.6 ppm to 1.2 ppm, adapted in accord with the amount of water consumed.[7]

B. Chemicals Used

1. *Sources.* Minerals from which the fluoride ion is derived are naturally occurring and are mined in various parts of the world. Examples of the common sources are fluorspar, cryolite, and apatite.
2. *Criteria for acceptance of a fluoride compound for fluoridation*
   a. Solubility to permit its regular use in a water plant.
   b. Relatively inexpensive.
   c. Readily available to prevent interruptions in maintaining the proper fluoride level.
3. *Compounds used*
   a. Dry compounds: sodium fluoride and sodium silicofluoride.
   b. Solution of hydrofluorosilicic acid.

EFFECTS AND BENEFITS OF FLUORIDATION

I. APPEARANCE OF TEETH

Teeth exposed to an optimum or slightly higher level of fluoride frequently are white, shining, opaque, and without blemishes. When the level is slightly more than optimum for the individual, white areas, such as bands or flecks, may be apparent. These areas can be seen professionally by drying the teeth and observing them under a dental light. Without such close scrutiny, such spots may blend with the overall appearance. Dental fluorosis associated with higher than optimum fluoride levels has been classified as shown in Table 29-1.

II. DENTAL CARIES: PERMANENT TEETH

Continuous use of fluoridated water from birth can result in as many as 40% to 65% fewer carious lesions. The effects are similar to those found in communities with optimum levels of natural fluoride in the water. Many more individuals are completely caries-free when fluoride is in the water.

A. Distribution

Anterior teeth, particularly maxillary, receive more protection from fluoride than do posterior teeth.[11] The anterior teeth are contacted by the drinking water as it passes into the mouth. Fluoride is added to the enamel after eruption.

B. Progression

Not only are the numbers of carious lesions reduced, but the caries rate is slowed. Caries progression is also reduced in the surfaces that receive fluoride for the first time after eruption.[12]

III. ROOT CARIES

Root caries experience of life-long residents of a community with fluoridated water is in direct proportion to the fluoride concentration in the water when compared with the experience of residents of a fluoride-free community.[13] The incidence of root caries is approximately 50% less in life-long residents of a fluoridated community.[14]

IV. DENTAL CARIES: PRIMARY TEETH

With fluoridation from birth, caries incidence is reduced up to 50% in the primary teeth. For example, children aged 6 to 9 years in Newburgh had five times as many caries-free primary teeth present as did the

TABLE 29-1 Descriptive Criteria and Scoring System for the Tooth Surface Index of Fluorosis (TSIF)

Numerical Score	Descriptive Criteria
0	Enamel shows no evidence of fluorosis.
1	Enamel shows definite evidence of fluorosis, namely areas with parchment-white color that total less than one third of the visible enamel surface. This category includes fluorosis confined only to incisal edges of anterior teeth and cusp tips of posterior teeth ("snow-capping").
2	Parchment-white fluorosis totals at least one third of the visible surface, but less than two thirds.
3	Parchment-white fluorosis totals at least two thirds of the visible surface.
4	Enamel shows staining in conjunction with any of the preceding levels of fluorosis. Staining is defined as an area of definite discoloration that may range from light to very dark brown.
5	Discrete pitting of the enamel exists, unaccompanied by evidence of staining of intact enamel. A pit is defined as a definite physical defect in the enamel surface with a rough floor that is surrounded by a wall of intact enamel. The pitted area is usually stained or differs in color from the surrounding enamel.
6	Both discrete pitting and staining of the intact enamel exist.
7	Confluent pitting of the enamel surface exists. Large areas of enamel may be missing and the anatomy of the tooth may be altered. Dark-brown stain is usually present.

From Horowitz, H.S., Driscoll, W.S., Meyers, R.J., Heifetz, S.B., and Kingman, A.K.: A New Method for Assessing the Prevalence of Dental Fluorosis—The Tooth Surface Index of Fluorosis, *J. Am. Dent. Assoc., 109,* 37, July, 1984.

children of Kingston, where fluoride was not present in the community drinking water.[15]

V. TOOTH LOSS

Both primary and permanent tooth loss are much greater in teeth without fluoride[15] because of increased dental caries, which progresses more rapidly.

VI. ADULTS

When a person resides in a fluoride area throughout life, benefits continue. In Colorado Springs, adults aged 20 to 44 years who had used water with natural fluoride showed 60% less caries experience than did adults in fluoride-deficient Boulder. In Boulder, adults also had had three to four times as many permanent teeth extracted.[16] In a survey of adults in Rockford (no fluoride), there were about seven times as many edentulous persons as there were in a comparable group in Aurora (natural fluoride).[17]

VII. PERIODONTAL DISEASES

Indirect favorable effects of fluoride on periodontal health can be shown. Improved bone density resulting from fluoride can affect the alveolar bone, along with all bones, and may have an effect on bone resorption and resistance to local factors.

Dental carious lesions favor plaque retention and, therefore, irritation to gingival tissues, particularly lesions adjacent to the gingival margin and proximal lesions, which favor food impaction. When dental caries, tooth loss, and malocclusion are decreased, a difference can be expected in the periodontal conditions because of lack of retentive areas for bacterial plaque.

The incidence of periodontal diseases increases with age because of the cumulative effects of etiologic factors and the disease processes. With the use of fluorides, particularly fluoridation, fewer teeth are lost because of dental caries at younger ages. Therefore, periodontal disease prevention and control must be emphasized in communities with fluoride in the drinking water.

PARTIAL DEFLUORIDATION

Several hundred communities in the United States have water supplies that contain more than twice the optimal level of fluoride. Water with excess fluoride does not meet the requirements of the United States Public Health Service.

Defluoridation can be accomplished by one of several chemical systems.[18] The efficacy of the methods has been shown. The water supply in Britton, South Dakota, has been reduced from almost 7 ppm to 1.5 ppm since 1948, and in Bartlett, Texas, from 8 ppm to 1.8 ppm since 1952. Examinations have shown a dramatic reduction in incidence of objectionable fluorosis in children born since defluoridation.[19,20]

SCHOOL FLUORIDATION

One satisfactory method for bringing the benefits of fluoridation to children living in areas lacking a central water system has been the fluoridation of a school water supply. Because of the intermittent use of the water (only part of each day for 5 days each week during the school year), the amount of fluoride added can be increased over the usual 1 ppm.

Although children are 5 or 6 years old before they go to school, definite benefits have been shown. The effect is about twice as great on late-erupting teeth because they receive the benefit of systemic fluoride and topical exposure. Early erupting teeth have topical benefits.

After 12 years of fluoride at 5 ppm in the school drinking water of Elk Lake, Pennsylvania, children who had attended that school regularly had 39% fewer decayed, missing, and filled teeth than did those in the control group. The greatest benefits were found on proximal tooth surfaces.[21]

The benefits increase with increased fluoride levels. In the schools of Seagrove, North Carolina, after 12 years with fluoride level at 6.3 ppm, the children experienced a 47.5% decrease in decayed, missing, and filled surfaces when compared with those in the control group.[21]

DISCONTINUED FLUORIDATION

The control of dental caries by fluorides can be clearly shown in a community when fluoride is removed. For example, in Antigo, Wisconsin, the action of antifluoridationists in 1960 brought about the discontinuance of fluoridation, which had been installed in 1949. Examinations in the years following 1960 revealed the marked drop in the number of children who were caries-free and the steep increases in caries rates. For example, from 1960 to 1966, the number of caries-free children in the second grade decreased by 67%.[22] Fluoridation was reinstated in 1966 by popular demand.

ECONOMIC BENEFITS

I. COST OF FLUORIDATION[23]

In the United States, costs after installation have been estimated to be as low as 15 cents per person per year. When the benefits are considered, and the fact that ALL children are reached, not just those whose parents make the effort to seek preventive professional care, there is little question about the need for fluoridation in all possible domestic water supplies.

No other method for the administration of fluorides has consistently shown equal benefits. All other methods require more professional time, more effort on the part of the individual, and/or more financial outlay.

II. COST OF PROFESSIONAL CARE

A. Influence of Fluoridation
Individual, family, and community costs of dental care can be reduced markedly. In addition, the number of dental appointments, the extent of individual restorations, and the number of dental extractions are all reduced.

B. Newburgh–Kingston Study[24]
Newburgh, New York, and the control city, Kingston (without fluoridation), have been used to demonstrate a specific program of dental care. After 6 years of dental clinic operation for the 5- and 6-year-old life-long residents of the poorest socioeconomic areas of the cities, the cost for care of the children exposed to fluoridation was shown to be less than half that required for the Kingston children.

At the initial examinations, 41% of the Newburgh children were caries-free, whereas only 17% of the Kingston children were. Of the needed restorations, about 75% of those for the Kingston children were compound; in Newburgh only about 55% involved more than one surface. At the annual maintenance appointment, the Kingston children consistently required more restorative services; the Newburgh children required only about one-half as many appointments. These findings have marked significance for all types of dental programs for all ages.

FLUORIDES IN FOODS

I. FOODS
Certain foods contain fluoride, but not enough to constitute a significant part of the day's need for caries prevention. Meat, eggs, vegetables, cereals, and fruits have very small but measurable amounts, whereas tea and fish have larger amounts.

II. SALT[25]
Fluoridated salt has been used, particularly in Switzerland, and although reduced incidence of dental caries has been shown, effects comparable to those gained by fluoridation of water have not been attained. The use of salt as it is currently available supplies about one-third to one-half of the amount of fluoride ingested daily from 1 ppm fluoridated water, when average amounts of water used by individuals are compared.

DIETARY FLUORIDE SUPPLEMENTS

Approximately 23% of the population of the United States live in areas that do not have central water systems. Without fluoride in the drinking water, individuals and communities must resort to other means for making fluoride available. One method is the use of dietary fluoride supplements. Supplements and other methods are not substitutes for fluoridation but are needed as follows:

- For people who use a private water supply that does not have natural fluoride and that is not practical to fluoridate.
- When the fluoride in the water is less than optimum level.
- For those whose community water supply has not yet been fluoridated.

I. ADMINISTRATION
A. A fluoride supplement can be administered as a pill, chewable tablet, lozenge, drop, or mouthrinse for swallowing after rinsing.
B. The supplement may be prescribed on an individual patient basis for daily use at home, or it may be administered to school classroom groups as part of a total public health program.
C. Chewing and rinsing with a supplement before swallowing results in a dual action: first, locally on the tooth surface, and second, systemically in teeth that have not erupted (see Figures 29-1 and 29-2, page 458). After chewing, the mixture should be swished over and between the teeth for 1 minute so that optimal benefit can be obtained. The person should not eat or drink for 30 minutes after chewing the tablet. The preferred time for using the tablet is after toothbrushing before going to bed. The maximum topical effect occurs on newly erupted teeth.

II. DETERMINE THE NEED
A. Review patient history to be certain the child is not receiving other fluoride in such preparations as vitamin–fluoride supplements.
B. Refer to list of fluoridated communities to determine patient's fluoride consumption level. Lists are available from state or local health departments.
C. Request water analysis when fluoride level in private water source has not been determined.

III. AVAILABLE FORMS OF SUPPLEMENTS
Products are classified by the American Dental Association, Council on Scientific Affairs.

A. Tablets and Lozenges
Tablets may be scored or unscored. They may be chewed, rinsed, and swallowed, or dissolved slowly in the mouth as a lozenge. The resulting mix with saliva should be swished over and between the teeth for 1 minute. For infants, the tablet can be crushed to add to food.

B. Mouthrinse
A measured amount of rinse contains pre-

scribed daily fluoride. The rinse is swished for at least 1 minute before swallowing.

C. Drops

The liquid is prepared in a concentrate with directions that specify the number of drops for the prescription equivalent. The liquid form has its primary use for the child from 6 months to 3 years; a drop can be placed directly into the child's mouth or in food. For other children, the tooth contact of the chewable tablet or mouthrinse is important to provide the enamel surface with protective fluoride.

IV. PRESCRIPTION

A. Adjust for No Fluoride in the Drinking Water[26]

1. *6 to 16 years:* 1.0 mg (prescription: 2.2 mg sodium fluoride; a 2.2-mg sodium fluoride tablet contains 1.0 mg fluoride ions).
2. *3 to 6 years:* 0.5 mg (one-half of a 2.2-mg tablet).
3. *6 months to 3 years:* 0.25 mg.

B. Adjust for Fluoride in the Water System up to 0.7 ppm

Table 29-2 shows the fluoride dosage necessary to supplement the different levels of fluoride in the drinking water.

C. Prescription for Breast-Fed Infant

The concentration of fluoride in breast milk is very low, even when the mother uses fluoridated community water. Infants who are totally breast-fed after 6 months need a daily fluoride supplement of 0.25 mg (Table 29-2).

In a fluoridated community, an infant who receives other sources of liquid, such as drinking water or supplemental formula feedings made with fluoridated water, does not need the prescription.

D. Limitation on Total Prescription

1. Prescribe no more than 264 mg of sodium

fluoride at a time; sufficient for 4 months when 2.2 mg is used daily.
2. The amount (264 mg) is below the toxic or lethal doses and therefore eliminates the hazard of storing large amounts in the home.

E. Storage

Tablets should be kept out of the reach of children.

F. Vitamins With Fluoride

1. Preparations are available in liquid and tablet form.
2. The American Dental Association has not considered for acceptance vitamin–fluoride combinations for several reasons:
   a. It is more difficult to adjust the prescribed fluoride to the amount already received through the water supply (Table 29-2).
   b. The preparation contains a fixed amount of fluoride.
   c. There is no evidence that the vitamins enhance the effectiveness of the fluoride.
   d. The expense of buying vitamins that are not needed or prescribed is unnecessary.

V. PATIENT INSTRUCTION

A. Individual

Patients who receive a prescription for fluoride tablets need instruction, motivation, and supervision. When prescribed on an individual basis, problems arise in the continued administration of the tablets over the years until all tooth crowns have mineralized, even when parents are conscientious and highly motivated.

B. Patient Follow-up

Maintenance appointments should be planned for the time when the patient's prescription will be in need of renewal so that encouragement and supervision can be provided.

TABLE 29-2 Fluoride Supplements Dosage Schedule (mg F/day)*			
	Water Fluoride Concentration (ppm)		
Age of Child (years)	Less than 0.3	Between 0.3 and 0.6	Greater than 0.6
Birth–6 mo	0	0	0
6 mo–3 yr	0.25 mg	0†	0†
3–6 yr	0.50 mg	0.25 mg	0
6–16 yr	1.0 mg	0.5 mg	0

*2.2 mg sodium fluoride provides 1 mg fluoride ions.
† Infants receiving their total diet from breast-feeding need a 0.25-mg supplement.
(Recommendations from the American Dental Association, Chicago, IL.)

TOPICAL FLUORIDE APPLICATIONS

Topical application of fluoride is an essential part of a total preventive program, particularly for patients at risk for dental caries. Topical fluoride applications are both professionally applied and self-applied by the patient. Professionally applied fluorides may be solutions, gels, foams, or varnishes. They will be described first, followed by self-applied fluorides.

I. INDICATIONS

The professional application of a fluoride preventive agent is a selective procedure. Routine application after scaling and debridement has definite advantages and can be considered a necessity for patients such as those listed in Table 29-3.

II. DEVELOPMENT

Research in topical applications has continued since the early 1940s, when Dr. Basil G. Bibby conducted the initial topical sodium fluoride study using Brockton, Massachusetts, schoolchildren.[27] More than one-third fewer new carious lesions resulted from a 0.1% aqueous solution applied at 4-month intervals for 2 years.

That research led to extensive studies by Dr. John W. Knutson and others sponsored by the United States Public Health Service. The aim was to determine the most effective concentration of sodium fluoride, the minimum time required for application, and procedural details.[28,29] Their results still provide the basis for applications used currently and described in following sections.

III. CLINICAL PROCEDURES

Table 29-4 provides a summary of the professionally applied topical agents with the concentrations used. Benefits from topical application of solution, gel, foam, and varnish are considered within the same general average of 25% to 35% reduction in incidence of dental caries. Because the caries-preventive effects are similar, the choice of method of application used may be based on convenience, patient age and acceptance, cost, or clinician's preference.

A. Objectives
1. *Remineralization of demineralized areas*
   a. White spots in the cervical third, especially under bacterial plaque.
   b. Exposed root surfaces after periodontal treatment.
2. *Prevention of dental caries.* Identify special problems including areas adjacent to restorations, orthodontic appliances; xerostomia; and other risk factors listed in Table 14-5, page 243.
3. *Desensitization.* Fluoride aids in blocking dentinal tubules (page 599). Varnish covers and protects a sensitive area, and fluoride is slowly released for uptake.

B. Preparation of the Teeth
When fluoride application is to be applied at a time other than following a routine dental hygiene scaling and debridement, a rubber cup polishing is not routinely necessary. Fluoride solution or gel application has been shown to provide the same benefits when applied with or without a prior polishing.[30] A toothbrush cleaning is recommended.

TABLE 29-3 Indications for Professional Topical Fluoride Application: Patients at Risk for Dental Caries

- Primary teeth
  - Infant/toddler: prevention baby bottle tooth decay
  - Parental oral care; parental caries pattern
- Posteruptive period
  - Rapid uptake of fluoride important for newly exposed enamel
- Active caries (new carious lesions at regular maintenance)
- Secondary/recurrent caries adjacent to previous restorations
- Wearing orthodontic appliances: bands, bonded brackets
- Compromised salivary flow
  - Radiation therapy to head and neck
  - Sjögren's syndrome or other condition that limits salivary excretion by the glands
  - Medication with side effect of xerostomia
- Teeth supporting an overdenture
- Exposed root surfaces following periodontal recession
- Lack of compliance and conscientious efforts for daily bacterial plaque removal
- Low or no fluoride in drinking water
- Early carious lesions:
  - Pit and fissure: restore caries; sealant for all others
  - Proximal surface: need fluoride application

TABLE 29-4 Professionally Applied Topical Fluorides

Agent	Form	Concentration	Mode Application	Special Notes
Sodium fluoride (NaF) pH = neutral	Solution 2%	9,040 ppm 0.90% F ion	Paint on	Cotton-roll isolation absorbs excess solution
	Gel 2%	9,040 ppm 0.90% F ion	Paint on or Tray	Take care not to overfill tray. Request patient not to swallow.
	Foam 2%	9,040 ppm 0.90% F ion	Tray	Less amount needed to fill tray Less risk of swallowing because of consistency
	Varnish 5%	22,600 ppm 2.3% F ion	Paint on	Sets promptly. No risk of swallowing excess F.
Acidulated phosphate fluoride (APF) pH = 3.0 to 3.5	Solution 1.23%	12,300 ppm	Paint on	Cotton-roll isolation absorbs excess solution. Avoid ceramic and composite resin restorations.
	Gel 1.23%	12,300 ppm	Paint on or Tray	Take care not to overfill tray. Avoid ceramic and composite resin restorations.
	Foam 1.23%	12,300 ppm	Tray	Smaller amount needed to fill tray; less F. Avoid ceramic and composite resin restorations.

1. *Toothbrush preparation.* Use patient instruction time to remove debris and bacterial plaque with toothbrush and floss. Patient should learn all methods of caries prevention and how they work together.
2. *Apply principles of selective polishing for stain removal* (page 607). After calculus removal when stains must be removed, use the rubber cup with paste selectively on the areas where the stains occur. A fluoride-containing polishing paste may be used (page 609). Although only small amounts of fluoride may be added to the tooth surface, the fluoride paste may replace, in part, the fluoride removed by the polishing abrasive.[31]

C. Patient Counseling
1. *Inform patient (and parent).* Let them understand the purposes and benefits as well as the limitation of topical applications. The limitation is that the fluoride is only part of the total prevention program, which includes daily bacterial plaque control and limitation of cariogenic foods.

2. *Appointment sequence*
   a. Schedule appointment to end 30 minutes before the patient's eating time.
   b. Prepare the patient for any discomfort, especially the 4-minute timing.
   c. Explain need not to swallow but to expectorate immediately after.
3. *After application.* Patient must not rinse, eat, drink, brush, or floss for at least 30 minutes for solution or gel and 2 hours for varnish. Rinsing immediately after an application has been shown to lessen the benefits.[32]

IV. PAINT-ON TECHNIQUE: SOLUTION OR GEL

A. Seat Patient
Upright to prevent fluoride from passing into the throat.

B. Area
1. *Two-step procedure.* Maxillary and mandibular one side; then the other without rinsing.
2. *Small child.* One step for maxillary and two for mandibular when small-sized cotton roll

holder is too large and cotton rolls are held by clinician.

C. Isolate

1. *Cotton-roll holder.* Figure 29-4 shows position of continuous cotton roll with short lengths (1¼- to 2-inch lengths) on lingual aspect.
2. *Saliva absorber (bibulous pad).* Place over opening to parotid duct in cheek.
3. *Activate saliva ejector.* Position opposite from cotton roll holder.

D. Quick Check Before Application

Make certain that

1. Cotton is not on teeth to absorb fluoride.
2. Oral tissues are protected from metal cotton roll holder.
3. Cotton rolls are not extended so far distally they can be readily displaced or cause coughing.

E. Dry the Teeth

Follow sequence shown in Figure 29-5.

F. Apply Fluoride Preparation

1. Moisten all teeth quickly, mandibular first.

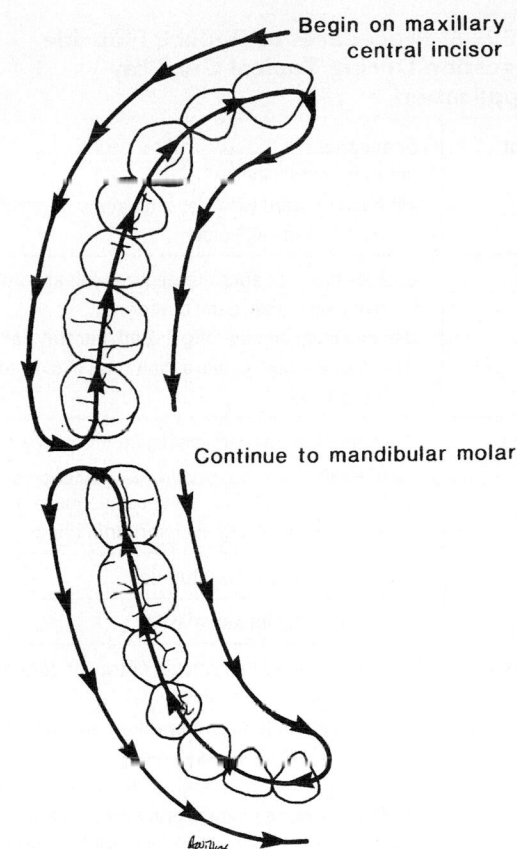

FIGURE 29-5 Procedure for Drying Teeth. After the teeth have been isolated using cotton in cotton-roll holder, a saliva ejector is positioned. The teeth are dried before applying the solution or gel. Because maxillary teeth can be maintained in a drier state longer, the mandibular teeth are dried with compressed air after the maxillary teeth have been dried. As shown by arrows, air is applied from the maxillary facial, over the occlusal, and then to the palatal surfaces. Proceed to the mandibular lingual surfaces, over the occlusal surfaces, and finally over the facial surfaces. Apply fluoride preparation to the mandibular teeth first (see text).

2. Start the 4-minute timing; patient may assist by turning on a timer.
3. Keep surfaces moistened throughout the timing; press solution or gel into interproximal areas.

G. Completion

1. Wipe teeth briefly to remove excess gel or solution.
2. Patient may expectorate but not rinse.
3. Proceed to other side.

V. TRAY TECHNIQUE: GEL OR FOAM

Procedures to prevent a young patient from ingesting fluoride are listed in Table 29-5.

A. Design of Tray: Shaped to hold the gel and prevent ingestion.

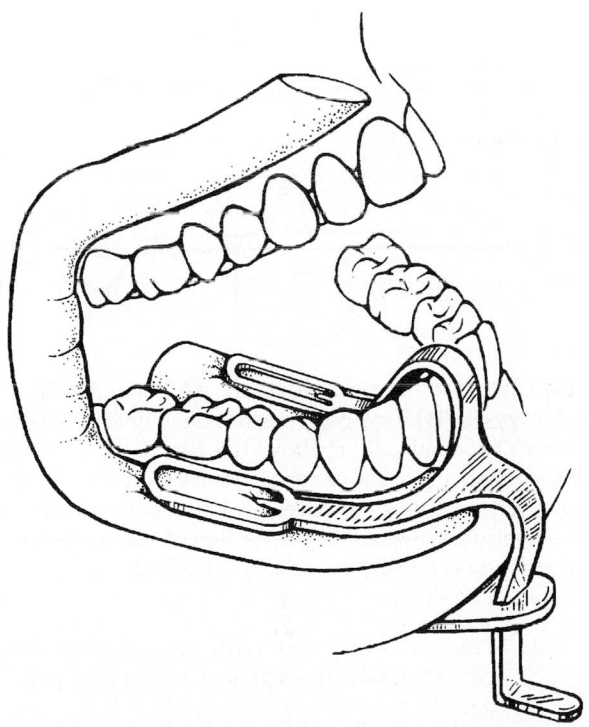

FIGURE 29-4 Isolation Using Cotton-Roll Holders. One half of the teeth are treated simultaneously. A continuous cotton roll extends from the mandibular anterior vestibule to the maxillary anterior vestibule. Bevel ends of cotton rolls to facilitate retention. Lingual prong holds cotton roll adjacent to tongue over floor of mouth. Care is taken to maintain cotton away from tooth surfaces to ensure maximum contact of fluoride solution or gel being applied.

TABLE 29-5 Procedures to Reduce Fluoride Ingestion During Topical Gel-Tray Application

Patient	Seat upright Instruct not to swallow Tilt head forward with trays; tilt away from side with cotton-roll holder
Trays	Custom-made or appropriate size with absorptive liners; post-dam; border rim Use minimum amount of gel: 2 mL per tray, less for small tray; no more than total of 5 mL for large trays
Isolation	Use saliva ejector with maximum efficiency suction Cotton-roll holder technique: position for security, stability; place saliva absorber in cheek
Attention	Do not leave patient unattended
Timing	Use a timer; do not estimate
Completion	Tilt head forward for removal of tray or cotton-roll holder Request patient to expectorate for several minutes; do not allow swallowing Wipe excess gel from teeth with gauze sponge Use high-power suction to draw out saliva and gel Instruct patient not to rinse, eat, drink, or brush teeth for at least 30 minutes

(Recommendations based on *Oral Health Policies for Children: Protocol for Fluoride Therapy,* American Academy of Pediatric Dentistry, 211 E. Chicago Avenue, Chicago, IL 60611.)

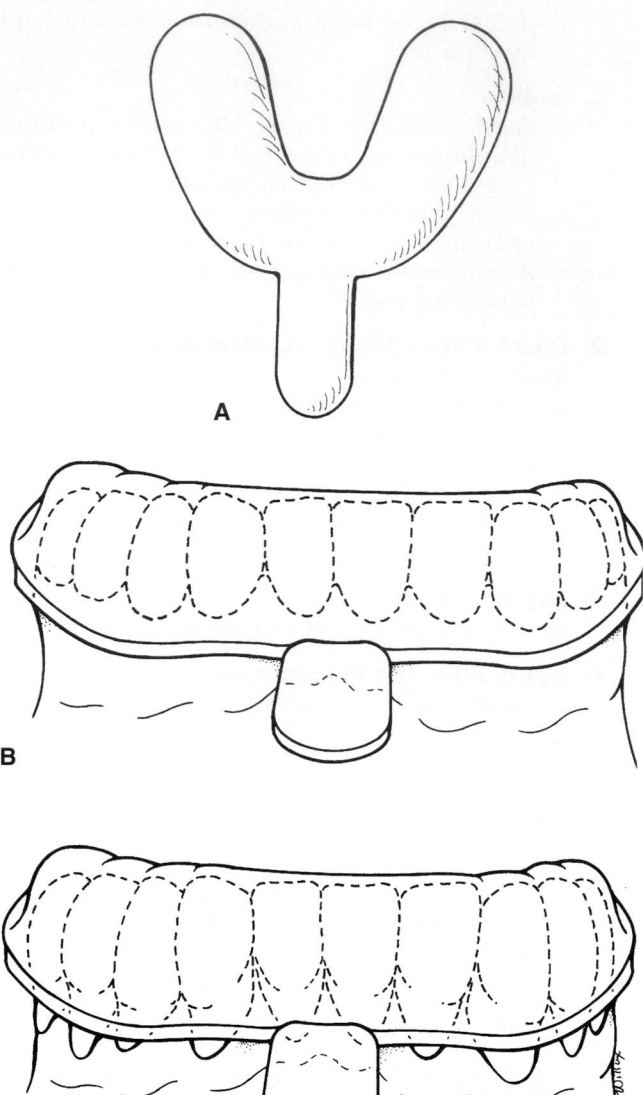

FIGURE 29-6 Tray Selection. (A) Mandibular tray held for try-in. **(B)** Tray over teeth is deep enough to cover the entire exposed enamel above the gingiva. **(C)** In patient with recession and areas of root surfaces exposed, the same tray is not deep enough to cover the important root surfaces where fluoride is needed for prevention of root caries or hypersensitivity. A custom-made tray is needed.

B. Coverage
1. Complete dentition must be covered.
2. Check for areas of recession; may need larger or custom-made tray (Figure 29-6).

C. Place Gel in Tray
1. Adult: 5 mL maximum
2. Child: 2 mL
3. Test measurement of quantity (Figure 29-7)

D. Seat Patient: Upright.

E. Dry the teeth: Prior to tray insertion
1. Insert saliva ejector between the trays.
2. Place cotton roll between trays on side opposite saliva ejector to prevent dislodging trays because of imbalance.

F. Time: Start the 4-minute timing; patient may assist.

G. Two-Step Procedure: Patient does not rinse but may expectorate before placement of second tray.

H. Completion
1. Request patient to expectorate but not swallow.

2. Wipe off extra gel with sponge; use high-power suction to evacuate saliva and gel.

VI. VARNISH

A. Dry Each Quadrant: Mandibular First
Use gentle compressed air; hold retraction with sponge during the application. The procedure is brief, but a saliva ejector may be necessary for selected patients.

B. Apply Varnish
Use a swab or disposable applicator brush; coating is yellow-brown.

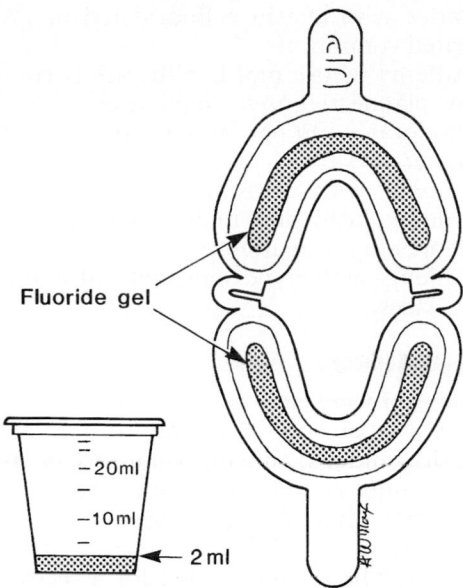

Fluoride gel

—20ml
—10ml
← 2 ml

■ **FIGURE 29-7 Measured Gel in Tray.** No more than 2 mL gel should be placed in each tray for small children, and no more than 2.5 mL for larger patients with permanent teeth. A medicine cup can be used to measure the amount once, so that the correct level of gel in the tray can be determined. A minimum amount of gel is indicated to prevent ingestion by the patient.

C. Adherence
Sets rapidly in the presence of saliva.

D. Instruction
1. *Do not disturb.* Instruct patient to avoid eating or drinking for 2 hours; avoid rough foods to allow fluoride uptake to continue undisturbed.
2. *Removal.* Patient removes with toothbrush and floss the day after.

E. Infant, Toddler, and Children Under 4 Years
1. *Position.* Figure 43-2 (page 662) shows the parent and clinician sitting knee-to-knee with the child held across the knees.
2. *Application.* Treat maxillary anterior first (site of initial baby bottle tooth decay); treat all teeth if possible.
3. *Instruct parent.* Avoid giving food or drink for at least 1 hour; toothbrush off the coating the next day.

SELF-APPLIED FLUORIDES

Self-applied fluorides include prescription and over-the-counter products. Self-applied products are available as dentifrices, mouthrinses, and gels. They may be applied by toothbrushing, rinsing, or trays that are custom made or disposable. A fluoride may also be used as an irrigation agent as described on page 383.

I. METHODS
The three methods for self-application are by mouth tray, rinsing, and toothbrushing.

A. Mouth Tray
1. *Custom-made or disposable tray.* The tray should be selected to fit the individual mouth. Patient must receive instruction not to overfill the tray.
2. *Overdenture patient.* Gel drops are placed in the impression surface at the location of the natural teeth; denture used as a tray (page 409).

B. Rinsing
The patient swishes for 1 minute with a measured amount of a fluoride rinse. Except when used as a fluoride supplement in a nonfluoridated community, the fluoride rinse is expectorated.

Certain patients will need to learn how to rinse properly to force the solution between the teeth. Table 24-1 (page 384) lists steps for rinsing.

C. Toothbrushing
A gel or paste is used for regular brushing two or three times daily. In addition, a brush-on gel may be used after regular brushing to provide special benefits. Use interdental brush to apply fluoride to proximal surfaces or open furca.

II. INDICATIONS
Indications for use of mouth tray, rinsing, and/or toothbrushing depend on the individual patient problems. Patient needs are determined as a part of total care planning. Certain patients need multiple procedures combined with professional applications at the regular maintenance appointments. Special indications are suggested as each method is described in the following sections.

TRAY TECHNIQUE: HOME APPLICATION

The original gel tray studies using custom-fitted polyvinyl mouthpieces compared the use of 1.1% acidulated NaF with plain NaF gel. The gel was applied daily over a 2-year period by schoolchildren aged 11 to 14 years during the school years. Dental caries incidence was reduced up to 80%.[33]

I. INDICATIONS FOR USE
A. Rampant enamel or root caries in persons of any age.
B. Xerostomia from any cause, particularly loss of salivary gland function.
C. Exposure to radiation therapy (pages 728 to 729).
D. Caries prevention under an overdenture (page 409).
E. Root surface hypersensitivity (page 600).

II. GEL USED

A. Concentrations[34]
APF 0.5%; NaF 1.1%.

B. Precautions
1. Do not dispense large quantities. Prescription of 24 to 30 mL of APF 0.5% in a dropper bottle that dispenses drops containing 0.1 mL F is suggested.
2. Do not use acidulated preparations on porcelain,[35] composite, or titanium restorations or filled sealants.

III. PROCEDURE: PATIENT INSTRUCTIONS

A. Brush and floss to remove thoroughly all bacterial plaque possible.
B. Use prepared custom-made polyvinyl tray. A disposable tray can be used if the appropriate fit can be obtained. Load the tray by distributing no more than 5 drops of the gel around each tray. Each drop is equivalent to 0.1 mL.
C. Dry the mouth by swallowing several times.
D. Apply the tray(s) over the teeth and close gently. Hold head upright.
E. Time by a clock for 4 minutes. *Do not swallow.*
F. Expectorate several times when the trays are removed.
G. Do not eat or drink for 30 minutes. One application should be made just before retiring.

FLUORIDE MOUTHRINSES

Mouthrinsing is a practical and effective means for self-application of fluoride. The only persons excluded from the practice of this method are children under 6 years of age and those of any age who cannot rinse because of oral and/or facial musculature problems or other disability. Rinsing can be part of an individual care plan or can be included in a group program conducted during school attendance.

Mouthrinses containing fluoride can be reviewed by the American Dental Association, Council on Scientific Affairs. Approved products are listed annually and bear the seal of the ADA (see Figure 24-15, page 389).

I. INDICATIONS

Mouthrinsing with a fluoride preparation may have particular meaning for the following:
A. General prevention of dental caries in
1. Young persons during the high-risk preteen and adolescent years.
2. Patients with areas of demineralization.
3. Patients with root exposure following recession and periodontal therapy.
4. Participants in a school health group program for all grades.
B. Patients with moderate to rampant dental caries who live in a fluoridated or nonfluoridated community.
C. Patients whose oral health care is complicated by plaque-retentive appliances, including orthodontics and partial dentures or space maintainers.
D. Patients with xerostomia from any cause, including head and neck radiation and saliva-depressing drug therapy.
E. Patients with hypersensitivity of exposed root surfaces.

II. LIMITATIONS

A. Alcohol Content
1. Use of alcohol-based mouthrinses should be discouraged; aqueous solutions are available.
2. Alcohol content of commercial preparations is not advisable for children.
3. Alcohol-containing preparations should never be recommended for a recovering alcoholic person.

B. Compliance
Motivation of patient and/or parent to carry out faithfully the recommended procedures. Daily rinse is better than weekly rinse when practiced on an individual home basis.

III. PREPARATIONS

Rinse preparations are referred to as *low-potency/high-frequency rinses, high-potency/low-frequency rinses,* and *oral rinse supplements.*[36] Certain low-potency rinses may be purchased directly over-the-counter (OTC); all others are provided by prescription.

A. Over-the-Counter: Neutral Sodium Fluoride 0.05%
1. *Fluoride content:* 0.025% fluoride ion; 225 ppm.
2. *Specifications*
   a. Single container must contain no more than 264 mg NaF (120 mg fluoride) dispensed at one time. A 500-mL bottle of 0.05% NaF rinse contains 100 mg fluoride.
   b. Bottle must have child-proof cap.
   c. Label must state that the rinse is not to be used by children under 6 years of age or by children with a disability involving oral and/or facial musculature. Young children do not have sufficient control to expectorate, and they tend to swallow quickly.
   d. Label must indicate that the rinse is not to be swallowed.
3. *Procedure for use*
   a. Rinse daily with 1 teaspoonful (5 mL) after brushing before retiring.
   b. Swish between teeth with lips tightly closed for 60 seconds; expectorate.

B. Prescription
1. *Fluoride content:* 0.20% F; 900 ppm (high potency).

2. *Use:* Weekly rinse using 5 mL (younger children) or 10 mL (older children) swished for 60 seconds and expectorated.

3. *School group program:* The use of the weekly rinse is the most common school-based program in the United States. Advantages are that it requires little time (about 5 minutes once weekly for an entire class), is inexpensive, is easy to learn and is well accepted by participants, and can be carried out by nondental personnel. Responsibility for providing the correctly mixed 0.2% solution and for locking the fluoride in an inaccessible place can be taken by school officials and a supervising dental hygienist.[36]

IV. BENEFITS

Benefits from fluoride mouthrinsing have been documented many times since the original research using various percentages of various fluoride preparations.[37,38] Frequent rinsing with low concentrations of fluoride has the following effects:

A. A 30% to 40% average reduction in dental caries incidence.

B. Greater benefit for smooth surfaces, but some benefit to pits and fissures.

C. Greatest benefit to newly erupted teeth (thus, the program should be continued through the teenage years to benefit the second and third permanent molars).

D. Added benefits for a community with fluoridation.[39]

E. Increase in post-treatment benefits as the length of time of rinsing increases.[33,40]

F. Primary teeth present in school-age children benefit by as much as 42.5% average reduction in dental caries incidence.[41]

FLUORIDE DENTIFRICES

Historically dentifrices have been tried with various compounds, including stannous fluoride, sodium fluoride, sodium monofluorophosphate, and amine fluoride. The main research objective has been to find fluoride and abrasive systems that are compatible. Early dentifrices had problems of stability and fluoride availability for uptake by the tooth surface.

A dentifrice containing stannous fluoride 0.4% was the first fluoride-containing dentifrice to gain approval by the Council on Dental Therapeutics.[42] An excellent review by Stookey that describes the development of present formulations and the extensive research over past years is recommended for reading.[43] Guidelines for the acceptance of dentifrices by the Council are frequently updated and call for laboratory and clinical efficacy of each product.[44]

I. INDICATIONS

A. Dental Caries Prevention

A fluoride dentifrice approved by the American Dental Association should be recommended for each patient as part of the complete preventive program.

B. Caries-Risk Patients

Patients with moderate to rampant dental caries should be advised to brush several times each day with a fluoride-containing dentifrice.

C. Desensitization

Certain dentifrices containing fluoride have desensitizing properties. These are included on page 600.

II. PREPARATIONS

Fluoride dentifrices are available as gels or pastes. Sodium fluoride and sodium monofluorophosphate dentifrices are approved currently. Amine fluorides have not been developed and promoted in the United States.

A. Current Constituents

1. Sodium fluoride (NaF) 0.24% (1100 ppm).

2. Sodium monofluorophosphate (Na_2PO_3F) 0.76% (1000 ppm). An "extra-strength" Na_2PO_3F contains 1500 ppm.

B. Specifications From Guidelines for Acceptance[44]

To gain acceptance by the American Dental Association and to use the seal of acceptance (see Figure 24-15, page 389), a product must meet certain criteria, including the following:

1. The active fluoride (F) agent must be chemically free and available in both fresh and aged samples to the end of the specified expiration date.

2. The ability to deliver and incorporate levels of F into both sound and demineralized enamel must be demonstrated.

3. The product must promote or enhance remineralization of enamel.

4. The product must reduce the rate of demineralization.

III. PATIENT INSTRUCTION: RECOMMENDED PROCEDURES

Instruction in the selection of a dentifrice, the need for frequent use, the method for application to the tooth surfaces, and the effects of fluoride can help the patient appreciate the significant role of fluoride in oral health.

A. Select an accepted fluoride-containing dentifrice.

B. Place a small amount of dentifrice on the toothbrush.

1. *Child.* Use only a small amount, the size of a small pea (Figure 29-8A). Demonstrate spreading this amount over the ends of the filaments, and explain that the child should not swallow excess amounts of

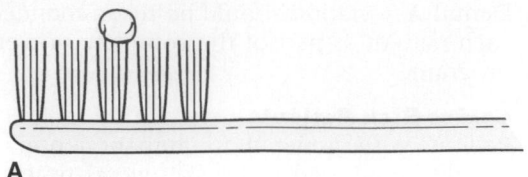

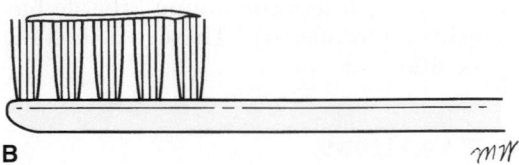

■ **FIGURE 29-8 Dentifrice for a Child.** To prevent ingestion of an excess amount of dentifrice, a parent must be instructed to place only a small portion of dentifrice on the brush. **(A)** The size can be compared to the size of a small pea. **(B)** For very small children, a little paste is spread over the brush surface.

dentifrice because that may cause white spots to develop in the enamel (page 456).
2. *Toddler and other small children.* About one-half the size of a small pea should be used and spread along the brushing plane (Figure 29-8*B*). The paste should then be spread over all the teeth before starting to brush so that all teeth benefit and large amounts are not available for swallowing.
3. *Older children and adults.* Use ½ inch or less.
C. Spread dentifrice over the teeth with a light touch of the brush.
D. Proceed with correct brushing for sulcular removal of bacterial plaque.
E. Keep dentifrice container out of reach of children.

IV. BENEFITS

Dentifrices are used often, at least once or twice each day as recommended. Caries-risk patients may use a dentifrice several times per day. The dentifrice is a continuing source of fluoride for the tooth surface in the control of demineralization and promotion of remineralization. Fluoride is deposited in demineralized white spots (see Figure 29-3).

Many research studies have shown that the incidence of dental caries can be reduced between 20% to 30% when NaF or Na_2PO_3F dentifrices are used regularly.

BRUSH-ON GEL

Brush-on gel has been used as an adjunct to the daily application of fluoride in a dentifrice and as a supplement to periodic professional applications.

I. PREPARATIONS

A. Sodium fluoride (NaF) 1.1%, neutral pH, (5000 ppm).
B. Stannous fluoride (SnF_2) 0.4% in glycerin base.

II. PROCEDURE

A. Use once a day, preferably at night after toothbrushing and flossing.
B. Place about 2 mg of the gel over the brush head and spread over all teeth.
C. Brush 1 minute, then swish before expectorating.

III. PATIENT INSTRUCTION

A. Gels of this category are not for use as dentifrices. Teeth are cleaned first with thorough brushing and flossing.
B. Regular use has been shown to help to control demineralization about orthodontic appliances,[45] and to provide protection against postirradiation caries in conjunction with other fluoride applications.[46]

COMBINED FLUORIDE PROGRAM

Most patients can benefit from more than one method of use of fluorides. When the preventive program is planned for an individual patient, the fluoride preparations and modes of application selected should provide the greatest possible protection against dental caries.

When self-administered methods are chosen, patient cooperation is a significant factor. Age and eruption pattern influence the method selected. Fluorides must be applied as soon after tooth eruption as possible and continued indefinitely to control demineralization.

Maintenance appointments can be scheduled for frequent topical applications and for continuing instruction and motivation. All methods are supplemented by the use of a dentifrice with fluoride.

FLUORIDE SAFETY

Fluoride preparations and fluoridated water have wide margins of safety. Fluoride is beneficial in small amounts, but it can be injurious if used without attention to correct dosage and frequency. All dental personnel should be familiar with recommended approved procedures, know potentials for toxic effects, and be prepared to administer emergency measures should accidental overdoses occur.

I. SUMMARY OF FLUORIDE MANAGEMENT

A. Use and recommend for patient use only approved fluoride preparations. Products have approval from the Food and Drug Administration and the American Dental Association in the United States.

B. Use only researched, recommended amounts and methods for delivery.

C. Know potential toxicity of the various products, and be prepared for administering emergency measures for treating an accidental toxic response.

D. Instruct patients in proper care of fluoride products.

1. Dentist prescribes no more than 264 mg of sodium fluoride at one time. Do not store large quantities in the home.

2. Request parental supervision of child's brushing or other fluoride administration. Rinses, for example, are not to be used by children under 6 years of age.

3. Fluoride products should have child-proof covers and should be kept out of reach of small children and other persons, such as the mentally handicapped, who may not understand limitations.

4. In school health programs, dispensing of the fluoride product must be supervised by responsible adults. Containers must be stored under lock and key when not in active use.

II. ACUTE TOXICITY

Acute refers to rapid intake of an excess dose over a short time, whereas *chronic* applies to long-term ingestion of fluoride in amounts that exceed the approved therapeutic levels. An accidental ingestion of a concentrated fluoride preparation can lead to a toxic reaction. Acute fluoride poisoning is rare.[47]

A. Certainly Lethal Dose (CLD)[48]

A lethal dose is the amount of a drug likely to cause death if not intercepted by antidotal therapy.

1. *Adult CLD:* 5 to 10 g of sodium fluoride taken at one time. The fluoride ion equivalent is 32 to 64 milligrams fluoride per kilogram body weight (mg F/kg; Table 29-6*A*).

2. *Child:* Approximately 0.5 to 1.0 g variable with size and weight of the child.

B. Safely Tolerated Dose (STD): One Fourth of the CLD

1. *Adult STD:* 1.25 to 2.5 g of sodium fluoride (8 to 16 mg F/kg).

2. *Child:* Table 29-6*B* shows STDs and CLDs for children. Weights given for each selected age are minimal, and calculations for the doses are conservative. As can be noted from the table, less than 1 g (1000 mg) may be fatal for children 12 years old and younger, and 0.5 g (500 mg) exceeds the STD for all ages shown. For children under 6 years of age, however, 500 mg would be lethal.[48]

TABLE 29-6 Lethal and Safe Doses of Fluoride

A. Lethal and safe dosages of fluoride for a 70-kg adult.

Certainly Lethal Dose (CLD)
5–10 g NaF
or
32–64 mg F/kg

Safely Tolerated Dose (STD) = ¼ CLD
1.25–2.5 g NaF
or
8–16 mg F/kg

B. CLDs and STDs of fluoride for selected ages

Age (years)	Weight (lbs)	CLD (mg)	STD (mg)
2	22	320	80
4	29	422	106
6	37	538	135
8	45	655	164
10	53	771	193
12	64	931	233
14	83	1,206	301
16	92	1,338	334
18	95	1,382	346

(From Heifetz, S.B. and Horowitz, H.S.: The Amounts of Fluoride in Current Fluoride Therapies: Safety Considerations for Children, *ASDC J. Dent. Child.*, 51, 257. July–August, 1984.)

III. SIGNS AND SYMPTOMS OF ACUTE TOXIC DOSE

Symptoms begin within 30 minutes of ingestion and may persist for as long as 24 hours.

A. Gastrointestinal Tract

Fluoride in the stomach is acted on by the hydrochloric acid to form hydrofluoric acid, an irritant to the stomach lining. Symptoms include

1. Nausea, vomiting, diarrhea.
2. Abdominal pain.
3. Increased salivation, thirst.

B. Systemic Involvement

1. *Blood.* Calcium may be bound by the circulating fluoride, thus causing symptoms of hypocalcemia.

2. *Central nervous system.* Hyperreflexia, convulsions, paresthesias.

3. *Cardiovascular and respiratory depression.* If not treated, may lead to death in a few hours from cardiac failure or respiratory paralysis.

IV. EMERGENCY TREATMENT

A. Induce Vomiting

1. *Mechanical.* Digital stimulation at back of tongue or in throat.
2. *Drug.* Ipecac syrup.

B. Second Person
Call emergency service; transport to hospital.

C. Administer Fluoride-Binding Liquid When Patient Is Not Vomiting
1. Milk.
2. Lime water (CaOH$_2$ solution 0.15%).

D. Support Respiration and Circulation (see Chapter 61, pages 900 to 906)

E. Additional Therapy Indicated at Emergency Room
1. Calcium gluconate for muscle tremors or tetany.
2. Gastric lavage.
3. Cardiac monitoring.
4. Endotracheal intubation.
5. Blood monitoring (calcium, magnesium, potassium, pH).
6. Intravenous feeding to restore blood volume, calcium.

V. CHRONIC TOXICITY

A. Skeletal Fluorosis[47]
Isolated instances of osteosclerosis result from chronic toxicity after long-term (20 or more years) use of water with 10 to 25 ppm fluoride or from industrial exposure. Methods for defluoridation have been developed, as described on page 462.

B. Dental Fluorosis
Naturally occurring excess fluoride in the drinking water can produce visible fluorosis only when used during the years of development of the crowns of the teeth, namely, from birth until ages 12 or 16 or when the crowns of the third permanent molars are completed. No systemic effects result from the fluoride, and the individual has protection against dental caries. A classification of fluorosis is found in Table 29-1, page 461.

C. Mild Fluorosis
1. *Clinical evaluation.* In its mild and very mild forms, dental fluorosis appears as white opacities in the enamel surface. No esthetic or health problem is involved. Many such white spots are not visible except when scrutinized under a dental light and the surface is dried. Because all white spots in the enamel are not related to fluoride intake, distinction must be made by reviewing the patient's dental and fluoride-intake history, by noting the location and distribution of the white spots, and by considering the sequence of tooth development.
2. *Relation to fluoride sources.* Mild fluorosis or white spots may result from inadvertent ingestion of excess fluoride by young children during topical procedures both self-applied and professional. No problem exists when care is taken to follow basic rules, such as

those listed in Table 29-5 for professional applications and shown in Figure 29-8 for daily use of dentifrice the size of a small pea. Mouthrinses are not indicated for children under 6 years of age.

Small amounts of dentifrice may be swallowed at each brushing. A child of 4 years who lives in a nonfluoridated community, uses a daily supplement (0.5 mg), and swallows two or three small amounts of dentifrice ingests far less than the STD of 106 mg shown in Table 29-6*B*.

VI. HOW TO CALCULATE AMOUNTS OF FLUORIDE[48–50]

Figure 29-9 is a flowchart that shows the steps necessary to determine the amount of fluoride in a fluoride compound. By doing so, one then can calculate the amount ingested by the patient.

First, the percentage of fluoride ion in the compound is multiplied by the molecular weight conversion ratio, as shown in Figure 29-9. The ratio was obtained by dividing the molecular weight of the compound by the atomic weight of fluoride. For example, the molecular weight of sodium fluoride is 42 (Na = 23, F = 19). When divided by 19, a 1 to 2.2 ratio results, as used in the example in Figure 29-9.

TECHNICAL HINTS

I. ALTERNATE ISOLATION PROCEDURES FOR TOPICAL APPLICATION

The procedure described on page 467 is for isolation of one-half of the dentition at one time. Objectives are to conserve time, to maintain as dry a field as possible, and to prevent the fluoride solution from being absorbed by cotton rolls and the saliva from contaminating or diluting the solution. Other systems that may be applied include:

A. Rubber Dam
1. *Use.* For application of fluoride following restorative procedures or sealant placement.
2. *Preparation.* When the rubber dam has not been fitted to include the entire quadrant, additional holes may be made in the dam with an explorer.
3. *Advantages*
   a. Better control of the patient during the application, particularly of a small child or disabled patient with special problems.
   b. Saves time. Dry teeth can be maintained.
   c. Helpful when general anesthesia is used, particularly for a hospitalized patient.
4. *Disadvantage.* When root surface exposure needs fluoride, retraction of rubber dam may be difficult or impossible.

B. Single Quadrant
Each quadrant can be done separately by holding the cotton rolls with the fingers. In a very

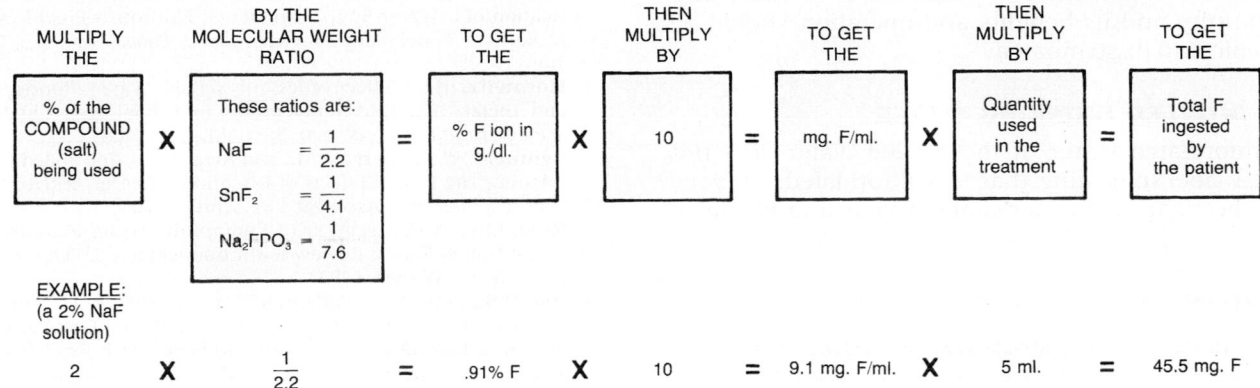

FIGURE 29-9 Fluoride Calculation. Flowchart shows steps in the calculation of the amount of fluoride in a compound used in treatment. The example shows that 5 mL of a 2% solution of NaF contains 45.5 mgF, an amount slightly greater than half of the safely tolerated dose (STD) for a 2-year-old child (Table 29-6B). (Data from Heifetz, S.B. and Horowitz, H.S.: The Amounts of Fluoride in Current Fluoride Therapies: Safety Considerations for Children, *ASDC J. Dent. Child., 51,* 257, July–August, 1984.)

small mouth, a No. 1 continuous cotton roll may be held around the entire maxillary arch to make the entire application in one step. This approach can be particularly useful for a small child.

II. FLUORIDE APPLICATION FOLLOWING POLISHING OF RESTORATIONS

Because abrasive stones and polishing agents remove a layer of surface enamel and polishing procedures extend over the margins of the restoration, a topical application of fluoride may be particularly important (page 632). The topical fluoride can help to promote remineralization.

III. COMMUNITIES WITH FLUORIDATION

Maintain list of communities. Update annually by contacting the state health department.

FACTORS TO TEACH THE PATIENT

I. PERSONAL USE OF FLUORIDES

A. Purposes, action, and expected benefits relative to the specific forms of fluoride treatment the patient will receive.
B. Specific instruction concerning self-applied techniques that will be performed at home. Prepared printed instruction materials can be especially useful.

II. NEED FOR PARENTAL SUPERVISION

A. Supervise daily care of child's teeth and mouth, including brushing of teeth using small, pea-sized quantity of dentifrice to prevent excess ingestion of fluoride.

B. Keep fluoride products out of reach of small children.
C. Brush teeth before using chewable dietary supplements. Avoid eating and drinking after use. Preferred time for use is just before going to bed.

III. DETERMINING NEED FOR FLUORIDE SUPPLEMENTS

A. Reference to list of communities with fluoride in the drinking water at optimum level.
B. Where to call to obtain information about fluoride in drinking water—health department, water department, or other community source.
C. Where to send private water source sample for fluoride analysis.

IV. PREPARATION FOR TOPICAL FLUORIDE APPLICATION

When the teeth are free from plaque and the gingival tissue is firm and healthy, uptake of fluoride by the teeth is greater and the possibility of a slight tissue reaction is lessened. When the gingiva is inflamed, the patient needs instruction to understand why the topical application must be postponed until the tissue has healed.

V. FLUORIDES ARE PART OF THE TOTAL PREVENTIVE PROGRAM

Control of cariogenic foods in the diet, particularly between meals, and professional care are still necessary to supplement fluoride treatment for caries control.

VI. FLUORIDATION

In a nonfluoridated community, information concerning the significance of fluoridation to the entire community and its benefits and operation should be available and disseminated.

VII. BOTTLED DRINKING WATER

Use fluoridated water. If the bottled water does not have a label indicating that it is fluoridated, fill your water bottle from a water supply that is fluoridated.

REFERENCES

1. **Ekstrand,** J.: Fluoride Metabolism, in Fejerskov, O., Ekstrand, J., and Burt, B.A., eds.: *Fluoride in Dentistry,* 2nd ed. Copenhagen, Munksgaard, 1996, pp. 55–67.
2. **Bhaskar,** S.N., ed.: *Orban's Oral Histology and Embryology,* 11th ed. St. Louis, Mosby, 1990, pp. 28–48, 75–105.
3. **Melfi,** R.C.: *Permar's Oral Embryology and Microscopic Anatomy,* 9th ed. Philadelphia, Lea & Febiger, 1994, pp. 43–83.
4. **Yoon,** S.H., Brudevold, F., Gardner, D.E., and Smith, F.A.: Distribution of Fluoride in Teeth from Areas with Different Levels of Fluoride in the Water Supply, *J. Dent. Res., 39,* 845, July–August, 1960.
5. **Rölla,** G. and Ekstrand, J.: Fluoride in Oral Fluids and Dental Plaque, in Fejerskov, O., Ekstrand, J., and Burt, B.A., eds.: *Fluoride in Dentistry,* 2nd ed. Copenhagen, Munksgaard, 1996, pp. 215–229.
6. **Rölla,** G., Øgaard, B., and deAlmeida Cruz, R.: Topical Application of Fluorides on Teeth. New Concepts of Mechanisms of Interaction, *J. Clin. Periodontol., 20,* 105, February, 1993.
7. **Richards,** L.F., Westmoreland, W.W., Tashiro, M., McKay, C.H., and Morrison, J.T.: Determining Optimum Fluoride Levels for Community Water Supplies in Relation to Temperature, *J. Am. Dent. Assoc., 74,* 389, February, 1967.
8. **Herschfeld,** J.J.: Classics in Dental History. Frederick S. McKay and the "Colorado Brown Stain," *Bull. Hist. Dent., 26,* 118, October, 1978.
9. **McKay,** F.S.: The Relation of Mottled Enamel to Caries, *J. Am. Dent. Assoc., 15,* 1429, August, 1928.
10. **Churchill,** H.V.: Occurrence of Fluorides in Some Waters of United States, *J. Indust. Engin. Chem., 23,* 996, 1931.
11. **Dean,** H.T., Arnold, F.A., Jr., and Elvove, E.: Domestic Water and Dental Caries. V. Additional Studies of the Relation of Fluoride Domestic Waters to Dental Caries Experience in 4425 White Children, Aged 12 to 14 Years, of 13 Cities in 4 States, *Public Health Rep., 57,* 1155, August 7, 1942.
12. **Backer Dirks,** O., Houwink, B., and Kwant, G.W.: Some Special Features of the Caries Preventive Effect of Water Fluoridation, *Arch. Oral Biol., 4,* 187, August, 1961.
13. **Burt,** B.A., Ismail, A.I., and Eklund, S.A.: Root Caries in an Optimally Fluoridated and a High-fluoride Community, *J. Dent. Res., 65,* 1154, September, 1986.
14. **Stamm,** J.W., Banting, D.W., and Imrey, P.B.: Adult Root Caries Survey of Two Similar Communities with Contrasting Natural Water Fluoride Levels, *J. Am. Dent. Assoc., 120,* 143, February, 1990.
15. **Ast,** D.B. and Fitzgerald, B.: Effectiveness of Water Fluoridation, *J. Am. Dent. Assoc., 65,* 581, November, 1962.
16. **Russell,** A.L. and Elvove, E.: Domestic Water and Dental Caries. VII. A Study of the Fluoride-Dental Caries Relationship in an Adult Population, *Public Health Rep., 66,* 1389, October 26, 1951.
17. **Englander,** H.R. and Wallace, D.A.: Effects of Naturally Fluoridated Water on Dental Caries in Adults, *Public Health Rep., 77,* 887, October, 1962.
18. **Murray,** J.J., Rugg-Gunn, A.J., and Jenkins, G.N.: *Fluorides in Caries Prevention,* 3rd ed. Oxford, Wright, Butterworth-Heinemann, 1991, pp. 94–99.
19. **Horowitz,** H.S., Maier, F.J., and Law, F.E.: Partial Defluoridation of a Community Water Supply and Dental Fluorosis, *Public Health Rep., 82,* 965, November, 1967.

20. **Horowitz,** H.S. and Heifetz, S.B.: The Effect of Partial Defluoridation of a Water Supply on Dental Fluorosis—Final Results in Bartlett, Texas, after 17 Years, *Am. J. Public Health, 62,* 767, June 1972.
21. **Horowitz,** H.S.: Effectiveness of School Water Fluoridation and Dietary Fluoride Supplements in School-aged Children, *J. Public Health Dent., 49,* 290, Special Issue, 1989.
22. **Lemke,** C.W., Doherty, J.M., and Arra, M.C.: Controlled Fluoridation: The Dental Effects of Discontinuation in Antigo, Wisconsin, *J. Am. Dent. Assoc., 80,* 782, April, 1970.
23. **Ripa,** L.W.: A Half-century of Community Water Fluoridation in the United States: Review and Commentary, *J. Public Health Dent., 53,* 17, Winter, 1993.
24. **Ast,** D.B., Cons, N.C., Pollard, S.T., and Garfinkel, J.: Time and Cost Factors to Provide Regular, Periodic Dental Care for Children in a Fluoridated and Nonfluoridated Area: Final Report, *J. Am. Dent. Assoc., 80,* 770, April, 1970.
25. **Burt,** B.A. and Marthaler, T.M.: Fluoride Tablets, Salt Fluoridation, and Milk Fluoridation, in Fejerskov, O., Ekstrand, J., and Burt, B.A., eds.: *Fluoride in Dentistry,* 2nd ed. Copenhagen, Munksgaard, 1996, pp. 291–310.
26. **Burrell,** K.H.: Systemic and Topical Fluorides, in American Dental Association, Council on Scientific Affairs: *ADA Guide to Dental Therapeutics.* Chicago, ADA Publishing Co., 1998, pp. 214–215.
27. **Bibby,** B.G.: Use of Fluorine in the Prevention of Dental Caries. II. The Effects of Sodium Fluoride Applications, *J. Am. Dent. Assoc., 31,* 317, March 1, 1944.
28. **Knutson,** J.W.: Sodium Fluoride Solutions: Technic for Application to the Teeth, *J. Am. Dent. Assoc., 36,* 37, January, 1948.
29. **Galagan,** D.J. and Knutson, J.W.: The Effect of Topically Applied Fluorides on Dental Caries Experience. VI. Experiments with Sodium Fluoride and Calcium Chloride . . . Widely Spaced Applications . . . Use of Different Solution Concentrations, *Public Health Rep., 63,* 1215, September 17, 1948.
30. **Ripa,** L.W.: Need for Prior Toothcleaning when Performing a Professional Topical Fluoride Application: Review and Recommendations for Change, *J. Am. Dent. Assoc., 109,* 281, August, 1984.
31. **Vrbic,** V., Brudevold, F., and McCann, H.G.: Acquisition of Fluoride by Enamel from Fluoride Pumice Pastes, *Helv. Odontol. Acta., 11,* 21, April, 1967.
32. **Stookey,** G.K., Schemehorn, B.R., Drook, C.A., and Cheetham, B.L.: The Effect of Rinsing with Water Immediately after a Professional Fluoride Gel Application on Fluoride Uptake in Demineralized Enamel: An *In Vivo* Study, *Pediatr. Dent., 8,* 153, June, 1986.
33. **Englander,** H.R., Keyes, P.H., and Gestwicki, M.: Clinical Anticaries Effect of Repeated Topical Sodium Fluoride Applications by Mouthpieces, *J. Am. Dent. Assoc., 75,* 638, September, 1967.
34. **Burrell:** op. cit., pp. 218–225.
35. **American Dental Association,** Council on Dental Materials, Instruments, and Equipment and Council on Dental Therapeutics: Status Report: Effect of Acidulated Phosphate Fluoride on Porcelain and Composite Restorations, *J. Am. Dent. Assoc., 116,* 115, January, 1988.
36. **Ripa,** L.W.: Fluoride Rinsing: What Dentists Should Know, *J. Am. Dent. Assoc., 102,* 477, April, 1981.
37. **Torell,** P. and Ericsson, Y.: The Potential Benefits Derived from Fluoride Mouth Rinses, in Forrester, D.J. and Schulz, E.M., eds.: *International Workshop on Fluorides and Dental Caries Reductions.* Baltimore, University of Maryland School of Dentistry, 1974, pp. 114–176.
38. **Birkeland,** J.M. and Torell, P.: Caries-preventive Fluoride Mouthrinses, *Caries Res., 12,* 38, Supplement 1, 1978.
39. **Driscoll,** W.S., Swango, P.A., Horowitz, A.M., and Kingman, A.: Caries-preventive Effects of Daily and Weekly Fluoride Mouthrinsing in a Fluoridated Community: Final Results after 30 Months, *J. Am. Dent. Assoc., 105,* 1010, December, 1982.
40. **Leske,** G.S., Ripa, L.W., and Green, E.: Posttreatment Benefits in a School-based Fluoride Mouthrinsing Program. Final Results after 7 Years of Rinsing by All Participants, *Clin. Prev. Dent., 8,* 19, September–October, 1986.

41. **Ripa,** L.W., Leske, G.S., and Varma, A.: Effect of Mouthrinsing with a 0.2 Percent Neutral NaF Solution on the Deciduous Dentition of First to Third Grade School Children, *Pediatr. Dent., 6,* 93, June, 1984.

42. **American Dental Association,** Council on Dental Therapeutics: Evaluation of Crest Toothpaste, *J. Am. Dent. Assoc., 61,* 272, August, 1960.

43. **Stookey,** G.K.: Are All Fluoride Dentifrices the Same? in Wei, S.H.Y., ed.: *Clinical Uses of Fluorides.* Philadelphia, Lea & Febiger, 1985, pp. 105–131.

44. **American Dental Association,** Council on Dental Therapeutics: Guidelines for the Acceptance of Fluoride-containing Dentifrices, *J. Am. Dent. Assoc., 110,* 545, April, 1985.

45. **Stratemann,** M.W. and Shannon, I.L.: Control of Decalcification in Orthodontic Patients by Daily Self-administrated Application of a Water-free 0.4 Percent Stannous Fluoride Gel, *Am. J. Orthod., 66,* 273, September, 1974.

46. **Wescott,** W.B., Starcke, E.N., and Shannon, I.L.: Chemical Protection Against Postirradiation Dental Caries, *Oral Surg. Oral Med. Oral Pathol., 40,* 709, December, 1975.

47. **Hodge,** H.C. and Smith, F.A.: Fluoride Toxicology, in Newbrun, E., ed.: *Fluorides and Dental Caries,* 3rd ed. Springfield, IL, Charles C Thomas, 1986, pp. 199–220.

48. **Heifetz,** S.B. and Horowitz, H.S.: The Amounts of Fluoride in Current Fluoride Therapies: Safety Considerations for Children, *ASDC J. Dent. Child., 51,* 257, July–August, 1984.

49. **Bayless,** J.M. and Tinanoff, N.: Diagnosis and Treatment of Acute Fluoride Toxicity, *J. Am. Dent. Assoc., 110,* 209, February, 1985.

50. **Lyon,** T.C.: Topical Fluorides: How Much Are You Using? *Dent. Hyg., 59,* 58, February, 1985.

SUGGESTED READINGS

Barbakow, F., Imfeld, T., and Lutz, F.: Enamel Remineralization: How to Explain It to Patients, *Quintessence Int., 22,* 341, May, 1991.

Bottenberg, P., Bultmann, C., and Gräber, H.G.: Distribution of Fluoride in the Oral Cavity after Application of a Bioadhesive Fluoride-releasing Tablet, *J. Dent. Res., 77,* 68, January, 1998.

Cirincione, U.K.: The Safe Use of Fluorides in Dental Hygiene Practice, *J. Dent. Hyg., 66,* 319, September, 1992.

FDI World Dental Federation: Position Statement on Fluorides and Dental Caries, *FDI World, 4,* 7, September/October, 1995.

Fluoride Supplement Dosage. British Dental Association, the British Society of Paediatric Dentistry and the British Association for the Study of Community Dentistry, *Br. Dent. J., 182,* 6, January 11, 1997.

Ong, Y.S., Williams, B., and Holt, R.: The Effect of Domestic Water Filters on Water Fluoride Content, *Br. Dent. J., 181,* 59, July 20, 1996.

Robinson, S.N., Davies, E.H., and Williams, B.: Domestic Water Treatment Appliances and the Fluoride Ion, *Br. Dent. J., 171,* 91, August 10/24, 1991.

Fluoridation

Brossok, G.E., McTigue, D.J., and Kuthy, R.A.: The Use of a Colorimeter in Analyzing the Fluoride Content of Public Well Water, *Pediatr. Dent., 9,* 204, September, 1987.

Edelstein, B.L., Cottrel, D., O'Sullivan, D., and Tinanoff, N.: Comparison of Colorimeter and Electrode Analysis of Water Fluoride, *Pediatr. Dent., 14,* 47, January/February, 1992.

Grembowski, D., Fiset, L., and Spadafora, A.: How Fluoridation Affects Adult Dental Caries. Systemic and Topical Effects Are Explored, *J. Am. Dent. Assoc., 123,* 49, February, 1992.

Horowitz, H.S.: Grand Rapids: The Public Health Story, *J. Public Health Dent., 49,* 62, Winter, 1989.

Horowitz, H.S.: The Effectiveness of Community Water Fluoridation in the United States, *J. Public Health Dent., 56,* 253, Special Issue, 1996.

Pakhomov, G.N.: The International Milk Fluoridation Programme, *FDI World, 5,* 8, July/August, 1996.

Weinberger, S.J., Johnston, D.W., and Wright, G.Z.: A Comparison of Two Systems for Measuring Water Fluoride Ion Level, *Clin. Prev. Dent., 11,* 19, September–October, 1989.

Supplements

Glass, R.G.: Water Purification Systems and Recommendations for Fluoride Supplementation, *ASDC J. Dent. Child., 58,* 405, September–October, 1991.

Ismail, A.I.: Fluoride Supplements: Current Effectiveness, Side Effects, and Recommendations, *Community Dent. Oral Epidemiol., 22,* 164, June, 1994.

Levy, S.M. and Muchow, G.: Provider Compliance with Recommended Dietary Fluoride Supplement Protocol, *Am. J. Public Health, 82,* 281, February, 1992.

McGuire, S.. Fluoride Content of Bottled Water (Correspondence), *N. Engl. J. Med., 321,* 836, September 21, 1989.

Pendrys, D.G. and Morse, D.E.: Use of Fluoride Supplementation by Children Living in Fluoridated Communities, *ASDC J. Dent. Child., 57,* 343, September–October, 1990.

Stannard, J., Rovero, J., Tsamtsouris, A., and Gavris, V.: Fluoride Content of Some Bottled Waters and Recommendations for Fluoride Supplementation, *J. Pedod., 14,* 103, Number 2, 1990.

Szpunar, S.M. and Burt, B.A.: Evaluation of Appropriate Use of Dietary Fluoride Supplements in the U.S., *Community Dent. Oral Epidemiol., 20,* 148, June, 1992.

Toumba, K.J., Levy, S., and Curzon, M.E.J.: The Fluoride Content of Bottled Drinking Water, *Br. Dent. J., 176,* 266, April 9, 1994.

Dental Fluorosis

Clark, D.C.: Evaluation of Aesthetics for the Different Classifications of the Tooth Surface Index of Fluorosis, *Community Dent. Oral Epidemiol., 23,* 80, April, 1995.

Clark, D.C., Hann, H.J., Williamson, M.F., and Berkowitz, J.: Influence of Exposure to Various Fluoride Technologies on the Prevalence of Dental Fluorosis, *Community Dent. Oral Epidemiol., 22,* 461, December, 1994.

Driscoll, W.S., Horowitz, H.S., Meyers, R.J., Heifetz, S.B., Kingman, A., and Zimmerman, E.R.: Prevalence of Dental Caries and Dental Fluorosis in Areas with Negligible, Optimal, and Above-optimal Fluoride Concentrations in Drinking Water, *J. Am. Dent. Assoc., 113,* 29, July, 1986.

Ellwood, R.P. and O'Mullane, D.: Enamel Opacities and Dental Esthetics, *J. Public Health Dent., 55,* 171, Summer, 1995.

Giambro, N.J., Prostak, K., and Den Besten, P.K.: Characterization of Fluorosed Human Enamel by Color Reflectance, Ultrastructure, and Elemental Composition, *Caries Res., 29,* 251, July–August, 1995.

Ishii, T. and Suckling, G.: The Severity of Dental Fluorosis in Children Exposed to Water with a High Fluoride Content for Various Periods of Time, *J. Dent. Res., 70,* 952, June, 1991.

Lalumandier, J.A. and Rozier, R.G.: Parents' Satisfaction with Children's Tooth Color: Fluorosis as a Contributing Factor, *J. Am. Dent. Assoc., 129,* 1000, July, 1998.

Lalumandier, J.A. and Rozier, R.G.: The Prevalence and Risk Factors of Fluorosis Among Patients in a Pediatric Dental Practice, *Pediatr. Dent., 17,* 19, January/February, 1995.

Lewis, D.W. and Banting, D.W.: Water Fluoridation: Current Effectiveness and Dental Fluorosis, *Community Dent. Oral Epidemiol., 22,* 153, June, 1994.

Lewis, H.A., Chikte, U.M.E., and Butchart, A.: Fluorosis and Dental Caries in Schoolchildren from Rural Areas with about 9 and 1 ppm F in the Water Supplies, *Community Dent. Oral Epidemiol., 20,* 53, February, 1992.

Nowjack-Raymer, R.E., Selwitz, R.H., Kingman, A., and Driscoll, W.S.: The Prevalence of Dental Fluorosis in a School-based Program of Mouthrinsing, Fluoride Tablets, and Both Procedures Combined, *J. Public Health Dent., 55,* 165, Summer, 1995.

Pendrys, D.G.: Risk of Fluorosis in a Fluoridated Population. Implications for the Dentist and Hygienist, *J. Am. Dent. Assoc., 126,* 1617, December, 1995.

Peterson, J.: Solving the Mystery of the Colorado Brown Stain, *J. Hist. Dent., 45*, 57, July, 1997.

Ripa, L.W.: A Critique of Topical Fluoride Methods (Dentifrices, Mouthrinses, Operator-, and Self-applied Gels) in an Era of Decreased Caries and Increased Fluorosis Prevalence, *J. Public Health Dent., 51*, 23, Winter, 1991.

Stookey, G.K.: Review of Fluorosis Risk of Self-applied Topical Fluorides: Dentifrices, Mouthrinses and Gels, *Community Dent. Oral Epidemiol., 22*, 181, June, 1994.

Whitford, G.M.: Acute and Chronic Fluoride Toxicity, *J. Dent. Res., 71*, 1249, May, 1992.

Infant and Preschool

Bentley, E.M., Ellwood, R.P., and Davies, R.M.: Factors Influencing the Amount of Fluoride Toothpaste Applied by the Mothers of Young Children, *Br. Dent. J., 183*, 412, December 13–27, 1997.

Heilman, J.R., Kiritsy, M.C., Levy, S.M., and Wefel, J.S.: Fluoride Concentrations of Infant Foods, *J. Am. Dent. Assoc., 128*, 857, July, 1997.

Levy, S.M., Kiritsy, M.C., Slager, S.L., Warren, J.J., and Kohout, F.J.: Patterns of Fluoride Dentifrice Use Among Infants, *Pediatr. Dent., 19*, 50, January/February, 1997.

Levy, S.M., Kiritsy, M.C., and Warren, J.J.: Sources of Fluoride Intake in Children, *J. Public Health Dent., 55*, 39, Winter, 1995.

Levy, S.M., Kohout, F.J., Guha-Chowdhury, N., Kiritsy, M.C., Heilman, J.R., and Wefel, J.S.: Infants' Fluoride Intake from Drinking Water Alone, and from Water Added to Formula, Beverages, and Food, *J. Dent. Res., 74*, 1399, July, 1995.

Levy, S.M., Kohout, F.J., Kiritsy, M.C., Heilman, J.R., and Wefel, J.S.: Infants' Fluoride Ingestion from Water, Supplements and Dentifrice, *J. Am. Dent. Assoc., 126*, 1625, December, 1995.

Levy, S.M., Maurice, T.J., and Jakobsen, J.R.: Feeding Patterns, Water Sources and Fluoride Exposures of Infants and 1-year-olds, *J. Am. Dent. Assoc., 124*, 65, April, 1993.

Margolis, M.Q., Hunt, R.J., Vann, W.F., and Stewart, P.W.: Distribution of Primary Tooth Caries in First-grade Children from Two Nonfluoridated U.S. Communities, *Pediatr. Dent., 16*, 200, May/June, 1994.

McKnight-Hanes, M.C., Leverett, D.H., Adair, S.M., and Shields, C.P.: Fluoride Content of Infant Formulas: Soy-based Formulas as a Potential Factor in Dental Fluorosis, *Pediatr. Dent., 10*, 189, September, 1988.

Robinson, C. and Kirkham, J.: The Effect of Fluoride on the Developing Mineralized Tissues, *J. Dent. Res., 69*, 685, February, 1990.

Rock, W.P.: Young Children and Fluoride Toothpaste, *Br. Dent. J., 177*, 17, July 9, 1994.

Shulman, J.D. and Wells, L.M.: Acute Fluoride Toxicity from Ingesting Home-use Dental Products in Children, Birth to 6 Years of Age, *J. Public Health Dent., 57*, 150, Summer, 1997.

Skotowski, M.C., Hunt, R.J., and Levy, S.M.: Risk Factors for Dental Fluorosis in Pediatric Dental Patients, *J. Public Health Dent., 55*, 154, Summer, 1995.

Van Winkle, S., Levy, S.M., Kiritsy, M.C., Heilman, J.R., Wefel, J.S., and Marshall, T.: Water and Formula Fluoride Concentrations: Significance for Infants Fed Formula, *Pediatr. Dent., 17*, 305, July/August, 1995.

Williams, J.E. and Zwemer, J.D.: Community Water Fluoride Levels, Preschool Dietary Patterns, and the Occurrence of Fluoride Enamel Opacities, *J. Public Health Dent., 50*, 276, Summer, 1990.

Periodontal Relationship

Bansal, G.S., Newman, H.N., and Wilson, M.: The Survival of Subgingival Plaque Bacteria in an Amine Fluoride-containing Gel, *J. Clin. Periodontol., 17*, 414, August, Part I, 1990.

Grembowski, D., Fiset, L., Spadafora, A., and Milgrom, P.: Fluoridation Effects on Periodontal Disease among Adults, *J. Periodont. Res., 28*, 166, May, 1993.

Mengel, R., Wissing, E., Schmitz-Habben, A., and Florès-de-Jacoby, L.: Comparative Study of Plaque and Gingivitis Prevention by AmF/SnF$_2$ and NaF, A Clinical and Microbiological 9-month Study, *J. Clin. Periodontol., 23*, 372, April, 1996.

Paine, M.L., Slots, J., and Rich, S.K.: Fluoride Use in Periodontal Therapy: A Review of the Literature, *J. Am. Dent. Assoc., 129*, 69, January, 1998.

Ravald, N. and Birkhed, D.: Factors Associated with Active and Inactive Root Caries in Patients with Periodontal Disease, *Caries Res., 25*, 377, September–October, 1991.

Topical Fluorides

Adair, S.M.: The Role of Fluoride Mouthrinses in the Control of Dental Caries: A Brief Review, *Pediatr. Dent., 20*, 101, March/April, 1998.

Cooper, M.D. and Kracher, C.M.: Topical Fluorides, *RDH, 18*, 26, February, 1998.

Øgaard, B., Seppä, L., and Rølla, G.: Professional Topical Fluoride Applications—Clinical Efficacy and Mechanism of Action, *Adv. Dent. Res., 8*, 190, July, 1994.

Ripa, L.W.: Review of the Anticaries Effectiveness of Professionally Applied and Self-applied Topical Fluoride Gels, *J. Public Health Dent., 49*, 297, Special Issue, 1989.

Wei, S.H.Y. and Chik, F.F.: Fluoride Retention Following Topical Fluoride Foam and Gel Application, *Pediatr. Dent., 12*, 368, November/December, 1990.

Varnish

Arends, J., Duschner, H., and Ruben, J.L.: Penetration of Varnishes into Demineralized Root Dentine *in vitro*, *Caries Res., 31*, 201, May–June, 1997.

Bravo, M., Baca, P., Llodra, J.C., and Osorio, E.: A 24-month Study Comparing Sealant and Fluoride Varnish in Caries Reduction on Different Permanent First Molar Surfaces, *J. Public Health Dent., 57*, 184, Summer, 1997.

Bravo, M., Garcia-Anllo, I., Baca, P., and Llodra, J.C.: A 48-month Survival Analysis Comparing Sealant (Delton) with Fluoride Varnish (Duraphat) in 6- to 8-year-old Children, *Community Dent. Oral Epidemiol., 25*, 247, June, 1997.

Clark, D.C.: A Review on Fluoride Varnishes: An Alternative Topical Fluoride Treatment, *Community Dent. Oral Epidemiol., 10*, 117, July, 1982.

Clark, D.C., Hanley, J.A., Geoghegan, S., and Vinet, D.: The Effectiveness of a Fluoride Varnish and a Desensitizing Toothpaste in Treating Dentinal Hypersensitivity, *J. Periodont. Res., 20*, 212, March, 1985.

Mandel, I.D.: Guest Editorial: Fluoride Varnishes—A Welcome Addition, *J. Public Health Dent., 54*, 67, Spring, 1994.

Petersson, L.G., Magnusson, K., Andersson, H., Deierborg, G., and Twetman, S.: Effect of Semi-annual Applications of a Chlorhexidine/Fluoride Varnish Mixture on Approximal Caries Incidence in Schoolchildren. A Three-year Radiographic Study, *Eur. J. Oral Sci., 106*, 623, April, 1998.

Petersson, L.G., Twetman, S., and Pakhomov, G.N.: The Efficiency of Semiannual Silane Fluoride Varnish Applications: A Two-year Clinical Study in Preschool Children, *J. Public Health Dent., 58*, 57, Winter, 1998.

Seppä, L., Leppänen, T., and Hausen, H.: Fluoride Varnish Versus Acidulated Phosphate Fluoride Gel: A 3-year Clinical Trial, *Caries Res., 29*, 327, September–October, 1995.

Seppä, L. and Tolonen, T.: Caries Preventive Effect of Fluoride Varnish Applications Performed Two or Four Times a Year, *Scand. J. Dent. Res., 98*, 102, April, 1990.

Dentifrices

Beltrán, E.D. and Szpunar, S.M.: Fluoride in Toothpastes for Children: Suggestion for Change, *Pediatr. Dent., 10*, 185, September, 1988.

Chan, J.C.Y. and O'Donnell, D.: Ingestion of Fluoride Dentifrice by a Group of Mentally Handicapped Children During Toothbrushing, *Quintessence Int., 27*, 409, June, 1996.

DenBesten, P. and Ko, H.S.: Fluoride Levels in Whole Saliva of Preschool Children After Brushing with 0.25g (pea-sized) as Compared to 1.0g (full-brush) of a Fluoride Dentifrice, *Pediatr. Dent., 18*, 277, July/August, 1996.

Horowitz, H.S.: The Need for Toothpastes with Lower than Conventional Fluoride Concentrations for Preschool-aged Children, *J. Public Health Dent., 52,* 216, Summer, 1992.

Jensen, M. and Kohout, F.: The Effect of a Fluoridated Dentifrice on Root and Coronal Caries in an Older Adult Population, *J. Am. Dent. Assoc., 117,* 829, December, 1988.

Levy, S.M.: A Review of Fluoride Intake from Fluoride Dentifrice, *ASDC J. Dent. Child., 60,* 115, March–April, 1993.

Naccache, H., Simard, P.L., Trahan, L., Brodeur, J.-M., Demers, M., and Lachapelle, D.: Factors Affecting the Ingestion of Fluoride Dentifrice by Children, *J. Public Health Dent., 52,* 222, Summer, 1992.

Rolla, G., Øgaard, B., and deAlmeida Cruz, R.: Clinical Effect and Mechanism of Cariostatic Action of Fluoride-containing Toothpastes: A Review, *Int. Dent. J., 41,* 171, June, 1991.

Fluoride Programs

Driscoll, W.S., Nowjack-Raymer, R., Selwitz, R.H., Li, S.-H., and Heifetz, S.B.: A Comparison of the Caries-preventive Effects of Fluoride Mouthrinsing, Fluoride Tablets, and Both Procedures Combined: Final Results after Eight Years, *J. Public Health Dent., 52,* 111, Winter, 1992.

Haugejorden, O., Lervik, T., Birkeland, J.M., and Jorkjend, L.: An 11-year Follow-up Study of Dental Caries after Discontinuation of School-based Fluoride Programs, *Acta Odontol. Scand., 48,* 257, August, 1990.

Heidmann, J., Poulsen, S., Arnbjerg, D., Kirkegaard, E., and Laurberg, L.: Caries Development after Termination of a Fluoride Rinsing Program, *Community Dent. Oral Epidemiol., 20,* 118, June, 1992.

Holland, T.J., Whelton, H., O'Mullane, D.M., and Creedon, P.: Evaluation of a Fortnightly School-based Sodium Fluoride Mouthrinse 4 Years Following Its Cessation, *Caries Res., 29,* 431, November–December, 1996.

Horowitz, H.S., Meyers, R.J., Heifetz, S.B., Driscoll, W.S., and Li, S.-H.: Combined Fluoride, School-based Program in a Fluoride-deficient Area: Results of an 11-year Study, *J. Am. Dent. Assoc., 112,* 621, May, 1986.

Sterritt, G.R., Frew, R.A., Rozier, R.G., and Brunelle, J.A.: Evaluation of a School-based Fluoride Mouthrinsing and Clinic-based Sealant Program on a Non-fluoridated Island, *Community Dent. Oral Epidemiol., 18,* 288, December, 1990.

Trubman, A., Silberman, S.L., and Meydrech, E.F.: Treatment Costs for Carious Primary Teeth Related to Fluoride Exposure, *ASDC J. Dent. Child., 58,* 69, January–February, 1991.

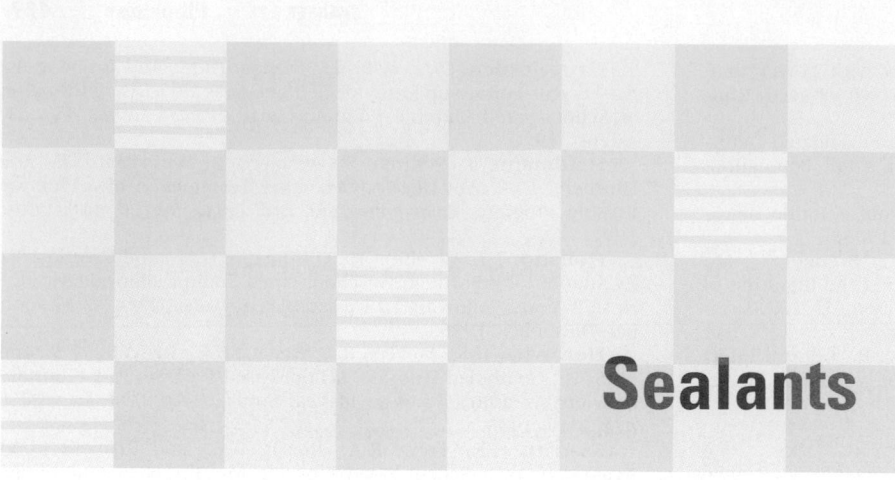
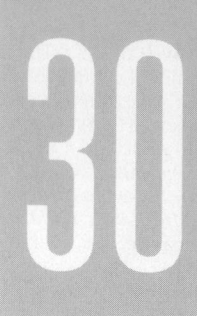

Sealants

As part of a complete preventive program, pit and fissure sealants are indicated for selected patients. Because topically or systemically applied fluorides protect smooth tooth surfaces more than occlusal surfaces, a method to reduce the incidence of occlusal dental caries is needed. The incidence of new pit and fissure caries can be lowered significantly by the application of adhesive sealants. Box 30-1 provides definitions and terminology relative to sealants and their application.

Other preventive measures used for and by the patient are necessary. Sealant application should be part of a complete prevention program, not an isolated procedure. As an isolated procedure, patient (and parent) may misunderstand the selected area of prevention that this measure represents. Other surfaces and other teeth still need other methods of preventive protection.

DEVELOPMENT OF SEALANTS

Sealants were developed by Dr. Michael Buonocore and the group of dental scientists at the Eastman Dental Center in Rochester, New York. The focus of the early research was on the need to prepare the enamel surface so that a dental material would adhere. They demonstrated that by using an acid etch process, the enamel could be altered to increase retention. The research proved to be a major breakthrough, particularly in esthetic and preventive dentistry.[1,2]

HOW SEALANTS WORK

I. DEFINITION

A pit and fissure sealant is an organic polymer (resin) that flows into the pit or fissure and bonds to the enamel surface mainly by mechanical retention.

II. ACTION

A. Purpose of the Sealant
  1. To provide a physical barrier to "seal off" the pit or fissure.
  2. To prevent oral bacteria and their nutrients from collecting within the pit or fissure to create the acid environment necessary for the initiation of dental caries.
  3. To fill the pit or fissure as deep as possible.

BOX 30-1 KEY WORDS AND ABBREVIATIONS: Pit and Fissure Sealants

Acid etchant: in sealant placement, the enamel surface is prepared by the application of phosphoric acid, which etches the surface to provide mechanical retention for the sealant.

Articulating paper: an inked ribbon held between teeth to determine tooth contacts.

Bibulous (bib'ū-lus): absorbent; a flat bibulous pad, placed in the cheek over the opening of Stensen's duct, is used to aid in maintaining a dry field while placing sealants.

Biocompatibility: the ability of things to exist together without harm.

Bis-GMA: bisphenol A-glycidyl methylacrylate; plastic material used for dental sealants.

Bonding (mechanical): physical adherence of one substance to another; the adherence of a sealant to the enamel surface is accomplished by an acid-etching technique that leaves microspaces between the enamel rods; the sealant becomes mechanically locked (bonded) in these microspaces

Bond strength: expression of the degree of adherence between the tooth surface and the sealant.

Conditioner (kon-dish'un-er): a substance added to another substance to increase its usability; in sealant placement, the acid etchant is added to the enamel to prepare it for bonding with the sealant.

Curing: the process by which plastic becomes rigid.

Incipient caries: beginning caries, caries limited to the enamel.

In vitro (vē'tro): under laboratory conditions.

In vivo (vē'vo): within the living body.

Micropores: tiny openings.

Polymer (pol'ĭ-mer): a compound of high molecular weight formed by a combination of a chain of simpler molecules (monomers).

Polymerization: a reaction in which a high-molecular-weight product is produced by successive additions of a simpler compound.

Photopolymerization: polymerization with the use of an external light source.

Autopolymerization (aw"tō-pol"ĭ-mer"ĭ-zā'shun): self-curing; a reaction in which a high-molecular-weight product is produced by successive additions of a simpler compound; hardening process of pit and fissure sealants.

Sealant: organic polymer that bonds to an enamel surface by mechanical retention accommodated by projections of the sealant into micropores created in the enamel by etching; the two types of sealants, filled and unfilled, both are composed of Bis-GMA.

Filled sealant: contains, in addition to Bis-GMA, microparticles of glass, quartz, silica, and other fillers used in composite restorations; fillers make the sealant more resistant to abrasion.

Viscosity: in general, the resistance to flow or alteration of shape by any substance as a result of molecular cohesion.

When sealant material is worn or cracked away on the surface around the pit or fissure, the sealant in the depth of the micropore can remain and provide continued protection.

B. Purpose of the Acid Etch
1. To produce irregularities or micropores in the enamel.
2. To allow the liquid resin to penetrate into the micropores and create a bond or mechanical locking. Figure 30-1 illustrates the sealant placed on a smooth enamel surface in contrast with placement on an etched surface with retention.

SEALANT MATERIALS

I. CRITERIA FOR THE IDEAL SEALANT[1]
A. Achieve prolonged bonding to enamel.
B. Be biocompatible with oral tissues.
C. Offer a simple application procedure.
D. Be a free-flowing, low viscosity material capable of entering narrow fissures.
E. Have low solubility in the oral environment.

II. CLASSIFICATION OF TYPES OF SEALANTS
A majority of sealants in clinical use are made of Bis-GMA (bisphenol A–glycidyl methylacrylate). The techniques of application vary slightly among available products.

The American Dental Association has a program for evaluation and acceptance of pit and fissure sealants.[3] The three types of sealants currently available are filled, unfilled, and fluoride-releasing filled. Sealants are also identified by the method required for polymerization.

A. Classification by Method of Polymerization
1. *Self-Cured or Autopolymerized*
   a. Preparation: the material is supplied in two parts. When the two are mixed they quickly polymerize (harden).

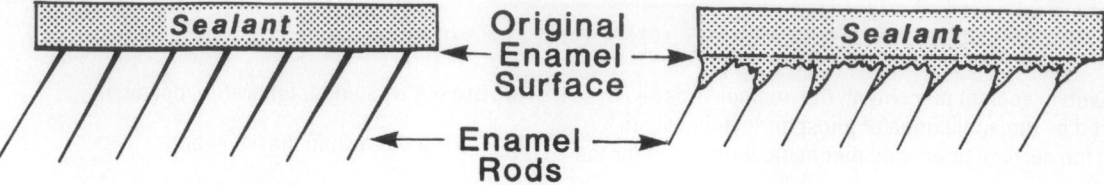

Non-Etched Surface   Etched Surface

■ **FIGURE 30-1 Enamel–Sealant Interface.** Diagram of enamel–sealant interface to compare nonetched surface with etched surface. Etching produces microscopic porosities in the enamel to increase the area of retention. The unpolymerized resin flows into the porosities and hardens in tag-like projections, as shown on the right. (Adapted from Buonocore, M.G., Matsui, A., and Gwinnett, A.J.: Penetration of Resin Dental Materials into Enamel Surfaces with Reference to Bonding, *Arch. Oral Biol., 13,* 61, 1968.)

b. Advantages: no special equipment required.
c. Disadvantages: mixing required; working time limited because polymerization begins when the material is mixed.
2. *Visible-Light-Cured or Photopolymerized*
  a. Preparation: the material hardens when exposed to a special curing light.
  b. Advantages: no mixing required; increased working time due to control over start of polymerization.
  c. Disadvantages: extra costs and disinfection time required for curing light, protective shields, and/or glasses.

B. Classification by Filler Content
1. *Filled*
  a. Purpose of filler: to increase abrasion resistance, bond strength, and wear.
  b. Fillers: glass and quartz particles.
  c. Effect: viscosity of the sealant is increased. Flow into the depth of a fissure varies.
2. *Unfilled*
3. *Fluoride-Releasing*
  a. Purpose: enhance caries resistance.
  b. Action: remineralization of incipient caries at base of pit or fissure.

D. Classification by Color
1. Available: clear, tinted, and opaque.
2. Purpose: quick identification for evaluation during maintenance assessment.
3. Effect: clear, tinted, or opaque sealants do not differ in retention.

INDICATIONS FOR SEALANT PLACEMENT

I. PATIENTS WITH RISK FOR DENTAL CARIES (ANY AGE)

A. Xerostomia: from medications or other reasons.
B. Patient undergoing orthodontics.

C. Incipient caries: when the caries is limited to the enamel.

II. TEETH

A. Newly erupted: as soon after eruption as possible.
B. Occlusal contour: when pit or fissure is deep and irregular.
C. Caries history: other teeth restored or have carious lesions.

III. CONTRAINDICATIONS

A. Radiographic evidence of proximal dental caries.
B. Pit and fissures are well coalesced and self-cleansing; low caries risk.

IV. SELECTION OF TEETH

Figure 30-2 is a flowchart to assist in decision making.

CLINICAL PROCEDURES

I. GENERAL RULES

A. Treat each quadrant separately.
B. Use four-handed method with assistant
  1. To ensure moisture control.
  2. To work efficiently and save time.
C. Follow manufacturer's directions for each product.
D. Success of treatment (retention) depends on the precision in each step of the application.
E. Retention of sealant depends on maintaining a dry field during etching and sealant placement.
F. Steps in procedure: follow the outline in Table 30-1.

II. PREPARATION OF TOOTH

A. Purposes
  1. Remove deposits and debris.

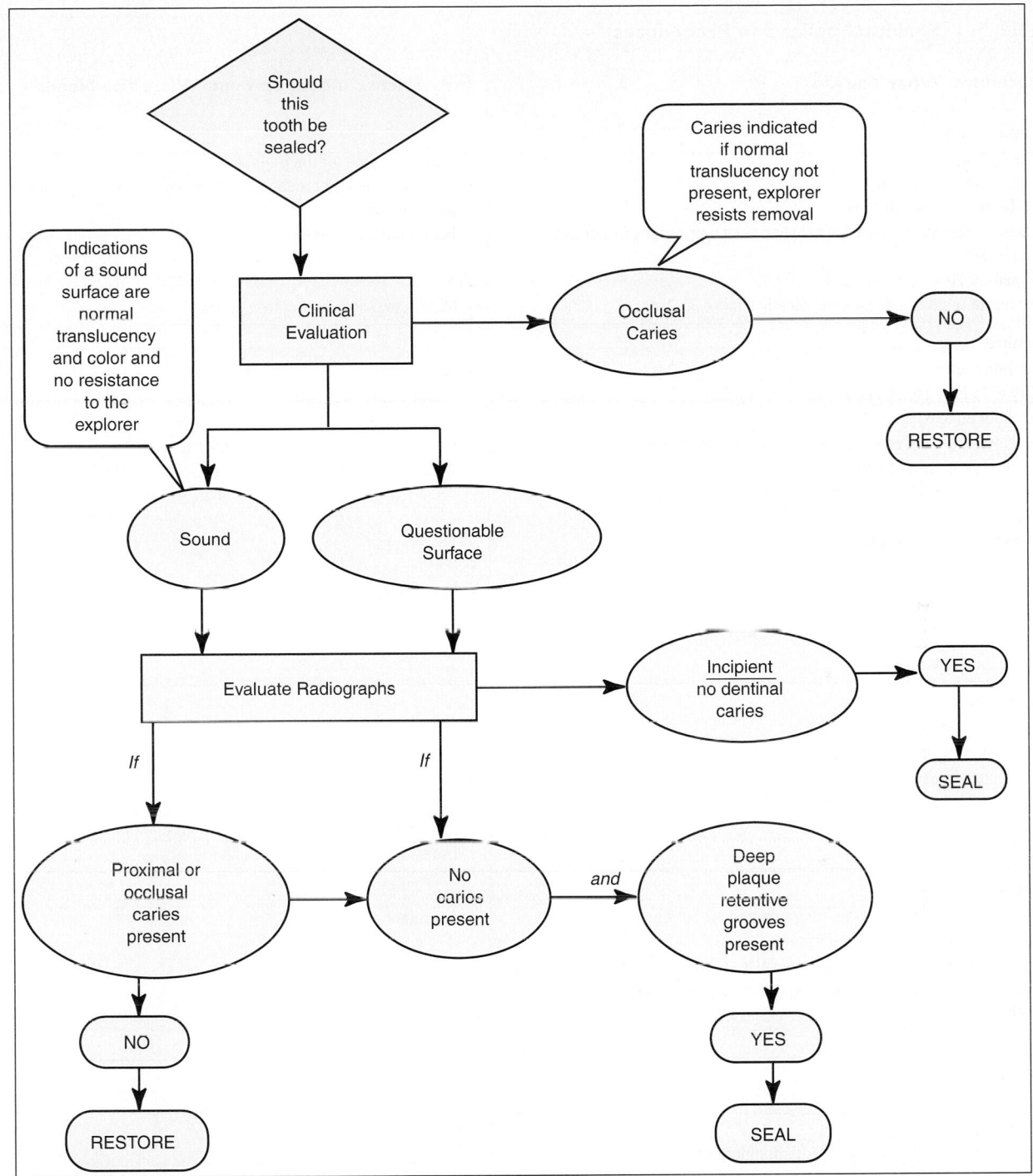

■ **FIGURE 30-2 Tooth Selection for Sealant Placement.** Flow chart to assist in decision-making for placement of sealants.

2. Permit maximum contact of the etch and the sealant with the enamel surface.
3. Encourage sealant penetration into the pit or fissure.

B. Examine the Surfaces: Remove calculus and heavy stains.

C. Patient With No Stain or Calculus
1. Request patient to brush; apply filaments straight into occlusal pits and fissures (see Figure 23-12A, page 364).
2. Suction the pits and fissures with high-velocity evacuator.
3. Use sharp explorer tip to dig out debris and bacteria from the pit or fissure.
4. Suction again to remove loosened material.
5. Evaluate for additional cleaning; the brushing may be sufficient.

TABLE 30-1 Sealant Application Procedures

Procedure: What You Do	Instruments and Equipment: What You Need
Preparation • Set up tray • Seat patient comfortably • **Debride** occlusal surface • Use toothbrush, air-powder polisher device or prophy brush and pumice • **Rinse** for 20 to 30 seconds • **Evaluate** teeth to be sealed clinically (Figure 30-2)	• Safety glasses for the patient • Prophy angle and brushes, tooth brush, or an air-powder polishing unit • Plain flour of pumice • Mirror, explorer, and cotton pliers

Etching
• **Isolate** area
• **Dry** area for 20 to 30 seconds with tri-syringe
• **Etch** for 30 to 60 seconds
• Gel: brush on surface and leave in contact without disturbing it
• Liquid: cover surface and continue to keep surface wet by adding additional etch throughout etch time
• *Do not rub*
• **Rinse** until surface is free of etch
• Gel: 60 seconds
• Liquid: 30 seconds
• **Re-isolate** area
• **Dry** for 20 seconds and check for chalky appearance
• *If not chalky, re-etch*
	• Isolation materials:
	    Rubber dam setup or
	    Cotton rolls and holders, bibulous pads
	• Brushes or cotton pellets to dispense etch
	• Acid etch material (15%–50%) phosphoric acid
	
	• Tri-syringe
	• High-speed suction
	• Saliva ejector

Application • **Apply** sealant material • Mix autopolymerized sealant material prior to placement • Light cured needs no mixing • **Cure** while maintaining a dry field	• Sealant material • Brushes or flow tubes or cannulas to dispense sealant material • Mixing sticks (if using self-cured) • Material tray or waxed paper pad • Ultraviolet safety glasses or shield for clinician • Timer or watch with a second hand
Evaluation • Evaluate the placed sealant for voids and air bubbles • Add additional sealant if necessary • Re-etch prior to placement of material if salivary contamination occurs • Check occlusion with articulating paper, adjust if sealant interferes with occlusion • Floss contact areas	• Articulation paper • Dental floss
Follow-up • Educate the patient • Administer fluoride treatment • Re-evaluate at each subsequent appointment	• Fluoride gel and trays

D. Cleansing Procedure: Choices:

1. Polishing cup and brush with pumice; low-speed handpiece
   a. Disadvantage: pumice particles become lodged in the pits and not rinsed out.
   b. Alternative: use bristle brush with clear water.
2. Air-powder polisher[4,5]

III. ISOLATION

A. Purposes of Isolation

1. Keep the tooth clean and dry for optimal action and bonding of the sealant.

2. Eliminate possible contamination by saliva and moisture from the breath.
3. Keep the materials from contacting the oral tissues, being swallowed accidentally, or being unpleasant to the patient because of flavor.

B. Rubber Dam

1. Rubber dam application is the method of choice because the most complete isolation is obtained. This method is especially helpful when more than one tooth must be sealed.
2. Rubber dam is essential when profuse saliva flow and overactive tongue and oral muscles

make retraction and consistent maintenance of a dry, clean field impossible.

3. Combined treatment should be planned. When a quadrant has a rubber dam and anesthesia for restoration of other teeth, teeth indicated for sealant may be treated.

4. Use anesthesia when application of the clamp can not be tolerated by the patient.

5. Rubber dam may not be possible when a tooth that is essential for holding the clamp is not fully erupted.

C. Cotton-Roll Isolation

1. Patient position: tilt head to allow saliva to pool on the opposite side of the mouth.

2. Position cotton roll holder (Garmer holder for mandibular arch; see Figure 29-4 page 467).

3. Place saliva ejector.

4. Apply triangular saliva absorber over the opening of the parotid duct in the cheek (bibulous pad).

5. Take great care to prevent contamination from entering the area to be etched.

IV. DRY THE TOOTH

A. Purposes

1. Prepare the tooth for acid etch.
2. Eliminate moisture and contamination.

B. Use Clean Air

1. Clear the air by releasing the spray into a sink.
2. Test for absence of moisture by blowing on a mirror or other dry surface.

C. Time: Air dry the tooth for at least 10 seconds.

V. ACID ETCHING

A. Action

1. Create micropores to increase the surface area and provide retention for the sealant.
2. Remove contamination from enamel surface.
3. Provide antibacterial action.

B. Etch Forms

1. *Phosphoric acid:* 15% to 50%, depends on product and manufacturer.
2. *Liquid:* Low viscosity allows good flow into pit or fissure but may be difficult to control.
3. *Gel:* Tinted gel with thick consistency allows increased visibility and control but may be difficult to rinse off the tooth surface.
4. *Semi-gel:* Tinted with viscosity between the gel form and the liquid allows good visibility, control, and rinsing ease.

C. Etch Timing: varies from 15 to 60 seconds. Follow manufacturer's instructions for each product.

D. Etch Delivery

1. Liquid etch

a. Use a small brush, sponge, or cotton pellet.

b. Apply continuously throughout the etch time to keep the surface moist.

2. Gel and semi-gel: use a syringe, brush, or manufacturer-supplied single-use cannula.

E. Completion of Etching

1. Rinse thoroughly; apply suction to prevent saliva from reaching the etched surface.
2. Dry, and examine the etched surface.
3. Repeat etching process if the surface does not appear white and chalky.
4. Dry for 15 to 20 seconds; maintain isolation ready for sealant application.

VI. SEALANT APPLICATION

A. Follow Manufacturer's Instructions

B. General Instructions

1. Avoid overmanipulation to prevent producing air bubbles.
2. Use disposable implement supplied.
3. Cover all pits and fissures but do not overfill to a high, flat surface.
4. After placement: leave in place for 10 seconds to allow for optimum penetration.

C. Curing

1. *Timing:* 20 to 30 seconds in accord with manufacturer's instructions. Longer curing time is related to increased retention.
2. *Apply curing light:* Use eye protection. Cover entire tooth surface to allow complete polymerization.
3. *Check for voids:* Material can be added if surface has not been contaminated or wet.

VII. OCCLUSION[6,7]

A. Use articulating paper to locate high spots; adjust as required.

B. Occlusal wear: unfilled sealants wear down to correct height; filled sealants require occlusal adjustment.

PENETRATION OF SEALANT

The penetration of a sealant depends on the configuration of the pit or fissure, the presence of deposits and debris within the pit or fissure, and the properties of the sealant itself.

I. PIT AND FISSURE ANATOMY

A review of the anatomy of pits and fissures may be helpful in understanding the effects of sealants in the prevention of dental caries. The shape and depth of pits and fissures vary considerably even within one tooth.

Long narrow pits and grooves reach to, or nearly to, the dentinoenamel junction. Others are *wide V-shaped* or *narrow V-shaped,* whereas still others may have a

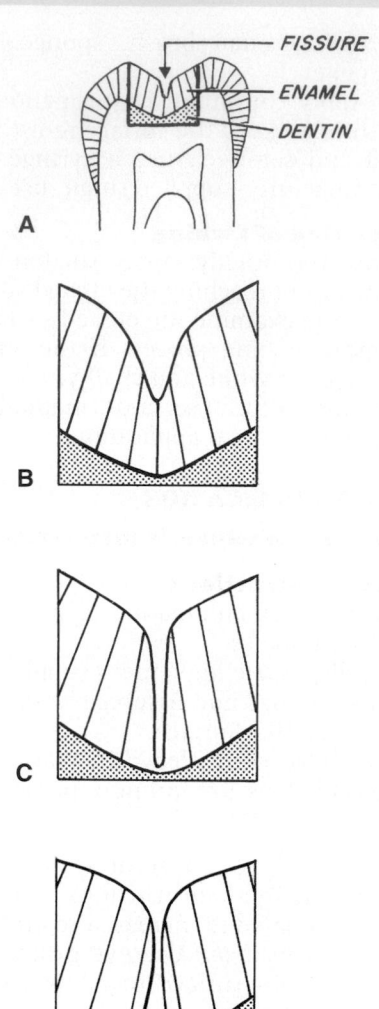

FIGURE 30-3 Occlusal Fissures. Drawings made from microscopic slides show variations in shape and depth of fissures. **(A)** Tooth with section enlarged for B, C, and D. **(B)** Wide V-shaped fissure. **(C)** Long narrow groove that reaches nearly to the dentinoenamel junction. **(D)** Long constricted form with a bulbous terminal portion.

long constricted form with a bulbous terminal portion (Figure 30-3). The pit or fissure may take a wavy course; thus, it may not lead directly from the outer surface to the dentinoenamel junction.

II. CONTENTS OF A PIT OR FISSURE

A pit or fissure contains bacterial plaque, pellicle, debris, and sometimes relatively intact remnants of tooth development.

III. EFFECT OF CLEANING

The narrow, long fissures are difficult to clean completely. Retained cleaning material can block the sealant from filling the fissure and can also become mixed with the sealant. Removal of pumice used for cleaning and thorough washing are necessary to the success of the sealant.

IV. AMOUNT OF PENETRATION

Wide V-shaped and shallow fissures are more apt to be filled by sealant (Figure 30-4B). Although ideally the sealant should penetrate to the bottom of a pit or fissure, such penetration is frequently impossible. Microscopic examination of pits and fissures after sealant application has shown that the sealant does not penetrate to the bottom because residual debris, cleansing agents, and trapped air prevent passage of the material (Figure 30-4C and D).

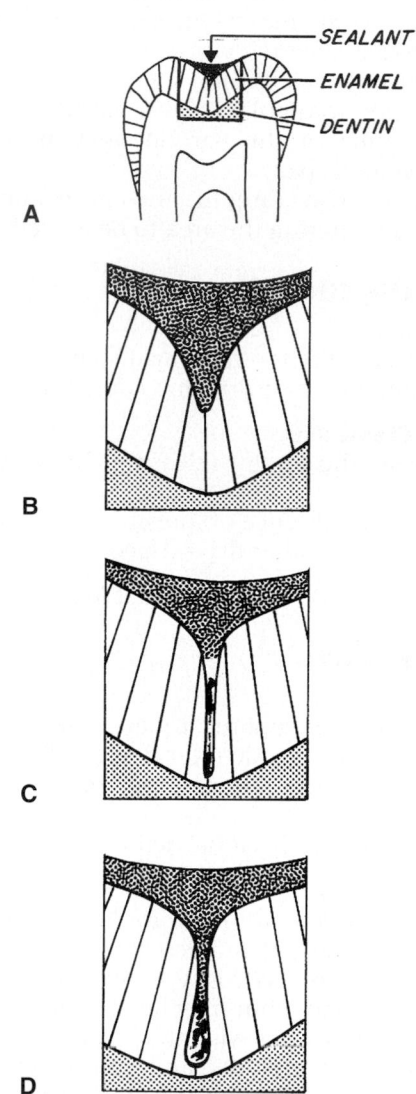

FIGURE 30-4 Pit and Fissure Sealant in Fissures. Drawings made from microscopic slides show extent to which sealant fills a fissure. **(A)** Tooth with section enlarged for B, C, and D. **(B)** Sealant fills wide V-shaped fissure and extends a short way up the slopes of surrounding cusps. **(C)** and **(D)** Fissures partially filled as a result of narrow constriction of the groove and blockage by trapped debris.

MAINTENANCE

I. RE-EXAMINATION

At each maintenance appointment, or at least every 6 months, each sealant should be examined for deficiencies that may have developed.

II. RETENTION

A. Retention Time

Sealants can be retained for many years.[8] Although surface sealant may be lost, sealant in the pits and fissures and sealant that penetrated into the microspaces of the enamel still remain and provide protection.[9]

B. Retention Factors

1. *During placement*
   a. Precision of technique.
   b. Exclusion of moisture and contamination during placement.
2. *Care of existing restorations.* Avoid using an air-powder polisher on intact existing sealants during maintenance appointments. Sealant wear increases with time of exposure to air-powder polisher abrasion.[10]

III. REPLACEMENT

A. Consult the manufacturer's instructions.
B. Tooth preparation: same as for original application.
C. Removal of sections of retained sealant is not usually necessary.
D. Re-etching of the tooth surface is always essential.

TECHNICAL HINTS

I. SEALANTS AND DENTAL CARIES

The effectiveness of sealants in prevention of dental caries is directly related to retention of the material, and the retention of the material is directly related to the precision of techniques during the placement. Precision of techniques is directly related to the conscientiousness and skills of the clinician.

II. RECORDS

Document in the patient's record the type of sealant used. Manufacturer's directions for replacement of a broken or lost sealant may vary.

III. UNIT DOSING

Sealant materials are available in multidose containers and unit dose containers. The risk of cross contamination is reduced with unit doses. Cleaning up at chairside is simplified with disposal of a unit dose container.

IV. EYE PROTECTION

The patient must wear safety eyewear for both protection from the chemicals of etching and sealant, but also from the light of the curing lamp.

V. CARE OF MATERIALS

Heed manufacturer's directions for care and storage of all materials.

FACTORS TO TEACH THE PATIENT

I. Sealants are part of a total preventive program. Sealants are not substitutes for other preventive measures, including limitations of dietary sucrose, use of fluorides, and bacterial plaque control.
II. What a sealant is and why such a meticulous application procedure is required.
III. What can be expected from a sealant; how long it lasts, how it prevents dental caries.
IV. Need for examination of the sealant at frequent, scheduled appointments, and need for replacement when indicated.

REFERENCES

1. **Handleman**, S.L. and Shey, Z.: Michael Buonocore and the Eastman Dental Center: A Historic Perspective on Sealants, *J. Dent. Res.,* 75, 529, January, 1996.
2. **Cueto**, E.I. and Buonocore, M.G.: Sealing of Pits and Fissures With an Adhesive Resin. Its Use in Caries Prevention, *J. Am. Dent. Assoc.,* 75, 121, July, 1967.
3. **American Dental Association**, Council on Access, Prevention and Interprofessional Relations: Council on Scientific Affairs: Dental Sealants, *J. Am. Dent. Assoc., 128,* 485, April, 1997.
4. **Scott**, L., Brockmann, S., Houston, G., and Tira, D.: Retention of Dental Sealants Following the Use of Airpolishing and Traditional Cleaning, *Dent. Hyg., 62,* 402, September, 1988.
5. **Brockmann**, S.L., Scott, R.L., and Eick, J.D.: A Scanning Electron Microscopic Study of the Effect of Air Polishing on the Enamel-sealant Surface, *Quintessence Int., 21,* 201, March, 1990.
6. **Stach**, D.J., Hatch, R.A., Tilliss, T.S., and Cross-Poline, G.N.: Change in Occlusal Height Resulting from Placement of Pit and Fissure Sealants, *J. Prosthet. Dent., 68,* 750, November, 1992.
7. **Tilliss**, T.S.I., Stach, D.J., Hatch, R.A., and Cross-Poline, G.N.: Occlusal Discrepancies after Sealant Therapy, *J. Prosthet. Dent., 68,* 223, August, 1992.
8. **Simonsen**, R.J.: Retention and Effectiveness of Dental Sealant after 15 years, *J. Am. Dent. Assoc., 122,* 34, October, 1991.
9. **Buonocore,** M.G.: Pit and Fissure Sealing, *Dent. Clin. North Am., 19,* 367, April, 1975.
10. **Huennekens,** S.C., Daniel, S.J., and Bayne, S.C.: Effects of Air Polishing on the Abrasion of Occlusal Sealants, *Quintessence Int., 22,* 581, July, 1991.

SUGGESTED READINGS

American Dental Association, Council on Access, Prevention and Interprofessional Relations: Caries Diagnosis and Risk Assessment, *J. Am. Dent. Assoc., 126,* 1S-24S, Supplement, June, 1995.

Daniel, S.J., Grose, M.D., Scruggs, R.R., and Stoltz, R.F.: Examiner Reliability in Evaluating Dental Sealants, *Dent. Hyg., 61,* 410, September, 1987.

Daniel, S.J., Scruggs, R.R., and Grady, J.J.: The Accuracy of

Student Self-evaluations of Dental Sealants, *J. Dent. Hyg., 64,* 339, September, 1990.

Llodra, J.C., Bravo, M., Delagado-Rodriguez, M., Baca, P., and Galvez, R.: Factors Influencing the Effectiveness of Sealants—A Meta-analysis, *Community Dent. Oral Epidemiol., 21,* 261, October, 1993.

Nathanson, D., Lertpitayaklin, P., Lamkin, M.S., Edalatpour, M., and Chou, L.C.: In Vitro Elution of Leachable Components from Dental Sealants, *J. Am. Dent. Assoc., 128,* 1517, November, 1997.

Ripa, L.W.: Sealants Revisited: An Update of the Effectiveness of Pit-and-fissure Sealants, *Caries Res., 27,* 77, Supplement 1, 1993.

Selwitz, R.H., Colley, B.J., and Rozier, R.G.: Factors Associated With Parental Acceptance of Dental Sealants, *J. Public Health Dent., 52,* 137, Spring, 1992.

Clinical Procedures

Carstensen, W.: The Effects of Different Phosphoric Acid Concentrations on Surface Enamel, *Angle Orthod., 62,* 51, Spring, 1992.

Ellingson, P. and Nickerson, A.: Successful Sealant Placement. Discussion of One Technique, *J. Practical Hyg., 1,* 9, November/December, 1992.

Feigal, R.J., Hitt, J., and Splieth, C.: Retaining Sealant on Salivary Contaminated Enamel, *J. Am. Dent. Assoc., 124,* 88, March, 1993.

Lehtinen, R. and Kuusilehto, A.: Absorption of UVA Light by Latex and Vinyl Gloves, *Scand. J. Dent. Res., 98,* 186, April, 1990.

Marcushamer, M., Neuman, E., and Garcia-Godoy, F.: Fluoridated and Nonfluoridated Unfilled Sealants Show Similar Shear Strength, *Pediatr. Dent., 19,* 289, May/June, 1997.

Poulos, J.G. and Styner, D.L.: Curing Lights: Changes in Intensity Output With Use Over Time, *Gen. Dent., 45,* 70, January–February, 1997.

Waggoner, W.F. and Siegal, M.: Pit and Fissure Sealant Application: Updating the Technique, *J. Am. Dent. Assoc., 127,* 351, March, 1996.

Other Sealant Techniques

Croll, T.P.: The Quintessential Sealant? *Quintessence Int., 27,* 729, November, 1996.

Croll, T.P. and Cavanaugh, R.R.: Direct Bonded Class I Restorations and Sealants: Six Options, *Quintessence Int., 28,* 157, March, 1997.

DeCraene, G.P., Martens, C., and Dermaut, R.: The Invasive Pit-and-Fissure Sealing Technique in Pediatric Dentistry: An SEM Study of a Preventive Restoration, *ASDC J. Dent. Child., 55,* 34, January–February, 1988.

doRego, M.A. and deAraújo, M.A.M.: A 2-Year Clinical Evaluation of Fluoride-containing Pit and Fissure Sealants Placed With an Invasive Technique, *Quintessence, Int., 27,* 99, February, 1996.

Feldens, E.G., Feldens, C.A., deAraújo, F., and Souza, M.A.L.: Invasive Technique of Pit and Fissure Sealants in Primary Molars: A SEM Study, *J. Clin. Pediatr. Dent., 18,* 187, Spring, 1994.

Garcia-Godoy, F., Summitt, J.B., and Donly, K.J.: Caries Progression of White Spot Lesions Sealed With an Unfilled Resin, *J. Clin. Pediatr. Dent., 21,* 141, Winter, 1997.

Kramer, P.F., Zelante, F., and Simionato, M.R.L.: The Immediate and Long-term Effects of Invasive and Noninvasive Pit and Fissure Sealing Techniques on the Microflora in Occlusal Fissures of Human Teeth, *Pediatr. Dent., 16,* 108, March/April, 1993.

Mertz-Fairhurst, E.J., Curtis, J.W., Ergle, J.W., Rueggeberg, F.A., and Adair, S.M.: Ultraconservative and Cariostatic Sealed Restorations: Results at Year 10, *J. Am. Dent. Assoc., 129,* 55, January, 1998.

V

TREATMENT

INTRODUCTION

Instrumentation for scaling, root planing, extrinsic stain removal, care of dental restorations, debonding, and postcare procedures are included in Part V. Placement and removal of dressings, removal of sutures, and treatment of hypersensitive teeth are described. Immediate evaluation of techniques and their effects, short-term follow-up, and maintenance assessment follow instrumentation. These procedures are all part of *nonsurgical periodontal therapy*.

The first objective of treatment is to create an environment in which the tissues can return to health. In the sequence of patient treatment, introduction to preventive measures occurs first, before professional instrumentation.

After health has been attained, the patient's self-care on a daily basis is essential to keep the teeth and gingival tissues free from new or recurrent disease caused by the microorganisms of bacterial plaque. Professional instrumentation makes a limited contribution to arresting the progression of disease without daily plaque control measures performed by the patient.

I. ORAL PROPHYLAXIS: DEFINITION DILEMMA

The term *oral prophylaxis* refers to those specific treatment procedures aimed at removing local irritants to the gingiva, including complete calculus removal with bacterial debridement. A smooth tooth surface resists the retention of dental deposits. The oral prophylaxis performed with these objectives is truly a *preventive periodontal treatment procedure*.[1]

There is a definite need for clarification and new terminology for the various services performed under the title "oral prophylaxis." Through common usage, oral prophylaxis has taken on a variety of meanings.

Because *prophylaxis* means *prevention of disease*, then *oral prophylaxis*, as the *prevention of oral disease*, should include such preventive procedures as restoring individual teeth, replacing missing teeth, adjusting the occlusion, correcting faulty proximal contacts, and many other procedures, the basic purposes of which are preventive.[2]

Unfortunately, the term "oral prophylaxis" also is sometimes used to mean a superficial 5- to 10-minute application of a rubber polishing cup with an abrasive paste to the enamel surfaces that appear above the gingival margin. The term "oral prophylaxis" obviously must be carefully and specifically defined if it is to be applied to the comprehensive treatment services of a dental hygienist.

In the development of a meaningful concept of the oral prophylaxis upon which the procedures and anticipated outcomes described in this book are based, the only acceptable definition is based on the preventive aspects of periodontal infections.

II. OBJECTIVES OF TREATMENT

Specific objectives for each type of instrumentation are included in the chapter that describes the details of the technique. General objectives of dental hygiene instrumentation are to

A. Create an environment in which the tissues can return to health and then be maintained in health.

B. Eliminate or suppress periodontal pathogenic microorganisms and control reinfection.

C. Aid in the prevention and control of gingival and periodontal infections by removal of factors that predispose to the retention of bacterial plaque. Factors particularly implicated are dental calculus and irregular and overhanging restorations.

D. Compose the total treatment needed for certain patients with uncomplicated disease, and the initial preparatory phase of treatment for others with more advanced disease.

E. Assist in the maintenance phase of care to prevent recurrence of disease.

F. Provide the patient with smooth tooth surfaces, which are easier to clean and to keep plaque-free by daily self-care procedures.

G. Assist in instructing the patient in the appearance and feeling of a thoroughly clean mouth as a motivation toward the development of adequate habits of personal oral care.

H. Prepare the teeth and gingiva for dental procedures, including those performed by the restorative dentist, prosthodontist, orthodontist, pedodontist, and oral surgeon.

I. Improve oral esthetics and sanitation.

REFERENCES

1. *World Workshop in Periodontics*. Ann Arbor, University of Michigan, 1966, p. 450.
2. **Bunting**, R.W.: *Oral Hygiene*, 3rd ed. Philadelphia, Lea & Febiger, 1957, p. 233.

Anxiety and Pain Control

Concern for patient anxiety and pain is an integral part of a dental hygiene appointment. Recognizing and managing a patient's anxiety and pain is an essential part of dental hygiene care planning. The decision to use a pharmacologic agent for management of anxiety and pain is dependent upon a number of factors. Periodontal health status, the treatment being rendered, and patient's pain threshold must all be considered. Pain threshold is highly individual and variable. Box 31-1 provides terminology and definitions relative to anxiety and pain and to their management.

COMPONENTS OF PAIN

There are two components of pain. Pain perception is primarily a neurologic experience of pain; pain reaction is the personal interpretation and response to the pain message.

I. PAIN PERCEPTION

   A. Relates to the physical process of receiving a painful stimulus and transmitting the information through the nervous system to the brain.
   B. In the brain it is interpreted as pain.
   C. There is little variability in pain perception between individuals with intact nervous systems.

II. PAIN REACTION

   A. The reaction is a combination of the interpretation and the response to the pain message.
   B. The reaction is highly variable between individuals and even in the same individual at different times.
   C. Accounts for much of the variability seen between patients in personal pain management needs.
   D. Many factors influence pain reaction. Factors included are age, fatigue, emotional state, and both cultural and ethnic learned behaviors.
   E. The presence of anxiety has special significance because with anxiety the patient is predisposed to feel pain.
   F. People with a strong or rapid reaction to pain are said to have a low pain threshold.

PAIN CONTROL MECHANISMS

Five pain control mechanisms are available. They are often combined for optimum effect. The five categories are:

I. REMOVE THE PAINFUL STIMULUS

   A. Affects pain perception.
   B. Examples: patient avoids dental appointment; clinician corrects faulty, pain-causing instrument technique.

II. BLOCK THE PATHWAY OF THE PAIN MESSAGE

   A. Affects pain perception.
   B. Examples: use of local anesthetic, topical anesthetic.

III. PREVENT PAIN REACTION BY RAISING PAIN REACTION THRESHOLD

   A. Affects pain reaction.
   B. Examples: use of nitrous oxide–oxygen conscious sedation; nonsteroidal anti-inflammatory drugs (NSAIDs).

IV. DEPRESS CENTRAL NERVOUS SYSTEM

   A. Affects pain reaction.
   B. Example: general anesthesia.

V. USE PSYCHOSOMATIC METHODS (ALSO CALLED IATROSEDATION)

   A. Affects both pain perception and pain reaction.
   B. Includes any nonpharmacologic technique that reduces patient anxiety, builds a trust relationship, or lets the patient feel more in control.
   C. May be used alone or may be combined with pharmacologic pain management.
   D. Examples: explain procedures carefully; allow patient to express concerns; use relaxation or distraction techniques.

NITROUS OXIDE–OXYGEN SEDATION

The gases nitrous oxide and oxygen, in combination, are widely used in dental and dental hygiene practice settings. A state of conscious sedation is produced with the patient awake, relaxed, responsive to commands, able to cooperate with treatment, and having intact protective reflexes. The patient has some degree of analgesia and a higher pain reaction threshold.

CHARACTERISTICS OF NITROUS OXIDE

I. ANESTHETIC AND ANALGESIC PROPERTIES

   A. Produces analgesia.
   B. Achieves optimum analgesia and patient cooperation at 30% to 40% nitrous oxide for most patients. The need for higher or lower concentrations depends on individual biologic variability.
   C. Reduces the intensity of pain but does not block it; only mildly potent as an anesthetic gas.
   D. Combines with local anesthetic when the patient experiences significant discomfort.

BOX 31-1 KEY WORDS: Anxiety and Pain Control

Ambient air: surrounding atmosphere.

Analgesia (an"al-je'ze-ah): diminution or elimination of pain in the conscious patient.

Anesthesia (an"es-the'zhah): loss of feeling or sensation, especially loss of tactile sensitivity, with or without loss of consciousness.

Block anesthesia: induced by injecting the anesthetic close to a nerve trunk; may be at some distance from the area to be treated.

General anesthesia: the elimination of all sensations, accompanied by the loss of consciousness.

Infiltration anesthesia: induced by injecting the anesthetic directly into or around the tissues to be anesthetized.

Local anesthesia: loss of sensation, especially pain, in a circumscribed area without loss of consciousness; also called regional anesthesia.

Topical anesthesia: a form of local anesthesia whereby free nerve endings in accessible structures are rendered incapable of stimulation by the application of an anesthetic drug directly to the surface of the area.

Anxiety: a negative, emotional response to an anticipated event, the outcome of which is unknown. This is a learned response from personal experience or the stories of others.

Aspiration: recommended technique for preventing injection of local anesthetic directly into circulatory system. Negative pressure is created in anesthetic cartridge. If needle tip is in artery or vein, blood will be visible in cartridge.

Conscious: state in which patient is capable of rational response to commands and protective reflexes are intact, including the ability to maintain a patent airway independently and continuously.

Conscious sedation: the calming or allaying of nervous excitement while maintaining a conscious state by pharmacologic, nonpharmacologic, or combined methods.

Epinephrine: a hormone secreted by the adrenal medulla that, among many functions, causes vasodilation of blood vessels of skeletal muscles, vasoconstriction of arterioles of skin and mucous membranes, and stimulation of heart action; used in local anesthetics for its vasoconstrictive action.

Hypoxia (hi-pok'se-ah): diminished availability of oxygen to body tissues.

Diffusion hypoxia: lack of adequate amounts of oxygen that can result from the rapid diffusion of nitrous oxide molecules from the blood stream into the lungs. Occurs if 100% oxygen is not administered at the conclusion of a nitrous oxide–oxygen sedation procedure.

Iatrosedation: reduction of anxiety as a result of the clinician's behavior or actions. A psychosomatic method of pain control.

Metered spray: a method for dispensing topical anesthetic that administers a fixed volume of drug and then stops automatically.

Occupational exposure: subject to an action or influence, usually negative, as a result of one's occupation or work environment.

Pain: a sensation in which a person experiences discomfort, distress, or suffering; may vary in intensity from mild discomfort to intolerable agony.

Pain threshold: point at which a sensation starts to be painful and a response results. Varies between individuals based on interpretation of sensation. May be altered by some drugs.

High pain threshold: a greater than average tolerance to a painful stimulus.

Low pain threshold: a strong or rapid reaction to a painful stimulus.

Potency: strength of a drug. Amount of a medication or drug necessary to achieve a desired effect.

Psychosomatic method: any nonpharmacologic technique that reduces anxiety and improves pain control. Effective because the mind influences the body's perception and interpretation of pain.

Scavenging device: that part of the nitrous oxide equipment that collects exhaled nitrous oxide and removes it. The main component is the scavenging nasal hood. Since 1980 the American Dental Association has recommended that effective scavenging devices be installed whenever nitrous oxide is used to reduce occupational exposure.

Sedation: one of the stages of anesthesia in which the patient is still conscious but is under the influence of a central nervous system depressant drug.

Titration: a technique for individualization of drug dose. Administration of small, incremental dose of a drug until the desired clinical action is observed.

Vasoconstrictor: a drug that constricts blood vessels. An additive to most local anesthetic solutions to offset the vasodilating actions of the local anesthetic.

II. CHEMICAL AND PHYSICAL PROPERTIES

A. Gas at room temperature and pressure.
B. Heavier than air; accumulates near the floor in a still room.
C. Colorless; sweet smelling.
D. Nonirritating and nonallergenic.
E. Nonflammable but will support the combustion of flammable substances.

III. BLOOD SOLUBILITY

A. Relatively insoluble in blood; primary saturation of blood occurs in 3 to 5 minutes.[1]
B. The gas molecules at the alveoli-blood interface and blood-brain interface pass readily to the tissue with the lowest concentration of nitrous oxide.
   1. Results in rapid onset and recovery.
   2. Results in potential diffusion hypoxia at completion of sedation procedure if 100% oxygen is not administered.

IV. PHARMACOLOGY OF NITROUS OXIDE

A. Is not metabolized in the body; remains unchanged in blood and tissues.
B. Enters and exits almost entirely through the lungs.

EQUIPMENT

The equipment for nitrous oxide–oxygen conscious sedation is available as a portable unit or a central storage system with gas piped to individual treatment rooms. Currently available units have several built-in safety features to ensure that a minimal level of oxygen is always delivered and that the two gases could not be reversed inadvertently in delivery. The equipment can be divided into three basic parts: gas storage cylinders, a gas delivery portion, and a scavenger system with the nasal hood (mask) having components of both the gas delivery and scavenger portions.

I. COMPRESSED GAS CYLINDERS

A. Nitrous Oxide
   1. *Color code:* Light blue.
   2. *Physical state:* Gas and liquid.
   3. *Pressure:* Constant at 750 pounds per square inch (psi) until almost empty.

B. Oxygen
   1. *Color code:* Green (international = white).
   2. *Physical state:* Gas.
   3. *Pressure:* Falls at a uniform rate with use from a full pressure of 2000 psi or 2200 psi for size E or H cylinders, respectively.
   4. *Use ratio:* About 2.5 cylinders of oxygen are used for each comparably sized one of nitrous oxide.

C. Handle Carefully
   1. Use no grease, oil, lubricant, or hand cream around the cylinder valves or any fittings that come in contact with the gases.
   2. Store vertically on a rack or in other stable and secure manner.
   3. Open cylinder valves slowly in a counterclockwise direction.

II. GAS DELIVERY SYSTEM

A. Regulator or Reducing Valve
   1. Converts high pressure of gas in the cylinders to a usable, lower level.
   2. Subject to extreme high temperature if compressed gas cylinders are opened quickly.

B. Flow Meter
   1. Visual indicator of liters per minute (lpm) flow of oxygen and nitrous oxide.
   2. Flow meter comes in two designs:
      a. Gas flow rates of nitrous oxide and oxygen are adjusted independently. The sum of the two is the total gas flow rate.
      b. A total combined gas flow rate is established and the respective concentrations of the two gases are adjusted concurrently.

C. Reservoir Bag
   1. Reservoir of gases to accommodate an exceptionally deep breath.
   2. Allows for visualization of respirations for monitoring.
   3. Degree of inflation can be used to help establish total flow rate of gas needed by the patient for comfortable respirations.
   4. May be used to provide oxygen in assisted ventilation if attached to a full face mask.

D. Conducting or Breathing Tubes

III. NASAL HOOD, NOSE PIECE, MASK

A. Deliver gas for patient inhalation.
B. Collect exhaled gas and direct it into scavenger system.
C. Good fit and seal around patient's nose are important in size selection.
D. Ideally a disposable item, or sterilize before each use.

IV. SCAVENGER SYSTEM

A. Removes exhaled gas to keep nitrous oxide levels low in the ambient air of the treatment room.
B. Connects to the office high-speed evacuation system.
C. Vents to outside of building and away from windows and air intakes.

V. SAFETY FEATURES

A. Universal color coding of tanks, hoses, flow controls for each gas.
B. Pin index and diameter index safety systems

physically prevent gas cylinders or hoses from being mistakenly interchanged between the gases.

C. Minimum oxygen flow, usually 2 to 3 lpm.

D. Oxygen fail-safe system automatically shuts off nitrous oxide if the oxygen falls below a minimum level.

E. Emergency air inlet to provide room air if system shuts down.

F. Oxygen flush button to supply 100% oxygen quickly.

VI. EQUIPMENT MAINTENANCE

A. Function Checks

Maintain working order and safe practice by periodic checking of equipment.

B. Gas Leaks

All equipment connections and rubber goods are subject to leaking. Figure 31-1 shows the places that should be examined for tight connections, defects, and wear. Apply soapy water to connections; bubbles will form if leaks are present.

PATIENT SELECTION

I. INDICATIONS

A. Patient with mild to moderate anxiety.

B. Medically compromised patient who would benefit from additional oxygen and/or anxiety reduction. Examples: patient with a cardiovascular or cerebrovascular disease, or with stress-induced bronchial asthma.

C. Procedures that are short in duration and cause a low level of pain. The analgesic effect is most pronounced on the soft tissues, making it especially useful during dental hygiene procedures.

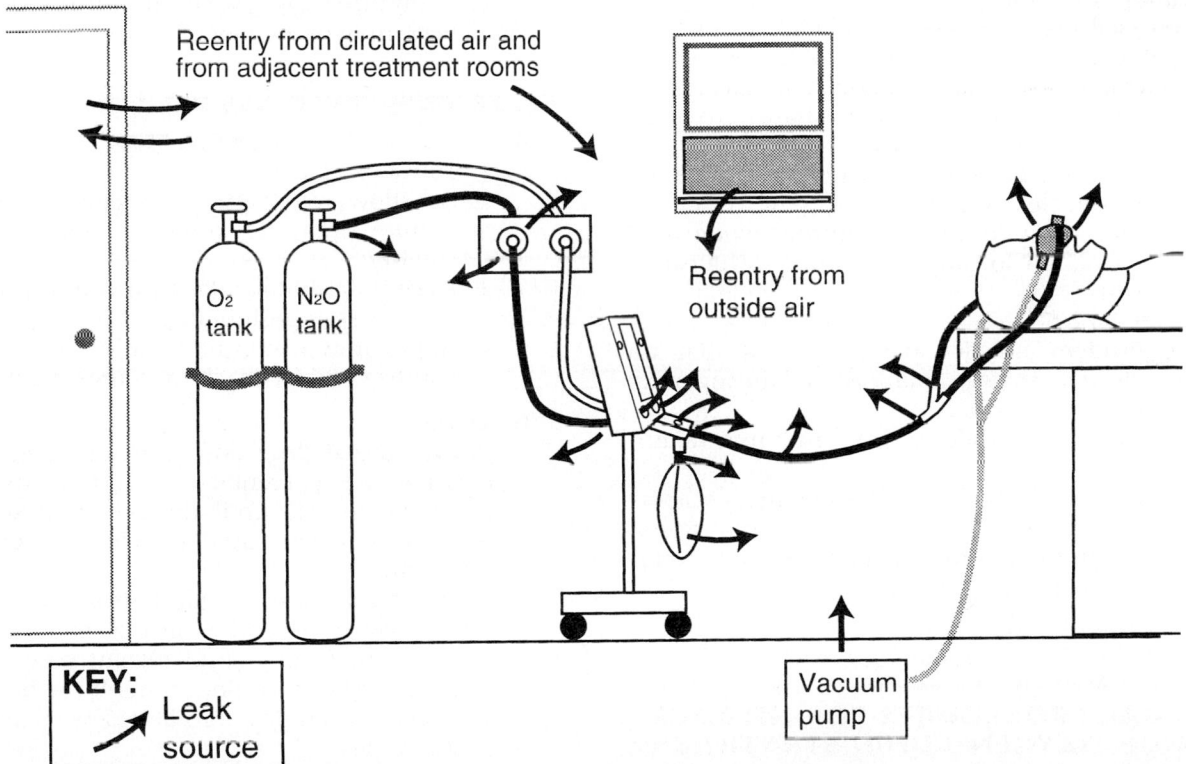

FIGURE 31-1 Potential Sources of Leaks from Nitrous Oxide–Oxygen Delivery Systems. Arrows show locations where regular inspection and testing is necessary. The most common sites of leakage are: *High-pressure connections:* from the gas delivery tanks, the wall connectors, the hoses connecting to the anesthesia machine, and the anesthesia machine itself (especially the on-demand valve). *Low-pressure connections:* from the anesthetic flow meter and the scavenging mask. Look for loose-fitting connections, loosely assembled or deformed slip joints and threaded connections, defective or worn seals, and gaskets. *Rubber goods:* hoses and reservoir bag. Look for cracks and tears. (Adapted from **NIOSH:** *Alert: Controlling Exposures to Nitrous Oxide During Anesthetic Administration.* [NIOSH Publication No. 94-100]. Cincinnati, U.S. Department of Health, Education, and Welfare, Public Health Service, Centers for Disease Control and Prevention, National Institute for Occupational Safety and Health, 1994, p. 5).

II. CONTRAINDICATIONS

There are no absolute contraindications to the use of nitrous oxide. It is nonirritating to the respiratory system and does not interact chemically or biotransform within the body. There are no known allergies.

There are a few relative contraindications or conditions for which nitrous oxide–oxygen sedation may not be either effective or the optimum choice for pain management. Individuals with the following conditions should be evaluated carefully before nitrous oxide–oxygen sedation:

A. Unable to cooperate and/or communicate
1. Unwilling to breathe through nose and/or leave nasal hood in place.
2. Claustrophobia.
B. Moderate to severe chronic obstructive pulmonary disease (COPD). Example: emphysema, chronic bronchitis.
C. Upper respiratory tract obstruction or infection if nose breathing would be difficult or breathing apparatus cannot be sterilized or replaced.
D. Conditions of confined air spaces within the body that would be adversely affected by increased pressure, such as middle ear or tympanic membrane problems, blockage of Eustachian tube or sinuses, bowel obstruction.
E. Severe personality disorders characterized by a tenuous grasp on reality.
F. Compulsive personalities who do not like the feeling of "losing control."
G. Patients who do not want nitrous oxide–oxygen sedation for any of a variety of personal reasons.
H. Pregnancy
1. Prudent practice would suggest that no elective drugs be administered during pregnancy.
2. Drug is considered safe and non-teratogenic.
3. Increased incidence of spontaneous abortion can result from chronic exposure but not from occasional patient exposure to nitrous oxide.

CLINICAL PROCEDURES FOR NITROUS OXIDE–OXYGEN ADMINISTRATION

I. PATIENT PREPARATION

A. Inform
1. Explain procedure in positive terms. Stress the pleasant sense of relaxation; the patient will be aware and in control at all times.
2. Establish informed consent.

B. Assess
1. Evaluate patient's medical status.
2. Take and record vital signs.

C. Other Instructions for Patient
1. No specific food limitations but generally avoid fasting or heavy meals just before the appointment.
2. Wear comfortable clothing and loosen tight collars.
3. Remove contact lenses, especially hard contacts. Gas leaks around nasal hood can cause extreme drying of the eyes.

II. EQUIPMENT PREPARATION

A. Nasal Hood
1. Select the appropriate size for optimum comfort and minimum gas leakage.
2. Attach to tubing.

B. Scavenger System
1. Connect, usually to high-speed volume evacuation, and activate system.
2. Adjust setting of scavenger system.

C. Turn on Gas Tanks
1. Open slowly, first oxygen, then nitrous oxide.
2. Centralized gas systems are turned on at the beginning of the day.

III. TECHNIQUE FOR GAS DELIVERY

A. Establish Volume of Gas Flow
1. 100% oxygen.
2. Gas flow rate between 5 and 7 liters per minute (lpm) for adults, 3 and 4 lpm for children.
3. Place nasal hood, adjust for comfort; patient may assist in positioning.
4. Adjust flow using the inflation of the reservoir bag and feedback from the patient.

B. Titration
Individualized drug dose is determined by increasing the percentage of nitrous oxide in small increments until the optimum sedation level is achieved based on clinical signs and symptoms.
1. *Initial Concentration.* Start titration at about 20% concentration of nitrous oxide. Because of the rapid uptake of nitrous oxide in the lungs and distribution through the body, the effect of each dose can be assessed after 1 to 2 minutes.
2. *Patient Response.* Observe the patient for signs of relaxation or other changes. Ask the patient what is felt. Use the patient's signs and symptoms to determine when the optimum level of sedation has been reached. Table 31-1 lists signs and symptoms for various levels of nitrous oxide–oxygen sedation.
3. *Adjust Dose.* Increase or decrease the nitrous oxide by 5% to 10% when the optimum individual dose has not been achieved. Wait 1 to 2 minutes and reassess. Repeat as needed.

TABLE 31-1   Correlation of Signs and Symptoms to Levels of N₂O-O₂ Sedation

Levels	Symptoms	Signs
1. Early to ideal sedation	Light-headedness (dizziness) Tingling of hands and feet Body warmth Feeling of vibration throughout body Numbness of hands and feet Numbness of soft tissues of oral cavity Feeling of euphoria Feeling of lightness or heaviness in extremities Analgesia	Blood pressure, heart rate slightly elevated early in procedure, then return to base-line values Respirations are normal Peripheral vasodilation Flushing of extremities, face Decreased muscle tone as anxiety decreases (arms and legs relax)
2. Heavier sedation/slight oversedation	Hearing, especially of distant sounds, becomes more acute Visual images become confused (patterns on ceiling begin to move) Sleepiness Laughing, crying Dreaming Nausea	Movement increases Heart rate, blood pressure increase Rate of respiration increases Sweating increases Possible tearing
3. Oversedation	Nausea	Vomiting Loss of consciousness

Adapted from Malamed, S.F.: *Sedation, A Guide to Patient Management*, 3rd ed. St. Louis, Mosby, 1995, p. 260.

a. Distribution of optimum sedation dose for different individuals follows a bell curve. For about 70% of patients, the ideal is in the 30% to 40% nitrous oxide range.[2]

b. At high altitudes, greater nitrous oxide concentrations will be needed because of the change in the partial pressure of the gases.

4. *Time.* Allow approximately 5 minutes for titration.

5. *Monitor.* Continue to monitor and adjust the concentration throughout the appointment. As the appointment proceeds or during less anxiety-producing parts of the appointment, a lower dose may be more comfortable. Avoid excessive fluctuations.

6. *Attend Patient.* Do not leave a sedated patient unattended; sedation can become deeper without some stimulation or interaction.

7. *Outcome.* Titration increases clinical success rate of nitrous oxide–oxygen conscious sedation and decreases adverse responses.

IV. COMPLETION OF SEDATION

A. Recovery

1. *Procedure.* At the completion of sedation, return the patient to 100% oxygen for at least 3 to 5 minutes or longer if needed for full recovery.

2. *Factors Affecting Recovery Time.* Biologic variation, duration of sedation procedure, and concentration of nitrous oxide administration. Generally, the more nitrous oxide administered, the longer the recovery time.

3. *Signs of Recovery.* Patient's report of feeling "back to normal," comparable presedation and postsedation vital signs, and the return of fine motor skills.

B. Diffusion Hypoxia

If patient is returned directly to room air rather than 100% oxygen, diffusion hypoxia can result.

1. Nitrous oxide diffuses into an area of lower concentration more rapidly than oxygen, causing inadequate oxygen in the alveoli if the patient is not given supplemental oxygen at the completion of sedation.

2. Hypoxia can result in patient discomfort or syncope.

C. Dismissal Follows Full Recovery

Usually the patient is able to return to all normal activities, including driving.

D. Record Keeping

1. Presedation and postsedation vital signs.

2. Concentrations of both nitrous oxide and oxygen administered.

3. Total liter per minute (lpm) flow of gas.

4. Length of time for sedation procedure.

5. Length of time on recovery oxygen.

6. Statement of patient's recovery status and postcare instructions given.

7. Summary of patient's response to nitrous oxide can be helpful for subsequent appointments.

POTENTIAL HAZARDS OF OCCUPATIONAL EXPOSURE[3,4]

Chronic occupational exposure to nitrous oxide may have deleterious effects on health. Overexposure must be prevented.

I. ISSUES OF OCCUPATIONAL EXPOSURE

A. Potential Health Problems
1. Reduced fertility with as little as 3 to 5 hours of unscavenged nitrous oxide exposure per week.[5]
2. Spontaneous abortion.[6]
3. Increased rate of neurologic, renal, and liver disease.[6]
4. Decreased mental performance, audiovisual ability, and manual dexterity.[3]

B. Recommended Exposure Levels
1. Consensus has not been reached on occupational exposure limits.
2. National Institute of Occupational Safety and Health (NIOSH) recommends no more than 25 parts per million (ppm) during administration.

II. METHODS FOR MINIMIZING OCCUPATIONAL EXPOSURE

A. Use an effective scavenging system.
B. Maintain equipment and inspect regularly for gas leaks, especially at the locations shown in Figure 31-1. Shut off and secure equipment at the end of each day's use.
C. Improve general air quality: introduce fresh air, use a nonrecycling air-conditioning system, or open a window. Vent the scavenger system gases outside the building and away from windows and air intakes.
D. Use an air sweep fan to direct nitrous oxide away from the clinicians' breathing zone; periodically monitor air quality in the clinicians' breathing zone.
E. Minimize patient conversations and mouth breathing; fit the nasal hood carefully to avoid leaks.
F. Set conservative limits on the duration and concentration of nitrous oxide use per patient.

ADVANTAGES AND DISADVANTAGES OF CONSCIOUS SEDATION ANESTHESIA

I. ADVANTAGES

A. Both a mild analgesic and sedative: reduces patient's perception of pain; increases relaxation and cooperation during treatment.

B. Reduces the gag reflex.
C. Very safe with few side effects and few medical contraindications.
D. Excellent for management of many medically compromised patients:
1. Provides oxygen enrichment as well as stress reduction.
2. Helps prevent emergencies because of anxiety and pain management.
E. Readily absorbed and excreted from the body; rapid onset and recovery from drug effect:
1. Able to titrate to optimum level.
2. Recovery complete so patient can be dismissed to return to normal activities.
F. Appointments less stressful for clinician because of relaxed, conscious, cooperative patient.

II. DISADVANTAGES

A. A low-potency analgesic drug
1. Not effective with all patients because of low potency; does not block all perception.
2. Severely distressed or phobic patient may need a more potent drug or combination of drugs.
B. Patient must be able and willing to breathe through the nose.
C. Equipment and gases are expensive.
D. Use of poor techniques such as failure to titrate or use a scavenger system results in undesirable patient experiences and potential staff health risks.
E. Potential for recreational abuse by health professionals.
F. May stimulate sexual fantasies in some patients and any resulting accusations can result in embarrassment, loss of reputation, and/or license.

LOCAL ANESTHESIA

Local anesthesia is the main modality for the management of dental pain. It blocks sensations, especially of pain, from teeth, soft tissues, and bone in the anesthetized area. Root instrumentation without discomfort requires a profound pulpal and periodontal tissue level of anesthesia.[7]

Dental hygiene treatment provided with the use of local anesthesia is a more comfortable and satisfying treatment for both the patient and clinician. Instrumentation can be comprehensive and definitive, and patient compliance can increase.

PHARMACOLOGY OF LOCAL ANESTHETICS[8,9]

Local anesthetics are the most frequently used drugs for dental and dental hygiene treatment. They are safe when administered in the recommended manner and amounts.

I. CONTENTS OF A LOCAL ANESTHETIC CARTRIDGE

A dental cartridge is prefilled by the manufacturer to include the following:

A. *Amide anesthetic:* Blocks the transfer of ions across the nerve membrane, which stops the transmission of pain messages.

B. *Vasoconstrictor:* Constricts local blood vessels to offset the vasodilation caused by the amide anesthetic. Cartridges without vasoconstrictor are available.

C. *Antioxidant:* Preservative for the vasoconstrictor, usually sodium metabisulfite or sodium bisulfite.

D. *Sterile water:* Diluent.

E. *Sodium chloride:* Creates an isotonic match with the body.

II. ESTER AND AMIDE ANESTHETIC DRUGS

Dental local anesthetic drugs can be divided chemically into two major groups: esters and amides. The first dental anesthetic was procaine (Novocain), an ester, which has not been available in dental cartridges in the United States since 1996. Currently used local anesthetic agents are almost exclusively amides. There are a number of available drugs in this group that are similar for safety and effectiveness.

A. General Characteristics of Ester Anesthetics

1. Widely used in topical anesthetic agents.
2. Have a higher incidence of allergic reactions; are less effective and shorter acting compared to amides.
3. Metabolized in the blood plasma by the enzyme cholinesterase. The medical condition atypical plasma cholinesterase may result in the slow removal of the drug from the body.

B. General Characteristics of Amide Anesthetics

1. Extremely low incidence of allergic reactions.
2. Potential for toxicity or drug overdose make attention to detail in technique of administration and total drug dose critical.
3. Metabolized by the liver (see specific medical considerations, page 502).
4. Cause vasodilation of local blood vessels.

III. CHARACTERISTICS OF SPECIFIC SHORT- AND MEDIUM-ACTING AMIDE DRUGS

A. Lidocaine

1. Proprietary names include: Xylocaine, Octocaine, Lignospan.
2. First amide and still most widely used dental anesthetic; also available as a topical.
3. Used with vasoconstrictor to give adequate working time.

B. Mepivacaine

1. Proprietary names include: Carbocaine, Polocaine, Isocaine.
2. Causes less vasodilation than lidocaine; therefore, can be used for short procedures without vasoconstrictor.
3. Mepivacaine 3%, also called mepivacaine plain, is often the drug of choice when vasoconstrictors or their sulfite antioxidants are contraindicated.

C. Prilocaine

1. Proprietary names are: Citanest Plain and Citanest Forte.
2. Least toxic of the amide anesthetics.
3. Metabolic by-products can cause transient methemoglobinemia, a condition that reduces the blood's oxygen-carrying capacity (see specific medical considerations, page 502).
4. Can be used without vasoconstrictor because it causes limited vasodilation.
5. When injected into tissues with limited vascularity, the duration of action is similar with and without vasoconstrictor. Example: inferior alveolar nerve block injection.

D. Articaine

1. Proprietary names are: Ultracaine and Septanest.
2. Not available in the United States.
3. Reported to diffuse through soft and hard tissues better than other amides.
4. Metabolic by-products can cause transient methemoglobinemia.

IV. CHARACTERISTICS OF SPECIFIC LONG-ACTING AMIDE DRUGS

A. Bupivacaine

1. Proprietary name: Marcaine
2. Long-lasting anesthetic with an extended period of analgesia for postcare pain management.
3. May have delayed onset of action.

B. Etidocaine

1. Proprietary name: Duranest
2. Long-lasting anesthetic with an extended period of analgesia for postcare pain management.

V. VASOCONSTRICTORS

A. Reasons for Use

1. *Safety.* Potential for toxic reaction (overdose) to anesthetic is reduced by slowing the rate at which it enters circulation.
2. *Longevity.* Duration of anesthetic effect is increased.
3. *Effectiveness.* Depth and profoundness of anesthetic is increased.
4. *Hemostasis.* Only if drug is locally injected directly into the area.

B. Potential Risks With Use of Vasoconstrictors
1. Hypersensitivity to the drugs.
2. Medical problems (see specific medical considerations, page 502).
3. Drug interactions (see potential drug interactions, page 502).
4. Degree of risk to medically compromised patients, including those with heart disease, varies. Use of vasoconstrictors in low doses is considered safe.[10]

C. Drugs Used
1. *Epinephrine*
   a. Potent sympathomimetic amine.
   b. Used in low concentrations, usually 1:100,000 or 1:200,000.
   c. Maximum recommended doses (MRDs) for healthy patients and for medically compromised, especially those with cardiac disease, are given in Table 31-2.
2. *Levonordefrin* (Neo-Cobefren)
   a. Half as potent as equal doses of epinephrine and with less cardiac effect.
   b. Used at higher concentration (1:20,000) to accomplish adequate vasoconstriction.
   c. Higher doses may result in greater increase in blood pressure than epinephrine.
   d. Maximum recommended doses (MRDs) for healthy patients and for medically compromised, especially those with cardiac disease, are given in Table 31-2.

VI. CRITERIA FOR DRUG SELECTION

Amide local anesthetics are safe and effective when employed properly.[11]
A. Length of time pain control is needed is a primary criterion for drug selection. Table 31-3 shows the typical duration of action for common local anesthetics.

B. Medical status of the patient.
C. Potential for prolonged discomfort after treatment.
D. Potential for self-inflicted injury before anesthetic wears off.

INDICATIONS

Local anesthesia is indicated for treatment that has the potential to cause discomfort or pain. Anesthesia prevents both the patient and the clinician from the anticipation of discomfort, thus allowing both to relax and to make treatment comfortable.

I. DENTAL HYGIENE PROCEDURES

A. Scaling and root planing in areas with probing depths of 4 mm or greater.
B. Extensive instrumentation with either manual or power-driven instruments.
C. Treatment in areas of challenging pocket topography, furcations, or other difficult root anatomy.
D. Instrumentation of sensitive root surfaces.
E. Instrumentation in areas of painful, inflamed soft tissue.
F. Treatments that involve soft tissue manipulation
   1. Gingival curettage
   2. Suture removal
   3. Removal of subgingival overhang
G. Treatment in areas of excessive hemorrhage.

II. PATIENT FACTORS

A. Extent of patient's disease and deposits directly influence the extent or rigor of the needed treatment.
B. Patient's pain reaction or pain threshold.

TABLE 31-2   Vasoconstrictors: Concentrations and Maximum Recommended Dose (MRD)

Vasoconstrictors and Concentrations	MRD, Healthy Patient		MRD, Medically Compromised Patient	
	Mg/appt	Cartridges/appt	Mg/appt	Cartridges/appt
Epinephrine				
1:50,000	Use Not Recommended		Use Not Recommended	
1:100,000 (0.018 mg/cart.)	0.2	10	0.04	2
1:200,000 (0.009 mg/cart.)	0.2	*	0.04	4
Levonordefrin				
1:20,000 (0.09 mg/cart.)	1.0	10	0.2	2

*Local anesthesia is the limiting drug.
Adapted from Biron, C.R.: Vasoconstrictors, *RDH, 13*, 40, May, 1993.

TABLE 31-3   Duration of Action of Common Local Anesthetics

Drug Name	Duration of Action	
Generic Name	Soft Tissue	Pulpal
Short Acting		
3% mepivacaine	2–3 hr	Infiltration: 20 min Block: 40 min
4% prilocaine	Infiltration: 1½ hr	Infiltration: 10 min
Medium Acting		
2% lidocaine w/epinephrine 1:100,000	3–5 hr	60 min
2% mepivacaine w/levonordefrin 1:20,000	3–5 hr	60–90 min
4% prilocaine	Block: 2–4 hr	Block: 60 min
4% prilocaine w/epinephrine 1:200,000	3–8 hr	60 90 min
4% articaine w/epinephrine 1:100,000	3–6 hr	60–75 min
Long Acting		
0.5% bupivacaine w/epinephrine 1:200,000	4–9+ hr	90–180 min
1.5% etidocaine w/epinephrine 1:200,000	4–9 hr	90–180 min

Adapted from Malamed, S.F.: *Handbook of Local Anesthesia,* 4th ed. St. Louis, Mosby, 1997, pp. 55–67.

PATIENT ASSESSMENT

The goal of patient assessment is to ensure an effective and safe local anesthesia experience. Pretreatment evaluation is the first and most important step for avoiding a medical emergency.

I. SOURCES OF INFORMATION FOR COMPLETE PREANESTHETIC ASSESSMENT

A. Vital signs.
B. Medical history, especially ASA status (page 104).
C. Current medications.
D. Emotional status/anxiety level.
E. Dental history related to local anesthesia.
F. Chief complaint and presence of inflammation.

II. TREATMENT OPTIONS BASED ON ASSESSMENT FINDINGS

Amide local anesthetics and the small amount of vasoconstrictor normally incorporated into the dental anesthetic cartridge can be administered safely to almost all patients.

A. Use local anesthetic without special precaution.
B. Avoid use of local anesthetic or of a specific local anesthetic because of high medical risk.
C. Select an alternative drug that will minimize or avoid risk.
D. Limit the dose of drug given at any specific appointment.
E. Use local anesthesia combined with maximum stress management; use in combination with nitrous oxide–oxygen conscious sedation.
F. Seek medical intervention, consult, or additional testing before proceeding.

III. GENERAL MEDICAL CONSIDERATIONS

A. ASA IV patients and some ASA III patients (especially those who are anxious about injections) may not have the functional reserve to tolerate the injection procedure and the subsequent treatment (ASA, Table 21-2, page 324).
B. Patients who are too medically compromised for local anesthesia may not be appropriate for any elective dental therapy.
C. When performing a risk-benefit analysis for use of local anesthesia, consider the potential for medical distress that can result from inadequate pain control.

D. Seek a medical consult when there is doubt about the safety of a local anesthetic choice.

IV. SPECIFIC MEDICAL CONSIDERATIONS

Most contraindications are relative, meaning that a case-specific evaluation needs to focus on the severity of the condition and treatment needs.

A. Allergy
1. *Amide anesthetics.* True allergy is rare. If confirmed, avoid all amide anesthetics.
2. *Ester anesthetics.* Allergy is fairly common. If confirmed, avoid all ester anesthetics, including injectable and topical anesthetics; and para-aminobenzoic acid (PABA) preservatives, such as methylparaben.
3. *Bisulfites.* Sodium metabisulfite, acetone sodium bisulfite, and sodium or potassium bisulfite are used as the preservatives for the vasoconstrictor. If allergy is known, avoid anesthetics containing vasoconstrictors.

B. Hyperthyroidism
1. *Uncontrolled:* Avoid vasoconstrictor.
2. *Controlled:* Normal local anesthesia.

C. Impaired Liver or Kidney Function
1. Only severe impairment is clinically relevant.
2. Half-life of amide anesthetic could be prolonged, which could result in overdose.

D. Malignant Hyperthermia
1. Trend is to consider amide anesthetics used in dentistry as safe.
2. Medical consult is indicated as this could be a life-threatening condition.

E. Methemoglobinemia
1. A congenital or acquired condition; hemoglobin molecule is converted to methemoglobin, which has less oxygen-carrying capacity. A cyanosis-like state may develop if a high percentage of molecules convert.
2. Prilocaine and articaine cause a dose-related methemoglobinemia. Avoid their use in patients with a pre-existing condition.

F. Heart Failure
1. Reduced circulation resulting from heart failure slows elimination of amide anesthetic, which increases potential for anesthetic overdose.
2. Patient is stress intolerant: pain and anxiety must be carefully managed. Consider use of nitrous oxide–oxygen sedation alone or in combination with local anesthesia.

G. Coronary Disease, Heart Attack, Recent Heart Surgery, Angina Pectoris, Hypertension, and Stroke
1. Concern is for use and amount of vasoconstrictor.
2. Decision based on patient ASA category, treatment and treatment time needs; possible medical consultation.
3. Usual treatment decision is to limit total amount of vasoconstrictor or, in some cases, to eliminate its use.

H. Hemophilia
1. Excessive bleeding may result from needle contact with blood vessel.
2. Decision, based on severity of condition, can range from treatment in hospital to avoiding injections into highly vascularized areas (for example, the posterior superior alveolar [PSA]).

I. Pregnancy
1. Local anesthetic and vasoconstrictors are not teratogens and may be safely administered.
2. It is prudent practice to limit any elective drug administration, especially during the first trimester.

J. Potential Drug Interactions
All medications reported in a patient's medical history need to be checked for potential drug interactions before selecting the pain control plan. Following are examples of frequently prescribed or otherwise used drugs that interact with an anesthetic or a vasoconstrictor. Precaution is needed.
1. Cimetidine and lidocaine.
2. Nonselective beta blockers and vasoconstrictors.
3. Tricyclic antidepressants and vasoconstrictors.
4. Phenothiazines and vasoconstrictors.
5. Cocaine and vasoconstrictors.

ARMAMENTARIUM

I. SYRINGE

A. Design Features
1. Durable metal or plastic can be sterilized and reused with the addition of a new needle and cartridge.
2. Single-use, disposable syringes have safety features to prevent inadvertent needle stick after use.

B. Provide Good Visibility of the Cartridge

C. Promote Easy Aspiration
1. Manual aspiration is the traditional design.
2. Self-aspirating syringe works well for small hands.

II. NEEDLE

A. Disposable
Intended for single patient use.

B. Parts and Lengths of the Needle (Figure 31-2)

1. *Short needle:* Approximately 1 inch or 25 mm. Used for most injections.
2. *Long needle:* Approximately 1½ inches or 40 mm.

C. Gauge or Needle Diameter

1. *Size:* Ranked from largest to smallest, 25-, 27-, and 30-gauge needles are used in dentistry.
2. *Rigidity:* 25-gauge needles are stiffer and deflect less as they penetrate the tissue. They are preferred for accuracy when a long needle is needed.

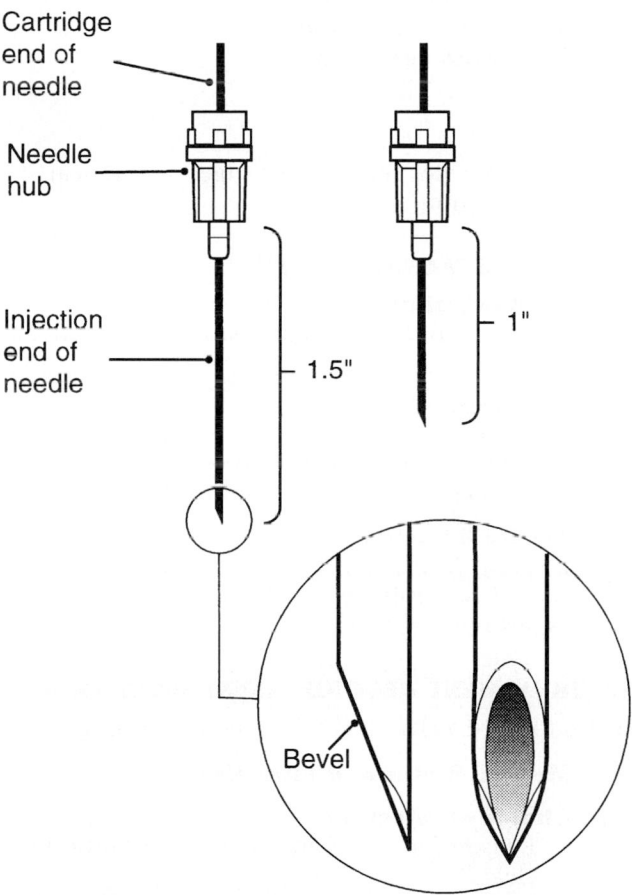

FIGURE 31-2 The Dental Anesthetic Needle. Dental needles are available in two lengths, *long* and *short.* Lengths vary slightly between manufacturers. The components of the needle are: *cartridge end,* which penetrates the rubber diaphragm of the dental cartridge, *hub,* which attaches the needle to the syringe (made of plastic or metal), *injection end* or *shank* or *shaft,* which penetrates the oral tissue so that anesthetic solution is deposited at the desired site. **INSERT:** Shows an enlargement of the tip of the needle with sharp terminus and bevel. When giving an injection, the needle is oriented so that the bevel is parallel to the bone to help prevent the needle from catching the periosteum, the sensitive covering over the bone.

3. *Aspiration:* Larger gauge needles provide easier and more accurate aspiration.

III. CARTRIDGE OR CARPULE

A. Volume: 1.8 mL of solution in the United States.
B. Storage
   1. Store at cool room temperature and away from the light.
   2. Do not store in an alcohol or disinfectant solution.
C. Label each cartridge: drug, manufacturer, and expiration date information.

IV. ADDITIONAL ARMAMENTARIUM

A. Topical antiseptic to prevent post-injection infections.
B. Topical anesthetic to increase patient comfort.
C. Cotton gauze to wipe the injection site to clean, dry, and remove the topical anesthetic. May also be used to improve grasp for lip or cheek retraction.
D. Needle recapping device.
E. Sharps disposal system to meet safe practice standards for used needle disposal.

V. SEQUENCE OF SYRINGE ASSEMBLY

Figure 31-3 illustrates the assembly of the conventional anesthetic syringe; sequence makes the attachment between the harpoon and rubber stopper easier without applying excess force to the glass cartridge.

VI. COMPUTER-CONTROLLED ANESTHESIA DELIVERY SYSTEM (WAND™)

A. Pressure, volume, and rate of speed of local anesthetic delivery are precisely regulated by a computer.
B. Device includes a light, pen-like handpiece attached to a computer-controlled, 2-speed motor that is activated by a foot control. Any gauge Luer-lock needle and standard anesthetic cartridge may be used.
C. Slow, controlled delivery of anesthesia solution promotes more comfortable injections, especially palatal and periodontal ligament (PDL) injections; allows unique injections, the anterior middle superior alveolar (AMSA) and the palatal anterior superior alveolar (P-ASA), as well as all traditional dental injections.

CLINICAL PROCEDURES FOR LOCAL ANESTHETIC ADMINISTRATION

I. INJECTION(S) SELECTION

A. Basic Injections
Table 31-4 lists injections with hard and soft tissues anesthetized, and the branches of the trigeminal nerve involved.

B. Areas Anesthetized: Shown in Figure 31-4.

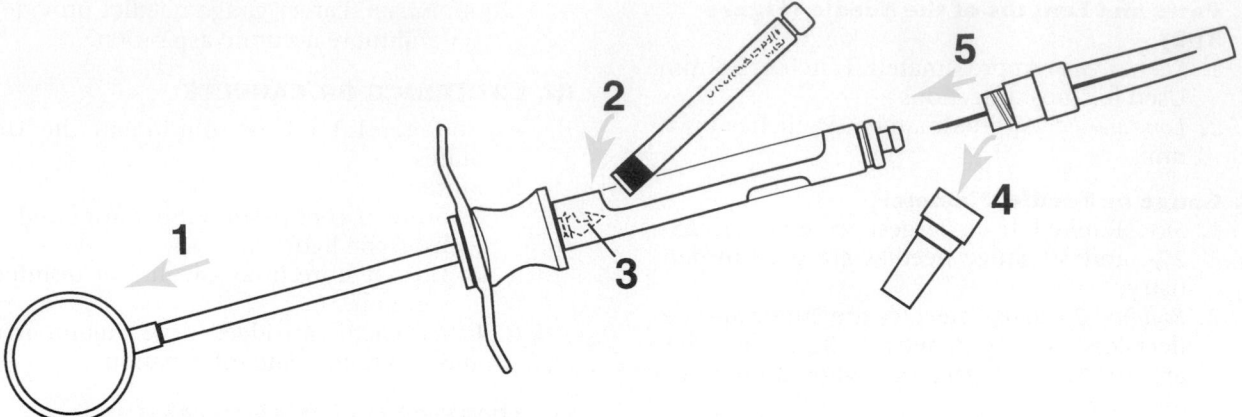

FIGURE 31-3 Sequence for Assembling a Breech-Loading Aspirating Syringe.
1. Pull back on thumb ring. **2.** Insert anesthetic cartridge, rubber stopper end first, toward the thumb ring, then the diaphragm end toward the needle opening. **3.** Set harpoon and test for lock into rubber stopper. **4.** Remove safety cap from needle. **5.** Screw needle onto the syringe.

C. Steps and Procedures
Table 31-5 outlines the sequence and procedures for the administration of local anesthesia.

II. ASPIRATION

A. Purpose
To determine if the tip of the needle is within a blood vessel. An anesthetic solution must be deposited extravascularly to be effective and to prevent toxicity.

B. When
Aspirate before depositing anesthetic solution.

C. Procedure
1. Hold the needle steady so that the tip does not change position.
2. Create negative pressure within the dental cartridge.
   a. *Standard harpoon-style syringe.* Pull back gently on the thumb ring. Movement is small, only 1 to 2 mm.
   b. *Self-aspirating syringe.* Stop applying positive pressure to the thumb ring.
3. Rotate the syringe by a quarter turn and repeat aspiration (prevent a false negative).
4. Repeat periodically throughout injection.

D. Interpretation
Any fluid at the tip of the needle will be drawn into the cartridge. If the tip of the needle is in an artery or vein, blood will become visible; it may only be a small amount at the needle end of the cartridge.
1. *Negative aspiration.* No blood in cartridge; proceed with injection.
2. *Positive aspiration.* Blood in the cartridge.
   a. A small amount of blood with most of the cartridge clear: move to a new location and reaspirate.
   b. Cartridge generally bloody: withdraw needle, replace cartridge, and repeat injection.

III. SHARPS MANAGEMENT[12]

A. No Manipulation
Do not manipulate needles; do not bend, break, or shear.

B. Recapping
1. A one-handed technique, also called "scoop" technique (Figure 31-5*A*).
2. A mechanical device (Figure 31-5*B* and *C*).

C. Needle Removal
Disposal containers for contaminated sharps should be easily accessible and located as close as possible to the area of use.

IV. TREATMENT RECORD: ANESTHESIA ENTRY
Goal is to have a clear but brief medical/legal record.

A. Medical Status and Vital Signs

B. Choice of Injection
1. Reason for use of anesthesia if not otherwise clear.
2. Injections given with location. Examples: (1) infiltration over no. 8; (2) right inferior alveolar.

C. Drug
1. Topical, local anesthetic, and vasoconstrictor.
2. Concentration of drugs. Example: lidocaine 2% with epinephrine 1:100,000.
3. Dose can be recorded in cartridges, milliliters, or milligrams.

D. Effects/Reactions
1. Effect or profoundness of anesthesia; anesthetic duration if unusual.
2. Patient acceptance or response, if significant.
3. Adverse drug reaction, if any.

TABLE 31-4 Common Local Anesthetic Injections for Dental Hygiene Procedures

Injection	Tissues Anesthetized	Branch of the Trigeminal Nerve Maxillary Division
Maxillary Arch Posterior superior alveolar (PSA)	*Hard tissue:* second and third molars; first molar excluding mesiobuccal root; associated supporting structures *Soft tissue:* overlying facial tissues	Posterior superior alveolar
Middle superior alveolar (MSA)	*Hard tissue:* first and second premolars, mesiobuccal root of first molar, and associated supporting structures *Soft tissue:* overlying facial tissues	Middle superior alveolar
Anterior superior alveolar (ASA)	*Hard tissue:* canine and incisors and associated supporting structures *Soft tissue:* overlying facial tissues and lip	Anterior superior alveolar
Infraorbital (IO)	*Hard tissue:* premolars, canine, incisors, and associated supporting structures *Soft tissue:* overlying facial tissues, cheek, and lip	Infraorbital (includes both anterior and middle superior alveolar)
Greater palatine (GP)	*Hard tissue:* none *Soft tissue:* palatal tissue from teeth to midline from distal of third molar to canine	Greater palatine
Nasopalatine (NP)	*Hard tissue:* none *Soft tissue:* palatal tissues from left canine to right canine	Nasopalatine
Infiltration (Inf)	*Hard tissue:* individual teeth associated supporting structures *Soft tissue:* facial tissue overlying individual teeth	Individual terminal branches
Mandibular Arch Long buccal (LB)	*Hard tissue:* none *Soft tissue:* facial tissue of molars	Buccal (long buccal)
Inferior alveolar with lingual (mandibular block) (IA)	*Hard tissue:* molars, premolars, canine, and incisors to midline, as well as associated supporting structures *Soft tissue:* facial tissue anterior to mental foramen, including lip	Inferior alveolar (includes dental, mental, and incisive branches)
	Hard tissue: none *Soft tissue:* lingual tissue from molar to midline, including anterior two thirds of tongue; floor of mouth	Lingual
Gow-Gates technique (GG)	*Hard tissue:* mandibular teeth to midline; body of mandible; inferior portion of ramus *Soft tissue:* facial and lingual tissue; anterior two thirds of tongue and floor of mouth; skin over the zygoma; posterior portion of the cheek and temporal regions	Third division nerve block (includes inferior alveolar, mental, incisive, lingual, mylohyoid, auriculotemporal, and buccal nerves)
Mental and incisive (M/I)	*Hard tissue:* premolars, canine, incisors, and associated supporting structures *Soft tissue:* facial tissue and lip anterior to mental foramen	Mental and incisive branch of inferior alveolar
Either Arch Interpapillary	*Hard tissue:* none *Soft tissue:* individual papilla	Free nerve endings
Periodontal ligament (PDL)	*Hard tissue:* individual tooth *Soft tissue:* adjacent	Terminal nerve endings

Adapted from Stach, D.J.: Pain and Pain Control: Topical and Local Anesthesia, in Woodall, I.R.: *Comprehensive Dental Hygiene Care,* 4th ed. St. Louis, Mosby, 1993, p. 688.

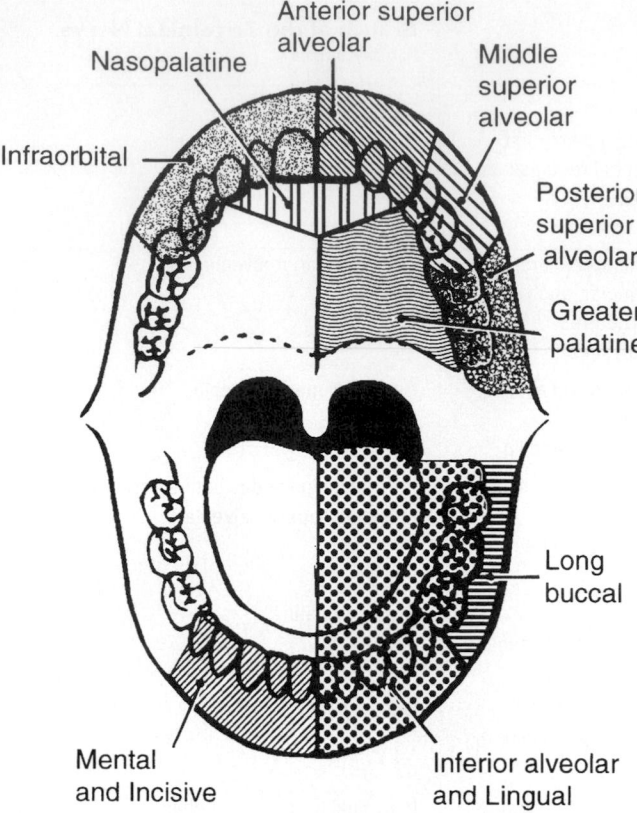

Anterior superior alveolar

Nasopalatine

Middle superior alveolar

Infraorbital

Posterior superior alveolar

Greater palatine

Long buccal

Mental and Incisive

Inferior alveolar and Lingual

■FIGURE 31-4 Diagrammatic Representation of Teeth and Soft Tissues Anesthetized by Common Dental Injections.

E. Comments As Appropriate
1. Instructions to patient.
2. Atypical occurrence or finding; positive aspiration.
3. Future alert or plan.

F. Example
Non-significant medical history, BP 120/80, pulse 68. Patient reports general root sensitivity. Administered 3.6 mL 2% lidocaine (Xyl) with epinephrine (epi) 1:100,000 for right anterior superior alveolar (ASA), middle superior alveolar (MSA), posterior superior alveolar (PSA), inferior alveolar (IA). Benzocaine topical. Anesthesia profound; procedure well tolerated.

G. Abbreviations
May be used and are acceptable when they are clearly understood and standardized in the dental practice or clinic.

POTENTIAL ADVERSE REACTIONS TO LOCAL ANESTHESIA PROCEDURES

Local anesthetics, like all drugs, have both desirable and potentially undesirable effects. Additional information on managing anesthetic reactions is listed in Table 61-5 (page 914).

I. ADVERSE DRUG REACTIONS

A. Toxic Drug Overdose
1. Overdose is the most common adverse drug reaction with amide anesthetics.
2. Occurs when the circulating blood level of the drug becomes too high and reaches a toxic level for the individual.
3. Typical causes of overdose
   a. *Intravascular injection:* Prevented by aspiration prior to deposition of the anesthetic drug.
   b. *Excessive total drug dose:* Affected by drug volumes; drug choice; patient's lean weight, age, physical/medical status.
   c. *Rapid absorption into the circulatory system:* Affected by rate of injection, presence or absence of a vasoconstrictor, or vascularity of injection site.
   d. *Reduced elimination and/or metabolism of drug:* Reduced kidney or liver function or reduced circulation as a result of congestive heart failure may reduce the rate at which the drug is removed from circulation.

B. Allergy
1. *Incidence:* Although often reported, incidence is rare with amide drugs. (Review allergy under specific medical considerations [page 502]).
2. *Definition:* Allergy is a hypersensitive state where a subsequent exposure to an allergen results in an exaggerated response. In local anesthesia, the most common allergens are the bisulfite antioxidant or ester topical anesthetic.
3. *Symptoms:* Response may range from mild, such as localized erythema or itching, to life threatening, such as generalized anaphylaxis or laryngeal edema.
4. *Onset:* May range from a few seconds to many hours.
5. *Management:* Table 61-5 presents procedures for managing an allergic reaction.

II. PSYCHOGENIC REACTIONS

A. Cause
Anxiety response to the injection procedure.

B. Symptoms
1. Vasodepressor syncope (fainting) and hyperventilation are most common.
2. Symptoms can be highly varied and may mimic drug reactions or other medical conditions.
3. Reactions reported by patients as allergies are often psychogenic in nature.

III. LOCAL COMPLICATIONS

A. Causes
1. *Varied Problems:* Exact cause is specific to

TABLE 31-5 Steps in the Administration of Local Anesthesia

1. Assess patient medical status, treatment, and pain control needs in order to select injection(s) and anesthetic drug.
2. Assemble and test the syringe set-up (Figure 31–3).
   a. Orient the needle so that the bevel will be toward the bone during the injection.
   b. Test the assembled syringe.
3. Position patient for good visibility and to prevent syncope with head level with or lower than heart.
4. Wipe injection site with gauze to clean and dry the area.
5. Use topical anesthetic.
   a. Apply to penetration site for the appropriate time. For benzocaine, 1 to 2 minutes is optimal.
   b. Remove residual topical with gauze or water spray.
6. Retract the lip or cheek for good visibility; stretch the tissue for easier needle penetration.
7. Keep the syringe out of the patient's sight.
8. Establish a fulcrum or hand rest for stability during the injection.
9. Insert the needle into the tissue and gently advance to desired site for administration of anesthetic.
10. Aspirate before depositing solution; reaspirate as needed throughout procedure.
11. Deposit the anesthetic solution slowly (1 to 2 min for full cartridge) to prevent patient discomfort and to reduce potential for a toxic reaction.
12. Withdraw the needle carefully at the completion of the injection, and recap the needle using a safe technique.
13. Remain with and observe the patient. Adverse drug reactions are most likely to occur during or shortly after the injection.
14. Record injection information in patient chart.
15. Use positive, supportive communication with the patient throughout the procedure.

each situation. Each is caused by the patient's reaction to the local anesthetic procedure.

2. *Prevention:* Use of excellent injection technique.

B. Symptoms

Vary with each complication. Examples:
1. *Trismus:* Spasm of the jaw muscles that restricts opening or makes it uncomfortable.
2. *Hematoma* (bruise): Blood from a breached artery or vein leaks into the surrounding tissue.
3. *Paresthesia:* Trauma to nerve results in persistent anesthesia, usually lasting a few days to weeks.
4. *Epithelial desquamation* (tissue sloughing): May follow prolonged application of topical anesthetic.

ADVANTAGES AND DISADVANTAGES OF LOCAL ANESTHESIA

I. ADVANTAGES

A. Patient experiences no pain or discomfort during treatment procedure; clinician has increased confidence to provide complete treatment when the patient is pain-free.
B. Local effect results in loss of sensation in area of treatment without a change in level of consciousness or patient cooperation.
C. Completely reversible without residual side effects.
D. Rapid onset of action.
E. Adequate duration of clinical action that is reasonably predictable and that can be varied by choice of commercially available drugs.
F. Relatively free of allergic reactions.
G. Hemostasis if injected directly into area of desired hemorrhage control.

II. DISADVANTAGES

A. Anticipating and receiving dental injections may cause high anxiety. Effects may include
   1. Need for special anxiety reduction technique.
   2. Undesirable psychogenic reactions.
   3. Avoidance of needed care.
B. Significant potential exists for toxicity (overdose) with amide drugs.
C. There are systemic side effects from both the local anesthetic drug and vasoconstrictor.
D. Where state law or skill levels preclude the dental hygienist from administering local anesthesia, it may be inconvenient or time consuming for the dentist to provide the injections.

TOPICAL ANESTHESIA

A topical anesthetic is a drug applied directly to the surface of the mucous membrane to produce a loss of sensation. A topical anesthetic is used with varying degrees of success for short-duration desensitization of the gingiva, but it does not influence sensations in the teeth. It is not a substitute for local anesthetic administered by injection.

Topical anesthetic applied to the tissue using the transoral patch method provides a profound level of

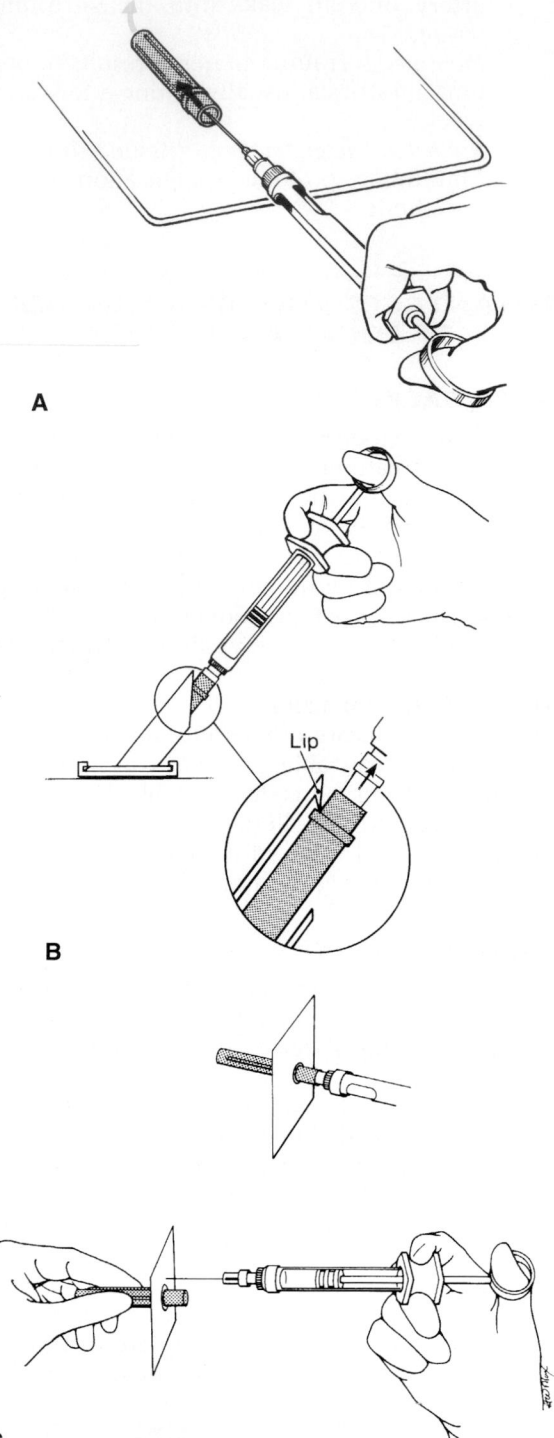

A

B

C

FIGURE 31-5 Prevention of Percutaneous Injury: Needle Recapping Methods. One-handed recapping or recapping with a safety mechanical device is required. **(A)** "Scoop" technique. Cap is placed on the tray and the needle is guided into it. **(B)** Example of commercially available holder for cap. Device is fastened to the tray, and cap is removed and recapped by directing the needle into the cap holder. **(C)** Cardboard shield retained on cap. During replacement of cap, protection is provided as shown. Needles must be discarded in a puncture-resistant container.

anesthesia to the soft tissues. It may provide slight loss of sensation to the teeth as well.

I. INDICATIONS FOR USE

A topical anesthetic can be used conservatively for selected dental hygiene and dental services, including the following:

A. Preparation for local anesthesia injection.

B. Prevention of gagging in radiographic techniques and impression taking.

C. Temporary relief of pain from localized diseased areas, such as oral ulcers, wounds, or inflammation.

D. During instrumentation for probing and scaling. When discomfort involves the teeth as well as gingiva, a local anesthetic usually is indicated.

E. Suture removal.

II. ACTION OF A TOPICAL ANESTHETIC

A. Purpose

The purpose of a topical anesthetic is to desensitize the mucous membrane by anesthetizing the terminal nerve endings. A superficial anesthesia is produced that is related to the amount of absorption of the drug by the tissue.

B. Absorption of Drug

The absorption varies with the thickness of the stratified squamous epithelial covering and the degree of keratinization. The skin, lips, and palatal mucosa are highly resistant; the attached gingival and buccal mucosa absorb drugs slowly; and the tissues without keratinization absorb promptly.

III. AGENTS USED IN SURFACE ANESTHETIC PREPARATIONS[13]

A. Benzocaine or Ethyl Aminobenzoate (Ester Type)

1. Used in 20% formulation; most widely used topical agent.
2. Available as liquid, gel, ointment, and spray.
3. Not readily absorbed into circulation; potential for toxicity is minimal.
4. May cause allergic reaction, especially with prolonged or repeated application.
5. Onset starts in 30 seconds; reaches optimum depth and intensity after several minutes.
6. A 1- to 2-minute application time is recommended before needle penetration; duration of 5 to 15 minutes.

B. Tetracaine Hydrochloride (Ester Type)

1. Available as part of a combination of drugs in liquid form and controlled-dose spray.
2. Most toxic of the dental topical anesthetics; rapidly absorbed.
3. Onset begins within 2 minutes; duration 20 to 60 minutes.

C. Lidocaine and Lidocaine Hydrochloride (Amide Type)

1. The only amide used as a topical.
2. Available in liquid, gel, ointment, spray, and transoral patch.
3. Toxicity unlikely from topical alone but would be additive with other amide anesthetics.

D. Lidocaine: Formulations Not Including Transoral Patch

1. Onset starts in 1 to 2 minutes; optimum effect may take 5 minutes; duration about 15 minutes.
2. A 3-minute application is recommended before needle penetration.

E. Lidocaine: Transoral Patch[14]

1. A delivery system that uses a bioadhesive patch to improve the duration of contact between the topical and oral soft tissue.
2. Provides profound soft tissue anesthesia as well as minimal pulpal anesthesia in some cases.
3. Onset is between 2½ and 5 minutes; maximum effect is after 15 minutes.[15]
4. Duration about 45 minutes based on 15-minute application.

F. Dyclonine Hydrochloride (Ketone Type)

1. Available as a liquid.
2. May be used as a rinse as well as usual method of application with cotton swab.
3. Onset varies between 2 and 10 minutes; duration about 30 minutes.

APPLICATION OF TOPICAL ANESTHETIC

I. PATIENT PREPARATION

A. Consult history and other records for pertinent information concerning a patient's previous experiences with anesthetics. A patient with an allergy to a local anesthetic may also be allergic to a topical anesthetic.
B. Determine the most appropriate anesthetic agent and method of application.
C. Explain purpose and anticipated effect to the patient.

II. APPLICATION TECHNIQUES

Several application techniques are available. Not all methods are applicable to all products. Select the most appropriate method from the following:

A. Surface Application

1. May be used with liquid, gel, or ointment formulations of any of the available topical agents.
2. Topical is applied with a cotton-tipped swab or cotton roll.
3. Time before becoming effective varies with the drug used.

4. After application, excess topical is removed by rinsing or gentle wiping.

B. Aerosol Spray

1. Prevent inhalation by avoiding spray preparations when another method would be as effective. A spray must never be directed toward the throat.
2. Use metered- or controlled-dose spray dispensers to prevent inadvertent overdose.

C. Oral Rinse

1. Used with dyclonine liquid (Dyclone).
2. Place approximately 5 mL of anesthetic liquid in mouth and swish for about 2 minutes.

D. Transoral Patch

1. Used with lidocaine transoral patch (Denti-patch).
2. Air dry the tissue for 30 seconds, apply the patch, and hold in place with firm finger pressure for an additional 30 seconds.
3. Apply for 5 to 10 minutes prior to most procedures; may be left in place for up to 15 minutes. Suggested application times for typical procedures are
   a. 5 minutes for most injections.
   b. 8 to 10 minutes for palatal injections.
   c. 15 minutes for most instrumentation (may be able to begin after 5 minutes).
4. Test tissue to confirm level of anesthesia after an appropriate application time. If adequate, remove the patch.
   a. Periodontal instrumentation may be started while the patch is in place if anesthesia is adequate; remove after 15 minutes.
   b. Injections should not be given through a patch.
5. Typical patch placement for scaling of the mandibular incisors is shown in Figure 31-6.

III. COMPLETION OF TOPICAL ANESTHETIC APPLICATION

A. Wait appropriate length of time for anesthetic to take effect before proceeding.
B. Limit drug exposure
   1. Apply only to the area of need.
   2. Use the smallest effective amount.
   3. Remove residual drug after application time.
C. Apply to a limited area at a time when using a drug with a short duration of action for a long procedure such as scaling.
D. Record topical anesthetic drug information in the patient's record.

TECHNICAL HINTS

I. Include decisions about anxiety and pain management during dental hygiene care planning.

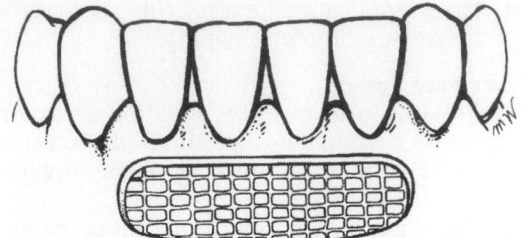

■ **FIGURE 31-6 Transoral Lidocaine Patch Placement.** In this example, for topical anesthesia to the mandibular incisors and facial tissues, patch is placed over the roots of the incisors with the upper edge 2 to 4 mm apical to the free gingival margin. Patch may be left in place during scaling and root planing for up to 15 minutes.

A. Match the pain control method to the patient's treatment needs and medical status.

B. Provide effective pain control before the patient experiences pain.

II. Administer the most comfortable injections possible by using gentle tissue manipulation, careful needle penetration, slow deposition of solution, and good patient communication.

III. Local anesthetics are less effective when injected into inflamed tissues because the low pH in those areas inhibits drug distribution.

IV. Use the minimum dose of drug that will be effective for nitrous oxide, local, and topical anesthesia.

V. Avoid directing spray toward the throat when using aerosol spray for topical anesthetic application.

VI. The administration and/or monitoring of nitrous oxide–oxygen conscious sedation is not universally legal; practitioners must know the state or province practice regulations.

FACTORS TO TEACH THE PATIENT

I. NITROUS OXIDE–OXYGEN CONSCIOUS SEDATION

A. The level of sedation should be adjusted individually for optimum relaxation and comfort. If the sedation becomes too strong or is too weak, the clinician should be informed so that adjustments can be made.

B. The gas will not result in unusual or undesirable behavior; the patient maintains control of all personal actions.

C. Eat normally before treatment; avoid fasting or heavy meals.

II. LOCAL AND TOPICAL ANESTHESIA

A. Be careful not to bite lip, cheek, or tongue while tissues are without normal sensations.

1. Children, especially, should be warned and monitored by their parents to prevent injury.

2. Do not test anesthesia by biting the lip.

B. Avoid chewing hard foods and avoid hot food and drinks until normal sensation has returned.

REFERENCES

1. **Malamed,** S.F.: *Sedation: A Guide to Patient Management,* 3rd ed. St. Louis, Mosby, 1995, p. 209.
2. **Malamed:** op. cit., p. 268.
3. **NIOSH:** *Alert: Controlling Exposures to Nitrous Oxide During Anesthetic Administration.* (NIOSH Publication No.94-100). Cincinnati, U.S. Department of Health, Education, and Welfare, Public Health Service, Centers for Disease Control, National Institute for Occupational Safety and Health, 1994, pp. 1–11.
4. **ADA Council on Scientific Affairs; ADA Council on Dental Practice:** Nitrous Oxide in the Dental Office, *J. Am. Dent. Assoc., 128,* 364, March, 1997.
5. **Rowland,** A.S., Baird, D.D., Weinberg, C.R., Shore, D.L., Shy, C.M., and Wilcox, A.J.: Reduced Fertility Among Women Employed as Dental Assistants Exposed to High Levels of Nitrous Oxide, *N. Engl. J. Med., 327,* 993, October 1, 1992.
6. **Cohen,** E.N., Gift, H.C., Brown, B.W., Greenfield, W., Wu, M.L., Jones, T.W., Whitcher, C.E., Driscoll, E.J., and Brodsky, J.B.: Occupational Disease in Dentistry and Chronic Exposure to Trace Anesthetic Gases, *J. Am. Dent. Assoc., 101,* 21, July, 1980.
7. **Sisty-LePeau,** N., Nielson-Thompson, N., and Lutjen, D.: Use, Need and Desire for Pain Control Procedures by Iowa Hygienists, *J. Dent. Hyg., 66,* 137, March, 1992.
8. **Malamed,** S.F.: *Handbook of Local Anesthesia,* 4th ed. St. Louis, Mosby, 1997, pp. 37–67.
9. **Requa-Clark,** B.S. and Holroyd, S.V.: *Applied Pharmacology for the Dental Hygienist,* 3rd ed. St. Louis, Mosby, 1995, pp. 151–155.
10. **Jastak,** J.T., Yagiela, J.A., and Donaldson, D.: *Local Anesthesia of the Oral Cavity,* Philadelphia, W.B. Saunders Co., 1995, pp. 69–78.
11. **Malamed,** S.F., Sykes, P., Kubota, Y., Matsuura, H., and Lipp, M.: Local Anesthesia: A Review, *Anesth. Pain Control Dent., 1,* 11, Winter, 1992.
12. **United States, Occupational Safety and Health Administration:** Rules and Regulations, *Fed. Reg., 56,* 64175, December 6, 1991.
13. **Jastak,** Yagiela, and Donaldson: op. cit., pp. 110–118.
14. **Noven Pharmaceuticals, Inc.,** Miami, Fl., 33186.
15. **Hersh,** E.V., Houpt, M.I., Cooper, S.A., Feldman, R.S., Wolff, M.S., and Levin, L.M.: Analgesic Efficacy and Safety of an Intraoral Lidocaine Patch, *J. Am. Dent. Assoc., 127,* 1626, November, 1996.

SUGGESTED READINGS

Bowen, D.M. and Paarmann, C.S.: Use of Pain Control Modalities, in Hodges, K.O.: *Concepts in Nonsurgical Periodontal Therapy.* New York, Delmar Publishers, 1997, pp. 227–252.

Dionne, R.A., Gordon S.M., McCullagh, L.M., and Phero, J.C.: Assessing the Need for Anesthesia and Sedation in the General Population, *J. Am. Dent. Assoc., 129,* 167, February, 1998.

McCarthy, F.M., Pallasch, T.J., and Gates, R.: Documenting Safe Treatment of the Medical-risk Patient, *J. Am. Dent. Assoc., 119,* 383, September, 1989.

Milgrom, P., Coldwell, S.E., Getz, T., Weinstein, P., and Ramsay, D.S.: Four Dimensions of Fear of Dental Injections, *J. Am. Dent. Assoc., 128,*756, June, 1997.

Raab, F.J., Schaffer, E.M., Guillaume-Cornelissen, G., and Halberg, F.: Interpreting Vital Sign Profiles for Maximizing Patient Safety During Dental Visits, *J. Am. Dent. Assoc., 129,* 461, April, 1998.

Tripp, D.A., Neish, N.R., and Sullivan M.J.L.: What Hurts During Dental Hygiene Treatment, *J. Dent. Hyg., 72,* 25, Fall, 1998.

Nitrous Oxide–Oxygen Conscious Sedation

ADA Council on Scientific Affairs, ADA Council on Dental Practice: Nitrous Oxide in the Dental Office, Appendix G, in *ADA Guide to Dental Therapeutics.* Chicago, ADA Publishing Co., Inc., 1998, pp. 554–556.

Clark, M.S. and Brunick, A.L.: *Handbook of Nitrous Oxide and Oxygen Sedation.* St. Louis, Mosby, 1998, pp. 1–242.

Clark, M.S., Renehan, B.W., and Jeffers, B.W.: Clinical Use and Potential Biohazards of Nitrous Oxide/Oxygen, *Gen. Dent., 45,* 486, September–October, 1997.

Howard, W.R.: Nitrous Oxide in the Dental Environment: Assessing the Risk, Reducing the Exposure, *J. Am. Dent. Assoc., 128,* 356, March, 1997.

Peretz, B., Katz, J., Zilburg, I., and Shemer, J.: Response to Nitrous-oxide and Oxygen Among Dental Phobic Patients, *Internat. Dent. J., 48,* 17, February, 1998.

Rohlfing, G.K., Dilley, D.C., Lucas, W.J., and Van Jr., W.F.: The Effect of Supplemental Oxygen on Apnea and Oxygen Saturation During Pediatric Conscious Sedation, *Pediatr. Dent., 20,* 8, January/February, 1998.

Stach, D.J.: Nitrous Oxide Sedation: Understanding the Benefits and Risks, *Am. J. Dent., 8,* 47, February, 1995.

Stach, D.J. and Dafoe, B.: Nitrous Oxide and Oxygen Conscious Sedation, in Woodall, I.R.: *Comprehensive Dental Hygiene Care,* 4th ed. St. Louis, Mosby, 1993, pp. 699–715.

Local and Topical Anesthesia

Clancy, M.S.: Clinical Overview of Anesthetic Use in Dentistry, *J. Pract. Hyg., 7,* 36, March/April, 1998.

Gargiulo, A.V., Bianco, C.P., Burns, G.M., and Majcina, L.: A Research Study Using Dyclonine Hydrochloride 0.5% as a Topical Anesthetic for Debridement, *J. Pract. Hyg., 7,* 2, March/April, Supplement, 1998.

Goulet, J.-P., Pérusse, R., and Turcotte, J.-Y.: Contraindications to Vasoconstrictors in Dentistry: Part III. Pharmacologic Interactions. *Oral Surg. Oral Med. Oral Pathol., 74,* 692, November, 1992.

Hersh, E.V.: Local Anesthetics in Dentistry: Clinical Considerations, Drug Interactions, and Novel Formulations, *Compend. Cont. Educ. Dent., 14,* 1020, August, 1993.

Houpt, M.I., Heins, P., Lamster, I., Stone, C., and Wolff, M.S.: An Evaluation of Intraoral Lidocaine Patches in Reducing Needle-insertion Pain, *Compend. Cont. Educ. Dent., 18,* 309, April, 1997.

Malamed, S.F.: Calculation of Local Anesthetic and Vasopressor Dosages, Appendix J, in *ADA Guide to Dental Therapeutics.* Chicago, ADA Publishing Co., Inc., 1998, p. 562.

Pallasch, T.J.: Anesthetic Management of the Chemically Dependent Patient, *Anesth. Prog., 39,* 157, Number 4/5, 1992.

Pérusse, R., Goulet, J.-P., and Turcotte, J.-Y.: Contraindications to Vasoconstrictors in Dentistry: Part I. Cardiovascular Diseases, *Oral Surg. Oral Med. Oral Pathol., 74,* 679, November, 1992.

Pérusse, R., Goulet, J.-P., and Turcotte J.-Y.: Contraindications to Vasoconstrictors in Dentistry: Part II. Hyperthyroidism, Diabetes, Sulfite Sensitivity, Cortico-dependent Asthma, and Pheochromocytoma, *Oral Surg. Oral Med. Oral Pathol., 74,* 687, November, 1992.

Rethman, J.: Local Anesthetic Administration. General Guidelines for Success, *J. Pract. Hyg., 7,* 40, March/April, 1998.

Stach, D.J.: Pain and Pain Control: Topical and Local Anesthesia, in Woodall, I.R.: *Comprehensive Dental Hygiene Care,* 4th ed. St. Louis, Mosby, 1993, pp. 676–698.

Yagiela, J. and Malamed, S.F.: Injectable and Topical Local Anesthetics, in *ADA Guide to Dental Therapeutics.* Chicago, ADA Publishing Co., Inc., 1998, pp. 1–16.

Computer-Controlled Anesthesia

Friedman, M.J. and Hochman, M.N.: A 21st Century Computerized Injection System for Local Pain Control, *Compend. Cont. Educ. Dent., 18,* 995, October, 1997.

Krochak, M. and Friedman, N.: Using a Precision-metered Injection System to Minimize Dental Injection Anxiety, *Compend. Cont. Educ. Dent., 19,* 137, February, 1998.

32

Instruments and Principles for Instrumentation

Instrumentation begins with the identification of the various types of instruments for specific services to be performed and knowledge of the parts of those instruments. The requirements for putting the instruments into action to accomplish a particular task are stabilization by means of a correct grasp and finger rest, adaptation, angulation, lateral pressure, and stroke. Key words related to basic instrumentation are defined in Box 32-1.

A study of oral and dental anatomy and histology necessarily accompanies learning instrumentation procedures and skills. Development of a thorough, efficient, and safe procedure for treatment depends on an understanding of the normal, healthy, and diseased characteristics of the dental and periodontal tissues being treated.

A high degree of skill in the care and use of the fine instruments is required. Skill depends on knowledge and understanding of the goals of therapy and of how the goals can be reached through application of the fundamental principles of instrumentation. The scope of nonsurgical therapy and the aims and expected outcomes are described on page 545.

INSTRUMENT FEATURES

I. RECOGNITION OF INSTRUMENTS

The instruments needed for examination and evaluation were described in Chapter 12, pages 204 to 218, and instruments for scaling and related procedures are described in this chapter.

Each instrument must be recognized by sight and distinguished at a glance by the profile of the instrument on the sterile tray. The clinician must be able to designate the names and numbers, and to associate each instrument promptly with the various phases of instrumentation. Such spot identification contributes to neatness of tray arrangement and efficiency of service rendered through prompt selection of the proper instrument for the service to be performed.

BOX 32-1 KEY WORDS: Principles for Instrumentation

Adaptation: relationship between the working end of an instrument and the tooth surface being treated.

Angulation: the angle formed by the working end of an instrument with the surface to which the instrument is applied for treatment.

Blade: working end of an instrument with special design for a particular clinical treatment.

Curet: a curved, rounded dental instrument utilized for scaling, root planing, and gingival curettage.

    Universal curet: a curet designed for use on any tooth surface where the adaptation, angulation, and other principles of instrument used can be correctly and effectively accomplished.

    Area-specific curet: a specialized instrument designed with specific angles in the shank for adaptation to a certain group of tooth surfaces.

Curettage: removal of inflamed soft tissue lining of the pocket wall.

Dominant hand: the hand generally used for performing fine tasks such as writing and holding instruments for scaling.

Finger rest: for an intraoral rest, the place on a tooth or teeth where the third or ring finger of the hand holding the instrument is placed to provide stabilization and control during activation of the instrument.

Fulcrum (ful'krum): the support upon which a lever rests while force intended to produce motion is exerted.

Indirect vision: use of a dental mouth mirror to view the area of instrumentation. Indirect lighting is provided by the mirror.

Lateral pressure: the minimal pressure that is required of an instrument against the tooth or soft tissue to accomplish the objective of the designated treatment.

Offset blade: the blade of an area-specific Gracey curet in which the lower shank is at a 70° angle to the face of the blade; contrasts with a universal curet blade, which is at a 90° angle with the lower shank (Figure 32-6).

Scaler: instrument with two cutting edges that meet at a point; designed for supragingival **scaling** (the removal of calculus).

Scaling: instrumentation of a tooth surface to remove supra- and subgingival calculus.

Shank: the part of the instrument between the handle and the working end.

    Lower or terminal shank: the part of the shank next to the blade.

Stroke: a single unbroken movement made by an instrument against a tooth surface during an examination or treatment procedure to accomplish a particular objective; the motion made for activation of an instrument.

A. Classification by Purpose and Use
1. *Examination Instruments:* Probe, explorer.
2. *Treatment Instruments:* Curets, scalers (sickle, hoe, chisel).

B. Description on the Instrument Handle
1. *Design Name:* The school or individual responsible for the design or development.
2. *Design Number:* The traditional number used to identify the specific instrument. The same instrument may be made by various manufacturers using the same number.

II. INSTRUMENT BALANCE

A. Definition
The working end of a balanced instrument is centered in line with the long axis of the handle (Figure 32-1).

B. Effect of Shank Length
The distance from the cutting edge (working end) of the blade to the junction of the shank and handle should not be greater than 35 to 40 mm (1½ inches). Too short a distance limits action; too long a distance may result in an unbalanced instrument.

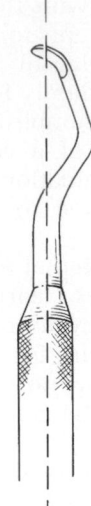

FIGURE 32-1 Instrument Balance. The working end of a balanced instrument is centered in line with the long axis of the instrument handle.

ting edge of a curet (see Figure 32-4, page 516).
2. *Lateral Surfaces:* The lateral surfaces meet or are continuous (as in the round back of a curet) to form the back of the instrument.

B. Nonsharp Instruments
The working end of a nonsharp instrument is a dull blade, or a *nib.* Although the term nib is most frequently applied to instruments for restorative dentistry, such as a condenser or burnisher, it may also apply to nonsharp ends, such as the wood point at the end of the porte polisher (page 620) and the rubber cup of the prophylaxis angle (page 611).

II. SHANK

The shank connects the working end with the handle, as shown in Figure 32-2. The shape and rigidity of the shank govern the access of the working end to accomplish the intended purpose for which the instrument was designed.

A. Shape
1. *Straight:* For adaptation to tooth surfaces

INSTRUMENT PARTS

The three major parts are the *working end,* the *shank,* and the *handle* or shaft. The relationship of these parts is illustrated by the scaler in Figure 32-2.

I. WORKING END

The working end refers to that part used to carry out the purpose and function of the instrument. Each working end is unique to the particular instrument.

A. Sharp Instruments
The working end of a sharp instrument is called a *blade.* The parts of a sharp blade are the following:
1. *Cutting Edge:* A very fine line where two surfaces meet. For example, the face and the lateral surfaces meet to form the sharp cut-

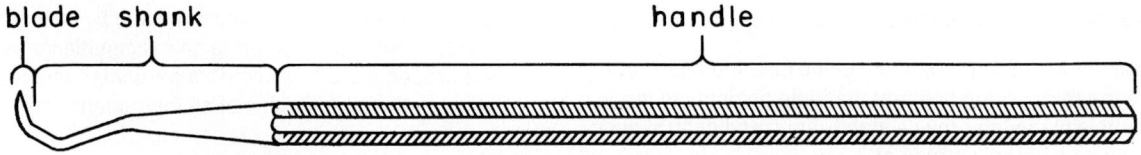

FIGURE 32-2 Parts of an Instrument. Scaler shows the relationship of the working end (blade), shank, and handle. The section of the shank next to the blade is referred to as the terminal or lower shank.

with unrestricted access, such as for anterior teeth. With many instruments, the straight shank can aid in correct positioning for treatment.

2. *Angled:* For adaptation to tooth surfaces with restricted access, such as proximal surfaces of posterior teeth. In general, the more restricted the access, the more angulated a shank must be and the sharper the bends of the angles. Examples are the Gracey curets nos. 11 and 12 and nos. 13 and 14, each of which has three bends. Because the *distal* surfaces of molars and premolars are much less accessible than are the mesial surfaces, the shank angles of the nos. 13 and 14 are designed with deeper bends to make access possible.

B. Lower or Terminal Shank

The section of the shank adjacent to the blade is called the lower or terminal shank.

1. *Instrument Positioning.* During positioning of a curet for treatment, the terminal shank is utilized to provide the clue to the appropriate blade adaptation and angulation for scaling and root planing.

2. *Elongated Terminal Shank.* Special instruments have been designed with terminal shanks longer than the traditional lengths. The purpose is to give better access to deep pockets.

C. Shank Flexibility

Instruments are made with shanks of varying degrees of thickness and rigidity that relate to the purpose for which they are used.

1. *Rigid, Thick Shank.* A thick shank is stronger and is able to withstand pressure without flexing when applied during instrumentation. Strong instruments are needed for removal of heavy calculus deposits.

2. *Less Rigid, More Flexible Shank.* A thinner shank may provide more tactile sensitivity and is used, for example, for removal of fine deposits of calculus and for root debridement.

III. HANDLE

The handle is the part of the instrument that is held (grasped) during activation of the working end.

A. Overall Design

1. Single-end instrument has one working end.
2. Double-ended instrument may have paired (mirror image) or complementary working ends. Paired working ends are used for access to proximal surfaces from the facial or lingual aspects.
3. Cone socket handles are separable from the shank and working end. They permit instrument exchanges and replacements.

B. Weight

Hollow handles are lighter and are preferred to solid handles because the lighter weight enhances tactile sensitivity and lessens fatigue.

C. Diameter

In general, four diameters of instruments are available. As shown in Figure 32-3, the most common diameters available from manufacturers are ⅜, 5⁄16, ¼, and 3⁄16 inch.

The ideal instrument for comfort and best tactile sensitivity has a lightweight, serrated, hollow handle with a ⅜ or 5⁄16-inch diameter.

D. Surface Texture: Serrations

Instrument handles may be smooth, ribbed, or knurled. For control and comfort without muscle fatigue, a smooth handle should be avoided.

THE INSTRUMENTS

Each instrument is designed for a specific type of application during treatment procedures. An instrument first can be categorized by whether it is designed primarily for supragingival treatment procedures (scalers) or for subgingival treatment (curets). Scalers and curets are then subdivided by their blade anatomy.

I. CATEGORIES

A. Curets

1. Universal.
2. Area specific.

B. Scalers

1. Sickle scaler
   a. Curved sickle scaler.
   b. Straight sickle scaler.
2. Hoe scaler.
3. Chisel scaler.
4. File scaler.

II. INSTRUMENT BLADE ANATOMY

The parts of the blade of a scaler or a curet are the *face* (inner surface), *lateral surfaces, back, tip* (scaler) or *toe*

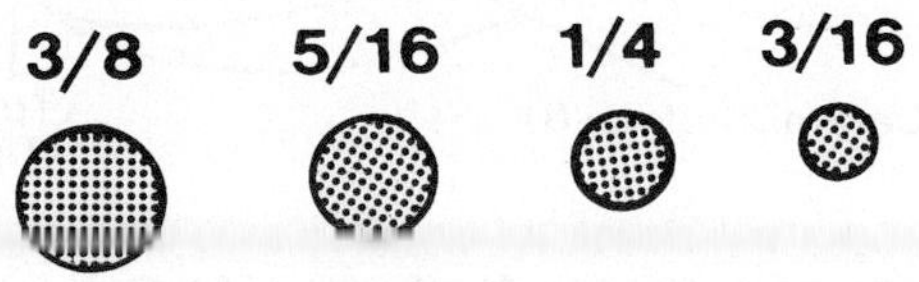

3/8 5/16 1/4 3/16

FIGURE 32-3 Diameters of Instrument Handles. The most common diameters are 3/8, 5/16, 1/4, and 3/16 inch. For comfort and tactile sensitivity, the widest diameter in a lightweight, hollow handle is recommended.

(curet), and *cutting edges*. A cutting edge is formed by the junction of the face and the lateral surface.

Figure 32-4 shows a curet with each part labeled. The parts of a scaler are the same. The differences are the pointed tip and the V-shaped back, shown in Figure 32-7. Each type of instrument is described in the next sections.

CURETS

I. CHARACTERISTICS

A. Blade
1. *Cutting Edges:* Two cutting edges on a curved blade (Figure 32-4A). The two cutting edges curve around to meet at the toe. In reality, a curet has one continuous cutting edge because the two sides are united without interruption by the rounded toe.
2. *Face:* Flat in cross section (Figure 32-4B) and curved lengthwise.
3. *Back or Undersurface:* Rounded.
4. *Cross Section of the Blade:* Shaped like a half circle.
5. *Internal Angles:* Angles of 70° to 80° are formed where the lateral surfaces meet the face. Figure 32-5 shows the cross section of a curet with the internal angles marked.

B. Shank
1. *Anterior Teeth.* Shank, blade, and handle may be in a relatively flat plane for curets primarily adaptable to anterior teeth.

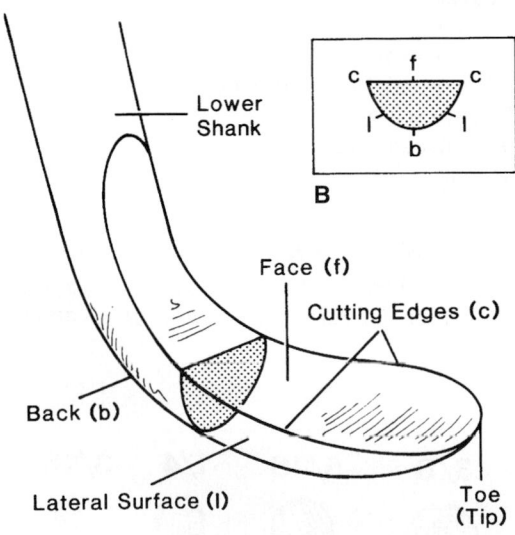

A

FIGURE 32-4 Parts of a Curet. (A) Curet with parts labeled. Lower shank is also called the terminal shank. The curet has a round toe, whereas the scaler has a pointed tip. **(B)** Cross section of a curet labeled *f* (face), *c* (cutting edges), *l* (lateral surfaces), and *b* (back).

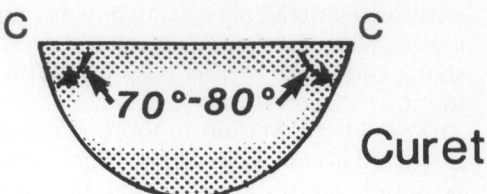

FIGURE 32-5 Internal Angles of a Curet. Cross section of a curet shows the 70° to 80° internal angles at the cutting edges.

2. *Posterior Teeth.* The shank is contra-angled for access to proximal surfaces.

C. Universal Curet
A universal curet can be adapted for instrumentation on any tooth surface.
1. Designed with paired mirror-image working ends usually placed on a single handle.
2. The face of the blade is perpendicular (at a 90° angle) to the lower shank (Figure 32-6A).
3. The cutting edge (continuous around the face), used on both sides, is sharpened on both sides and around the toe. Angulation and adaptation determine the side that is correct for the surface being treated.

D. Area-Specific Curet
The Gracey curets are area specific, which means that each curet is designed for adaptation to specific surfaces.
1. Designed with paired mirror-image working ends usually placed on a single handle. The original seven pairs are numbers 1–2, 3–4, 5–6, 7–8, 9–10, 11–12, and 13–14.
2. The face of the blade is "offset" (at an angle of approximately 70°) in relation to the lower shank (Figure 32-6B).
3. The cutting edge is continuous around the face.

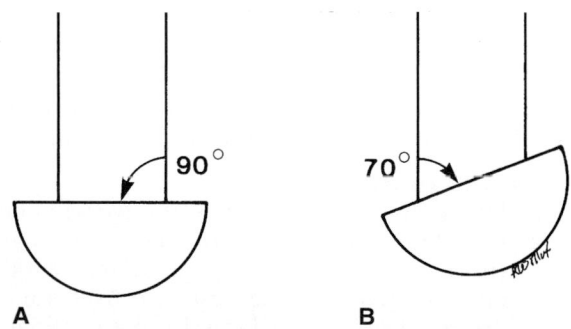

A   **B**

FIGURE 32-6 Curet Design. (A) A universal curet with the blade at a 90° angle to the lower shank. **(B)** Offset blade of an area-specific curet at a 70° angle to the lower shank.

4. Only the longer, outer cutting edge is used during instrumentation.

E. Variations

Variations of area-specific curets have been introduced to provide clinicians with greater opportunities to complete subgingival instrumentation with improved skills.

1. *Shank:* Terminal (lower) shank elongated by three millimeters to adapt in deeper pockets. The total length of the shank from blade to handle is not changed.
2. *Blade:* Reduced length, half the length of a standard Gracey blade, for special adaptation to narrow root surfaces and line angles otherwise difficult to access. Facilitates adaptation to narrow pockets and furcation areas.

II. PURPOSES AND USES

A. Standard instrument for subgingival scaling and root planing (see also pages 550 to 554).
B. After ultrasonic or sonic scaling to complete the procedure as needed.
C. Removal of supragingival calculus, especially the fine supragingival calculus close to the gingival margin. The rounded instrument is best adapted to the cervical area; round back does not traumatize the gingival margin.
D. Curettage of the inflamed lining of the gingival wall of a pocket.
E. Useful for obtaining a sample of subgingival plaque to place on a glass slide for the phase microscope or for microbiologic tests.

III. APPLICATION

A. Angulation

Blade is applied to the tooth so that the face is at an angle of 70° (between 60° and 80°).

B. Adaptation

Adaptation is described on page 524 in this chapter. The lower third of the cutting edge of a curet (the part nearest the toe) is maintained on the tooth surface at all times to minimize soft tissue trauma from extension of the toe away from the tooth in the narrow pocket. Changes in tooth surface contour require constant attention to accomplish proper contact. On line angles, only 1 or 2 mm near the toe may be used (see Figure 33-5, page 552).

C. Curet Selection

Universal curets are used for subgingival scaling for removal of as much of the calculus as possible, followed by area-specific curets for fine scaling and root planing.

D. Design

The design of the curet allows easy entrance into the sulcus, and the curved blade with rounded end permits access to the base of the sulcus or pocket. The slender shank permits entrance to the sulcus with minimal tissue distention. The round back minimizes possible trauma at the base of the sulcus or pocket.

E. Stroke

Pull stroke only; applied in vertical, horizontal, or oblique directions (see Figure 32-18, page 526).

SCALERS

I. SICKLE SCALER

By usual definition a sickle is considered curved. The shapes of sickle scalers vary, however, and in some forms the blade and cutting edges are straight. When reference is made to a specific instrument with either a curved or a straight blade, the types usually are called "curved sickle" or "straight sickle."

A. Curved Sickle Scaler

1. Two cutting edges on a curved blade (Figure 32-7).
2. Face is flat in cross section and curved lengthwise.
3. The face converges with the two lateral surfaces to form the *tip* of the scaler, which is a sharp point.
4. In cross section, some blades are triangular (Figure 32-7B), whereas others are trapezoidal.

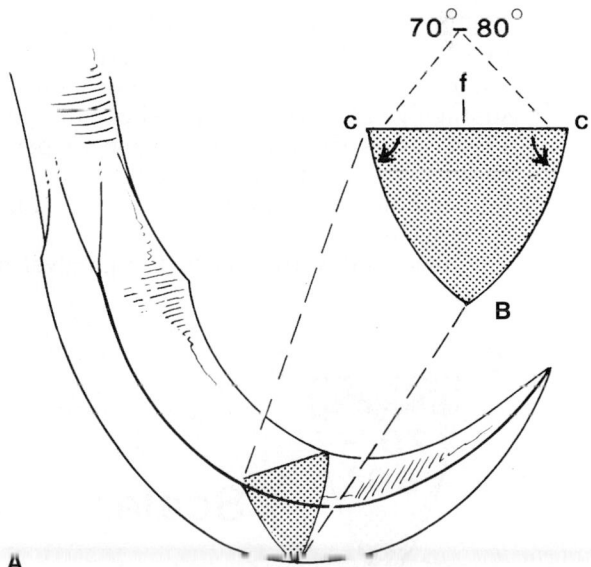

FIGURE 32-7 Curved Sickle Scaler. (A) The curved blade terminates in a point. **(B)** Cross section shows the face *(f)* and the two cutting edges *(c)* formed where the lateral surfaces meet the face at 70° to 80° angles.

5. Internal angles of 70° to 80° are formed where the lateral surfaces meet the face at the cutting edges. Figure 32-8 shows the cross section of a scaler with the internal angles marked.

B. Straight Sickle Scaler

1. Two cutting edges on a straight blade (Figure 32-9).
2. Face (between the cutting edges) is flat.
3. The face converges with the two lateral surfaces to form the tip of the scaler, which is a sharp point.
4. Cross section of the blade is triangular (Figure 32-9B).
5. Internal angles of 70° to 80° are formed where the lateral surfaces meet the face at the cutting edges (Figure 32-8).

C. Angulation of the Shank

Both curved and straight sickle scalers are available with angulated or straight shanks.

1. *Straight:* Single instrument in which the relationships of the shank, blade, and handle are in a flat plane; adaptable primarily for anterior teeth, although may be used for scaling premolars when the lips and cheeks permit retraction for correct angulation.
2. *Modified or Contra-Angle:* Paired instruments that are mirror images of each other to provide access to the proximal surfaces of posterior teeth; one adapts from the facial and the other from the lingual and palatal aspects.

D. Purposes and Uses of Sickle Scalers

1. Principally for the removal of supragingival calculus.
2. May be useful for removal of gross calculus that is slightly below the gingival margin when the calculus is continuous with the supragingival calculus, and when the gingival tissue is spongy and flexible to permit easy insertion of the instrument.
3. Contraindications for use of sickle scalers subgingivally:
   a. Cause undue trauma to the gingival tis-

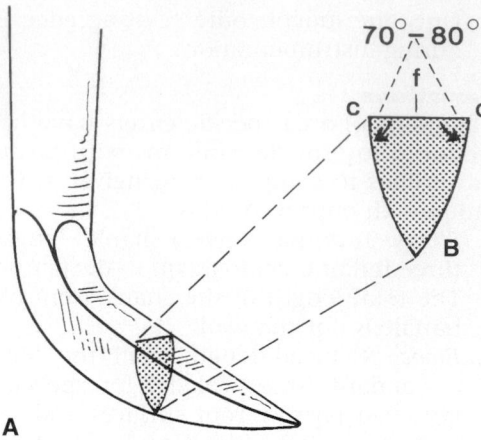

A

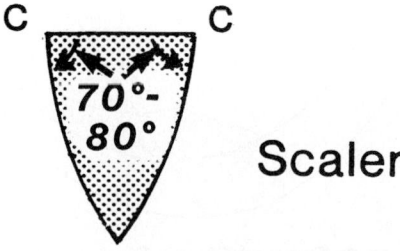

FIGURE 32-9 Straight Sickle Scaler. (A) The straight blade converges to a point where the two cutting edges meet at the tip. **(B)** Cross section of the scaler shows the face *(f)*, the two cutting edges *(c)*, and the 70° to 80° internal angles. This type of sickle scaler is also known as the Jacquette scaler.

sue because of the large size, thickness, and length of the blade.
   b. Pointed tip and straight cutting edges cannot be adapted to the curved tooth surfaces. Risk of grooving or scratching the cemental surface is greater.
   c. Tactile sensitivity decreased with larger, heavier blades.
4. Small sickle scalers can be useful for removal of fine supragingival deposits directly under contact areas and between overlapping teeth.

E. Application

1. *Angulation.* The face of the blade is adapted to the tooth surface at an angle of approximately 70° (60° to 80°).
2. *Stroke.* Pull stroke only for this type of blade.

II. HOE SCALER

A. Characteristics

1. Single, straight cutting edge (Figure 32-10).
2. Blade turned at a 99° to 100° angle to the shank.
3. Cutting edge beveled at a 45° angle to the end of the blade (Figure 32-10B).
4. Shank variously angulated for adaptation of cutting edges to accessible tooth surfaces; some are paired.

B. Purposes and Uses of a Hoe Scaler

1. Removes supragingival calculus, particularly large, accessible, tenacious pieces.
2. Contraindications for use subgingivally:
   a. Insertion of the thick-bladed instrument into the sulcus causes distention of the pocket wall.

FIGURE 32-8 Internal Angles of a Scaler. Cross section of a scaler shows the 70° to 80° internal angles. These angles are restored by sharpening techniques.

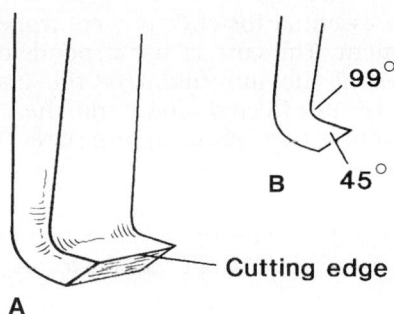

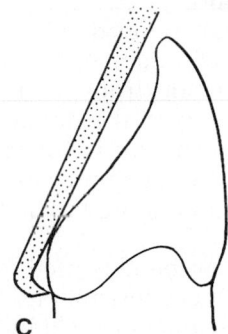

FIGURE 32-10 Hoe Scaler. (A) The hoe has a single cutting edge. **(B)** The blade is turned at an angle of 99° to the shank, and the cutting edge is beveled at a 45° angle. **(C)** Adaptation to a tooth for removal of calculus is with a two-point contact where possible.

  b. Lack of adaptability of the wide straight cutting edge to the curved root surface.

  c. Difficulty of use without gouging the cemental surface. The sharp "corners" should be rounded (as shown in Figure 32-36, page 540).

  d. Lack of sensitivity because of the bulk of the instrument and the marked angulation of the shanks of some hoes.

  e. Impossibility of reaching the bottom of the pocket without stretching and tearing the gingival pocket wall unnecessarily because of the size and shape of the blade.

C. Application

 1. Full width of the cutting edge is in contact with the calculus, and when possible, a two-point contact is maintained with the tooth to stabilize the instrument during the positioning and activation. Two-point contact means contact of the cutting edge and the side of the shank with the tooth (Figure 32-10C).

 2. Hoes are not generally applied to proximal surfaces except the surface adjacent to an edentulous area.

 3. Pull stroke is used toward occlusal or incisal surfaces.

III. CHISEL SCALER

A. Characteristics

 1. Single straight cutting edge (Figure 32-11).

 2. Blade is continuous with a slightly curved shank.

 3. End of blade is flat and beveled at 45° (Figure 32-11B).

B. Purposes and Uses of a Chisel Scaler

 1. Useful for removal of supragingival calculus from exposed proximal surfaces of anterior teeth where interdental gingiva is missing.

 2. Well suited for quick dislodgement of heavy calculus from the proximal areas of mandibular anterior teeth. When the calculus on the lingual surfaces forms a continuous bridge across several teeth, the chisel can be pushed horizontally from the facial aspect to break up the large masses of calculus.

 3. Useful for proximal surfaces of premolars when flexibility of the lips and cheeks permits retraction for proper positioning of the cutting edge.

C. Application

 1. Full width of cutting edge should be applied, as the sharp corners can nick and groove the tooth surface. The sharp "corners" should be rounded during sharpening (page 540).

 2. Stroke is horizontal only, from facial to lingual on proximal surfaces of anterior, particularly mandibular, teeth.

IV. FILE SCALER

A. Characteristics

 1. Multiple cutting edges lined up as a series of miniature hoes on a round, oval, or rectangular base (Figure 32-12A).

 2. The multiple blades are at a 90° or 105° angle with the shank (Figure 32-12B).

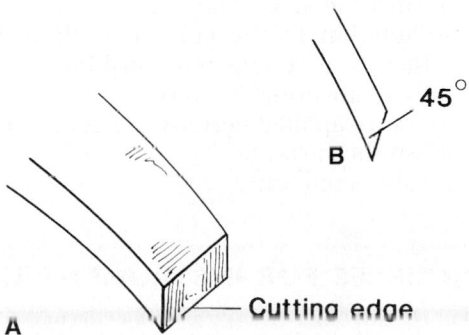

FIGURE 32-11 Chisel Scaler. (A) A chisel scaler has a single cutting edge, and the blade is continuous with a slightly curved shank. **(B)** A 45° bevel is at the cutting edge.

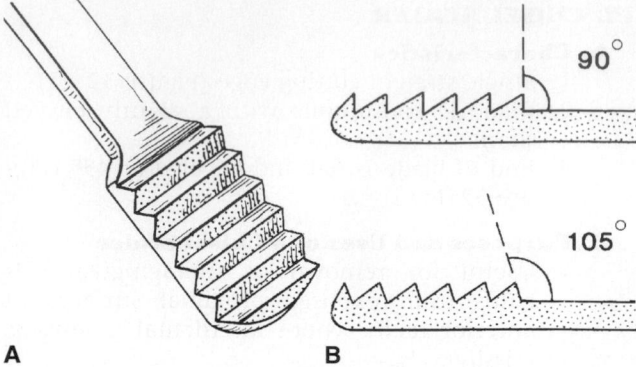

■ **FIGURE 32-12 File Scaler. (A)** A file has multiple cutting edges. **(B)** Each blade is at a 90° or a 105° angle with the shank.

3. Shanks are variously angulated, similar to the hoes; some are paired instruments, others single.
4. Reduced tactile sensitivity because of the size and shape; files are wide, flat, and bulky.

B. Purposes and Uses of a File Scaler

In general, the file can be considered a supplementary instrument rather than a definitive instrument for routine use during scaling and root planing.

Although never used by some dental hygienists, the file is used by others for one or more of the following purposes:

1. Removal of calculus (accomplished by crushing or fragmentation).
2. Smoothing of the tooth at the cemento-enamel junction.
3. Root planing, primarily the exposed root surface following periodontal surgery.
4. Smoothing down of overextended or rough amalgam restorations, particularly on proximal surfaces or in the cervical areas.

C. Application

1. The entire working surface is placed flat against the area to be treated.
2. Adaptation to the curved tooth surfaces is difficult. In certain relationships the file has only a tangential contact.
3. Pressure applied permits the cutting edges to grasp the surface.
4. Stroke is pull only.

PRINCIPLES FOR INSTRUMENT USE

Understanding the purpose of each instrument and development of dexterity in the effective use of the instruments are basic to clinical dental hygiene practice. The clinical results obtained for the patient depend in part on the proficiency and thoroughness with which the instrumentation is accomplished.

Stability is essential for effective, controlled action of an instrument. The correct use depends on maintaining *control* of the movement of the instrument through use of an effective *grasp* and the establishment and maintenance of an appropriate, firm, fulcrum *finger rest*.

INSTRUMENT GRASP

I. FUNCTIONS OF THE INSTRUMENT GRASP

A. Dominant Hand

The right hand is the dominant hand for the right-handed clinician. A few rare people are completely ambidextrous, and others are partially dexterous with the nondominant hand, a useful accomplishment when carrying out dental and dental hygiene procedures. Exercises for developing dexterity are provided on pages 526 to 528.

The dominant hand is used to hold and activate the treatment instrument. The manner in which the instrument is held influences the entire procedure.

A rigid grasp, in which the instrument is gripped tightly, lessens the tactile sensitivity and, hence, the effectiveness of instrumentation. The appropriate grasp is controlled, displays the confidence of the clinician in the work being done, and provides the following effects:

1. Increased fingertip tactile sensitivity.
2. Positive control of the instrument with balance and flexibility during motion.
3. Decreased hazard of trauma to the dental and periodontal tissues, which in turn results in less postcare discomfort for the patient.
4. Prevention of fatigue to clinician's fingers, hand, and arm.

B. Nondominant Hand

The right-handed clinician uses the left hand and the left-handed clinician uses the right hand for essential supplementary functions to assist the dominant hand. Figure 32-13 shows the recommended modified pen grasp (described later) for each hand. The mouth mirror is frequently held by the nondominant hand. With the appropriate grasp and finger rest, the following effects can be provided:

1. Control of the position of the mirror for indirect vision, indirect lighting, and retraction.
2. Assistance in providing the dominant hand with an auxiliary finger rest.

II. TYPES

A. Modified Pen Grasp

1. *Description.* The modified pen grasp is a three-finger grasp with the tips of the thumb, index finger, and middle (second) finger all in con-

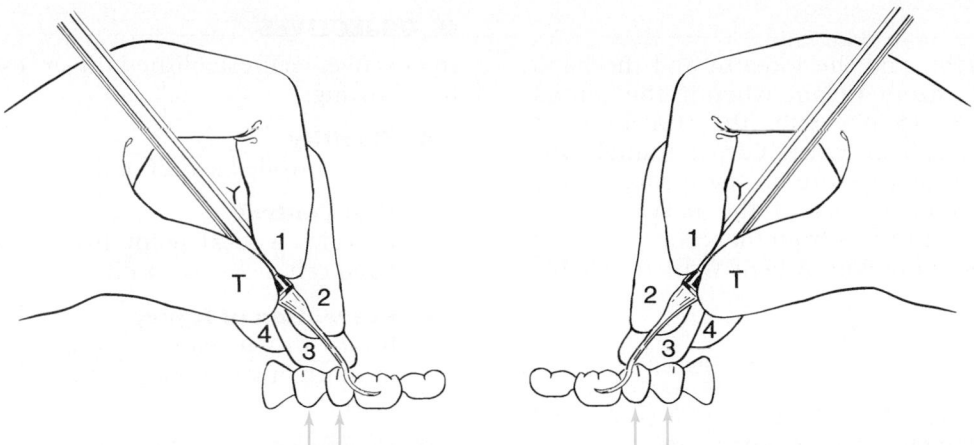

FIGURE 32-13 Modified Pen Grasp for Left and Right Hands. An instrument is held by the thumb *(T)*, index finger *(I)*, and the second, or "middle," finger *(2)*, which also provides support. The third, or "ring," finger *(3)* serves as the finger rest, and the fourth, or "little," finger *(4)* is positioned beside the ring finger to supplement the finger rest.

tact with the instrument. The ring finger is the finger rest. The instrument is held by the thumb and index finger at the junction of the shank and handle. The middle (second) finger is placed on the shank to hold and guide the movement (Figure 32-13).

2. *Role of Middle Finger.* The shank of the instrument is held against the pad of the middle finger. The instrument is not held across the nail or the side of the middle finger, as in a pen grasp usually used for writing. The specific position of the middle finger is extremely important to instrument control in preventing the instrument from slipping during adaptation and activation.

B. Palm Grasp

1. *Description.* The handle of the instrument is held in the palm by cupped index, middle, ring, and little fingers. The thumb is free to serve as the fulcrum (Figure 32-14).

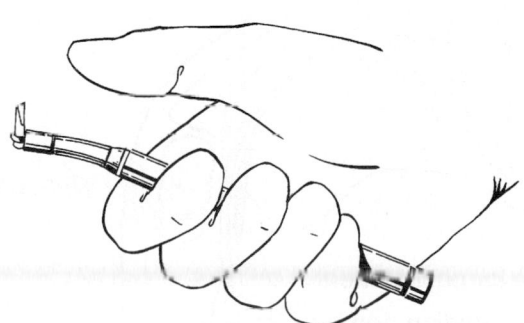

FIGURE 32-14 Palm Grasp of Instrument. The instrument handle is held in the palm by cupped index, middle, ring, and little fingers. Thumb is free and serves as the finger rest.

2. *Limitations of Use.* Instruments for calculus removal and root debridement are not used with a palm grasp. The possible exception is a chisel scaler when it is used to remove gross calculus by a push stroke (page 519). The palm grasp limits operation in that there is less tactile sensitivity and less flexibility of movement.

3. *Examples of Uses for Palm Grasp*
   a. Air syringe.
   b. Rubber dam clamp holder.
   c. Handpiece for instrument sharpening (see Figure 32-33, page 539, for holding the Nievert whittler).
   d. Porte polisher for facial surfaces. A porte polisher is shown in Figure 32-14.

WRIST, ARM, ELBOW, SHOULDER: NEUTRAL POSITIONS

Neutral positions for the wrist, forearm, elbow, and shoulder are basic to efficient performance directed at the prevention of occupational pain risks, particularly for those risks related to cumulative trauma disorders. Clinical activities to prevent cumulative trauma disorders, particularly prevention of carpal tunnel syndrome, are considered later in this chapter (pages 528 to 529).

General clinician and dental chair positioning were described in Chapter 5. Principles of the 90° 90° 90° body position for the clinician were illustrated in Figures 5-1 and 5-2 (page 76). Correct seating includes a right angle at each of the hips, knees, and ankles. In this section, the neutral positions for the hand, wrist, elbow, and shoulder can be related directly to the grasp and finger rest for instrumentation.[1]

I. WRIST

The wrist is straight, and the forearm and the hand are in the same horizontal plane when in the neutral position. Figure 32-15 illustrates the straight wrist and the effect of a bent wrist. Carpal tunnel syndrome, brought on by pressure on the median nerve in the carpal tunnel, is one of the nerve entrapment conditions that results from inappropriate work habits, such as working with a bent wrist (see Table 32-2, page 530).

II. ELBOW

The neutral elbow is at 90°, the forearm is positioned horizontally, and the hand is straight ahead.

III. SHOULDER

In neutral, both shoulders are level and relaxed to their lowest position. The arms are straight down to the elbow.

FULCRUM: FINGER REST

A fulcrum must always be used when instruments are applied to the teeth and gingiva.

I. DEFINITION

A. Fulcrum
The support, or point of rest, on which a lever turns in moving a body.

B. Finger Rest
The support, or point of finger rest on the tooth surface, on which the hand turns in moving an instrument.

II. OBJECTIVES

An effective, well-established finger rest is essential to the following:

A. Stability
For controlled action of the instrument.

B. Unit Control
Provides a focal point from which the whole hand can move as a unit.

C. Prevention of Injury
Injury to the patient's oral tissues can result from irregular pressure and uncontrolled movement.

D. Comfort for the Patient
Confidence in clinician's ability, which results from the feeling of securely applied instruments.

E. Control of Length of Stroke
With instrument grasp, the finger rest limits the instrumentation to where it is needed.

III. CONVENTIONAL INTRAORAL RESTS

The intraoral finger rest is essentially a total hand co-ordinated effort to provide stabilization. Figure 32-13 shows the fingers grouped together with the fulcrum where the ring finger (no. 3 in Figure 32-13) maintains its position on a tooth near the tooth being treated.

A. Digits Used for Finger Rest
1. *Modified Pen Grasp:*
   a. Ring finger. Little finger is held close beside ring finger (finger nos. 3 and 4 in Figure 32-13).
   b. Supplementary. Pad of middle finger rests lightly on incisal or occlusal surface of tooth to which instrument is applied; ring

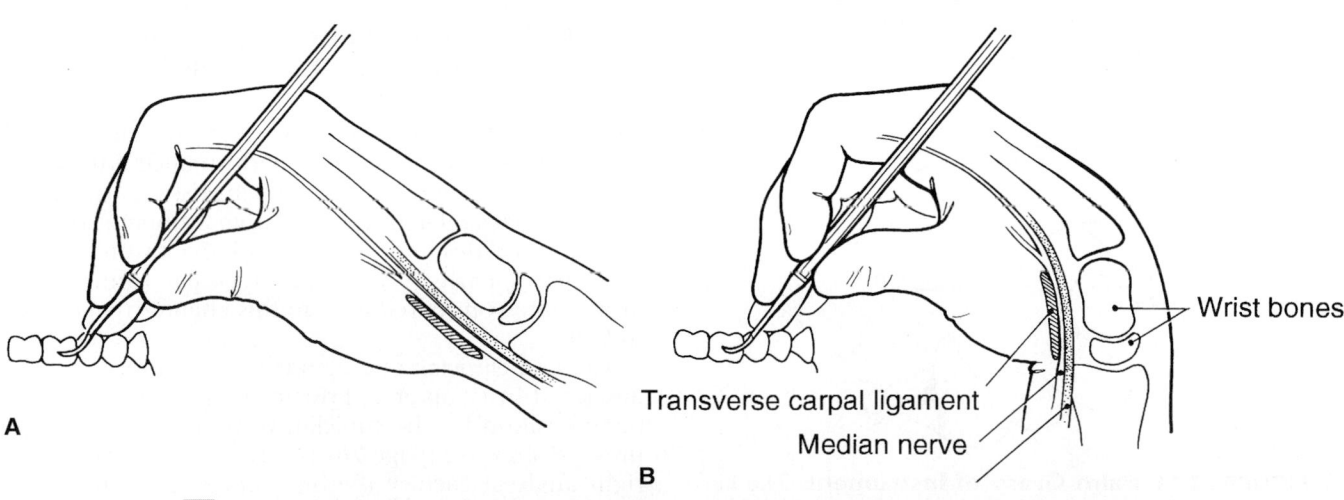

A   **B**

FIGURE 32-15 Effect of Wrist Position. (A) Wrist in neutral position in straight line with forearm. **(B)** Bent wrist shows cramping of median nerve in the carpal tunnel of the wrist. Repeated pressure on the median nerve can cause carpal tunnel syndrome.

finger maintains regular fulcrum position, and middle finger maintains its grasp on instrument.

2. *Palm Grasp:* Thumb.

B. Location of Finger Rest

1. *Purposes.* The location of a finger rest is selected for the following reasons:
   a. Convenience to area of instrumentation.
   b. Ease in instrument adaptation.
   c. Maintenance of an effective grasp.
   d. Application of the appropriate angulation.
   e. Stability and control of instrument during the activation (strokes).
   f. Safety of the clinician. A finger rest placed in line of the stroke direction could result in a rubber glove puncture and/or a finger stab if the patient moved suddenly or the instrument slipped for any reason.

2. *Principles*
   a. The first choice for a rest is usually the tooth adjacent to the tooth being treated.
   b. Maintain the rest on firm stable tooth or teeth. The patient's chin, lips, and checks are mobile and flexible and therefore less reliable for stability.
   c. Where possible, the rest should be on the same arch, maxillary or mandibular, as the instrumentation; also, where possible, the rest should be in the same quadrant.

IV. VARIATIONS OF FINGER REST

A basic fulcrum location cannot always be used or may require supplementation.

A. Problems

1. A patient's facial musculature; oral anatomic features, such as size of tongue or mouth opening (microstomia); arrangement of the teeth or malocclusions of individual teeth; or physical disability affecting the oral cavity indirectly may interfere with customary positioning for instrumentation.

2. Tenacious calculus in difficult-access areas may not be removed and root surfaces may not be planed by the usual procedures. Greater support and pressure to the instrument are required.

3. When the problem in instrumentation seems to be related to space and accessibility, the height and position of the patient's oral cavity should be checked. Also, a change in the clinician's working position may be necessary.

B. General Categories of Variations[2]

When a variation in finger rest is used, basic rules for stability and control are applied, and rests on movable tissues are avoided. Three types of variations are suggested here: *substitute,* *supplementary,* and *reinforced* finger rests. Any of these variations may require an external position.

1. *Substitute*
   a. Missing teeth where finger rest is usually applied. For an edentulous area, a cotton roll or gauze sponge may be packed into the area to provide a dry finger rest. Otherwise, a rest across the dental arch or in the opposite arch may be required to provide stability.
   b. Mobile teeth, or teeth with inadequate bony support. Avoid mobile teeth for finger rests or use only with minimal pressure for brief periods. Not only would the rest on a mobile tooth be unstable, but pressure, movement, and undue stress on the tooth could traumatize and tear the periodontal ligament fibers.
   c. Index finger of nondominant hand may be placed in the vestibule over a cotton roll. The usual finger rest can be placed on the index finger to aid retraction and visibility, particularly in the mouth of a small child.

2. *Supplementary.* Place the index finger of the nondominant hand on the occlusal surfaces of teeth adjacent to the working area. The finger rest can then be applied to the index finger. Such supplements are not useful for distal surfaces where the mouth mirror is essential for vision.

3. *Reinforced*
   a. In this type, a support is placed between the instrument handle and the working end to provide additional strength and force, particularly for hard, tenacious calculus in pockets. Greater control of the instrument can result and, when applied correctly, reduce the danger of instrument breakage. A definite rest for both hands is needed to distribute the pressure.
   b. Index finger of nondominant hand can be rested on the tooth adjacent to the one being scaled, while the thumb is placed on the instrument shank (or handle) for a reinforcement.

V. TOUCH OR PRESSURE APPLIED TO FINGER REST

A. Balance

The fulcrum finger maintains a firm hold with moderate pressure to balance the action of the instrument being applied.

B. Effects of Excess Pressure

1. Decreased stability.
2. Diminished control.
3. Overtightened grasp to accommodate.
4. Fatigue of patient caused by use of mandibu-

lar fulcrums. Heavy pressure on the movable mandible can cause fatigue in the temporomandibular joint and related muscles and, thus, discomfort for the patient.

5. Fatigue in clinician's fingers and hand.

ADAPTATION

With an appropriate grasp and finger rest, the instrument is next ready for application. The working end of the instrument is adapted to the surface of the tooth or tissue where instrumentation is to take place.

I. RELATION TO TOOTH SURFACE

The side of the tip or toe is maintained in close approximation to the surface being examined or treated. Figure 33-4 (page 551) shows the divisions of a curet blade.

II. CHARACTERISTICS OF A WELL-ADAPTED INSTRUMENT

A. Working End

1. The working end of the instrument is correctly positioned for the task to be accomplished. For example, when scaling, the angle formed by the face of the instrument and the tooth surface is crucial for effective calculus removal. Angulation is described in a following section.

2. The instrument is adapted for maximum usefulness of the working end. For example, 2 to 3 mm of the end of a curet may be adaptable when on a "flat" surface, whereas at a line angle or convex surface of a narrow root, less than 2 mm may be adaptable.

3. The working end is applied to conform to the contour of the tooth surface.

4. As the instrument is activated, it can be adjusted to changes required by variations in the surface topography.

B. Soft Tissue

A properly adapted instrument harms neither the tissue being treated nor the surrounding or adjacent tissues.

III. PROBLEM AREAS

Areas where instrument adaptation is most difficult and requires more attention, time, and careful application of skill include the following:

A. Line Angles

All line angles require that the instrument be rolled between the fingers to turn the working end as the instrument is activated. At each change of direction around a line angle, the instrument must be rolled to keep it adapted to the surface. Figure 32-16 shows the adaptation of an explorer tip to a line angle.

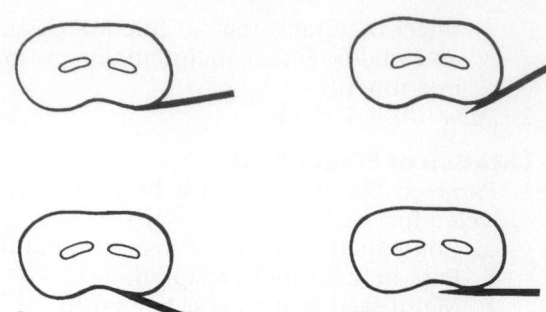

■ FIGURE 32-16 Instrument Adaptation. Cross section of maxillary first permanent premolar to show adaptation of the tip of an explorer. **(A)** Appropriate adaptation in which the tip of the explorer is maintained on the tooth surface in a series of strokes to explore around a line angle. **(B)** Incorrect adaptation with the tip of the explorer extended away from the tooth surface.

B. Convex and Rounded Surfaces
Particularly of narrow roots.

C. Cervical Area
Where the root is constricted.

D. Proximal Root Surfaces
Root surfaces may be concave, have longitudinal grooves, and have open furcations.

ANGULATION

A factor closely related to and directly influencing instrument adaptation is angulation. Angulation refers to the angle formed by a working end of an instrument with the surface to which the instrument is applied. Each instrument is applied to a surface in a specific manner for optimum adaptation and angulation.

I. PROBE

The usual adaptation of a probe is to maintain the side of the working tip on the tooth, with the long axis of the working end nearly parallel with the tooth surface (pages 208 to 209).

As used for a bleeding index, the tip is placed inside the pocket wall and pressed lightly on the wall as the probe is moved horizontally around the tooth (see Figure 19-9, page 307).

II. EXPLORER

An explorer is held with the tip at a right angle to the occlusal surface when detecting occlusal pit or fissure caries. On other surfaces, the side of the tip is kept on the tooth at all times. The angle is 5° or less. Figure 12-15, page 217, illustrates the use of the subgingival explorer.

III. SCALERS AND CURETS

Angulation for a scaler or a curet means the angle

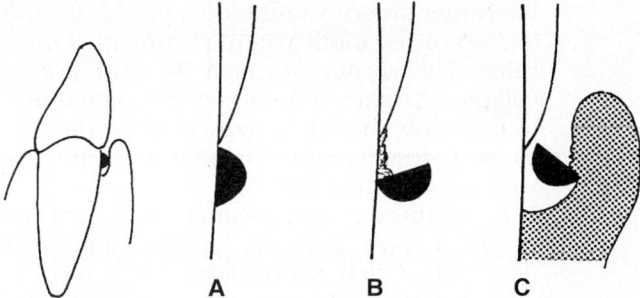

FIGURE 32-17 Instrument Angulation. Enlargement of pocket area from the tooth on the left shows cross section of a curet blade in black. **(A)** The curet is angulated at 0° with the tooth surface when used in an exploratory or insertion stroke. At 0° the face of the blade is flat against the tooth surface. **(B)** Blade angulated at approximately 70° with the tooth surface for scaling and root planing. **(C)** Open blade angulated toward the pocket wall in position for gingival curettage. The face of the blade forms an angle of approximately 70° with the soft tissue pocket wall.

formed by the face of the instrument with the surface to which the instrument is applied. Figure 32-17 shows the various angles for curet adaptation. At zero angulation the curet face is flat against the tooth surface (Figure 32-17*A*).

A. Scaling and Root Planing

An angle of less than 90° but not less than 45° permits effective calculus removal. The preferred angulation is between 60° and 80° (Figure 32-17*B*). Using a markedly closed angulation of less than 45° may result in burnishing the calculus to produce a smooth veneer.

B. Gingival Curettage

The face is turned toward the soft tissue wall of the pocket. The angle formed by the face of the curet blade and the soft tissue pocket wall being treated is less than 90° but more than 45° (Figure 32-17*C*).

LATERAL PRESSURE

Lateral pressure means the pressure of the instrument against the tooth surface during activation. It is described as light, moderate, or heavy pressure.

I. DETECTION INSTRUMENTS

Explorers and probes are used with a light pressure to maximize the sense of touch in detecting irregularities.

II. TREATMENT INSTRUMENTS

A. Placement Stroke

A light but secure pressure is applied as a curet is passed over the tooth surface to the edge of the calculus deposit or lower border of a rough root surface.

B. Scaling Stroke

A definite, controlled stroke of moderate to heavy pressure is used for calculus removal.

C. Root Planing Stroke

A lighter pressure is applied progressively as the root surface becomes smooth (page 553).

ACTIVATION: STROKE

A stroke is an unbroken movement made by an instrument; it is the action of an instrument in the performance of the task for which it was designed.

Strokes may be identified by the instrumentation being performed. Examples are the "probing stroke," "scaling stroke," or "root planing stroke." Technique for each type is described in the chapters covering the specific procedures.

I. CHARACTERISTICS OF STROKES

A. Types of Strokes by Action

1. *Pull.* Example: scaler removing calculus.
2. *Placement.* Example: exploratory stroke when a curet is being positioned.
3. *Combined Push and Pull.* Example: explorer in a walking stroke, which is moving the instrument up and down with equal pressure on the surface (see Figure 12-15, page 217).
4. *Walking Stroke.* Example: probe is moved up and down, touching the coronal border of the periodontal attachment with each down stroke (see Figure 12-6, page 209).

B. Types of Strokes by Function

1. *Assessment Stroke:* The stroke used to detect irregularities of the tooth surface such as the presence of calculus, a carious lesion, or a rough overhanging margin. The probe is used with an assessment stroke to locate the attachment at the bottom of the periodontal pocket. An ultrasonic tip is used with the power turned off to examine the surface being treated to estimate the thoroughness of the calculus removal. The assessment stroke is also called an exploratory stroke. The touch and pressure is light so that tactile sense is magnified.
2. *Working Stroke:* The stroke applied to accomplish a task such as calculus removal or reshaping an overhanging margin.

C. Types of Strokes by Direction (Figure 32-18)

1. *Diagonal or Oblique:* Stroke that is diagonal across the surface being treated (Figure 32-18A).
2. *Vertical:* Strokes parallel with the long axis of the tooth being treated (Figure 32-18B).
3. *Horizontal:* Strokes parallel with the occlusal

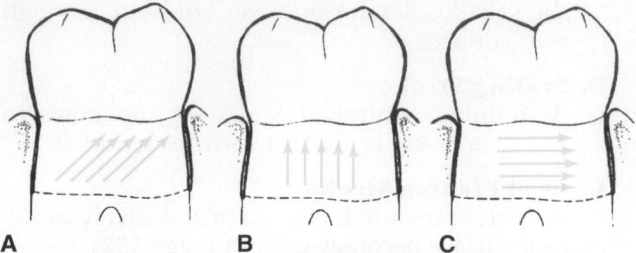

FIGURE 32-18 Directions of Instrument Strokes.
Arrows on root surface represent **(A)** diagonal or oblique stroke, **(B)** vertical stroke, **(C)** and horizontal stroke.

surface of the tooth (Figure 32-18*C*) being treated. They are sometimes called circumferential, which should not be interpreted to mean that a stroke can be made to go around a tooth or large segment of a tooth. A horizontal stroke necessarily must be a short stroke because of the constant changes in the topography of the tooth surface.

4. *Circular:* Stroke used with a porte polisher. A small circular stroke 1 to 2 mm in diameter is used with pressure, for example, to apply desensitizing paste (page 621).

II. FACTORS THAT INFLUENCE SELECTION OF STROKE

A. Size, contour, and position of gingiva.
B. Surface and section of surface where the instrument is used.
C. Probing depth.
D. Size and shape of instrument used.
E. Procedure objective, for example, nature of the deposit to be removed.

III. NATURE OF STROKE

A. Grasp

The grasp of a scaler or curet is light while the working end is positioned for the stroke, and then the instrument is held more firmly during movement. An explorer and a probe should be held lightly for tactile sensitivity at all times.

B. Hand Stability

During a stroke, the whole hand pivots or rotates on the fulcrum.

C. Motion

The motion for a stroke is generated by a unified action of the shoulder, arm, wrist, and hand.

D. Length

1. The length of the scaling stroke is limited by the extent of calculus deposit and by the anatomic features of the area where the deposit is located.
2. The stroke is short, controlled, decisive, and directed to protect the tissues from trauma.

3. Instrumentation should be applied to the section of the tooth where treatment is indicated. This section is called the *instrumentation zone*. Strokes should not be long enough to pass over the whole crown when the calculus represents only a small area at the cervical third of the tooth.
4. The length of a stroke varies with each instrument and purpose. A description of strokes for each instrument is included in the respective chapters. The probe is described on pages 208 to 209; the explorer, page 217; scalers and curets, page 552; and the ultrasonic scaler, page 559.

VISIBILITY AND ACCESSIBILITY

I. EFFECTS OF ADEQUATE VISION AND ACCESSIBILITY

A. Instrumentation is more thorough with minimal trauma to the oral tissues.
B. Length of time required is lessened, thereby lessening fatigue for patient and clinician.
C. Patient cooperation is increased because of shortened treatment time and less discomfort.

II. CONTRIBUTING FACTORS

A. Patient and clinician positions (pages 75 to 76).
B. Efficient use of direct or reflected (by mouth mirror) illumination for each tooth surface.
C. Adequate, yet gentle, retraction of lips, cheeks, and tongue with consideration for the patient's comfort and clinician's convenience.

DEXTERITY DEVELOPMENT

The dental hygiene student and the dental hygienist returning to practice after a temporary leave of absence can appreciate the need for exercises to develop dexterity and strength for the efficient and effective use of instruments. In addition, all students, returning retirees, and dental hygienists continuing in practice need an understanding of preventive measures that can preserve the health of their hands, arms, shoulders, and all muscles and joints involved when undertaking patient care.

However generally dexterous a person may be, the use of new or unusual instruments requires different procedures for coordination. Control is essential, and guided strength contributes to control.

Proficiency during procedures comes from repeated correct use of the instruments. Exercises for the fingers, hands, and arms supplement experience. Directed exercises are needed for both hands, separately and together. A regular period of time each day during the training period should be set aside for exercises.

I. SQUEEZING THERAPY PUTTY OR A SOFT BALL

A. Purpose
To develop strength and control.

B. Procedure
1. Hold putty in palm of hand; grip with thumb and all fingers (Figure 32-19A).
2. Tighten and release grip at regular intervals.
3. One hand rests while other is exercising.
4. Use a ball in each hand at the same time.

II. STRETCHING

A. Purposes
1. To strengthen finger and hand muscles.
2. To develop control of finger movements.

B. Rubber Band on Finger Joints
1. Place band at joint between first phalanx and second phalanx.
2. Stretch band by separating middle and ring fingers (Figure 32-19B).
3. Place band at joint between second phalanx and third phalanx and proceed as before.
4. Place bands on both hands and do exercises together.

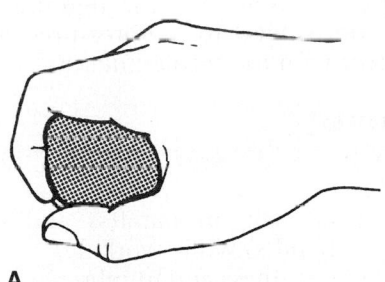

A

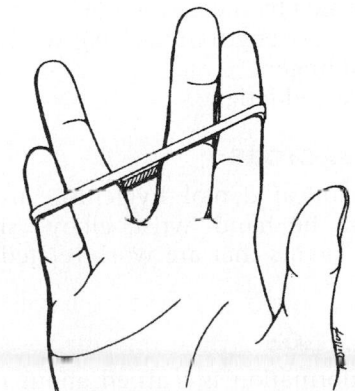

B

FIGURE 32-19 Exercises for Dexterity Development. (A) Squeezing therapy putty can aid in developing strength and control. **(B)** Stretching a rubber band can be applied at each group of finger and thumb joints.

C. Rubber Band on Finger Joints With Use of Fulcrum
1. Place band on joint between first phalanx and second phalanx.
2. Establish fulcrum (ring finger) on tabletop with little finger closely adjacent to it; elbow and forearm are free, as they are during instrumentation. Keep wrist straight, in same horizontal line as the forearm, and hold elbow at 90°. Stretch band by separating middle and ring fingers.
3. Touch thumb and index and middle fingers to simulate a modified pen grasp for holding an instrument. Stretch band by separating middle and ring fingers.
4. Variations
   a. Hold instrument in modified pen grasp while doing the exercise.
   b. Do writing exercise with rubber band in place.
5. Rest one hand while other is being exercised.

III. WRITING

A. Purposes
1. To develop correct modified pen grasp.
2. To propel instrument by activation from wrist and arm, without moving fingers.
3. To practice use of instruments when mouth mirror is required.
4. To develop control and precision.

B. Circles and Vertical Lines
1. Hold long, well-sharpened pencil with modified pen grasp.
2. Establish fulcrum (ring finger) on a piece of paper on tabletop. Keep wrist straight in line with forearm; elbow is at 90°, and shoulder is in neutral position. Forearm and elbow are free.
3. Inscribe counterclockwise small circles and vertical lines on paper, rapidly and lightly at first, slowly and with more pressure later.
4. Accomplish writing by activation of the hand by the upper arm, without flexing or extending the thumb and fingers holding the pencil.
5. Practice with each hand separately at first; then use a pencil in each hand at the same time, alternating writing action to simulate adaptation of the mirror first and then the explorer or scaler.

C. Using Mouth Mirror
1. Hold mouth mirror with modified pen grasp in nondominant hand close to pencil while practicing writing exercises (previous section) through the mirror. Reverse hands.
2. Using engineer's graph paper and modified pen grasp with fulcrum as described earlier, follow the lines of the small squares while looking in mirror held with opposite hand.

D. Everyday Penmanship

1. Use modified pen grasp whenever possible for writing.
2. Practice word writing with the left hand (with the right hand for left-handed person) to increase dexterity for handling instruments.

IV. MOUTH MIRROR, COTTON PLIERS, AND EXPLORER

A. Purposes

1. To develop ability to turn mouth mirror at various angles.
2. To develop dexterity in holding objects with cotton pliers.
3. To establish desired grasp of explorer to assure maximum touch sensitivity.

B. Mouth Mirror

1. Hold mouth mirror with modified pen grasp, ring finger on tabletop as fulcrum finger with little finger closely adjacent to it; elbow and forearm are free. The mirror is most frequently used in the nondominant hand.
2. Practice turning mirror with fingers, adjusting as to the several surfaces of the tooth.
3. Hold a small object in the dominant hand for viewing in mirror held in nondominant hand.
4. Practice crossing the mirror over fulcrum finger as in position for retracting lower lip while viewing lingual surfaces of mandibular anterior teeth in mouth mirror.

C. Cotton Pliers

1. Make small, tight cotton pellets with thumb and index and middle fingers of each hand; then make one in each hand simultaneously.
2. Hold cotton pliers with modified pen grasp and establish fulcrum finger on tabletop; elbow and forearm are free.
3. Practice picking up cotton pellets using mirror vision.
   a. Use in wiping motion on tabletop or other object.
   b. Move to different area to release pellet.

V. TACTILE SENSITIVITY

A. Explorer

1. Hold explorer with modified pen grasp, and establish fulcrum finger on tabletop with upper arm and forearm free.
2. Mount small pieces of fine-grain sandpaper of varying abrasiveness. With eyes closed, compare roughness.
3. Use extracted teeth to feel with explorer tip until a light grasp permits maximum security of grasp and maximum sense of touch. Extracted teeth can be used to provide a contrast between exploring enamel, cementum,

calculus, or other rough area of tooth surface (page 229).

B. Probe

1. Repeat exercises described for explorer.
2. Compare with explorer.

PREVENTION OF CUMULATIVE TRAUMA

Of the many types of cumulative trauma, carpal tunnel syndrome is most common and well known. Surveys have shown that as many as 6% to 7% of dental hygienists have been diagnosed with carpal tunnel syndrome, and many more have reported pain and other symptoms related to cumulative trauma.[3–5] Box 32-2 defines key words relating to cumulative trauma.

I. ANATOMY OF THE MEDIAN NERVE

The symptoms of carpal tunnel syndrome are caused by compression of the median nerve within the carpal tunnel. Figure 32-20 shows the anatomic parts of the wrist. The tunnel is formed by the concave arch of the carpal wrist bones and roofed over by the transverse carpal ligament.

The median nerve passes through the tunnel and emerges to send branches to the thumb, index, and second fingers, and to the medial aspect of the ring finger, as illustrated in Figure 32-21. Distribution of the ulnar and radial nerves is also shown. The ulnar and radial nerves do not pass through the carpal tunnel and are not subject to the pressures of compression that occur with the median nerve.

II. SYMPTOMS[5]

A. Pain in hand, wrist, shoulder, neck, lower back.
B. Nocturnal pain in hand(s) and forearm(s); pain in hand(s) while working.
C. Morning stiffness and numbness.
D. Daytime numbness and tingling in areas innervated by median nerve.
E. Loss of strength in hand(s); weakened grip.
F. Cold fingers.
G. Increased fatigue.

III. RISK FACTORS

Practicing clinical dental hygienists are at risk for problems of the hand, wrist, elbow, shoulder, and back.[5] Risk factors that are work related are listed in Table 32-1.

IV. PREVENTION

As more information is learned about the effects of clinical practice habits on the development of carpal tunnel syndrome, detrimental habits can be prevented and corrected. New students will learn from the start how to prevent and control individual risk factors.

BOX 32-2 KEY WORDS: Cumulative Trauma

Carpal tunnel syndrome: the most common type of cumulative trauma; combination of symptoms that results from compression of the median nerve in the transverse carpal tunnel; also called compression neuropathy.

Cumulative trauma: refers to disorders of the musculoskeletal, autonomic, and peripheral nervous systems caused by repeated stresses to tendons, muscles, or nerves. Repeated stresses include awkward postures, forceful grasps, as well as exposure to mechanical stresses, vibration, and cold temperatures.

Flexion (flek'shun): act of bending, such as the forearm bent at the elbow and raised toward shoulder.

Hypesthesia (hīp"es-thē'zhah): abnormally diminished sensitivity.

Median nerve: mixed nerve with both sensory and motor fibers; passes under the transverse carpal ligament at the wrist and branches to supply the thumb, first two fingers, and the medial aspect of the ring finger (Figure 32-21).

Median nerve compression: nerve entrapment and compression within the carpal tunnel resulting from increased pressure from injury or inflammation.

Paresthesia (par"es-thē'zhah): abnormal sensation, such as burning, prickling, or tingling.

Phelan's test (Fā'lanz): a test for carpal tunnel syndrome in which the hands are placed back to back with wrists flexed at 90° and held for 1 minute; if tingling or numbness occurs, the test is positive.

Tinel's sign (Tī nelz'): nerve compression in the carpal tunnel can be diagnosed by tapping over the median nerve on the ventral side of the wrist; if the median nerve is compressed, tingling or electric shooting pain will result.

A. Clinical Procedures[5-8]

Table 32-2 provides a comprehensive list of recommendations for decreasing the incidence of cumulative trauma.

Each dental hygienist needs to analyze the daily clinical routine to identify the potential activities that can contribute to symptoms of cumulative trauma. By taking necessary precautions, later problems may be avoided.

B. Exercises

Stretching exercises for stress release, improvement of posture, and counteracting the repetitive movements used during patient care are shown in Figure 32-22.

1. *Hand muscles.* Special exercises for the hand muscles can be important. A variety of exercises have been devised using therapy putty, as suggested in Figure 32-19.[7,8]

    Stretching exercises performed between patients during working hours can contribute to less fatigue. One exercise to practice is shown in Figure 32-23. Each time an instrument is returned to the tray, fingers can be stretched before retrieval of the next instrument.

2. *Time Spent on Exercises*
    a. Time spent on exercises should be sufficient in any one period to cause moder-

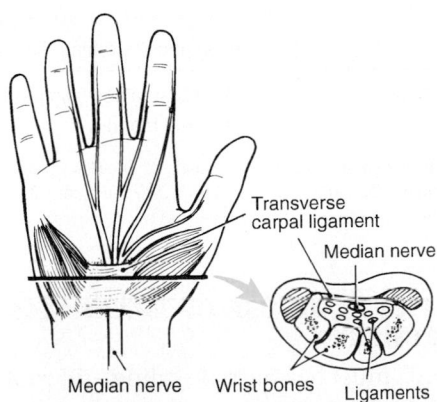

FIGURE 32-20 Anatomy of the Wrist. *Left,* the median nerve passes through the transverse carpal tunnel of the wrist and branches to innervate the thumb, the index and middle fingers, and the medial aspect of the ring finger. ***Right,*** cross section of wrist shows the median nerve passing through the carpal tunnel. The tunnel is formed by the concave arch of the carpal (wrist) bones and roofed over by the transverse carpal ligament.

Transverse carpal ligament
Median nerve
Median nerve   Wrist bones   Ligaments

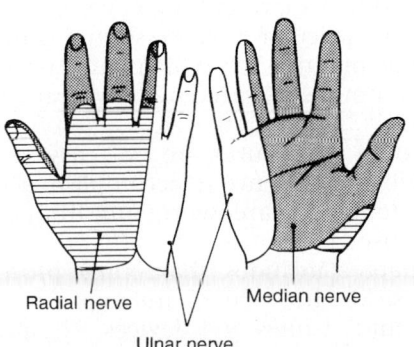

Radial nerve   Median nerve
Ulnar nerve

FIGURE 32-21 Distribution of the Median Nerve Fibers. Back of hand on left and palm on right show distribution of radial, ulnar, and median nerves.

TABLE 32-1 Risk Factors for Cumulative Trauma

Repetition	Constant wrist and forearm flexion, extension, rotation Constant tight grasping with thumb and fingers
Force	Firm grasp on instrument handle during scaling and root planing Firm grasp on ultrasonic instrument
Awkward posture	Back and shoulders rounded Arms elevated Elbows bent more than 90° Wrist flexed or deviated while fingers grasp
Static posture	Maintaining same position for long period
Vibration	Cumulative use of instruments with vibration (ultrasonic and sonic handpieces)
Mechanical stress	Instruments pressing on nerves or blood vessels in fingers
Cold temperature	Handwashing with cold water Cold room temperature Cold constricts blood flow

(From Martha Sanders, Occupational and Sports Medicine Center, Meriden, CT. Used by permission.)

TABLE 32-2 Recommendations to Decrease the Incidence of Cumulative Trauma

Hand use	Use proper instrumentation Keep wrist in neutral during forearm rotation Vary between intraoral and extraoral fulcrums Avoid thumb hypertension Wear proper-fitting gloves; avoid glove constriction at thumb joint
Instruments	Select balanced instruments Use wide-diameter handles Use instruments with handle serrations Keep instruments sharp Dampen vibration components (ultrasonic, sonic, handpieces) Minimize drag on hose; keep hose untangled
Posture	Use alternate work positions Keep neutral positions for shoulders, elbow, wrist Use properly adjusted clinician's stool with lumbar support Use indirect vision (mouth mirror) to avoid awkward, twisted positions Stretch forearm, neck, shoulders, and back periodically
Workplace practices	Alternate scheduling of heavy- and light-calculus patients Allot adequate time per patient; haste tenses fingers and general posture Eliminate wasted motions; minimize reach distances Utilize selective polishing to minimize use of handpiece Add buffer time to schedule for relaxation and stretching
Body signals	Pay attention to body signals, such as pain and fatigue

(Adapted from Atwood, M.J. and Michalak, C.: The Occurrence of Cumulative Trauma in Dental Hygienists, *WORK, 2,* 17, Summer, 1992.)

ate (but never severe) strain and fatigue of hand muscles.

    b. To relax the muscles of the hands during a practice session, wash hands in warm water.

INSTRUMENT SHARPENING

Objectives for techniques of sharpening emphasize the *preservation of the original shape* of the instrument while restoring a sharp cutting edge. Instruments designed for a particular purpose should continue to be used in the manner for which they were designed and should not be distorted by inaccurate sharpening techniques.

Sharpening procedures are not easy to learn and require skill and patience to accomplish. More instruments undoubtedly are worn out from sharpening than from use.

This chapter includes sharpening procedures for the curet, sickle, hoe, chisel, and explorer, using various sharpening stones and devices. The principles of sharpening that are outlined and illustrated here may be applied to various types of sharpening stones and instruments. Terms related to instrument sharpening are defined in Box 32-3.

I. BENEFITS FROM USE OF SHARP MANUAL INSTRUMENTS

Instruments must be sharp if scaling and root debridement are to be completed efficiently with minimal trauma to the tissues. When the instrument blade is maintained with its original contour and sharp cutting edges, the following may be expected:

    A. Greater precision of treatment, improved quality of results, and less working time involved.

    B. Increased tactile sensitivity during instrumentation. A sharp instrument does not have to be gripped as firmly as a dull one.

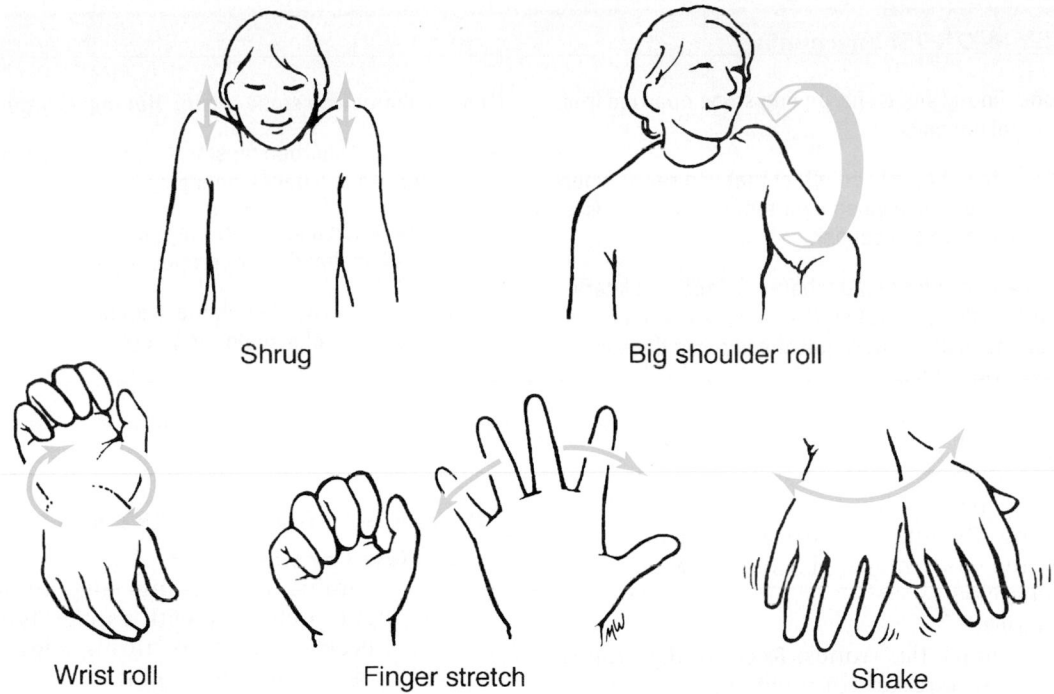

Shrug   Big shoulder roll

Wrist roll   Finger stretch   Shake

■ **FIGURE 32-22 Chairside Stretching Exercises.** Stretching exercises to relax the back, shoulders, and neck are shown with the shrug, and rolling the head around with the big shoulder roll. Hand and finger rolls, stretches, and shaking can be performed anytime, even while attending a patient.

C. Greater control of the instrument because of the lighter grasp needed; less pressure on the tooth being scaled or planed and decreased pressure on the finger rest are required.

D. Fewer strokes required.

E. Less possibility of burnishing rather than removing the calculus.

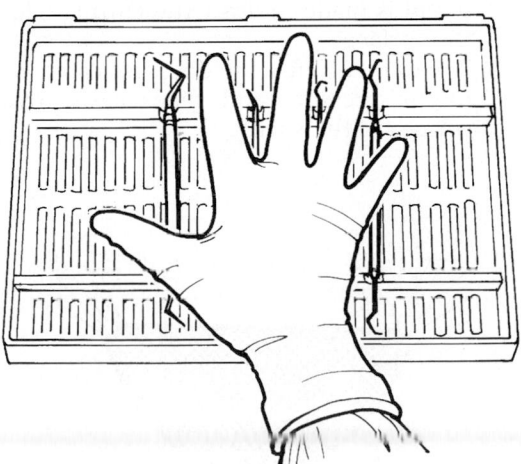

■ **FIGURE 32-23 Stretching Fingers Prior to Instrument Retrieval.** One of the exercises that can be used during actual clinical practice.

F. Prevention of unnecessary trauma to gingival tissues and, therefore, less discomfort experienced by the patient.

G. Decreased possibility of nicking, grooving, or scratching the tooth surfaces.

H. Less fatigue for the clinician.

II. SHARPENING STONES

A. Materials and Their Sources

1. *Natural Abrasive Stones.* Quarried from mineral deposits, the hard Arkansas stone is used for dental instruments because of its fine abrasive particle size.

2. *Artificial Materials*

   a. Hard, nonmetallic substances impregnated with aluminum oxide, silicon carbide, or diamond particles. Examples: ruby stone, carborundum stones, and the diamond hone.

   b. Ceramic aluminum oxide.

   c. Steel alloys are metals that are harder than most dental instrument steel and, therefore, are capable of sharpening the instrument. Example: tungsten carbide steel used in the Neivert whittler.

B. Categories

Sharpening stones as they are manufactured for use may be classified into two general groups: those for manual (unmounted) sharpening and

BOX 32-3 KEY WORDS: Sharpening

Arkansas stone: fine-grained sharpening stone quarried from natural mineral deposits.

Burnish: to smooth and polish; an effect that can result when a dull scaler or curet is passed over tenacious calculus in an attempt to remove the deposit.

Cutting edge: the fine line formed where the face and lateral surfaces of a scaler or curet meet when the instrument is sharp; when the instrument is dull, the line has thickness and may even reflect light.

Hone: a sharpening stone (noun). **Honing:** sharpening (verb).

Rotary stone: a sharpening stone mounted on a metal mandrel for use in a dental handpiece.

Sharpness: when a scaler or curet is sharp, the cutting edge is a fine line that does not reflect light.

Testing stick: plastic ¼-inch rod, 3 inches long, used to test the sharpness of a scaler or a curet.

---

those for power-driven (mandrel-mounted) sharpening. Examples of procedures using both unmounted and mounted stones are supplied in this chapter.

1. *Unmounted*
   a. Stationary flat stones: Rectangular stones with square or rounded edges, or with one side grooved for the special adaptation of curved blades.
   b. Hand stones: Cylindrical (tapered or straight) or rectangular with rounded edges.
   c. Other types: Sharpening devices, such as the Neivert whittler.
2. *Mandrel Mounted.* Cylindrical (straight or tapered) small stones of various diameters designed to fit the various sizes of instrument blades.

III. DYNAMICS OF SHARPENING

A. Sharpening Stone Surface

A sharpening stone acts as an abrasive to reshape a dulled blade by grinding the surface until the cutting edge is restored. The surface of the stone is made up of masses of minute crystals, which are the abrasive particles that accomplish the grinding of the instrument. A smaller particle size or a finer grain, as it is generally called, abrades or reduces more slowly and produces a finer cutting edge.

B. Cutting Edge

The cutting edge is a very fine *line* formed where the face and lateral surface meet at an angle. The edge is a line and, therefore, has length but no thickness. The edge becomes dull when pressed against a hard surface (the tooth), or it may be nicked when drawn over a rough surface. A dull edge is rounded and therefore has thickness. *The object in sharpening is to reshape the cutting edge to a line.*

C. Sharpening

Sharpening is accomplished by grinding the surface or surfaces that form the cutting edge.

IV. TESTS FOR INSTRUMENT SHARPNESS

A. Visual or Glare Test

1. Examine the cutting edge under adequate light, preferably with a magnifying glass.
2. Because the sharp cutting edge is a fine *line,* it does not reflect light.
3. The dull cutting edge presents a rounded, shiny *surface,* which reflects light. Figure 32-24 shows the cross section of a dull universal curet. The cutting edges are tiny surfaces that reflect light. Compare the cutting edges with Figure 32-5 (page 516), which shows the sharp cutting edges, at the points labelled "c," of a universal curet.

B. Plastic Testing Stick[9]

1. Use a sterile plastic or acrylic ¼-inch rod, 3 inches long.
2. Apply the instrument blade to the plastic stick at the correct angle for scaling; press lightly but firmly.
3. The sharp cutting edge engages or grips the plastic and moves with resistance if an attempt is made to draw the cutting edge over the surface.
4. The dull cutting edge does not catch without undue pressure and slides easily over the surface of the stick.

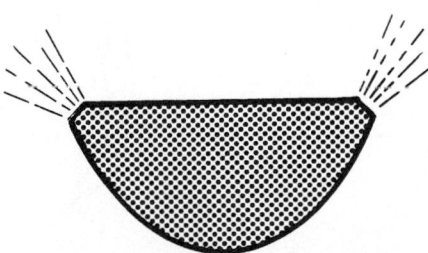

■ **FIGURE 32-24 Cross Section of a Dull Curet.** A sharp curet has a fine line at the cutting edge that will not reflect light. A dull cutting edge is a like a small surface and reflects light as shown.

5. Test each area along an entire cutting edge because the edge is not uniformly dulled during use.

SOME BASIC SHARPENING PRINCIPLES

I. STERILIZATION OF THE SHARPENING STONE

A sterile sharpening stone and testing stick should be a part of the basic clinic set-up for a scaling appointment. Instruments then may be sharpened throughout the procedure as they show signs of dullness. Efficiency increases, and the patient benefits from receiving a more thorough treatment in less time.

Sterilization of stones may be accomplished by any of the acceptable sterilization methods described in Chapter 4 (pages 60 to 64). The steam autoclave may dry out an Arkansas stone and lead to chipping or breakage.

II. INSTRUMENT HANDLING

All instruments must be handled with care to preserve sharpness and prevent accidental damage to the cutting edges.

III. PREPARATION OF STONE FOR SHARPENING

A. Dry Stone
Because of the problems related to maintaining a sterile stone and preventing contamination when oil, tap water, or a lubricant is applied, the use of a dry stone provides a particular advantage.

A dry stone contributes to the following effects:
1. Sharpens the cutting edge without nicks in the blade; nicks can be created from particles of metal suspended in a lubricant.
2. Allows the stone to be completely sterilized without the problem of interference by the oil left in and on the stone.

B. Water on Stone
Ceramic stones may be used dry or with water.

C. Lubricated Stone
Certain quarried stones need lubrication to prevent drying out. Instruments are autoclaved before sharpening, and then stone and instruments are sterilized again after nonsterile lubricant is used.

When it is necessary to sharpen during a treatment, a sterile swab is used to apply a thin layer of water-soluble lubricant to the sterile stone. The lubricant must be kept in a clinically clean covered jar or tube and reserved expressly for that purpose.

The lubricant can provide the following effects:
1. Facilitate the movement of the instrument blade over the stone and prevent scratching of the stone.
2. Suspend the metallic particles removed during sharpening and so help to prevent clogging of the pores of the stone (glazing).

IV. SHARPENING

A. Objectives
The objectives during sharpening are to produce a sharp cutting edge and to preserve the original shape of the blade.

B. When to Sharpen
Sharpen at the first sign of dullness during an appointment. When instruments become grossly dulled, recontouring wastes the instrument. Restoration of the original contour while maintaining a strong blade is difficult to achieve.

C. Angulation
Before starting to sharpen, analyze the cutting edge and establish the proper angle between the stone and the blade surface. Maintain the angle through the firm grasp, secure finger rest, moderate pressure, short stroke, and other features of the technique appropriate to the individual instrument.

D. Maintain Control
Maintain control so that the entire surface is reduced evenly. Care must be taken not to create a new bevel at the cutting edge.

E. Prevent Grooving
Prevent grooving of the sharpening stone by varying the areas for instrument placement. Cleaning and stain removal procedures are described on page 541.

V. AFTER SHARPENING

Gently hone or burnish the nonbeveled surface adjacent to the cutting edge.

A. Honing
Honing means sharpening, but in common usage, honing has been applied to the process whereby the "bur" or "wire edge" is removed from the side of the cutting edge that was not reduced.

B. How the Wire Edge Is Produced
During sharpening, some of the metal particles removed during grinding remain attached to the edge of the instrument and create the wire edge. If allowed to remain, the tiny particles may be removed when the instrument is applied to the tooth surface during treatment.

By sharpening into, toward, or against the cutting edge, the production of a wire edge is minimized.

C. Removal of Wire Edge

Using an even and light pressure, pass a sharpening stone along the side of the cutting edge. One or two strokes are usually sufficient. If heavy pressure is applied, the bevel of the cutting edge can be altered.

SHARPENING CURETS AND SICKLES

I. SELECTION OF CUTTING EDGE TO SHARPEN

The cutting edge is formed at the junction of the lateral surface and the face of the blade. Figure 32-25 shows the cutting edges to sharpen for a universal curet (two sides), an area-specific curet (one side), and a scaler (two sides). These instruments were described on pages 516 to 518.

To determine which side of an area-specific instrument to sharpen, hold the instrument upright with the back of the blade directed to the floor, and look into the face of the curet. In general, the cutting edge farthest from the handle (the one closest to the floor, the longest edge) is the correct edge to use for treatment and to sharpen.

II. SELECTION OF SHARPENING PROCEDURE

Sharpening of both the lateral surfaces and the face preserves the original contour of the blade. For both curets and sickles, the internal angle at the cutting edge is 70° to 80° (see Figures 32-5 and 32-8). To preserve or restore this angle, the sharpening stone must be placed and activated precisely.

Manual sharpening procedures are the methods of choice so that the blade is not reduced unnecessarily by a rapid-cutting mounted stone. Procedures in this section show the use of a flat stone for manual sharpening of lateral surfaces. When sharpening lateral surfaces, the flat stone may be used in one of two ways: the stone may be moved while the instrument is stationary, or the stone may be stationary while the instrument is moved.

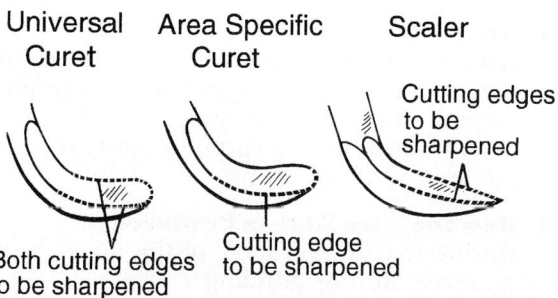

Universal Curet — Both cutting edges to be sharpened

Area Specific Curet — Cutting edge to be sharpened

Scaler — Cutting edges to be sharpened

FIGURE 32-25 Selection of Cutting Edge to Sharpen. Both cutting edges and the rounded toe are sharpened for a universal curet *(left)*. An area-specific curet is sharpened on the longer cutting edge and the rounded toe. A scaler is sharpened on the two sides and the tip is brought to a point.

MOVING FLAT STONE: STATIONARY INSTRUMENT

The side of the cutting edge formed by the lateral surface is reduced by this method. The technique described applies to both curets and sickles. Because the sickle has a pointed tip and the curet has a round toe end, a variation is necessary in the adaptation of the sharpening stone to that portion of the blade.

I. EXAMINE THE CUTTING EDGE TO BE SHARPENED

Test for sharpness to determine specific areas that are dull.

II. STABILIZE THE INSTRUMENT

A. Grasp the instrument in a palm grasp, and hold the hand against the edge of an immovable workbench or table under adequate light (Figure 32-26A). The instrument should be low enough to allow the clinician to see clearly the cutting edges and the angle formed by the instrument and the sharpening stone.

B. Turn the face of the instrument up and parallel with the floor. Point the toe toward the clinician to provide better access for moving the stone.

III. APPLY SHARPENING STONE

A. Apply the stone in a vertical position to the lateral surface at the end of the cutting edge nearest the terminal shank. Figure 32-26B shows the position for one side of the blade, and Figure 32-26C shows the position for the other side.

B. Look into the face of the scaler or curet (Figure 32-27).
 1. *Curet.* The cutting edges of the curet (c and c) are parallel from the terminal shank until they curve around to form the round toe. Both c and c-1 are sharpened for a universal curet, but only the longer cutting edge is sharpened for a Gracey curet (see Figure 32-25).
 2. *Scaler.* The cutting edges of the scaler (c and c-1) are parallel from the terminal shank until they curve in to form the pointed tip. All scalers are universal so are used and sharpened on both sides.

C. Adjust the angle at which the stone is held to maintain the internal 70° to 80° of the blade. The angle on the outside, between the instrument and the stone, is 100° to 110° (Figure 32-28A and B).

IV. ACTIVATE THE SHARPENING STONE

A. Keep the stone in contact with the blade and at the proper angle throughout the proce-

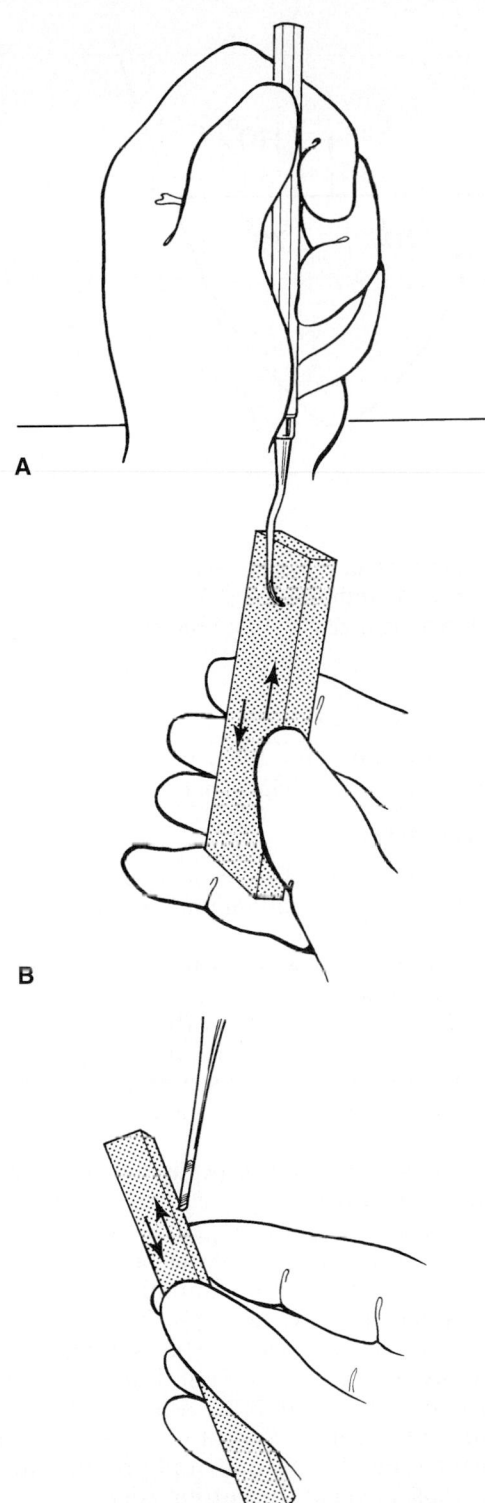

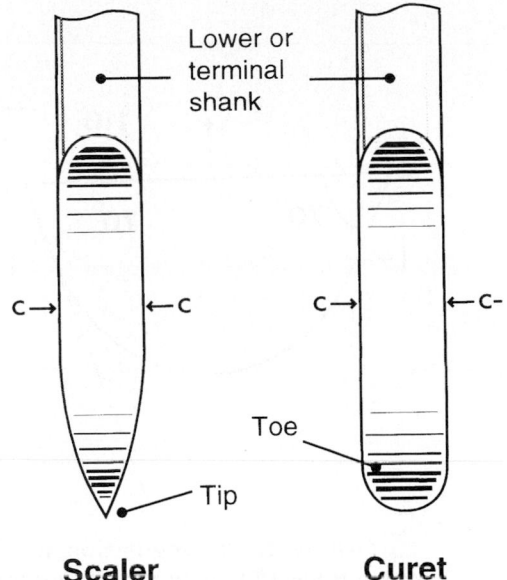

Lower or terminal shank

c→ ←c   c→ ←c-1

Toe

Tip

Scaler   **Curet**

▢ **FIGURE 32-27 View of a Scaler and a Curet Looking into the Face.** The cutting edges (*c* and *c-1*) are parallel until they curve in to form the pointed tip (scaler) or the round toe (curet).

A

B

C

▢ **FIGURE 32-26 Stationary Instrument—Moving Stone Technique. (A)** Grasp the instrument with the nondominant hand. Stabilize the hand on the edge of a stationary table or bench and provide good light on the instrument. **(B)** The stone is angled with the face of the instrument at 100° to 110° (Figure 32-28) to maintain the internal angle of the blade at 70 to 80°. **(C)** Stone reversed to sharpen the opposite cutting edge of a universal curet.

dure. The broken line in Figure 32-28 represents the flat surface of the sharpening stone.

B. Move the stone up and down with short rhythmic strokes about ⅛ to ¼ inch high. Put more pressure on the down stroke.

C. Follow the cutting edge from heel to toe, applying several strokes to each millimeter.

D. Do not change the angle of the stone with the face of the instrument. When the angle is varied, an irregularity is ground into the cutting edge.

E. Keep the wrist straight and use the whole arm to standardize the stroke and the adaptation of the stone to the instrument.

F. Variation at the toe end
   1. For a sickle scaler, the stone is held straight as it nears the pointed tip.
   2. For the curet, the position of the stone is adapted so that sharpening continues around the round toe. The same angle between the stone and the face is maintained.

G. Finish with a down stroke.

V. TEST FOR SHARPNESS

Determine whether to repeat the first side before starting the second.

STATIONARY FLAT STONE: MOVING INSTRUMENT

I. CURET

A. Place the stone flat on a steady surface.

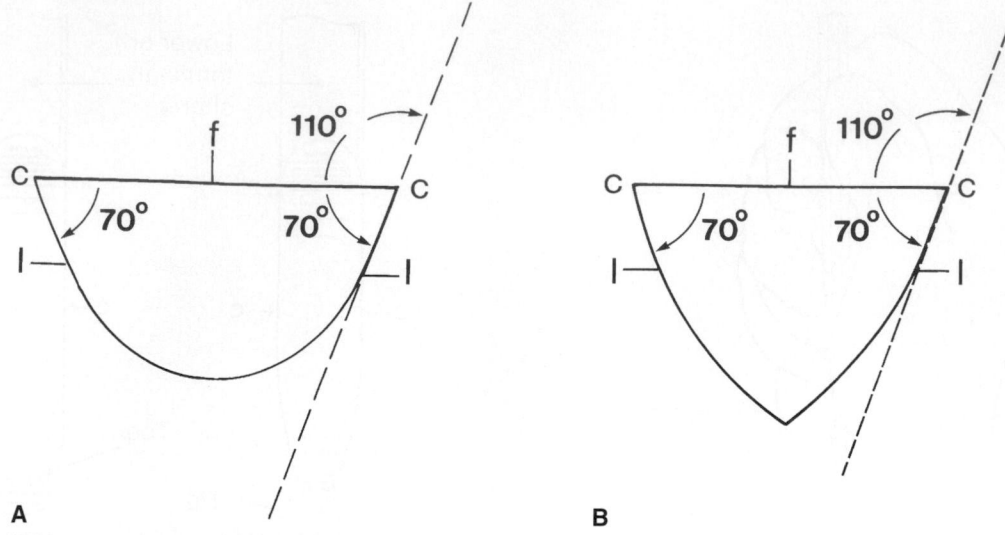

A **B**

■ FIGURE 32-28 **Angulation for Sharpening.** Cross sections of a curet **(A)** and a sickle scaler **(B)** show correct angulation of the face of the blade with the flat sharpening stone (broken line) to reproduce the internal angle of the instrument at 70°. Note the cutting edges (c) and the lateral surfaces (l).

B. Examine the cutting edges to be sharpened. Test for sharpness.
C. Hold the instrument in a modified pen grasp, and establish a secure finger rest (Figure 32-29A).
D. Apply the cutting edge to the stone. An angle of 110° is formed by the stone and face.
   1. Because the curet is curved, only a small section of the cutting edge can be applied at one time.
   2. Sharpening is performed in a *series* of applications of the cutting edge to the stone, each overlapping the previous, as the instrument is turned and drawn steadily along the stone.
   3. The portion of the cutting edge nearest the shank is applied first (Figure 32-29B, a).
E. Apply moderate to light but firm pressure while the instrument is activated.
F. Use a slow steady stroke to maintain control and to ensure that each portion of the cutting edge receives equal treatment.
G. Move the blade forward into the cutting edge. Turn the instrument continuously until the center of the round end of the blade is reached (Figure 32-29B, b).
H. Test for sharpness along the entire cutting edge; reapply to stone as necessary for ideal sharpness.
I. Turn the instrument to sharpen the second cutting edge. Overlap at the center of the round toe. Universal curets are sharpened on both sides and around the toe. Gracey curets are sharpened on one side only and around the toe (see Figure 32-25).
J. Use the manual sharpening cone (described in the next section) or the Neivert whittler (page

538) for removing the wire edge or for sharpening from the facial aspect.

II. SICKLE SCALER

A. Place the stone flat on a firm table or bench top under adequate light. Do not tilt the stone while sharpening.
B. Examine cutting edges to be sharpened. Test for sharpness.
C. Hold the instrument with a firm pen grasp, using thumb, index, and middle (second) fingers to prevent the instrument from rotating or changing angles during sharpening (Figure 32-30A).
D. Establish finger rest on side of stone using ring and little fingers.
E. Stabilize stone with fingers of opposite hand.
F. Apply cutting edge to be sharpened to the stone. Maintain 70° to 80° internal angle of the instrument (Figure 32-28B). The portion of the cutting edge nearest the shank is applied first.
G. Apply moderate to light but firm pressure while instrument is in motion. Heavy pressure can reduce control of instrument, cause scratching of the stone, and produce an unfavorable bevel at the cutting edge.
H. Use a short, slow stroke to maintain the exact relation of the cutting edge to the stone.
   1. Pull blade forward, toward the cutting edge.
   2. All fingers move with the arm as a unit.
   3. Use a slow, steady stroke to maintain control and to ensure that each portion of the cutting edge receives equal treatment.
   4. Turn the instrument continually to follow the arclike shape of the blade to the pointed tip.

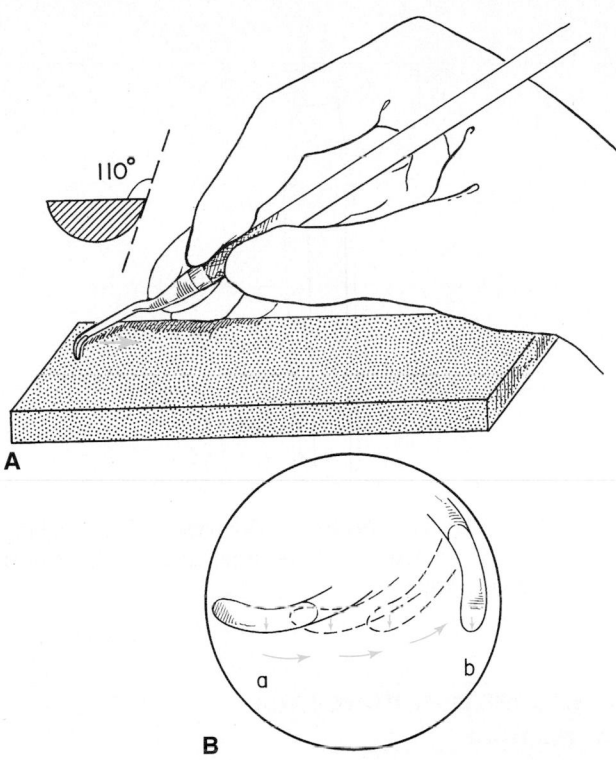

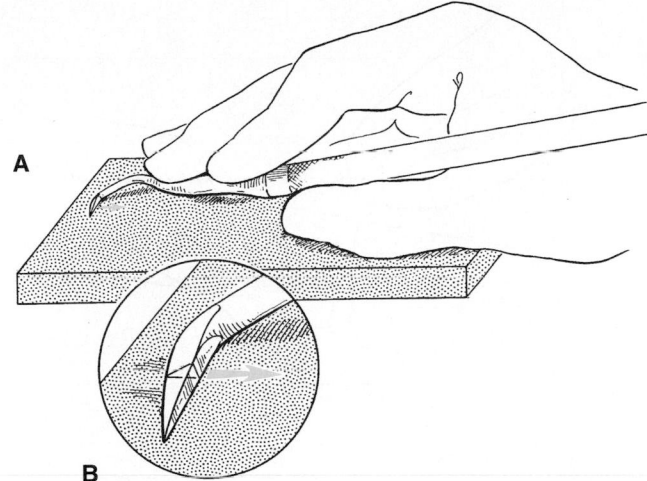

FIGURE 32-30 Stationary Stone Technique for a Scaler. (A) With a modified pen grasp and a finger rest established on the side of the stone, the scaler is positioned for sharpening. **(B)** The portion of the cutting edge nearest the lower shank is applied first with an angle of 100° to 110° between the face and the stone. The instrument is turned continuously to follow the arc-like shape of the blade. The cutting edges are sharpened to the pointed tip.

FIGURE 32-29 Stationary Stone—Moving Instrument Technique. (A) Stone placed flat with blade in position at the beginning of the sharpening stroke. With the finger rest stabilized on the edge of the stone, the cutting edge is maintained at the proper angulation (110°) as the instrument is drawn along the stone with an even moderate pressure. **(B)** The movement of the blade is shown by the arrows, which indicate each portion of the cutting edge as the blade is turned on the stone from the beginning (a) to the completion (b) of the stroke at the center of the round toe of the curet. For a universal curet, the instrument is turned over and the opposite cutting edge is sharpened.

I. Test for sharpness after one or two strokes. Repeat as needed for ideal sharpness.

J. Turn instrument and proceed to sharpen other lateral surface. When instrument placement is awkward for a modified contra-angle sickle, use a narrow side of the stone.

SHARPENING CONE

I. DESCRIPTION

A. Types

Stones are cylindrical Arkansas cones (tapered or straight), or rectangular with rounded edges, and tapered carborundum stones.

B. Uses

1. *Arkansas.* Tapered cone is recommended for curved cutting edges of sickles and curets.
2. *Carborundum.* Coarser grain is useful for pre-

liminary shaping or sharpening of excessively dulled instruments. Use of a finer stone follows to refine the cutting edge.

II. SHARPENING PROCEDURE

A. Position

1. Hold instrument in nondominant hand across palm with fingers and thumb grasping firmly. Direct blade toward self, with face of the blade up and parallel with the floor.
2. For additional support, place instrument over the edge of a firm hard block and maintain rigidly (Figure 32-31).
3. Stabilize arms between the wrists and elbows on the edge of a solid table or bench top.
4. Use the following procedure for a tapered cone:
   a. With a firm grasp of the sharpening cone, position the appropriate diameter of the cone to fit the curvature of the surface to be sharpened.
   b. Apply the stone straight across the face so that an even pressure can be applied to both cutting edges simultaneously to produce an evenly sharpened instrument (Figure 32-31).

B. Motion

1. Rotate stone counterclockwise over the instrument with even, firm pressure.
2. Continue rotation of stone upward (as in a circle) when approaching the end of the

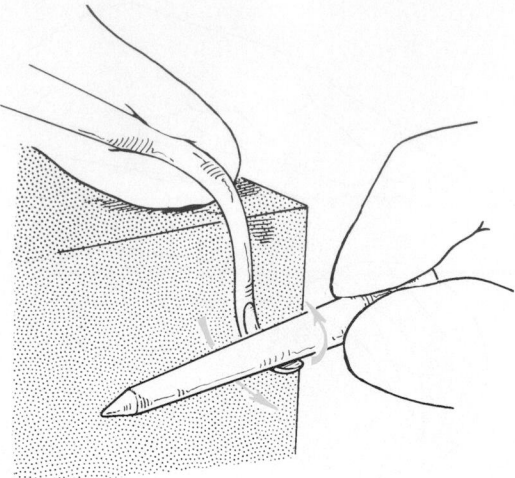

FIGURE 32-31 **Sharpening Cone.** A cylindrical stone is applied to the face of a curet. The instrument is stabilized over a firm block, and the stone is positioned to fit the curvature of the surface to be sharpened. An even pressure is applied across the face of the instrument so that both cutting edges will be sharpened on the same plane.

curet to prevent tapering off and reshaping (flattening) the curvature of the tip. (Figure 32-34*B* illustrates this motion for the mounted stone.)

C. Test for Sharpness
Test for sharpness after a few applications. Repeat as necessary to obtain ideal sharpness.

THE NEIVERT WHITTLER

I. DESCRIPTION

A. Working End
The working end consists of five sharpening edges and a rounded burnishing edge of tungsten carbide steel.

B. Handle
The handle, which is made of stainless steel, is bulky and hexagonal for comfortable grasping (Figure 32-32).

II. USES
A. Manufacturer's instructions describe the procedure used for sharpening straight and curved blades, including those of dental instruments, scissors, and knives.
B. Particularly useful for the face of a curved scaler or curet.
C. The outer rounded edge is designed for honing.

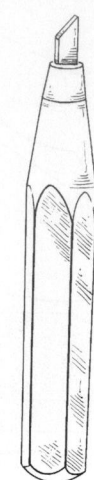

FIGURE 32-32 **The Neivert Whittler.** The working end is made of tungsten carbide steel and the handle is made of stainless steel.

III. SHARPENING PROCEDURE

A. Position
Stability and control are most important.
1. Hold instrument to be sharpened firmly in the nondominant hand, across palm, grasping with all fingers and the thumb, with the surface to be sharpened turned toward self. The instrument can also be stabilized over the edge of a firm, hard surface, as shown for the cone in Figure 32-31.
2. Stabilize arms between the wrists and the elbows on the edge of an immovable table or bench top.
3. Whittler is held in a palm grasp with thumb under handle adjacent to the working end. At the same time, the thumb rest is applied beneath the instrument blade on the nondominant hand (Figure 32-33*A*).
4. Apply working end to the curvature of the surface to be sharpened straight across so that even pressure can be applied to both cutting edges simultaneously, thereby producing an evenly sharpened instrument (Figure 32-33*B*).

B. Motion
1. Draw the whittler edge across the length of the face with a moderate, even pressure.
2. As the end is approached, continue in an upward motion to prevent tapering off and reshaping curvature of the tip.

C. Test for Sharpness
Test for sharpness after a few applications.

D. Hone
Hone the lateral surfaces of blade next to cutting edges.

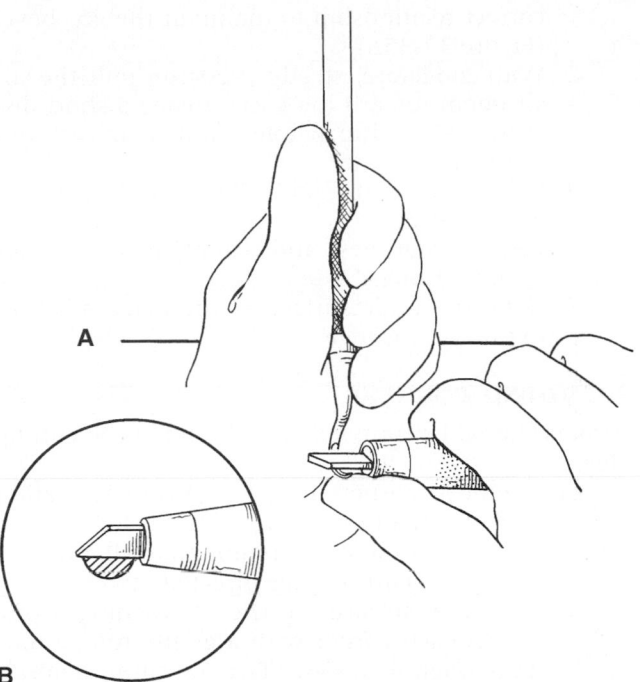

FIGURE 32-33 Sharpening with a Neivert Whittler. (A) The instrument is stabilized in the nondominant hand, and the whittler is held in a palm grasp with the thumb rest close to the instrument to be sharpened. **(B)** Close-up shows position of the blade of the sharpener across the face of the curet.

MANDREL-MOUNTED STONES

I. DESCRIPTION

A. Types
1. *Arkansas:* Fine grain.
2. *Ruby Stone:* Coarser grain, especially useful for recontouring excessively dull instrument. When used for routine sharpening, the ruby stone should be applied conservatively.

B. Shapes
The stones are cylindrical with flat end or cone shape.

C. Use
1. Applicable to most cutting edges. Various sizes and grains of stones are selectively utilized.
2. Coarse-grained ruby stone may be useful for reshaping.
3. Stones are sterilized and may be used with water for cooling.

II. SHARPENING PROCEDURE

A. Select Stone
Select a sharpening stone with a diameter appropriate to fit the blade of the instrument to be sharpened.

B. Position
1. Hold instrument to be sharpened in a palm grasp with blade face up.
2. Hold handpiece in other hand using a palm grasp with the thumb securely placed against the thumb of the hand holding the instrument (Figure 32-34*A*).
3. Stabilize arms between wrists and elbows on the edge of a solid table or bench top.
4. Apply stone to surface to be sharpened straight across so that light, even pressure can be applied to both cutting edges simultaneously, thereby producing an evenly sharpened instrument.

C. Motion
1. Use low speed to
   a. Minimize heat production (alteration of the temper of the steel can result with repeated use).
   b. Allow complete control of position of sharpening stone on blade.
2. Apply light pressure to prevent undue reduction of instrument. Pressure, however, should be sufficiently heavy to create a smooth surface.
3. Maintain blade shape. Pass the rotating stone upward when approaching the end of the blade to prevent tapering off and reshaping the tip (Figure 32-34*B*).

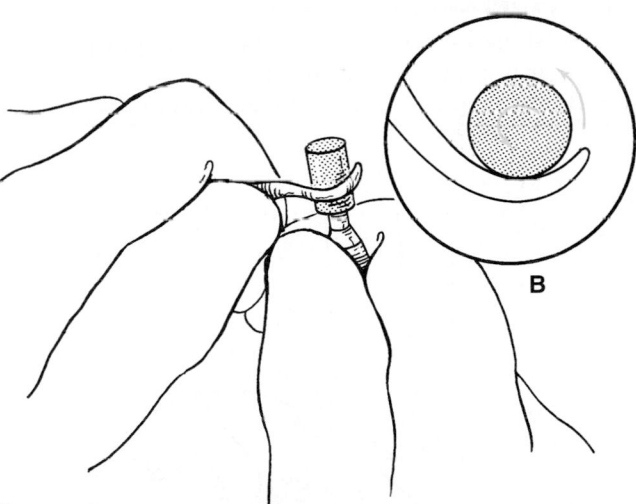

FIGURE 32-34 Mandrel-Mounted Sharpening Stone. (A) A mounted stone with a diameter appropriate for the curved blade to be sharpened is positioned across the face for even sharpening of the cutting edges. Hands and arms are stabilized for precision and control. **(B)** With low speed to minimize heat production, the rotating stone is passed along the face of the instrument. Near the toe, the stone is moved upward to prevent flattening of a curved instrument.

D. Test for Sharpness

Test for sharpness after one or two applications. Repeat when necessary.

E. Hone

Hone the lateral borders of the cutting edges.

III. DISADVANTAGES OF POWER-DRIVEN SHARPENING

A. Inconsistent results because of variations in speed and difficulty of stabilization of instrument and sharpening stone.

B. Excess reduction of instrument during shorter period of use; less conservation of instruments than by manual methods.

C. Frictional heat may affect the temper of the steel.

SHARPENING THE HOE SCALER

Characteristics of the hoe scaler are described on page 518. The hoe has only one surface to be ground. Because placement of the small surface on the flat stone is difficult to visualize, use of a magnifying glass can be particularly helpful.

I. SURFACE TO BE GROUND

Examine surface to be ground (Figure 32-35A). Test for sharpness.

II. SHARPENING PROCEDURE

A. Hold instrument in modified pen grasp. Establish finger rest on the stone.

B. Apply the surface to be ground to the stone in

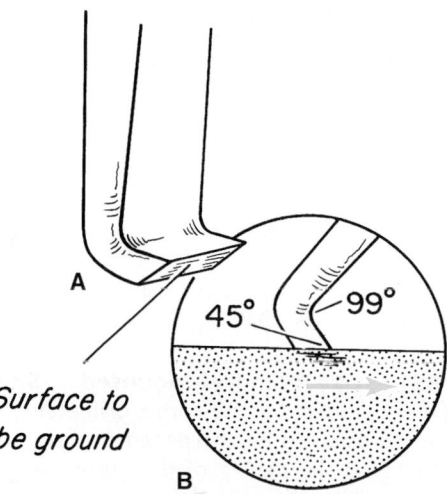

A

45°   **99°**

Surface to be ground

B

■ **FIGURE 32-35 Sharpening a Hoe Scaler. (A)** Surface to be ground. **(B)** Hoe adapted to the surface of a stationary flat stone at the proper angle to maintain the original bevel of 45°. Arrow indicates direction of the sharpening stroke leading into the cutting edge.

correct relationship to maintain the 45° bevel (Figure 32-35B).

C. With moderate, steady pressure, pull the instrument toward the cutting edge a short distance. Allow the whole hand to move with the arm as a unit.

D. Release pressure and slide the instrument back. Repeat.

E. Test for sharpness and reapply as needed for ideal sharpness.

F. Hone the undersurface of the blade adjacent to the cutting edge.

III. ROUND CORNERS

Corners should be rounded at each end of the cutting edge.

A. Rounded corners help to prevent laceration of soft tissue or grooving of tooth surface.

B. Hold instrument in nondominant hand with corners of cutting edge directed inward.

C. Rub the surface of the sharpening stone across each corner with a gentle rolling motion (Figure 32-36). Two or three applications are usually sufficient.

SHARPENING THE CHISEL SCALER

Sharpening procedures for the chisel are similar to those for the hoe. Again, the surface is small, the angulation is difficult to visualize, and the use of a magnifying glass is recommended. Review the characteristics of the chisel scaler on page 519.

I. SURFACE TO BE GROUND

Examine surface to be ground (Figure 32-37A). Test for sharpness.

II. SHARPENING PROCEDURE

A. Hold instrument with a modified pen grasp, establish finger rest, and apply the surface to be ground to the stone in the correct relationship to maintain the 45° bevel (Figure 32-37B).

B. With moderate, steady pressure, push the instrument forward, toward the cutting edge,

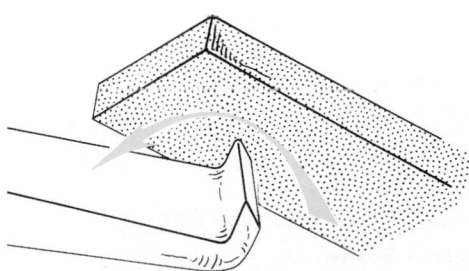

■ **FIGURE 32-36 Rounding a Hoe Scaler.** To round the sharp corners of the hoe scaler, a flat stone is rubbed over the instrument with a gentle rolling motion.

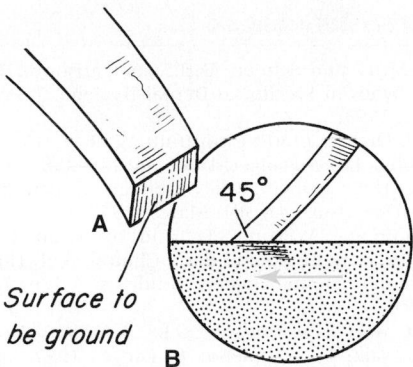

FIGURE 32-37 Sharpening a Chisel Scaler. (A) Surface to be ground. **(B)** Chisel is adapted to the surface of a stationary flat stone at the proper angle to maintain the original bevel of 45°. Arrow indicates direction of the sharpening stroke leading into the cutting edge.

without changing the relationship with the stone.

C. After two or three applications, test for sharpness and reapply as necessary for an ideal cutting edge.

D. Hone the nonbeveled surface.

III. ROUND CORNERS

Round the corners at each end of the cutting edge. In a manner similar to that shown in Figure 32-36 for the hoe scaler, rub the surface of the flat stone across each corner of the chisel with a gentle, even, rolling motion. Two or three applications are usually sufficient.

SHARPENING EXPLORERS

I. TESTS FOR SHARPNESS

A. Visual

When examined under concentrated light, a dull explorer tip appears rounded.

B. Plastic Testing Stick

A sharp explorer grips the plastic tester on light pressure and moves with resistance when pulled over the surface. A dull explorer does not catch. It slides.

II. RECONTOUR

Small-nosed pliers can be used to straighten a bent tip.

III. SHARPENING PROCEDURE

A. Use flat stone.

B. Instrument is held with a modified pen grasp. Finger rest is established on side of stone.

C. Placement and movement of the tip over the stone resemble somewhat the procedure for the curet on the stone (see Figure 32-29, page 537).

1. Place side of tip on stone at approximately a 15° to 20° angle of stone with shank of explorer.

2. As tip is moved over the surface, the handle is rotated so that even pressure can be applied to each part of the tip.

CARE OF SHARPENING STONES

I. FLAT ARKANSAS STONE

A. Prepare for Sterilization

Submerge in ultrasonic cleaner or scrub with soap and hot water to remove metal particles left from sharpening. Wrap and seal for sterilization or place in cassette.

B. Stain Removal

Periodically clean with ammonia, gasoline, or kerosene when stone becomes discolored. If the stone becomes "glazed" by metal particles ground into the surface, rub the stone over emery paper placed on a flat, solid surface.

C. Storage

Keep in sealed, sterilized package until needed for sharpening.

II. MOUNTED STONES

A. Arkansas Mounted Stones

Same basic procedures as those for the flat stone.

B. Ruby Stone

1. Clean by scrubbing with soap and water.

2. Maintain an ungrooved surface by frequently applying the stone to a Joe Dandy disc (Figure 32-38). A sandpaper disc is too flexible for this purpose.

3. Sterilize in a sealed bag.

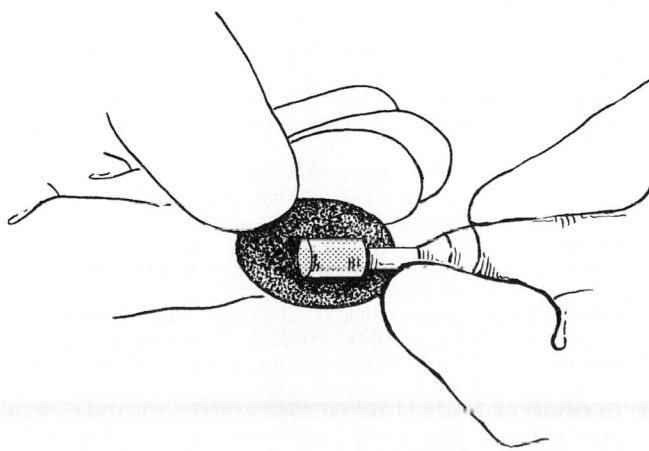

FIGURE 32-38 Care of a Mounted Stone. A Joe Dandy disc is used to maintain a smooth surface on the stone. Repeated sharpenings tend to make grooves in a stone.

III. MANUFACTURER'S DIRECTIONS

Follow manufacturer's directions for all artificial stones.

TECHNICAL HINTS

I. Prevent unnecessary dulling of instruments by applying the following suggestions:

A. When handling instruments for cleaning, sterilizing, or other reasons, keep blades from hooking, bumping, or pressing against each other, as cutting edges become dull from contact with hard metal surfaces. Thinner instruments, such as explorers and probes, are subject to bending and breaking.

B. During instrumentation, utilize instruments at the appropriate angulation to the teeth. Avoid pressing instrument against hard surface of metallic restorations.

C. Autoclave sterilization does not dull sharp instruments.

II. Discard instruments that have been reduced so much by frequent sharpening that even moderate to slight pressure flexes the blade. A tip could break off in a pocket or interproximally during instrumentation.

III. Sharpening of files has not been included in this chapter for several reasons. Sharpening of files is a difficult procedure owing to the several parallel cutting edges. When sharpening of a file is required, a jeweler's tang file may be obtained for that purpose. Use of a professional sharpening service or return of the files to the manufacturer for sharpening is highly recommended.

REFERENCES

1. **Meador,** H.L.: The Biocentric Technique: A Guide to Avoiding Occupational Pain, *J. Dent. Hyg., 67,* 38, January, 1993.

2. **Pattison,** A.M. and Pattison, G.L.: *Periodontal Instrumentation,* 2nd ed. Norwalk, CT, Appleton & Lange, 1992, pp. 166, 232, 371.

3. **MacDonald,** G., Robertson, M.M., and Erickson, J.A.: Carpal Tunnel Syndrome among California Dental Hygienists, *Dent. Hyg., 62,* 322, July/August, 1988.

4. **Osborn,** J.B., Newell, K.J., Rudney, J.D., and Stoltenberg, J.L.: Carpal Tunnel Syndrome among Minnesota Dental Hygienists, *J. Dent. Hyg., 64,* 79, February, 1990.

5. **Atwood,** M.J. and Michalak, C.: The Occurrence of Cumulative Trauma in Dental Hygienists, *WORK, 2,* 17, Summer, 1992.

6. **Dobias,** M.T.: Carpal Tunnel Syndrome: Can It Be Prevented? *DentalHygienistNews, 5,* 1, Winter, 1992.

7. **Gerwatowski,** L.J., McFall, D.B., and Stach, D.J.: Carpal Tunnel Syndrome, Risk Factors and Preventive Strategies for the Dental Hygienist, *J. Dent. Hyg., 66,* 89, February, 1992.

8. **McFall,** D.B., Stach, D.J., and Gerwatowski, L.J.: Carpal Tunnel Syndrome: Treatment and Rehabilitation Therapy for the Dental Hygienist, *J. Dent. Hyg., 67,* 126, March–April, 1993.

9. **Hu-Friedy Manufacturing Co.,** 3232 N. Rockwell Street, Chicago, IL 60618.

SUGGESTED READINGS

Barata, M.-C. and Schoen, D.H.: Comparison of Two Instructional Approaches in Preclinical Dental Hygiene, *J. Dent. Educ., 57,* 766, October, 1993.

Hard, D.: Oral Prophylaxis, in Bunting, R.W.: *Oral Hygiene,* 3rd ed. Philadelphia, Lea & Febiger, 1957, pp. 249–258.

Hirschfeld, L.: Subgingival Curettage in Periodontal Treatment, *J. Am. Dent. Assoc., 44,* 301, March, 1952.

MacDonald, G., Wilson, S.G., and Waldman, K.B.: Physical Characteristics of the Hand and Early Clinical Skill. Their Relationship in a Group of Dental Hygiene Students, *J. Dent. Hyg., 65,* 380, October, 1991.

Pattison, A.M. and Pattison, G.L.: *Periodontal Instrumentation,* 2nd ed. Norwalk, CT, Appleton & Lange, 1992, pp. 129–154, 288–300.

Tondrowski, V.E.: Preclinical Procedures for the Dental Hygiene Student, *J. Dent. Educ., 20,* 321, November, 1956.

Cumulative Trauma Disorders

Coady, C.D.: The Alexander Technique. Postural and Neuromuscular Re-education, *DentalHygienistNews, 7,* 12, Spring, 1994.

Conrad, J.C., Conrad, K.J., and Osborn, J.B.: Median Nerve Dysfunction Evaluated During Dental Hygiene Education and Practice (1986–1989), *J. Dent. Hyg., 65,* 283, July–August 1991.

Conrad, J.C., Conrad, K.J., and Osborn, J.B.: A Short-term Epidemiological Study of Median Nerve Dysfunction in Practicing Dental Hygienists, *J. Dent. Hyg., 66,* 76, February, 1992.

Huntley, D.E. and Shannon, S.A.: Carpal Tunnel Syndrome, A Review of the Literature, *Dent. Hyg., 62,* 316, July/August, 1988.

Nunn, P., Hart, C., and Gaulden, F.: Perfect Instrumentation Can Be Hazardous to Your Health! or Ergonomic Applications for the Prevention of Carpal Tunnel Syndrome, *Access, 9,* 37, January, 1995.

Oberg, T., Karsznia, A., Sandsjö, L., and Kadefors, R.: Work Load, Fatigue, and Pause Patterns in Clinical Dental Hygiene, *J. Dent., Hyg., 69,* 223, September–October, 1995.

Poindexter, S.M.: All the Right Moves: Ergonomics and the Dental Hygienist at Work, *Access, 9,* 18, January, 1995.

Sanders, M.J. and Michalak-Turcotte, C.: Preventing Cumulative Trauma Disorders in Dental Hygienists, in Sanders, M., ed.: *Management of Cumulative Trauma Disorders.* Newton, Mass., Butterworth Heinemann, 1997, pp. 283–296.

Instruments

Balevi, B.: Engineering Specifics of the Periodontal Curet's Cutting Edge, *J. Periodontol., 67,* 374, April, 1996.

Biller, I.R. and Karlsson, U.L.: SEM of Curet Edges, *Dent. Hyg., 53,* 549, December, 1979.

Burns, S.: Partners in Practice, *RDH, 9,* 23, October, 1989.

Glenner, R.A.: The Scaler, *Bull. Hist. Dent., 38,* 31, April, 1990.

Long, B.A. and Singer, D.L.: A New Curet Series: The Gracey Curvettes, *RDH, 12,* 46, February, 1992.

McKechnie, L.B.: Instrumentation, Selection and Care, in Genco, R.J., Goldman, H.M., and Cohen, D.W., eds.: *Contemporary Periodontics.* St. Louis, Mosby, 1990, pp. 525–539.

Nunn, P.J.: Getting a Handle on Ergonomic Periodontal Instrument Design, *Access, 11,* 16, March, 1997.

Tal, H., Kozlovsky, A., Green, E., and Gabbay, M.: Scanning Electron Microscope Evaluation of Wear of Stainless Steel and High Carbon Steel Curettes, *J. Periodontol., 60,* 320, June, 1989.

Sharpening Procedures

Green, E. and Seyer, P.C.: *Sharpening Curets and Sickle Scalers,* 2nd ed. Berkeley, CA, Praxis Publishing Co., 1972, 40 pp.

Huntley, D.E.: A Fine Edge: Instrument Sharpening, Part I, *RDH, 2,* 15, July/August, 1982.

Huntley, D.E.: Honing Your Technique. Instrument Sharpening, Part II, *RDH, 2,* 51, September/October 1982.

Marquam, B.J.: Keep Eye on Sharpening Techniques to Prevent Disease Transmission, *RDH, 12,* 20, August, 1992.

Marquam, B.: Redi-Reference: Sharpening Tips, *DentalHygienistNews, 6,* 17, Fall, 1993.

Murray, G.H., Lubow, R.M., Mayhew, R.B., Summitt, J.B., and Usseglio, R.J.: The Effects of Two Sharpening Methods on the Strength of a Periodontal Scaling Instrument, *J. Periodontol., 55,* 410, July, 1984.

Nield-Gehrig, J.S. and Houseman, G.A.: *Fundamentals of Periodontal Instrumentation,* 3rd ed. Baltimore, Williams & Wilkins, 1996, pp. 453–466.

Parkes, R.B. and Kolstad, R.A.: Effects of Sterilization on Periodontal Instruments, *J. Periodontol., 53,* 434, July, 1982.

Rappold, A.P., Ripps, A.H., and Ireland, E.J.: Explorer Sharpness as Related to Margin Evaluations, *Oper. Dent., 17, 2,* January–February, 1992.

Rossi, R. and Smukler, H.: A Scanning Electron Microscope Study Comparing the Effectiveness of Different Types of Sharpening Stones and Curets, *J. Periodontol., 66,* 956, November, 1995.

Sasse, J.: Cutting Edges of Curets. Effect of Repeated Sterilization, *Dent. Hyg., 61,* 14, January, 1987.

Schulze, M.B.: Instrument Sharpening—"The Flat Stone in Motion," *DentalHygienistNews, 3,* 7, Summer, 1990.

Smith, B.A., Setter, M.S., Caffesse, R.G., and Bye, F.L.: The Effect of Sharpening Stones upon Curet Surface Roughness, *Quintessence Int., 18,* 603, September, 1987.

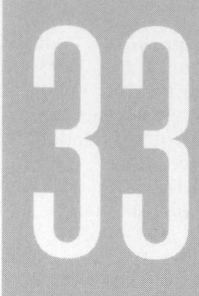

Nonsurgical Periodontal Instrumentation

Basic treatment for inflammatory gingival and periodontal infections is the removal of bacterial plaque, bacterial toxic materials (endotoxins), and supra- and subgingival calculus. The term debridement has been applied to the group of procedures involved and includes scaling (manual and power driven), planing to smooth the tooth surface, as well as the procedures carried out by the patient daily, when using a toothbrush and proximal plaque-removal devices.

Such debridement can provide the definitive or complete treatment for many patients with less advanced infections. For those with more advanced disease it is the preparatory or initial therapy. The progress and success of treatment can be influenced by host factors.

Dental hygiene care aims to *prevent, arrest, control,* or *eliminate* the infection in the gingiva (Case type I) or periodontal tissues (Case types II, III, IV, page 225). The ultimate goals of the instrumentation are to eliminate pathogenic microorganisms that cause the infection and promote continuing health in the periodontal tissues. Box 33-1 contains key words related to nonsurgical therapy.

The long-range success of treatment depends on the *control* of the bacterial plaque by the patient on a daily basis. Therefore, instruction and monitoring plaque-control procedures must precede, continue simultaneously with, and follow professional mechanical instrumentation.

THE SCOPE OF NONSURGICAL THERAPY

The current chapter will be devoted to techniques for the removal of supra- and subgingival deposits using manual and power-driven scaling procedures. The following chapter (34) includes a variety of adjunctive interventions also considered within the scope of nonsurgical periodontal therapy. The indication for each procedure is assessed on an individual patient basis. Nonsurgical therapy may include a combination of the following procedures:

I. Removal of bacterial plaque, endotoxins, other bacterial products, and calculus.
II. Root planing to create a smoother tooth surface.
III. Irrigation using an antimicrobial agent.
IV. Sustained release antibiotic or antimicrobial agent particularly for refractory infections.
V. Removal of iatrogenic plaque retainers.
   A. Overhanging margins of restorations (pages 624 to 627).
   B. Unfinished, poorly contoured, or unpolished restorations.
VI. Concurrent dental procedures. Examples include:
   A. Restore to arrest advanced carious lesions to aid gingival healing by preventing food impaction and making personal plaque removal possible.
   B. Analysis and correction of occlusal irregularities.

PREPARATION OF THE CLINICIAN

Skill in procedures for disease control in a patient requires more than the development of manual techniques for applying instruments to the tooth surfaces. In these refined and exacting techniques, knowledge of the anatomic, histopathologic, and physiologic characteristics of the teeth and supporting tissues is

---

BOX 33-1 KEY WORDS: Nonsurgical Instrumentation

Bacteremia (bak"ter-ē'mē-ah): presence of bacteria in the blood.

Debridement (de-brēd'ment): a form of nonsurgical periodontal therapy accomplished by the mechanical removal of tooth surface irritants using manual and/or power-driven methods.

Endotoxin (en"dō-tok'sin): lipopolysaccharide (LPS) complex found in the cell wall of many gram-negative microorganisms; contained superficially within periodontally involved cementum.

Furcation (fur-kā'shun): anatomic area of a multirooted tooth where the roots diverge

   Furcation invasion: pathologic resorption of bone within a furcation.

Instrumentation zone: area on tooth where instrumentation is confined; area where calculus and altered cementum are located and treatment is required.

Nonsurgical periodontal therapy: bacterial plaque removal and control, supra- and subgingival scaling, root planing, and adjunctive treatments such as the use of chemotherapy; the basic objectives are to restore periodontal health; arrest or slow the progression of early periodontal disease; or, for more advanced disease, to prepare the tissues for more complex periodontal therapy.

Root planing: a definitive treatment procedure designed to remove altered cementum or surface dentin that is rough, impregnated with calculus, or contaminated with toxins or microorganisms.

Scaling: instrumentation of the crown or root surfaces to remove bacterial plaque and calculus.

necessary. Such knowledge must be tied together with recognition of the clinical manifestations of the tissues in disease and then in health as the effects of treatment become apparent.

The needs of the individual patient are identified through patient assessment, and the course of treatment is defined by the dental hygiene diagnosis and care plan. The length and number of appointments, the special management required for the individual patient, the treatment sequence, and selection of instruments to accomplish each task are carefully organized.

FOCUS OF TREATMENT

The focus of clinical treatment is on the elimination of the causes of the infection. Bacterial plaque, endotoxins and other bacterial products, cementum, and calculus are all involved.

I. BACTERIAL PLAQUE

A. Gingival inflammation and periodontal destruction result from the action of pathogenic microorganisms and their endotoxins.
B. Microorganisms are attached to the surfaces of the teeth, to calculus, and to the gingiva and may become embedded in the cemental surface and exposed dentinal tubules.

II. ENDOTOXINS

A. Lipopolysaccharides or endotoxins, derived from the cell walls of gram-negative pathogenic microorganisms, are toxic to human tissue and cause inflammation and destruction of the periodontal attachment.
B. Endotoxins are embedded on the cemental surface and in the superficial bacterial plaque and can be removed readily.[1–4]

III. CEMENTUM

A. The cementum is thin at the cervical third of the root. Some or even complete removal of the cementum during instrumentation for calculus removal is inevitable.
B. Excess removal of the cementum and vigorous root planing is not necessary.[5,6] However, a smooth surface is significant, since the microorganisms collect and colonize on a rough surface much more rapidly than on a smooth surface.[7,8]

IV. CALCULUS

A. Calculus is not directly a cause of gingival inflammation, but the irregular surface provides a nexus for bacterial plaque collection.
B. Calculus must be removed to provide a healing environment for the periodontal tissues.

AIMS AND EXPECTED OUTCOMES

The effects and benefits of complete, carefully performed nonsurgical pocket therapy are summarized here.

I. INTERRUPT OR STOP THE PROGRESS OF DISEASE.

II. CREATE AN ENVIRONMENT THAT ENCOURAGES THE TISSUE TO HEAL AND THE INFLAMMATION TO BE RESOLVED.

A. Convert pocket (disease) to sulcus (health).
B. Shrink previously enlarged spongy tissue.
C. Reduce probing depths.
D. Eliminate bleeding on probing.
E. Regenerate the gingival tissues to normal color, size, and contour (see Table 11-1, pages 194 to 195).
F. Change the quality of the tissues from spongy to firm.
G. Improve the integrity of the clinical attachment.

III. INDUCE POSITIVE CHANGES IN THE QUALITY AND QUANTITY OF THE SUBGINGIVAL BACTERIAL FLORA.

A. Before instrumentation, the predominant microorganisms are anaerobic, gram-negative, motile forms with many spirochetes and rods, high counts of all types of microorganisms, and many leukocytes.
B. After instrumentation, the composition of the bacterial flora shifts to a predominance of aerobic, gram-positive, nonmotile, coccoid forms with lowered total counts and fewer leukocytes (see Table 33-2, page 562).

IV. DELAY REPOPULATION OF MICROORGANISMS IN THE POCKET; HENCE PREVENT OR POSTPONE DISEASE RECURRENCE.

V. PROVIDE INITIAL PREPARATION (TISSUE CONDITIONING) FOR COMPLICATED PERIODONTAL THERAPY REQUIRED FOR ADVANCED DISEASE.

A. Reduce or eliminate etiologic and predisposing factors.
B. Permit re-evaluation. Surgical procedures may be lessened in extent.

VI. MOTIVATE THE PATIENT.

A. To appreciate the values of a healthy mouth.
B. To make a commitment to perform daily personal bacterial plaque control measures.

OVERALL APPOINTMENT SYSTEMS

Whether a single or multiple appointment plan is required, the initial step is patient instruction. The overall care plan must be described and the consent of the patient, parent, or guardian obtained. Treatment begins with the patient's own treatment (pages 322 to 327). In this chapter the segment of the appointments devoted to instrumentation for the removal of calculus, bacterial plaque, and endotoxins is described.

I. WHEN A SINGLE APPOINTMENT MAY BE ADEQUATE

A. The diagnosis is Case type I or even Case type II with small areas of deposits readily accessible; anesthesia usually is not needed.

B. Only a few teeth present; limited areas of anesthesia may be needed.

C. Patient presents with a good plaque score, evidence of reasonable personal care without need for time for extended instruction and motivation.

D. Patient acts responsibly in keeping appointments for maintenance and continued monitoring for disease control.

II. PLANNED MULTIPLE APPOINTMENTS

The extent of periodontal involvement (Case types II, III, IV, Table 13-1, page 225), probing measurements, distribution and extent of calculus deposits, and oral cleanliness that shows evidence of the patient's personal care or lack of it are major determinants in the number of appointments needed. The patient should never be promised that the treatment will be completed in a given number of appointments.

A. Quadrant Scaling Appointments

The most efficient system for appointment planning is by quadrant with anesthesia, at 1-week intervals to permit patient learning and progressive healing.

With less severe periodontitis and a compliant patient, two quadrants of the same side may be completed at an appointment. The patient is informed that a final appointment for evaluation will be needed.

B. Tissue Conditioning

At the initial appointment basic bacterial plaque removal is introduced. Interdental devices to complement the use of a toothbrush can be added as the patient demonstrates readiness. At each successive appointment a plaque score is shown to the patient and procedures are reviewed.

Each week the tissues will show changes toward a healthy state. In this manner, the patient *conditions* the tissue for the clinician so there is less debris, less bleeding, and fewer bacteria for contaminating the aerosols created during instrumentation. The effect is a cleaner environment in which the clinician can carry out the treatment procedures.

C. Evaluation

1. At each appointment the quadrants previously treated are examined for evidence of healing. Calculus left inadvertently can be removed by remedial scaling procedures.

2. Final evaluation: 10 days to 2 weeks after the final scaling, healing of the tissues is expected. Restoration of the clinical attachment permits probing.

III. PROBLEMS OF INCOMPLETE SCALING

One system that has been used by some clinicians involves an initial "gross scaling" or "prescaling." A series of appointments then is planned for deep scaling by quadrants. "Gross" scaling is not recommended for a number of reasons. Before using such a plan, the following should be considered:

A. Healing at the Gingival Margin

When the irritants are removed around the opening of the pocket, the tissue heals and the gingival margin can close tight around the tooth. The marginal tissue may take on a color and shape that appears normal to the patient, but underneath the probing depth and bleeding on probing have not changed. With tightening of the opening of the pocket, insertion of curets for additional deep instrumentation can be difficult.

B. Potential for Abscess Formation[9]

1. Predisposing factors:
   a. Deep suppurating pockets; advanced periodontal infection.
   b. Pockets extending into furcation areas or intrabony defects.
   c. Patient susceptible to infection, such as with uncontrolled diabetes, with immunodeficiency disease, or being treated with an immunosuppressive drug.

2. Sequence: With partial scaling, healing can begin, the tissue at the gingival margin tightens, the pocket closes, microorganisms multiply within, an abscess develops (pages 582 to 583).

C. Patient Instruction

When supragingival calculus and bacterial plaque are removed from the crowns of the teeth, the visible lesson is taken away. When treatment is carried out quadrant by quadrant, the patient has unscaled areas with which to compare the healing quadrants. The patient can see and feel changes and improvements that contrast with untreated areas.

D. Roughened Calculus

Calculus roughened by partial removal may be a source of increased subgingival plaque collections. Bacteria readily collect and colonize on a rough surface thus providing more sources for infection in the surrounding gingival tissues.[7,8]

E. Patient Misunderstanding

For the patient with limited understanding of the seriousness and extent of periodontal infection, the mouth may feel good and look good after a gross "cleaning." As a result, the patient may not realize the need to return for the continuing appointments to complete the deep scaling. The personal objective of "clean teeth" had been fulfilled.

Later, when severe periodontitis develops, the patient may claim that incomplete treatment was provided originally. By receiving repeated information at each successive quadrant treatment and by seeing the changes, the patient can gain a better understanding of the seriousness of the disease in the periodontal tissues.

PREPARATION FOR INSTRUMENTATION

I. REVIEW THE PATIENT'S RECORD

A. Study the data from the complete assessment.
B. Note special needs from medical history and plan accordingly.
C. Identify systemic or physical problems with potential for emergency.

II. REVIEW RADIOGRAPHIC FINDINGS

A. Note findings applicable during instrumentation, such as
  1. Anatomic features of roots, furcations, and bone level, which may need special adaptations of curets.
  2. Overhanging restorations that must be removed.
B. Leave radiographs on lighted viewbox throughout the treatment for reference.

III. PATIENT PREPARATION

A. Premedication requirements for patient at risk (pages 101 to 104)
  1. Transient bacteremia can occur during and immediately after scaling procedures.
  2. Frequency and duration of bacteremia depends on severity of periodontal infection and inflammation and the degree of trauma during the instrumentation.[10,11]
  3. Check that the patient has taken the medication as prescribed (see Table 6-4, page 102).
B. Provide preprocedural bactericidal rinse (page 68).
C. Prepare for anesthesia as indicated.

IV. SUPRAGINGIVAL EXAMINATION

A. **Visual**
Gross deposits and tooth surface irregularities can be seen by direct vision. Fine, unstained, white or yellowish calculus is frequently invisible when wet with saliva. Observe tooth surfaces closely while a gentle stream of compressed air is applied. Dry calculus is seen more readily than wet calculus (see pages 279 to 280 for calculus detection).

B. **Tactile**
Without deposits or anatomical irregularities, the enamel surface is smooth. An explorer passed over the surface slides freely, smoothly, and quietly. When rough calculus deposits are present, the explorer does not slide freely, but meets with resistance and produces a scratchy sound.

V. SUBGINGIVAL EXAMINATION

A. **Visual**
  1. *Gingiva.* The clinical appearance suggestive of underlying calculus may be:
    a. Soft, spongy, bluish-red gingiva, with enlargement of the interdental papillae over proximal surface calculus.
    b. Dark-colored area beneath relatively translucent marginal gingiva.
  2. *Calculus.* A loose, resilient pocket wall can be deflected from the tooth surface with a gentle stream of compressed air. Dark, subgingival calculus can be seen within the pocket on the root.

B. **Tactile**
  1. *Periodontal charting.* Use probing depth recordings as basic guide.
  2. *Identify shallow pockets (sulci).* Scaling in shallow pockets of fewer than 3 mm can lead to loss of periodontal attachment.[12–14] Research has shown that repeated use of a curet when no calculus is present can result in detachment of periodontal ligament fibers and that healing does not bring them back.[14]
  3. *Determine distribution and extent of deposits.* Figure 33-1 illustrates probing. As the probe passes over the surface it may be intercepted by calculus (Figure 33-1*B*). Use an explorer for distinction of fine hard deposits.
  4. *Evaluate tooth topography.*
    a. Detect grooves and furcations using a horizontal stroke (Figure 33-1*C*).
    b. Use a furcation probe to examine furcations (see Figure 12-8, page 211).
    c. Note root and furcation variations (Figure 33-2).

CALCULUS REMOVAL

I. PREREQUISITES

A. Position of Clinician to Prevent Cumulative Trauma (pages 75 to 77)

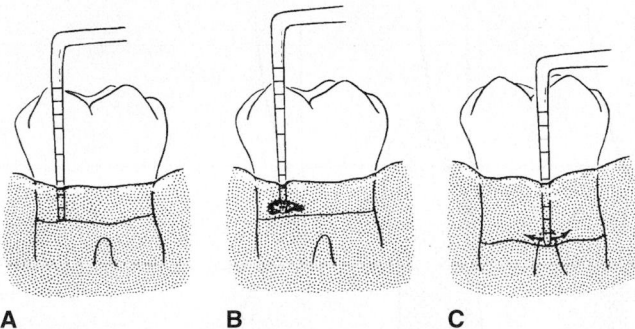

FIGURE 33-1 Subgingival Examination Using a Probe. (A) Probe inserted to the bottom of a pocket for complete examination prior to subgingival scaling. **(B)** As the probe passes over the root surface, it may be intercepted by a hard mass of calculus. **(C)** Using a horizontal probe stroke to examine the topography of a furcation area. Keep the side of the tip of the probe on the tooth surface and slide over one root, into the furcation, and across to the other root.

    B. Clear Visibility with Excellent Lighting
    C. Sharp Instruments

II. LOCATION OF INSTRUMENTATION

Figure 33-3 illustrates the location of instrumentation. Instrumentation and the selection of the correct instrument depend on:
    A. Type of pocket (gingival or periodontal).
    B. Location of calculus (on crown or root surface).
    C. Position of gingival margin (recession or covering cementoenamel junction).
    D. Level of clinical attachment (no loss of attachment or on root).

III. THE SCALING PROCESS

The process is the series of procedures and events that lead to achievement of a specific result. The proce-

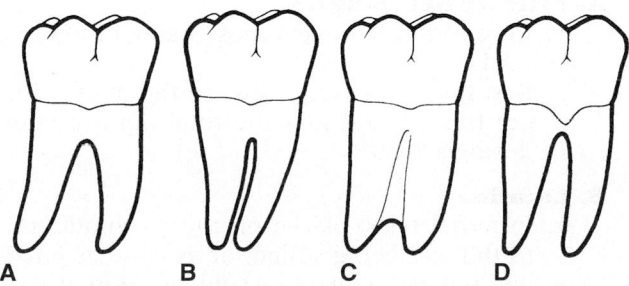

FIGURE 33-2 Anatomic Variations of Furcations. (A) Widely separated. **(B)** Separated but close together. **(C)** Fused roots separated only in the apical portion. **(D)** Presence of an enamel projection that may be conducive to an early furcation involvement. (From Carranza, F.A. and Newman, M.G.: *Clinical Periodontology,* 8th ed., W.B. Saunders Co., 1996, page 641.)

dures involve a systematic removal of calculus and soft deposits from tooth to tooth and section to section of the deposit on each tooth surface. Each stroke overlaps the previous stroke as the instrument is positioned progressively along the area of the deposit, which is the *instrumentation zone.*[15]

Scaling is not a fine shaving process in which layers are removed. Such a procedure tends to make the surface of the calculus smooth and burnished and sometimes indistinguishable from the tooth surface when explored.

The oldest calculus, located next to the tooth surface, is the hardest calculus. The outermost calculus is covered with a layer of bacterial plaque that has not yet started to mineralize.

IV. SPECIAL SUBGINGIVAL CONSIDERATIONS

Although the basic steps described for calculus removal apply to both supra- and subgingival deposits, subgingival techniques are unique and complicated by several significant factors. The instrumentation is more complex and difficult than supragingival calculus removal. Some of the variables are included here.

    A. Subgingival Anatomy
        1. Tooth Surface Pocket Wall
           As shown in Figure 33-3B,C, and E, some subgingival instrumentation is on the crown (enamel), and some on the root(cementum or dentin). In the cervical third of the root, the cementum is thin (0.03 to 0.06 mm) and may have been removed during previous instrumentation.
        2. Soft Tissue Pocket Wall
          a. The pocket wall hugs closely to the tooth surface covered with rough calculus which in turn is covered with bacterial plaque. Only a narrow area is available for manipulation of instruments. The pocket narrows in the deeper area next to the clinical attachment.
          b. Bleeding during instrumentation is inevitable because of the inflammation in the wall of the pocket.
        3. Variations in Depths of Pockets
           The periodontal charting is a primary guide to subgingival instrumentation. Probing depths must be recorded about each tooth because the depths can vary on a single surface.

    B. Accessibililty and Visibility
        1. Pocket is a confined area; instrumentation is necessary in areas where access is difficult.
        2. Techniques must depend almost entirely on tactile sensitivity.
        3. Soft tissue pocket wall limits freedom of movement. Careful adaptation to tooth surface configurations is essential.

    C. Subgingival Calculus
        1. Location

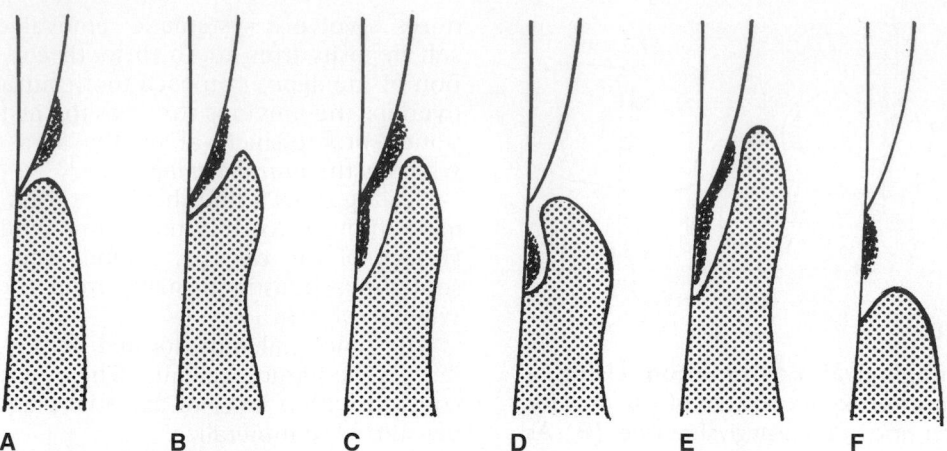

A   B   C   D   E   F

■ FIGURE 33-3 Location of Instrumentation. The location of calculus depositis, level of periodontal atachment, depth of pocket, and position of the gingival margin determine the site of instrumentation. **(A)** Supragingival calculus on the enamel. **(B)** Gingival pocket with both supra- and subgingival calculus on enamel. **(C)** Periodontal pocket with both supra- and subgingival calculus. **(D)** Periodontal pocket with subgingival calculus only on cementum. **(E)** Periodontal pocket with subgingival calculus only on both enamel and cementum. **(F)** Calculus on cementum exposed by gingival recession.

Subgingival calculus may be located on the enamel, the root, or both (Figure 33-3B, C,D,E).

2. Attachment

Calculus attaches to the cementum in minute irregularities and in areas of cemental resorption. It is more tenacious than on the enamel and requires a different technique. On the enamel it is attached primarily by means of an acquired pellicle, which makes calculus removal much easier.

3. Morphology of Calculus

Subgingival calculus is irregularly deposited. It occurs in nodular, ledge, smooth veneer, and other forms (see Table 17-1, page 279).

MANUAL SCALING STEPS

Types of instruments and the basic principles for their use were included in Chapter 32 (pages 515 to 526). This chapter continues from Chapter 32 to describe the use of the instruments for deposits removal. Table 33-1 summarizes the steps.

I. SELECT CORRECT CUTTING EDGE

A. Curets are paired and usually mounted on double-ended handles. Single-ended handles may be selected for certain patients or procedures.

B. Correct blade for scaling: when positioned on the tooth surface, only the back of the blade can be seen.

C. Incorrect blade adaptation: the open face of the blade will be seen. The open blade is in the

correct position for gingival curettage to remove the inner soft tissue lining of the pocket wall.

II. INSTRUMENT GRASP

A. Apply a modified pen grasp (see Figure 32-13, page 521).

B. Use a light grasp while instrument is positioned and at the completion of a stroke.

C. Use a slightly tighter grasp for hard deposit removal.

D. Apply a light grasp with light lateral pressure after calculus removal.
   1. To remove small irregularities.
   2. To leave the treated area smooth.

III. STABILIZATION: ESTABLISH THE FINGER REST

A. Primary Rest Fingers
   1. Ring and little fingers (nos. 3 and 4 in Figure 32-13).
   2. Rest fingers are kept close to the middle finger (no. 2) and join the total hand motion during activation.

B. Location
   1. Intraoral rests: placed on the tooth adjacent to the one being scaled, or as close as possible and convenient. Avoid position in the path of the strokes to protect from accidental glove and finger cut.
   2. Distance rests: long stretches between the rest and the point of instrument application can decrease control.
   3. Variations: substitute, supplementary, and reinforced rests are described on page 523.

TABLE 33-1 Steps for Calculus Removal Using Manual Instruments

1. Probe to determine pocket/sulcus characteristics.
2. Explore to determine location and extent of deposits and tooth surface irregularities.
3. Select correct instrument for areas being treated.
4. Hold instrument with a modified pen grasp.
*5. Establish stable finger rest.
*6. Identify correct cutting edge of blade for surface being scaled.
    For area-specific curets: terminal shank parallel with surface being scaled.
7. Insert. Use placement or exploratory stroke to locate apical edge of deposit.
8. Adjust working angulation (average at 70°).
9. Activate for working stroke.
    a. Apply moderate to firm lateral pressure for calculus removal.
    b. Apply light lateral pressure to smooth the surface.
    c. Control length and direction of stroke.
    d. Maintain continuous adaptation throughout the stroke.
10. Continue channel scaling with overlapping strokes.
    a. Apply placement stroke to reposition blade for next stroke.
    b. Activate instrument circumferentially around line angles to treat the entire surfaces that require instrumentation.
11. Use explorer to determine end point of treatment.

*For deep pockets associated with posterior teeth, steps 5 and 6 may be reversed to determine whether access can be attained best using an intraoral or extraoral rest.

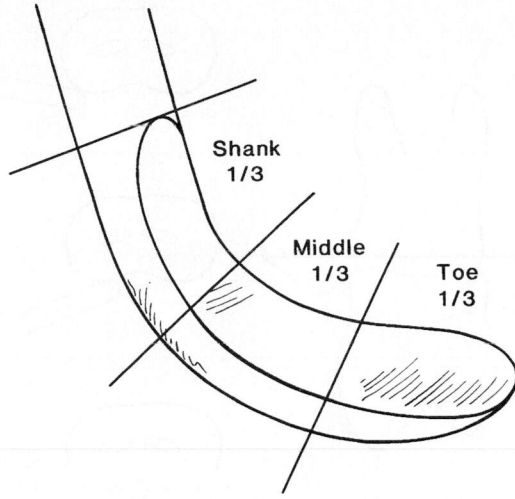

FIGURE 33-4 Curet Divided Into Thirds. The toe third is kept in contact with the tooth surface during instrumentation. Because of tooth contours, most strokes for scaling and root planing are accomplished using the toe third. Adaptation of the toe third is shown in Figure 33-5.

C. Dry the Rest Position
Bacterial plaque and saliva make tooth surfaces slippery. Use compressed air or dry with gauze sponge.

IV. ADAPTATION OF THE CUTTING EDGE

A. Apply blade (working end) to conform to tooth surface being treated. Because of tooth contours, only a portion of a blade can be adapted.
The toe and middle thirds of a curet blade are used most frequently (Figure 33-4).

B. Adaptation of the Toe of a Curet (Figure 33-5)
After the toe is adapted, as much of the cutting edge is used as can be applied without traumatizing the adjacent soft tissue in a pocket.

C. Maintain Adaptation
Around line angles and other tooth curvatures; rolling the handle between the fingers of the grasp helps to maintain the neutral position and keep the correct adaptation.

V. ANGULATION

A. Insertion
Close the angle to nearly flat against the tooth

surface (0°) as the instrument is inserted to the base of a pocket (Figure 33-6A and B).

B. Optimal Angle for Scaling
A 60° to 80° (average 70°) angle is effective for deposit removal using a scaler or a curet.

VI. LATERAL PRESSURE

A. Degree of Pressure of Blade Against Tooth
Whether a light, moderate, or heavy pressure is needed will depend on the nature of the deposit. When the instrument is sharp, a minimum pressure allows the cutting edge to "grab" the calculus; when dull, the blade can slide over the deposit.

B. Balance of Pressure During Stroke
Careful control is accomplished by a balance of pressure between the grasp of the instrument, the pressure on the finger rest, and the lateral pressure.

VII. ACTIVATION: STROKE

A. Tighten the Grasp
1. Renew the stability of the rest position; move the instrument firmly and deliberately.
2. Wrist and arm bear the weight during the stroke, rather than flexing the fingers in the grasp.

B. Maintain Cutting Edge Evenly During the Stroke
1. Maintain the angulation.
2. Maintain the adaptation.

C. Motion Control
Without independent finger movement, the

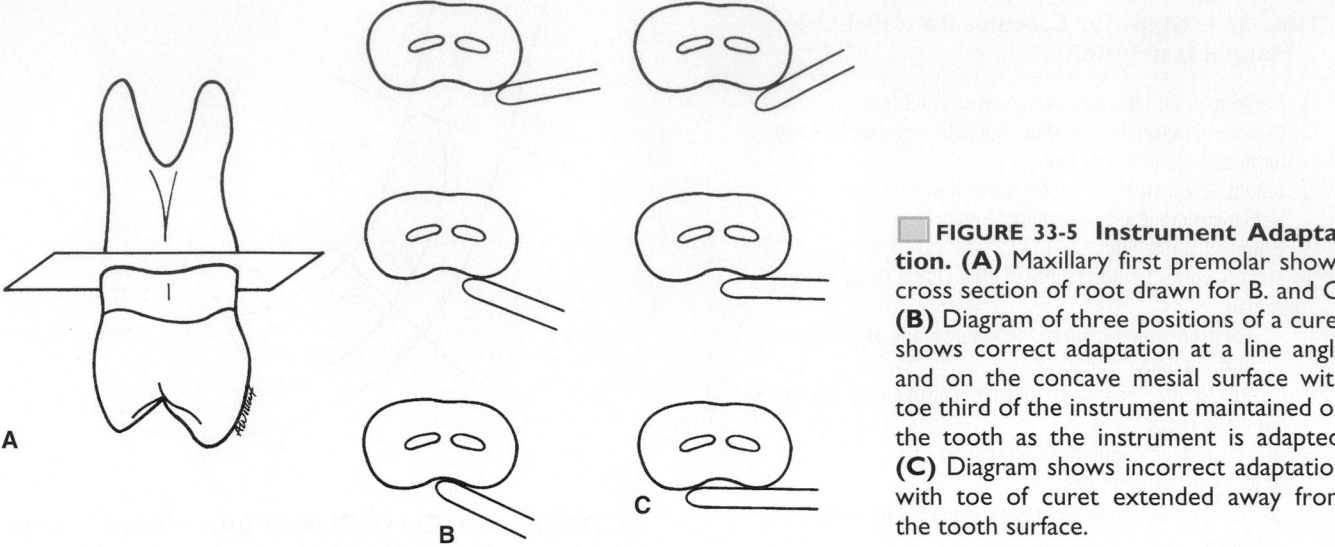

FIGURE 33-5 Instrument Adaptation. (A) Maxillary first premolar shows cross section of root drawn for B. and C. **(B)** Diagram of three positions of a curet shows correct adaptation at a line angle and on the concave mesial surface with toe third of the instrument maintained on the tooth as the instrument is adapted. **(C)** Diagram shows incorrect adaptation with toe of curet extended away from the tooth surface.

hand, wrist, and arm act as a continuum to activate the instrument.

D. Direction of Strokes

1. Overlapping vertical, oblique (diagonal), or horizontal strokes are selected to accommodate the anatomical features of the tooth surfaces (see Figure 32-18, page 526).
2. Strokes are applied systematically, not haphazardly.
3. Horizontal strokes should not be used at the

bottom of a pocket to avoid damage to the clinical attachment.

E. Length of Stroke: Within Instrumentation Zone

1. Short, smooth, decisive strokes permit accommodation of the cutting edges to changes in the topography of the tooth surface.
2. Confine the strokes within a pocket to prevent the need for repeated removal and

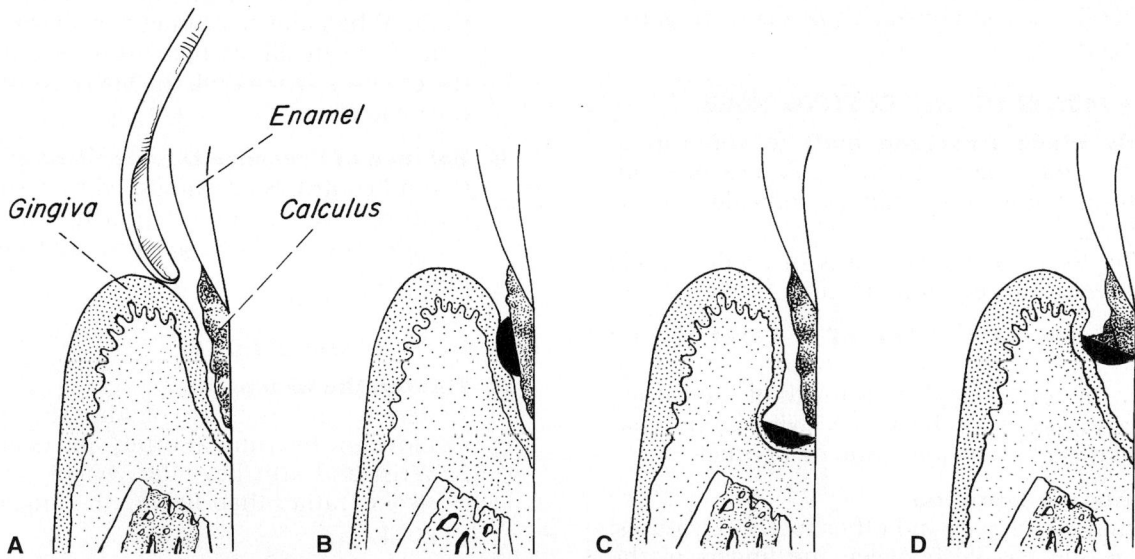

FIGURE 33-6 Subgingival Scaling and Root Planing. (A) The curet is inserted gently under the gingival margin. **(B)** With a placement stroke, the blade is passed over the surface of the tooth or calculus. Note 0° angle of the face of the curet with the calculus. **(C)** The curet is lowered to the base of the pocket until the tension of the soft tissue is felt with the rounded back of the curet. The curet then is positioned at an angle of 70° to 80° with the tooth surface beneath the calculus deposit. **(D)** The blade is moved along the root surface in a scaling stroke to remove the calculus.

reinsertion of the curet, to prevent trauma to the gingival margin.

3. Extending the blade up the side of the tooth in unnecessarily long strokes
   a. Decreases control by the clinician.
   b. Causes trauma to the pocket wall.
   c. Wastes time.
   d. Dulls the instrument.

VIII. CHANNELS OF STROKES (FIGURE 33-7)

A. At the completion of each stroke, move the instrument laterally to the adjacent part of the deposit; maintain the same finger rest.

B. Overlap strokes in channels: ensure complete surface coverage for thorough removal of deposits.

C. Repeat strokes until surface has been completely debrided.

IX. PLANE THE ROOT SURFACE

Finishing techniques for smoothing the tooth surfaces to lessen immediate recolonization of bacteria are ba-

sically the same as for scaling. Techniques are applied only where deemed necessary after subgingival exploration with a fine subgingival explorer.

A. Adaptation

Instrument control, adaptation, directions for strokes, and other principles are not essentially different from scaling. Some clinicians prefer to close the angulation slightly after the calculus is believed to be removed.

B. Touch and Pressure

1. Specific differences in technique are related to touch and pressure. A lighter grasp must be used to increase tactile sensitivity. Because increased pressure is not needed, a lighter shaving-like stroke can be used for smoothing the root surface.

2. Light lateral pressure is applied for maximum sensitivity to minute irregularities of the surface.

C. Strokes

1. Smooth strokes with even lateral pressure that systematically overlap are used. As the surface becomes smoother, longer strokes with reduced pressure help to remove small lines, scratches, or grooves without gouging the surface.

2. Vertical, then oblique, strokes are used. When applicable away from the attachment epithelium, horizontal strokes may be used (Figure 33-8).

3. Careful application is needed to adapt the

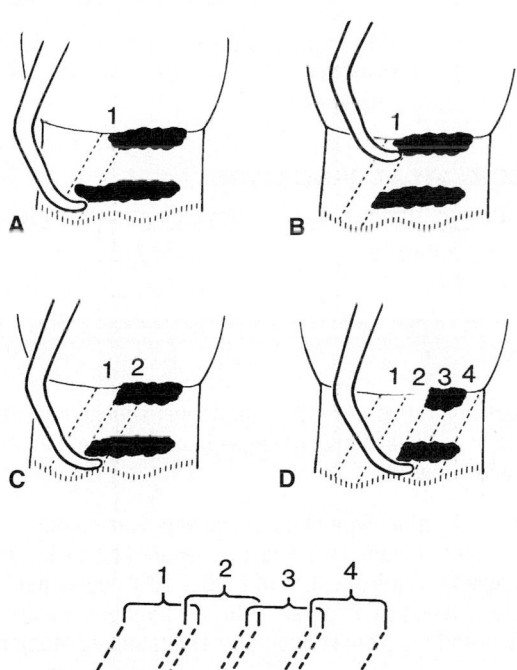

FIGURE 33-7 Channel Scaling. (A) Curet adapted in position for channel 1 stroke from the base of the pocket under the calculus deposit. **(B)** Completion of stroke for channel 1. **(C)** Using an exploratory stroke, the curet is lowered into the pocket and is positioned for calculus removal in channel 2. **(D)** Curet positioned for channel 3. Several strokes in each channel may be needed to ensure complete calculus removal. **(E)** Strokes of each channel must overlap strokes of the previous channel. (Adapted from Parr, R.W., Green, E., Madsen, L., and Miller, S.: *Subgingival Scaling and Root Planing.* Berkeley, CA, Praxis Publishing Co., 1976.)

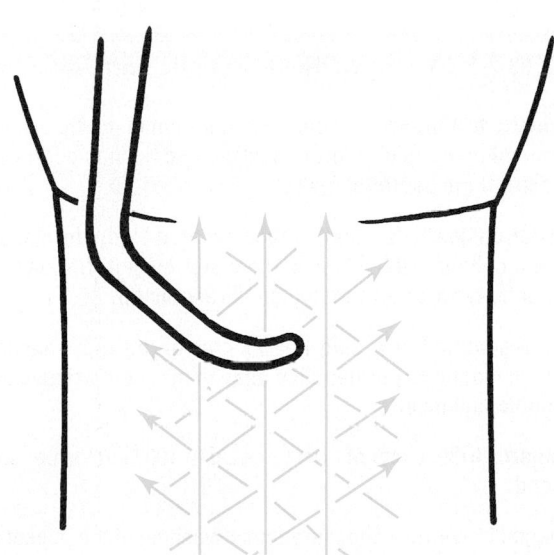

FIGURE 33-8 Root Surface Strokes. The use of strokes in vertical and oblique directions with light lateral pressure can eliminate grooves left after scaling. A smooth surface results. (Adapted from Parr, R.W., Green, E., Madsen, L., and Miller, S.: *Subgingival Scaling and Root Planing.* Berkeley, CA, Praxis Publishing Co., 1976, p. 42.)

curet to the unique anatomic features of the roots. The convex surfaces, the constricted cervical areas, the concavities and grooves of the proximal surfaces, and the variations in furcations all require precise adaptation.

4. As a surface area becomes smooth, a gradual change in the sound of the instrument may occur. At the completion, the instrument may be as quiet as when used on polished enamel.

X. EVALUATION

A. Use subgingival explorer to examine for completion of calculus removal and smoothness of the treated surfaces.

B. Apply explorer in both vertical and diagonal strokes to detect irregularities (Figure 33-8).

C. Refine slight spots of roughness with a sharp curet.

D. Adapt curet with light lateral pressure for maximum sensitivity to minute irregularities of the surface. Avoid grooving the treated surface.

E. Postcare patient instructions are described on page 560.

ULTRASONIC AND SONIC SCALING

Manual instrumentation was the only method available for the safe removal of supragingival and subgingival calculus until the ultrasonic scaling device was introduced in the 1950s.[16,17] The power-driven scaling device converted high-frequency electrical energy into mechanical energy in the form of rapid vibrations.

Technologic advances in ultrasonics allowed for rapid calculus removal and resulted in much less hand fatigue on the part of the clinician. Later sonic scalers were developed that worked on the same principle but utilized an air turbine as an energy source. Terminology related to power-driven instrumentation is defined in Box 33-2.

For many years, power-driven scaling devices were recommended for supragingival scaling only. Because of advances in design and efficiency of the devices, they are now recommended for both supragingival and subgingival treatment.

Slimmer ultrasonic instrument tips have been designed to provide better access to subgingival deposits. Changes in the understanding of the role of microorganisms and their by-products in the progression of periodontal disease have led to an increased use of ultrasonic and sonic instruments for periodontal debridement.

MODE OF ACTION

Although the main action of the ultrasonic scaler is mechanical, cavitation and irrigation also play important roles in debridement.

I. MECHANICAL VIBRATION

A. Power-driven scaling devices convert electrical

BOX 33-2 KEY WORDS: Ultrasonic and Sonic Instrumentation

Acoustic turbulence (a-koos′tik): agitation in the fluids surrounding a rapidly vibrating ultrasonic tip; has potential to disrupt the bacterial matrix.

Cavitation (kav″ĭ-tā′shun): action created by the formation and collapse of bubbles in the water by high-frequency sound waves surrounding an ultrasonic tip.

Ferromagnetic (fer″o-mag-net′ik): type of rod with unusually high magnetic permeability used in magnetostrictive ultrasonic unit inserts.

Kilohertz (kHz): a unit of energy equal to 1000 cycles per second.

Lavage (lah-vahzh′): the therapeutic washing of the pocket and root surface to remove endotoxins and loose debris.

Magnetic field: space occupied by magnetic lines of force.

Magnetostrictive: ultrasonic scaling device that generates a magnetic field and produces tip vibrations by the expansion and contraction of a metal stack or rod.

Piezoelectric (pi-e″zo-e-lek′trik): ultrasonic scaling device activated by dimensional changes in crystals housed in the handpiece.

Sonic scaler (son′ik): type of mechanical power-driven scaler that functions from energy delivered by a vibrating working tip in the frequency of 2500 to 7000 cycles per second; driven by compressed air, the handpiece connects directly to a conventional rotary handpiece tubing.

Stack: inserts made up of flat metal strips stacked, or sandwiched, together; metal in stack acts like an antennae to pick up magnetic field and cause vibration.

Transducer (trans-doo′ser): a device that converts energy or power from one form to another.

Ultrasonic scaler: power-driven scaling instrument that operates in a frequency range between 25,000 to 50,000 cycles per second to convert a high-frequency electrical current into mechanical vibrations.

energy or air pressure into high-frequency sound waves.

B. Sound waves produce rapid vibrations in the specially designed scaling tips.

C. Calculus is shattered from the tooth surface when the vibrations are applied to the deposit.

II. CAVITATION

A. Water is required to dissipate the heat produced at the vibrating tip.

B. Cavitation occurs when the water meets the vibrating tip, creating minute bubbles that collapse and release energy.[18]

C. Effect of cavitation. Although the cavitation has little influence on hard deposit removal, it can destroy bacteria[19] and remove endotoxin from the root surface.[20]

III. IRRIGATION

The water spray penetrates to the base of the pocket[21] to provide a continuous flushing of debris, bacteria, and endotoxin. Oscillation of the ultrasonic tip causes hydrodynamic waves to surround the tip. This acoustic turbulence is believed to disrupt bacteria.[22,23]

TYPES OF POWER-DRIVEN SCALING DEVICES

There are three types of powered scaling devices available: magnetostrictive ultrasonic scalers, piezoelectric ultrasonic scalers, and the less powerful sonic scalers.

I. MAGNETOSTRICTIVE ULTRASONIC SCALERS

A. **Unit:** Consists of an electric generator, a handpiece assembly, a set of interchangeable scaling tip inserts, and a foot control.

B. **Activation:** Vibrations in the tip occur when electric current is applied to the handpiece, resulting in the creation of a magnetic field and thus expansion and contraction of metal in the handpiece.
   1. Conventional magnetostrictive units utilize a stack of metal strips in the handpiece.
   2. Ferromagnetic units utilize a ferric rod that generates less heat than the conventional metal stack.

C. **Tip Movement**
   1. Conventional tip moves in an elliptical pattern; all surfaces of the tip are active.
   2. Ferromagnetic tip rotates 360° in three different planes; equal effectiveness on all sides of the tip.

D. **Frequency:** Number of cycles per second (cps) the tip moves
   1. Conventional units range from 25,000 to 50,000 cps. Older units are designed to oper-

ate at 25,000 cps and are called 25-kilohertz (kHz) machines; newer units are designed to operate at 30,000 cps and are called 30-kHz machines.
   2. Ferromagnetic units operate at 42,000 cps.

E. **Water Source:** The units require a water source so that water can be delivered to the handpiece and through or around the instrument tip.

II. PIEZOELECTRIC ULTRASONIC SCALERS

A. **Unit:** Consists of an electric generator, a handpiece assembly, a set of interchangeable scaling tip inserts, and a foot control.

B. **Activation:** By dimensional changes in quartz or metal alloy crystal transducers housed in the handpiece.

C. **Tip Movement:** Moves in a linear pattern; only two sides of the tip are active, limiting adaptation.

D. **Frequency:** Varies according to manufacturer; range from 25,000 to 50,000 cps.

E. **Water Source:** Although the unit generates less heat than a magnetostrictive unit, a water source is still required to cool the friction produced between the instrument tip and the tooth surface.

III. SONIC SCALERS

A. **Unit:** Consists of a handpiece and interchangeable scaling tips. The handpiece attaches directly to the dental unit and is activated with the conventional handpiece foot control.

B. **Activation:** Driven by compressed air from the dental unit rather than electrical energy.

C. **Tip Movement:** Moves in an elliptical pattern; all surfaces of the tip are active.

D. **Frequency:** Less powerful than ultrasonic scalers; producing vibrations at the tip; range between 2,500 and 6,300 cps. Because of fewer vibrations produced, calculus removal is more difficult.

E. **Water Source:** While heat is not generated, water is required to cool the friction between the instrument tip and the tooth surface.

PURPOSES AND USES

I. INDICATIONS FOR USE

A. Removal of supragingival calculus and tenacious stains.

B. Subgingival periodontal debridement, including removal of calculus, attached plaque, and endotoxins from the root surface, and unattached plaque from the sulcular space.[24]

C. Initial debridement for a patient with necrotizing ulcerative gingivitis or other condition that can be relieved by removal of deposits. Loose debris, materia alba, and microorganisms must first be removed by rinsing, brushing, and flossing during patient instruction to prevent contaminated aerosol production.

D. Debridement of furcation areas.[25,26]

E. Debridement of deposits prior to oral surgery.

F. Removal of orthodontic cement; debonding.

G. Removal of overhanging margins of restorations.

II. CONTRAINDICATIONS AND PRECAUTIONS

A. General Health Conditions

1. *Communicable Disease.* Patient with a communicable disease that can be transmitted by aerosols, such as tuberculosis.

2. *Susceptibility to Infection.* Compromised patient with marked susceptibility to infection. Examples: immunosuppression from disease or chemotherapy, uncontrolled diabetes, debilitation, and kidney and other organ transplant.

3. *Respiratory Risk.* Patient with a respiratory risk. Septic material and microorganisms from bacterial plaque and periodontal pockets can be aspirated into the lungs.[27]
   a. History of chronic pulmonary disease, including asthma, emphysema, or cystic fibrosis.
   b. History of cardiovascular disease with secondary pulmonary disease or breathing problem.

4. *Swallowing Difficulty.* Patient with a swallowing problem or prone to gagging. Examples: amyotrophic lateral sclerosis, muscular dystrophy, paralysis, multiple sclerosis.

5. *Cardiac Pacemaker.* Although no case has ever been reported in which an ultrasonic scaler disrupted a pacemaker, theoretically it is possible. Some newer devices have protective coverings. Consultation with the patient's cardiologist is necessary.

B. Oral Conditions

1. *Demineralized Areas.* Ultrasonic vibrations can remove the delicate remineralizing cover of a demineralized area.

2. *Exposed Dentinal Surfaces.* Tooth structure can be removed in excess and create sensitivity. The smear layer can be removed and dentinal tubules uncovered, which can increase sensitivity or aggravate existing sensitivity.

3. *Restorative Materials.* Certain restorative materials can be damaged (porcelain and amalgam) or removed altogether (composite resins, laminate veneers) by ultrasonic instrumentation.

4. *Titanium Implant Abutments.* Ultrasonic instrumentation will damage titanium surfaces unless the tip insert is covered with a specially designed plastic sheath.

5. *Narrow Periodontal Pockets.* Narrow subgingival pockets interfere with proper angulation and impede visibility.

C. Children

1. Young, growing, developing tissues are sensitive to ultrasonic vibrations.

2. Primary and newly erupted permanent teeth have large pulp chambers. The vibrations and heat from the ultrasonic scaler may damage pulp tissue.

INSTRUMENT TIP DESIGN

The parts of the ultrasonic handpiece insert are illustrated in Figure 33-9. The design of the instrument tip will vary according to the intended use. Figure 33-10 shows examples of various tip designs.

I. SHAPE

A. Straight: Tip slightly curved in only one direction; designed to be used throughout the mouth. Also called universal.

B. Contra-Angled: Instrument tips designed to be used on specific surfaces of the teeth.

C. Beavertail: Designed to be used on supragingi-

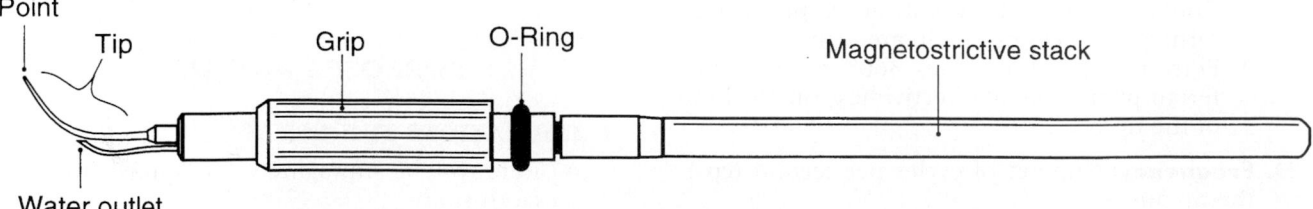

Point   Tip   Grip   O-Ring   Magnetostrictive stack

Water outlet

■ **FIGURE 33-9 Ultrasonic Handpiece Insert.** With parts labeled, showing design with external water delivery tube.

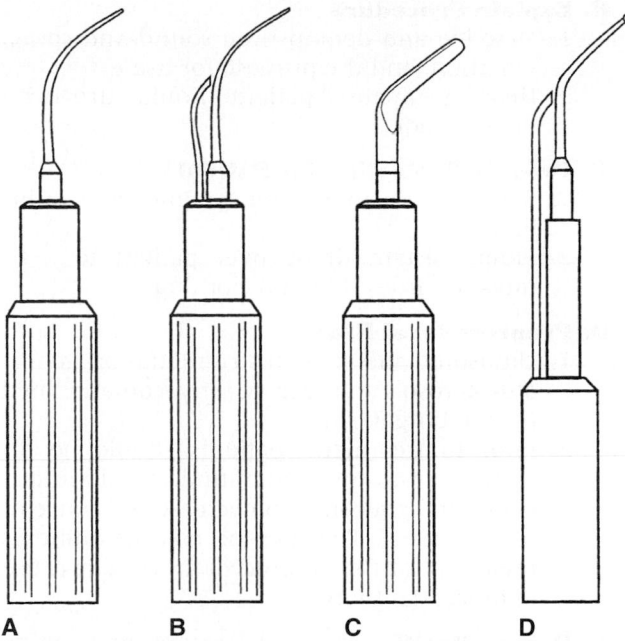

FIGURE 33-10 Ultrasonic Tip Designs. (A) Straight tip with internal flow water delivery. **(B)** Thinner tip with external water delivery. **(C)** Beavertail for supragingival surfaces needing removal of heavy calculus or cement. **(D)** 0.8-mm ball-end design for adaptation in furcation areas.

val surfaces for the removal of heavy calculus and stain and orthodontic cement.

D. Periodontal Probe: Thin, straight tip designed for subgingival instrumentation.

E. Chisel: Designed for supragingival calculus on anterior teeth or premolar teeth. Also used for removal of overhanging restorations.

F. Ball Point: An 0.8-mm sphere found on the tip designed for use in furcations.[25]

II. SIZE

A. Conventional: Traditional ultrasonic and sonic tips, bulkier than most curet tips, and generally used for moderate to heavy deposit removal supragingivally.

B. Periodontal: Thinner tips now designed to provide better access to subgingival surfaces.

III. WATER DELIVERY

A. External Tube. An external tube delivers the water to the tip of the instrument (Figure 33-10).

B. Internal Tube. Water is delivered from the unit to cool the tip through the internal structure of the insert.

IV. PLASTIC TIP[28,29]

A. Close-Fitting Plastic Sheath. The sheath fits over the metal working end.

B. Dentin and Titanium. Plastic tip is used with a light, gentle activation on dentin and titanium surfaces to remove soft and mineralizing deposits.

CLINICAL PREPARATION

I. DENTAL HYGIENE CARE PLAN

A. Examination. Review the care plan, radiographs, and chart to determine the following:
1. Location of deposits.
2. Depth of pockets.
3. Furcations.

B. Instrumentation Plan
1. Plan a systematic sequence.
2. Complete one quadrant before starting another.

II. INFECTION CONTROL MEASURES

A. Personal Protective Equipment
1. The clinician and assistant must wear protective eyewear or face shield, gloves, and protective outerwear.
2. A high efficiency bacterial filtration face mask is worn even in the presence of a face shield because of the aerosols produced during instrumentation. Masks should be changed often.

B. Flush Water Lines[30,31]
1. Opportunistic pathogens can colonize and replicate on the internal surfaces of dental tubing, as found in the dental unit and ultrasonic unit.
2. To reduce bacterial contamination, water lines are flushed for 2 to 3 minutes at the beginning of each day, for 20 to 30 seconds between patients, and before sterile insert is placed in the handpiece.

C. High-Volume Evacuation
1. Deposition of tooth-associated materials into the pulmonary system during ultrasonic scaling can result in pulmonary infection.[27]
2. The use of high-volume evacuation will reduce aspiration of contaminated aerosols by both the patient and clinician.
3. An assistant is required when a high-volume evacuator is used.
4. A special high-volume evacuator attachment provides suction around the handpiece tip and reduces aerosol contamination in the treatment room.[32,33]

III. ULTRASONIC UNIT PREPARATION

A. Establish Power and Water Connections.

B. Fill Handpiece With Water. This is done before placing the insert to eliminate trapped air and reduce heat.

C. Select Insert
1. Insert must be compatible with ultrasonic unit available.
2. The metal stacks in the 30-kHz inserts are much shorter than the 25-kHz inserts.
3. The tip should be appropriate for the intended use.

D. Set Power Level
1. Select the lowest power setting that is effective.[34]
2. Consistent use of the unit on the highest power setting will increase the aerosols produced and the potential for thermal damage without necessarily increasing efficiency.
3. Using a low to medium power setting for normal treatment procedures should produce adequate vibration for the removal of plaque, calculus, and endotoxins.

E. Adjust Water
1. Water provides cooling and irrigation.
2. Proper water setting should create a fine mist at the tip of the instrument.
3. Increase water if heat is produced.

F. Use of an Antimicrobial Solution
1. Some ultrasonic units have reservoirs so an antimicrobial solution can be used as the coolant since the lavage of ultrasonics can penetrate to the base of the pocket.[21]
2. When 0.12% chlorhexidine is used as the coolant/irrigant, there is a greater reduction in clinical probing depth.[35,36]
3. Antimicrobial solutions will provide control of aerosol contamination.

IV. SONIC UNIT PREPARATION

A. Flush water lines in slow-speed-handpiece line for 2 minutes.
B. Attach sonic handpiece to slow-speed-handpiece line.
C. Select and screw sonic tip into handpiece.

V. PATIENT PREPARATION

A. Review Health History
1. Check to ensure that the patient who requires preprocedural antibiotic has taken the prescribed medication. Bacteremia is produced in a high percentage of patients treated by powered instrumentation, as well as manual instrumentation.[37]
2. Identify any contraindications to ultrasonic instrumentation.

B. Explain Procedure
1. Describe and demonstrate sound and spray, vibration, and the purpose for use.
2. Hearing impaired patient should turn off a hearing aid.

C. Provide Protection for Patient
1. Safety glasses to prevent eye infections or injury.
2. Fluid-resistant drape over patient to keep moisture from skin and clothing.

D. Preprocedural Rinse
1. Ultrasonic and sonic instrumentation generates aerosols that are heavily contaminated by microorganisms.[38]
2. Prior to treatment, patients should be directed to rinse with an antimicrobial mouthrinse for 30 seconds to decrease incidence of bacteremia.[39] The use of chlorhexidine is preferred for the preprocedural rinse because of its substantivity.

E. Patient Position. Place the patient in a supine position for maximum visibility and to slightly close the airway.

F. Pain Control. Prepare to use topical or local anesthetic as necessary.

G. Water Control. Prepare to use evacuation with saliva ejector or high-volume evacuator with assistant as indicated by the severity and degree of sepsis[27] and communicability of infection from the patient.
1. Evacuation system must be properly disinfected before use.
2. Shape and position saliva ejector so that the patient can hold it in place and collect water that is pooling in the mouth.

INSTRUMENTATION

As with manual instrumentation, ultrasonic instrumentation also depends on tactile sensitivity and knowledge of tooth morphology to debride periodontal pockets efficiently and safely.

I. ULTRASONIC SCALING

A. Grasp
1. Use a pen or modified pen grasp.
2. A light grasp will increase tactile sensitivity.
3. The weight of the cord tends to pull on the handpiece and place additional strain on the wrist. This can be managed by looping the cord and holding it between the ring finger and little finger or hanging the cord over the shoulder.

B. Fulcrum
1. A hard tissue fulcrum is not required be-

cause force and pressure against the tooth surface are not indicated.

2. A gentle finger rest is used to stabilize and guide the instrument tip.
3. Extraoral and soft tissue rests may be used if necessary.

C. Adaptation (Figure 33-11)
1. Keep the side of the instrument tip parallel to or at no more than a 15° angle with the tooth surface.
2. Do not hold the tip perpendicular to the tooth surface because damage to the tooth surface can result.

D. Stroke
1. Keep the instrument tip moving at all times to prevent the following:
   a. Scratches on the tooth surface.
   b. Excessive heat build-up.
   c. A shock effect to the patient.
2. Use light featherlike pressure to prevent tooth damage. Excessive lateral pressure can result in the following:
   a. Damage to the tooth surface.
   b. Deactivation of the tip vibrations.

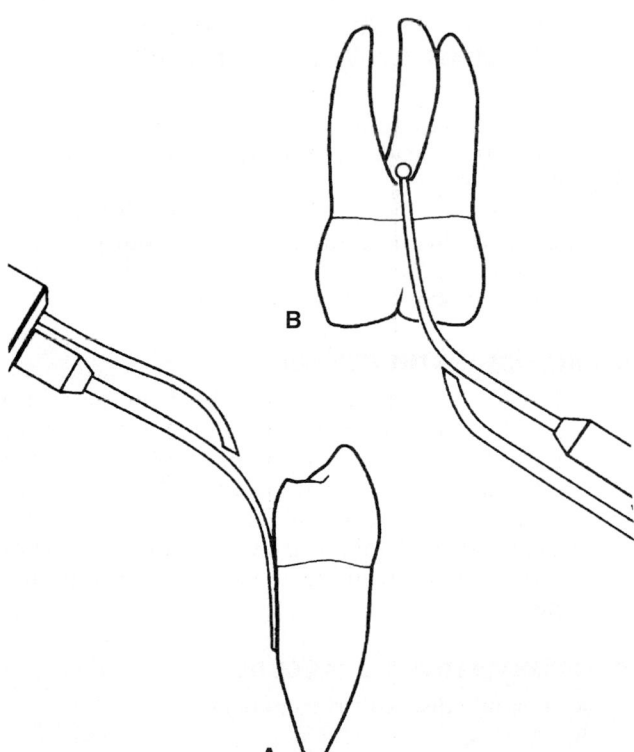

FIGURE 33-11 Adaptation of Ultrasonic Tip. (A) The side of the point of a tip is placed parallel to the tooth surface to prevent damage to the tooth structure. Damage occurs when the point is held perpendicular to the surface. **(B)** Ball end of tip designed for adaptation in furcation areas.

3. Overlap strokes to cover all surfaces of the root. Strokes may be horizontal, vertical, oblique, or a combination.
4. Instrument tip may bind when inserted interproximally. If so, deactivate the power, remove the instrument tip, and reactivate the instrument.

E. Evaluation. Use the instrument without power as a probe or explorer to evaluate surface.

II. WATER CONTROL
A. Release the foot pedal or rheostat at regular intervals to aid in water control. Stop periodically to evaluate tooth surfaces.
B. Mirror use
1. Water is continuously sprayed onto the mirror surface, making indirect vision difficult.
2. The clinician can wipe the wet surface of the mirror with a gloved finger to coalesce the drops into a clear wet surface. When water is allowed to pool on the surface in this manner, a clearer image of the working area can be seen through the water.

III. MANUAL SCALING
Complete the procedure with manual instruments directly following ultrasonic instrumentation.
A. Check subgingival areas with a subgingival explorer.
B. Remove remaining subgingival irregularities and smooth the surface with curets.
C. Manual scaling is especially important following the use of conventional ultrasonic tips, which are bulky and provide limited application subgingivally.

RISK CONSIDERATIONS

I. CLINICIAN

A. Cumulative Trauma
It has been estimated that dental hygienists apply over 32 tons of scaling forces per year using over 25,000 scaling strokes for calculus removal.[40,41] Many dental hygienists suffer from symptoms related to cumulative trauma.

Powered scaling actually reduces the force needed to remove deposits, and it can reduce the risk of carpal tunnel syndrome.

B. Magnetic Fields
Ultrasonic scalers produce weak, time-varying magnetic fields similar to those produced by common household appliances. There is no scientific evidence that cumulative exposure to weak, time-varying magnetic fields has caused any biological harm to any dental personnel.[42]

II. PATIENT

A. Heat Production

Potential damage to the pulp tissue should be kept in mind during instrumentation.[43,44] Constant motion of the instrument, correct angulation, and ample water for cooling are essential to operation.

B. Hearing Shifts

Extended exposure to noises above a certain level, such as the noise of a high-speed handpiece or an ultrasonic scaler, may be potentially damaging. Temporary hearing shifts have been demonstrated for a group of patients.[45]

III. DAMAGE TO THE INTEGRITY OF RESTORATIONS

A. Porcelain: fracturing; loss marginal integrity.[46,47]

B. Amalgam: surface defects; loss marginal integrity.[48,49]

C. Composites: surface alterations.[50]

IV. TITANIUM IMPLANT ABUTMENTS

Metal scratches titanium.[28,51]

COMPLETION OF NONSURGICAL INSTRUMENTATION

After each treatment using nonsurgical instrumentation, an immediate evaluation is made and special instructions are given to the patient for the initial tissue healing period. Adequate personal therapeutic bacterial plaque control is critical to the outcome of treatment.

After health has been attained, it must be maintained. Planning long-term maintenance programs is described in Chapter 42.

IMMEDIATE EVALUATION

I. OBJECTIVES

A. Teeth

Observation and exploration reveal the immediate effects of instrumentation on the teeth. An objective has been to produce a smooth tooth surface, free from deposits. The effect of specific instrumentation is to facilitate the patient's self-care by removing local factors, particularly calculus and overhanging fillings, that encourage plaque retention.

B. Gingiva

The gingival changes are not apparent immediately after instrumentation. Tissue regeneration and healing take approximately 1 week to 10 days for initial healing and even longer for maturation of connective tissue and keratinization of epithelium.

The objective at the treatment appointment is to *create an environment in which the gingival tissue can heal and be maintained in health by the patient.*

II. EXAMINATION

When scaling is accomplished over a series of appointments, each previously scaled quadrant or area is examined and rescaled as needed at each appointment. For the final evaluation, visual and tactile methods are applied carefully to each tooth surface.

A. Visual

1. Compressed air should be used with a mouth mirror and adequate lighting to examine the supragingival areas and just below the gingival margins.

2. Transillumination methods are applied.

B. Tactile

An evaluation by exploring immediately after completion of instrumentation is made to ascertain that the tooth surfaces are smooth and that all detectable calculus has been removed. The real evaluation, the true test of successful treatment, cannot be made until 1 to 2 weeks after the initial scaling and root planing. At that time, the response of the gingival tissue is apparent.

PATIENT INSTRUCTIONS AFTER SCALING AND ROOT PLANING

Personalized instructions are provided for each patient at the end of each dental hygiene and periodontal appointment.

Instruction pertaining to periodontal dressings is outlined in Table 36-1 on page 593. Many of the same principles can be applied for postcare instruction when a dressing has not been applied.

I. PRINTED INSTRUCTIONS

A. Printed instructions help to give the patient a handy reference. An added personal note or underlining of significant parts of the printed materials can let a patient sense the caring attitude of the professional team.

B. Verbal instructions can be forgotten or misinterpreted by even the most conscientious patient.

II. INFORMATION TO INCLUDE

A. Possible discomfort to expect

B. Rinsing

C. Toothbrushing

D. Eating

III. RINSING

A warm solution is soothing to the tissues and improves the circulation, thereby helping healing. A suggested solution provides the appropriate concentration for osmotic balance of the salts of the solution with the salts of the oral tissue fluids.

A. Solutions Suggested for Use

1. *Hypertonic Salt Solution:* Level ½ teaspoonful of table salt in ½ cup (4 ounces) of warm water.
2. *Sodium Bicarbonate Solution:* Level ½ teaspoonful of baking soda in 1 cup (8 ounces) of warm water.
3. *Chlorhexidine 0.12%.* Following instrumentation for NUG, NUP, and advanced periodontitis, chlorhexidine rinsing may prove helpful. It must be made clear that it is not a substitute for personal bacterial plaque removal with toothbrush and interdental aids.

B. Directions for Rinsing

1. Every 2 hours; after eating; after toothbrushing; before retiring.
2. Use the rinse mouthful by mouthful, forcing the solution between the teeth (page 384).

IV. TOOTHBRUSHING

The use of a soft brush is recommended after scaling and root planing. The patient must clearly understand the importance of bacterial plaque removal.

V. EATING

Dietary and nutritional factors may be discussed. The temporary use of bland foods lacking in strong, spicy seasonings, as well as continuing use of nutritional foods to promote healing, are basic.

EFFECTS OF NONSURGICAL INSTRUMENTATION

The essential components of successful nonsurgical instrumentation are thorough subgingival debridement by the clinician and effective bacterial plaque control by the patient. The focus of treatment and the aims and expected outcomes are specified on page 546 at the beginning of this chapter.

Tissue response is the most important measure of success in periodontal debridement. Tissue response is manifested by clinical features commonly referred to as the endpoints of therapy.

I. CLINICAL ENDPOINTS

A. Bleeding on probing: eliminated
B. Probing depths: reduced
C. Attachment levels: same or improved
D. Inflammation: resolved
E. Gingival appearance: size reduced, color normal
F. Subgingival microflora: lowered in numbers, delay in repopulation
G. Bacterial plaque control record: improvement

in plaque scores approaching 100% plaque-free
H. Tooth surface: smooth, free from plaque-retentive irregularities

II. HEALING

A. Factors Affecting Healing

1. Severity of the infection and clinical features at the start of treatment.
2. Non-compliance of the patient
   a. To bacterial plaque control.
   b. To follow the complete treatment plan.
3. Tobacco use: smoking.[52]
4. Systemic influences
   a. Diabetes.
   b. Lowered defense: immunocompromised as, for example, in HIV/AIDS, cancer chemotherapy.
5. Root surface irregularities from incomplete debridement: retained calculus, endotoxins, and microorganisms.

B. Healing Process

1. *Resolution of Inflammation.* Edema recedes, necrotic cells are cleared away, and tissue regenerates.
2. *Sequence.* Within 2 days after scaling, epithelial regeneration starts. New attachment to the tooth surface can appear as early as 5 days, and regeneration of epithelium by approximately 2 weeks.
3. *Clinical Attachment.* A long epithelial attachment can be expected.

III. EFFECT ON MICROORGANISMS

A. Changes in Pocket Flora[53,54]

The subgingival bacterial flora is changed after debridement, as shown in Table 33-2. Prior to instrumentation for treatment of periodontitis, the subgingival microorganisms are primarily anaerobic, gram-negative, motile forms.

After scaling and root planing, the total number of subgingival organisms decreases substantially. A shift to aerobic, gram-positive, nonmotile forms occurs.

With the conversion of the disease-producing gram-negative pocket microorganisms to a health-producing gram-positive flora, the gingiva reflects the changes. Gingival bleeding on probing is lessened, and the color, size, shape, and other characteristics assume a normal appearance.

B. Repopulation

Without personal daily plaque control, the microorganisms can return to pretreatment levels within an average of 42 days.[55] With plaque control, the repopulation of the pocket takes longer, even in susceptible patients. In many patients, nonsurgical periodontal therapy re-

TABLE 33-2 Effect of Instrumentation on Pocket Microflora

Periodontal Infection Before Treatment	Periodontal Health After Treatment
Predominant flora is	Predominant flora is:
Anaerobic	Aerobic
Gram-negative	Gram-positive
Motile	Nonmotile
Spirochetes, motile rods; pathogenic	Coccoid forms; nonpathogenic
Very high total count of all types of microorganisms	Much lower total counts of all types of microorganisms
Many leukocytes	Lower leukocyte counts

sults in a gingival condition that can be maintained free from reinfection.

C. Endotoxins

Endotoxins are lipopolysaccharides (LPSs) released from gram-negative bacterial cell walls. They occur in the bacteria covering the cementum and superficially in the cementum itself. Endotoxins have been shown to be toxic to human cells.[56] Endotoxins do not penetrate deeply into cemental surfaces.[1,2]

Retained endotoxins are held by calculus not removed during instrumentation as well as by new microorganisms recolonizing on the surfaces.

D. Effectiveness in Furcations

Manual and ultrasonic instruments were equally effective in Class I furcations in debriding and altering the bacterial flora. However, ultrasonic instruments were shown superior in Class II and III furcations in at least one research study.[26]

IV. COMPARISON OF MANUAL AND POWER-DRIVEN INSTRUMENTATION

Ultrasonic and manual nonsurgical instrumentation produce equivalent results in calculus and bacterial plaque removal. Long-term goals of therapy are accomplished by both.[13,24,57,58]

TECHNICAL HINTS

I. PREVENTIVE INSTRUMENTATION

A. Primary aims are to accomplish debridement with
1. Minimal damage to tooth surface.
2. Minimal discomfort to patient.

B. Minimize root surface damage
1. *Use probe and explorer.* Analyze before instrumentation for distribution of soft and hard deposits and at intervals during treatment for thoroughness to avoid overinstrumentation.
2. *Ultrasonic instrumentation.* Use slimmer insert tip with careful adaptation, featherlike strokes, and low power setting.
3. *Manual curet instrumentation.* Select a sharp instrument designed for the given tooth surface, adapt at appropriate angulation, and control strokes with finger rest and lateral pressure.

II. INSTRUMENT MAINTENANCE

A. Ultrasonic Tips
1. Avoid dry heat sterilization; use steam or chemical vapor autoclave. Pre-dipping in antirust emulsion may be advisable to prevent corrosion.
2. Insert tips wear with use and can cause damage to tooth surfaces. Check at intervals (appropriate to extent of use) and replace.

B. Manual Scalers and Curets
1. Examine for wear while sharpening. Reserve thinned or shortened curets to use for conscientious, motivated maintenance patients with shallow sulci and minimal calculus.
2. Handle all instruments with care. Avoid damage, breakage, and dulling of sharp cutting edges.

III. BROKEN INSTRUMENT

The procedure to follow when an instrument blade tip breaks in a patient's mouth during treatment should be in accord with the dentist's own policy. Therefore, the procedure should be discussed and clarified before an accident happens.

The principal objective in the location of a broken instrument tip is to know positively that the tip has been removed. With this in mind, rinsing, use of suction or compressed air, or initiation of other procedures that could cause the removal of the tip unknowingly would be out of order. A general procedure is suggested here.

A. Cease procedure, retain retraction without moving the patient's head unnecessarily, and isolate with gauze or cotton roll.

B. Do not alarm the patient by describing the accident.

C. Examine the immediate area, the floor of the mouth, and the mucobuccal fold. Blot the gingival tissue dry with a cotton roll and examine around the tooth.

D. Apply transilluminator or mouth light when available.

E. The gingival sulcus can be gently examined using a curet in a spooninglike stroke, but take care not to push the tip into the base of the sulcus (should the tip be there).

F. Consult the dentist for assistance in accord with previously discussed policy.

G. When the tip is not removed by any means mentioned thus far, make a periapical radiograph of the area.

FACTORS TO TEACH THE PATIENT

I. The nature, occurrence, and etiology of calculus.

II. The importance of the complete removal of calculus to the health of the oral tissues in the prevention of periodontal infections.

III. Relationship of the accumulation of bacterial plaque to the patient's personal oral hygiene procedures.

IV. Basic reasons for need and advantages of multiple appointments to complete the scaling and root planing.

V. Needed frequency of maintenance appointments in relation to oral health.

REFERENCES

1. **Nakib**, N.M., Bissada, N.F., Simmelink, J.W., and Goldstine, S.N.: Endotoxin Penetration Into Root Cementum of Periodontally Healthy and Diseased Human Teeth, *J. Periodontol.*, 53, 368, June, 1982.
2. **Moore**, J., Wilson, M., and Kieser, J.B.: The Distribution of Bacterial Lipopolysaccharide (Endotoxin) in Relation to Periodontally Involved Root Surfaces, *J. Clin. Periodontol.*, 13, 748, September, 1986.
3. **Smart**, G.J., Wilson, M., Davies, E.H., and Kieser, J.B.: The Assessment of Ultrasonic Root Surface Debridement by Determination of Residual Endotoxin Levels, *J. Clin. Periodontol.*, 17, 174, March, 1990.
4. **Chiew**, S.Y.T., Wilson, M., Davies, E.H., and Kieser, J.B.: Assessment of Ultrasonic Debridement of Calculus-associated Periodontally-involved Root Surfaces by the Limulus Amoebocyte Lysate Assay. An *in vitro* Study, *J. Clin. Periodontol.*, 18, 240, April, 1991.
5. **Nyman**, S., Westfelt, E., Sarhed, G., and Karring, T.: Role of "diseased" Root Cementum in Healing Following Treatment of Periodontal Disease: A Clinical Study, *J. Clin. Periodontol.*, 15, 464, August, 1988.
6. **Corbet**, E.F., Vaughan, A.J., and Kieser, J.B.: The Periodontally-involved Root Surface, *J. Clin. Periodontol.*, 20, 402, July, 1993.
7. **Quirynen**, M. and Bollen, C.M.L.: The Influence of Surface Roughness and Surface-free Energy on Supra- and Subgingival Plaque Formation in Man: A Review of the Literature, *J. Clin. Periodontol.*, 22, 1, January, 1995.
8. **Leknes**, K.N.: The Influence of Anatomic and Iatrogenic Root Surface Characteristics on Bacterial Colonization and Periodontal Destruction: A Review, *J. Periodontol.*, 68, 507, June, 1997.
9. **Perry**, D.A. and Taggart, E.J.: Occurrence Rate of Acute Periodontal Abscess Following Scaling Procedures, *J. Dent. Res.*, 76, 335, Abstract 2569, Special Issue, 1997.
10. **Bender**, I.B., Naidorf, I.J., and Garvey, G.J.: Bacterial Endocarditis: A Consideration for Physician and Dentist, *J. Am. Dent. Assoc.*, 109, 415, September, 1984.
11. **Pallasch**, T.J. and Slots, J.: Antibiotic Prophylaxis and the Medically Compromised Patient, *Periodontol. 2000*, 10, 107, 1996.
12. **Ramfjord**, S.P., Caffesse, R.G., Morrison, E.C., Hill, R.W., Kerry, G.J., Appleberry, E.A., Nissle, R.R., and Stults, D.L.: Four Modalities of Periodontal Treatment Compared over Five Years, *J. Periodontal Res.*, 22, 222, May, 1987.
13. **Badersten**, A., Nilvéus, R., and Egelberg, J.: Effect of Nonsurgical Periodontal Therapy. I. Moderately Advanced Periodontitis, *J. Clin. Periodontol.*, 8, 57, February, 1981.
14. **Lindhe**, J., Nyman, S., and Karring, T.: Scaling and Root Planing in Shallow Pockets, *J. Clin. Periodontol.*, 9, 415, September, 1982.
15. **Pattison**, G.L. and Pattison, A.M.: Principles of Periodontal Instrumentation, in Carranza, F.A. and Newman, M.G.: *Clinical Periodontology*, 8th ed. Philadelphia, W.B. Saunders Co., 1996, p. 463.
16. **Zinner**, D.D.: Ultrasonic Studies in Dentistry: A Preliminary Report, American Institute of Ultrasonics in Medicine; Proceedings of the Fourth Annual Conference on Ultrasonic Therapy; Library of Congress Number 55-12257, August 27, 1955, pp. 6–16.
17. **Johnson**, W.N. and Wilson, J.R.: The Application of the Ultrasonic Dental Unit to Scaling Procedures, *J. Periodontol.*, 28, 264, October, 1957.
18. **Walmsley**, A.D., Laird, W.R.E., and Williams, A.R.: A Model System to Demonstrate the Role of Cavitational Activity in Ultrasonic Scaling, *J. Dent. Res.*, 63, 1162, September, 1984.
19. **Baehni**, P., Thilo, B., Chapuis, B., and Pernet, D.: Effects of Ultrasonic and Sonic Scalers on Dental Plaque Microflora in Vitro and in Vivo, *J. Clin. Periodontol.*, 19, 455, August, 1992.
20. **Walmsley**, A.D., Walsh, T.F., Laird, W.R.E., and Williams, A.R.: Effects of Cavitational Activity on the Root Surface of Teeth During Ultrasonic Scaling, *J. Clin. Periodontol.*, 17, 306, May, 1990.
21. **Nosal**, G., Scheidt, M.J., O'Neal, R., and Van Dyke, T.E.: The Penetration of Lavage Solution into the Periodontal Pocket During Ultrasonic Instrumentation, *J. Periodontol.*, 62, 554, September, 1991.
22. **McInnes**, C., Engel, D., and Martin, R.W.: Fimbria Damage and Removal of Adherent Bacteria After Exposure to Acoustic Energy, *Oral Microbiol. Immunol.*, 8, 277, October, 1993.
23. **McInnes**, C., Engel, D., Moncla, B.J., and Martin, R.W.: Reduction in Adherence of *Actinomyces viscosus* After Exposure to Low-frequency Acoustic Energy, *Oral Microbiol. Immunol.*, 7, 171, June, 1992.
24. **Copulos**, T.A., Low, S.B., Walker, C.B., Trebilcock, Y.Y., and Hefti, A.F.: Comparative Analysis Between a Modified Ultrasonic Tip and Hand Instruments on Clinical Parameters of Periodontal Disease, *J. Periodontol.*, 64, 694, August, 1993.
25. **Takacs**, V.J., Lie, T., Perala, D.G., and Adams, D.F.: Efficacy of 5 Machining Instruments in Scaling of Molar Furcations, *J. Periodontol.*, 64, 228, March, 1993.
26. **Leon**, L.E. and Vogel, R.I.: A Comparison of the Effectiveness of Hand Scaling and Ultrasonic Debridement in Furcations as Evaluated by Differential Dark-field Microscopy, *J. Periodontol.*, 58, 86, February, 1987.
27. **Suzuki**, J.B. and Delisle, A.L.: Pulmonary Actinomycosis of Periodontal Origin, *J. Periodontol.*, 55, 581, October, 1984.
28. **Gantes**, B.G. and Nilvéus, R.: The Effects of Different Hygiene

Instruments on Titanium Surfaces: SEM Observations, *Int. J. Periodontics Restorative Dent.*, 11, 225, Number 3, 1991.

29. **Gantes**, B.G., Nilvéus, R., Lie, T., and Leknes, K.N.: The Effect of Hygiene Instruments on Dentin Surfaces: Scanning Electron Microscopic Observations, *J. Periodontol.*, 63, 151, March, 1992.

30. **Barbeau**, J., Tanguay, R., Faucher, E., Avezard, C., Trudel, L., Cote, L., and Prevost, A.P.: Multiparametric Analysis of Waterline Contamination in Dental Units, *Appl. Environ. Microbiol.*, 62, 3954, November, 1996.

31. **American Dental Association**, Council on Scientific Affairs and the Council on Dental Practice: Infection Control Recommendations for the Dental Office and the Dental Laboratory, *J. Am. Dent. Assoc.*, 127, 672, May, 1996.

32. **Harrel**, S.K., Barnes, J.B., and Rivera-Hidalgo, F.: Reduction of Aerosols Produced by Ultrasonic Scalers, *J. Periodontol.*, 67, 28, January, 1996.

33. **King**, T.B., Muzzin, K.B., Berry, C.W., and Anders, L.M.: The Effectiveness of an Aerosol Reduction Device for Ultrasonic Scalers, *J. Periodontol.*, 68, 45, January, 1997.

34. **Chapple**, I.L.C., Walmsley, A.D., Saxby, M.S., and Moscrop, H.: Effect of Instrument Power Setting During Ultrasonic Scaling Upon Treatment Outcome, *J. Periodontol.*, 66, 756, September, 1995.

35. **Reynolds**, M.A., Lavigne, C.K., Minah, G.E., and Suzuki, J.B.: Clinical Effects of Simultaneous Ultrasonic Scaling and Subgingival Irrigation with Chlorhexidine. Mediating Influence of Periodontal Probing Depth, *J. Clin. Periodontol.*, 19, 595, September, 1992.

36. **Taggart**, J.A., Palmer, R.M., and Wilson, R.F.: A Clinical and Microbiological Comparison of the Effects of Water and 0.02% Chlorhexidine as Coolants During Ultrasonic Scaling and Root Planing, *J. Clin. Periodontol.*, 17, 32, January, 1990.

37. **Bandt**, C.L., Korn, N.A., and Schaffer, E.M.: Bacteremias from Ultrasonic and Hand Instrumentation, *J. Periodontol.*, 35, 214, May–June, 1964.

38. **Legnani**, P., Checchi, L., Pelliccioni, G.A., and D'Achille, C.: Atmospheric Contamination During Dental Procedures, *Quintessence Int.*, 25, 435, June, 1994.

39. **Fine**, D.H., Mendieta, C., Barnett, M.L., Furgang, D., Meyers, R., Olshan, A., and Vincent, J.: Efficacy of Preprocedural Rinsing With an Antiseptic in Reducing Viable Bacteria in Dental Aerosols, *J. Periodontol.*, 63, 821, October, 1992.

40. **White**, D. J., Cox, E.R., Arends, J., Nieborg, J.H., Leydsman, H., Wieringa, D.W., Dijkman, A.G., and Ruben, J.R.: Instruments and Methods for the Quantitative Measurement of Factors Affecting Hygienist/Dentist Efforts During Scaling and Root Planing of the Teeth, *J. Clin. Dent.*, 7, 32, Number 2, 1996.

41. **Liskiewicz**, S.T. and Kerschbaum, W.E.: Cumulative Trauma Disorders: An Ergonomic Approach for Prevention, *J. Dent. Hyg.*, 71, 162, Summer, 1997.

42. **Bohay**, R.N., Bencak, J., Kavaliers, M., and MacLean, D.: A Survey of Magnetic Fields in the Dental Operatory, *J. Can. Dent. Assoc.*, 60, 835, September, 1994.

43. **American Dental Association**, Council on Dental Materials, Instruments, and Equipment: Status Report on Professional Scaling and Stain-removal Devices, *J. Am. Dent. Assoc.*, 111, 801, November, 1985.

44. **Abrams**, H., Barkmeier, W.W., and Cooley, R.L.: Temperature Changes in the Pulp Chamber Produced by Ultrasonic Instrumentation, *Gen. Dent.*, 27, 62, September–October, 1979.

45. **Möller**, P., Grevstad, A.O., and Kristoffersen, T.: Ultrasonic Scaling of Maxillary Teeth Causing Tinnitus and Temporary Hearing Shifts, *J. Clin. Periodontol.*, 3, 123, May, 1976.

46. **Lee**, S.-Y., Lai, Y.-L., and Morgano, S.M.: Effects of Ultrasonic Scaling and Periodontal Curettage on Surface Roughness of Porcelain, *J. Prosthet. Dent.*, 73, 227, March, 1995.

47. **Vermilyea**, S.G., Prasanna, M.K., and Agar, J.R.: Effect of Ultrasonic Cleaning and Air Polishing on Porcelain Labial Margin Restorations, *J. Prosthet. Dent.*, 71, 447, May, 1994.

48. **Rajstein**, J. and Tal, M.: The Effects of Ultrasonic Scaling on the Surface of Class V Amalgam Restorations—A Scanning Electron Microscope Study, *J. Oral Rehabil.*, 11, 299, May, 1984.

49. **Sivers**, J.E. and Johnson, G.K.: Comparison of Effects of Ultra-

sonic and Sonic Instrumentation on Amalgam Restorations, *Gen. Dent.*, 37, 130, March–April, 1989.

50. **Bjornson**, E.J., Collins, D.E., and Engler, W.O.: Surface Alteration of Composite Resins After Curette, Ultrasonic, and Sonic Instrumentation: An *in vitro* Study, *Quintessence Int.*, 21, 381, May, 1990.

51. **Rapley**, J.W., Swan, R.H., Hallmon, W.W., and Mills, M.P.: The Surface Characteristics Produced by Various Oral Hygiene Instruments and Materials on Titanium Implant Abutments, *Int. J. Oral Maxillofac. Implants*, 5, 47, Number 1, 1990.

52. **Preber**, H. and Bergström, J.: The Effect of Non-surgical Treatment on Periodontal Pockets in Smokers and Non-smokers, *J. Clin. Periodontol.*, 13, 319, April, 1986.

53. **Listgarten**, M.A. and Helldén, L.: Relative Distribution of Bacteria at Clinically Healthy and Periodontally Diseased Sites in Humans, *J. Clin. Periodontol.*, 5, 115, May, 1978.

54. **Slots**, J., Mashimo, P., Levine, M.J., and Genco, R.J.: Periodontal Therapy in Humans. I. Microbiologic and Clinical Effects of a Single Course of Periodontal Scaling and Root Planing, and of Adjunctive Tetracycline Therapy, *J. Periodontol.*, 50, 495, October, 1979.

55. **Mousqués**, T., Listgarten, M.A., and Phillips, R.W.: Effects of Scaling and Root Planing on the Composition of the Human Subgingival Microbial Flora, *J. Periodont. Res.*, 15, 144, March, 1980.

56. **Aleo**, J.J., DeRenzis, F.A., Farber, P.A., and Varboncoeur, A.P.: The Presence and Biologic Activity of Cementum-bound Endotoxin, *J. Periodontol.*, 45, 672, September, 1974.

57. **Oosterwaal**, P.J.M., Matee M.I., Mikx, F.H.M., van't Hof, M.A., and Renggli, H.H.: The Effect of Subgingival Debridement with Hand and Ultrasonic Instruments on the Subgingival Microflora, *J. Clin. Periodontol.*, 14, 528, October, 1987.

58. **Badersten**, A., Nilvéus, R., and Egelberg, J.: Effect of Nonsurgical Periodontal Therapy. II. Severely Advanced Periodontitis, *J. Clin. Periodontol.*, 11, 63, January, 1984.

SUGGESTED READINGS

Boretti, G., Zappa, U., Graf, H., and Case, D.: Short-term Effects of Phase I Therapy on Crevicular Cell Populations, *J. Periodontol.*, 66, 235, March, 1995.

Campbell, P.R.: Redi-Reference: Patient Instructions Following Scaling and Root Planing, *DentalHygienistNews*, 7, 14, Summer, 1994.

Cobb, C.M.: Non-surgical Pocket Therapy: Mechanical, in American Academy Periodontology, 1996 World Workshop in Periodontics, *Annals of Periodontology*, 1, 443–490, November, 1996.

Kaldahl, W.B., Kalkwarf, K.L., Patil, K.D., Molvar, M.P., and Dyer, J.K.: Long-term Evaluation of Periodontal Therapy: I. Response to 4 Therapeutic Modalities, *J. Periodontol.*, 67, 93, February, 1996.

Kaldahl, W.B., Kalkwarf, K.L., Patil, K.D., Molvar, M.P., and Dyer, J.K.: Long-term Evaluation of Periodontal Therapy: II. Incidence of Sites Breaking Down, *J. Periodontol.*, 67, 103, February, 1996.

Lembariti, B.S., van der Weijden, G.A., and van Palenstein Helderman, W.H.: The Effect of a Single Scaling With or Without Oral Hygiene Instruction on Gingival Bleeding and Calculus Formation, *J. Clin. Periodontol.*, 25, 30, January, 1998.

Lowenguth, R.A. and Greenstein, G.: Clinical and Microbiological Response to Nonsurgical Mechanical Periodontal Therapy, *Periodontol. 2000*, 9, 14, 1995.

Miller, C.S., Leonelli, F.M., and Latham, E.: Selective Interference With Pacemaker Activity by Electrical Dental Devices, *Oral Surg. Oral Med. Oral Pathol. Oral Radiol. Endod.*, 85, 33, January, 1998.

Nunn, P.J.: Root Instrumentation: How Much Is Enough? *Access*, 10, 30, September–October, 1996.

Otero-Cagide, F.J. and Long, B.A.: Comparative in Vitro Effectiveness of Closed Root Debridement With Fine Instruments on Specific Areas of Mandibular First Molar Furcations. I. Root Trunk and Furcation Entrance, *J. Periodontol.*, 68, 1093, November, 1997.

Otero-Cagide, F.J. and Long, B.A.: Comparative *in Vitro* Effectiveness of Closed Root Debridement With Fine Instruments on Specific Areas of Mandibular First Molar Furcations. II. Furcation Area, *J. Periodontol., 68*, 1098, November, 1997.

Schwartz, M.: The Prevention and Management of the Broken Curet, *Compend. Cont. Educ. Dent., 19*, 418, April, 1998.

Manual and Ultrasonic Compared

Cross-Poline, G.N., Stach, D.J., and Newman, S.M.: Effects of Curet and Ultrasonics on Root Surfaces, *Am. J. Dent., 8*, 131, June, 1995.

Drisko, C.H.: Periodontal Debridement. Hand Versus Power-driven Scalers, *DentalHygienistNews, 8*, 18, Special Issue, Spring, 1995.

Jacobson, L., Blomlof, J., and Lindskog, S.: Root Surface Texture after Different Scaling Modalities, *Scand. J. Dent. Res., 102*, 156, June, 1994.

Ritz, L., Hefti, A.F., and Rateitschak, K.H.: An *in vitro* Investigation on the Loss of Root Substance in Scaling with Various Instruments, *J. Clin. Periodontol., 18*, 643, October, 1991.

Ultrasonic Scaling

Anderson, G.B., Plotzke, A.E., Morrison, E.C., and Caffesse, R.G.: Effectiveness of an Irrigating Solution Utilized During Ultrasonic Scaling, *Quintessence Int., 26*, 849, December, 1995.

Bray, K.K.: Challenging the Fundamental Principles of Ultrasonics, *DentalHygienistNews, 8*, 14, Number 3, 1995.

Clark, S.M.: The Influence of Two Ultrasonic Tips on Root Surfaces—*in Vivo*, *Gen. Dent., 38*, 125, March–April, 1990.

Ewen, S.J. and Tascher, P.J.: Clinical Uses of Ultrasonic Root Scalers, *J. Periodontol., 29*, 45, January, 1958.

Flemmig, T.F., Petersilka, G.J., Mehl, A., Hickel, R., and Klaiber, B.: Working Parameters of a Magnostrictive Ultrasonic Scaler Influencing Root Substance Removal *in vitro, J. Periodontol., 69*, 547, May, 1998.

Forabosco, A., Galetti, R., Spinato, S., Colao, P., and Casolari, C.: A Comparative Study of a Surgical Method and Scaling and Root Planing Using the Odontoson,® *J. Clin. Periodontol., 23*, 611, July, 1996.

Hawkins, P.: Micro Ultrasonics. Contemporary Periodontal Instrumentation, *Access, 10*, 25, July, 1996.

Lee, A., Heasman, P.A., and Kelly, P.J.: An *in Vitro* Comparative Study of a Reciprocating Scaler for Root Surface Debridement, *J. Dent., 24*, 81, January/March, 1996.

Peterson, C.A., Lutz, E.R., and Mauriello, S.M.: A Task Analysis for Ultrasonic Instrumentation, *J. Practical Hyg., 4*, 11, March/April, 1995.

Schlageter, L.,Rateitschak-Plüss, E.M., and Schwarz, J.-P.: Root Surface Smoothness or Roughness Following Open Debridement: An *in Vivo* Study, *J. Clin. Periodontol., 23*, 460, May, 1996.

Stach, D.J.: Perspectives on Ultrasonics, Sonics. Their Role in Periodontal Debridement, *Dent. Teamwork, 7*, 22, March–April, 1994.

Sonic Scaling

Grant, D.A., Lie T., Clark, S.M., and Adams, D.F.: Pain and Discomfort Levels in Patients During Root Surface Debridement With Sonic Metal or Plastic Inserts, *J. Periodontol., 64*, 645, July, 1993.

Jotikasthira, N.E., Lie, T., and Leknes, K.N.: Comparative *in Vitro* Studies of Sonic, Ultrasonic and Reciprocating Scaling Instruments, *J. Clin. Periodontol., 19*, 560, September, 1992.

Kocher, T., Rühling, A., Herweg, M., and Plagman, H.-C.: Proof of Efficacy of Different Modified Sonic Scaler Inserts Used for Debridement in Furcations—A Dummy Head Trial, *J. Clin. Periodontol., 23*, 662, July, 1996.

Leknes, K.N. and Lie, T.: Influence of Polishing Procedures on Sonic Scaling Root Surface Roughness, *J. Periodontol., 62*, 659, November, 1991.

Reed, K.L.: Sonic Scalers: A Review, *Gen. Dent., 40*, 34, January–February, 1992.

Shah, S., Walmsley, A.D., Chapple, I.L.C., and Lumley, P.J.: Variability of Sonic Scaling Tip Movement, *J. Clin. Periodontol., 21*, 705, November, 1994.

Ultrasonics/Aerosol Production

Allison, C., Simor, A.E., Mock, D., and Tenenbaum, H.C.: Prosol-chlorhexidine Irrigation Reduces the Incidence of Bacteremia During Ultrasonic Scaling With the Cavi-Med: A Pilot Investigation, *J. Can. Dent. Assoc., 59*, 673, August, 1993.

Barnes, J.B., Harrel, S.K., and Rivera-Hidalgo, F.: Blood Contamination of the Aerosols Produced by *in vivo* Use of Ultrasonic Scalers, *J. Periodontol., 69*, 434, April, 1998.

Gross, K.B.W., Overman, P.R., Cobb, C., and Brockman, S.: Aerosol Generation by Two Ultrasonic Scalers and One Sonic Scaler: A Comparative Study, *J. Dent. Hyg., 66*, 314, September, 1992.

Swanson, S.J. and Tobian, M.L.: Facts about Aerosols, *Access, 10*, 42, January, 1996.

Ultrasonics/Restorative Materials

Cutler, B.J., Goldstein, G.R., and Simonelli, G.: The Effect of Dental Prophylaxis Instruments on the Surface Roughness of Metals Used for Metal Ceramic Crowns, *J. Prosthet. Dent., 73*, 219, February, 1995.

Meschenmoser, A., d'Hoedt, B., Meyle, J., Elbner, G., Korn, D., Hämmerle, H., and Schulte, W.: Effects of Various Hygiene Procedures on the Surface Characteristics of Titanium Abutments, *J. Periodontol., 67*, 229, March, 1996.

Nonsurgical Periodontal Therapy: Supplemental Care Procedures

34

The two essential components of successful nonsurgical therapy are complete subgingival scaling with root debridement and effective microbial plaque control. The objective is to eliminate or at least suppress the pathologic microorganisms in the subgingival area to promote healing and hence control the infection.

Supplemental care procedures are selected in accord with the special needs of the patient. The need, the procedures, and the expected outcomes are carefully explained to the patient. The patient must accept responsibility and understand that the success of all periodontal therapy depends on the daily personal plaque control by the patient.

In this chapter purposes and procedures for professional irrigation and local delivery of antimicrobials are described. Box 34-1 defines key words and related terminology.

I. PATIENT NEEDS

For the patient with uncomplicated gingivitis, complete scaling and patient compliance in personal daily plaque removal usually can bring about a reversal of inflammation, and health can be maintained. Likewise, for the patient with early periodontitis, control of infection also may be attained through nonsurgical periodontal therapy. Maintaining the healthy state requires continuing routine appointments for professional scaling and supervision of the patient's plaque removal methods.

On the other hand, for patients with moderate to advanced periodontal conditions, or refractory patients with poor response to routine therapy, supplemental therapeutic measures usually are required. Certain periodontal conditions of patients of all degrees of disease severity will require surgical or other advanced therapeutic procedures and will be referred to a periodontist.

II. SUPPLEMENTAL CARE PROCEDURES

Examples of supplemental care procedures that are carried out by the dental hygienist described in other chapters of this book include:
A. Smoking cessation assistance (Chapter 27)
B. Desensitization of teeth (Chapter 37)
C. At-home rinsing, irrigation, use of dentifrice, and other selective use of antimicrobials (Chapter 24)
D. Care for dental implants (Chapter 26)

BOX 34-1 KEY WORDS: Nonsurgical Periodontal Therapy*

Antibiotic: a form of antimicrobial agent, produced by or obtained from microorganisms that can kill other microorganisms or inhibit their growth; may be specific for certain organisms or may cover a broad spectrum.

Antimicrobial therapy: use of specific chemical or pharmaceutical agents for the control or destruction of microorganisms, either systemically or at specific sites.

Attachment: with reference to the *clinical attachment level,* which is the position of the periodontal attached tissue at the base of a sulcus or pocket as measured from a fixed point (pages 209 to 210).

New attachment: the union of connective tissue or epithelium with a root surface that has been deprived of its original attachment apparatus; the new attachment may be epithelial adhesion and/or connective tissue adaptation or attachment, and it may include new cementum.

Reattachment: the reunion of epithelial and connective tissues with root surfaces and bone such as occurs after an incision or injury.

Biodegradable (bi"o-de-grād'ah-bul): susceptible of degradation by biological processes, as by bacterial or other enzymatic action.

Cannula (kan'ū-lah): tubular instrument placed in a cavity to introduce or withdraw fluid.

Chemotherapy (ke'mō-ther'ah-pē): treatment by means of chemical or pharmaceutical agents.

Controlled release: local delivery of a chemotherapeutic agent to a site-specific area; may be a patch to be worn on the skin or a polymeric fiber, such as that used to deliver an agent to a periodontal pocket.

Infection (in-fek'shun): invasion and multiplication of microorganisms in body tissues.

Endogenous infection (en-doj'ĕ-nus): caused by microorganisms that are part of the normal microbiota of the skin, nose, mouth, and intestinal and urogenital tracts.

Exogenous infection (ek-soj'ĕ-nus): caused by organisms acquired from outside the oral cavity or the host.

Opportunistic infection: occurs in a systemically or locally impaired host; opportunistic pathogens may not be highly virulent, but they can cause disease when the host defense is altered.

Open scaling and root planing: instrumentation performed after the area has been exposed by tissue removal or the tissue is separated and laid back as a flap; visibility and accessibility allow more thorough treatment.

Refractory periodontitis: clinical attachment loss despite optimal subgingival debridement and performance of acceptable oral hygiene by the patient.

*Other definitions pertaining to irrigation may be found in Box 24-1, page 371.

E. Dental caries prevention: fluoride applications and other preventive measures, especially for root caries prevention for the patient with periodontal recession (Fluorides, Chapter 29; Sealants, Chapter 30)

F. Correction of plaque-retaining irregularities; overhang removal when not included in the routine tooth preparation procedures (Chapter 40)

G. Dietary analysis for all special needs (Chapter 28)

H. Personal counseling for patients with systemic conditions for which periodontal infection is a risk factor (Chapters 43 [Pregnancy], 58 [Cardiovascular], 60 [Diabetes])

ANTIMICROBIAL TREATMENT

The use of antimicrobial agents for supplemental or adjunctive treatment of gingival and periodontal infections may be local or systemic.

I. OBJECTIVES OF ANTIMICROBIAL THERAPY

By arresting the infection using antimicrobial drugs, further loss of periodontal attachment and other periodontal tissue destruction caused by microorganisms can be prevented. Treatment using antimicrobials aims to suppress and eliminate pathogenic microorganisms to allow the recolonization of the microbiota that are compatible with health.

II. TYPES OF DELIVERY OF ANTIMICROBIALS

The types will be described in the following order in this chapter.

A. Systemic Administration

Systemic administration of antibiotics is well known and highly successful in the world of medical care. Antibiotics have saved the lives of many people with generalized infectious diseases.

B. Local Delivery

The knowledge that periodontal diseases are site-specific infections has led to the development of methods for placing antimicrobials directly at the site of the infection—the pocket. Irrigation and controlled-release methods will be described.

SYSTEMIC

I. ACTION OF SYSTEMICALLY ADMINISTERED ANTIBIOTIC

In contrast to locally applied agents placed directly into a pocket, antibiotics administered systemically reach the pathogenic organisms in the pocket through the circulation. The antibiotic is absorbed into the circulation from the intestine. From the blood stream the drug is passed into the body tissues. It enters the periodontal tissues and passes into the pocket by way of the gingival sulcus fluid. The systemically administered drug is in a diluted form by the time it reaches the pathogenic microorganisms, where the destruction is taking place.

II. SELECTION OF ANTIBIOTIC

Ideally the specific microorganism that is causing a certain periodontal disease should be determined first, and the antibiotic that is selected should be specific for that organism.[1] Microbiological testing is available and can be used to guide clinical decisions. Examples of specific treatment in current practice are the use of tetracyclines and metronidazole in combination with mechanical debridement to treat *Actinobacillus actinomycetemcomitans* in juvenile periodontitis and refractory periodontal conditions.[2,3]

Periodontal diseases are caused by mixed infections of microorganisms. The pathogens tend to work in clusters, that is, in combination with other organisms. Selective identification of specific organisms that match with specific antibiotics has been accomplished only to a limited degree.

III. LIMITATIONS

The precautions and adverse effects, as well as the acquisition of antibiotic resistance by the organisms, preclude the widespread use of systemic antibiotics for periodontal problems. Limitations include the following:

A. Side effects of certain antibiotics.
B. Potential for the development of resistant strains.
C. Local concentration diluted by the time the drug reaches the pathogens; drug is "wasted" in that it covers a large area not needing the treatment.
D. Superimposed infection can develop, such as candidiasis.
E. Low compliance of the patient in following the prescription for the required number of days.

IV. USE OF SYSTEMIC THERAPY

Most periodontal infection does not require systemic therapy except when there is systemic involvement shown by generalized symptoms such as fever. Examples are an acute inflammation in necrotizing ulcerative gingivitis or abscess formation. Treatment using systemic antibiotics is a selective procedure.[1]

PROFESSIONAL SUBGINGIVAL IRRIGATION

Professional subgingival irrigation is based on the premise that delivery of antimicrobial agents may enhance the effects of treatment by scaling and root planing. Irrigation into a pocket can disrupt the numbers of microorganisms left behind following instrumentation.

Studies have shown that repopulation of the subgingival microflora can occur within weeks after treatment.[4] In addition, the reduction of the subgingival flora depends on the ability of the clinician to remove subgingival plaque and calculus definitively; clearly, total removal is difficult in deep pockets.

Irrigation with an antimicrobial agent provides a supplemental therapeutic step and results in additional clinical benefits.[5]

I. DELIVERY METHOD

A presterilized disposable cannula, with a side port, multiple side ports, or end release (Figure 34-1A), is used with one of the following:

A. Disposable hand syringe.
B. Specially designed jet irrigator.
C. Air-driven irrigation handpiece.

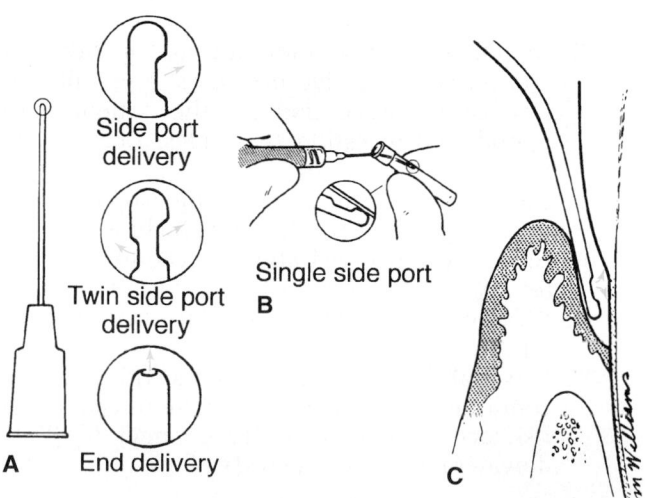

FIGURE 34-1 Professional Irrigation. (A) Types of cannula tips with side-port or end-delivery openings. **(B)** Prepare the cannula for use by bending the sterile tip within the encasement to make the insertion easier. **(C)** With knowledge of each probing depth, insert the cannula gently to near the bottom of a pocket. No force should be used.

II. PROCEDURE

A. Prepare the cannula by bending it slightly as it is uncovered (Figure 34-1*B*).

B. Insert the cannula subgingivally (Figure 34-1*C*).

C. Allow the irrigant to fill the pocket.

D. Apply circumferentially, releasing solution at three points on the facial surface and three on the lingual surface.

E. Irrigate all teeth, quadrants, or specific selected sites as dictated by the patient's need.

III. RECOMMENDATIONS FOR USE

A. Preprocedural Delivery

An antimicrobial agent can aid in reducing the numbers of microorganisms to prevent aerosol contamination during instrumentation.

B. Preanesthesia Application

Used to reduce microorganisms before application of topical anesthetic in preparation for local anesthetic injection.

C. Maintenance Phase: Postprocedure Irrigation

1. Patient with site(s) not responding to traditional periodontal care.
2. Patient with gingivitis superimposed on periodontitis.
3. Patient with areas inaccessible to mechanical instrumentation because of root contour, furcations, or depth of pocket where open scaling and root planing are not alternatives.

IV. ANTIMICROBIAL AGENTS

A variety of antimicrobial agents, saline solution, and water have been researched for professional irrigation with varying results. Products used include chlorhexidine gluconate and stannous fluoride.[5–8]

V. SPECIAL CONSIDERATIONS

A. Antibiotic Premedication

Subgingival irrigation can produce a bacteremia. Professional irrigation requires premedication in patients susceptible to the effects of bacteremia. When irrigation is selected as a specific form of treatment for a patient susceptible to bacterial endocarditis, the periodontal tissues should be brought to health first. The usual procedure for all dental appointments should be followed.

B. Irrigation Pressure

Professional irrigation systems usually control the amount of pressure. Caution must be exercised, however, when irrigating with a disposable syringe because pressure may exceed the safety level for the oral tissues.

LOCAL DELIVERY OF ANTIMICROBIALS

Local delivery means that the medication used to treat the periodontal infection is concentrated at the site of the infection. The infecting pathogenic microorganisms are located in the depths of the pockets and the surrounding tissue. Irrigation does deliver the medication to the pocket, but the action is temporary because of the constant turnover and cleansing that is going on in the pocket.

Controlled delivery refers to providing the medication over an extended period of time by being held in the pocket and released slowly. Slow-release methods are used in a variety of ways. The nicotine patch, used to assist a person trying to break a smoking addiction, is an example described in Chapter 27.

I. REQUIREMENTS

A local delivery method can place high concentrations of the antimicrobial in an infected pocket. To be successful the medication must:[9]

A. Be of a concentration that will act on the microorganisms causing the infection.

B. Reach all areas of the pocket to the very bottom and into furcations.

C. Stay in contact long enough at the effective concentration for the antimicrobial action to take place.

D. Comparison with systemic: When systemic treatment is used, much less of the antimicrobial medication reaches the actual site of the infection where the pathogens are concentrated because the agent becomes diluted as it passes through the system.

II. USES FOR SLOW-RELEASE LOCAL DELIVERY[10]

A. At Initial Therapy

Periodontal diseases result from local infection with a pathogenic microflora. The periodontal pocket is generally teeming with microorganisms and may also contain subgingival calculus, which further adds to harbor bacteria. Scaling and root planing are highly effective procedures for controlling periodontal infections, reducing inflammation, and reducing probing depths.

The adjunctive use of local antimicrobials may enhance the effect of the mechanical instrumentation. Research has shown that the adjunctive use of a controlled-release antimicrobial increases the effect of scaling and root planing.[11]

B. Adjunctive Treatment: At Re-evaluation

For the minority of sites that do not respond to basic therapy and may be classified as refractory periodontal disease, a local delivery method can be selected. At the completion of periodontal therapy, a re-evaluation is made at the first maintenance appointment, and areas that do not respond to additional scaling and root planing may be selected for a local drug delivery treatment.

C. Recurrent Disease
Over time during the maintenance phase of therapy, pockets can recolonize. Recurrence of periodontal infection usually occurs in localized pockets, particularly in areas most difficult for the patient to carry out complete bacterial plaque removal on a daily basis.

D. Peri-Implantitis
The ailing or failing implant may respond to a localized slow-release antimicrobial.

E. Periodontal Abscess
After incision and drainage has been established, a locally delivered, sustained-release antimicrobial may aid the healing process. When a tetracycline fiber is used it may serve as a wick in the drainage of the abscess.

F. Preparation for Periodontal Surgery
Preconditioning the tissue and lessening the severity of the infection can contribute to less bleeding during surgery and smoother, more rapid healing.

III. TYPES OF LOCAL DELIVERY AGENTS
Available for treatment of periodontal infections are a tetracycline fiber; a chlorhexidine chip; and antibiotic gels, metronidazole, minocycline, and doxycycline.

Subgingival drug therapy should always be applied as a supplement or adjunctive procedure after meticulous scaling and root debridement has been completed and the results evaluated. Special features of each type and procedures for clinical application will be presented. For all products, the manufacturer's advice and directions should be followed.

TETRACYCLINE FIBER

The concept of a controlled local delivery for treatment of periodontal pathogens in a pocket infection was developed over many years by Goodson and co-workers.[12]

Use of the fiber has shown significant clinical improvement in probing depth, clinical attachment level, and bleeding on probing[13–15] and reduction of sites with periodontal pathogenic microorganisms.[16]

I. DESCRIPTION
A. Monolithic fiber: 9 inches (23 cm) long, 0.5 mm diameter; flexible.
B. Composition of fiber: ethylene/vinyl acetate, biocompatible copolymer.
C. Contents: 12.7 mg tetracycline hydrochloride (25%) mixed with the polymer; imparts a yellow color to the fiber.
D. Controlled delivery; nonbiodegradable; maintains high concentration over full 10-day period of application.

II. ACTION
A. Slow-Release
The pocket moisture dissolves the drug from the fiber.

B. Amount Released
Depends on the length of fiber used; higher dose in deep pockets where more fiber length is used.

C. Comparison With Systemically Administered Antibiotic
1. *Prescription:* 250-mg tablets taken four times per day for 10 days results in total dose of 10,000 mg.
2. *Fiber:* total dose 12.7 mg possible when a whole fiber is used.

D. Suggested Contraindications
1. Sensitivities or allergies to tetracycline or the cyanoacrylate used for dressings.
2. Immunocompromized patient susceptible to infection related to overgrowth of fiber-resistant bacteria or *Candida.*
3. Pregnant or breast-feeding women. The amount of tetracycline is small, but prudent practice suggests that no elective drugs be administered during pregnancy or lactation.
4. Patient with inadequate self-care who does not comply with routine maintenance must be informed of the potential for limited success.

III. PLACEMENT PROCEDURES
A. Site Selection
Probing depth of 5 mm or more is best for fiber retention.

B. Fiber Preparation
1. *Length needed.* Depends on probing depth; more efficient to work with 2- to 3-inch lengths.
2. *Number of teeth treated.* More than one pocket can be treated in the same appointment on the same side, preferably the same quadrant for convenience and comfort of patient's postcare. Chewing, brushing, and other disturbances increase chances of displacement.
3. *Sterility of the fiber.* Once the package is opened, extra fiber not used cannot be kept for a future appointment.

C. Steps in Placement
1. *Anesthesia.* Anesthesia is not usually needed for fiber placement. When scaling is performed at the same appointment, anesthesia may have been administered already.
2. *Isolation.* Cotton rolls and saliva ejector are indicated.

3. *Fiber placement*
   a. Place fiber around the tooth first to aid retention; thread under contact areas by looping fiber with dental floss or using a floss threader.
   b. Use a gingival retraction cord packing instrument or other dull instrument to pack the fiber down; pass the fiber to the bottom of the pocket.
   c. Fold the fiber back and forth on itself (Figure 34-2A).
   d. Furcation area. Use a small piece of fiber to pack the furca first; then fill the rest of the pocket.
   e. Interdental pocket. Pack from either or both facial and lingual or palatal.
   f. Fill to within 1 mm of the gingival margin. Anticipate that the tissue will shrink.
   g. When the pocket is filled, trim ends of fiber that extend above gingival margin and pack down (Figure 34-2B).
4. *Place adhesive dressing*
   a. Isolate, dry gently with gauze square or light air blast.
   b. Apply the adhesive dressing all around the margin in small amounts to hold the fiber in place.
   c. Adhesive sets rapidly. May cover with water-soluble lubricant to smooth the surface and prevent sticking.
5. *Additional recommendation.* Cover with periodontal dressing to ensure that the fiber cannot be displaced. Periodontal dressing placement is described on page 591.

6. Make appointment for fiber removal in 7 to 14 days.

D. Patient Instruction
1. Prevent accidental removal:
   a. Do not touch with fingers or tongue.
   b. Avoid coarse, rough, or sticky foods.
   c. Brush and floss all other teeth; avoid area of fiber.
2. Rinse with chlorhexidine 0.12% twice daily.
3. Call for appointment if fiber is lost before 7 days; must be replaced for complete treatment.

E. Fiber Removal
1. Provide patient with preprocedural antimicrobial mouthrinse.
2. Isolate, dry the surface, tease the fiber out using a curet; cut the fiber that crosses through the interdental area.
3. Examine tissue. There may be a small gap between margin and tooth; it will close in a short time. Check for and remove any newly formed calculus.
4. Instruct patient to resume regular self-care procedures to control bacterial plaque; advise patient to continue chlorhexidine rinsing for a few more days.

F. Evaluation
Examine in 2 to 3 weeks to ensure that tissue has responded and that the patient is maintaining the area. Proceed to 3-months' maintenance.

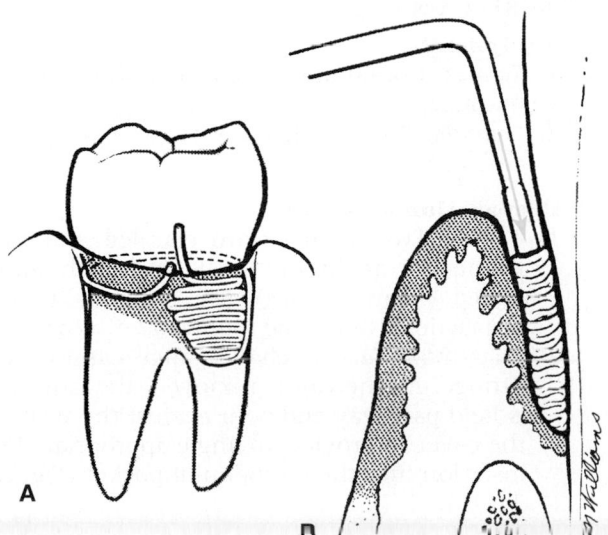

FIGURE 34-2 Tetracycline Fiber. (A) The fiber is first placed around the tooth to provide retention. Then starting at the very bottom of the pocket, the fiber is layered on itself until the pocket is filled. **(B)** Pack the fiber down with a dull instrument.

CHLORHEXIDINE CHIP

The chlorhexidine chip benefits periodontal health by significant improvements in probing depths, gain of clinical attachment, and reduced subgingival bacteria.[17]

The chlorhexidine chip is intended for use as an adjunctive therapy with scaling and root debridement. Chlorhexidine as an agent for local delivery has the advantage over the antibiotics in that there is no potential for the development of bacterial resistance.

I. DESCRIPTION
A. Size: 4 by 5 mm and 0.35 mm thick (Figure 34-3A).
B. Shape: rectangular, rounded at one end (resembling a baby's fingernail).[10]
C. Contents: matrix of hydrolyzed gelatin with 2.5 mg chlorhexidine gluconate incorporated; color is orange-brown.
D. Controlled delivery; biodegradable; maintains high level chlorhexidine for 7 to 10 days. The gingival sulcus fluid concentration is greater than 125 μg/mL for 8 days.

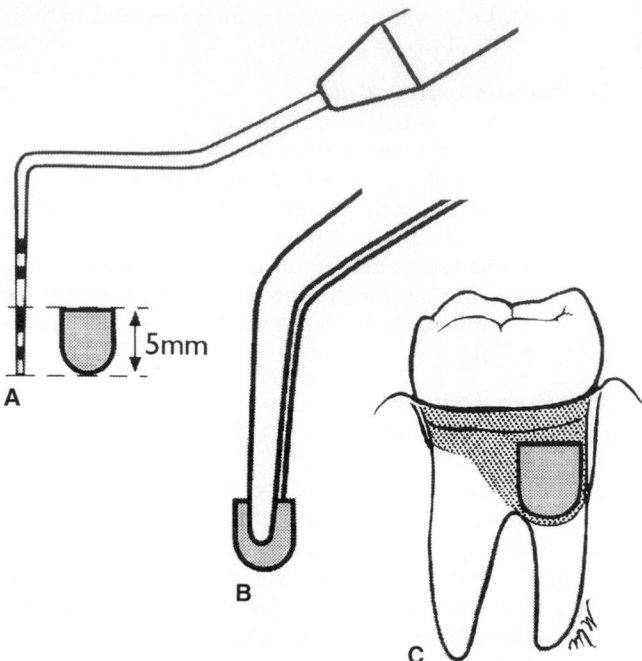

FIGURE 34-3 **Chlorhexidine Chip. (A)** The chip is 5 mm × 4 mm rounded at one end. **(B)** For insertion, the chip is grasped by cotton pliers on the square side. **(C)** The chip is inserted to the very base of the pocket where the periodontal pathogens are concentrated.

II. PLACEMENT PROCEDURE

A. Site Selection

1. *Pocket Depth.* The chip should be contained within the pocket, so since the chip is 5 mm long, pockets of more than 5 mm are indicated for treatment.
2. *Chips Placed.* More than one pocket can be treated in the same appointment on the same side, preferably in the same quadrant for the comfort and convenience of the patient's postcare.

B. Chip Care and Preparation

1. Store chips in a refrigerator (2° to 8°C, 36° to 46°F).
2. Package contains 10 chips. Each chip is packaged individually in a separate compartment of an aluminum blister pack.

C. Steps in Placement

1. *Isolation*
   a. Position cotton rolls and saliva ejector.
   b. Dry the area with a sponge to prevent wetting chip during placement. Chip may start to soften and become more difficult to place if it gets wet before placement in the pocket.
2. *Insertion*
   a. Hold chip with cotton pliers; position chip with round side away from the cotton pliers (Figure 34-3*B*).

b. Insert the chip to the bottom of the pocket; position at the deepest part (Figure 34-3*C*).

C. Action

1. Chip biodegrades in 7 to 10 days.
2. Approximately 40% of the chlorhexidine may be released within the first 24 hours, and the rest over the following 7 to 10 days.

D. Patient Instructions

1. Avoid disturbing the area. Do not use dental floss at the site of the insertion for 10 days.
2. Brush all other teeth and clean interdentally as usual.
3. Although some mild to moderate sensitivity may be expected during the first week after placement, contact the clinic or office promptly if pain, swelling, or other problem occurs.

E. Maintenance Appointments

1. Place a chip in pockets 5 mm or deeper at each 3-months' maintenance appointment.
2. Evaluate probing depth and clinical attachment levels.
3. Ascertain that patient is maintaining a high level of bacterial plaque control.

DOXYCYCLINE POLYMER

Biodegradable doxycycline polymer in liquid form is delivered by cannula into a pocket and solidifies on contact with the dampness of the sulcus fluid. Beneficial effects include reduction of probing depths, gain of attachment, and destruction of periodontal pathogenic microorganisms.[18,19]

I. DESCRIPTION

A. Equipment

1. *Syringe.* Containing liquid 10% doxycycline hyclate.
2. *Cannula.* Blunt ended, 23 gauge, narrow diameter.

B. Preparation of Agent

1. *Mixing.* Two syringes are coupled and the substances are passed back and forth until mixed (Figure 34-4*A*). The manufacturer's instructions should be followed with care.
2. *Adapt cannula.* Attach 23-gauge cannula to syringe. As the cap is removed, the cannula is held part way and bent against the wall of the cover to provide an angle appropriate for insertion into the periodontal pocket (Figure 34-4*B*).

II. DELIVERY

A. Insert Cannula to Base of Pocket. Express the agent to just over the gingival margin; withdraw cannula (Figure 34-4C).

B. Packing. Use a blunt instrument to pack the

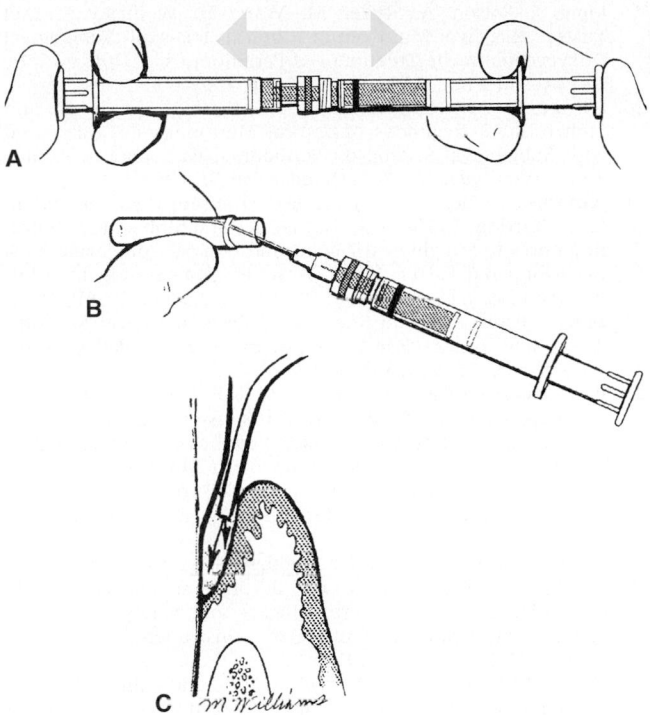

FIGURE 34-4 Doxycycline Polymer Gel. (A) Syringes are coupled and the contents passed back and forth until mixed. **(B)** The cannula is attached to the syringe with the agent; as the cap is removed, the cannula is pressed against the side to bend it to an angle appropriate for accessing the pocket to be treated. **(C)** The cannula is inserted to the base of the pocket, and the agent is released to fill the pocket.

agent down. Add more if necessary to fill the pocket. Wet the instrument to prevent sticking to the agent.

C. Hardening of Agent. On contact with the moisture of the pocket, the agent will harden.

D. Periodontal Dressing
Placing a dressing over the area aids retention.

E. Patient Instruction
1. Prevent accidental removal. Care of area with dressing is described in Table 36-1, page 593.
2. Routine brushing and other self-care on all other areas.

F. Appointment for Removal of Dressing
1. Dressing removal is outlined on page 592.
2. Evaluate tissue; evaluate plaque removal.
3. Plan routine maintenance.

METRONIDAZOLE GEL

Metronidazole in the form of a suspension is delivered by cannula for periodontal pocket therapy. As a biodegradable product with sustained release, its bene-fits have been shown to include probing depth and bleeding on probing reduction, clinical attachment gain, and reduced incidence of periodontal pathogenic organisms.[20–22] An advantage that metronidazole has is a specific activity against anaerobic microorganisms without generalized destruction of all aerobes as well.

I. DESCRIPTION
A. Composition: oil-based gel with 25% metronidazole in glyceryl mono-oleate and sesame oil.
B. Sustained release: 24 to 36 hours.

II. DELIVERY
A. Delivered by cannula in a viscous consistency; liquifies by body heat, and then hardens when in contact with fluids of the pocket to form crystals.
B. Two applications 1 week apart are recommended.

MINOCYCLINE GEL

A minocycline ointment applied as an adjunct to scaling and root debridement requires several applications but has beneficial outcomes. A reduction in periodontal pathogenic microorganisms and reductions in probing depths and other clinical parameters have been demonstrated.[23–25]

I. DESCRIPTION
A. Composition: gel suspension with 2% minocycline hydrochloride.
B. Sustained release: biodegradable.
C. Care of gel: refrigerate.

II. DELIVERY
A. Delivered by cannula with blunt tip.
B. Administered weekly; different reports used different numbers of applications.

III. MAINTENANCE
A. Probe carefully to test results of treatments.
B. Repeat gel treatment as needed.

FACTORS TO TEACH THE PATIENT

I. What a periodontal pocket is and why it needs to be treated.
II. How the treatment using tetracycline fiber, chlorhexidine chip, or doxycycline polymer (whichever is being used to treat the patient) affects the infection in the pocket.
III. How to use the home irrigator; relation between home irrigation and the irrigation in the dental office.
IV. The success of all periodontal therapy depends

on the daily personal bacterial plaque control by the patient.

REFERENCES

1. **van Winkelhoff**, A.J., Rams, T.E., and Slots, J.: Systemic Antibiotic Therapy in Periodontics, *Periodontology 2000, 10,* 45, 1996.
2. **Slots**, J. and Rosling, B.G.: Suppression of the Periodontopathic Microflora in Localized Juvenile Periodontitis by Systemic Tetracycline, *J. Clin. Periodontol., 10,* 465, September, 1983.
3. **Loesche**, W.J., Schmidt, E., Smith, B.A., Morrison, E.C., Caffesse, R., and Hujoel, P.P.: Effect of Metronidazole on Periodontal Treatment Needs, *J. Periodontol., 62,* 247, April, 1991.
4. **Mousquès**, T., Listgarten, M.A., and Phillips, R.W.: Effect of Scaling and Root Planing on the Composition of the Human Subgingival Microbial Flora, *J. Periodont. Res., 15,* 144, March, 1980.
5. **Southard**, S.R., Drisko, C.L., Killoy, W.J., Cobb, C.M., and Tira, D.E.: The Effect of 2% Chlorhexidine Digluconate Irrigation on Clinical Parameters and the Level of *Bacteroides gingivalis* in Periodontal Pockets, *J. Periodontol., 60,* 302, June, 1989.
6. **Schmid**, E., Kornman, K.S., and Tinanoff, N.: Changes of Subgingival Total Colony Forming Units and Black Pigmented Bacteroides after a Single Irrigation of Periodontal Pockets with 1.64% SnF_2, *J. Periodontol., 56,* 330, June, 1985.
7. **Mazza**, J.E., Newman, M.G., and Sims, T.N.: Clinical and Antimicrobial Effect of Stannous Fluoride on Periodontitis, *J. Clin. Periodontol., 8,* 203, June, 1981.
8. **Schlagenhauf**, U., Stellwag, P., and Fiedler, A.: Subgingival Irrigation in the Maintenance Phase of Periodontal Therapy, *J. Clin. Periodontol., 17,* 650, October, 1990.
9. **Goodson**, J.M.: Controlled Drug Delivery: A New Means of Treatment of Dental Diseases, *Compend. Cont. Educ. Dent., 6,* 27, January, 1985.
10. **Killoy**, W.J. and Polson, A.M.: Controlled Local Delivery of Antimicrobials in the Treatment of Periodontitis, *Dent. Clin. North Am., 42,* 263, April, 1998.
11. **Greenstein**, G. and Polson, A.: The Role of Local Drug Delivery in the Management of Periodontal Diseases: A Comprehensive Review, *J. Periodontol., 69,* 507, May, 1998.
12. **Goodson**, J.M., Haffajee, A., and Socransky, S.S.: Periodontal Therapy by Local Delivery of Tetracycline, *J. Clin. Periodontol., 6,* 83, April, 1979.
13. **Newman**, M.G., Kornman, K.S., and Doherty, F.M.: A 6-month Multicenter Evaluation of Adjunctive Tetracycline Fiber Therapy Used in Conjunction with Scaling and Root Planing in Maintenance Patients: Clinical Results, *J. Periodontol., 65,* 685, July, 1994.
14. **Kerry**, G.: Tetracycline-loaded Fibers as Adjunctive Treatment in Periodontal Disease, *J. Am. Dent. Assoc., 125,* 1199, September, 1994.
15. **Vandekerckhove**, B.N.A., Quirynen, M., and van Steenberghe, D.: The Use of Tetracycline-containing Controlled-release Fibers in the Treatment of Refractory Periodontitis, *J. Periodontol., 68,* 353, April, 1997.
16. **Lowenguth**, R.A., Chin, I., Caton, J.G., Cobb, C.M., Drisko, C.L., Killoy, W.J., Michalowicz, B.S., Pihlstrom, B.L., and Goodson, J.M.: Evaluation of Periodontal Treatments Using Controlled-release Tetracycline Fibers: Microbiological Response, *J. Periodontol., 66,* 700, August, 1995.
17. **Stabholz**, A., Sela, M.N., Friedman, M., Golomb, G., and Soskolne, A.: Clinical and Microbiological Effects of Sustained Release Chlorhexidine in Periodontal Pockets, *J. Clin. Periodontol., 13,* 783, September, 1986.
18. **Polson**, A.M., Garrett, S., Stoller, N.H., Bandt, C.L., Hanes, P.J., Killoy, W.J., Southard, G.L., Duke, S.P., Bogle, G.C., Drisko, C.H., and Friesen, L.R.: Multi-center Comparative Evaluation of Subgingivally Delivered Sanguinarine and Doxycycline in the Treatment of Periodontitis. II. Clinical Results, *J. Periodontol., 68,* 119, February, 1997.
19. **Garrett**, S., Adams, D., Bandt, C., Beiswanger, B., Bogle, G., Caton, J., Donly, K., Drisko, C., Hallmon, W., Hancock, B., Hanes, P., Hawley, C., Johnson, L., Kiger, R., Killoy, W., Mel-lonig, J., Polson, A., Ryder, M., Wang, H., Wolinsky, L., and Yukna, R.: Two Multi-center Clinical Trials of Subgingival Doxycycline in the Treatment of Periodontitis, *J. Dent. Res., 76,* 153 (Abstract no. 1113), Special Issue, 1997.
20. **Klinge**, B., Attström, R., Karring, T., Kisch, J., Lewin, B., and Stoltze, K.: 3 Regimens of Topical Metronidazole, Compared with Subgingival Scaling on Periodontal Pathology in Adults, *J. Clin. Periodontol., 19,* 708, October, Part II, 1992.
21. **Ainamo**, J., Lie, T., Ellingsen, B.H., Hansen, B.F., Johansson, L.-A., Karring, T., Kisch, J., Paunio, K., and Stoltze, K.: Clinical Responses to Subgingival Application of a Metronidazole 25% Gel Compared to the Effect of Subgingival Scaling in Adult Periodontitis, *J. Clin. Periodontol., 19,* 723, October, Part II, 1992.
22. **Lie**, T., Bruun, G., and Böe, O.E.: Effects of Topical Metronidazole and Tetracycline in Treatment of Adult Periodontitis, *J. Periodontol., 69,* 819, July, 1998.
23. **van Steenberghe**, D., Bercy, P., Kohl, J., DeBoever, J., Adriaens, P., Vanderfaeillie, A., Adriaenssen, C., Rompen, E., DeVree, H., McCarthy, E.F., and Vandenhoven, G.: Subgingival Minocycline Hydrochloride Ointment in Moderate to Severe Chronic Adult Periodontitis: A Randomized, Double-blind, Vehicle-controlled, Multicenter Study, *J. Periodontol., 64,* 637, July, 1993.
24. **Timmerman**, M.F., van der Weijden, G.A., van Steenbergen, T.J.M., Mantel, M.S., de Graaff, J., and van der Velden, U.: Evaluation of the Long-term Efficacy and Safety of Locally-applied Minocycline in Adult Periodontitis Patients, *J. Clin. Periodontol., 23,* 707, August, 1996.
25. **Graca**, M.A., Watts, T.L.P., Wilson, R.F., and Palmer, R.M.: A Randomized Controlled Trial of a 2% Minocycline Gel as an Adjunct to Non-surgical Periodontal Treatment, Using a Design with Multiple Matching Criteria, *J. Clin. Periodontol., 24,* 249, April, 1997.

SUGGESTED READINGS

Drisko, C.H.: Non-surgical Pocket Therapy: Pharmacotherapeutics, *Annals Periodontol., 1,* 491–506, November, 1996.

Finkelman, R.D. and Williams, R.C.: Local Delivery of Chemotherapeutic Agents in Periodontal Therapy: Has Its Time Arrived? *J. Clin. Periodontol., 25,* 943, November, 1998 (Part II).

Goodson, J.M.: Antimicrobial Strategies for Treatment of Periodontal Diseases, *Periodontology 2000, 5,* 142, 1994.

Killoy, W.J.: Chemical Treatment of Periodontitis: Local Delivery of Antimicrobials, *Int. Dent. J., 48,* 305, June, Supplement 1, 1998.

Larsen, T. and Fiehn, N.-E.: Development of Resistance to Metronidazole and Minocycline *in vitro, J. Clin. Periodontol., 24,* 254, April, 1997.

Systemic Antibiotics

American Academy of Periodontology: Position Paper. Systemic Antibiotics in Periodontics, *J. Periodontol., 67,* 831, August, 1996.

Greenstein, G.: Clinical Significance of Bacterial Resistance to Tetracyclines in the Treatment of Periodontal Diseases, *J. Periodontol., 66,* 925, November, 1995.

Pallasch, T.J.: Pharmacokinetic Principles of Antimicrobial Therapy, *Periodontology 2000, 10,* 5, 1996.

Walker, C.B.: Selected Antimicrobial Agents: Mechanisms of Action, Side Effects and Drug Interactions, *Periodontology 2000, 10,* 12, 1996.

Walker, C.: Antibiotics, in American Dental Association: *ADA Guide to Dental Therapeutics.* Chicago, ADA Publishing Co., 1998, pp. 134–163.

Walker, C.B.: The Acquisition of Antibiotic Resistance in the Periodontal Microflora, *Periodontology 2000, 10,* 79, 1996.

Professional Irrigation

Allison, C., Simor, A.E., Mock, D., and Tenenbaum, H.C.: Prosol-chlorhexidine Irrigation Reduces the Incidence of Bacteremia During Ultrasonic Scaling with the Cavi-Med.: A Pilot Investigation, *J. Can. Dent. Assoc., 59,* 673, August, 1993.

Chapple, I.L.C., Walmsley, A.D., Saxby, M.S., and Moscrop, H.: Effect of Subgingival Irrigation with Chlorhexidine During Ultrasonic Scaling, *J. Periodontol., 63,* 812, October, 1992.

Chaves, E.S., Kornman, K.S., Manwell, M.A., Jones, A.A., Newbold, D.A., and Wood, R.C.: Mechanism of Irrigation Effects on Gingivitis, *J. Periodontol., 65,* 1016, November, 1994.

Fine, J.B., Harper, D.S., Gordon, J.M., Hovliaras, C.A., and Charles, C.H.: Short-term Microbiological and Clinical Effects of Subgingival Irrigation with an Antimicrobial Mouthrinse, *J. Periodontol., 65,* 30, January, 1994.

Greenstein, G.: Supragingival and Subgingival Irrigation: Practical Application in the Treatment of Periodontal Diseases, *Compend. Cont. Educ. Dent., 13,* 1098, December, 1992.

Lofthus, J.E., Waki, M.Y., Jolkovsky, D.L., Otomo-Corgel, J., Newman, M.G., Flemmig, T., and Nachnani, S.: Bacteremia Following Subgingival Irrigation and Scaling and Root Planing, *J. Periodontol., 62,* 602, October, 1991.

Rams, T.E. and Slots, J.: Local Delivery of Antimicrobial Agents in the Periodontal Pocket, *Periodontology 2000, 10,* 139, 1996.

Reynolds, M.A., Lavigne, C.K., Minah, G.E., and Suzuki, J.B.: Clinical Effects of Simultaneous Ultrasonic Scaling and Subgingival Irrigation with Chlorhexidine. Mediating Influence of Periodontal Probing Depth, *J. Clin. Periodontol., 19,* 595, September, 1992.

Schlagenhauf, U., Horlacher, V., Netuschil, L., and Brecx, M.: Repeated Subgingival Oxygen Irrigations in Untreated Periodontal Patients, *J. Clin. Periodontol., 21,* 48, January, 1994.

Shiloah, J. and Patters, M.R.: DNA Probe Analysis of the Survival of Selected Periodontal Pathogens Following Scaling, Root Planing, and Intra-pocket Irrigation, *J. Periodontol., 65,* 568, June, 1994.

Stabholz, A., Kettering, J., Aprecio, R., Zimmerman, G., Baker, P.J., and Wikesjö, U.M.E.: Retention of Antimicrobial Activity by Human Root Surfaces after *in situ* Subgingival Irrigation with Tetracycline HCL or Chlorhexidine, *J. Periodontol., 64,* 137, February, 1993.

Tetracycline Fiber

Carlson-Mann, L.D.: Use of Tetracycline Fibre to Treat Localized Unstable Periodontitis, *Can. Dent. Hyg. Assoc./PROBE, 29,* 150, July/August, 1995.

Ciancio, S.G., Cobb, C.M., and Leung, M.: Tissue Concentration and Localization of Tetracycline Following Site-specific Tetracycline Fiber Therapy, *J. Periodontol., 63,* 849, October, 1992.

Davis, M.W.: Techniques to Enhance Success in Placement of Tetracycline Fibers as a Periodontal Therapy, *Gen. Dent. 46,* 62, January–February, 1998.

Latner, L.: Patient Selection and Clinical Applications of Periodontal Tetracycline Fibers, *Gen. Dent., 46,* 58, January–February, 1998.

Mombelli, A., Lehmann, B., Tonetti, M., and Lang, N.P.: Clinical Response to Local Delivery of Tetracycline in Relation to Overall and Local Periodontal Conditions, *J. Clin. Periodontol., 24,* 470, July, 1997.

Morrison, S.L., Cobb, C.M., Kazakos, G.M., and Killoy, W.J.: Root Surface Characteristics Associated with Subgingival Placement of Monolithic Tetracycline-impregnated Fibers, *J. Periodontol., 63,* 137, February, 1992.

Radvar, M., Pourtaghi, N., and Kinane, D.F.: Comparison of 3 Periodontal Local Antibiotic Therapies in Persistent Periodontal Pockets, *J. Periodontol., 67,* 860, September, 1996.

Rapley, J.W., Cobb, C.M., Killoy, W.J., and Williams, D.R.: Serum Levels of Tetracycline During Treatment with Tetracycline-containing Fibers, *J. Periodontol., 63,* 817, October, 1992.

Tonetti, M.S.: Local Delivery of Tetracycline: From Concept to Clinical Application, *J. Clin. Periodontol., 25,* 969, November, 1998 (Part II).

Tonetti, M., Cugini, M.A., and Goodson, J.M.: Zero-order Delivery with Periodontal Placement of Tetracycline-loaded Ethylene Vinyl Acetate Fibers, *J. Periodont. Res., 25,* 243, July, 1990.

Tonetti, M.S., Pini-Prato, G., and Cortellini, P.: Principles and Clinical Applications of Periodontal Controlled Drug Delivery with Tetracycline Fibers, *Int. J. Periodont. Restorative Dent., 14,* 421, October, 1994.

Wilson, T.G., McGuire, M.K., Greenstein, G., and Nunn, M.: Tetracycline Fibers Plus Scaling and Root Planing Versus Scaling and Root Planing Alone: Similar Results After 5 Years, *J. Periodontol, 68,* 1029, November, 1997.

Chlorhexidine Chip

Friedman, M. and Golomb, G.: New Sustained Release Dosage Form of Chlorhexidine for Dental Use. I. Development and Kinetics of Release, *J. Periodont. Res., 17,* 323, Number 3, 1982.

Jeffcoat, M.K., Bray, K.S., Ciancio, S.G., Dentino, A.R., Fine, D.H., Gordon, J.M., Gunsolley, J.C., Killoy, W.J., Lowenguth, R.A., Magnusson, N.I., Offenbacher, S., Palcanis, K.G., Proskin, H.M., Finkelman, R.D., and Flashner, M.: Adjunctive Use of a Subgingival Controlled-release Chlorhexidine Chip Reduces Probing Depth and Improves Attachment Level Compared with Scaling and Root Planing Alone, *J. Periodontol., 69,* 989, September, 1998.

Killoy, W.J.: The Use of Locally Delivered Chlorhexidine in the Treatment of Periodontitis: Clinical Results, *J. Clin. Periodontol., 25,* 953, November, 1998 (Part II).

Soskolne, W.A., Heasman, P.A., Stabholz, A., Smart, G.J., Palmer, M., Flashner, M., and Newman, H.N.: Sustained Local Delivery of Chlorhexidine in the Treatment of Periodontitis: A Multicenter Study, *J. Periodontol., 68,* 32, January, 1997.

Soskolne, A., Golomb, G., Friedman, M., and Sela, M.N.: New Sustained Release Dosage Form of Chlorhexidine for Dental Use. II. Use in Periodontal Therapy, *J. Periodont. Res., 18,* 330, May, 1983.

Stabholz, A., Soskolne, W.A., Friedman, M., and Sela, M.N.: The Use of Sustained Release Delivery of Chlorhexidine for the Maintenance of Periodontal Pockets: 2-year Clinical Trial, *J. Periodontol., 62,* 429, July, 1991.

Metronidazole

Greenstein, G.: The Role of Metronidazole in the Treatment of Periodontal Diseases, *J. Periodontol., 64,* 1, January, 1993.

Hitzig, C., Charbit, Y., Bitton, C., Fosse, T., Teboul, M., Hannoun, L., and Varonne, R.: Topical Metronidazole as an Adjunct to Subgingival Debridement in the Treatment of Chronic Periodontitis, *J. Clin. Periodontol., 21,* 146, February, 1994.

Magnusson, I.: The Use of Locally Delivered Metronidazole in the Treatment of Periodontitis. Clinical Results, *J. Clin. Periodontol., 25,* 959, November, 1998 (Part II).

Pedrazzoli, V., Kilian, M., and Karring, T.: Comparative Clinical and Microbiological Effects of Topical Subgingival Application of Metronidazole 25% Dental Gel and Scaling in the Treatment of Adult Periodontitis, *J. Clin. Periodontol., 19,* 715, October, Part II, 1992.

Somayaji, B.V., Jariwala, U., Jayachandran, P., Vidyalakshmi, K., and Dudhani, R.V.: Evaluation of Antimicrobial Efficacy and Release Pattern of Tetracycline and Metronidazole Using a Local Delivery System, *J. Periodontol., 69,* 409, April, 1998.

Stelzel, M. and Flores-de-Jacoby, L.: Topical Metronidazole Application Compared with Subgingival Scaling. A Clinical and Microbiological Study on Recall Patients, *J. Clin. Periodontol., 23,* 24, January, 1996.

Minocycline Gel

Jones, A.A., Kornman, K.S., Newbold, D.A., and Manwell, M.A.: Clinical and Microbiological Effects of Controlled-release Locally Delivered Minocycline in Periodontitis, *J. Periodontol., 65,* 1058, November, 1994.

Preus, H.R., Lassen, J., Aass, A.M., and Ciancio, S.G.: Bacterial Resistance Following Subgingival and Systemic Administration of Minocycline, *J. Clin. Periodontol., 22,* 380, May, 1995.

Saito, A., Horaka, Y., Nakagawa, T., Seida, K., Yamada, S., and Okuda, K.: Locally Delivered Minocycline and Guided Tissue Regeneration to Treat Post-juvenile Periodontitis. A Case Report, *J. Periodontol., 65,* 835, September, 1994.

Vandekerckhove, B.N.A., Quirynen, M., and van Steenberghe, D.: The Use of Locally Delivered Minocycline in the Treatment of Chronic Periodontitis: A Review of the Literature, *J. Clin. Periodontol., 25,* 964, November, 1998 (Part II).

Acute Periodontal Conditions

35

The dental hygienist frequently participates in clinical treatment procedures for acute gingival lesions. Key words for acute conditions are defined in Box 35-1.

NECROTIZING ULCERATIVE GINGIVITIS/PERIODONTITIS

Necrotizing ulcerative gingivitis (NUG) and necrotizing ulcerative periodontitis (NUP) are acute, inflammatory, destructive diseases of the periodontium. Other names that have been used include necrotizing gingivitis (NG), acute necrotizing ulcerative gingivitis (ANUG), trench mouth, Vincent's infection, Vincent's disease, and ulceromembranous gingivitis. The condition may be superimposed over existing periodontitis.

Although NUG may occur at any age, it is usually seen among young people between ages 15 and 30 years. It is rare in children under 10 years of age in the United States, but it is not uncommon in young children from low socioeconomic groups studied in South America and in some developing countries.[1,2] Malnutrition and lowered resistance to infection are significant predisposing factors. Individuals with Down's syndrome have been shown to have an increased incidence of NUG, as described on page 815.

TYPES OF NECROTIZING PERIODONTAL CONDITIONS

I. NECROTIZING ULCERATIVE GINGIVITIS (NUG)

A. Basic Characteristics
Gingival inflammation limited to the free gingiva with ulceration of one or more interdental papilla tips. Other clinical signs include pain and bleeding.

B. HIV-Positive Patient
Linear gingival erythema with ulceration of tips of interdental papillae.[3]

II. NECROTIZING ULCERATIVE PERIODONTITIS

A. Basic Characteristics
Destructive infection of periodontal tissues with

BOX 35-1 KEY WORDS: Acute Periodontal Conditions

Abscess (ab′ses): localized collection of pus in a circumscribed or walled-off area formed by the disintegration of tissues.

  Acute: runs a relatively short course; produces pain and local inflammation.

  Chronic: slow development with little evidence of inflammation; usually an intermittent pus discharge; may follow an acute abscess.

  Periapical: circumscribed collection of pus around the apex of a tooth root; results from pulpal necrosis.

  Periodontal: localized in the periodontal tissues; also called **lateral** or **parietal.**

Fetor oris (fe′tor ō′ris): foul, offensive odor from the mouth; halitosis.

Fistula (fis′tū-lah): a pathologic sinus or abnormal passage that leads from an abscess to the surface of the gingiva or mucosa.

Gum boil: a lay term for a circumscribed swelling in the tissue over the alveolar process, usually at the level of the root apices; may break and drain periodically, thus preventing pain.

Linear gingival erythema: gingivitis in the HIV-positive patient; characterized by a well-demarcated band of intense erythema at the gingival margin, not associated with bacterial plaque, and which does not respond to conventional plaque-removal procedures.[x]

Malaise (mal-āz′): feeling of general indisposition, uneasiness, discomfort; may be early indication of illness.

Necrosis (nĕ-krō′sĭs): death of tissue; morphologic changes indicative of cell death caused by enzymatic degradation.

Necrotizing ulcerative periodontitis (NUP): severe and rapidly progressive disease that has a distinctive erythema of the free gingiva, attached gingiva, and the alveolar mucosa; extensive soft tissue necrosis that usually starts with the interdental papillae; marked loss of periodontal attachment; deep probing depths may not be evident because of marked recession.

Parenteral (pah-ren′ter-al): not administered by way of the alimentary canal, but, for example, subcutaneous, intramuscular, or intravenous.

Pericoronitis: gingival inflammation around the crown of an incompletely erupted tooth; most frequently occurs about a mandibular third molar.

Pseudomembrane (soo″dō-mem′brān): false membrane; false layer of tissue that covers a surface.

Purulent (pu′roo-lent): accompanied by or containing pus.

Sinus tract (sī′nus): a channel that connects with an abscess or suppurating area.

Ulceration (ul″sĕr-ā′shun): formation or development of an ulcer with loss of epithelial surface and sloughing of necrotic inflammatory tissue.

*From Greenspan, J.S.: Periodontal Complications of HIV Infection, *Compend. Cont. Educ. Dent., 15,* S604, Suppl. Nov. 10, 1994.

---

ulceration of interdental papillae, cratering of interdental bone and soft tissue, and clinical attachment loss.

B. HIV-Positive Patient

An increased incidence of NUG/NUP has been diagnosed in HIV-positive patients. A more severe, rapidly progressive breakdown of the periodontium occurs with ulceration of interdental papillae, cratering of interdental bone, clinical attachment loss, and presence of exposed bone with sequestration in the most severe involvement. Because of the rapid breakdown, necrosis, and tissue recession with severe attachment loss, the condition usually is not associated with deep pockets.[3]

III. NECROTIZING STOMATITIS

Necrosis may extend beyond the tooth-supporting tissues and cause bone destruction and sequestration. Severe disease may resemble noma or cancrum oris.

IV. CANCRUM ORIS (NOMA)

Orofacial gangrenous necrosis is believed to be an extension of untreated NUP. It is predisposed by malnutrition and debilitating systemic illness.[1,2]

CLINICAL RECOGNITION

I. INITIAL SIGNS AND SYMPTOMS

The patient with NUG or NUP reports
  A. Sudden onset.
  B. Pain and soreness caused by slight pressure, such as during chewing and toothbrushing; may be intensified by hot or highly seasoned foods. Gentle probing may produce an exaggerated pain response.

C. Bleeding that occurs spontaneously or on slight pressure.
D. Poor appetite.
E. Metallic or other unpleasant taste.
F. Fetid odor.

II. CHARACTERISTIC CLINICAL FINDINGS

A. Interdental Necrosis
Ulceration of the papillae produces craterlike defects in the col area. In early disease, only the tips of papillae are involved, followed by progressive destruction of entire papillae and extension to the marginal gingiva facially and lingually (Figure 35-1).

B. Pseudomembrane
Forms over the necrotic area. It is a gray, loose, necrotic slough that, when wiped off, exposes a red and shiny hemorrhagic gingiva. The pseudomembrane consists primarily of fibrin, necrotic tissue, leukocytes, and masses of microorganisms.

C. Extent
The membranous ulceration may be seen locally, that is, between two or three teeth, or it may be generalized throughout both maxillary and mandibular arches.

D. Other Clinical Findings
1. Debris, materia alba, and plaque that collect profusely because the patient avoids brushing the sensitive teeth and gingiva.
2. Fetor oris (bad breath) that is often severe. It is caused by necrotic tissue, stagnant saliva, and breakdown products of blood and debris.
3. Increased salivation.

E. Signs of Systemic Involvement
Examination should always be made to detect the presence of the following:
1. Malaise.
2. Lymphadenopathy of submandibular and cervical nodes.
3. Possible slight elevation of body temperature.

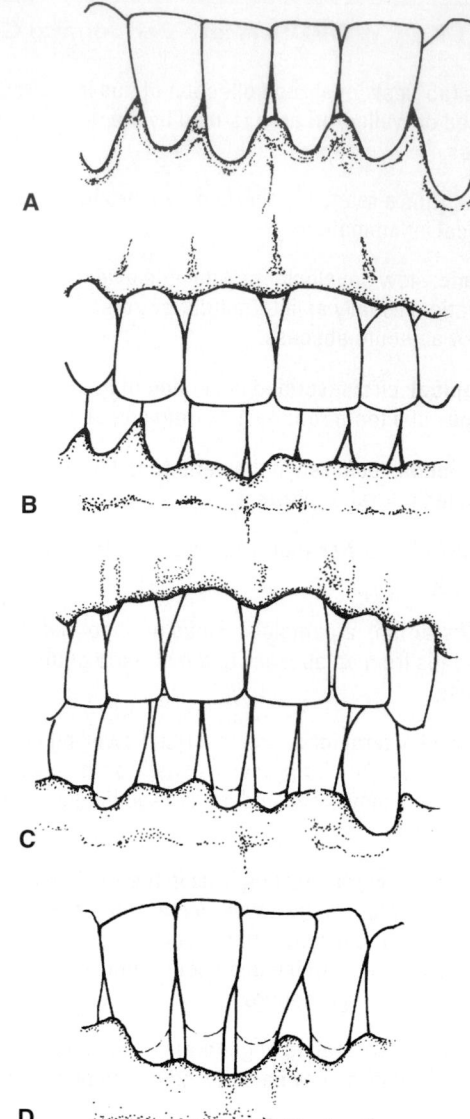

FIGURE 35-1 Necrotizing Ulcerative Gingivitis/Periodontitis. (A) Early lesion with blunted papillae and interdental necrosis. **(B)** Increased destruction with loss of interdental tissue; rolled margins of the gingiva. **(C)** More advanced destruction with recession and interdental cratering. **(D)** Very advanced lesions, with loss of attached gingiva, recession, and tooth mobility.

RISK FACTORS

NUG is an infectious disease caused by a fusospirochetal complex of microbes that develops and increases in association with predisposing factors that have lowered the body's defenses. Major predisposing factors are stress, neglected oral hygiene, inadequate diet, and tobacco smoking.

I. LOCAL FACTORS

NUG is rarely, if ever, seen in a clean, healthy, cared-for, and professionally supervised mouth. Many of the factors that can be considered predisposing are the same as those that predispose to chronic marginal gingivitis.

Predisposing factors include
A. Pre-existing gingivitis and/or periodontitis.
B. Inadequate personal oral care with general neglect.
C. Tobacco use.
D. Factors related to retention of microorganisms and deposits (pages 231 to 233).

II. STRESS FACTORS

A. Acute anxiety related to life situations is a common characteristic of patients with NUG. In susceptible people, the condition has been found to occur or recur during periods of stress. Examples include students during examination periods, military men in combat, and people during important decision-making times.

B. Emotional stress is frequently accompanied by poor oral care, improper diet, excessive smoking, overexertion, interrupted sleep, and other deviations in health habits.

III. SYSTEMIC: DISEASE-RESISTANCE FACTORS

A. Dietary and nutritional inadequacies; vitamin deficiencies.

B. Recent illnesses; frequent upper respiratory infections, infectious mononucleosis, pernicious anemia, hepatitis, and HIV infection.

C. Side effects of chemotherapy and radiation.

D. Fatigue; insufficient sleep.

ETIOLOGY

Bacteriologic and immunologic factors are implicated. For many years, bacteriologic smears were made from the NUG lesion and examined by microscope for the presence of fusiform bacilli and spirochetes. The smear test is no longer considered significant for making a diagnosis.

I. MICROBIOLOGY[4]

Of the many types of organisms found in NUG lesions, fusiform bacilli and medium-sized spirochetes predominate. The constant flora has been shown to include *Treponema* and *Selenomonas* species, *Prevotella intermedia, Porphyromonas gingivalis,* and *Fusobacterium* species.

II. COURSE OF DEVELOPMENT

A. Description of the Lesion

1. NUG is superimposed on gingivitis or periodontitis.
2. Ulceration and necrosis begin in the col area.
3. Both epithelial tissue and connective tissue are involved.
4. The disease process progresses to involve the entire papilla and, eventually, the marginal gingiva on the facial and lingual surfaces.
5. The pseudomembrane covering the lesion is a necrotic slough of the surface epithelium. It contains leukocytes, bacteria, epithelial cells, and fibrin.
6. Connective tissue shows the signs of acute inflammation. It is hyperemic and filled with leukocytes, and its capillaries are engorged. When the pseudomembrane is lifted, the red inflamed connective tissue can be seen.

B. Microscopic Examination

Four layers in the lesion have been described from observations made by electron microscopy.[5] All layers contain spirochetes.

1. *Bacterial Zone.* The most superficial zone consists primarily of a mass of varied bacteria, including a few spirochetes.
2. *Neutrophil-rich Zone.* Under the bacterial zone is a layer of leukocytes, predominantly neutrophils. Microorganisms, including many spirochetes, are found among the leukocytes.
3. *Necrotic Zone.* This zone contains disintegrating tissue cells, many spirochetes, and other bacteria.
4. *Spirochetal Infiltration Zone.* In this nonnecrotized layer where tissue components are still preserved, spirochetes have invaded, but other microorganisms have not. The action of toxins and other bacterial products was described with pocket formation on pages 225 to 227.

DENTAL HYGIENE CARE

Patient instruction and motivation for self-care are needed along with skillful subgingival instrumentation. After the initial symptoms have subsided, complete therapy must be carried out. The tissue destruction usually has left the gingiva deformed, with interdental flattening or cratering. Surgical treatment may be needed to restore a physiologic form that can be maintained by the patient in the plan to prevent recurrence of the disease.

I. PREPARATION FOR DIAGNOSIS

Initially, certain data must be collected for making the diagnosis and care plan. Basic information needed is suggested by the steps described here.

A. History

1. *Record the Chief Complaint.* The history of the current disease is described by date of onset, duration, symptoms as reported, and what self-treatment the patient has already performed.
2. *Record Whether This Is a Recurrence.* If so, note details of previous episodes, and the treatment given.
3. *Obtain Information Needed for Preliminary Treatment*
   a. Conditions needing medical consultation.
   b. Need for premedication for prevention of infective endocarditis (pages 101 to 104).
   c. Allergies.
4. *Use Knowledge of Predisposing Factors for NUG to Gather Pertinent Information*
   a. Tobacco habits.
   b. Recent illnesses or types of therapy may explain a lowered resistance.
   c. Record of immediately previous 24-hour

food intake. When the mouth has been sore and eating has been painful, a diet recording may not be typical of the patient's usual intake. Later, a 5-day or week-long food record will be requested as part of the continuing prevention program (pages 444 to 449).

   d. Variations of normal sleeping hours and routine.

B. Examination

1. *Record the Patient's Temperature* (page 107)
2. *Extraoral Examination*
   a. Palpate submandibular and cervical nodes (see Figure 8-4, page 120).
   b. Observe face and skin to determine whether flushed, damp.
   c. Observe signs of malaise.
3. *Oral Examination.* Without instrumentation, a preliminary examination can be made and the overall appearance of the gingival tissue recorded. The dentist may prefer to see the gingiva as it appears initially, before instrumentation or rinsing, to make the diagnosis and prepare the treatment plan. Instrumentation will be temporarily delayed for patients requiring premedication.

II. CARE PLAN

The dental hygiene care plan is formulated within the total treatment plan. Only a partial treatment plan is made until after the acute phase of the disease has passed.

A. Systemic Treatment

1. Directions concerning diet, rest, and other systemic influences.
2. Multivitamin supplements are sometimes prescribed.
3. After the diagnosis is made, the dentist determines whether systemic antibiotic therapy is indicated. Except for a patient who requires antibiotic coverage to prevent infective endocarditis, antibiotics are prescribed conservatively.

B. Relief of Acute Symptoms

1. Personal care instructions for rinsing, brushing, and limiting use of tobacco.
2. Debridement of teeth and gingiva.
3. Subgingival scaling and root planing started.
4. Chlorhexidine 0.12% rinse twice daily.

C. Basic Therapy

1. *Preventive program*
   a. Instruction for prevention of recurrence of NUG; eliminate tobacco use.
   b. Dietary analysis and counseling.
   c. Self-care fluoride, professional application when indicated.
2. *Complete scaling and debridement.*

3. *Reduction or elimination of predisposing factors to NUG*
   a. Removal of overhanging margins and other plaque retention factors.
   b. Restoration of teeth and contact areas.
4. *Evaluation for periodontal surgery.* Need for restoration of tissue contour and elimination of craters.
5. *Restoration of occlusion.* Prosthetic replacements and all other dental needs.

CARE FOR THE ACUTE STAGE

A series of appointments for a typical patient with NUG is outlined here. The number of appointments and the exact procedure at each appointment depend on the severity of the disease and the response of the gingiva as treatment progresses.

Four or five appointments may be needed during the acute stage, depending on the probing depths and the extent of calculus deposits. The basic objective is to debride the teeth thoroughly to encourage soft tissue healing. When the acute stage has subsided, a regular appointment plan is established for continued supervision.

I. ACUTE PHASE: FIRST APPOINTMENT

A. Patient Instruction

1. Explain local causes and control measures.
2. Demonstrate plaque with a disclosing agent.
3. Show plaque removal procedures, using a soft brush moistened with warm water.

B. General Debridement

1. Apply hydrogen peroxide (3% solution mixed with equal parts of water) with cotton pellets at proximal areas; request patient to rinse. Avoid use of compressed air or water spray to prevent dispersion of contaminated aerosols.
2. Apply topical anesthetic, or when painful, treat by quadrants, using block anesthesia.
3. Use power-driven or manual instruments or a combination for scaling. Use warm water for frequent irrigation while scaling.

C. Subgingival Instrumentation

The gingiva responds sooner when scaling can be started at the first visit.
1. Perform instrumentation carefully to prevent tissue damage.
2. Have assistant evacuate continuously when a power-driven instrument is used to prevent contaminated aerosols and to protect the patient from inhaling microorganisms.
3. Irrigate and evacuate frequently to clear all debris and calculus removed during instrumentation.

D. Patient Instruction

1. *Instructions for Home Use.* Instructions for home procedures must be carefully explained. Written directions are needed.
2. *Instructions for Continuing Care.* Inform the patient that treatment will not be complete when the pain is eliminated. Explain the underlying gingival or periodontal infection and how NUG recurs if the periodontal condition is not treated.
3. *Rinsing Directions.* Vigorous rinsing with warm water or weak saline solution (pages 560 to 561) is necessary every hour during the period of acute symptoms. Using 3% hydrogen peroxide with equal parts of water is preferred by some clinicians. If used, it should be recommended for only a few days and then discontinued.

    Rinsing with chlorhexidine (0.12%) twice daily continues: use 0.5 ounce after brushing after breakfast, and after brushing and flossing before retiring; swish between the teeth for 1 minute.
4. *Toothbrushing.* Use a soft nylon brush gently, but thoroughly. Clean the teeth as much as possible after each meal and before going to bed. When a brush is not given the patient at the clinic or office, write down the names of specific brushes for the patient to purchase.

F. Introduce Tobacco Cessation

1. *Inform Patient.* Describe the effect of smoked or smokeless tobacco on the oral cavity, with special emphasis on facts about the gingival tissues.
2. *Avoiding Tobacco Products.* The heavy smoker who is not ready for cessation can be requested to limit the use while treatment for NUG is underway.

G. Diet[6]

1. Recommend frequent, small, nutritious meals that incorporate daily requirements from the Food Guide Pyramid (see Figure 28-2, page 445).
2. A liquid or soft bland diet is advised for the first day, particularly for the patient with systemic symptoms or pronounced sensitivity when chewing. A diet of soft solids can be used on the second day. Examples of foods to include in a liquid and a soft solid diet are listed on pages 717 to 718.
3. The choice of foods should include increased amounts of meat and milk groups and of fruits and juices.
4. Avoid highly seasoned foods and alcoholic beverages.

II. ACUTE PHASE: SECOND APPOINTMENT

A. Patient Examination

1. *Changes.* A remarkable improvement usually can be seen within 24 hours, with pain and discomfort lessened, the pseudomembrane gone, and tissue enlargement reduced.
2. *Toothbrushing.* Apply disclosing agent and show patient missed areas. Emphasize thorough coverage of the entire dentition, using sulcular brushing.

B. Scaling and Root Planing

Continue procedures from the previous appointment after checking areas previously treated. The objective is to be as thorough as possible, because plaque retained over residual calculus and altered cementum can keep the tissues from healing completely.

C. Instruction: Second Day

1. *Rinsing.* When healing is progressing favorably, change rinsing schedule to every 2 hours.
2. *Proximal Surfaces.* The use of floss is advised and should be emphasized at this or the third appointment, depending on the readiness of the patient and the tissue. Other proximal cleaning devices may be useful. When the interdental embrasures are open as a result of papillary necrosis (Figure 35-1C and D), an interdental brush or other device is indicated. The importance of complete plaque removal must be explained.
3. *Diet.* A liquid diet is not usually indicated after the first day, and the patient can use the soft solids diet or a regular diet adapted with bland foods that will not irritate the healing tissues.
4. *Instructions.* Provide specific written instructions.

III. SUCCESSIVE APPOINTMENTS

After the acute stage, regular appointments for basic treatment are planned. The gingiva is evaluated, and repeated scaling and root planing are performed as needed to complete that part of the treatment.

A. Complete Assessment

The complete plan for dental care is prepared, and the patient is instructed for continued treatment.

B. Recurrence of NUG/NUP

When the gingival and bony craters that remain after the initial healing phase are not treated, they are vulnerable to continuing disease and recurrence of NUG. Plaque and debris can collect readily in the misshapen proximal areas, and these areas are difficult to clean with plaque control techniques. Gingival craters invite further tissue breakdown, leading to periodontal pocket formation.

Surgical treatment is explained to the patient. When bony craters exist, treatment may involve flap surgery with osseous reshaping.

PERIODONTAL ABSCESS

Gingival and periodontal abscesses occur within the periodontal tissues. An abscess is called *gingival* when it is located in the marginal area, and *periodontal* when it is in the deeper periodontal tissues. They may also be known as *lateral abscesses* because they occur along the lateral surfaces of a tooth, in contrast to a periapical abscess, which is associated with the apex.

I. DEVELOPMENT OF A PERIODONTAL ABSCESS

Pus collects in the tissue as a result of bacterial infection. The infection may be a complication of an existing periodontal disease, or it may be an immediate result of microorganisms forced into the tissue by some form of trauma. The body's reaction is to send large numbers of defense cells to the area, particularly polymorphonuclear leukocytes (PMNs), which are major constituents of the purulent exudate (pus) that collects.

Pus is a thick fluid product of inflammation. It contains many living and dead PMNs mixed with debris from cells and tissues that have been destroyed by the enzymes released by the PMNs. Unless there is a means for drainage, the pus collects and forms an abscess.

A sinus or fistula may form. Drainage may occur through the sinus and release the pressure within the abscess, thereby relieving the pain the patient may experience.

II. ETIOLOGIC FACTORS

A. Periodontal Pockets

Deep pockets of chronic inflammatory periodontal infection provide an environment for abscess formation. Special anatomic variations predispose to abscess formation. Instrumentation applied within the pocket and the effects of the instrumentation may be the precipitating factors that initiate abscess formation.

1. *Anatomic Features.* Intrabony pockets, pockets that extend into bi- or trifurcation areas, and complex pockets that develop in winding or irregular shapes are particularly susceptible to becoming closed and, therefore, susceptible to abscess formation.
2. *Instrumentation.*[7] Incomplete scaling in the depth of a pocket may allow the tissue at the opening of the pocket to heal, tighten, and prevent drainage from the infectious material deep in the pocket. Plaque and calculus remaining in the sealed off part of the pocket attract the collection of more bacteria and PMNs, and an abscess develops.

B. Trauma

Foreign objects may enter by way of the sulcus or pocket and become embedded along with microorganisms. The infection leads to abscess formation.

1. *Implanted or Impacted Material*[8]
   a. Popcorn husk, small fish bone or shellfish fragment, seeds, seed coverings, or other material from food.
   b. Oral hygiene devices include toothbrush bristle or filament or a sliver from a toothpick.
2. *Instrumentation.* Trauma during subgingival instrumentation may force infectious material into the pocket wall.

C. Patient Susceptibility to Infection

The possibility for abscess formation within the gingival tissue is increased from any of the etiologic factors that have been mentioned when the patient's resistance to infection is lowered. Patients with uncontrolled diabetes or who are receiving immunosuppressive medication are examples of those at greater risk.

III. CLINICAL SIGNS AND SYMPTOMS

Even though clinical manifestations may vary, the classic signs and symptoms are listed here.

A. Clinical Appearance

The area of the abscess is enlarged, with a red, shiny, smooth surface. It may appear domelike or pointed, and on slight digital pressure, pus may appear.

B. The Tooth

1. *Sensitivity.* The tooth may be sensitive to percussion. When extruded, it may be sensitive to touching the tooth in the opposing jaw. It may be slightly mobile.
2. *Pulp Vitality Test.* Pulp testing usually reveals a vital tooth, responding within the normal range (page 249).
3. *Radiographs.* A radiolucency may be noted along the lateral wall beside the tooth, but such a finding is variable. No bone loss shows in early lesions. The amount of bone destruction and the location of the abscess influence the possible radiographic findings.

C. General Physical Condition

Occasionally, a patient shows evidence of systemic involvement, such as a slight elevation in body temperature, malaise, and lymphadenopathy.

D. Chronic Abscess

In the chronic state, a sinus tract usually opens on the gingival surface and drains periodically. Before drainage, the patient may have a dull pain from the pressure of the fluid within the abscess area. Acute symptoms may be expected from time to time unless definitive periodontal therapy is completed.

IV. COMPARISON OF PERIAPICAL AND PERIODONTAL ABSCESSES

The dentist must often differentiate between a periapical and a periodontal abscess. Certain signs and symptoms are nearly the same for both. A few of the potentially distinguishing findings are noted here.

A. Pulp Test
The tooth with a periapical lesion does not respond normally to a pulp tester (pages 249 to 250).

B. Sinus Tract Formation
The opening of a sinus tract from a periapical abscess usually is positioned more apically, whereas the opening from a periodontal abscess is more coronal.

C. Pain
Sharp steady pain is typical of a periapical lesion, whereas the pain from a periodontal abscess varies.

D. Periodontal Examination
A tooth with a periapical lesion is not necessarily periodontally involved. Probing may reveal no probing depth of note, and no bone loss may be apparent in the radiograph.

Occasionally, a combined periodontic and endodontic lesion occurs. Communication between a deep periodontal pocket and an apical lesion is not unusual. Communication may also exist from a periodontal pocket into the pulp by way of a lateral or accessory canal through the dentin.

E. Dental Caries
A diseased pulp leading to a periapical abscess is caused by either trauma to the tooth or dental caries extending inward until the pulp becomes infected. A carious lesion may also be present with a periodontal abscess and may complicate the differential diagnosis.

F. Radiographic Examination
Early stages of either a periapical or a periodontal abscess are not evident in a radiograph. A widening of the periodontal ligament space may appear.

V. CARE PLAN

Two phases of treatment are used for the patient with a periodontal abscess. The first is for immediate relief of acute symptoms, and the second is the definitive treatment followed by preventive maintenance. The entire plan should be explained to the patient at the outset.

A. Objectives of Emergency Treatment
1. Relieve pain.
2. Establish drainage.
3. Determine need for systemic antibiotic therapy.

B. Review Medical History
Determine necessary preappointment precautions, such as the need for antibiotic premedication (pages 101 to 104).

C. Examination for Systemic Involvement
Antibiotic medication is frequently prescribed by the dentist when systemic involvement is definite.
1. Determine and record the patient's body temperature (page 107).
2. Examine submandibular and neck nodes for lymphadenopathy.

D. Provide Anesthesia
When the abscess is confined to the gingival area, and the drainage may be expected to cause little if any discomfort, a topical anesthetic may suffice. Usually, block anesthesia is indicated.

E. Methods for Drainage
1. *Via Pocket or Sulcus Opening.* Isolate the area, swab with a topical antiseptic, and use a probe to gain admission into the sulcus or pocket. Gently probe circumferentially until an opening into the abscess is found. Drainage usually begins promptly.
2. *Curet Area.* Use a curet to open the area, and locate and remove a foreign body irritant when it is known to be present from the history obtained from the patient. Scaling and root planing are performed as needed.

F. Postoperative Instructions
Rinsing with hot saline solution every 2 hours is advised. The patient should return for observation in 24 to 48 hours. Relief from pain and discomfort can be expected and appointments for definitive treatment planned. Plaque control instruction is initiated or continued, and scaling and root planing are completed.

G. Anticipated Results
1. Acute symptoms are resolved.
2. Pain relief occurs within a short time following the initiation of drainage, because the pressure is released from within the abscessed area.
3. Extruded tooth returns to its normal position.
4. Swelling is reduced.
5. Temporary comfort is obtained for the patient; the lesion is reduced to a standard chronic lesion that requires additional treatment.
6. If drainage is not complete, an acute lesion may develop into a lesion with a chronic sinus.

VI. DEFINITIVE THERAPY

Whatever pocket elimination procedures are indicated should be completed within a reasonable time to prevent further complications. Careful and regular bacterial plaque control with scaling and root planing are usually needed.

TECHNICAL HINTS

I. Provide explicit directions concerning rinsing when hydrogen peroxide is prescribed. Extended use of oxygenating drugs can cause undesirable tissue changes.

II. Instructions for patients can be printed or written. Because instructions change each day during the acute phase, individual slips should be prepared, using paper of different colors. Printed instructions can be personalized with added written notations.

FACTORS TO TEACH THE PATIENT

I. Premature discontinuation of treatment for NUG because acute signs have subsided can lead to recurrence of the infection.

II. The role of diet, rest, and bacterial plaque control in the prevention of NUG.

III. The avoidance of an oral irrigating device in the presence of acute inflammatory conditions. Microorganisms may be forced into the tissues beneath a pocket, and bacteremia can be produced.

REFERENCES

1. **Enwonwu,** C.O.: Infectious Oral Necrosis (cancrum oris) in Nigerian Children: A Review, *Community Dent. Oral Epidemiol., 13,* 190, June, 1985.

2. **Taiwo,** J.O.: Oral Hygiene Status and Necrotizing Ulcerative Gingivitis in Nigerian Children, *J. Periodontol., 64,* 1071, November, 1993.

3. **Greenspan,** J.S.: Periodontal Complications of HIV Infection, *Compend. Cont. Educ. Dent., 15,* S694, Supplement Number 18, 1994.

4. **Loesche,** W.J., Syed, S.A., Laughon, B.E., and Stoll, J.: The Bacteriology of Acute Necrotizing Ulcerative Gingivitis, *J. Periodontol., 53,* 223, April, 1982.

5. **Listgarten,** M.A.: Electron Microscopic Observations on the Bacterial Flora of Acute Necrotizing Ulcerative Gingivitis, *J. Periodontol., 36,* 328, July–August, 1965.

6. **Davis,** J.R. and Stegeman, C.A.: *The Dental Hygienist's Guide to Nutritional Care.* Philadelphia, W.B. Saunders Co., 1998, pp. 382–386.

7. **Armitage,** G.C.: *Biologic Basis of Periodontal Maintenance Therapy.* Berkeley, CA, Praxis Publishing Co., 1980, pp. 154–159.

8. **Gillette,** W.B. and Van House, R.L.: Ill Effects of Improper Oral Hygiene Procedures, *J. Am. Dent. Assoc., 101,* 476, September, 1980.

SUGGESTED READING

Necrotizing Ulcerative Gingivitis

Barr, C.E. and Robbins, M.R.: Clinical and Radiographic Presentations of HIV-1 Necrotizing Ulcerative Periodontitis, *Spec. Care Dentist., 16,* 237, November/December, 1996.

Cutler, C.W., Wasfy, M.O., Ghaffar, K., Hosni, M., and Lloyd, D.R.: Impaired Bactericidal Activity of PMN from Two Brothers with Necrotizing Ulcerative Gingivo-periodontitis, *J. Periodontol., 65,* 357, April, 1994.

Glick, M., Muzyka, B.C., Salkin, L.M., and Lurie, D.: Necrotizing Ulcerative Periodontitis: A Marker for Immune Deterioration and a Predictor for the Diagnosis of AIDS, *J. Periodontol., 65,* 393, May, 1994.

Haring, J.L.: Case #1 Acute Necrotizing Ulcerative Gingivitis, *RDH, 15,* 13, January, 1995.

Horning, G.M.: Necrotizing Gingivostomatitis: NUG to Noma, *Compend. Cont. Educ. Dent., 17,* 951, October, 1996.

Horning, G.M. and Cohen, M.E.: Necrotizing Ulcerative Gingivitis, Periodontitis, and Stomatitis: Clinical Staging and Predisposing Factors, *J. Periodontol., 66,* 990, November, 1995.

Murayama, Y., Kurihara, H., Nagai, A., Dompkowski, D., and Van Dyke, T.E.: Acute Necrotizing Ulcerative Gingivitis: Risk Factors Involving Host Defense Mechanisms, *Periodontology 2000, 6,* 116, 1994.

Osuji, O.O.: Necrotizing Ulcerative Gingivitis and Cancrum Oris (Noma) in Ibadan, Nigeria, *J. Periodontol., 61,* 769, December, 1990.

Riviere, G.R., Weisz, K.S., Simonson, L.G., and Lukehart, S.A.: Pathogen-related Spirochetes Identified Within Gingival Tissue from Patients with Acute Necrotizing Ulcerative Gingivitis, *Infect. Immun., 59,* 2653, August, 1991.

Robinson, P.G., Winkler, J.R., Palmer, G., Westenhouse, J., Hilton, J.F., and Greenspan, J.S.: The Diagnosis of Periodontal Conditions Associated with HIV Infection, *J. Periodontol., 65,* 236, March, 1994.

Rowland, R.W., Mestecky, J., Gunsolley, J.C., and Cogen, R.B.: Serum IgG and IgM Levels to Bacterial Antigens in Necrotizing Ulcerative Gingivitis, *J. Periodontol., 64,* 195, March, 1993.

Tolle-Watts, L.: ANUG—Dental Hygiene Intervention, *DentalHygienistNews, 4,* 1, Summer, 1991.

Periodontal Abscess

Carranza, F.A. and Newman, M.G.: *Clinical Periodontology,* 8th ed. Philadelphia, W.B. Saunders Co., 1996, pp. 292–294, 483–485.

Dello Russo, N.M.: The Post-prophylaxis Periodontal Abscess: Etiology and Treatment, *Int. J. Periodontics Restorative Dent., 5,* 28, Number 1, 1985.

Fedi, P.F. and Vernino, A.R.: *The Periodontic Syllabus,* 3rd ed. Baltimore, Williams & Wilkins, 1995, pp. 187–189.

Flood, T.R., Samaranayake, L.P., MacFarlane, T.W., McLennan, A., MacKenzie, D., and Carmichael, F.: Bacteremia Following Incision and Drainage of Dento-alveolar Abscesses, *Br. Dent. J., 169,* 51, July 21, 1990.

Hafström, C.A, Wikstrom, M.B., Renvert, S.N., and Dahlén, G.G.: Effect of Treatment on Some Periodontopathogens and Their Antibody Levels in Periodontal Abscesses, *J. Periodontol., 65,* 1022, November, 1994.

Haring, J.I.: Case #4 Periodontal Abscess, *RDH, 16,* 12, April, 1996.

McLeod, D.E., Lainson, P.A., and Spivey, J.D.: Tooth Loss Due to Periodontal Abscess: A Retrospective Study, *J. Periodontol., 68,* 963, October, 1997.

Taani, D.S.Q.: An Effective Treatment for Chronic Periodontal Abscesses, *Quintessence Int., 27,* 697, October, 1996.

36

Sutures and Dressings

Many periodontal surgical procedures require sutures and dressings. When the dental hygienist participates in initial preparation of a patient and is involved with his/her postcare, knowledge of the surgical procedures required adds to the continuity of treatment. Key words related to sutures and dressings are defined in Box 36-1.

SUTURES

A suture is a strand of material used to ligate blood vessels and approximate tissue. Sutures are necessary in many oral surgical procedures whenever the surgical wound must be closed, a flap positioned, or tissue grafted.

Through the centuries a wide range of suture materials has been used including silk, cotton, linen, and animal tendons and intestines. Current suture materials are designed for specific procedures thereby decreasing potential for postsurgical infections while providing patient comfort and convenience.

I. PURPOSES OF SUTURES
  A. Close periodontal wounds and secure grafts in position
  B. Assist in maintaining hemostasis
  C. Reduce posttreatment discomfort
  D. Promote primary intention healing
  E. Prevent underlying bone exposure
  F. Protect surgically treated tissue from foreign debris and trauma

BOX 36-1 KEY WORDS: Sutures and Dressings

Border mold: the shaping of the peripheries of a dressing by manual manipulation of the tissue adjacent to the borders (for example, lips, cheeks) to duplicate the contour and size of the vestibule.

Chemical cure (kem′ĭ-kul): mode of self-cure or setting of a dressing in which the ingredients unite in a chemical process that starts as soon as the blending is complete; the setting time is influenced by warm temperature and the addition of an accelerator.

Coapt (kō-apt′): to approximate, as the edges of a wound; bring edge to edge with no overlap.

Dressing (dres′ing): any of various materials used for covering and protecting a wound; in dentistry, may sometimes be called a pack.

Pressure dressing: for maintaining pressure to control bleeding or to hold a particular flap or graft in position.

Protective dressing: to shield the area from injury or trauma.

Eugenol (ū′jĕn-ol): constituent of clove oil; used in early periodontal dressings with zinc oxide for its alleged antiseptic and anodyne properties; more recently found to be toxic, to elicit allergic reactions, and to hinder, more than promote, healing.

Hemostasis (hē″mō-stā′sĭs): arrest of the escape of blood by either natural (clot formation or vessel spasm) or artificial (compression or ligation) means.

Suture (sū′chur): a stitch or series of stitches made to secure apposition of the edges of a surgical or traumatic wound.

Absorbable suture: becomes dissolved in body fluids and disappears, for example, catgut and tendon.

Interrupted suture: one in which each stitch is made with a separate piece of material; in contrast with a **continuous suture** made with an uninterrupted length that connects each stitch with the previous one.

Surgical gut suture: an absorbable suture prepared from submucous connective tissue of the small intestine of healthy sheep.

Swage (swāj): to fuse, as suture material to the end of a suture needle.

Tensile strength: amount of strength the suture material will retain throughout the healing period. As the wound gains strength, the suture loses strength.

Visible-light cure: light activation using a photocure system; shorter curing time than self-cure (chemical cure); does not start setting until the light is activated, thereby allowing longer working time for adapting the dressing material.

II. SUTURE CHARACTERISTICS

The suture material is expected to do the following:
A. Be handled comfortably and easily
B. Pass through tissue with minimal trauma
C. Cause little or no tissue reaction throughout healing
D. Possess a high tensile strength

III. CLASSIFICATION OF SUTURE MATERIALS

A. By Number of Strands
1. *Monofilament sutures:* Made of a single strand of material.
2. *Multifilament suture:* Consists of several strands usually twisted or braided together.

B. By Material Used
1. *Natural:* Capable of causing adverse tissue reaction.
2. *Synthetic:* Recently developed to reduce tissue reactions and unpredictable rates of absorption commonly found in natural sutures.

C. By Absorption Properties
1. *Absorbable sutures:* Approximate tissue until wound heals sufficiently to endure normal stress.
   a. Natural absorbable sutures: digested by body enzymes.
      Example: surgical gut, chromic gut
   b. Synthetic absorbable sutures: broken down by hydrolysis.
      Example: sutures made from raw materials of homopolymer of glycolic acid or copolymers of polyglycolic acid (eg, coated Vicryl™)
2. *Nonabsorbable sutures:* Must be removed within specific time period.
   a. Natural nonabsorbable
      Example: silk
   b. Synthetic nonabsorbable
      Example: nylon, propylene polytetrafluoroethylene, polyester

D. By Diameter of Material
1. Suture material: diameters from 1-0 to 11-0
2. More zeros, the smaller the diameter
3. Fewer zeros, the larger the diameter
   Example: 3-0 is larger than 5-0

NEEDLES

Many types of suturing needles are available. Their use and selection are based on specific procedures, location for use, and clinician's preference.

I. NEEDLE COMPONENTS

A. Swaged End (Eyeless)
Swaged (eyeless) to allow suture material and needle to act as one unit (Figure 36-1).

B. Body
1. *Shape/curvature:*
   a. Straight.
   b. Half-curved.
   c. Curved ¼, ½, ⅜, ⅝ (Figure 36-2).
2. *Diameter:* Gauge or size; finer for delicate surgeries.
3. *Grasp with needle holder:* At widest part of the body.

C. Point
1. *Conventional cutting:* Triangular at the tip, third cutting edge inside the curvature; tapers back to flat body (Figure 36-3).
2. *Reverse cutting:* Third cutting edge on back or bottom side of the body.
3. *Tapered:* Sharp point and round body.

II. NEEDLE CHARACTERISTICS

A. Material
Most needles are made of stainless steel formulated and sterilized for surgical use.

B. Attachment
Majority of needles are permanently attached

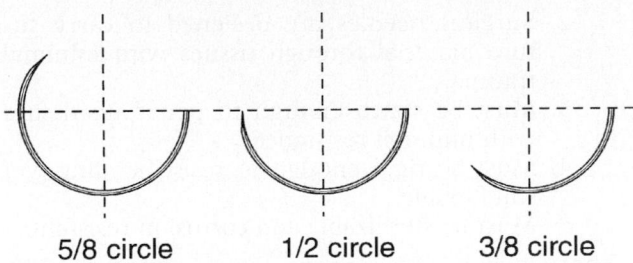

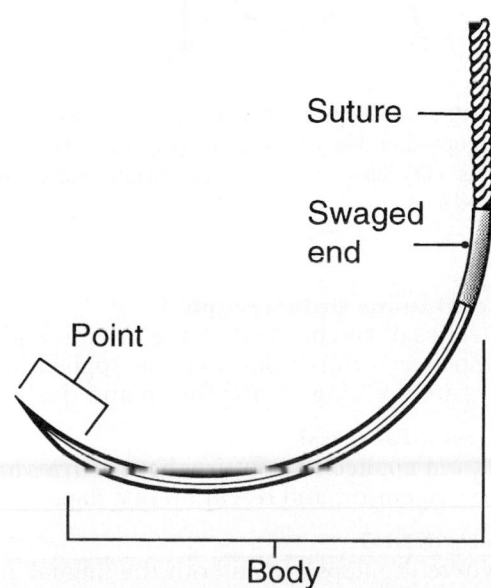

to suture material; eliminates need for threading and unnecessary handling.

C. Cutting Edge
1. *Reverse cut:* Has two opposing cutting edges with a third located on outer convex curve of needle.
2. *Conventional cut:* Consists of two opposing cutting edges and a third within the concave curvature of the needle.

D. Requirements
1. Needle point is chosen according to specific surgical procedure.

5/8 circle   1/2 circle   3/8 circle

■ **FIGURE 36-2 Suture Needles. Body Curvatures.** A curved needle is manipulated with a needleholder. The 3/8 curve is most effective for closure of skin and mucous membranes, and is a needle of choice in many dental and periodontal surgeries.

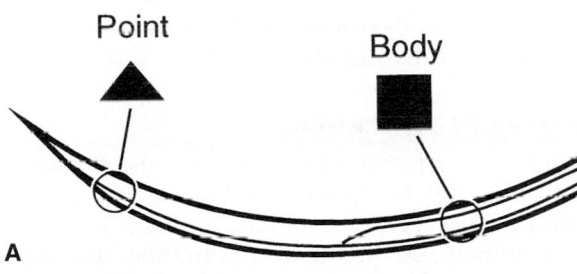

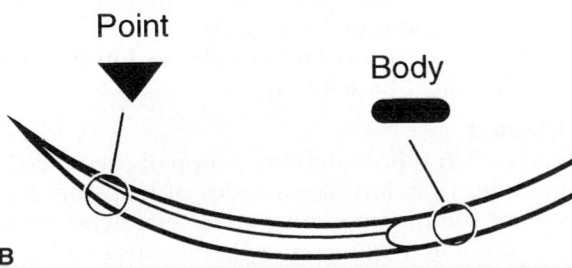

■ **FIGURE 36-3 Suture Needles. Shapes of Points.** Triangle shows cross section of needle point. **(A)** Conventional cutting with third cutting edge on the inside of the needle curvature. **(B)** Reverse cutting with third cutting edge on the outer curvature of the needle used for difficult-to-penetrate tissue such as skin.

■ **FIGURE 36-1 Suture Needle Components.**

2. Surgical needles are designed to carry suture material through tissues with minimal trauma.
3. Must be sharp enough to penetrate tissues with minimal resistance.
4. Must be rigid enough to resist bending, yet still flexible.
5. Must be sterilizable and corrosion resistant.

KNOTS

The Encyclopedia of Knots describes more than 1400 knots. Only a few are used in dentistry. The type of knot used depends on the specific procedure, location of the incision, and the amount of stress the wound will endure. Most common knots used in dentistry are the surgeons and square knots.

I. KNOT CHARACTERISTICS

A. Knot should be tied as small as possible.
B. Completed knot should be firm to reduce slipping.
C. Excessive tension should be avoided so the material will not break nor the tissue be injured.

II. MANAGEMENT

A. Tie knots on facial aspect for access in removal.
B. Leave 2- to 3-mm suture "tail" to assist in locating at the time of removal.

III. SUTURING PROCEDURES

Many different patterns of suturing are used. Assisting and observing at the time of the surgical procedure can be especially educational.

At the time of the treatment, the number and type or description of the sutures placed should be recorded in the patient's record. At the time of removal, the information is necessary, because during healing, sutures may become loosened, misplaced, or sometimes covered with tissue. All sutures should be accounted for at the time of removal.

General types of sutures frequently used in the oral cavity are described here briefly.

A. Blanket

Each stitch is brought over a loop of the preceding one, thus forming a series of loops on one side of the incision and a series of stitches over the incision (Figure 36-4A). It is also called a continuous lock. This stitch is used, for example, to approximate the gingival margins after alveolectomy.

B. Interrupted

Figure 36-4B shows a series of interrupted sutures.

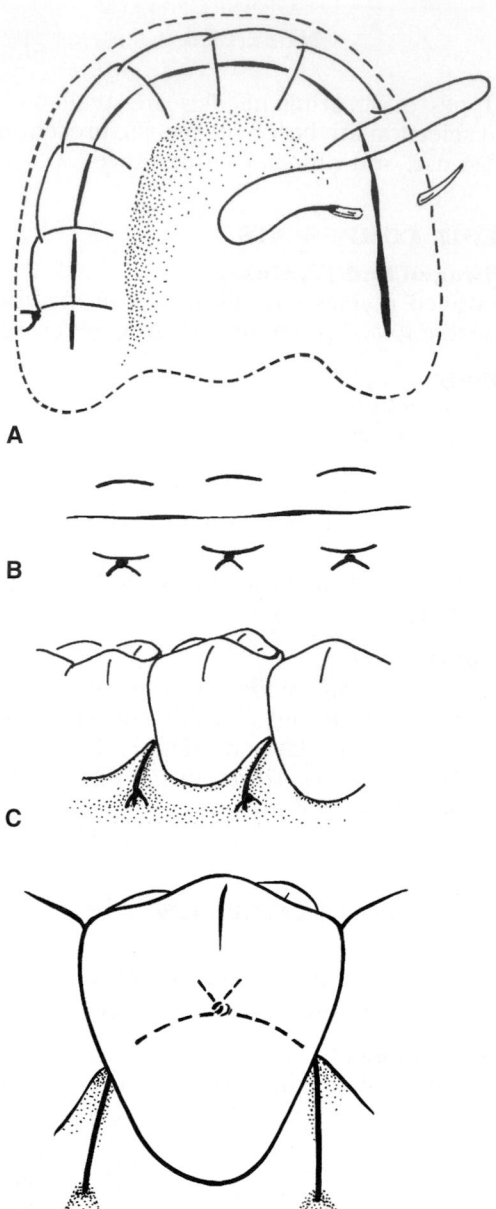

FIGURE 36-4 Types of Sutures. (A) Blanket stitch. **(B)** Interrupted, individual sutures. **(C)** Interdental individual sutures. **(D)** Sling or suspension suture tied on the lingual (*dotted line*).

C. Continuous Uninterrupted

A series of stitches tied at one or both ends. Examples of sutures that may be applied in a series are the sling or suspension and the blanket.

D. Circumferential

A term applied to a suture that encircles a tooth for suspension and retention of a flap.

E. Interdental

Where the flaps are on both the lingual and facial sides, interdental ligation joins the two by passing the suture through each interdental area (Figure 36-4*C*). Coverage for the interdental area can be accomplished by coapting the edges of the papillae.

F. Sling or Suspension

When a flap is only on one side, facial or lingual, the sutures are passed through the interdental papilla, through the interdental area, around the tooth, and then into the adjacent papilla (Figure 36-4*D*). The suture is adjusted so that the flap can be positioned for correct healing.

PROCEDURE FOR REMOVAL

When a dressing has been placed over sutures, the steps overlap with the procedure described in "Dressing Removal," page 592. A suture can become caught in dressing material and may need to be cut and removed while the dressing is being removed. The same principles for removal are to be observed.

I. SUPPLIES FOR SUTURE REMOVAL

Mouth mirror
Cotton pliers
Curved sharp scissors with pointed tip (suture scissors)
Gauze sponge
Topical anesthetic: Use type that can be applied safely on an abraded or incompletely healed area (pages 507 to 508)
Topical antiseptic
Cotton pellets
Saliva ejector tip

II. PREPARATION OF PATIENT

A. Patient History Check

Suture removal can cause bacteremia.[1,2] High-risk patients need antibiotic premedication for suture removal (pages 101 to 104).

B. Patient Examination

1. Observe healing tissue around the suture(s).
2. Record any deviations of color, size, shape of the tissue, adaptation of a flap, or coaptation of an incision healing by first intention.

C. Preparation of the Sutured Area

1. Debride area; rinse the area and remove debris particles, using a cotton-tipped applicator or a cotton pellet dipped in 3% peroxide. Follow with another rinse, or wipe gently with a gauze sponge.
2. Place and adjust saliva ejector.
3. Retract and pat area with gauze sponge to remove surface moisture.
4. Swab area with topical antiseptic. Maintain retraction to prevent dilution.
5. Apply topical anesthetic.

D. Retraction

Three hands are really needed: one for retraction, one for cotton pliers to hold and remove the suture, and one for cutting the suture.

When an assistant is not available, a cotton roll placed in the vestibule may provide enough retraction along with the finger rest and little finger of the nondominant hand holding the cotton pliers.

III. STEPS FOR REMOVAL

The suture removal procedure described here and illustrated in Figure 36-5 is for a single interrupted suture. The same principles apply for the ends and each segment of a continuous suture, wherever septic suture material could pass through the soft tissue.

    A. Grasp the suture knot with the cotton plier held in the nondominant hand. Gently draw

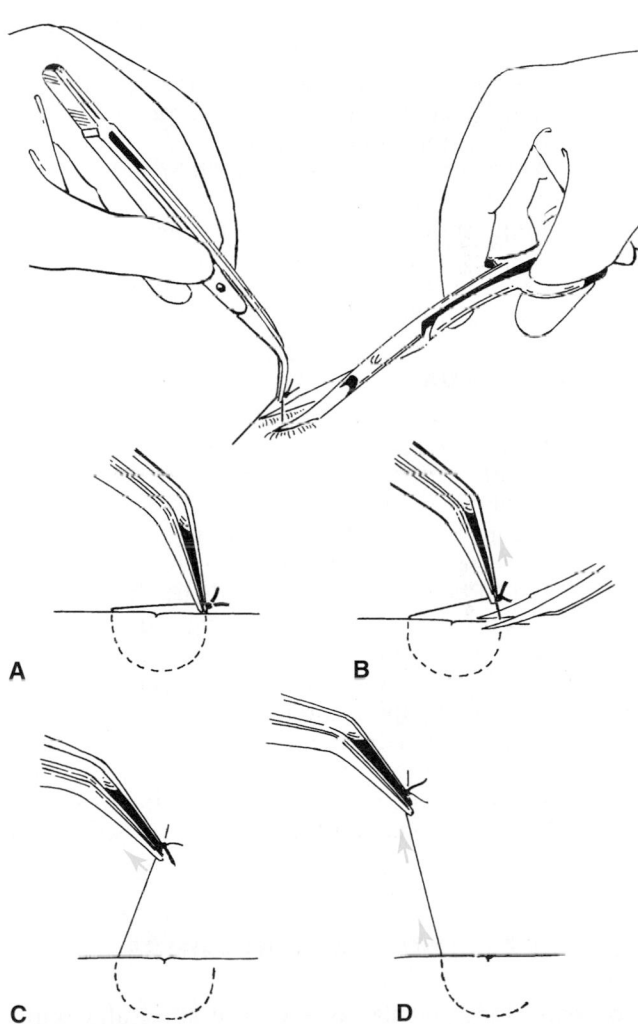

■ **FIGURE 36-5 Suture Removal. (A)** Suture grasped by pliers near the entrance into tissue. **(B)** Suture pulled gently up while scissor is inserted close to the tissue. Suture is cut in the part previously buried in the tissue. **(C)** Suture is held up for vertical removal. **(D)** Suture is pulled gently to bring it out on the side opposite from where it was cut. The object is to prevent the external part of the suture from passing through the tissue and introducing infectious material.

the suture up about 2 mm and hold with slight tension (Figure 36-5A). A finger rest is needed for control.

B. Insert tip of sharp scissors under the suture, slightly depress the tissue with the back of the scissor blade, and cut the suture in the part that was previously buried in the tissue (Figure 36-5B).

C. Hold knot end up with the cotton plier and pull gently to allow suture to come out through the side opposite where it was cut (Figure 36-5C). This prevents any part of the external segment of the suture from passing through the tissue and introducing infectious material.

D. Withdraw gently and steadily (Figure 36-5D).

E. Place each suture on a sponge for final counting, and proceed to remove the next suture.

F. Count total sutures and confirm with the patient's record of the surgical procedures of the previous appointment.

G. Apply gauze sponge with slight pressure on bleeding spots.

H. Request dentist to observe the area.

I. Request patient to close on the sponge while dressing is readied (when a dressing replacement is indicated).

IV. PRECAUTIONS

In summary of the points brought out in the preceding description, precautions are as follows:

A. Count sutures; record number placed and number removed.

B. Record all observations of the tissues and note any adverse reactions or bleeding problems. Record comments made by the patient.

C. Sutures should not be left longer than 5 to 10 days. Make special arrangements for removal for the patient who cannot return for a scheduled appointment.

D. Take care when removing a periodontal dressing to prevent ripping out a suture that may have become embedded in the dressing.

E. Provide proper postappointment instructions for the patient.

PERIODONTAL DRESSINGS

A dressing may be placed over the surgical wound following periodontal surgery. Dressings are used for all surgical procedures by some clinicians, used occasionally by others, and used rarely by still others.

I. PURPOSES AND USES

A. Provide protection for the surgical wound against external irritation or trauma.

B. Help to prevent posttreatment bleeding by maintaining the initial clot in place.

C. Support mobile teeth during healing.

D. Assist in shaping or molding the newly formed tissues; aid in holding a flap in place or immobilizing a graft.

E. Retain site-specific fibers for slow-release chemotherapy in pockets.

II. CHARACTERISTICS OF ACCEPTABLE DRESSING MATERIAL

An acceptable periodontal dressing should have the following characteristics:

A. Be conveniently prepared, placed, and removed with minimal discomfort for the patient.

B. Be adhesive to itself, the teeth, and adjacent tissues, and maintain retention in interdental areas.

C. Provide stability and flexibility to withstand distortion and displacement without fracturing.

D. Be nontoxic and nonirritating to the oral tissues.

E. Have a smooth surface that resists accumulation of bacterial plaque.

F. Not damage or stain the teeth or restorative materials.

G. Be esthetically acceptable.

TYPES OF DRESSINGS

Traditionally, dressings were classified into two groups: those that contained eugenol and those that did not contain eugenol. With the development of new products, the "non-eugenol-containing" dressings have been reclassified into chemical-cure and visible-light-cure systems. They may be available as ready-mix, paste-paste, or paste-gel preparations.

Products are reviewed by the American Dental Association, Council on Scientific Affairs. Approved products use the ADA seal (see Figure 24-15, page 389).

I. ZINC OXIDE WITH EUGENOL DRESSING

A. Basic Ingredients

1. *Powder:* Zinc oxide, powdered rosin, and tannic acid. Formerly, asbestos fiber was used as a binder in some formulas. Because airborne asbestos is a recognized pulmonary health hazard, dental team members responsible for mixing periodontal dressings frequently may become overexposed. Asbestos fiber is no longer an acceptable ingredient of dressings.

2. *Liquid:* Eugenol, with an oil, such as peanut or cottonseed, and thymol.

B. Examples

Well-known dressings are Ward's Wonderpack and Kirkland Periodontal Pack.

C. Advantages

1. *Consistency:* Firm and heavy; provides support for tissues and flaps.
2. *Slow setting:* Good working time.
3. *Preparation and storage:* Can be prepared in quantity and stored (frozen) in work-size pieces.

D. Disadvantages

1. *Taste:* Sharp, unpleasant taste.
2. *Tissue reaction:* Irritating to membranes; sensitivity reactions can occur.
3. *Consistency:* Dressing is hard, brittle, and breaks easily. Rough surface encourages bacterial plaque retention.

II. CHEMICAL-CURED DRESSING

The ingredients of commercial products are trade secrets, but some general information about available dressings can be found. Two examples of chemical-cured dressings are PerioCare and Coe-Pak.

A. Basic Ingredients[3]

1. *PerioCare:* Paste-gel.
   a. Paste: zinc oxide, magnesium oxide, calcium hydroxide, vegetable oils.
   b. Gel: resins, fatty acids, ethyl cellulose, lanolin, calcium hydroxide.
2. *Coe-Pak:* Paste-paste.
   a. Base: rosin, cellulose, natural gums and waxes, fatty acid, chlorothymol, zinc acetate, alcohol.
   b. Accelerator: zinc oxide, vegetable oil, chlorothymol, magnesium oxide, silica, synthetic resin, coumarin.

B. Advantages

1. *Consistency:* Pliable, easy to place with light pressure.
2. *Smooth surface:* Comfortable to patient; resists plaque and debris deposits.
3. *Taste:* Acceptable.
4. *Removal:* Easy, often comes off in one piece.

III. VISIBLE-LIGHT-CURED DRESSING

Visible-light-cured (VLC) dressing (Barricaid) is available in a syringe for direct application, when appropriate, or from a mixing pad for indirect application. The same light-curing unit is used that is available in most dental practices for composite restorations and sealants.

A. Basic Ingredients[3]

Gel ingredients include polyether urethane dimethacrylate resin, silanated silica, visible-light cure photo initiator and accelerator, stabilizer, and colorant.

B. Advantages

1. *Color:* More like gingiva than are most other dressings.
2. *Setting:* Does not start until activated by the light-curing unit. (Exposure before placement should be limited because daylight in a room can activate it slightly.)
3. *Removal:* Easy, often comes off in one piece.

IV. COLLAGEN DRESSINGS

Absorbable collagen dressings have particular uses in promoting wound healing. They are available in individual sterile packages.

One special use in periodontal surgery for a collagen patch dressing is for protection during healing of graft sites of the palate. One form is prepared in a bullet shape to use for deep biopsy sites. In general, the collagen dressing may be placed on clean moist or bleeding wounds.

CLINICAL APPLICATION

I. DRESSING PLACEMENT

A. General Procedure

For all types of dressing, the first rule is to follow the manufacturer's instructions. Each product has properties that require special handling.

B. Retention

1. Mold the dressing by pressing at each interproximal site; do not extend over the height of contour of each tooth.
2. Border mold to prevent displacement by the tongue, cheeks, lips, or frena.
3. Check the occlusion and remove areas of contact.

II. CHARACTERISTICS OF A WELL-PLACED DRESSING (FIGURE 36-6)

Dressings placed in keeping with biologic principles contribute to healing and yet are tolerated by the patient. A satisfactory dressing has the following characteristics:

A. Is secure and rigid. A movable dressing is an irritant and can promote bleeding.
B. Has as little bulk as possible, yet is bulky enough to give strength.

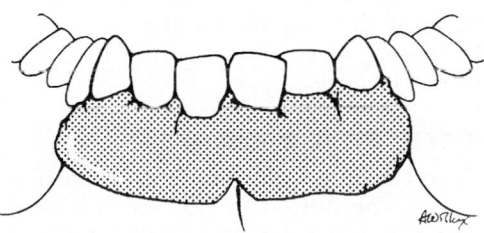

FIGURE 36-6 Periodontal Dressing. A dressing must cover the surgical wound without unnecessary overextension and fill interdental areas to lock the dressing between the teeth. It should be molded in the vestibule and around frena to allow movement of the lips, cheeks, and tongue with no displacement of the dressing.

C. Is locked mechanically interdentally and cannot be displaced by action of tongue, cheek, or lips.

D. Covers all the surgical wound without unnecessary overextension.

E. Fills interdental area to cover the treated area and discourage retention of debris and bacterial plaque.

F. Has a smooth surface to prevent irritation to cheeks and lips and to discourage debris and plaque retention.

III. PATIENT DISMISSAL AND INSTRUCTIONS

A. Patient must not be dismissed until bleeding or oozing from under the dressing has ceased.

B. Written instructions are more effective than verbal. Table 36-1 lists items for which instructions should be given to a patient who has a periodontal dressing. Printed instructions can be prepared from these items. Other instructions for the patient after general oral surgery or tooth removal may be found on pages 710 to 711.

DRESSING REMOVAL AND REPLACEMENT

During healing, epithelium covers a wound in 5 to 6 days, and complete restoration of epithelium and connective tissue can be expected by 21 days. The dressing may be left in place from 7 to 10 days as predetermined by the surgeon.

If the dressing breaks or falls off before the appointed time for removal, the healing tissue should be evaluated. After 4 or 5 days, dressing replacement may not be needed, and the patient should proceed with daily frequent plaque removal and rinsing with an antimicrobial agent. When replacement is indicated, the dressing should be wholly replaced rather than patched because the remaining segment usually is loose.

I. PATIENT EXAMINATION

A. Question patient about and record posttreatment effects or discomfort. Record length of time the dressing stayed in place.

B. Examine the mucosa around the dressing and record its appearance.

II. PROCEDURE FOR REMOVAL

A. Insert a large scaler, hoe, or plastic instrument under the border of the dressing (coronal or apical border, or both); apply lateral pressure.

B. Watch for sutures that may be caught in the dressing. They may need to be cut for release. Use principles for suture removal as described on page 589.

C. Remove pieces of dressing gently with cotton pliers to avoid scratching the thin epithelial covering of the healing tissue with the rough edges of the dressing.

D. Observe tissue and record its appearance. Note any deviations from the normal healing expected in the length of time since the treatment.

E. Use a scaler for removal of pieces attached to tooth surfaces; use curet for particles near the gingival margin. All calculus and roughness should be eliminated to prevent new bacterial plaque retention.

F. Syringe with a gentle stream of *warm* water, and provide *warm* diluted mouthrinse for the patient's comfort.

III. PROCEDURAL SUGGESTIONS FOR DRESSING REPLACEMENT

A. Use a topical anesthetic to prevent patient discomfort (pages 507 to 508).

B. Use a soft dressing with minimal pressure during application over a partly healed area.

IV. BACTERIAL PLAQUE CONTROL FOLLOW-UP

Plaque control follow-up is essential after the final dressing removal.

A. Use a soft brush on the treated area, paying careful attention to plaque removal at the gingival margin. Use usual methods for all other areas of the mouth.

B. Increase intensity of care on the treated area each day, with a return to complete procedures by 3 or 4 days.

C. Rinse with chlorhexidine 0.12% during the healing period twice daily. Force the liquid between the teeth to encourage healing.

D. Use a dentifrice with sodium fluoride for root caries prevention regularly and indefinitely.

E. When teeth are sensitive, a dentifrice containing a desensitizing agent may be advisable on a temporary basis. Other suggestions for coping with sensitivity may be found on page 600.

V. FOLLOW-UP

Return for observation of complete healing in 1 week to 1 month, depending on the individual patient's progress and total treatment plan.

TECHNICAL HINTS

I. Sutures placed without a dressing may have a crust over them at the time of removal. Apply a water-based gel with a cotton swab or pellet, and in a short time, the crust will soften and can be wiped away. Removing the suture with the crust can cause unnecessary discomfort for the patient.

II. When prolonged or excessive bleeding occurs (or may be anticipated because of occurrences

TABLE 36-1 Instructions for Postoperative Care

Factor	Instructions to Patient	Purpose of Instruction
Information about the dressing	Dressing to protect the surgical wound and to help it heal Do not disturb it; keep it on until the next appointment	Understanding and cooperation by the patient
Care during the first few hours	Dressing will not be hard for a few hours; do not eat anything that requires chewing Use only cool liquids Keep quiet; get rest	Dressing must harden and be undisturbed
Anesthesia	Be careful not to bite the lip or cheek Avoid foods that require chewing until the anesthesia has worn off	Prevent trauma to lip or cheek
Discomfort after the anesthesia wears off	When a prescription is given, have the prescription filled and follow the directions for taking the medication; do not take more than directed Do not take aspirin	Pain control Aspirin can interfere with blood clotting
Ice pack or cold compress	Use as directed only Apply every 30 minutes for 15 minutes; or 15 minutes on and 15 minutes off	Prevent swelling from edema
Bleeding	Slight temporary bleeding within the first few hours is not unusual Do not suck on the area or use straws, the blood clot should be left undisturbed Persistent or excessive bleeding should be reported to the dentist for treatment	Alleviate patient alarm over small amount of bleeding, but assure patient of help as needed
Dressing care and retention	Avoid pressing the dressing with the tongue or trying to clean under it Small particles may chip off during the week: no problem, unless the sharp edge bothers the tongue or the dressing seems to have loosened Call the dentist if the whole dressing or a large portion of it falls off before the 5th day; it should be replaced. If after the 5th day, call for an early replacement appointment when area is unusually sensitive; otherwise rinse with saline solution and chlorhexidine 0.12% twice daily	Dressing needed for wound protection Epithelium covers wound by 5th or 6th day in normal healing
Use of tobacco and tobacco products	Do not smoke, avoid all tobacco products A heavy smoker should make every effort to decrease quantity of tobacco used	Heat and smoke irritate the gingiva and delay healing
Rinsing	Do not rinse on the day of the treatment Second day: use saline solution made with ½ teaspoon (measured) in ½ cup of warm water every 2 to 3 hours Start chlorhexidine 0.12% twice daily	Might disturb clot Saline cleanses and aids healing
Toothbrushing and flossing	Use better-than-usual brushing and flossing procedures on untreated areas Brush occlusal surface over dressing Use soft brush with water carefully on surface of dressing to clean off debris and film Brush the tongue	Bacterial plaque control Oral sanitation Odor and taste control Reduce number of oral microorganisms
Eating	Highly nutritious food is needed during healing. Check the food guide pyramid (Figure 28–2, page 445) Use soft-textured diet Omit foods that are highly seasoned, spicy, hot Avoid sticky, crunchy, or coarse foods that could break the dressing	Healing Protect the dressing from breakage or displacement
Mastication	Avoid foods that require excessive chewing. Use ground meat, or cut meat into small pieces Chew only on untreated side Take small bite-sized pieces at a time	Dressing protection

during previous appointments), an extra-stiff dressing should be placed.

FACTORS TO TEACH THE PATIENT

I. Care of the mouth during the period of treatment while wearing dressings (see Table 36-1).
II. Smoking is detrimental and delays healing.
III. Maintenance and follow-up care after treatment is formally over.

REFERENCES

1. **King**, R.C., Crawford, J.J., and Small, E.W.: Bacteremia Following Intraoral Suture Removal, *Oral Surg. Oral Med. Oral Pathol.,* 65, 23, January, 1988.
2. **Giglio**, J.A., Rowland, R.W., Dalton, H.P., and Laskin, D.M.: Suture Removal-induced Bacteremia: A Possible Endocarditis Risk, *J. Am. Dent. Assoc., 123,* 65, August, 1992.
3. **von Fraunhofer**, J.A. and Argyropoulos, D.C.: Properties of Periodontal Dressings, *Dent. Materials, 6,* 51, January, 1990.

SUGGESTED READINGS

Carranza, F.A. and Newman, M.G.: *Clinical Periodontology,* 8th ed. Philadelphia, W.B. Saunders Co., 1996, pp. 571–574; 596–600.

Fedi, P.F., ed.: *The Periodontic Syllabus,* 3rd ed. Philadelphia, Lea & Febiger, 1995, pp. 101–110.

Pattison, A.M. and Pattison, G.L.: *Periodontal Instrumentation,* 2nd ed. Norwalk, CT, Appleton & Lange, 1992, pp. 441–451, 452–457.

Sutures

Chu, C.C. and Kizil, Z.: Quantitative Evaluation of Stiffness of Commercial Suture Materials, *Surg., Gynecol., Obstet., 168,* 233, March, 1989.

Dietz, E.R.: Suture Preparation and Removal, *Dent. Assist., 60,* 9, January–February, 1991.

Hutchens, L.H.: Periodontal Suturing: A Review of Needles, Materials, and Techniques, *Postgrad. Dent., 2,* 3, Number 4, 1995.

Levin, M.P.: Periodontal Suture Materials and Surgical Dressings, *Dent. Clin. North Am., 24,* 767, October, 1980.

Meyer, R.D. and Antonini, C.J.: A Review of Suture Materials, Part I. *Compend. Cont. Educ. Dent., 10,* 260, May, 1989; Part II. *Compend. Cont. Educ. Dent., 10,* 360, June, 1989.

Rockwood, D.P. and Miller, R.I.: Characteristics of Currently Available Suture Materials, *Gen. Dent., 36,* 489, November–December, 1988.

Shaw, R.J., Negus, T.W., and Mellor, T.K.: A Prospective Clinical Evaluation of the Longevity of Resorbable Sutures in Oral Mucosa, *Br. J. Oral Maxillofac. Surg., 34,* 252, June, 1996.

Dressings

Checchi, L. and Trombelli, L.: Postoperative Pain and Discomfort With and Without Periodontal Dressing in Conjunction With 0.2% Chlorhexidine Mouthwash After Apically Positioned Flap Procedure, *J. Periodontol., 64,* 1238, December, 1993.

Cheshire, P.D., Griffiths, G.S., Griffiths, B.M., and Newman, H.N.: Evaluation of the Healing Response Following Placement of Coe-pak and an Experimental Pack After Periodontal Flap Surgery, *J. Clin. Periodontol., 23,* 188, March, 1996.

Eber, R.M., Shuler, C.F., Buchanan, W., Beck, F.M., and Horton, J.E.: Effect of Periodontal Dressings on Human Gingival Fibroblasts *In Vitro, J. Periodontol., 60,* 429, August, 1989.

Geiger, B., Goral, V., and Meister, F.: Periodontal Dressings: Rationale and Procedures, *Dent. Hyg., 55,* 21, September, 1981.

Gilbert, A.D., Lloyd, C.H., and Scrimgeour, S.N.: The Effect of a Light-cured Periodontal Dressing Material on HeLa Cells and Fibroblasts in Vitro, *J. Periodontol., 65,* 324, April, 1994.

Hume, W.R.: The Pharmacologic and Toxicological Properties of Zinc Oxide-eugenol, *J. Am. Dent. Assoc., 113,* 789, November, 1986.

Jorkjend, L. and Skoglund, L.A.: Effect of Non-eugenol- and Eugenol-containing Periodontal Dressings on the Incidence and Severity of Pain after Periodontal Soft Tissue Surgery, *J. Clin. Periodontol., 17,* 341, July, 1990.

Nezwek, R.A., Caffesse, R.G., Bergenholtz, A., and Nasjleti, C.E.: Connective Tissue Response to Periodontal Dressings, *J. Periodontol., 51,* 521, September, 1980.

Othman, S., Haugen, E., and Gjermo, P.: The Effect of Chlorhexidine Supplementation in a Periodontal Dressing, *Acta Odontol. Scand., 47,* 361, December, 1989.

Rubinoff, C.H., Greener, E.H., and Robinson, P.J.: Physical Properties of Periodontal Dressing Materials, *J. Oral Rehabil., 13,* 575, November, 1986.

Sachs, H.A., Farnoush, A., Checchi, L., and Joseph, C.E.: Current Status of Periodontal Dressings, *J. Periodontol., 55,* 689, December, 1984.

Samuelson, G., Rakes, G., and Aiello, A.: Visible-light-polymerized Periodontal Dressing for Treatment of Trauma from Orthodontic Appliances, *J. Clin. Orthod., 24,* 564, September, 1990.

Skoglund, L.A. and Jorkjend, L.: Postoperative Pain Experience after Gingivectomies Using Different Combinations of Local Anaesthetic Agents and Periodontal Dressings, *J. Clin. Periodontol., 18,* 204, March, 1991.

Smeekens, J.P.A.M., Maltha, J.C., and Renggli, H.H.: Histological Evaluation of Surgically Treated Oral Tissues after Application of a Photocuring Periodontal Dressing Material. An Animal Study, *J. Clin. Periodontol., 19,* 641, October, 1992.

Thorstensen, A.E.R., Duguid, R., and Lloyd, C.H.: The Effects of Adding Chlorhexidine and Polyhexamethylene Bisguanide to a Light-cured Periodontal Dressing Material, *J. Oral Rehabil., 23,* 729, November, 1996.

37

Dentin Sensitivity

Hypersensitivity, which can produce considerable discomfort, occurs when dentin is exposed. Care must be taken during instrumentation and use of air to minimize hypersensitive reactions.

Patients are appreciative of clinical procedures directed at desensitizing an involved area. Several chemical and mechanical means have been used successfully to reduce or eliminate pain. Methods available are not consistently effective for all patients. Box 37-1 provides definitions for terms relating to hypersensitivity.

FACTORS CONTRIBUTING TO HYPERSENSITIVITY

A careful history, along with radiologic and clinical assessment, is needed to identify the cause of sensitivity. More than one factor can be contributing.

I. LOSS OF GINGIVA

A. Steps in Exposure of Dentinal Tubules
1. Loss of clinical attachment produces actual and visible recession.
2. Root surface is uncovered; dentinal tubules exposed; hypersensitivity can result.

B. Causes of Gingival Recession[1,2]
1. *Periodontal Infection.* Actual recession occurs with migration of the junctional epithelium (see Figure 11-12, page 197). Inflammation causes breakdown in the connective tissue, which leads to loss of periodontal attachment.
2. *Instrumentation.* Initial therapy
   a. Main objective of instrumentation for root surface debridement is resolution of the inflammation and shrinkage of edematous tissues.

BOX 37-1 KEY WORDS: Dentin Sensitivity

Abfraction (ab-frak'shun): the dynamic stresses that occur in the mouth during interocclusal activity, such as chewing or bruxing, create a cyclic tension and compression that occur in the cervical region of the tooth, resulting in flexing, cracking, or breakage of the tooth structure. The bending of the tooth from side to side results in fracture of the most flexed zone, the cervical surface layer, affecting enamel, cementum, or dentin.

Dentin hypersensitivity: transient pain arising from exposed dentin typically in response to chemical, thermal, tactile, osmotic stimuli, which cannot be explained as arising from any other form of dental defect or pathology and subsides quickly when stimulus is removed.

Hydrodynamic mechanism: stimuli applied to dentinal tubules cause movement of dentinal fluid, which then stimulates nerve processes in the more pulpal areas of the dentin and/or nerves in the pulp itself; pain impulse transmission results.

Idiopathic (id"ē-ō-path'ĭk): a disease or condition of unknown origin or cause, arising spontaneously with no apparent external cause; self-originated.

Intratubular dentin: mineralized, hypercalcified lining of the dentinal tubule that increases in thickness with age and results in sclerotic dentin.

Iontophoresis (i-on"tō-fah-rē'sĭs): introduction of ions of soluble salts into the body by electric current; a means of applying medications with the assistance of a small electric current.

Osmosis (oz-mō'sĭs): the phenomenon of the passage of certain fluids and solutions of lesser concentration through a selective membrane to one of greater solute concentration; adj., osmotic.

Patent (pa'tent): open, unobstructed.

Permeability (per"mē-a-bil'-ĭ-tē): ability of permitting passage of a substance; permeability of dentin refers to passage of fluid through the tubules.

Reparative dentin: a type of secondary dentin formed along the pulpal wall as a protective mechanism; has fewer, less regular dentinal tubules; may form throughout life in response to extensive wear, erosion, dental caries, or restorative procedures.

Smear layer: thin, tenacious, amorphous layer of microcrystalline particles that remains on instrumented dentinal surfaces whenever they are cut with a dental bur or root planed; the particles are burnished together and onto the underlying surface in a manner that prevents the layer from being rinsed off or scrubbed away; layer is removed during acid-etch; the particles may cover the dentinal surface and obturate the tubules.

---

b. Tissue shrinkage exposes the root surface when clinical attachment loss has occurred.

c. In shallow pockets, attachment loss can be initiated by instrumentation (page 548).

d. Smear layer left after use of instruments protects the tooth from sensitivity at first, but the smear can be readily removed.

3. *Periodontal Surgery.* Removal of tissue allows root surface exposure; healing leads to subsequent tissue shrinkage.

4. *Restorative Procedures and Oral Surgery.* Changes following restorative procedures and oral surgery can result in recession.

5. *Orthodontic Treatment*[3,4]

a. Moving teeth in the presence of contributing factors can lead to loss of attachment and isolated gingival recession.

b. Contributing factors include bacterial plaque, inflammation, poor quality and quantity of radicular bone, and minimal width of attached gingiva.

6. *Patient Self-Care*

a. Overvigorous or incorrect toothbrushing traumatizes the gingival tissues and can lead to recession.

b. Abrasive dentifrice ingredients can be detrimental.

II. LOSS OF CEMENTUM

A. Anatomy of the Cementoenamel Junction[5]

1. *Thickness of Cementum.* Cementum at the cervical third is only about 0.05 mm thick.

2. *Enamel-Cementum Relationship.* A zone of dentin occurs between the enamel and the cementum in approximately 10% of teeth (see Figure 13-2, page 229).

B. Effects of Treatment Procedures

1. *Instrumentation.* The thin layer of cementum can be removed in the process of calculus removal and root surface debridement.

2. *Stain Removal From Root Surfaces.* Dentinal tubules may be exposed after use of an abrasive agent with rubber cup or air-powder polisher.

C. Effects of Self-Care

1. *Toothbrush Abrasion.*
2. *Incomplete Daily Plaque Removal.* When brushing causes a sensitivity reaction, patient avoids brushing sensitive areas; the patient's discomfort reduces the effectiveness of plaque removal and compromises gingival health.

D. Root Caries

1. Root caries sensitivity can occur simultaneously with dentinal hypersensitivity.
2. Root caries exposes dentinal tubules.

III. LOSS OF ENAMEL

A. Noncarious Physical and Chemical Dental Lesions[6]

Abrasion, attrition, erosion, and abfraction contribute to exposure of dentinal tubules and dentinal hypersensitivity.

B. Erosion

1. *Exposure to Stomach Acids.* Erosion may result from conditions such as gastric reflux, morning sickness, self-induced vomiting (bulimia).
2. *Exposure to Acidic Industrial Aerosols.*
3. *Dietary Erosion.* Dietary sources of excess acid include sucking on citrus fruits, excessive intake of carbonated beverages, or other acidic liquids.

IV. ROLE OF SMEAR LAYER

A. Location

The smear layer is an amorphous or crystalline layer present on exposed dentinal surfaces after instrumentation. The layer attaches to the underlying surface in a manner that prevents the layer from being rinsed off or readily washed away.[7]

B. Blockage of Dentinal Tubules

The thicker and more amorphous the smear layer, the less sensitivity is experienced by the individual.

C. Removal of Smear Layer

With a thinner or missing smear layer, sensitivity increases; dentinal tubules appear more numerous and wider.

V. OTHER DENTAL FACTORS

Dental or pulpal sensitivity can result from a variety of pathologic and traumatic causes.

A. Comparison of Pain Symptoms

1. *Dentinal Hypersensitivity:* Sharp, brief, localized pain usually of short duration but occasionally will linger as a dull ache.
2. *Acute Pulpal Pain:* Constant and severe.
3. *Chronic Pulpitis:* Recurring episodes of pain; may be confused with dentin hypersensitivity.

B. Dental Conditions With Pain Symptoms

Conditions with pain symptoms similar to dentinal hypersensitivity include the following:

1. Cracked tooth syndrome
2. Defective restorations with marginal leakage
3. Fractured or chipped teeth or restorations
4. Dental caries
5. Sensitivity after restorative treatment
6. Incomplete polymerization of restorative materials

DENTIN STRUCTURE[8,9]

Dentin is composed of calcified tissue surrounding dentinal tubules. Normally it is covered by enamel on the crown and by cementum on the root.

I. TUBULES

A. Number

Millions of tubules penetrate the dentin. They follow pathways laid down by the odontoblasts during dentin formation. Significantly more tubules, and more patent tubules, are present within a hypersensitive tooth than in a nonsensitive tooth.

B. Direction

In the crown and cervical areas the tubules follow an "S" line from the pulp to the dentinoenamel and dentinocemental junctions. In the root the tubules are in straighter lines (Figure 37-1A).

C. Branching

The tubules branch near the dentinoenamel and dentinocemental junctions (Figure 37-1B). Cross-connections (anastomoses) also exist between the tubules.

D. Diameter

The tubules are wider at the dentinoenamel and dentinocemental junctions in hypersensitive teeth than in nonsensitive teeth. Tubules tend to narrow with age.

E. Content

Tubules are filled with a plasma-like fluid. When tubules are patent, the fluid is in constant movement.

II. ODONTOBLASTIC PROCESSES

Each dentinal tubule contains a cytoplasmic cell process that extends from the odontoblast cell body at the edge of the pulp. In young teeth each process extends the entire distance, whereas in older teeth processes may be withdrawn.

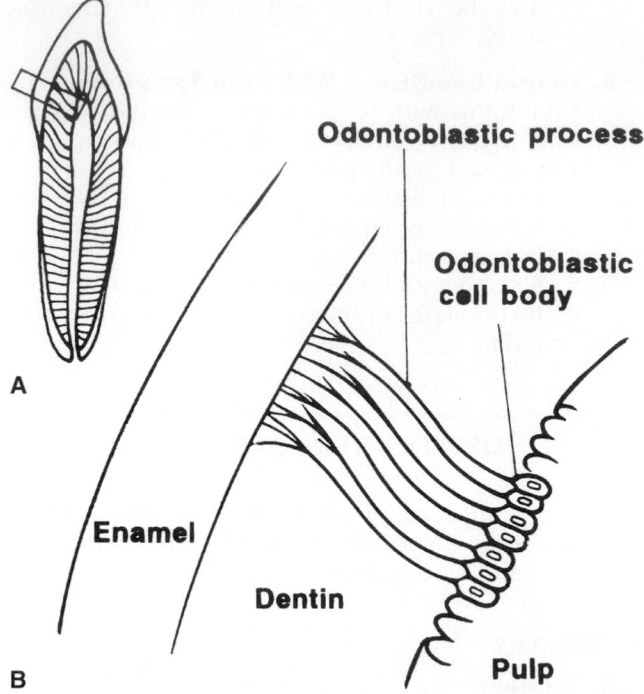

FIGURE 37-1 Odontoblasts. Cell body of an odontoblast is on the edge of the pulp. Each cell has an odontoblastic process that extends from the cell to the dentinoenamel junction. **(A)** In the crown, the processes run in an "S" line, whereas in the root they are straight across. **(B)** The processes may branch near the dentinoenamel and cementoenamel junctions to give more exposure when enamel or cementum is lost. (Redrawn from Brand, R.W. and Isselhard, D.E.: *Anatomy of Orofacial Structures*, 3rd ed. St. Louis, Mosby, 1986.)

TYPES OF PAIN STIMULI[10]

I. TACTILE (MECHANICAL)

Mechanical stimulation that can lead to pain can be caused by:
  A. Toothbrush filaments or bristles
  B. Eating utensils; periodontal and dental instruments
  C. Friction from denture clasps or other prostheses
  D. Oral habits

II. CHEMICAL

Other sources of pain stimuli are chemical:
  A. Acids present in many foods and beverages, such as citrus fruits, condiments, spices, wine, and carbonated beverages.
  B. Acids formed by breakdown of cariogenic foods by bacteria in plaque.
  C. Acid from gastric regurgitation acts on teeth.

III. THERMAL

Changes in temperature can cause pain reaction:

  A. Thermal stimulation can be caused by hot or cold foods and beverages.
  B. Air entering the oral cavity.
  C. Dehydration of oral fluids by high-volume evacuation or drying the tooth with blasts of air during dental and dental hygiene appointments.

IV. OSMOTIC

  A. Osmotic flow within the dentinal tubules is stimulated by concentrated solutions of sugar and/or salt on the dentin surface.
  B. The fluid movement stimulates the nerve endings.

V. BACTERIAL

The acid products of the bacteria that cause root demineralization and dental caries contribute to sensitivity. Bacteria on dentinal surfaces under defective restorations and in carious lesions can increase sensitivity.

PAIN IMPULSE CONDUCTION: THEORIES[11]

The exact mechanism of pain transmission from the tooth surface to the pulp has not been completely defined. Several theories have been the subjects of extensive research. Two of the theories are most commonly applied in the management of hypersensitivity.

I. HYDRODYNAMIC MECHANISM[12]

The hydrodynamic theory has been the most widely accepted.

  A. Fluid Movement in Dentinal Tubules
  Stimuli such as heat, cold, or air blast on the surface of the exposed dentin set up rapid movement of the fluid in the dentinal tubules. The fluid may expand with heat and contract with cold. The fluid then stimulates nerve endings in the pulp.

  B. Nerve Endings in the Dentin[13]
  Nerve endings extend from the pulp and end near the cells of the odontoblasts (Figure 37-2).

II. NEUROPHYSIOLOGY RELATED TO DENTAL PAIN[11,13]

There are two primary types of nerve fibers triggered in dental pain. The fibers are characterized by different types of pain: a sharp, short-duration sensation (A-type), or a dull ache of long duration (C-type). The sensations help to differentiate between pulpal sensitivity and dentinal sensitivity.

  A. A-Type Fibers
  1. Myelinated with a fast conduction velocity.
  2. Activated by stimulation of open dentinal

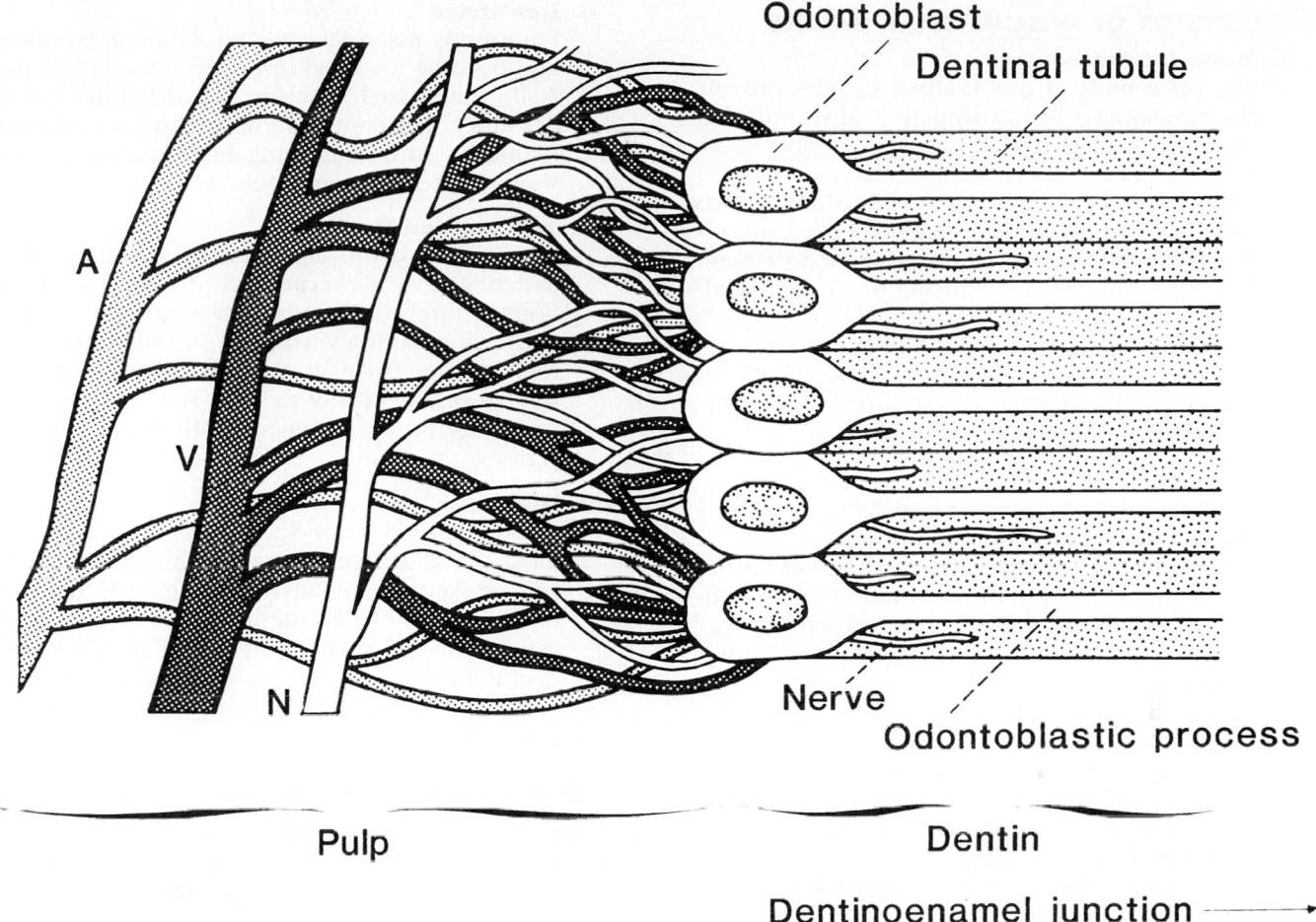

Odontoblast

Dentinal tubule

A

V

N

Nerve

Odontoblastic process

Pulp

Dentin

Dentinoenamel junction ⟶

FIGURE 37-2 Relationship of Odontoblasts and Nerve Endings. Nerve endings from the pulp lie side by side with odontoblasts lined up at the edge of the pulp. A few nerve endings extend short distances beside the dentinal tubules. (Adapted from Bennett, C.R.: *Monheim's Local Anesthesia and Pain Control in Dental Practice*, 7th ed. St. Louis, Mosby, 1984.)

tubules (tactile, chemical, thermal, and osmotic stimuli) and produce effects by induction of fluid flow in the dentinal tubules (hydrodynamic mechanism).

3. Produce sharp, well-localized, transient pain typical of dentinal sensitivity.

B. C-Type Fibers

1. Unmyelinated with a slow conduction velocity.
2. Activated by the chemical mediators of inflammation; do not respond to dentinal (hydrodynamic) stimulation.
3. Produce dull, poorly localized, aching pain.

DESENSITIZATION

I. UNTREATED: SPONTANEOUS REMISSION

A. Patient Education

1. Inform the patient before dental and dental hygiene procedures that may result in postcare sensitivity.
2. Alleviate anxiety by educating the patient about the causes and management of discomfort.

B. Factors Contributing to Gradual Lessening of Sensitivity

1. Formation of reparative and/or secondary dentin in response to irritation and trauma to the dentin or pulp.
2. Deposition of minerals at the openings of the dentinal tubules includes fluoride and minerals from the diet, dentifrice, and saliva, or fluorides from drinking water.
3. Formation of calculus that covers patent tubules of the sensitive area.
4. Dietary changes: limiting foods and beverages to those that do not provide a pain stimuli; avoiding acidic and carbonated beverages, sharp flavors or spices, and extremes of hot or cold.

II. SELECTION OF DESENSITIZING AGENTS

A. Modes of Action

The open ends of the dentinal tubules provide the mechanism for transmission of stimuli that cause the sensitivity. By covering or closing the open tubules, a mechanical blockage for transmission of sensations is created. Many agents have been tried with varying degrees of success in blocking the tubules. Preventive treatment has been directed at producing the following effects:

1. Surface coating over the tubule entrance.
2. Intratubular mineralization or precipitation.
3. Irritation and stimulation to encourage the formation of secondary dentin.
4. Interruption of nerve transmission.

B. Characteristics of an Acceptable Desensitizing Agent

The American Dental Association has established guidelines for the evaluation of the efficacy of agents for the reduction of sensitivity.[14] An acceptable agent is characterized by the following properties:[15]

1. Rapidity of action.
2. Ease of application.
3. Biologic acceptance by the body tissues.
4. Long-lasting or permanent effects.
5. No side effects, such as tooth discoloration, gingival irritation, or pulpal changes.
6. No pain to patient during application.
7. Consistent effectiveness.

DENTAL HYGIENE CARE

Few patients respond to a single form of treatment. For all, keeping the teeth free of bacterial plaque, particularly at the gingival third where sensitive areas are likely to occur, and using a form of self-applied topical fluoride are basic procedures. Specific agents can be selected on an individual basis for professional application to persistent areas of sensitivity.

I. SELF-CARE BY THE PATIENT[16]

A. Bacterial Plaque Control

Root surfaces subjected to vigorous plaque control measures by brushing, flossing, and the use of other selected aids can develop a smooth hard surface with less hypersensitivity. The dentinal tubules may be blocked off by increased mineralization.

When bacterial plaque is retained at the cervical third of the tooth, the root surfaces may develop root caries and may be hypersensitive because of bacterial toxins and acid formed from cariogenic substances. A concentrated program of adequate personal care and dietary limitations can reverse the process.

B. Dentifrice

Fluoride is essential for root caries prevention and must be included in the recommendations. A fluoride-based desensitizing dentifrice, or a dentifrice that contains fluoride in combination with another desensitizing agent such as potassium nitrate, is recommended.[17]

C. Self-Applied Fluoride

In addition to the desensitizing dentifrice, the patient's care plan can include daily applications of fluoride by mouth rinsing, custom tray with gel, brushing with a gel, or other mode for regular use. The various procedures were described on pages 469 to 472. With an increase in surface fluoride, hypersensitivity usually decreases.

D. Diet

A food diary kept for 5 to 7 days, from which a dietary assessment is made with the patient, can be valuable. Foods that aggravate the hypersensitivity can be identified, and substitutes can be selected with the patient. Excessive cariogenic foods, citrus fruits, or condiments with pronounced flavors may initiate the sensitivity reaction.

II. PROFESSIONAL APPLICATIONS[18,19]

Without effective personal plaque removal measures, professional applications have limited, and frequently temporary, effects. A variety of products are in current use to seal the dentinal tubules or protect the dentin surface against irritants, with the goal of reducing hypersensitivity.

A. Preparation for Desensitization

When teeth are too sensitive for application of an agent, a local anesthetic may be needed. Note specific areas where a desensitizing agent is to be applied before the anesthetic is administered.

B. Most Commonly Used Agents

1. *Fluorides.* Fluoride agents found to be effective include sodium and/or stannous fluoride in solution, gel, or varnish forms.
2. *Metallic Salts.* Agents with metallic salts crystallize and create a precipitate on the tooth surface that occludes the dentinal tubules. Agents include strontium chloride, potassium oxalate, and ferric oxalate.
3. *Varnishes, Bonding Adhesives, and Resins.* Varnishes, sealant materials, and restorative bonding agents are used to create physical blocks to external stimuli. More aggressive treatment may include placement of resin restorations in areas of lost tooth structure that react to stimuli.

C. Other Methods

1. *Iontophoresis.*[20,21] Iontophoresis is the impregnation of the tooth with ions from dissolved

salts with the aid of an electric current. A direct current is utilized to promote ionic transport of fluoride, a negatively charged ion, onto the tooth surface. The actual mechanism of action may be deposition of fluoride ions deeper into the dentin to obtain more extensive protoplasmic precipitation or formation of secondary dentin.

2. *Sodium Fluoride Desensitizing Paste*[22]
   a. Composition: 33% sodium fluoride, 33% kaolin, 33% glycerin.
   b. Application: On the clean dry area, a small amount of the paste is massaged into the sensitive area. A wood point (in porte polisher) or the handle of a cotton applicator is used to massage for 3 minutes. Excess paste is removed with a cotton pellet.
3. *Dental laser.*[23,24]
4. *Hypnosis.*[25]

TECHNICAL HINTS

I. Do not use compressed air on sensitive teeth. Dry only with cotton pellets or cotton roll.
II. Integrate desensitization therapies into preventive and maintenance care plans for each patient.
III. Consult American Dental Association's annual *Products of Excellence* for approved products. The listing is available on the Internet at http://www.ada.org.
IV. Agents and products for desensitization change as research progresses. The dental hygiene professional needs to keep current on available products.

FACTORS TO TEACH THE PATIENT

I. General causes of gingival recession.
II. Causes of hypersensitivity of teeth.
III. Importance of correct personal care techniques such as using a soft brush and avoiding vigorous brushing that encourages recession.
IV. Probability that the hypersensitivity will subside in time with daily bacterial plaque removal whether a desensitizer is applied or not.
V. Connection between acidic diet and sensitivity; specific foods that should and should not be used in the diet if relief from sensitivity is to be obtained.

REFERENCES

1. **Grant,** D.A., Stern, I.B., and Listgarten, M.A., eds.: *Periodontics,* 6th ed. St. Louis, Mosby, 1988, pp. 460–467.
2. **Carranza,** F.A. and Newman, M.G.: *Clinical Periodontology,* 8th ed. Philadelphia, W.B. Saunders Co., 1996, pp. 228–231.
3. **McComb,** J.L.: Orthodontic Treatment and Isolated Gingival Recession: A Review, *Br. J. Orthod., 21,* 151, May, 1994.
4. **Bimstein,** E., Machtei, E., and Becher, A.: The Attached Gingiva in Children: Diagnostic, Developmental and Orthodontic Considerations for Its Treatment, *ASDC J. Dent. Child., 55,* 351, September–October, 1988.
5. **Melfi,** R.C.: *Permar's Oral Embryology and Microscopic Anatomy,* 9th ed. Philadelphia, Lea & Febiger, 1994, pp. 151–164.
6. **Grippo,** J.O. and Simring, M.: Dental 'Erosion' Revisited, *J. Am. Dent. Assoc., 126,* 619, May, 1995.
7. **Rimondini,** L., Baroni, C., and Carrassi, A.: Ultrastructure of Hypersensitive and Non-sensitive Dentine: a Study on Replica Models, *J. Clin. Periodontol., 22,* 899, December, 1995.
8. **Melfi:** op. cit., pp. 113–133.
9. **Holland,** G.R.: Morphological Features of Dentine and Pulp Related to Dentine Sensitivity, *Arch. Oral Biol., 39,* 3S, Supplement, 1994.
10. **Grant,** Stern, and Listgarten: op. cit., p. 638.
11. **Pashley,** D.H.: Mechanisms of Dentin Sensitivity, *Dent. Clin. North Am., 34,* 449, July, 1990.
12. **Brännström,** M., Lindén, L.Å., and Åström, A.: The Hydrodynamics of the Dental Tubule and of Pulp Fluid: a Discussion of Its Significance in Relation to Dentinal Sensitivity, *Caries Res., 1,* 310, No. 4, 1967.
13. **Närhi,** M., Yamamoto, H., Ngassapa, D., and Hirvonen, T.: The Neurophysiological Basis and the Role of Inflammatory Reactions in Dentine Hypersensitivity, *Arch. Oral Biol., 39,* 23S, Supplement, 1994.
14. **American Dental Association,** Ad Hoc Advisory Committee on Dentinal Hypersensitivity, Council on Dental Therapeutics: Recommendations for Evaluating Agents for the Reduction of Dentinal Hypersensitivity, *J. Am. Dent. Assoc., 112,* 709, May, 1986.
15. **Grossman,** L.I.: A Systematic Method for the Treatment of Hypersensitive Dentin, *J. Am. Dent. Assoc., 22,* 592, April, 1935.
16. **Zappa,** U.: Self-applied Treatments in the Management of Dentine Hypersensitivity, *Arch. Oral Biol., 39,* 107S, Supplement, 1994.
17. **Silverman,** G., Berman, E., Hanna, C.B., Salvato, A., Fratarcangelo, P., Bartizek, R.D., Bollmer, B.W., Campbell, S.L., Lanzalaco, A.C., MacKay, B.J., McClanahan, S.F., Perlich, M.A., and Shaffer, J.B.: Assessing the Efficacy of Three Dentifrices in the Treatment of Dentinal Hypersensitivity, *J. Am. Dent. Assoc., 127,* 191, February, 1996.
18. **Trowbridge,** H.O. and Silver, D.R.: A Review of Current Approaches to In-office Management of Tooth Hypersensitivity, *Dent. Clin. North Am., 34,* 561, July, 1990.
19. **Scherman,** A. and Jacobsen, P.L.: Managing Dentin Hypersensitivity: What Treatment to Recommend to Patients, *J. Am. Dent. Assoc., 123,* 57, April, 1992.
20. **Gillam,** D.G. and Newman, H.N.: Iontophoresis in the Treatment of Cervical Dentinal Sensitivity—A Review, *J. West. Soc. Periodont./Periodont. Abstr., 38,* 129, No. 4, 1990.
21. **McBride,** M.A., Gilpatrick, R.O., and Fowler, W.L.: The Effectiveness of Sodium Fluoride Iontophoresis in Patients with Sensitive Teeth, *Quintessence Int., 22,* 637, August, 1991.
22. **Hoyt,** W.H. and Bibby, B.G.: Use of Sodium Fluoride for Desensitizing Dentin, *J. Am. Dent. Assoc., 30,* 1372, September 1, 1943.
23. **Renton-Harper,** P. and Midda, M.: NdYAG Laser Treatment of Dentinal Hypersensitivity, *Br. Dent. J., 172,* 13, January 11, 1992.
24. **Stabholz,** A., Rotstein, I., Neev, J., Moshonov, J., and Stabholz, A.: Efficacy of XeCl 308-nm Excimer Laser in Reducing Dye Penetration Through Coronal Dentinal Tubules, *J. Endod., 21,* 266, May, 1995.
25. **Starr,** C.B., Mayhew, R.B., and Pierson, W.P.: The Efficacy of Hypnosis in the Treatment of Dentin Hypersensitivity, *Gen. Dent., 37,* 13, January–February, 1989.

SUGGESTED READINGS

Addy, M. and Pearce, N.: Aetiological, Predisposing and Environmental Factors in Dentine Hypersensitivity, *Arch. Oral Biol., 39,* 33S, Supplement, 1994.

Carlson-Mann, L.D.: Dentin Hypersensitivity, *Canad. Dent. Hyg. Assoc., PROBE, 29*, 226, November/December, 1995.

Cuenin, M.F., Scheidt, M.J., O'Neal, R.B., Strong, S.L., Pashley, D.H., Horner, J.A., and Van Dyke, T.E.: An *In Vivo* Study of Dentin Sensitivity: The Relation of Dentin Sensitivity and the Patency of Dentin Tubules, *J. Periodontol., 62*, 668, November, 1991.

Fogel, H.M. and Pashley, D.H.: Effect of Periodontal Root Planing on Dentin Permeability, *J. Clin. Periodontol., 20*, 673, October, 1993.

Holland, G.R.: Odontoblasts and Nerves; Just Friends, *Proc. Finn. Dent. Soc., 82*, 179, Number 4, 1986.

Holland, G.R., Närhi, M.N., Addy, M., Gangarosa, L., and Orchardson, R.: Guidelines for the Design and Conduct of Clinical Trials on Dentine Hypersensitivity, *J. Clin. Periodontol., 24*, 808, November, 1997.

McAndrew, R. and Kourkouta, S.: Effects of Toothbrushing Prior and/or Subsequent to Dietary Acid Application on Smear Layer Formation and the Patency of Dentinal Tubules: An SEM Study, *J. Periodontol., 66*, 443, June, 1995.

Muzzin, K.: Redi-Reference: Dentinal Hypersensitivity, *Dental-HygienistNews, 7*, 21, Number 2, 1994.

Napiorkowski, D.M.: Redi-Reference: Management of Dentinal Hypersensitivity, *DentalHygienistNews, 10*, 7, Number 2, 1997.

Pashley, D.H.: Dentine Permeability and Its Role in the Pathobiology of Dentine Sensitivity, *Arch. Oral. Biol., 39*, 73S, Supplement, 1994.

Seltzer, S. and Boston, D.: Hypersensitivity and Pain Induced by Operative Procedures and the "Cracked Tooth" Syndrome, *Gen. Dent., 45*, 148, March–April, 1997.

Wichgers, T.G. and Emert, R.L.: Dentin Hypersensitivity, *Gen. Dent., 44*, 225, May–June, 1996.

Treatment Agents

Addy, M., Loyn, T., and Adams, D.: Dentine Hypersensitivity—Effects of Some Proprietary Mouthwashes on the Dentine Smear Layer: A SEM Study, *J. Dent., 19*, 148, June, 1991.

Gillam, D.G., Bulman, J.S., Jackson, R.J., and Newman, H.N.: Efficacy of a Potassium Nitrate Mouthwash in Alleviating Cervical Dentine Sensitivity (CDS), *J. Clin. Periodontol., 23*, 993, November, 1996.

Hack, G.D. and Thompson, V.P.: Occlusion of Dentinal Tubules with Cavity Varnishes, *Arch. Oral Biol., 39*, 149S, Supplement, 1994.

Lawson, K., Gross, K.B.W., Overman, P.R., and Anderson, D.: Effectiveness of Chlorhexidine and Sodium Fluoride in Reducing Dentin Hypersensitivity, *J. Dent. Hyg., 65*, 340, September, 1991.

Mazor, Z., Brayer, L., Friedman, M., and Steinberg, D.: Topical Varnish Containing Strontium in a Sustained-release Device as Treatment for Dentin Hypersensitivity, *Clin. Prev. Dent., 13*, 21, May–June, 1991.

Dentifrices

Gillam, D.G., Bulman, J.S., Jackson, R.J., and Newman, H.N.: Comparison of 2 Desensitizing Dentifrices with a Commercially Available Fluoride Dentifrice in Alleviating Cervical Dentine Sensitivity, *J. Periodontol., 67*, 737, August, 1996.

Kuroiwa, M., Kodaka, T., Kuroiwa, M., and Abe, M.: Dentin Hypersensitivity. Occlusion of Dentinal Tubules by Brushing With and Without an Abrasive Dentifrice, *J. Periodontol., 65*, 291, April, 1994.

Lavigne, S.E., Gutenkunst, L.S., and Williams, K.B.: Effects of Tartar-control Dentifrice on Tooth Sensitivity: A Pilot Study, *J. Dent. Hyg., 71*, 105, May–June, 1997.

Plagmann, H.-C., König, J., Bernimoulin, J.-P., Rudhart, A.C., and Deschner, J.: A Clinical Study Comparing Two High-Fluoride Dentifrices for the Treatment of Dentinal Hypersensitivity, *Quintessence Int., 28*, 403, June, 1997.

West, N.X., Addy, M., Jackson, R.J., and Ridge, D.B.: Dentine Hypersensitivity and the Placebo Response. A Comparison of the Effect of Strontium Acetate, Potassium Nitrate and Fluoride Toothpastes, *J. Clin. Periodontol., 24*, 209, April, 1997.

Extrinsic Stain Removal

After treatment by scaling, root planing, and other dental hygiene care, the teeth are assessed for the presence of stains. The use of polishing agents for stain removal is a selective procedure that not every patient needs, especially on a routine basis.

Stains on the teeth are not etiologic factors for any disease or destructive process. Therefore, the removal of stains is for esthetic, not for health, reasons. The need to remove stains by polishing should be evaluated after the plaque is under control, because some stains are incorporated in plaque and can be removed during brushing and flossing by the patient.

The objectives for stain removal may need to be clarified, because "polishing" has been a routine procedure in many offices and clinics. Information

should be provided for each patient concerning individual needs.

When the assessment is made, several factors must be taken into consideration. These factors are described in this chapter. Key words related to stain removal, instruments, coronal polishing, and air-powder polishing are defined in Box 38-1.

EFFECTS OF POLISHING

Because of the potentially detrimental effects, the needs of an individual patient must be reviewed before stain removal. *Professional judgment based on pa-*

BOX 38-1 KEY WORDS AND ABBREVIATIONS: Extrinsic Stain Removal

Abrasion (ah-bra′zhun): wearing away of surface material by friction.

Abrasive (ah-bra′siv): a material composed of particles of sufficient hardness and sharpness to cut or scratch a softer material when drawn across its surface; available in various particle sizes.

Air-powder polisher: air-powered device using air and water pressure to deliver a controlled stream of specially processed sodium bicarbonate slurry through the handpiece nozzle; also called airabrasive, airpolishing, air-powered abrasive, or airbrasive.

Binder: substance used to hold abrasive particles together; examples are ceramic bonding used for mounted abrasive points, electroplating for binding diamond chips for rotary instruments, and rubber or shellac for soft discs.

Coronal polishing: polishing of the anatomic crowns of the teeth to remove bacterial plaque and extrinsic stains; does not involve calculus removal.

Glycerin (glis′er-in): clear, colorless, syrupy fluid used as a vehicle and sweetening agent for drugs and as a solvent and vehicle for abrasive agents.

Grit: with reference to abrasive agents, grit is the particle size.

Polishing: the production, especially by friction, of a smooth, glossy, mirrorlike surface that reflects light; a very fine agent is used for polishing after a coarser agent is used for cleaning.

p.s.i: pounds per square inch.

r.p.m.: revolutions per minute

Slurry: thin, semifluid suspension of a solid in a liquid.

---

tient need determines when a service is to be included in a treatment plan.

I. BACTEREMIA

Because bacteremia can be created during the use of power-driven stain removal instruments, the *medical history* must be recorded initially and then reviewed and updated at succeeding appointments.

Bacteremias result from manipulation of the gingival tissues. In one research study, 11 of 39 children (mean age, 9 years) developed bacteremia following application of a rubber cup with a prophylaxis paste.[1] It is recommended that use of a rubber cup be withheld until the plaque is under control and the gingiva do not bleed when the patient brushes.

For patients at risk, particularly those with damaged or abnormal heart valves, prosthetic valves, joint replacements, rheumatic heart disease, and other conditions listed on pages 101 to 104, antibiotic prophylaxis as outlined by the American Heart Association is needed.

II. ENVIRONMENTAL FACTORS

A. Aerosol Production

Aerosols are created during use of all rotary instruments, including a prophylaxis handpiece with a polishing paste and the air and water sprays used during rinsing.[2] The biologic contaminants of aerosols stay suspended for long periods and provide a means for disease transmission to dental personnel, as well as to succeeding patients (page 18).

The use of power-driven instruments should be limited when a patient is known to have a communicable disease. Universal precautions are routine.

B. Spatter

Protective eyewear is needed for all dental team members and for the patient. Serious eye damage has occurred as a result of spatter in the eye from a polishing paste or from instruments. Constituents of commercial prophylaxis pastes may include various chemicals, such as oils, that can aggravate a severe inflammatory response.[3]

III. EFFECT ON TEETH

A. Removal of Tooth Structure

Polishing for 30 seconds with a pumice paste may remove as much as 4 μm of the outer enamel.[4] If performed repeatedly over the years, the tooth loss could be substantial. The effect has particular significance for children because the surfaces of young, newly erupted teeth are incompletely mineralized.

Cementum and dentin are softer and more porous, so greater amounts of these can be removed during polishing than of the enamel.[5,6] When cementum is exposed because of gingival recession, polishing of the exposed surfaces should be avoided. Also to be avoided are areas of demineralization. Nearly three times more surface enamel is lost from abrasive polishing over demineralized white spots than over intact enamel.[7]

B. Increased Roughness

A coarse abrasive may create a rougher tooth surface than existed before polishing. Grooves and scratches created by an abrasive applied with a rubber cup have been studied microscopically.[8,9] A smooth surface is needed. Microorganisms collect and colonize on a rough surface much more rapidly than on a smooth surface.[9]

C. Areas of Thin Enamel

Certain patients have teeth with thin enamel, such as those with amelogenesis imperfecta (page 289). The enamel over a demineralized area is also thin (see Figure 29-3, page 459).

Removal of tooth structure in the cervical portion of the tooth, where enamel is thin and cementum is exposed, can create unnecessary sensitivity. Special treatment problems may follow. The areas should not be polished with an abrasive because dentinal tubules can be exposed.

D. Removal of Fluoride-Rich Surface

More important than the amount of enamel lost during polishing is that the outermost layer of tooth structure contains the greatest amounts of fluoride.[10] The surface fluoride protects against dental caries. The concentration of fluoride drops quickly inward toward the dentin, so that, if the surface layer is polished away, the protection is greatly diminished.

The *fluoride-rich surface* is important and should not be removed. Certain conditions increase caries susceptibility and therefore preclude the removal of this surface through polishing.

Patients with *xerostomia* from any cause, for example drug or radiation therapy, cannot afford to have the enamel surface weakened by polishing. In contrast, their therapy must include daily addition of concentrated fluoride, usually through self-applied methods, such as rinsing or gel tray.

When, upon assessment, stain removal is shown to be required, the loss of the fluoride-rich surface may be unavoidable. Topical fluoride (gel or solution) must be applied in an attempt to replace the lost protection.[11]

Fluoride uptake is minimal from prophylaxis pastes as compared with that from topical solutions or gels. Use of a paste for stain removal is not a substitute for a non-fluoride agent. In addition to topical application, daily self-applied fluoride should be recommended and prescribed. All patients need a fluoride-containing dentifrice, and in addition, a rinse, chewable tablet, or gel tray can be used, depending on the patient's age and caries susceptibility.

E. Heat Production

Steady pressure with a rapidly revolving rubber cup or bristle brush and a minimum of wet abrasive agent can create sufficient heat to cause pain and discomfort for the patient. Damage to the pulp by the heat has not been documented, but the pulps of young people are large and may be more susceptible to heat. The rule is light pressure, a slow-motion instrument, and plenty of moisture mixed with the abrasive agent.

IV. EFFECT ON GINGIVA

Trauma to the gingival tissue can result, especially when the prophylaxis angle is run at a high speed and the rubber cup is applied for an extended period. In one study, a rubber cup with pumice rotated for 2 minutes caused a total removal of the epithelium inside the crest of the free gingiva.[12] Complete healing from such a wound takes from 8 to 14 days. The soreness and sensitivity of the tissues could prevent adequate plaque removal by the patient during that time, and a severe inflammation could result, along with calculus reformation.

With the fast rotation of a rubber cup, particles of a polishing agent can be forced into the subepithelial tissues and create a source of irritation. Stain removal after gingival and periodontal treatments, including scaling and root planing, is not recommended on the same day. The diseased lining of the pocket usually has been removed, and the pocket wall is wide open and can receive particles that may become embedded out of reach of the most careful irrigation and rinsing.

Rotation of the rubber cup can force microorganisms into the tissues. An inflammatory response can be expected, and bacteria may gain access to the blood stream to create a bacteremia.

Foreign-body reactions to abrasives have been tested. Several agents have been shown to have potential for creating reactions. Some explanation for delayed healing following tissue trauma may be found in this concept.[13]

V. EFFECT ON RESTORATIONS

A. Existing Restorations

Abrasive pastes can leave rough surfaces on various types of restorative materials, including gold, amalgam, and composites.[14]

B. Newly Placed Restorations

Procedures for finishing and polishing newly placed restorations are described in Chapter 40, pages 627 to 632. In the polishing process, a coarse abrasive is used first, followed by abrasives of finer grits. The tooth surface around the restoration must be left as intact as possible. Remineralization of the surface with fluoride is necessary after polishing the restoration.

INDICATIONS FOR STAIN REMOVAL

I. TO REMOVE EXTRINSIC STAINS NOT OTHERWISE REMOVED DURING TOOTHBRUSHING AND SCALING

A. Scaling and Root Planing

When the stain is to be removed, as much stain as possible must first be removed with plaque control instruction and then with the calculus during scaling. Certain stains can be scaled away readily even without being incorporated within calculus.

Black line stain, for example, has been identified as a type of calculus. It resembles calculus in that it is composed of microorganisms, has a similar mode of attachment to enamel, and similar signs of mineralization under a microscope.[15] Another reason why black line stain should be scaled rather than polished is that it is most commonly found on the teeth of children. Newly erupted teeth are more porous and less mineralized and should not be damaged by polishing agents. The effect of heat created by power-driven instruments is not completely known, except that excess heat can produce pulp damage.

For stains on adult teeth that are not removed with calculus, the least abrasive paste should be selected. The toothpaste manufactured for daily home use may be amply abrasive for professional use when very little stain removal is needed.

B. Patient Instruction

The source of an extrinsic stain should be discussed with the patient and a preventive plan initiated. When the recurrence of a stain is preventable, or when the etiologic factor is controllable, the patient should be encouraged to make the necessary habit changes to prevent the stain from collecting again.

Improved techniques of personal plaque removal and more frequent attention to oral hygiene can result in significant improvement. An example of a patient's own stain removal is the use of a toothpick for daily removal of brown stain associated with chlorhexidine rinsing.[16] The toothpick holder is shown in Figure 24-11, page 379.

II. TO PREPARE THE TEETH FOR CARIES-PREVENTIVE AGENTS

A. Pit and Fissure Sealant

Although the manufacturer's directions should be followed relative to preparation of the teeth for sealant application, research has shown that sealants have been successfully placed without the initial cleaning of the teeth. Because commercial prophylaxis pastes contain oils, flavoring substances, or other agents that may interfere with the integrity of the sealant, a plain, fine pumice with water is indicated when precleaning is determined to be necessary (pages 482 to 484).

B. Professional Application of Fluoride Solutions or Gels

1. *Individual*

   Traditionally, tooth polishing after scaling has preceded topical application of fluoride because of the original history-making research of Knutson.[17] Research has since shown that plaque and debris removal can be accomplished adequately by the patient using a toothbrush and dental floss, rather than requiring the more drastic means of professional polishing with a rubber cup and abrasive cleaning agent. The pellicle on the tooth surface does not act as a barrier to fluoride, and fluoride uptake in the enamel from a fluoride application is similar whether the teeth are brushed by the patient or polished with pumice.[18]

   Having a patient brush and floss prior to a topical application provides an excellent opportunity to combine patient instruction with treatment and to utilize the educational principle of participation of the learner. Such an objective has unquestionable value.

2. *Community Program*

   Excellent benefits for caries prevention, many similar to or better than those accomplished by professional topical applications, have been obtained from home and school fluoride-rinsing programs.[19,20] When considering whether the use of a rubber cup with prophylaxis paste is necessary before topical application, the effects of rinsing on a weekly or daily basis without prior polishing should be recognized.

3. *Use of Fluoride Paste*

   A stain removal procedure may be deemed necessary prior to professional fluoride application when stains are not removed during scaling. In that case, a fluoride-containing prophylaxis paste with minimal abrasiveness may be used. Although limited, the fluoride from the paste may replace in part that removed by the abrasive action.[4]

III. TO CONTRIBUTE TO PATIENT MOTIVATION

Removal of plaque must be a *daily* procedure carried out *by the patient*. It must be accomplished thoroughly at least once or twice daily, and for some patients three times daily, if infection is to be controlled and the sanitation of the mouth maintained.

A one-time removal of soft deposits from the teeth at a dental hygiene appointment does not accomplish any long-range preventive purpose because deposits return promptly. It is known that pellicle returns to cover the teeth within minutes after complete polishing; plaque bacteria begin to collect on the pellicle within 1 or 2 hours, increasing in thickness until, by 12 to 24 hours, plaque is thick enough to show clearly when a disclosing agent is applied. Undisturbed, plaque may begin to calcify within a few days in a calculus-susceptible patient (page 280).

The effect of stain removal as a preventive measure for gingival disease or dental caries has not been proven. Smooth polished tooth surfaces may contribute in part to the following effects:

A. Help the instructed patient to obtain more satisfactory results from self-care procedures. A smooth surface should be easier to clean.

B. Show the patient the appearance and feeling of a clean mouth for motivational purposes. The greatest change in behavior, or the true learning, however, can usually be obtained through patient participation in the use of a disclosing agent and personal removal of plaque with floss and toothbrush.

CLINICAL APPLICATION OF SELECTIVE STAIN REMOVAL

Stain removal polishing procedures should never be a substitute for complete calculus removal and root planing as a means for making the tooth surfaces smooth. Smoothing of tooth surfaces is a part of the basic instrumentation and is performed during the final series of strokes for scaling and planing.

Because of the numbers of health and safety factors involved, as have been described, the decision to "polish" should be based on consideration for the individual patient. Instruction for stain prevention is important, as is minimizing for all patients, or omitting for selected ones, the use of the abrasive paste with the rubber cup.

I. SUMMARY OF CONTRAINDICATIONS FOR POLISHING

The following list suggests some of the specific instances in which polishing either should be postponed or is contraindicated indefinitely.

A. No Unsightly Stain
The principle of selective polishing is not to polish unless necessary. Appearance is important to patients, but maintaining the integrity of the tooth surface for disease prevention is also important. When stain is noted on specific tooth surfaces, a stain removal procedure can be applied to selected areas without having to cover all the teeth in a generalized procedure.

B. Characteristics of Patients at Risk for Dental Caries
1. Rampant caries, nursing caries, root caries, all ages.
2. Thin enamel, amelogenesis imperfecta.
3. Demineralized areas.

4. Radiation to head, particularly involving the salivary glands.
5. Xerostomia for any reason.

C. Patients With Respiratory Problems
Power-driven instruments are contraindicated for such conditions as asthma or emphysema when breathing is a problem.

D. Tooth Sensitivity
Abrasive agent uncovers ends of dentinal tubules on area of thin cementum or dentin.

E. Restorations
Restorations and titanium implants may be scratched by polishing abrasive.

F. Newly Erupted Teeth
Incomplete mineralization of surface.

G. Conditions Requiring Postponement for Later Evaluation
1. When instruction for personal plaque removal (daily care) has not yet been given or when the patient has not demonstrated adequate plaque control.
2. Soft spongy tissue that bleeds on brushing or gentle instrumentation.
3. Immediately following deep subgingival scaling and root planing, because abrasive particles can become embedded in the pocket wall and interfere with healing.
4. Communicable disease potentially disseminated by aerosol.

II. SUGGESTIONS FOR CLINIC PROCEDURE

A. Give Instruction First
1. Daily bacterial plaque removal to assist in dental stain control.
2. Tobacco cessation introduction when stain is primarily from tobacco use (see Chapter 27, pages 434 to 438).

B. Remove Stain by Scaling
Whenever possible, stains can be removed during scaling. Unsightly stains can be removed for the new patient initially. At that time, an explanation of the selective polishing principle can be presented and assistance given for a preventive plan for stain control.

C. Remove Stain During Root Planing
The end product of root planing is a smooth, hard surface that does not need further polishing. Abrasive action of polishing paste can scratch the finely planed surface.

D. Minimize Instrumentation
Use a light, intermittent stroke with the rubber cup. Factors affecting the rate of abrasion are described in the next section.

E. Substitute Nonabrasive Agent
Use over-the-counter toothpaste with very light

pressure when stain is missing or minimal but the patient requests the treatment in spite of education.

CLEANING AND POLISHING AGENTS

Traditionally, abrasive agents have been applied with polishing instruments to remove extrinsic dental stains. Abrasives selected should produce smooth tooth surfaces but should not remove tooth structure and surface fluoride or abrade gingival epithelium.

I. FACTORS AFFECTING ABRASIVE ACTION

During polishing, sharp edges of abrasive particles are moved along the surface of a material, abrading it by producing microscopic scratches or grooves. The rate of abrasion, or speed with which structural material is removed from the surface being polished, is governed by characteristics of the abrasive particles, as well as by the manner in which they are applied.

A. Characteristics of Abrasive Particles[21]

1. *Shape.* Irregularly shaped particles with sharp edges produce deeper grooves and thus abrade faster than do rounded particles with dull edges.
2. *Hardness.* Particles must be harder than the surface to be abraded; harder particles abrade faster.
3. *Body Strength.* Particles that fracture into smaller sharp-edged particles during use are more abrasive than are those that wear down with use and become dull and rounded.
4. *Attrition Resistance.* Effective abrasive particles do not dull or become embedded in the surface being abraded; particles with greater attrition resistance abrade faster.
5. *Particle Size (Grit)*
   a. The larger the particles, the more abrasive they are and the less polishing ability they have. Finer abrasive particles achieve a glossier finish.
   b. Abrasive and polishing agents are graded from coarse to fine based on the size of the holes in a standard sieve through which the particles will pass. The finer abrasives are called powders or flours and are graded in order of increasing fineness as F, FF, FFF, and so on. Particles embedded in papers are graded 0, 00, 000, and so on.

B. Principles for Application of Abrasives

1. *Quantity Applied.* The more particles applied per unit time, the faster the rate of abrasion.
   a. Particles suspended in water or other vehicles are present in quantities proportional to the thickness of the paste. These vehicles act as lubricants to reduce the amount of frictional heat produced.
   b. Dry powders or flours represent the greatest quantity that can be applied per unit of time. Frictional heat produced is proportional to the rate of abrasion; therefore, the use of *dry agents* is *contraindicated* for polishing natural teeth because of the potential danger of thermal injury to the dental pulp.
2. *Speed of Application.* The greater the speed of application, the faster the rate of abrasion.
   a. With increased speed of application, pressure must be reduced.
   b. *Rapid abrasion* is *contraindicated* because it increases frictional heat.
3. *Pressure of Application.* The heavier the pressure applied, the faster the rate of abrasion.
   a. Particles to which pressure is applied produce deep grooves at first, but they fracture according to their impact strength. With sufficient pressure, the particles may disintegrate.
   b. *Heavy pressure* is *contraindicated* because it increases frictional heat.
4. *Summary.* When cleaning and polishing are indicated after patient evaluation, the following should be observed:
   a. Use wet agents.
   b. Apply a rubber polishing cup, using low speed.
   c. Use a light, intermittent touch.

II. ABRASIVE AGENTS[21]

The abrasives listed here are examples of commonly used agents. Some are available in several grades, and the specific use varies with the grade. For example, while a superfine grade might be used for polishing enamel surfaces and metallic restorations, a coarser grade would be used for laboratory purposes only.

Abrasives for use daily in a dentifrice must necessarily be of a finer grade than those used for professional polishing accomplished a few times each year. Dentifrice abrasives are described on page 387.

A. Silex (Silicon Dioxide)

1. *XXX Silex:* Fairly abrasive.
2. *Superfine Silex:* Can be used for stain removal from enamel.

B. Pumice

Powdered pumice is of volcanic origin and consists chiefly of complex silicates of aluminum, potassium, and sodium. The specifications for particle size are listed in the *National Formulary*[22] as follows:

1. *Pumice Flour or Superfine Pumice:* Least abrasive, and may be used to remove stains from enamel.
2. *Fine Pumice:* Mildly abrasive.
3. *Coarse Pumice:* Not for use on natural teeth.

C. Calcium Carbonate (Whiting, Calcite, Chalk)
Various grades are used for different polishing techniques.

D. Tin Oxide (Putty Powder, Stannic Oxide)
Polishing agent for teeth and metallic restorations.

E. Emery (Corundum)
Not used directly on the enamel.
1. *Aluminum Oxide (Alumina):* The pure form of emery. Used for composite restorations and margins of porcelain restorations.
2. *Levigated Alumina:* Consists of extremely fine particles of aluminum oxide, which may be used for polishing metals but are destructive to tooth surfaces.

F. Rouge (Jeweler's Rouge)
Iron oxide is a fine red powder sometimes impregnated on paper discs. It is useful for polishing gold and precious metal alloys in the laboratory.

G. Diamond Particles
Constituent of diamond polishing paste for porcelain surfaces.

CLINICAL APPLICATIONS

I. PREPARATION OF ABRASIVES
Agents used for stain removal from the natural teeth and for polishing restorations are mixed with water or other lubricant to facilitate particle movement across the tooth surface and to reduce frictional heat. A quantity of paste can be prepared in advance and kept in a closed jar. Glycerin is added to help as a spreading factor and to prevent splashing during application of the polishing cup.

A. Preparation of Single Quantity
1. Place water or flavored mouthrinse in a dappen dish. Some agents require a specific amount of water.
2. Add the dry agent to saturation and stir.

B. Consistency
The paste should be as moist as possible, but transportable between dappen dish and the teeth.

C. Containers
Two separate containers and rubber cups are used when a cleaning abrasive is used first and followed by a polishing agent.

II. COMMERCIAL PREPARATIONS
Numerous dental prophylactic cleaning and polishing preparations are available. Clinicians need more than one type available to meet the requirements of individual patients.

A. Constituents
Most commercially prepared polishing pastes contain an abrasive; water; a humectant; a binder; and agents for sweetening, flavoring, and color. Approximate proportions and purposes of each constituent with examples are as follows:
1. *Abrasive:* 50% to 60%, main ingredient. Examples: pumice, silicon dioxide.
2. *Water:* 10% to 20%, solvent, provides desired consistency.
3. *Humectant:* 20% to 25%, moisture retainer, stabilizes the ingredients. Examples: glycerin, sorbitol.
4. *Binder:* 1.5% to 2.0%, prevents separation, nonsplatter. Examples: agar, sodium silicate powder.
5. *Sweetener:* Artificial, noncariogenic.
6. *Flavoring and Coloring Agents.*

B. Packaging
Commercial preparations are in the forms of pastes, powders, or tablets. Some are available in measured amounts contained in small plastic or other individual packets that contribute to the cleanliness and sterility of the procedure.

Selection of a preparation has been based on its qualities of abrasiveness, consistency for convenient use, or flavor for patient pleasure.

C. Fluoride Prophylaxis Pastes
1. *Limited Caries Prevention.* Application of fluoride by pastes cannot be considered a substitute for conventional topical application on the basis of present-day research. Although reviews of the research show that moderate caries-preventive effects have been demonstrated, other studies have had minimal or no statistically significant results.[23,24]

    Evaluation of fluoride preparations that become available on the market requires a continuing review of the new research as additional studies are reported. Because the caries prevention that can be expected from the use of prophylaxis pastes is minimal, other means for applying fluoride must be used if the patient is to receive optimum protection by fluorides.
2. *Enamel Surface.* A limitation of the paste preparations is that certain abrasives can remove a thin layer of enamel during polishing.[11] With the removal of the enamel, the outer layer of fluoride is also removed, possibly as fast as it is added from the paste, but this concept has not been researched.
3. *Clinical Application.* Use only an amount sufficient to accomplish stain removal to prevent a child patient from swallowing unnecessary fluoride. The paste may contain 4,000 to 20,000 ppm fluoride ion.[25]

PROCEDURES FOR STAIN REMOVAL (CORONAL POLISHING)

I. PATIENT PREPARATION FOR STAIN REMOVAL

Preparation of the patient includes instruction in plaque control procedures, complete scaling and root planing, and overhang removal. The patient should be informed that polishing is a cosmetic procedure, not a therapeutic one.

A. Bacterial Plaque Control
Stain removal should be withheld until the patient's plaque removal on a daily basis is adequate, so that the deposition of stains can be controlled. When a patient is informed of the relationship between self-care and the recurrence of stains, cooperation may be obtained.

B. Scaling
As much stain as possible should be removed during scaling for calculus removal from the enamel. All stain can be removed during root planing, because the stain is located within the altered cementum.

C. Evaluation
After scaling and other periodontal treatment, an evaluation is made to determine the need for stain removal of teeth and polishing restorations and dental prostheses.

II. ENVIRONMENTAL PREPARATION

Environmental factors were described in Chapters 3 and 4. A topical summary is provided here.

A. Procedures to Lessen the Extent of Contaminated Aerosols
1. Clear the water that will be used for rinsing. Flush water through the tubing for 2 minutes at the beginning of each work period, and for 30 seconds after each appointment.
2. Request patient to rinse with an antimicrobial mouthrinse to reduce the numbers of oral microorganisms before starting instrumentation.
3. Use high-velocity evacuation.

B. Protective Barriers
Protective eyewear and coverall are necessary for the patient. The clinician wears the usual barrier protection, namely, eyewear, mask, gloves, and clinic gown to cover clothing.

III. INSTRUMENTS

Both power-driven and manual instruments may be useful when polishing. All instruments should be used with discretion and in a manner requiring minimal abrasion of the tooth surface. Because tooth structure is removed when an abrasive is used on the enamel, and still more is removed when it is used on dentin or cementum, only a mild abrasive agent is appropriate.

Power-driven implements, floss, and finishing strips are described first, followed by procedures for cleaning a removable prosthesis. In Chapter 41, the removal of bonding agents is presented, and in Chapter 40, the finishing of restorations is described.

THE INSTRUMENTS

I. HANDPIECE

A handpiece is used to hold rotary instruments in the dental unit. It is connected by an arm, cable, belt, or tube to the source of power. The three basic designs are straight, contra-angle, and right angle. Rotary instruments have been classified according to their rotational speeds, designated by revolutions per minute (r.p.m.) as high speed and low (or slow) speed.

A. Ultra or High Speed
1. *Speed:* 100,000 to 800,000 r.p.m.
2. *Uses:* For cavity preparation and other restorative preparations.
3. *Fiberoptic Light:* Better visibility is provided when a fiberoptic light is built into the head of the handpiece. The beam of light is projected onto the field of operation when the handpiece is activated.

B. Low Speed
Typical range is 6,000 to 10,000 r.p.m. Lowest speeds are used for polishing and finishing procedures.

II. PROPHYLAXIS ANGLE

Contra- or right-angle attachment for the handpiece to which polishing devices (rubber cup, bristle brush) are attached.

Many types of prophylaxis angles are available. Some are disposable and others are made of stainless steel and may have hard chrome, carbon steel, or brass bearings. Unless they are disposable, only instruments that can be sterilized should be selected.

III. PROPHYLAXIS ANGLE ATTACHMENTS

A. Rubber Polishing Cups
1. *Types* (Figure 38-1)
   a. Slip-on: With ribbed cup to aid in holding polishing agent.
   b. Slip-on: With bristles inside cup.
   c. Threaded (screw type): With plain ribbed cup or flange (webbed) type.
   d. Mandrel mounted.
2. *Materials*
   a. Natural rubber: More resilient; adapts readily to fit the contours of the teeth.
   b. Synthetic: Stiffer than natural rubber.

B. Bristle Brushes
1. *Types*

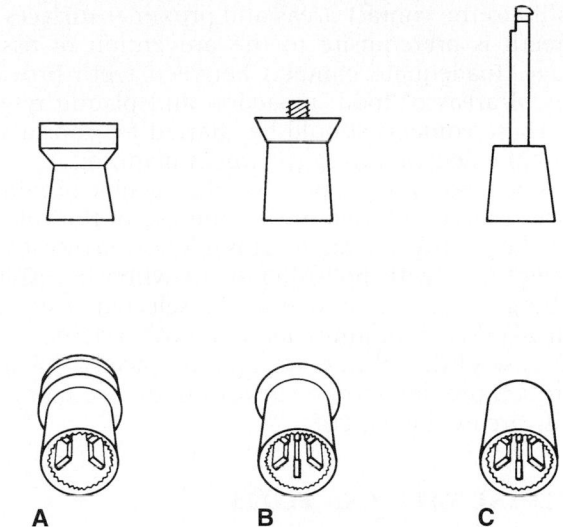

FIGURE 38-1 Rubber Cup Attachments. (A) Slip-on or snap-on for button-end prophylaxis angle. **(B)** Threaded for direct insertion in right angle. **(C)** Mandrel stem for latch-type angle.

  a. For prophylaxis angle: Slip-on or screw type.
  b. For handpiece: Mandrel mounted.
 2. *Materials:* Synthetic.

IV. USES FOR ATTACHMENTS

A. Handpiece With Straight Mandrel
1. Dixon bristle brush (type C, soft) for polishing removable dentures (page 616).
2. Mounted stone for sharpening instruments (page 539).
3. Rubber cup on mandrel for polishing facial surfaces of anterior teeth.

B. Prophylaxis Angle With Rubber Cup or Brush
1. *Rubber Cup:* For removal of stains from the tooth surfaces and polishing restorations.
2. *Brush*
 a. For removing stains from deep pits and fissures and enamel surfaces away from gingival margin. A brush is not recommended for use on exposed cementum or dentin, because they are easily grooved by such an instrument.
 b. For preliminary polishing of amalgam restorations.

USE OF THE PROPHYLAXIS ANGLE

I. EFFECTS ON TISSUES: PRECAUTIONS

The use of power-driven instruments can cause discomfort for the patient if care and consideration for the oral tissues are not exercised to prevent unnecessary trauma.

Awareness of the potential tissue damage is important. Tactile sensitivity of the clinician while using a thick, bulky handpiece is diminished, and unnecessary pressure may be applied inadvertently. Frictional heat may cause pain or discomfort.

Some loss of tooth structure occurs during polishing when an abrasive agent is used. Research on the effects on tooth structure was reviewed on pages 604 to 605.

The greater the speed of application of a polishing agent, the faster the rate of abrasion (page 608). Therefore, the handpiece should be operated at a low r.p.m.

Trauma to the gingival tissue can result from too high a speed, extended application of the rubber cup, or use of an abrasive polishing agent. Tissue damage and the need for antibiotic premedication for risk patients were described on page 604.

II. PROPHYLAXIS ANGLE PROCEDURE

The first technique principle is to apply the polishing agent only where it is needed, that is, where there is unsightly stain. Contraindications were listed on page 607.

As with all oral procedures, a systematic order should be followed. A variety of skills must be learned in using and caring for the equipment.

A. Instrument Grasp
Modified pen grasp (Figure 32-13, page 520).

B. Finger Rest (page 522)
1. Establish firmly on tooth structure.
2. Use a wide fulcrum area when practical to aid in the balance of the large instrument. For example, place cushion of fulcrum finger across occlusal surfaces of premolars while polishing the molars.
3. Avoid use of mobile teeth as finger rests.

C. Speed of Handpiece
1. Use lowest available speed to minimize frictional heat.
2. Adjust r.p.m. by changing the position of the rheostat foot pedal.

D. Use of Rheostat Pedal
1. Apply steady pressure with foot to produce an even, low speed.
2. Keep sole of the foot that activates rheostat pedal flat on the floor. Use toe to activate rheostat pedal.

E. Rubber Cup: Stroke and Procedure
1. Observe where stain removal is needed to prevent unnecessary rubber cup application.
2. Fill rubber cup with polishing agent, and distribute agent over tooth surfaces to be polished.
3. Establish finger rest and bring rubber cup almost in contact with tooth surface before activating power source.
4. Using slowest r.p.m., apply revolving cup

lightly to tooth surface for 1 or 2 seconds. Use a light pressure so that the edges of the rubber cup flare slightly.

5. Move cup to adjacent area on tooth surface; use a patting or brushing motion.

6. Replenish supply of polishing agent frequently.

7. Turn handpiece to adapt rubber cup to fit each surface of the tooth, including proximal surfaces and gingival surfaces of fixed partial dentures.

8. Start with the distal surface of the most posterior tooth of a quadrant and move forward toward the anterior. For each tooth, work from the gingival third toward the incisal third of the tooth.

9. When two polishing agents of different abrasiveness are to be applied, use a separate rubber cup for each.

10. Cups that cannot be sterilized are used only once. Disposable one-use cups are preferred.

F. Bristle Brush

Bristle brushes should be used selectively and limited to occlusal surfaces. Lacerations of the gingiva and grooves and scratches in the tooth surface, particularly the roots, can result.

1. Soak stiff brush in hot water to soften bristles.

2. Distribute mild abrasive polishing agent over occlusal surfaces of teeth to be polished.

3. Place fingers of nondominant hand in a position that both retracts and protects cheek and tongue from the revolving brush.

4. Establish a firm finger rest and bring brush almost in contact with the tooth before activating power source.

5. Using slowest r.p.m., apply revolving brush lightly to the occlusal surface only, avoiding contact of bristles with soft tissues.

6. Use a short stroke in a brushing motion; follow the inclined planes of the cusps.

7. Move from tooth to tooth to prevent generation of excessive frictional heat. Avoid overuse of the brush unnecessarily. Replenish supply of polishing agent frequently.

G. Irrigation

Teeth and interdental areas should be irrigated thoroughly several times with water from the syringe to remove abrasive particles. The rotary movement of the rubber cup or bristle brush tends to force the abrasive into the gingival sulci, thereby creating a potential source of irritation to the soft tissues.

POLISHING PROXIMAL SURFACES

Considerable care must be exercised in the use of floss, tape, and finishing strips. Understanding the anatomy of the interdental papillae and their relationship to the contact areas and proximal surfaces of the teeth is prerequisite to the prevention of tissue damage. Inadequate contacts between teeth provide potential areas of food impaction and plaque retention. These contacts should be charted for consideration by the dentist during treatment planning.

As much polishing as possible of accessible proximal surfaces is accomplished during the use of the rubber cup in the prophylaxis angle. This is followed by the use of dental tape with polishing agent when necessary. Finishing strips are used only in selected instances when all other techniques fail to remove a stain.

The use of dental floss or tape for bacterial plaque control on proximal tooth surfaces is an essential part of self-care by the patient.

I. DENTAL TAPE AND FLOSS

A. Features

Floss and tape were described on pages 372 to 374. The wax covering affords some protection for the tissues, facilitates the movement of the floss or tape, prevents excessive absorption of moisture, and helps to prevent shredding.

Tape is flat and has relatively sharp edges, whereas floss is round. Either floss or tape may injure the tissue when used incorrectly or carelessly.

B. Uses

1. *Tape for Polishing*
   a. Proximal tooth surfaces.
   b. Gingival surface of fixed partial denture.
2. *Floss for Removing*
   a. Debris and food particles. Patient instruction with toothbrush and floss at the beginning of appointment prepares the teeth for scaling.
   b. Particles of polishing agents at completion of polishing procedures.
      i. From interproximal areas and gingival sulci.
      ii. From gingival surface of fixed partial dentures.
   c. Retained abrasive particles after use of finishing strips.

C. Technique for Dental Floss and Tape

Techniques for tape and floss application are described on pages 372 to 374 and illustrated in Figures 24-1, 24-2, and 24-3. The same principles apply whether the patient or the clinician is using the floss. Finger rests must be used to prevent snapping through contact areas.

1. *Polishing With Dental Tape.* Polishing agent is applied to the tooth, and the tape is moved gently back and forth over the area where stain was observed.

2. *Polishing Gingival Surface of a Fixed Partial Denture.* A floss threader is used to position the floss or tape over the gingival surface. Floss threaders are described and illustrated on

page 401. Polishing agent is applied under the pontic, and the floss or tape is moved back and forth.

3. *Flossing After Polishing.* Particles of abrasive agent should be removed by irrigation and by using a clean length of floss applied in the usual manner.

4. *Rinsing and Irrigation.* Irrigate with water-spray syringe to clean out all abrasive agent.

II. FINISHING STRIPS

A. Description

Finishing strips are also known as linen abrasive strips. They are thin, flexible, and tape-shaped, and they are available in four widths—extra narrow, narrow, medium, and wide.

Finishing strips are made of linen or plastic, with one smooth side and the other side that serves as a carrier for abrasive agents bonded to that side. "Gapped" strips are available with an abrasive-free portion to permit sliding the strip through a contact area without abrading the enamel.

They are available in extra fine, fine, medium, and coarse grit. *Only extra narrow or narrow strips with fine grit are suggested for stain removal and then only with discretion.*

B. Use

1. *For Stain Removal on Proximal Surfaces of Anterior Teeth.* When other polishing techniques are unsuccessful.

2. *Precautions for Use*
   a. Edge of strip is sharp and may cut gingival tissue or lip.
   b. Rough working side of strip is capable of removing tooth structure and may make nicks or grooves, particularly in the cementum.
   c. Use of a finishing strip should be limited to enamel surfaces.

C. Technique for Finishing Strip

1. *Grasp and Finger Rest.* A strip no longer than 6 inches is most conveniently applied. The grasp and fulcrum must be well controlled. Protection of the lip by retraction with the thumb and index finger holding the strip is mandatory.

2. *Positioning*
   a. Direct the abrasive side of strip toward the proximal surface to be treated, as the strip is worked slowly and gently between the teeth with a slight sawing motion. Bring strip just through the contact area. If the strip breaks, immediately use floss to remove particles of abrasive.
   b. When a space is clearly visible through an interproximal area and the interdental papilla is missing, a narrow finishing strip may be threaded through. Prepare strip

by cutting the end on a diagonal to facilitate threading.

3. *Stain Removal*
   a. Press abrasive side of strip against tooth. Draw back and forth in a ⅛-inch arc two or three times, rocking on the established fulcrum.
   b. Remove strip. Do not attempt to turn the strip while it is in the interdental area.

4. *Dental Floss.* Follow each application of a finishing strip with dental floss to remove abrasive particles.

AIR-POWDER POLISHING

Principles of selective stain removal are applied to the use of the air-powder polishing system. After plaque control instruction, scaling, and root planing are completed, and follow with an evaluation of a need for stain removal.

I. PRINCIPLES OF APPLICATION

Air-powder polishing is an efficient and effective method for mechanical removal of stain and plaque.[26,27] Air-powder polishing systems use air, water, and sodium bicarbonate to deliver a controlled stream that propels specially processed sodium bicarbonate particles to the tooth surface.[28] The equipment, manufactured by several companies, is operated using inlet air pressure between 40 to 100 psi and inlet water pressure between 20 and 60 psi.

The orifice of the handpiece nozzle should be kept in a constant circular motion, with the nozzle tip 4 to 5 mm away from the enamel surface. The spray is angled away from the gingival margin. The periphery of the spray may be near the gingival margin, but the center should be directed at an angle less than 90° away from the margin.

Complete directions for care of equipment and preparation for use of the device are provided by the various manufacturers.

II. USES OF AIR-POWDER POLISHING

A. Requires less time and physical exertion by the clinician and generates no heat.[29]

B. Sodium bicarbonate is less abrasive than traditional prophylaxis pastes, which makes the air-powder polisher ideal for stain and plaque removal.[30]

C. Removal of heavy, tenacious tobacco stain and chlorhexidine-induced staining.[27,28]

D. Stain and plaque removal from orthodontically banded and bracketed teeth[29,31] and dental implants.[32,33]

E. Prior to bonding procedures.[34]

F. Root detoxification for periodontally diseased roots.[35,36]

III. TECHNIQUE

Proper angulation of the air-powder polishing handpiece is essential to reduce the amount of inherent aerosols created[37-39] and to remove stain and plaque without iatrogenic soft tissue trauma.

A. For Anterior Teeth (Figure 38-2A)
The handpiece nozzle should be placed at a 60° angle to the facial and lingual surfaces of anterior teeth.

B. For Posterior Teeth (Figure 38-2B)
The handpiece nozzle should be placed at an 80° angle to the facial and lingual surfaces.

C. For Occlusal Surfaces (Figure 38-2C)
The handpiece nozzle should be placed at a 90° angle to the occlusal plane.

D. Incorrect Angulation
Incorrect angulation of the handpiece is probably the single most common cause of excess aerosol production. When a clinician directs the handpiece at a 90° angle toward a facial, buccal, and some lingual surfaces, the result is an immediate reflux of the aerosolized spray back onto the clinician. Changing the angle of incidence to the proper angulations of 60° and 80° will result in a change in the angle of the reflection, thus reducing the amount of reflux of aerosolized spray.

IV. RECOMMENDATIONS AND PRECAUTIONS

A. Aerosol Production
A copious spray containing oral debris and microorganisms is produced. As with all contaminated aerosols, a health hazard can exist. Suggestions for minimizing contamination and the effects of the aerosols include the following:
1. Patient uses a preprocedural antibacterial mouthrinse.
2. High-volume evacuation is needed, using a wide tip held near the tooth where the spray is released from the nozzle.[37] A saliva ejector has been shown to be insufficient to reduce bacterial counts in the aerosol.[39]

B. Protective Patient and Clinician Procedures
1. Use protective eyewear, coverall, and hair cover.
2. Lubricate patient's lips to prevent drying effect of the sodium bicarbonate.
3. Do not direct the spray on the gingiva, directly into the gingival sulcus or other soft tissues, which creates patient discomfort and undue tissue trauma.
4. Avoid directing the spray into the periodontal pockets with bone loss or into extraction sites as a facial emphysema can be induced.[40]

V. RISK PATIENTS: AIR-POWDER POLISHING CONTRAINDICATED

The information from the patient's medical history must be reviewed and appropriate applications made. Antibiotic premedication is indicated for all the same patients who are at risk for any dental hygiene procedure (pages 101 to 104).

A. Contraindications
1. Physician-directed sodium-restricted diet.
2. Respiratory disease or other condition that limits swallowing or breathing.
3. Patients with end-stage renal disease.

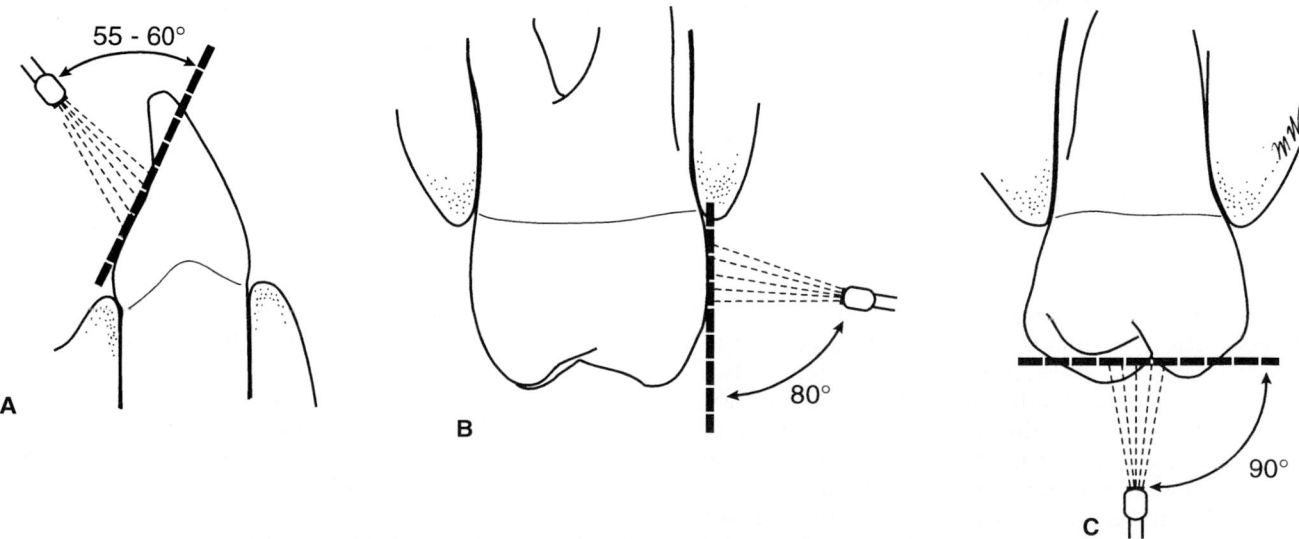

FIGURE 38-2 Air-Powder Polishing. Direct the aerosolized spray for **(A)** the anterior teeth at a 60° angle, **(B)** the posterior teeth facial and lingual or palatal at an 80° angle, and **(C)** the occlusal surfaces at a 90° angle to the occlusal plane.

4. Communicable infection that can contaminate the aerosols produced.

B. Other Contraindications

1. *Root Surfaces.* Routine polishing of cementum and dentin should be avoided. They can be removed readily during air-powder polishing.[35,41,42]
2. *Soft, Spongy Gingiva.* The air-powder can irritate the free gingival tissue, especially if not used with the recommended technique. When heavy stain calls for the use of an air-powder polisher, the patient should be instructed in daily bacterial plaque removal, scaling and root planing should be completed, and the stain removal should be postponed until soft tissue has healed.
3. *Restorative Materials.* The use of air-powder polishing on composite resins, cements, and other nonmetallic materials can cause removal or pitting.[28,43–45] Significant damage to margins of dental castings has been shown.[45]

CLEANING THE REMOVABLE DENTURE

A complete patient service includes the care of the natural teeth and cleaning and polishing of replacements. Complete and partial dentures may accumulate calculus, soft deposits, and stains that may affect the adaptation of the dentures in the mouth, as well as afford a source of irritation to adjacent mucous membranes. The parts of a complete denture are illustrated in Figure 25-13, page 403; the parts of a partial denture are in Figure 25-11, page 402.

A learning experience in the proper care of the dentures can be provided for the patient while the dentures are cleaned professionally. Specific instruction for the patient is described on pages 402 to 407.

I. OBJECTIVES

With professional cleaning of a removable denture, the following benefits can be expected:

A. Patient provided with a review of how to clean and maintain the denture.
B. Aid in preserving the natural teeth associated with a removable partial denture.
C. Removal of calculus and stains, thereby smoothing the surfaces of the denture to lessen plaque and debris retention.
D. Improvement of the appearance and sanitation of the denture.
E. Patient provided with the feeling of complete oral cleanliness.
F. Understanding by the patient of the importance of routine personal and professional care of the denture.

II. REMOVAL OF DENTURE

Usually, the patient removes the denture. The clinician may have occasion to remove dentures for certain patients, particularly those who may be disabled, helpless, or in an emergency situation.

Although denture removal may be complicated by anatomic features of an individual mouth, a general procedure is outlined here. The clinician wears gloves as with all intra-oral procedures.

A. Complete Maxillary Denture

1. Clinician is positioned at 11 to 12 o'clock; left-handed clinician is at 12 to 1 o'clock (see Figure 5-5, page 77).
2. Grasp the denture firmly with the thumb on the facial surface at the height of the border of the denture under the lip and the index finger on the palatal surface.
3. With the other hand, elevate the lip to expose the border of the denture to break the seal.
4. Remove the denture gently in a downward and forward direction.
5. If the retention of the denture cannot be overcome by elevation of the lip, request the able patient to blow into the mouth with the lips closed. This usually breaks the seal.

B. Complete Mandibular Denture

1. Clinician is positioned at 8 to 9 o'clock; left-handed clinician is at 3 to 4 o'clock.
2. Grasp the denture firmly on the facial surface with the thumb and on the lingual surface with the index finger.
3. With the other hand, retract the lower lip forward and remove the denture gently.

C. Partial Denture With Clasps

Exert an even pressure on both sides of the denture simultaneously as the clasps are lifted over their abutment teeth. Usually, the line of insertion and removal of a partial denture is designed and constructed for an even, vertical movement.

III. CARE OF DENTURES DURING INTRA-ORAL PROCEDURES

A. Provide a cleansing tissue for the patient's use when requesting the patient to remove or insert the denture.
B. Receive removable denture in a paper cup or container with a fitted cover. Rinse without splashing.
C. Immerse in antimicrobial solution.
D. Place container in a safe place away from working area to minimize hazard of breakage.

IV. PROCEDURE FOR CLEANING

Ultrasonic cleaning is the procedure of choice for the safety of the denture; for the preservation of the surface finish; for the elimination of the possibility of scratching the denture surface through the use of scalers, polishing agents, or other devices; and for the time saved. When ultrasonic equipment is not available, manual and power-driven instruments must be used.

A. Ultrasonic

1. Principles and procedures were described on page 59.
2. Use the solution designated for stain and calculus removal and follow the manufacturer's directions specifically.
3. Rinse thoroughly and scrub free of solution and loosened debris with a moderately stiff brush before returning the denture to the patient. Brushes reserved for this purpose should be sterilized.

B. Manual and Power-Driven

1. *Removal of Calculus.* Remove calculus by careful scaling. Care must be taken not to scratch the denture.
2. *Method for Holding Denture.* Grasp firmly and securely in the palm of the nondominant hand (see Figures 25-12, page 403 and 25-14, page 406); avoid excessive pressure on a partial denture bar or clasps to prevent bending.
3. *Polishing the Denture.* Polish only the external polished surface of a denture; abrasive applied to the internal impression surface could alter the fit of the denture.
4. *Polishing at the Dental Chair*
   a. Polishing over a cuspidor (lined with a towel) is convenient in some settings. Focus the dental light over the work area.
   b. Polish nonmetal parts with a mounted brush (Dixon C softened in warm water), and use very wet superfine pumice or other appropriate abrasive. The finger rest is maintained on the denture.
   c. Polish metal parts lightly with a rubber polishing cup. A fine polishing agent should be used to prevent scratching the metal.
5. *Polishing on the Dental Lathe in the Laboratory*
   a. Prevention of cross-contamination in the laboratory:
      i. Wear a mask and protective eyewear while working over a lathe.
      ii. Use sterile rag wheel and pumice.
   b. Use a wet rag wheel with fine wet abrasive for nonmetal parts, and use whiting or tin oxide on a separate rag wheel for the metal parts other than clasps. Keep denture and polishing agent wet at all times.
   c. Hold the denture in a two-handed grip. Cover the clasps and denture teeth with fingers to prevent abrasive from scratching the teeth and the clasps from hooking into the rag wheel. The clasps are cleaned later with a wood point in the porte polisher.
   d. Run the lathe at low speed and apply denture carefully. Constantly change the surface applied to the rag wheel to prevent excess frictional heat.
6. *Rinsing the Denture.* Rinse the denture thoroughly under warm (never hot) running water.
   a. Line the sink with a towel, or fill half-full with water, to avoid breakage in case the denture is dropped.
   b. Brush the internal impression surface of the denture using a mild soap or a detergent; rinse thoroughly.
7. *Evaluation.* Evaluate the cleanliness of the denture; examine under bright light and apply compressed air stream to detect calculus or denture plaque.
8. *Disinfection.* Soak the prosthesis in a disinfectant and rinse in water before returning it to the patient. The solution should be fresh for each patient.
9. *Return Denture.* Return the denture to the patient on a paper towel. The denture should be wet for comfortable insertion.

FACTORS TO TEACH THE PATIENT

I. How plaques and stains form on the natural teeth and their replacements.
II. The meaning of selective polishing and why it is not necessary to polish all teeth at every appointment when daily care is effective.
III. Stains and bacterial plaque removed by polishing can return promptly if plaque is not removed faithfully on a schedule of two or three times each day.
IV. Polishing agents utilized during professional coronal polishing are too abrasive for daily home use.
V. The need for adapting toothbrushing and flossing techniques to clean abutment teeth.
VI. The importance of regular cleaning of dentures with special attention to clasps.
VII. How to handle and clean a denture.

REFERENCES

1. **De Leo,** A.A.: The Incidence of Bacteremia Following Oral Prophylaxis on Pediatric Patients, *Oral Surg., 37,* 36, January, 1974.
2. **Micik,** R.E., Miller, R.L., Mazzarella, M.A., and Ryge, G.: Studies on Dental Aerobiology: I. Bacterial Aerosols Generated During Dental Procedures, *J. Dent. Res., 48,* 49, January–February, 1969.
3. **Hartley,** J.L.: Eye and Facial Injuries Resulting from Dental Procedures, *Dent. Clin. North Am., 22,* 505, July, 1978.
4. **Vrbic,** V., Brudevold, F., and McCann, H.G.: Acquisition of Fluoride by Enamel from Fluoride Pumice Pastes, *Helv. Odontol. Acta, 11,* 21, April, 1967.
5. **Kontturi-Närhi,** V., Markkanen, S., and Markkanen, H.: Effects of Airpolishing on Dental Plaque Removal and Hard Tis-

sues as Evaluated by Scanning Electron Microscopy, *J. Periodontol., 61,* 334, June, 1990.

6. **Stookey,** G.K.: *In Vitro* Estimates of Enamel and Dentin Abrasion Associated with a Prophylaxis, *J. Dent. Res., 57,* 36, January, 1978.

7. **Zuniga,** M.A. and Caldwell, R.C.: The Effect of Fluoride-containing Prophylaxis Pastes on Normal and "White-Spot" Enamel, *ASDC J. Dent. Child., 36,* 345, September–October, 1969.

8. **Jefferies,** R.W.: Polishing Dental Enamel, *N.Z. Dent. J., 69,* 167, July, 1973.

9. **Leknes,** K.N.: The Influence of Anatomic and Iatrogenic Root Surface Characteristics on Bacterial Colonization and Periodontal Destruction: A Review, *J. Periodontol., 68,* 507, June, 1997.

10. **Brudevold,** F., Gardner, D.E., and Smith, F.A.: The Distribution of Fluoride in Human Enamel, *J. Dent. Res., 35,* 420, June, 1956.

11. **Vrbic,** V. and Brudevold, F.: Fluoride Uptake from Treatment with Different Fluoride Prophylaxis Pastes and from the Use of Pastes Containing a Soluble Aluminum Salt Followed by Topical Application, *Caries Res., 4,* 158, Number 2, 1970.

12. **Löe,** H.: Reactions of Marginal Periodontal Tissues to Restorative Procedures, *Int. Dent. J., 18,* 759, December, 1968.

13. **Miller,** W.A.: Experimental Foreign Body Reactions to Toothpaste Abrasives, *J. Periodontol., 47,* 101, February, 1976.

14. **Roulet,** J.F. and Roulet-Mehrens, T.K.: The Surface Roughness of Restorative Materials and Dental Tissues after Polishing with Prophylaxis and Polishing Pastes, *J. Periodontol., 53,* 257, April, 1982.

15. **Theilade,** J., Slots, J., and Fejerskov, O.: The Ultrastructure of Black Stain on Human Primary Teeth, *Scand. J. Dent. Res., 81,* 528, Number 7, 1973.

16. **Tilliss,** T.S.I., Stach, D.J., and Cross-Poline, G.N.: Use of Toothpicks for Chlorhexidine Staining, *J. Clin. Periodontol., 19,* 398, July, 1992.

17. **Knutson,** J.W.: Sodium Fluoride Solutions: Technique for Application to the Teeth, *J. Am. Dent. Assoc., 36,* 37, January, 1948.

18. **Tinanoff,** N., Wei, S.H.Y., and Parkins, F.M.: Effect of a Pumice Prophylaxis on Fluoride Uptake in Tooth Enamel, *J. Am. Dent. Assoc., 88,* 384, February, 1974.

19. **Jones,** J.C., Murphy, R.F., and Edd, P.A.: Using Health Education in a Fluoride Mouthrinse Program: The Public Health Hygienist's Role, *Dent. Hyg., 53,* 469, October, 1979.

20. **Birkeland,** J.M. and Torell, P.: Caries-preventive Fluoride Mouthrinses, *Caries Res., 12,* 38, Supplement 1, 1978.

21. **Anusavice,** K.J.: *Phillips' Science of Dental Materials,* 10th ed. Philadelphia, W.B. Saunders Co., 1996, pp. 673–677.

22. **United States Pharmacopeia.** *The National Formulary,* January 1, 1995. United States Pharmacopeial Convention, Inc., 12601 Twinbrook Parkway, Rockville, MD 20852, p. 1342.

23. **Wei,** S.H., Ngan, P.W.K., Wefel, J.S., and Kerber, P.: Evaluation of Fluoride Prophylaxis Pastes, *J. Dent. Res., 60,* 1297, July, 1981.

24. **Ripa,** L.W.: The Roles of Prophylaxis and Dental Prophylaxis Pastes in Caries Prevention, in Wei, S.H.Y., ed.: *Clinical Uses of Fluorides.* Philadelphia, Lea & Febiger, 1985, pp. 45–49.

25. **Burrell,** K.H.: Systemic and Topical Fluorides, in American Dental Association, Council on Scientific Affairs: *ADA Guide to Dental Therapeutics.* Chicago, ADA Publishing Co., 1998, p. 220.

26. **Weaks,** L.M., Lescher, N.B., Barnes, C.M., and Holroyd, S.V.: Clinical Evaluation of the Prophy-jet as an Instrument for Routine Removal of Tooth Stain and Plaque, *J. Periodontol., 55,* 486, August, 1984.

27. **Orton,** G.S.: Clinical Use of an Air-powder Abrasive System, *Dent. Hyg., 61,* 513, November, 1987.

28. **Barnes,** C.M., Hayes, E.F., and Leinfelder, K.F.: Effects of an Airabrasive Polishing System on Restored Surfaces, *Gen. Dent., 35,* 186, May–June, 1987.

29. **Barnes,** C.M., Russell, C.M., Gerbo, L.R., Wells, B.R., and Barnes, D.W.: Effects of an Air-powder Polishing System on Orthodontically Bracketed and Banded Teeth, *Am. J. Orthod. Dentofac. Orthop., 97,* 74, January, 1990.

30. **Lehne,** R.K. and Winston, A.E.: Abrasivity of Sodium Bicarbonate, *Clin. Prev. Dent., 5,* 17, January–February, 1983.

31. **Gerbo,** L.R., Barnes, C.M., and Leinfelder, K.F.: Applications of the Air-powder Polisher in Clinical Orthodontics, *Am. J. Orthod. Dentofac. Orthop., 103,* 71, January, 1993.

32. **Barnes,** C.M., Fleming, L.S., and Mueninghoff, L.A.: An SEM Evaluation of the In-vitro Effects of an Air-abrasive System on Various Implant Surfaces, *Int. J. Oral Maxillofac. Implants, 6,* 463, Number 4, 1991.

33. **Parham,** P.L., Cobb, C.M., French, A.A., Love, J.W., Drisko, C.L., and Killoy, W.J.: Effects of an Air-powder Abrasive System on Plasma-sprayed Titanium Implant Surfaces: An *in vitro* Evaluation, *J. Oral Implantol., 15,* 78, Number 2, 1989.

34. **Scott,** L. and Greer, D.: The Effect of an Air Polishing Device on Sealant Bond Strength, *J. Prosthet. Dent., 58,* 384, September, 1987.

35. **Atkinson,** D.R., Cobb, C.M., and Killoy, W.J.: The Effect of an Air-powder Abrasive System on *in vitro* Root Surfaces, *J. Periodontol., 55,* 13, January, 1984.

36. **Toevs,** S.E.: Root Topography Following Instrumentation, A SEM Study, *Dent. Hyg., 59,* 350, August, 1985.

37. **Barnes,** C.M.: The Management of Aerosols with Airpolishing Delivery Systems, *J. Dent. Hyg., 65,* 280, July August, 1991.

38. **Glenwright,** H.D., Knibbs, P.J., and Burdon, D.W.: Atmospheric Contamination During Use of an Air Polisher, *Br. Dent. J., 159,* 294, November 9, 1985.

39. **Worrall,** S.F., Knibbs, P.J., and Glenwright, H.D.: Methods of Reducing Bacterial Contamination of the Atmosphere Arising from Use of an Air-polisher, *Br. Dent. J., 163,* 118, August 22, 1987.

40. **Finlayson,** R.S. and Stevens, F.D.: Subcutaneous Facial Emphysema Secondary to Use of the Cavi-jet, *J. Periodontol., 59,* 315, May, 1988.

41. **Willmann,** D.E., Norling, B.K., and Johnson, W.N.: A New Prophylaxis Instrument: Effect on Enamel Alterations, *J. Am. Dent. Assoc., 101,* 923, December, 1980.

42. **Galloway,** S.E. and Pashley, D.H.: Rate of Removal of Root Structure by the Use of the Prophy-jet Device, *J. Periodontol., 58,* 464, July, 1987.

43. **Cooley,** R.L., Lubow, R.M., and Patrissi, G.A.: The Effect of an Air-powder Abrasive Instrument on Composite Resin, *J. Am. Dent. Assoc., 112,* 362, March, 1986.

44. **Lubow,** R.M. and Cooley, R.L.: Effect of Air-powder Abrasive Instrument on Restorative Materials, *J. Prosthet. Dent., 55,* 462, April, 1986.

45. **Felton,** D.A., Bayne, S.C., Kanoy, B.E., and White, J.T.: Effect of Air Abrasives on Marginal Configurations of Porcelain-fused-to-metal Alloys: An SEM Analysis, *J. Prosthet. Dent., 65,* 38, January, 1991.

SUGGESTED READINGS

American Dental Association, Council on Dental Materials, Instruments and Equipment, and American Association of Oral and Maxillofacial Surgeons: Air-driven Handpieces and Air Emphysema, *J. Am. Dent. Assoc., 123,* 108, January, 1992.

American Dental Hygienists' Association: Position on Polishing Procedures, *Access, 11,* 29, August, 1997.

Banford, M.: To Polish or Not to Polish? *Can. Dent. Hyg. Assoc./Probe, 24,* 72, Summer, 1990.

Barnes, C.M., Fleming, L.S., and Russell, C.M.: An *in vitro* Evaluation of Commercially Available Disposable Prophylaxis Angles, *J. Dent. Hyg., 65,* 438, November–December, 1991.

Barnes, C.M., Fleming, L.S., and Russell, C.M.: Evaluation of Performance Characteristics of Four Commercially Available Disposable Prophylaxis Angles, *J. Pract. Hyg., 2,* 18, March/April, 1993.

Dean, M.-C., Barnes, D.M., and Blank, L.W.: A Comparison of Two Prophylaxis Angles: Disposable and Autoclavable, *J. Am. Dent. Assoc., 128,* 444, April, 1997.

Fleming, L.S., Barnes, C.M., and Russell, C.M.: An *in vivo* Comparison of Commercially Available Disposable Prophylaxis Angles, *J. Dent. Hyg., 65,* 441, November–December, 1991.

LaBrie, M.: Considerations in Stain Removal from Teeth and Restorations, *DentalHygienistNews, 4,* 13, Summer, 1991.

Landry, D.: Routine Dangers, (Editorial) *Can. Dent. Hyg. Assoc./ Probe, 29,* 117, July/August, 1995.

Nordstrom, N.K., Uldricks, J.M., and Beck, F.M.: Selective Polishing. An Educational Trend in Dental Hygiene, *J. Dent. Hyg., 65,* 428, November–December, 1991.

Nunn, P.F.: "Selective Polishing"—Time for a Change? *Access, 11,* 38, January, 1997.

Parton, B.J.: Selective Polishing, *DentalHygienistNews,* 7, 16, Summer, 1994.

Air-Powder Polishing

Bay, N.L., Overman, P.R., Krust-Bray, K., Cobb, C., and Gross, K.B.W.: Effectiveness of Antimicrobial Mouthrinses on Aerosols Produced by an Air Polisher, *J. Dent. Hyg., 67,* 312, September–October, 1993.

Berkstein, S., Reiff, R.L., McKinney, J.F., and Killoy, W.J.: Supragingival Root Surface Removal During Maintenance Procedures Utilizing an Air-powder Abrasive System or Hand Scaling, An *in vitro* Study, *J. Periodontol., 58,* 327, May, 1987.

Boyde, A.: Airpolishing Effects on Enamel, Dentine, Cement, and Bone, *Br. Dent. J., 156,* 287, April 21, 1984.

Brown, F.H., Ogletree, R.C., and Houston, G.D.: Pneumoparotitis Associated with the Use of an Air-Powder Prophylaxis Unit, *J. Periodontol., 63,* 642, July, 1992.

Dederich, D.N., Gulevich, T., and Reid, A.: The Effect of Rubber Cup vs. an Air-powder Abrasive System on Root Surfaces, *Can. Dent. Hyg. Assoc./Probe, 23,* 135, Fall, 1989.

Gerbo, L.R., Lacefield, W.R., Barnes, C.M., and Russell, C.M.: Enamel Roughness After Air-powder Polishing, *Am. J. Dent., 6,* 98, April, 1993.

Gilman, R.S. and Maxey, B.R.: The Effect of Root Detoxification on Human Gingival Fibroblasts, *J. Periodontol., 57,* 436, July, 1986.

Gutmann, M.E.: Air Polishing: A Comprehensive Review of the Literature, *J. Dent. Hyg., 72,* 47, Summer, 1998.

Logothetis, D.D., Gross, K.B.W., Eberhart, A., and Drisko, C.: Bacterial Airborne Contamination with an Air-polishing Device, *Gen. Dent., 36,* 496, November–December, 1988.

Mishkin, D.J., Engler, W.O., Javed, T., Darby, T.D., Cobb, R.L., and Coffman, M.A.: A Clinical Comparison of the Effect on the Gingiva of the Prophy-jet and the Rubber Cup and Paste Techniques, *J. Periodontol., 57,* 151, March, 1986.

Strand, G.V. and Raadal, M.: The Efficiency of Cleaning Fissures with an Air-polishing Instrument, *Acta Odontol. Scand., 46,* 113, Number 2, 1988.

White, S.L. and Hoffman, L.A.: A Practice Survey of Hygienists Using an Air-powder Abrasive System, an Investigation, *J. Dent. Hyg., 65,* 433, November–December, 1991.

Restorative Materials

Cooley, R.L. and Lubow, R.M.: Effect of Air-powder Abrasive on Glass Ionomer Microleakage, *Gen. Dent., 37,* 16, January–February, 1989.

Cooley, R.L., Lubow, R.M., and Brown, F.H.: Effects of Air-power Abrasive Instrument on Porcelain, *J. Prosthet. Dent., 60,* 440, October, 1988.

Elaides, G.C., Tzoutzas, J.G., and Vougiouklakis, G.J.: Surface Alterations on Dental Restorative Materials Subjected to an Airpowder Abrasive Instrument, *J. Prosthet. Dent., 65,* 27, January, 1991.

Gutmann, M.S.E., Marker, V.A., and Gutmann, J.L.: Restoration Surface Roughness After Air-powder Polishing, *Am. J. Dent., 6,* 99, April, 1993.

Homiak, A.W., Cook, P.A., and DeBoer, J.: Effect of Hygiene Instrumentation on Titanium Abutments: A Scanning Electron Microscopy Study, *J. Prosthet. Dent., 67,* 364, March, 1992.

Huennekens, S.C., Daniel, S.J., and Bayne, S.C.: Effects of Air Polishing on the Abrasion of Occlusal Sealants, *Quintessence Int., 22,* 581, July, 1991.

Kakaboura, A., Vougiouklakis, G., and Mountouris, G.: The Effect of an Air-powder Abrasive Device on the Bond Strength of Glass Ionomer Cements to Dentin, *Quintessence Int., 20,* 9, January, 1989.

Koka, S., Han, J.-S., Razzoog, M.E., and Bloem, T.J.: The Effects of Two Air-powder Abrasive Prophylaxis Systems on the Surface of Machined Titanium: A Pilot Study, *Implant Dent., 1,* 259, Number 2, 1992.

Vermilyea, S.G., Prasanna, M.K., and Agar, J.R.: Effect of Ultrasonic Cleaning and Air Polishing on Porcelain Labial Margin Restorations, *J. Prosthet. Dent., 71,* 447, May, 1994.

Tooth Whitening

Berry, J.H.: What About Whiteners? Safety Concerns Explored, *J. Am. Dent. Assoc., 121,* 223, August, 1990.

Byrne, B.E.: Bleaching Agents, in American Dental Association Council on Scientific Affairs: *ADA Guide to Dental Therapeutics.* Chicago, ADA Publishing Co., 1998, pp. 235–239.

Croll, T.P.: Enamel Microabrasion for Removal of Superficial Dysmineralization and Decalcification Defects, *J. Am. Dent. Assoc., 120,* 411, April, 1990.

Gegauff, A.G., Rosenstiel, S.F., Langhout, K.J., and Johnston, W.M.: Evaluating Tooth Color Change from Carbamide Peroxide Gel, *J. Am. Dent. Assoc., 124,* 65, June, 1993.

Howard, W.R.: Patient-applied Tooth Whiteners, *J. Am. Dent. Assoc., 123,* 57, February, 1992.

Lee, C.Q., Cobb, C.M., Zargartalebi, F., and Hu, N.: Effect of Bleaching on Microhardness, Morphology, and Color of Enamel, *Gen. Dent., 43,* 158, March–April, 1995.

McCracken, M.S. and Haywood, V.B.: Effects of 10% Carbamide Peroxide on the Subsurface Hardness of Enamel, *Quintessence Int., 26,* 21, January, 1995.

Rethman, J.: Tooth Whitening: The Future Looks Bright, *J. Pract. Hyg., 6,* 31, July/August, 1997.

Sterrett, J., Price, R.B., and Bankey, T.: Effects of Home Bleaching on the Tissues of the Oral Cavity, *J. Can. Dent. Assoc., 61,* 412, May, 1995.

Tipton, D.A., Braxton, S.D., and Dabbous, M.K.: Role of Saliva and Salivary Components as Modulators of Bleaching Agent Toxicity to Human Gingival Fibroblasts *in vitro, J. Periodontol., 66,* 766, September, 1995.

Tong, L.S.M., Pang, M.K.M., Mok, N.Y.C., King, N.M., and Wei, S.H.Y.: The Effects of Etching, Micro-abrasion, and Bleaching on Surface Enamel, *J. Dent. Res., 72,* 67, January, 1993.

The Porte Polisher

The porte polisher is a prophylactic hand instrument constructed to hold a wood point at a contra-angle. Figure 39-1A shows an assembled porte polisher.

Manual stain removal is accomplished by applying pressure with the wood point on the tooth surfaces as a moist abrasive is applied. The firm, carefully directed, rhythmic strokes impart a vigorous massage to the periodontal tissues. This is considered beneficial to the periodontal ligament because the periodontal fibers serve as a cushion for the slight movement of the tooth that occurs with the pressure of the instrument.

Fones described the beneficial effects to the gingival margin.[1] He suggested that the gentle bumping of the wood point on the tissue causes a light pressure and release that have a massaging effect in producing a stimulation of the peripheral circulation.

I. PURPOSES AND USES

The entire stain removal procedure may be accomplished with the porte polisher, although such an approach is unusual in routine practice because of the time factor. The porte polisher and the prophylaxis angle are compared in Table 39-1.

Patients can be highly appreciative of smooth, quiet, manual instrumentation. For certain patients, under particular circumstances and for selected procedures, porte polishing is specifically indicated. Functions, purposes, and uses of the porte polisher are suggested as follows:

A. Removes stains from the natural and restored surfaces of the teeth.
B. Effective for cervical areas and exposed cementum or dentin of teeth that are hypersensitive to the heat produced by even a slowly revolving rubber polishing cup. A superfine, unflavored abrasive mixed with water only is appreciated by the patient and may cause less abrasion of tooth structure.
C. Effective for care of titanium implant abutments.
D. Adapts to tooth surfaces that may be inaccessible to a prophylaxis angle, such as the following:
   1. Exposed proximal surfaces of the teeth of patients who have undergone periodontal surgery.
   2. Lingual surfaces of lingually inclined mandibular molars, or distal surfaces of maxillary third permanent molars.
E. Indicated for a patient with an infectious disease to prevent aerosol production and hence disease dissemination.
F. Instrument of choice for application of certain desensitizing agents for exposed cementum and dentin (page 600).
G. Useful for the homebound or bedridden patient when portable power-driven equipment is not available (Chapter 51, pages 761 to 763).
H. Helpful for orientation of small children, disabled patients, or other patients apprehensive of power-driven equipment.

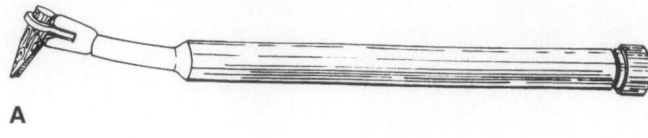

A

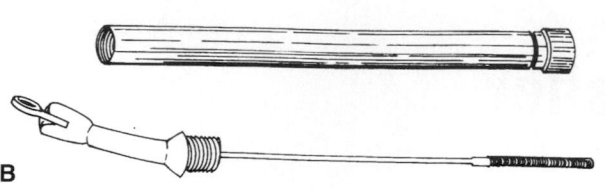

B

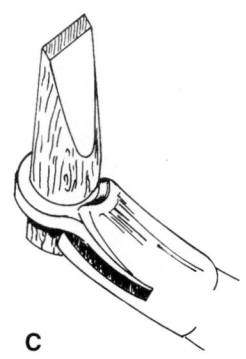

C

■ **FIGURE 39-1 Porte Polisher. (A)** Assembled instrument shows position of wood point ready for instrumentation. **(B)** Disassembled, ready for autoclave. **(C)** Working end shows wedge-shaped wood point inserted.

II. CHARACTERISTICS OF A PORTE POLISHER

Several types of porte polishers are available for use. Practical features that influence selection follow.

A. Can be taken apart conveniently for cleaning and sterilization (Figure 39-1*B*).

B. Does not rust or discolor when given ordinary care.

C. Has convenient adjustment for attachment of wood points of various widths.

D. Is lightweight for comfort of the clinician during use.

E. Has handle of diameter convenient to type of instrument grasp required.

F. Has handle with a finish that resists slipping in the hand during application.

III. SELECTION AND PREPARATION OF WOOD POINTS

Although several kinds of wood, including cedar, maple, and hard pine, have been used for polishing points, orangewood is preferred because it is hard enough to withstand pressure without fraying readily, yet is porous enough to hold polishing agents. Ready-made wood points are available commercially in standard sizes and shapes.

A supply of wood points of routinely used sizes and shapes should be cut, sterilized, and stored in small sealed packages. Wood points should be included in a package or tray for sterilization.

A. Length
1. *Short*
   a. To maintain rigidity of wood.
   b. To prevent unnecessary retraction of cheek and tongue.
2. *Long:* Sufficient length to gain access to tooth surfaces without interference of shank of the porte polisher.

B. Width
1. *Narrow*
   a. To adapt to the variety of tooth surfaces and contours.
   b. To prevent damage to the gingival margins as the point is adapted to the curved tooth surfaces.
2. *Wide:* Sufficient width for efficiency in stain removal.
3. *Recommended Width:* Equal to the diameter of the circular wood point holder of the porte polisher.

C. Shape
1. *Wedge:* For facial, lingual, and proximal surfaces and inclined planes of cusps. Figure 39-1*C* shows a wedge-shaped wood point.
2. *Cone (Pointed):* For occlusal pits and grooves.

D. Position in Handle
Place wood point flush with porte polisher attachment to prevent possible irritation to cheek, lip, or tongue.

IV. USE OF PORTE POLISHER

The principles of technique described in Chapter 32 are applied during manual instrumentation. A systematic order of procedure from one tooth surface to the next surface is prerequisite to thoroughness. Applications of the general principles are included here.

A. Instrument Grasps (pages 520 to 521)
1. *Modified Pen*
   a. Recommended for all surfaces except maxillary anterior facial.
   b. Hold middle finger as near working end of instrument as possible as a guide and support.
2. *Palm* (see Figure 32-14, page 521)
   a. Recommended for maxillary anterior facial surfaces.
   b. Adapt to posterior maxillary facial surfaces when indicated by existing stains.

B. Finger Rest
Securely maintained on firm tooth.

TABLE 39-1 Comparison of the Porte Polisher and the Prophylaxis Angle

Characteristic	Porte Polisher	Prophylaxis Angle
Aerosol production	None; useful for special cases, especially infectious disease	Aerosols produced, as with all powered instruments
Protection of gingiva from trauma	Easy because accomplished by use of slow, even strokes	Difficult to control because of speed at which rubber cup is moving
Danger of abrading enamel and cementum	Minimized	Greater because of faster speed and decreased sense of touch
Stain removal	Removes all stains	Time saved in the removal of gross stains, but steady application of rubber cup could produce heat and remove excess tooth-surface fluoride
Heat	None	Much heat produced
Accessibility to tooth surface	Readily adapted to all surfaces	Limited because of size and weight of handpiece
Clinician's sense of touch	Greater control of instrument is possible because sense of touch is present	Sense of touch is decreased because of weight and size of handpiece
Comfort to patient	Increased because of quietness and lack of discomfort from heat	Decreased because of noise, vibration, and heat produced
Comfort to clinician	Light instrument, less tiring to trained hands	Heavy instrument is tiring to hold
Polishing agent	Less damage because of fewer strokes; agent must be applied wet	Only very fine grain powder should be used; must be applied very wet
Portability	Is portable, therefore useful at any time (for example, for bedridden patient)	Useful only in dental office or with portable motor with power source
Care of instrument	Simple to sterilize	More time required for sterilization and maintenance

C. Strokes

1. *Circular:* Diameter $\frac{1}{16}$ to $\frac{1}{8}$ inch. Apply at cervical third and when adjacent to gingival margin.
2. *Linear*
   a. Horizontal: Back and forth on facial and lingual surfaces of posterior teeth and to proximal surfaces as applicable.
   b. Vertical: Up and down over facial and lingual surfaces of anterior teeth.
3. *Selection of Type and Size*
   a. Provide greatest protection for gingiva.
   b. Provide greatest efficiency in technique in accord with the anatomy of the tooth and the nature and location of the stains.

D. Manner of Operation

1. Apply appropriate grasp and finger rest, then position wood point on the tooth surface.
2. Hand, wrist, and arm rotate to propel the porte polisher.
   a. Fulcrum remains positioned as hand pivots around it.
   b. Fingers remain immobile, except to roll the instrument for adaptation.

E. Pressure Applied

1. Apply a directed, firm, moderate pressure with slow deliberate strokes.
2. Apply increased pressure when circular stroke is directed away from the free gingiva; decrease pressure when the stroke is directed toward the free gingiva.
3. Vary pressure with the tenacity of the deposit or stain to be removed.
4. Balance pressure applied to wood point with finger rest pressure.
5. Effect of excess pressure
   a. Increases hazard of injury to the margin of the free gingiva.
   b. Decreases stability and control during stroke.

SELECTIVE STAIN REMOVAL

I. EVALUATION

A. Preliminary Bacterial Plaque Control

1. Instruction precedes scaling procedures. As

much debridement of plaque as possible is accomplished by the patient during instruction with demonstration.

2. Practice brushing serves to decrease oral microorganisms; object is to make aerosols (produced during instrumentation) less contaminated.

B. Complete Calculus Removal

1. Scaling can remove stains that are incorporated within calculus.
2. Post-treatment procedures include thorough rinsing and irrigation.

C. Evaluation for Need for Stain Removal

1. Principles of selective stain removal are applied (pages 606 to 607).
2. Identify areas with unsightly stain.
3. When no stain remains after instruction, practice, and scaling, apply disclosing agent to determine areas with remaining microbial plaque that warrant professional removal.

II. CLINICAL PROCEDURES

A. Position saliva ejector or prepare for assisted evacuation.
B. Apply paste only to teeth where stain is to be removed.
C. Change wood point as necessary to prevent using one that is splintered or misshaped.
D. Use a fresh wood point when using more than one polishing agent; prevent mixing the abrasives.
E. Rinse and check frequently to determine removal of stain. Do not overpolish.
F. Complete the treatment with a topical fluoride application.

TECHNICAL HINTS

I. Edges of wood points should be trimmed and the wood grain smoothed to minimize splinters that may harm the gingival tissues.

II. As always, thorough flossing and irrigation of sulci following instrumentation with the use of abrasive agent are important because retained particles of polishing agent can be a source of irritation to the gingiva and increase post-treatment discomfort.

III. An iodine disclosing solution applied to green stain prior to polishing tends to facilitate its removal.

FACTORS TO TEACH THE PATIENT

I. The nature, occurrence, and causes of stains.
II. Reasons for dental stain removal: cosmetic but not therapeutic.
III. Benefits of manual instrumentation.
IV. Relationship of plaque and stain accumulation to the frequency and thoroughness of patient's personal oral care habits.

REFERENCE

1. **Fones,** A.C.: *Mouth Hygiene,* 4th ed. Philadelphia, Lea & Febiger, 1934, p. 277.

SUGGESTED READINGS

Alper, M.N.: An Evaluation of Tooth Polishing Techniques, *J. Am. Dent. Hyg. Assoc., 43,* 137, 3rd Quarter, 1969.

Carranza, F.A.: *Glickman's Clinical Periodontology,* 7th ed. Philadelphia, W.B. Saunders Co., 1990, pp. 606–607.

Fones, A.C.: *Mouth Hygiene,* 4th ed. Philadelphia, Lea & Febiger, 1934, pp. 277–289.

Hard, D.: Oral Prophylaxis, in Bunting, R.W.: *Oral Hygiene,* 3rd ed. Philadelphia, Lea & Febiger, 1957, pp. 255–258.

Miller, S.C.: *Textbook of Periodontia,* 3rd ed. Philadelphia, Blakiston Co., 1950, pp. 278–280.

Nield-Gehrig, J.S. and Houseman, G.A.: *Fundamentals of Periodontal Instrumentation,* 3rd ed. Baltimore, Williams & Wilkins, 1996, pp. 477–479.

Sorrin, S., ed.: *The Practice of Periodontia.* New York, The Blakiston Co., Division, McGraw-Hill, 1960, pp. 182–183.

Care of Dental Restorations

Continuing care of dental restorations and supervision of the patient's own care is a significant responsibility during the total dental hygiene preventive service. For a new patient entering the practice for the first time, irregularities of existing restorations are charted and the care plan is prepared to include necessary improvements.

The production and maintenance of smooth dental restorations contribute to the health of the gingiva and periodontal supporting tissues. Bacterial plaque collects and colonizes on a rough surface much more rapidly than on a smooth surface.[1]

Characteristics of an acceptable ideally finished restoration are listed in Table 40-1. With such characteristics and with personal daily care by the patient, the restoration can be expected to contribute to the patient's oral health for a long time.

Suggested care for composite resins, dental ceramics, and dental amalgam is included in this chapter. For all types of restorations the manufacturer's direc-

tions are followed. The research on dental materials is ongoing, and dental professionals are constantly on the alert for changes in procedures and requirements. Box 40-1 defines key words relating to finishing and polishing restorations.

I. RATIONALE FOR FINISHING AND POLISHING

Finishing and polishing restorations contribute to the following effects:

A. Improved gingival health because of less plaque retention by restorative irregularities.
B. Improved compatibility of the restorative material with the oral soft tissues.
C. Increased integrity of the junction of tooth surface and restoration.
D. Improved maintenance by the patient; plaque is more easily removed by brush and floss from smooth surfaces.
E. Increased length of service of the restoration

TABLE 40-1 Characteristics of an Acceptable Finished Restoration

Normal smooth anatomic contours
Contact areas intact with normal form
Embrasures spaced correctly
Refined margins
Smooth resistant surfaces
Functional effectiveness
Acceptable appearance
No plaque-retaining irregularities
Restored health of the gingival tissues

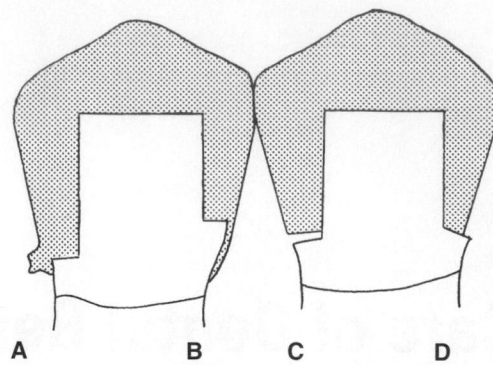

FIGURE 40-1 Proximal Irregularities. (A) Overhang. **(B)** Flash. **(C)** Open or deficient margin. **(D)** Undercontoured margin that can result from an improperly placed matrix band or misdirected carving.

by eliminating factors that lead to surface changes and recurrent dental caries.
F. Improved appearance of the restorations.

II. LONGEVITY OF RESTORATIONS

The initial factors that influence the length of time a restoration maintains its form and function include the following:
A. Design of the cavity preparation.
B. Mix and manipulation of the dental material.
C. Prevention of contamination during insertion.
D. Finishing and polishing.
E. Care of the completed restoration by a daily preventive program of bacterial plaque control, low cariogenic diet, and fluoride application, combined with maintenance supervision at professional appointments.

MARGINAL IRREGULARITIES

A restoration should follow the normal contours of the tooth. Excesses and deficiencies must be recognized and differentiated, so that finishing and polishing procedures can be carried out effectively. Certain deficiencies must be corrected by replacement of the restoration.

Common irregularities and defects of restorations are defined and described here.

I. OVERHANGING MARGIN

An overhang is illustrated in Figure 40-1A. Proximal overhangs result primarily from improper placement of the matrix band and wedge. Overhangs may occur on any tooth surface, supra- or subgingivally, in any class of cavity. They may be caused by errors of manipulation and finishing.

II. FLASH

A. Occlusal
Figure 40-2A illustrates an occlusal feather ledge or flash that was left during carving. When performed correctly, carving brings the cavosurface margin into view and makes the filling material flush with the enamel.

B. Proximal-Gingival
A proximal-gingival flash-type overhang can result when a restoration is packed between a matrix band and the tooth surface below the cavity preparation (Figure 40-1B). The irregularity can occur when a proximal wedge is not used or not positioned to adapt the matrix tightly against the tooth surface. A tooth with a concave proximal surface is most vulnerable to flash.

III. OPEN MARGIN

An open margin is found when there is a distinct space between the restoration and the wall of the cavity preparation (Figure 40-1C).

IV. UNDERCONTOURED

The opposite of an overhang is a deficiency of restorative material between the margin and the cavity wall, as shown in Figure 40-2D. On the proximal surface, causes may be related to improper placement of the matrix or wedge.

Undercontouring also is exemplified by missing contact areas, flattened cervical ridges, incomplete marginal ridges, and incomplete filling of the cavity preparation.

V. OVERCONTOURED

An overcontoured restoration has an excess of material in such a position as to change the normal anatomic form of the restoration. Interproximally overcontoured surfaces may widen the contact area or narrow the embrasure. When the crown is overcontoured, the effect can be plaque retention and pressure on the gingival margin.

In Figure 26-1C (page 413), overcontoured crowns of a double abutment have narrowed the embrasure. Problems of plaque control for the overcontoured crowns are illustrated in Figure 26-4 (page 416).

BOX 40-1 KEY WORDS: Care of Restorations

Abrasion: a wear process.

Amalgam: an alloy of one or more metals in combination with mercury. A dental amalgam contains silver, copper, tin, and other metals.

Burnishing: process of smoothing a surface by rubbing lightly with a specially designed instrument or cotton pellet. The effects are improved marginal adaptation and increased hardness.

Carving: the removal of excess filling material, using special instruments. The goal is to produce accurate anatomic contours and restore form and function to the tooth.

Cavosurface junction: the junction of any wall of a cavity preparation with the unprepared tooth structure.

Ceramics: compounds containing one or more metals and a non-metal that yield substances that are strong, brittle, hard, and inert conductors.

Composites: filled resins that are chemically cured, light cured, or light activated and chemically cured. Used for tooth-colored esthetic restorations.

Macrofilled: small particle resin filled with glass or quartz. Strong, but not easily polished.

Hybrid: mix of macrofill and microfill particles. Used in both anterior and posterior applications. Most are wear and fracture resistant, very polishable.

Microfilled: very finely ground silica filler, not as strong and tend toward brittleness. Anterior use due to high luster and polishability.

Corrosion: chemical and electrochemical deterioration on the surface and the subsurface of an amalgam restoration that usually begins as a tarnish. Caused by environmental factors, such as air, moisture, acid or alkaline solutions, or other chemicals. Corrosion at the margin can cause deterioration and fracturing, resulting in plaque accumulation. By-products can be carried to the dentin and show a discoloration around the restoration.

Direct restoration: placed and formed in the cavity preparation; includes amalgam, composite resins, and glass-ionomer cement.

Ditching: formation of a gap or groove between the cavity preparation margin and the restorative material.

Finishing: process that involves removing marginal irregularities, defining anatomic contours, and smoothing away surface roughness of a restoration.

Flash: type of overhang in which a thin layer of restoration extends beyond the cavosurface junction; also called a feather ledge.

Glass-ionomer: combines glass-ionomer cement with light curing resins. Good thermal expansion, strength, bonding ability. Exhibits anti-caries activity.

Indirect restoration: formed on a die reproduction of prepared tooth; includes porcelain, gold inlays, and porcelain crowns.

Margination: process of removing excess restorative material and applying finishing techniques to re-establish a smooth, well-adapted cavosurface margin. The resultant junction should conform in shape and normal anatomic characteristics.

Overcontour: an excess of restorative material such that the normal anatomic form is altered.

Overhang: area of a restoration where the restorative material extends outward past the cavosurface margin of the cavity preparation. Associated with gingival and periodontal disease, due to mechanical impingement and plaque retention.

Polishing: process carried out after placement of a restoration to remove minute scratches from the surface of a restoration and obtain a smooth, shiny luster. Also applied after other refinishing techniques to produce unscratched, homogeneous surface. Uses abrasive agents to remove roughness, eliminate pits or grooves, and make the surface more resistant to bacterial accumulation.

Porcelain: ceramic material bonded to the facial surface of teeth, as in a veneer.

Recontour: instrumentation to reshape and remove marginal excess and to restore the natural anatomic form.

Resin: organic paste, filled or unfilled. Filled contains glass or silica particles; unfilled has no filler particles.

Tarnish: a discoloration of the surface of a metal restoration, usually from sulfides. Caused by lack of cleanliness, plaque accumulation, and certain foods.

Veneer: a porcelain or composite facing that is applied to the facial surfaces of anterior teeth for esthetic reasons.

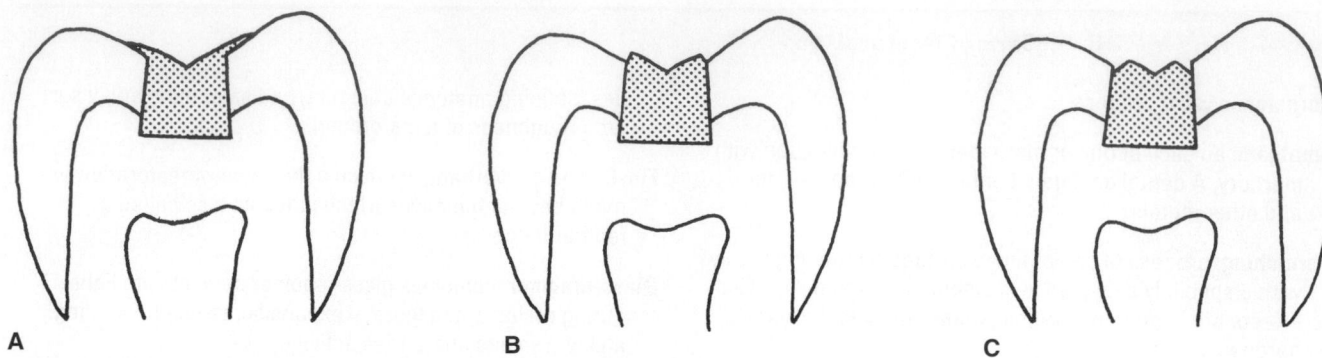

A   B   C

■ **FIGURE 40-2 Marginal Irregularities. (A)** Flash on the occlusal surface related to a Class I restoration. Flash refers to a thin layer of restoration that extends over the margin of the cavity preparation. **(B)** Irregular margin results when the flash breaks off. **(C)** Ditching results from broken off flash.

VI. DITCH OR GROOVE

Figure 40-2*C* shows a gap on the occlusal surface, where either the flash broke off or contraction of the material caused the restoration to pull away from the tooth structure. Plaque retention can lead to recurrent caries in such an area.

OVERHANGING RESTORATIONS

Recontouring overhanging restorations is an essential part of dental and periodontal treatment. Care planning for initial therapy, or Phase I periodontal therapy, must include the correction of overhangs if gingival and periodontal health is to be restored.[2]

I. IDENTIFICATION

A. Clinical

An overhang is identified by its relation to the gingival margin (supra- or subgingival), its location on a specific tooth surface (enamel, cementum, or dentin), its size or extent, and questioning the patient regarding floss breakage and food impaction. From these data, the required finishing procedures can be selected for a specific care plan.

B. Radiographic Examination

Overhangs on surfaces other than proximal are rarely visible on radiographic examination. Visibility of proximal surface overhangs depends on angulation of the x ray. In other words, radiographic examination for extent and location confirmation of overhangs should be a supplementary procedure to examination using an explorer. The entire outline of each restoration must be explored.

A magnifying glass is recommended for examining radiographs for Type I overhangs. Adjacent and undermining carious lesions are seen more definitively when magnification is used.

II. EFFECTS OF OVERHANGS

A. Relation to Periodontal Disease

Because overhanging restorations harbor plaque and hinder plaque removal by the patient, they are considered significant iatrogenic contributing factors in periodontal disease development. In the presence of overhangs, plaque collects in greater amounts and inflammation is more severe than in teeth that do not have overhangs.[3–5] Increased bone loss adjacent to overhangs has been demonstrated.[3,6]

Removal of overhangs is beneficial to the periodontal tissues. Combined with scaling and plaque control, a marked improvement in the periodontal condition has been shown after overhang removal.[4,7]

B. Problems of Bacterial Plaque Control

1. *Irregular Margins.* Overhangs catch and tear dental floss.
2. *Areas Inaccessible for Brush.* Under the ledge of a proximal overhang is inaccessible for the direct application of a toothbrush and other plaque removal aids.
3. *Gingival Enlargement.* Inflammation caused by bacterial plaque held by the overhang.
4. *Debris Retention.* Contributes to halitosis and a general lack of oral sanitation.

C. Dental Caries

Marginal irregularities harbor microorganisms in an environment conducive to the formation of secondary caries.

III. INDICATIONS AND CONTRAINDICATIONS FOR REMOVAL OF OVERHANGS

All overhanging restorations should be corrected, or removed and replaced for the health of the periodontium. Whether a certain overhang can be removed by finishing procedures or whether it must be replaced with a new restoration is a professional decision that must be made.

Guidelines for selection of the correct procedure are suggested here. Contraindications for finishing procedures apply to all restorations of any size or location.

A. Indications for Maintaining the Restoration

1. Tooth anatomy can be maintained or improved to conform with normal contour.
2. The overhang is small or moderate in size.
3. Proximal contact is intact.
4. No adjacent secondary dental caries is present.
5. There are no fractures at the cavity margin of the tooth or the filling, and no large fractures of the restoration.
6. The overhang is accessible for the instrumentation necessary for finishing and polishing without damaging the adjacent tooth structure or traumatizing the gingival tissues.

B. Indications for Removal and Restoration

1. The overhang is extensive and would require a long time to recontour completely.
2. Secondary marginal or undermining dental caries is present.
3. The contact area must be restored.
4. Fractures, chips, cracks, or broken margins are apparent.
5. If replacement will be delayed, a gross overhang should be reshaped and smoothed to make plaque control possible.

CONSIDERATIONS DURING INSTRUMENTATION

I. ANATOMIC

A. Cementum
When a restoration extends near or into the cementum, care must be taken to prevent ditching or grooving the cementum. Cementum is softer than enamel and therefore can be damaged more easily.

B. Tooth Form and Position
Concave surfaces such as the mesial surfaces of the maxillary first premolars and the mesial surfaces of the mandibular first molars, require special adaptations of instruments. Other problem areas are created by tooth rotations, inclinations, and other malpositions.

C. Gingival Tissues
Restorations may be partially or wholly covered by enlarged gingival tissue related to bacterial plaque accumulation.

When the papillae are bulbous, enlarged, and bleed easily on manipulation, plaque control and supervision should be provided first to improve the health of the tissue before undertaking margination procedures. Waxed floss can be used by the patient so that less tearing and shredding will occur when the floss is passed under the overhang.

II. INSTRUMENTATION

A. Finger Rests
Use secure finger rests to allow precision techniques. Prevention of damage to surrounding tooth structure, as well as preservation of tooth anatomy, is essential.

B. Contact Area
Avoid the contact area. It was created for a new restoration by a smooth, polished matrix band and requires no additional smoothing. Polishing agents can remove a layer of restorative material, which would alter the contour and contact.

COMPOSITE RESINS

Composite resins are filled resins composed of an organic resin matrix and an inorganic filler of differing particle size (macrofilled, microfilled, or hybrid). They are chemically cured, light cured, or light activated and chemically cured.

I. USES

A. Class III, IV, and V restorations (see Table 14-3, page 241)
B. Veneers for teeth that have been intrinsically stained by drugs or chemicals
C. Fill spaces such as diastemas
D. Enhance the size or contour of small or misshapen teeth
E. Pit and fissure sealants, filled and unfilled

II. CHARACTERISTICS

When explored, composites feel softer than enamel or porcelain. Composites are esthetic, fracture and wear resistant, color stable, and they come in a range of shades.

III. FINISHING COMPOSITES

Composite resins are finished, and polishing is completed at the time of insertion of the restorative material. Each manufacturer of composite material has recommended finishing and polishing materials and procedures. The systems are used in sequence from most abrasive to least abrasive. The manufacturer's product guidelines are to be followed.

A. Margination
Accomplished through sequenced finishing burs, diamond stones, and carbide burs.

B. Manual Instruments
Knives and carbide-tipped carving instruments may be used.

C. Power-Driven Instruments

1. *Types:* Selected according to the type of resin used:
   a. Abrasive finishing discs
   b. Ultrafine diamonds
   c. Medium grit burs
   d. Carbide burs
   e. White and green stones
   f. Flexible wheels and points
   g. Reciprocating action device
3. *Shapes*
   a. Discs fit broad, flat surfaces and incisal edges.
   b. Bullets or flame points fit lingual aspects of anteriors and occlusal surfaces of posteriors.
   c. Cups fit gingival margins and posterior occlusal surfaces.
   d. Pointed cone shape fits subgingival flash and tight proximal surfaces.

IV. POLISHING COMPOSITES

A. Debridement

1. *Examine.* Identify the dental material so mistakes cannot be made by using the incorrect treatment.
2. *Debridement.* Use sharp curets with a gentle stroke; avoid unnecessary pressure that could gouge the restoration.

B. Use Selective Polishing Only

1. *Plaque Removal.* Have patient clean the teeth using a soft toothbrush to remove bacterial plaque; combine with personal instruction.
2. *Examine for Stain.* If no stain, no polishing is needed.
3. *Polishing Indicated.* Use slow-speed handpiece in a wet environment; apply with light pressure for no longer than 30 seconds.
4. *Polishing Paste.* Use aluminum oxide paste only; never use diamond polishing agent on a composite resin restoration.
5. *Proximal Surfaces.* Apply paste to proximal surfaces using dental floss.

C. Heavier Stain Removal

1. *Avoid.* Ultrasonic and sonic scaling, and air-powder polishing devices.
2. *Graded Materials.* Use fine to coarser, and after stain is removed use fine again to smooth the surface.
3. *Rinse.* Between graded particles, rinse away larger particles before applying smaller to prevent continuing abrading of the surface.

D. Follow With a Neutral Sodium Fluoride Application

PORCELAIN

A ceramic or porcelain restoration is an indirect restoration and is completed in the laboratory before insertion.

I. TYPES

There are several types of porcelain. A high-fusing material is used for denture teeth, medium-fusing for ceramic restorations, and low-fusing in metal-ceramic restorations.

II. USES

A. Inlays, onlays, crowns
B. Laminate veneers
C. Porcelain fused to metal crowns

III. CHARACTERISTICS

The restorations are characterized by their tooth-colored, esthetic appearance; chemical inertness; high hardness; brittleness; and susceptibility to tensile or flexural fracture. They are generally more esthetic than composites due to stain and abrasion resistance, as well as luster retention over time.

IV. POLISHING PORCELAIN

Since porcelain restorations are cast in a laboratory and finished during placement, margination or finishing using stones or burs during the dental hygiene appointment should be unnecessary.

A. Debridement

1. *Curet.* Debride deposits with sharp curets for better tactile sensitivity.
2. *Avoid.* Sickle scalers, ultrasonics, and air polishers can scratch the glaze of porcelain and damage the bonding cement. Also avoid ordinary polishing agents.

B. Polishing Agent

Polish with porcelain polishing paste unless resin cement or cementum are exposed. In that case, use aluminum oxide polishing paste.

C. Routine Maintenance Procedure

1. Use a low-speed handpiece.
2. Apply special paste for porcelain with a cotton-tipped applicator to the restoration.
3. Put a drop of water in a soft, flexible rubber cup or on a felt disc; polish for 15 to 30 seconds.
4. Dilute the paste with water as the polishing progresses.
5. Floss the paste on proximal surfaces.
6. Rinse and dry, then evaluate.
7. If proximal stain is present, aluminum oxide polishing strips may be used conservatively.

D. Follow With a Neutral Sodium Fluoride Application.

AMALGAM RESTORATIONS

Amalgam has been a leading restorative material for many years. The extent of finishing necessary for a new restoration depends on the carving and burnishing performed at the time the restoration was placed.

The restoration that fulfills ideal, normal anatomic and functional requirements needs little smoothing of margins and surfaces before polishing. On the other hand, an "old" filling may have many irregularities of the margins from changes over the years.

I. PROPERTIES AND AGE CHANGES

A. Surface Changes

1. *Tarnish.* Tarnish is primarily a sulfide caused by lack of oral cleanliness, plaque collection, and certain foods containing sulfur; occurs less frequently on properly finished and polished restorations.
2. *Corrosion.* Corrosion is caused by environmental factors such as air, moisture, acid or alkaline solutions, and other chemicals. Polished amalgam resists corrosion.

   Corrosion at the margin of the restoration can cause deterioration and fracture, leaving an open gap where plaque collects and recurrent dental caries can occur. The products of corrosion may be carried into the dentinal tubules, and the entire area around the restoration may appear bluish-black.

B. Dimensional Changes

1. *Expansion.* The amalgam appears extruded above the cavosurface margin; caused by incomplete trituration and condensation or moisture contamination during mixing and placing.
2. *Contraction.* The amalgam pulls away from the cavosurface margin. Contraction is a cause of ditching (page 626).

C. Strength Changes

Fractures are a result of insufficient strength. A fracture may be seen as a gross irregularity, a crack line across an entire restoration, or a marginal chip. Several factors can contribute to amalgam fractures, including the following:

1. Manipulation of the filling material.
2. Overload of pressure on a restoration before setting is complete.
3. Inadequate strength of surrounding tooth structure.
4. Improper carving of the restoration.
5. Occlusal pressures.
6. Finishing procedures.

II. FINISHING

Amalgam is finished and carved, but at least 24 hours setting time is required before polishing. Dental hygienists frequently complete the finishing and polishing at the second appointment.

After the amalgam is condensed, excess material is removed and the anatomic form of the tooth is restored by carving and contouring. When the setting time is completed, margination follows, in preparation for polishing. All of the steps of margination and polishing apply to the renewal of an old restoration as well as the newly placed one.

MARGINATION

I. PROCEDURES SUMMARIZED

A. Remove excess amalgam and overhangs.
B. Finish all cavosurface margins to ensure continuous, uninterrupted, smooth relationships.
C. Smooth all surfaces of the restoration.

II. MANUAL INSTRUMENTS

A. General Suggestions for Use

1. *Instrument Selection.* Select on basis of accessibility, amount of reduction required, and surface finish desired.
2. *Sharp.* Maintain sharp instruments. The object is to remove, not burnish, excess amalgam in small increments and prevent amalgam fracture.
3. *Technique.* Work deliberately and carefully to prevent damage to gingival tissue and uninvolved tooth surfaces, especially cementum.
4. *Follow Tooth Anatomy.* Use the tooth surface as a guide to the contour of the restoration. The instrument is moved parallel with or diagonal to the margin.

B. Amalgam Knife (Figure 40-3)

1. Hold the knife blade across the tooth structure and amalgam, and activate the knife diagonally across the junction.
2. Use short, overlapping shaving strokes to remove amalgam in small increments. Prevent risk of fracture of the margins.
3. For proximal adaptation, move the knife away from the gingiva to prevent amalgam bits from being pushed into the gingiva. Continuous evacuation is recommended.

C. File (Figure 40-3)

1. Determine from the design of each file whether it is intended for a pull or a push stroke, and position the file accordingly.
2. Remove the bulk of the amalgam with coarser files; refine marginal smoothness with finer files.
3. Overlap tooth and amalgam together during a stroke to prevent ditching, gouging, or leaving a deficiency.
4. Begin on the outermost portion of the margin, and work inward toward the contact area.
5. Use short, controlled pull strokes with light to moderate pressure.

D. Cleoid and Discoid Carvers (Figure 40-3)

1. Refine fossae and fissures with a small sharp cleoid (the pointed tip). The discoid is not used in occlusal fossae because the effect

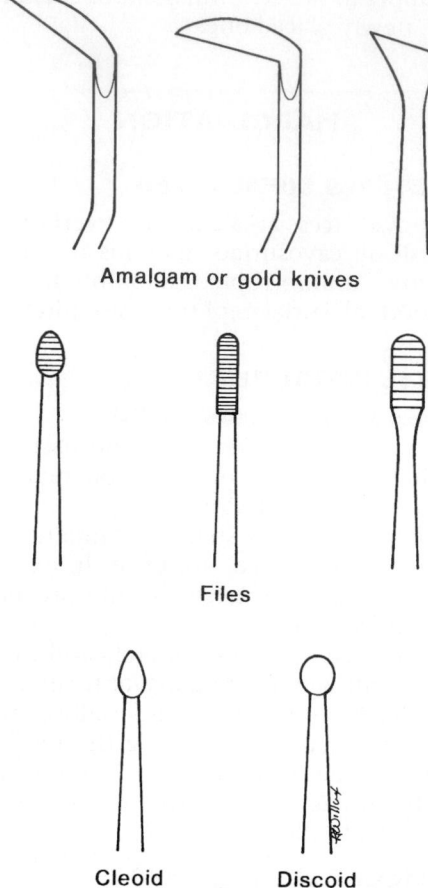

Amalgam or gold knives

Files

Cleoid   Discoid

FIGURE 40-3 Instruments for Margination. Amalgam and gold foil knives; various shapes of files; and the amalgam carvers, cleoid and discoid, especially useful for margination.

would be one of scooping out and making a rounded channel.

2. Use the discoid as an aid for redefining cavo-surface margins.

E. Finishing Strips

1. Use narrow, fine or medium strips after gross amalgam has been removed by amalgam knife or file.
2. Avoid contact area with abrasive finishing strip.
   a. Cut end of strip on diagonal to thread the strip through an embrasure.
   b. Strips with a gap or middle area without abrasive are available to make it possible to position the strip from the occlusal or incisal aspect.
3. Position strip over the amalgam at the cavo-surface margin. Avoid pressure of the abrasive strip on the adjacent tooth structure, especially cementum, to avoid making grooves.

F. Scaler

Only a strong scaler should be used. A scaler tip

can be broken easily if applied with much force. Using a metal cutting edge on the amalgam dulls the instrument rapidly.

G. Curet

A universal curet can smooth a proximal surface further. Use in oblique, horizontal, and vertical directions, overlapping the strokes.

III. POWER-DRIVEN INSTRUMENTS

A. General Suggestions for Use

Power-driven instruments can create heat, which is detrimental. Pressure and heat can produce vapors and aerosols. With careful techniques, detrimental effects will be minimized.

1. *Effects of Overheating*
   a. Irreversible pulp damage.
   b. Alteration of the chemical structure of the restorative material can occur, and the longevity of the restoration can be compromised.
   c. Patient discomfort from tooth sensitivity.
2. *Margins.* Use caution along the gingival margins, so that no damage is caused to adjacent soft tissues.
3. *Low Speed.* Use only low-speed handpiece, with intermittent, light strokes in a multi-directional motion.
4. *Keep Cool.* Use water and/or air for cooling.
5. *Evacuation.* Use high-velocity evacuation.

B. Finishing Burs and Stones

1. Select the shape appropriate for accessibility and visibility:
   a. Flame recommended for narrow embrasures.
   b. Round recommended for fossae and grooves.
   c. Pear recommended for cusp inclines.
2. Green stones are more abrasive than white stones:
   a. Green stones are used for removing excess.
   b. White stones are used for marginal discrepancies and fine, limited surface reduction.
3. Position the bur or stone to permit the remaining enamel to guide the contour produced. The instrument is held across the cavosurface margin and then moved diagonally to prevent fracture or ditching.
4. Keep the bur or stone in constant motion with a light, sweeping movement to reduce the possibility of leaving marks and grooves.

C. Discs (Figure 40-4)

1. Select abrasivity of discs in accord with objective. Coarse discs remove bulk more readily, but they also may be more damaging to surrounding tissues and tooth structure. The most commonly used are garnet (coarse) and cuttle (fine).

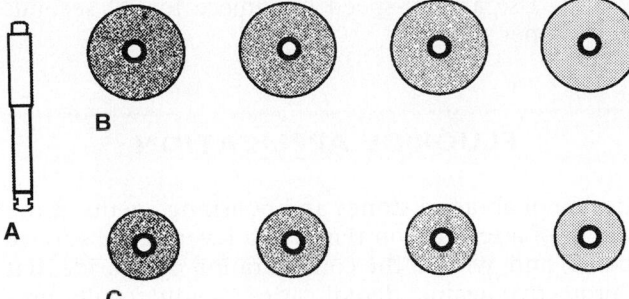

FIGURE 40-4 Use of Discs. Discs are available in several sizes, some with moisture-resistant backings. Abrasive devices are used in sequence in descending order of abrasiveness, coarse to fine. The mildest possible should be selected at the start to prevent unnecessary removal of material or tooth structure. **(A)** Mandrel for holding discs. **(B)** and **(C)** Two sizes of discs shaded to represent coarse to fine.

2. Do not reduce tooth structure.
3. Activate the disc for contouring and smoothing the proximal surface in a position that prevents flattening of the restoration and removing restorative material near the contact area.
4. Use short, overlapping strokes with a sweeping motion diagonally across the cavosurface margin. Rotate the disc from the tooth structure to the restoration to reduce chance of ditching.
5. Move discs away from the gingival tissues.

D. Reciprocating Action Device[8]
1. *Description.* A reciprocating motion handpiece has a variety of wedge-shaped abrasive tips that fit into a cylindrical piston of the friction grip handpiece head. The handpiece operates in a fixed mode or a self-steering mode to allow flexibility and adaptability.
2. *Inserts.* Variously shaped and sized, color-coded, autoclavable tips are used for shaping and recontouring.
3. *Abrasiveness.* Each tip has one side embedded with diamond particles ranging in abrasiveness from supercoarse to superfine. The opposite side is smooth to prevent tooth or gingival tissue damage.
4. *Polishing.* Disposable, hollow plastic polishing tips come in various sizes and allow filling with polishing paste.
5. *Procedure*
   a. Removal of the overhang is accomplished by choosing appropriate abrasive tips in descending order of abrasiveness as the bulk is reduced. Place the abrasive side against the restoration. Activate using light, consistent pressure and a firm fulcrum, moving constantly, adapting to the contours of the restorations.

b. Begin at the most cervical area and move toward the contact. Check frequently with explorer until tooth and restoration are flush.
c. Polishing is accomplished with a series of progressively finer abrasives, beginning with a wet slurry of fine pumice in the disposable polishing tip, rinsing, and repeating the process with a tin oxide slurry. Interproximal polishing can also be accomplished using dental tape with the sequenced abrasives.
d. Rinse and evacuate to ensure complete debris removal.

E. Ultrasonics
Certain models of ultrasonic machines have special tips designed for removal of overhanging margins. The device can be helpful for removal of gross overhangs prior to the use of finer instruments. The precautions for use of ultrasonic instruments are listed on page 556.

F. Re-evaluation
Gingival and periodontal tissues are ideally re-evaluated 4 to 6 weeks after the margination procedure. Status is recorded in the patient's chart.

POLISHING

After margination and surface smoothing, the amalgam is polished.

I. GENERAL SUGGESTIONS

A. Use Very Wet Polishing Agents
1. Avoid overheating.
2. Avoid dry polishing powders and discs.
3. Separate rubber polishing cups and points from the tooth and/or restoration by a wet abrasive agent.

B. Do Not Overpolish
Overpolishing, even with a fine abrasive agent, can alter the contour of the restoration, destroy the contact area, and remove excess surrounding tooth structure, especially when cementum is involved.

C. Use Low Speed
Use light, intermittent strokes.

D. Do Not Extend Polishing Brushes or Cups Over the Cementum
The abrasive polishing agent can groove and scratch the cementum.

II. INSTRUMENTS

A. Bristle brushes (pointed, cup-shaped, disc-shaped).

B. Rubber cups, points, wheels or discs.
C. Waxed dental tape.

III. PROCEDURES

A. Initial Polish

1. *Rubber Cups and Points.* Brown and green rubber cups and points have abrasives incorporated into the rubber; additional abrasive agents are not needed. They are excellent for smoothing after conventional burs, stones, or discs are used.
   a. Use points for occlusal.
   b. Use cups for proximal.
   c. Use brown first, then follow with green.
   d. Use light, quick, intermittent strokes under wet conditions.
   e. Cups and points are reusable and reshapable.
   f. Sterilize after use.
2. *Bristle Brushes*
   a. Prepare by soaking them in warm water.
   b. Use fine pumice or fine silex in a very wet slurry with water.
   c. Apply the agent over the tooth and restoration before starting the power-driven instrument. With each succeeding change in abrasive, rinse the previous one from the area.
   d. Use the pointed brush in the pits and fissures, and use cup-shaped brush or rubber cup for convex surfaces.
   e. Keep the brush or cup in constant motion with light, intermittent strokes to prevent heat generation.
   f. Use slow to moderate speed.
   g. Apply polishing agent to proximal surfaces with waxed dental tape. Avoid the contact area. Curve the tape around the tooth to prevent damage to the interdental gingival tissue.
3. *Examination.* Rinse and evaluate frequently to prevent overpolishing. Check to ensure a smooth surface.

B. Final Polish

1. Use a new rubber cup, and floss or tape to prevent mixing the agents.
2. Apply tin oxide in a thin, wet slurry with water.
3. Apply with light, intermittent strokes.
4. Rinse and evaluate to prevent overpolishing.

C. Fluoride

Follow the finishing and polishing by providing a fluoride treatment.

D. High Copper Alloys

To obtain a smooth surface on high copper alloy amalgams, polishing can be completed 8 to 12 minutes after placement.
1. Use a creamy paste of extra fine silex.
2. Use an unwebbed rubber cup.

3. Use a slow-speed handpiece for 30 seconds per surface.

FLUORIDE APPLICATION

The use of abrasive stones and polishing agents at the margin of a restoration removes a layer of the surface enamel and, with it, the concentration of fluoride that is protective against dental caries. Commercially prepared paste containing fluoride may restore in part the lost fluoride and can be used during the polishing procedure.

After polishing, a topical application of fluoride should be made, followed by periodic applications at succeeding maintenance appointments, depending on individual needs. Self-application on a daily basis, using a mouthrinse, custom tray, or brush-on gel, also may be recommended to supplement fluoride derived from the use of a dentifrice.

Neutral sodium fluorides are to be used on all tooth-colored restorations and sealants. Acidulated fluorides can change the surface texture and appearance.[9]

THE MAINTENANCE APPOINTMENT

For all types of restorations, concerns are for continuing care. The patient expects restorations to last a long time and the esthetic features to be maintained.

Procedures for a maintenance appointment are described in Chapter 42, page 644. Items included here are selected to highlight the care of restorations.

I. ASSESSMENT

A. Review of History

B. Study Previous Records

1. *Tooth-Color Restorations:* Locations, specific materials.
2. *Instruments and Agents:* Previous professional care for tooth-color restorations.
3. *Patient Counseling:* Personal care of restorations; advice given for stain prevention; smoking history past and present.

C. Clinical Examination

1. *Soft Tissue:* Gingiva adjacent to restorative materials.
2. *Probing:* Complete probing with special note of the gingiva and probing depths adjacent to restorations.
3. *Dental Examination*
   a. Exploration of all margins of restorations.
   b. Check documentation of new restorations placed since previous dental hygiene appointment; record the dental materials and determine care needed.

II. PATIENT COUNSELING

Instruction in personal care procedures and how to preserve the dental materials and the teeth must be an integral part of the dental hygiene health service.

A. Evaluate Patient's Personal Care

To review oral hygiene a disclosing agent is not used when there are tooth color restorations since the surface absorption characteristics cannot be fully realized. However, plaque can be detected by running a probe over the surfaces while the patient watches in a mirror; appropriate instruction is provided.

B. Tobacco Use

For the user, discussion of cessation attempts, or introduction of a cessation assist program, can be made (pages 436 to 438).

C. Dietary Review

1. Prevention of dental caries; effect on margins and recurrent caries.
2. Sources of foods that may discolor the esthetic restorations.

III. CLINICAL PROCEDURES

At the maintenance appointments the dental hygienist uses instruments and procedures that cannot alter or otherwise harm the surfaces and margins of the dental materials.

TECHNICAL HINTS

I. CONCERNING POLISHING AGENTS

- Do not use conventional polishing pastes on tooth-color restorations. They can scratch, roughen, and dull the surfaces of restorations.
- Only use aluminum oxide for polishing plastic restorations. Aluminum oxide polishing strips are available for proximal surfaces.
- Diamond polishing agent or aluminum oxide can be used for ceramic materials.
- Avoid air-powder polishers and sonic or ultrasonic scalers.

II. FLUORIDE

Use only neutral pH sodium fluoride preventive agents. Acidulated fluoride damages the surfaces of porcelain and composite resin.[9]

III. MERCURY HYGIENE

Amalgam is still an important restorative material even though the esthetic plastic and ceramic restorative materials have grown in selectability.

- Wear mask, protective eyewear, and gloves for protection from exposure to mercury vapor and amalgam dust.
- Work in well-ventilated areas.
- Handle amalgam with caution and without direct contact; clean up spilled mercury promptly.

- Use water stream and high-volume evacuation when removing or finishing amalgam restorations.
- Avoid carpeting or porous materials for treatment room floors.
- Store mercury in unbreakable, tightly sealed containers away from heat sources.
- Keep amalgam scrap in a tightly sealed container.
- Avoid heating mercury, amalgam, or mercury-containing solutions.

FACTORS TO TEACH THE PATIENT

I. The importance of the patient's self-care in the maintenance of restorations. Advise using a sulcular brushing technique with soft end-rounded filaments, dental floss, and a mild nonabrasive dentifrice.

II. The advantages of limiting cariogenic foods.

III. The detrimental effects of rough restorations, relating to plaque retention, gingival health, and dental caries.

IV. The softening effects of alcohol on plastic restorations.

V. Causes of discolorations of plastic and ceramic restorative materials.

VI. For the tobacco user, the need to quit and enter a cessation program.

VII. The adverse effects of oral habits that can chip or fracture the restorations.

VIII. The advantages of having restorations smooth and well finished.

IX. The reasons for having to wait 24 to 48 hours to have finishing procedures completed for a newly placed amalgam restoration.

X. The need for daily and/or professional applications of neutral sodium fluoride to promote remineralization around each restoration. Daily mouthrinse, brush-on gel, gel in a tray, or other forms of fluoride may be advised.

REFERENCES

1. **Quirynen**, M. and Bollen, C.M.L.: The Influence of Surface Roughness and Surface-free Energy on Supra- and Subgingival Plaque Formation in Man. A Review of the Literature, *J. Clin. Periodontol., 22,* 1, January, 1995.

2. **Schmid**, M.O.: Preparation of the Tooth Surface, in Carranza, F.A. and Newman, M.G.: *Clinical Periodontology,* 8th ed. Philadelphia, W.B. Saunders, 1996, pp. 488–490.

3. **Gilmore**, N. and Sheiham, A.: Overhanging Dental Restorations and Periodontal Disease, *J. Periodontol., 42,* 8, January, 1971.

4. **Highfield**, J.E. and Powell, R.N.: Effects of Removal of Posterior Overhanging Metallic Margins of Restorations Upon the Periodontal Tissues, *J. Clin. Periodontol., 5,* 169, August, 1978.

5. **Pack**, A.R.C., Coxhead, L.J., and McDonald, B.W.: The Prevalence of Overhanging Margins in Posterior Amalgam Restorations and Periodontal Consequences, *J. Clin. Periodontol., 17,* 145, March, 1990.

6. **Jeffcoat**, M.K. and Howell, T.H.: Alveolar Bone Destruction Due to Overhanging Amalgam in Periodontal Disease, *J. Periodontol., 51,* 599, October, 1980.

7. **Rodriguez-Ferrer**, H.J., Strahan, J.D., and Newman, H.N.: Effect on Gingival Health of Removing Overhanging Margins of

Interproximal Subgingival Amalgam Restorations, *J. Clin. Periodontol., 7,* 457, December, 1980.
8. **Sheaffer,** J.K.: Amalgam Overhang Removal Using Reciprocating Motor-driven Instrumentation, *Access, 7,* 28, December, 1993.
9. **American Dental Association,** Council on Dental Materials, Instruments, and Equipment and Council on Dental Therapeutics: Status Report: Effect of Acidulated Phosphate Fluoride on Porcelain and Composite Restorations, *J. Am. Dent. Assoc., 116,* 115, January, 1988.

SUGGESTED READINGS

Brown, R.S. and Johnson, C.D.: Corrosion of Dental Gold Restorations from Inhalation of "Crack" Cocaine, *Gen. Dent., 42,* 242, May–June, 1994.

Chen, J.J., Burch, J.G., Beck, F.M., and Horton, J.E.: Periodontal Attachment Loss Associated with Proximal Tooth Restorations, *J. Prosthet. Dent., 57,* 416, April, 1987.

Fruits, T.J., Coury, T.L., Miranda, F.J., and Duncanson, M.G.: Uses and Properties of Current Glass Ionomer Cements: A Review, *Gen. Dent., 44,* 410, September–October, 1996.

Hodsdon, K.A.: Postoperative Care for Aesthetic Restorations: A Challenge to Dental Hygienists, *J. Pract. Hyg., 7,* 19, March/April, 1998.

Jansson, L., Ehnevid, H., Lindskog, S., and Blomlöf, L.: Proximal Restorations and Periodontal Status, *J. Clin. Periodontal, 21,* 577, October, 1994.

McGuire, M.K. and Miller, L.: Maintaining Esthetic Restorations in the Periodontal Practice, *Int. J. Periodont. Restorative Dent., 16,* 231, June, 1996.

Miller, B.H.: Dental Restorative Materials. An Update on Care, *DentalHygienistNews, 8,* 9, Winter, 1995.

Miller, L.M.: *Maintaining Esthetic Restorations.* Houston, Realty Publishing Co., 1989, 114 pp.

Safar, J.A.: Subcutaneous Emphysema During Removal of an Overhang, *Gen. Dent., 43,* 424, September–October, 1995.

Swift, E.J. and Perdigao, J.: Effects of Bleaching on Teeth and Restorations, *Compend. Cont. Educ. Dent., 19,* 815, August, 1998.

Troendle, K., Nicholson, J., and Berry, T.: Adhesive Restorative Materials. A New Era in Dentistry, *Dent. Teamwork, 9,* 18, November–December, 1996.

Yap, A.U.J., Lye, K.W., and Sau, C.W.: Surface Characteristics of Tooth-colored Restoratives Polished Utilizing Different Polishing Systems, *Oper. Dent., 22,* 260, November/December, 1997.

Composites

Ashe, M.J., Tripp, G.A., Eichmiller, F.C., George, L.A., and Meiers, J.C.: Surface Roughness of Glass-ceramic Insert-composite Restorations: Assessing Several Polishing Techniques, *J. Am. Dent. Assoc., 127,* 1495, October, 1996.

Berastegui, E., Canalda, C., Brau, E., and Miguel, C.: Surface Roughness of Finished Composite Resins, *J. Prosthet. Dent., 68,* 742, November, 1992.

Dodge, W.W., Dale, R.A., Cooley, R.L., and Duke, E.S.: Comparison of Wet and Dry Finishing of Resin Composites with Aluminum Oxide Discs, *Dent. Mater., 7,* 18, January, 1991.

Goldstein, G.R. and Waknine, S.: Surface Roughness Evaluation of Composite Resin Polishing Techniques, *Quintessence Int., 20,* 199, March, 1989.

Harvey, H.L. and Swift, E.J.: Effects of a Calculus Scaling Gel on Microhardness of Composite Resins, *J. Pract. Hyg., 4,* 32, May/June, 1995.

Liebenberg, W.H.: Posterior Composite Resin Restorations: Assuring Restorative Integrity, *F.D.I. World, 6,* 12, March/April, 1997.

Nadarajah, V., Neiders, M.E., and Cohen, R.E.: Local Inflammatory Effects of Composite Resins, *Compend. Cont. Educ. Dent., 18,* 367, April, 1997.

Nash, L.B.: Maximizing Aesthetic Restorations: The Hygienist's Role, *J. Pract. Hyg., 1,* 23, March, 1992.

Papagiannoulis, L., Tzoutzas, J., and Eliades, G.: Effect of Top-

ical Fluoride Agents on the Morphologic Characteristics and Composition of Resin Composite Restorative Materials, *J. Prosthet. Dent., 77,* 405, April, 1997.

Settembrini, L., Penugonda, B., Scherer, W., Strassler, H., and Hittleman, E.: Alcohol-containing Mouthwashes: Effect on Composite Color, *Oper. Dent., 20,* 14, January/February, 1995.

Stoddard, J.W. and Johnson, G.H.: An Evaluation of Polishing Agents for Composite Resins, *J. Prosthet. Dent., 65,* 491, April, 1991.

Strassler, H.E. and Moffit, W.: The Surface Texture of Composite Resin After Polishing with Commercially Available Toothpastes, *Compend. Cont. Educ. Dent., 8,* 826, November/December, 1987.

Wilson, F., Heath, J.R., and Watts, D.C.: Finishing Composite Restorative Materials, *J. Oral Rehabil., 17,* 79, January, 1990.

Glass Ionomer

Arcoria, C.J., Gonzalez, J.P., Vitasek, B.A., and Wagner, M.J.: Effects of Ultrasonic Instrumentation on Microleakage in Composite Restorations with Glass Ionomer Liners, *J. Oral Rehabil., 19,* 21, January, 1992.

El-Badrawy, W.A. and McComb, D.: Effect of Home-use Fluoride Gels on Resin-modified Glass-ionomer Cements, *Oper. Dent., 23,* 2, January–February, 1998.

Helpin, M.L. and Rosenberg, H.M.: Resin-modified Glassionomers in Pediatric Dentistry, *J.Pract.Hyg., 5,* 33, January/February, 1996.

Hotta, M., Hirukawa, H., and Aono, M.: The Effect of Glaze on Restorative Glass-ionomer Cements, *J. Oral Rehabil., 22,* 197, March, 1995.

Liberman, R. and Geiger, S.: Surface Texture Evaluation of Glass Ionomer Restorative Materials Polished Utilizing Poly (Acrylic Acid) Gel, *J. Oral Rehabil., 21,* 87, January, 1994.

Momoi, Y., Hirosaki, K., Kohno, A., and McCabe, J.F.: *In Vitro* Toothbrush-dentifrice Abrasion of Resin-modified Glass Ionomers, *Dent. Mater., 13,* 82, March, 1997.

Ceramics

Anusavice, K.J.: Reducing the Failure Potential of Ceramic-based Restorations, Part 1: Metal-ceramic Crowns and Bridges, *Gen. Dent., 44,* 492, November–December, 1996.

Anusavice, K.J.: Reducing the Failure Potential of Ceramic-based Restorations. Part 2: Ceramic Inlays, Crowns, Veneers, and Bridges, *Gen. Dent., 45,* 30, January–February, 1997.

Goldstein, G.R., Barnhard, B.R., and Penugonda, B.: Profilometer, SEM, and Visual Assessment of Porcelain Polishing Methods, *J. Prosthet. Dent., 65,* 627, May, 1991.

Kourkouta, S., Walsh, T.T., and Davis, L.G.: The Effect of Porcelain Laminate Veneers on Gingival Health and Bacterial Plaque Characteristics, *J. Clin. Periodontol., 21,* 638, October, 1994.

Miller, L.M.: Porcelain Ceramic Systems: New, Quick, and Effective Techniques for Maintaining the Beauty of Porcelain Restorations, *J. Pract. Hyg., 1,* 17, September, 1992.

Nash, L.B.: Improving Aesthetics with Porcelain Laminate Veneers, *J. Pract. Hyg., 5,* 21, May–June, 1996.

Amalgam

Calley, K.H.: Polishing Amalgam Restorations, *DentalHygienistNews, 8,* 9, Number 3, 1995.

Eid, M.: Relationship Between Overhanging Amalgam Restorations and Periodontal Disease, *Quintessence Int., 18,* 775, November, 1987.

Fayyad, M.A. and Ball, P.C.: Bacterial Penetration Around Amalgam Restorations, *J. Prosthet. Dent., 57,* 571, May, 1987.

Holmstrup, P.: Reactions of the Oral Mucosa Related to Silver Amalgam, *J. Oral Pathol. Med., 20,* 1, January, 1991.

Paarman, C.: Finishing, Recontouring, and Polishing Amalgam Restorations, *J. Pract. Hyg., 2,* 9, January/February, 1993.

Pack, A.R.C.: The Amalgam Overhang Dilemma: A Review of Causes and Effects, Prevention and Removal, *N.Z. Dent. J., 85,* 55, April, 1989.

Rogo, E.J.: Overhang Removal: Improving Periodontal Health

Adjacent to Class II Amalgam Restorations, *J. Pract. Hyg.*, 4, 15, May/June, 1995.

Air Polisher on Restorations

Eliades, G.C., Tzoutzas, J.G., and Vougiouklakis, G.J.: Surface Alterations on Dental Restorative Materials Subjected to an Air-powder Abrasive Instrument, *J. Prosthet. Dent.*, 65, 27, January, 1991.

Gutmann, M.E.: Air Polishing: A Comprehensive Review of the Literature, *J. Dent. Hyg.*, 72, 47, Summer, 1998.

Vermilyea, S.G., Prasanna, M.K., and Agar, J.R.: Effect of Ultrasonic Cleaning and Air Polishing on Porcelain Labial Margin Restorations, *J. Prosthet. Dent.*, 71, 447, May, 1994.

41

Debonding

Brackets bonded to the teeth are used widely in orthodontic treatment. The brackets serve to retain arch wires and to aid in the application and control of the applied forces needed to accomplish the necessary tooth movement and bone remodeling for orthodontic therapy. Terminology used in conjunction with debonding is defined in Box 41-1.

I. COMPARISON OF CEMENTED BANDS AND BONDED BRACKETS

Formerly, fixed appliances mainly were circumferential stainless steel bands cemented to the teeth. Bands are illustrated in Figure 25-2, page 397. Cemented bands may be placed on molars and premolars, whereas bonded brackets are placed on anterior teeth. Banding may be recommended for maxillary and mandibular first permanent molars because of the need for their strength to hold orthodontic auxiliaries for palatal bars, elastics, or other special devices.

A. Advantages of Bonded Appliances
1. Improved esthetics.
2. Improved gingival condition because they provide access for control of bacterial plaque at the cervical third of the teeth.
3. Proximal surface dental caries can be detected and treated without band removal.

4. Patient can be aware immediately when a bracket loosens, whereas undermining of a band can go undetected.
5. Placement factors
   a. No need for tooth separation (as required for band placement) and no band spaces to close at the end of treatment.
   b. Bonded appliances can be placed on partially erupted teeth, so no wait for tooth eruption is necessary before treatment can be started.
   c. Lingual brackets ("invisible braces") may be used for specially selected cases.

B. Disadvantages of Bonded Brackets
1. Attachment may be weaker because less surface area is in contact with tooth. Bracket may detach more readily than a band.
2. Rebonding a loose bracket is more time consuming and requires more tooth preparation than does recementing a loose band.
3. Debonding at the end of treatment is more time consuming than debanding, with more potential danger of damage to the tooth surface because of the higher bond strength.
4. Lower fracture toughness; subject to cracks.[1]

BOX 41-1 KEY WORDS: Debonding

Arch wire: curved wire positioned in the brackets around the dental arch and held in place by elastomeres or ligatures.

Band: preformed stainless steel ring fitted around a tooth and cemented in place; available in shapes for each tooth form; each band has a bracket attached on the facial side, which is the mode of attachment for the arch wire.

Bonding: process by which orthodontic brackets are affixed to the tooth surface; a fluoride-releasing light-activated resin is frequently used.

  Direct bonding: a single-step intra-oral procedure in which orthodontic attachments are oriented and bonded individually.

  Indirect bonding: a two-step process by which orthodontic attachments are affixed temporarily to the teeth of a study cast from which they are transferred to the mouth at one time by means of a template or tray that preserves the predetermined orientation and permits them to be bonded simultaneously.

Bracket: attachment that is bonded to the enamel for the purpose of holding the arch wire.

Ceramic (sĕ-ram′ĭk): alumina (Al_2O_3) used as a single-crystal material or as a polycrystalline material.

Debonding: removal of brackets and residual adhesive after which the tooth surface is returned to its normal contour.

Elastomere: elastoplastic ring or latex elastic used to hold an arch wire in a bracket wing.

Fracture toughness: ability of bracket material to resist fracture.

Ligature: cord, thread, or stainless steel wire used to secure the arch wire to the bracket.

Tensile: susceptible to extension; capable of being stretched.

  Tensile strength: maximum stress that a material is capable of sustaining; usually expressed in pounds per square inch.

II. FIXED APPLIANCE SYSTEM

Figure 41-1 shows the bonded brackets with arch wire held in place by elastomeres.

A. Brackets
  1. *Materials*
     a. Metal (stainless steel).
     b. Plastic (polycarbonate).
     c. Plastic with metal reinforcements.
     d. Ceramic.
  2. *Forms.* Brackets are made in many styles, shapes, and sizes for different teeth, each designed to accomplish a specific objective of treatment. The basic forms are *single* or *twin* (Figure 41-2).
  3. *Base.* The base of the bracket is prepared with a mesh backing to assist in retaining the acrylic bonding agent. The mesh backing, or bonding pad as it is also called, is made to the exact size of the bracket so that no area of tooth is left uncovered where demineralization can occur.

     Mesh backings retain less bacterial plaque than do other types of backings.[2,3]

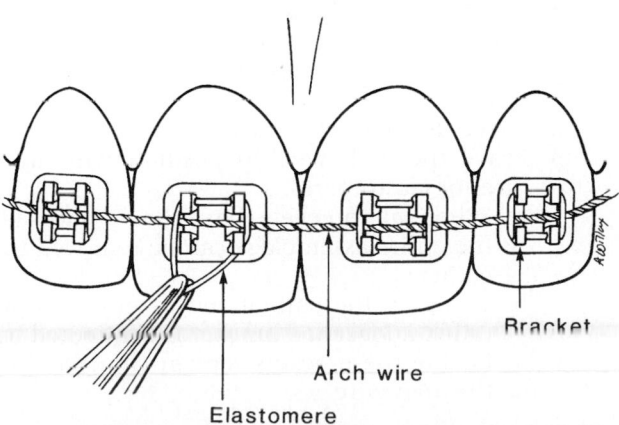

FIGURE 41-1 Fixed Appliance System. Bonded brackets with arch wire held in place by elastomeres.

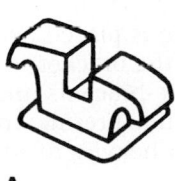 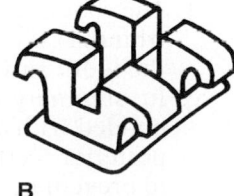

A   **B**

FIGURE 41-2 Orthodontic Brackets. (A) Single bracket with an incisal and a cervical wing. **(B)** Twin, or Siamese, with two wings on each side of the central groove where the arch wire is held. The shape and style of each bracket vary with the tooth on which the bracket will be located.

B. Arch Wire

The arch wire is used to generate or distribute forces that cause or guide orthodontic tooth movement. Arch wires are made of stainless steel or an alloy of chromium or titanium, and they may be round, rectangular, or multistranded (Figure 41-1).

C. Elastomere

An elastomere is used to
1. Hold wires in the brackets (Figure 41-1).
2. Apply force to close spaces between teeth.

III. CLINICAL PROCEDURES FOR BONDING[4,5]

The principles described in Chapter 30 (pages 480 to 486) for pit and fissure sealants apply for bonding orthodontic brackets. Details are not included here.

The basic procedural steps are *cleaning the tooth surface, conditioning the enamel surface,* and *applying the bonding agent.* After the bonding, the area around the bracket must be cleaned of excess resin.

A. Characteristics of Bonding Relating to Debonding

1. *Nature of the Bond*

   The acid etch exposes the prism structure and creates microclefts (Figure 30-1, page 482). The average depth of the microclefts ranges from 50 to 80 μm.[6-8] Some fine tag extensions have been observed to depths of 100 to 170 μm.[8] On the bracket side, the resin becomes locked into the mesh base.

2. *Effect of Filling Particles*

   a. Physical property values increase from unfilled to heavily filled resins. Fillers increase bond strength, hardness, and wear resistance.

   b. Heavily filled resins (composites) perform better for the posterior teeth because posterior attachments are subject to high forces of mastication.

   c. Ease of debonding can be related to the type of resin. Heavily filled composites are thicker and less viscous; they may be the more difficult to remove.

   d. The bond is stronger when a smaller (thinner) layer of resin is placed between the tooth surface and the bracket.

   e. In summary, anterior brackets may be bonded with a lightly filled resin, whereas posterior teeth need a heavily filled resin to prevent detachment.

B. Use of Fluoride-Releasing Bonding System

Demineralization around brackets can be a serious problem for even the most conscientious patient. Use of a fluoride-releasing bonding system has been shown to have positive preventive results.[9-11]

CLINICAL PROCEDURES FOR DEBONDING

Debonding can be divided into three basic steps, namely, bracket removal, reduction of the resin bulk, and restoration of the pretreatment characteristics of the tooth surface. After debonding, anticaries preventive care and patient instruction are essential.

I. RESEARCH

The aim in debonding is to remove the bracket and the residual resin with minimal damage to the enamel surface and minimal discomfort for the patient. Scratches and gouges of the enamel surface, as well as fractures of the enamel, have resulted from improperly applied techniques. An efficient and effective procedure is needed to minimize enamel damage.

Mechanical, electrothermal, and ultrasonic methods have been used in the attempt to determine which method is the most efficient, provides the least discomfort for the patient, and causes the least damage to the enamel.[12-14] To evaluate effects, studies have been made to measure the amount of enamel lost during each step of debonding. The appearance of the enamel surface after debonding with various bond-removing pliers, scalers, discs, rubber wheels, diamond and carbide burs, and pumice has been observed by scanning electron microscope, stereoscopic microscope, and other methods.

When debonding, each clinician must keep in mind that all the instruments and materials can lead to scratches, grooves, or other irregularities of the tooth surface, and that rotary instruments create heat that affects the pulp. Careful application of the instruments, as well as frequent visual and tactile examination of the surface, is necessary.

II. BRACKET REMOVAL[12,15]

A. Technique Objectives

1. Create a fracture within the resin bonding material or between the bracket and the resin.
2. Leave the enamel surface intact.
3. Leave the arch wire in position with ligatures or elastomeres.
   a. When all brackets have been released, the entire assemblage can be removed together.
   b. Threat of the patient swallowing or aspirating a loosened bracket is eliminated by having the brackets remain connected to the arch wire.

B. The "Squeeze-Release" Technique[12,15]

1. Use a small plier with blunt beaks.
2. Apply the beaks to outside edges of the

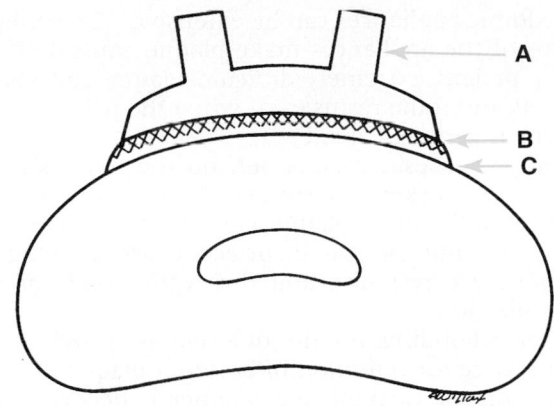

FIGURE 41-3 Cross Section of a Bracket. Viewed from the incisal aspect of a tooth. **A** Bracket wing. **B** Junction of bracket and mesh backing with resin at the adhesive-bracket interface. **C** Junction of resin and enamel. (Adapted from Bennett, C.G., Shen, C., and Waldron, J.M.: The Effects of Debonding on the Enamel Surface, *J. Clin. Orthod.*, 18, 330, May, 1984.)

mesial and distal bracket wings (arrow A, Figure 41-3).

3. Squeeze the beaks together; do not twist.
   a. The wings bend together and cause the mesial and distal edges of the bracket base to pull away.
   b. The break is at the adhesive–bracket interface, thereby leaving the enamel undisturbed.
   c. Varying amounts of adhesive are left on the tooth surface; some may be attached to the mesh bracket base.

C. Precautions
1. *For Mechanical Removal.* Do not twist in a shearing stroke for the following reasons:
   a. Potential fracture of enamel. The fragile projections of the etched enamel are susceptible to breaking.
   b. Traumatic for patient. Teeth following orthodontic treatment are often mobile. Twisting can be painful.
   c. Potential damage to periodontal ligament. Twisting stretches the fibers.
2. *For Selection and Positioning of Pliers*
   a. Dull pliers are preferred to prevent scratching or gouging.
   b. Pliers should be positioned for the A and B sites in Figure 41-3, at the adhesive–bracket interface. When cutting pliers are placed between the resin adhesive and the tooth (arrow C, in Figure 41-3) and used in a cutting stroke, the damage to the enamel can be severe.

III. REMOVAL OF RESIDUAL ADHESIVE

A. Procedure Objectives
1. Remove resin bulk.

2. Minimize damage to pulpal tissue.
3. Avoid damage to enamel surface.
4. Prevent excess enamel loss.

B. Examination
Varying amounts of resin remain after the bracket is removed, particularly in normal anatomic grooves. During debonding, frequent examination is necessary using visual and tactile methods.
1. *Identification of Residual Resin*
   a. Patient reports feeling roughness.
   b. Visual. When dry, the resin appears dull and opaque, as compared with clean, shiny enamel.
   c. Tactile. Application of an explorer reveals a rough surface, sometimes with catches along the margin of a resin tag.
2. *Use of Loupes for Magnification of the Tooth Surface.* A more accurate evaluation of enamel surface can be made.

C. Removal of Resin From Tooth Surface[16,17]
1. *Bur Selection.* Use a tapered, plain-cut, tungsten carbide finishing bur with low-speed handpiece.
2. *Speed.* Use low speed to control heat.
3. *Stroke.* Use a smooth, evenly applied, light brush stroke in one direction to prevent faceting.
4. *Direction.* Work systematically from cervical portion of the resin; move toward incisal third. The resin is removed in fine white shavings.
5. *Evaluate frequently.* To prevent overinstrumentation, rinse frequently, dry, and evaluate the surface. The resin will appear opaque in contrast to the glossy enamel.

IV. FINAL FINISH

A. Objective
Restore pretreatment enamel surface finish.

B. Examination
1. Perform visual and tactile examination for areas of normal enamel and irregularities.
2. Request patient to examine by rubbing the tongue over the surface.

C. Application of Rubber Cup
1. Use fine pumice water slurry.
2. Polish in a wet field to prevent overheating.
3. Adapt interrupted application of rubber cup, and move from area to area.
4. Check progress by rinsing and drying. Avoid overinstrumentation.

D. Finishing
For a final polish use points and cups impregnated with aluminum oxide to produce a glossy surface.

POST-DEBONDING EVALUATION

Each step of bonding and debonding has an effect on the enamel surface. Realization that the enamel surface can be damaged can help the clinician avoid unnecessary trauma during the various procedures.

I. ENAMEL LOSS

Total enamel loss from etching, bracket removal, residual resin removal, surface finishing, and application of pumice averages approximately 55 to 80 μm.[8,18] Enamel loss is greater when filled resins (composites) are used for bonding than when unfilled resins are used. The loss is also greater when a rotating bristle brush rather than a rubber cup is used with the abrasive for finishing.

The outer layer of enamel is the most significant. The fluoride-rich surface enamel is approximately 50 μm deep. Therefore, the entire protective layer can be removed. When multiple bonding and debonding procedures are done, such as when a bracket becomes detached, the enamel loss is compounded. As much as 72 μm of enamel may be lost during a complete multiple procedure.[19]

The need for careful selection of instruments and abrasives, along with minimal instrumentation, to prevent unnecessary enamel loss is apparent.

II. WHITE SPOTS (DEMINERALIZATION)

White spots or dental caries have been relatively common findings after orthodontic treatment. Patients with teeth that have been banded or bonded tend to develop the spots significantly more often than do patients who have not had orthodontic therapy.

Bacterial plaque retention by the appliances and the resin, along with the difficulty of plaque removal by the patient, contribute to demineralization and dental caries.

III. ETCHED ENAMEL NOT COVERED BY ADHESIVE

Surface areas etched but not covered with adhesive resin become remineralized when the fluoride contact is high through personal and professional applications. Etched enamel has a high fluoride uptake.

POST-DEBONDING PREVENTIVE CARE

I. PERIODONTAL EVALUATION

A complete examination with careful probing and charting is necessary, because many changes take place during treatment. Calculus removal should be completed as needed.

II. DENTAL CARIES

Examination for demineralization (white spots) and dental caries is essential. Bacterial plaque retention by

orthodontic appliances can be extensive. The configurations of the appliances make plaque control efforts by the patient extremely difficult. Plaque collects on brackets and some resins even when the patient's oral hygiene is generally good.[2]

Composite resin may be left on the tooth surface around the bracket. The surface of resins is difficult to make smooth; thus, plaque collects. The bacteria of the plaque, not the rough surface, cause the gingival inflammatory response and the white spots, or demineralization.

After debonding, the use of a retainer provides another source for retention of bacterial plaque. Special instruction for cleaning the retainer is needed (page 397).

III. FLUORIDE THERAPY[20]

A complete program of fluoride treatments, professionally at frequent maintenance appointments and by the patient on a daily basis, is prerequisite. With the loss of the fluoride-rich enamel surface during bonding and debonding procedures, the need for remineralization and replenishment of fluoride is clear.

TECHNICAL HINTS

I. Document any irregularities of the patient's teeth, such as white spots or cracks, before orthodontic treatment begins and appliances are affixed, to prevent misunderstanding by the patient after debonding.[21]
II. Take periodic photographs to compare gingival tissue changes and teeth before and after disclosing agent application for documentation and patient instruction.

FACTORS TO TEACH THE PATIENT

I. The significance of bacterial plaque around orthodontic appliances and the teeth.
II. How to apply the toothbrush and auxiliary devices to remove plaque from the bracket, the arch wire, and the teeth (Chapters 24 and 25).
III. How, when, and why to use fluoride rinse, toothpaste, and brush-on gel.
IV. The frequency for professional follow-up after debonding.

REFERENCES

1. **American Dental Association,** Council on Dental Materials, Instruments, and Equipment: Ceramic Orthodontic Brackets: How and When to Use Them, *J. Am. Dent. Assoc., 123,* 243, July, 1992.
2. **Gwinnett,** A.J. and Ceen, R.F.: Plaque Distribution on Bonded Brackets: A Scanning Microscopic Study, *Am. J. Orthod., 75,* 667, June, 1979.
3. **Zachrisson,** B.U. and Brobakken, B.O.: Clinical Comparison of

Direct Versus Indirect Bonding With Different Bracket Types and Adhesives, *Am. J. Orthod., 74,* 62, July, 1978.

4. **Gwinnett,** A.J. for the American Dental Association, Council on Dental Materials, Instruments, and Equipment: State of the Art and Science of Bonding in Orthodontic Treatment, *J. Am. Dent. Assoc., 105,* 844, November, 1982.

5. **Proffit,** W.R.: *Contemporary Orthodontics,* 2nd ed. St. Louis, Mosby, 1993, pp. 353–357.

6. **Buonocore,** M.G., Matsui, A., and Gwinnett, A.J.: Penetration of Resin Dental Materials into Enamel Surfaces with Reference to Bonding, *Arch. Oral Biol., 13,* 61, January, 1968.

7. **Retief,** D.H.: Effect of Conditioning the Enamel Surface with Phosphoric Acid, *J. Dent. Res., 52,* 333, March–April, 1973.

8. **Diedrich,** P.: Enamel Alterations from Bracket Bonding and Debonding: A Study with the Scanning Electron Microscope, *Am. J. Orthod., 79,* 500, May, 1981.

9. **Chan,** D.C.N., Swift, E.J., and Bishara, S.E.: *In Vitro* Evaluation of a Fluoride-releasing Orthodontic Resin, *J. Dent. Res., 69,* 1576, September, 1990.

10. **Bishara,** S.E., Swift, E.J., and Chan, D.C.N.: Evaluation of Fluoride Release from an Orthodontic Bonding System, *Am. J. Orthod. Dentofacial Orthop., 100,* 106, August, 1991.

11. **Basdra,** E.K., Huber, H., and Komposch, G.: Fluoride Released from Orthodontic Bonding Agents Alters the Enamel Surface and Inhibits Enamel Demineralization in Vitro, *Am. J. Orthod. Dentofacial Orthop., 109,* 466, May, 1996.

12. **Everett,** M.S.: Debonding Orthodontic Adhesives, *Dent. Hyg., 59,* 364, August, 1985.

13. **Bishara,** S.E. and Trulove, T.S.: Comparisons of Different Debonding Techniques for Ceramic Brackets: An *In Vitro* Study, Part I. Background and Methods, *Am. J. Orthod. Dentofacial Orthop., 98,* 145, August, 1990.

14. **Bishara,** S.E. and Trulove, T.S.: Comparisons of Different Debonding Techniques for Ceramic Brackets: An *In Vitro* Study. Part II. Findings and Clinical Implications, *Am. J. Orthod. Dentofacial Orthop., 98,* 263, September, 1990.

15. **Bennett,** C.G., Shen, C., and Waldron, J.M.: The Effects of Debonding on the Enamel Surface, *J. Clin. Orthod., 18,* 330, May, 1984.

16. **Gutmann,** M.E.: Composite Adhesive Resin Removal Following Orthodontic Treatment, *J. Pract. Hyg., 5,* 16, May–June, 1996.

17. **Campbell,** P.M.: Enamel Surfaces After Orthodontic Bracket Debonding, *Angle Orthod., 65,* 103, Number 2, 1995.

18. **Pus,** M.D. and Way, D.C.: Enamel Loss Due to Orthodontic Bonding with Filled and Unfilled Resins Using Various Clean-up Techniques, *Am. J. Orthod., 77,* 269, March, 1980.

19. **Thompson,** R.E. and Way, D.C.: Enamel Loss Due to Prophylaxis and Multiple Bonding/Debonding of Orthodontic Attachments, *Am. J. Orthod., 79,* 282, March, 1981.

20. **Boyd,** R.L.: Comparison of Three Self-applied Topical Fluoride Preparations for Control of Decalcification, *Angle Orthod., 63,* 25, Spring, 1993.

21. **Zachrisson,** B.U., Skogan, Ö., and Höymyhr, S.: Enamel Cracks in Debonded, Debanded, and Orthodontically Untreated Teeth, *Am. J. Orthod., 77,* 307, March, 1980.

SUGGESTED READINGS

Barcroft, B.D., Childers, K.R., and Harris, E.F.: Effects of Acidulated and Neutral NaF Solutions on Bond Strengths, *Pediatr. Dent., 12,* 180, May–June, 1990.

Boyd, R.L. and Baumrind, S.: Periodontal Considerations in the Use of Bonds or Bands on Molars in Adolescents and Adults, *Angle Orthod., 62,* 117, Summer, 1992.

Carstensen, W.: Direct Bonding with Reduced Acid Etchant Concentrations, *J. Clin. Orthod., 27,* 23, January, 1993.

Ehrlich, A. and Torres, H.O.: *Essentials of Dental Assisting.* Philadelphia, W.B. Saunders Co., 1992, pp. 465–476.

Flores, D.A., Caruso, J.M., Scott, G.E., and Jeiroudi, M.T.: The Fracture Strength of Ceramic Brackets: A Comparative Study, *Angle Orthod., 60,* 269, Winter, 1990.

Frazier, M.C., Southard, T.E., and Doster, P.M.: Prevention of Enamel Demineralization During Orthodontic Treatment: An *in vitro* Study Using Pit and Fissure Sealants, *Am. J. Orthod. Dentofacial Orthop., 110,* 459, November, 1996.

Gange, P.: Orthodontic Bonding, *Dent. Assistant, 64,* 5, Third Quarter, 1995.

Gwinnett, A.J. and Gorelik, L.: Microscopic Evaluation of Enamel After Debonding: Clinical Application, *Am. J. Orthod., 71,* 651, June, 1977.

Howell, S. and Weekes, W.T.: An Electron Microscopic Evaluation of the Enamel Surface Subsequent to Various Debonding Procedures, *Aust. Dent. J., 35,* 245, June, 1990.

Øgaard, B., Rezk-Lega, F., Ruben, J., and Arends, J.: Cariostatic Effect and Fluoride Release from a Visible Light-curing Adhesive for Bonding of Orthodontic Brackets, *Am. J. Orthod. Dentofacial Orthop., 101,* 303, April, 1992.

Retief, D.H. and Denys, F.R.: Finishing of Enamel Surfaces After Debonding of Orthodontic Attachments, *Angle Orthod., 49,* 1, January, 1979.

Rouleau, B.D., Marshall, G.W., and Cooley, R.O.: Enamel Surface Evaluations After Clinical Treatment and Removal of Orthodontic Brackets, *Am. J. Orthod., 81,* 423, May, 1982.

Staggers, J.A. and Margeson, D.: The Effects of Sterilization on the Tensile Strength of Orthodontic Wires, *Angle Orthod., 63,* 141, Summer, 1993.

Debonding Procedures

Bishara, S.E. and Fehr, D.E.: Comparisons of the Effectiveness of Pliers with Narrow and Wide Blades in Debonding Ceramic Brackets, *Am. J. Orthod. Dentofacial Orthop., 103,* 253, March, 1993.

Chate, R.A.C.: Safer Orthodontic Debonding with Rubber Dam, *Am. J. Orthod. Dentofacial Orthop., 103,* 171, February, 1993.

Gorbach, N.R.: Heat Removal of Ceramic Brackets, *J. Clin. Orthod., 25,* 247, April, 1991.

Krell, K.V., Courcy, J.M., and Bishara, S.E.: Orthodontic Bracket Removal Using Conventional and Ultrasonic Debonding Techniques, Enamel Loss, and Time Requirements, *Am. J. Orthod. Dentofacial Orthop., 103,* 258, March, 1993.

Oliver, R.G. and Griffiths, J.: Different Techniques of Residual Composite Removal Following Debonding—Time Taken and Surface Enamel Appearance, *Br. J. Orthod., 19,* 131, May, 1992.

Rinchuse, D.J.: Pain-free Debonding With Occlusal Rim Wax, *J. Clin. Orthod., 28,* 587, October, 1994.

Storm, E.R.: Debonding Ceramic Brackets, *J. Clin. Orthod., 24,* 91, February, 1990.

Strobl, K., Bahns, T.L., Willham, L., Bishara, S.E., and Stwalley, W.C.: Laser-aided Debonding of Orthodontic Ceramic Brackets, *Am. J. Orthod. Dentofacial Orthop., 101,* 152, February, 1992.

Tocchio, R.M., Williams, P.T., Mayer, F.J., and Standing, K.G.: Laser Debonding of Ceramic Orthodontic Brackets, *Am. J. Orthod. Dentofacial Orthop., 103,* 155, February, 1993.

Zachrisson, B.U.: Bonding in Orthodontics, in Graber, T.M. and Vanarsdall, R.L.: *Orthodontics, Current Principles and Techniques,* 2nd ed. St. Louis, Mosby, 1994, pp. 570–583.

Maintenance for Oral Health: Dental Hygiene Continuing Care

42

The overall purposes of treatment are to arrest disease and provide oral health, function, and comfort for the patient (Table 42-1). After a series of active treatments when evaluation shows that the soft tissue is in optimum health and the dentition has been restored in function, the patient enters a new phase of treatment for continuing supervision and care.

The primary objective of dental hygiene maintenance is to continue the healthy state attained during active therapy. The patient must realize that oral diseases do recur, but *control* is possible by combined personal and professional care. Life-long preservation of the teeth and their supporting structures is a realistic goal.

Initially the success of the program depends on the understanding by the patient of the maintenance procedure. One way to help the patient become aware is by including the concept of the maintenance phase in the initial care plan (page 326). Terms associated with preventive maintenance are defined in Box 42-1.

I. PURPOSES OF THE MAINTENANCE PROGRAM

A. Prevent new disease from starting.
B. Prevent recurrence of previous infections.
C. Monitor educational and behavioral changes.
D. Monitor clinical signs of health and disease
  1. Periodontal infections.
  2. Dental carious lesions.

  3. Oral mucosal lesions.
E. Provide specialized instruction for new implants, prostheses, and orthodontic appliances.
F. Offer motivational encouragement.

II. APPOINTMENT INTERVALS

A. Frequency Planning
No fixed schedule by which all patients can be maintained in oral health is possible because the frequency depends on the needs of each patient. Appointments may vary from 2 to 6 months. The time interval must be re-evaluated periodically and changed in accord with changing needs.

B. Maintenance Frequency: Contributing Factors
1. Risk for periodontal disease activity.
2. Risk for dental carious lesions.
3. Risk for oral cancer: tobacco and alcohol users.
4. Predisposing diseases, conditions, and behaviors for periodontal diseases: diabetes, HIV/AIDS, host genetic factors, smoking, and stress.[1]
5. Compliance: keeping appointments, personal daily plaque control.
6. Previous treatment: patient who has had previous disease, either dental caries or peri-

TABLE 42-1 Purposes and Outcomes of Dental Hygiene Periodontal Therapy

- Resolve inflammation
- Eliminate bleeding on probing
- Restore lost tissues to normal contour and texture
- Create environment for healing
- Arrest disease progression
- Preserve esthetics
- Provide patient comfort
- Encourage patient self-care
- Create environment that deters recurrence of infection
- Motivate patient to cooperate in continuing care

odontal infection, is at a greater risk for recurrence.

7. Local factors: rate of calculus formation.
8. Restorative complications: implants, prosthetic replacements.

C. Special Appointment Requirements

Intervals of 2 or 3 months are required for many patients. Examples of patients in this category are described throughout the book. A few are mentioned here.

1. *Patient Undergoing Extensive Dental Care.* The gingival or periodontal treatment may be completed or nearly completed by the time appointments for restorative phases of treatment are under way. The first maintenance appointment should be dated from the completion of the initial gingival and periodontal treatment. When extensive restorative, prosthetic, or other treatment is in progress, frequent tissue maintenance during long-term therapy is essential.

2. *Rampant Dental Caries.* Appointment for continuation of a caries control effort includes topical fluoride applications, dietary supervision, and personal care factors for bacterial plaque control.

3. *Orthodontic Therapy.* Appliances make cleaning and plaque control difficult; frequent topical fluoride applications may be indicated; response of gingival tissue to irritants can be marked.

4. *Mentally or Physically Disabled.* Managing the toothbrush may be difficult; when the disability involves the mouth area, opening the mouth may be a problem.

5. *Diabetes.* Diabetes or other disease can predispose patients to lowered resistance to infection; tissues must not be allowed to develop advanced disease.

6. *Cardiovascular Disease or Other Condition.* Brushing is a difficult procedure to carry out and only short appointments at the dental office can be tolerated because of the fatigue factor.

D. Periodontal Maintenance Therapy (PMT)[2]

Any of the types of patients who have been

BOX 42-1 KEY WORDS AND ABBREVIATIONS: Maintenance

Compliance: action in accordance with request; extent to which a person's health behaviors coincide with dental/medical health advice. Also called **adherence.**

Consultation: the joint deliberation, usually for diagnostic purposes, between two or more practitioners, or a patient and a practitioner.

Disease activity: ongoing dynamic process that results in loss of clinical attachment and alveolar supporting bone; an area is quiescent when a diseased site becomes inactive or stable without treatment.

End points: criteria for completion of a particular procedure; therapeutic end points generally have been reached when the clinical signs of the treated pathologic condition have been eliminated or reduced.

PMT: periodontal maintenance therapy; also called preventive maintenance, supportive periodontal treatment.

Recall: system of appointments for the long-term maintenance phase of patient care; the system is carried out by computer, telephone, and/or mail.

Refractory: resistant, not responding to routine therapy.

Remission (re-mish'un): diminution or abatement of the symptoms of a disease; the period during which the diminution occurs.

Response diagnosis: the diagnosis made at a re-evaluation spaced for a period of time after treatment (or a series of treatments); diagnosis that shows the response to prior treatment.

Risk factor: a characteristic, habit, or predisposing condition that makes an individual susceptible to, or in danger of acquiring, a certain disease or disability.

SPT: supportive periodontal therapy; procedures performed at selected intervals as an extension of periodontal therapy to assist the patient in maintaining oral health; includes complete assessment, review of and/or additional instruction in bacterial plaque control, and such clinical procedures as scaling and root planing; also called preventive maintenance, periodontal maintenance therapy.

mentioned and any of the "special" patients to be described in "Part VI" following this chapter may have a potentially recurrent periodontal infection or may have had periodontal corrective surgical therapy. Four categories of PMT have been defined:

1. *Preventive PMT:* To prevent the initiation of disease in individuals without periodontal infection.
2. *Trial PMT:* To provide an interim study period for borderline patients with conditions that must be observed and further evaluated before a decision can be made as to whether corrective surgery may be necessary or whether maintenance is possible without further advanced disease therapy.
3. *Compromise PMT:* To slow the progress of disease in patients for whom corrective surgery and other advanced treatment are indicated but cannot be implemented for reasons of health, economics, or other personal factors.
4. *Post-Treatment PMT:* To prevent the recurrence of disease and maintain the state of periodontal health attained during periodontal therapy. Such therapy may have been nonsurgical or surgical.

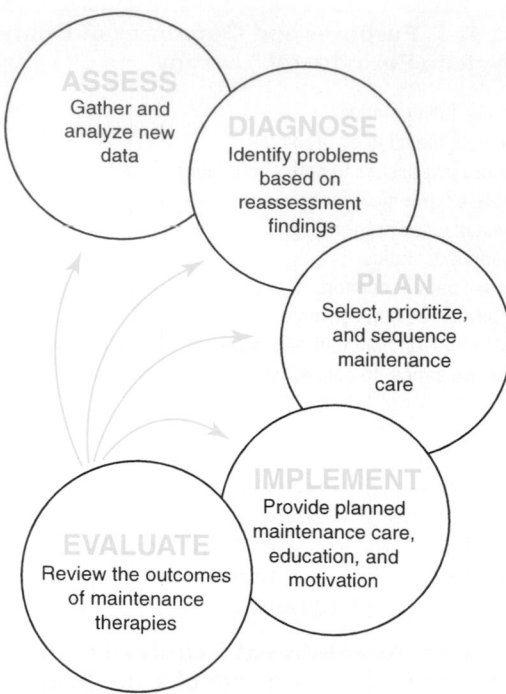

FIGURE 42-1 Components of the Dental Hygiene Process of Care. Planning for dental hygiene maintenance care unites all of the interrelated components.

MAINTENANCE APPOINTMENT PROCEDURES

The dental hygiene process of care was described in Chapter 1 and is illustrated in Figure 42-1. As with preparation of the initial dental hygiene care plan (Chapter 21, pages 320 to 322), the steps in the process of care apply for the *maintenance dental hygiene care plan*.

I. ASSESSMENT

Preparation of data follows the same plan as that for a new patient. Every patient needs a medical history review; an intra-oral and extra-oral examination for soft tissue lesions, particularly for cancer; and a blood pressure determination.

At every appointment, whether at 3, 6, or any other number of months, a patient of any age needs a complete probing and special evaluations for the particular problems of previous treatments.

Basic to all examinations are the periodontal examination (pages 204 to 213, 318) and the dental examination (pages 246 to 249) with charting.

Steps in preparation of a maintenance appointment work-up include the following:

A. Review of Patient History
Supplementary questions are asked to determine the present state of health, recent illnesses, present medications, and other pertinent data (pages 93 to 101).

B. Blood Pressure Determination (pages 111 to 114)

C. Extra-Oral and Intra-Oral Examination
A thorough extra-oral and intra-oral examination for oral disease, particularly cancer (see pages 124 to 126 and Table 8-1, pages 118 to 121), must be made and recorded.

D. Radiographs
The frequency of radiographic surveys is in accord with the dentist's determination of an individual patient's need (see Table 9-6, page 150).[3]

E. Periodontal Examination
1. Observe and record: gingival color, size, shape, position, recession
2. Complete probing: compare with previous probings
3. Mucogingival lines; attached gingiva
4. Occlusion, fremitus, mobility
5. Calculus: distribution, amount
6. Plaque score

F. Examination of the Teeth
1. Restorations
2. Sealants
3. Carious lesions
4. Sensitivity

G. Evaluation of Oral Cleanliness and Adequacy of Self-Care Measures

Relate plaque on teeth as observed after applying a disclosing agent to areas of gingival redness, enlargement, and other signs of infection.

H. Examination of Specific Areas

Areas of special problems include endodontically treated teeth, postsurgical areas, implants, occlusal factors, and prosthetic appliances.

I. Microbial Monitoring

Of the more than 300 species of bacteria that reside in the oral cavity, only a few, singly or in clusters, are responsible for periodontal infection leading to tissue destruction. Table 16-3 (page 274) lists major pathogens involved in destructive periodontal diseases. Tests for periodontal pathogens have been developed to aid in the diagnosis and treatment of infections.

1. *Possible Purposes for Testing*
   a. Select treatment procedures: certain bacteria respond to certain treatments.
   b. Monitor treated patients: determine pathogens present before treatment and test again after treatment to determine whether the pathogens have been eradicated.
   c. Screening: to determine sites that are at risk for periodontal infection.
2. *Types of Tests*
   a. Dark-field and phase-contrast microscope: show shifts in size, shape, and motility, but not specific organisms.
   b. Bacterial culture: most accurate method for identifying and quantifying specific organisms.
   c. Immunoassay and nucleic acid probe assay: target certain species by using specific antisera or antibody.
   d. Enzyme assays: test for collagenase, peptidases, and other enzymes specific to certain periodontal pathogens.
   e. DNA probes: identify specific organisms by their DNA.

II. MAINTENANCE CARE PLAN

A care plan is outlined, based on the new dental hygiene diagnosis and evaluation of the patient's oral condition. A patient in any of the maintenance categories will require the basic care plan below. Supplemental procedures may be needed.

A. Oral Hygiene Instruction/Motivation

During continuing care, the patient is considered a co-therapist. Compliance in faithful personal daily care is a major feature in the total program if etiologic factors are to be kept under control.

B. Periodontal Scaling and Debridement

C. Dental Caries Control

Prevention with attention to root caries; fluoride applications, dietary assessment, and diet modifications.

D. Supplemental Care Procedures

1. Smoking cessation assistance (pages 436 to 438)
2. Desensitization of sensitive areas
3. Special care for implants or fixed prostheses
4. Local delivery of antimicrobials for isolated persistent deep pockets (pages 569 to 573)

E. Referral for Retreatment Evaluation

III. CRITERIA FOR REFERRAL DURING MAINTENANCE

There are three points during patient care when the dental hygienist in a general practice must confer with the dentist to determine the need for referral to a periodontist. The decision can be made initially when the patient is first examined and severe periodontitis is evident, later during the reevaluation of initial scaling, or even later during the maintenance therapy. Criteria for referral during maintenance include:

A. Pocket depth that prohibits access for debridement or maintenance.
B. Furcation involvements and other deep or complex anatomical areas that cannot be instrumented successfully.
C. Mucogingival problems.

RECURRENCE OF PERIODONTAL DISEASE

Recurrence of signs and symptoms of periodontal infection indicates recolonization of periodontal pathogens. Recolonization of a pocket can occur within an average of 42 days.[4]

Without daily personal bacterial plaque control and regular professional supervision and maintenance procedures, infection can recur. How soon after the completion of treatment it may reappear will vary with each patient depending on a number of contributing factors.

I. CONTRIBUTING FACTORS

A. Inadequate or Insufficient Personal Bacterial Plaque Control

B. Lack of Compliance With Maintenance Appointments

1. *Patient Decision:* Misunderstanding of importance; personal reasons.
2. *Professional Laxity:* Insufficient patient counseling; inadequate recall system.

C. Incomplete Professional Treatment

1. *Scaling and Debridement:* Incomplete, espe-

cially in areas of difficult access such as furcations and deep proximal pockets.

  2. *Plaque Retention:* Neglect to remove or replace overhanging restorations and other areas that trap plaque and foster bacterial growth.

D. Tobacco Use[5]

E. Systemic Diseases

Diabetes mellitus,[6] HIV/AIDS, and certain other systemic diseases influence healing and control factors related to bone loss and severity of infections.

F. Genetic Factors[7,8]

Risk assessment includes testing for genetic factors.

II. RE-INFECTION

Transmission of periodontal microorganisms has been shown.[9,10] Colonization in the recipient depends on the number, frequency of exposure, and the virulence of the organisms.

TECHNICAL HINTS

Methods for administration of a maintenance plan vary. For any plan, individual file information includes name, address, telephone numbers, and instructions concerning appointment frequency and available or preferred day and time. The data may be kept on 3 × 5 or 4 × 6–inch file cards or in a computer.

I. PREBOOK METHOD

Make each patient's appointment before the patient leaves the current appointment. An appointment card is given the patient, who is asked to enter it on the calendar ahead of time. An envelope is prepared for mailing a duplicate card 10 days to 1 week before the scheduled appointment. The card should request the patient to call to confirm. For unconfirmed appointments, a call to the patient the day before must be made.

II. MONTHLY REMINDERS

By this system, individual data are filed alphabetically by the last name of the patient under the month when the patient is due. Each month the cards are pulled and reminders are mailed or telephoned well in advance.

III. COMPUTER ASSISTED

Computers can be helpful in maintaining appointment systems. Either the prebook or the monthly reminders can be used in combination with a computer.

Data stored on a computer can be readily accessible. Computers are capable of printing address labels so that postal cards can be mailed monthly or envelopes containing the prebook appointment card can be sent at the appropriate time.

FACTORS TO TEACH THE PATIENT

  I. Purposes of follow-up and maintenance appointments.
  II. Relationship of personal oral care habits to the maintenance of cleanliness provided through professional scaling and debridement.
  III. Importance of keeping all maintenance appointments.

REFERENCES

1. **Stamm**, J.W.: Periodontal Diseases and Human Health: New Directions in Periodontal Medicine, *Annals Periodontol., 3,* 1, July, 1998.
2. **Schallhorn**, R.G. and Snider, L.E.: Periodontal Maintenance Therapy, *J. Am Dent. Assoc., 103,* 227, August, 1981.
3. **American Dental Association,** Council on Dental Materials, Instruments, and Equipment: Recommendations in Radiographic Practices: An Update, 1988, *J. Am Dent. Assoc., 118,* 115, January, 1989.
4. **Mousqués**, T., Listgarten, M.A., and Phillips, R.W.: Effects of Scaling and Root Planing on the Composition of the Human Subgingival Microbial Flora, *J. Periodont. Res., 15,* 144, March, 1980.
5. **MacFarlane**, G.D., Herzberg, M.C., Wolff, L.F., and Hardie, N.A.: Refractory Periodontitis Associated with Abnormal Polymorphonuclear Leukocyte Phagocytosis and Cigarette Smoking, *J. Periodontol., 63,* 908, November, 1992.
6. **Grossi**, S.G., Skrepcinski, F.B., DeCaro, T., Zambon, J.J., Cummins, D., and Genco, R.J.: Response to Periodontal Therapy in Diabetics and Smokers, *J. Periodontol., 67,* 1094, Supplement, October, 1996.
7. **Hart**, T.C. and Kornman, K.S.: Genetic Factors in the Pathogenesis of Periodontitis, *Periodontol. 2000, 14,* 202, 1997.
8. **Kornman**, K.S. and diGiovine, F.S.: Genetic Variations in Cytokine Expression: A Risk Factor for Severity of Adult Periodontitis, *Annals Periodontol., 3,* 327, July, 1998.
9. **Von Troil-Lindén**, B., Torkko, H., Alaluusua, S., Wolf, J., Jousimies-Somer, H., and Asikainen, S.: Periodontal Findings in Spouses: A Clinical, Radiographic and Microbiological Study, *J. Clin. Periodontol., 22,* 93, February, 1995.
10. **Zambon**, J.J.: Periodontal Diseases: Microbial Factors, *Annals Periodontol., 1,* 904–908, November, 1996.

SUGGESTED READINGS

American Academy of Periodontology, Committee on Research, Science, and Therapy: Position Paper. Supportive Periodontal Therapy (SPT), *J. Periodontol., 69,* 502, April, 1998.

Axelsson, P. and Lindhe, J.: The Significance of Maintenance Care in the Treatment of Periodontal Disease, *J. Clin. Periodontol., 8,* 281, August, 1981.

DeVore, C.H., Hicks, M.J., and Claman, L.: A System for Insuring Success of Long-term Supportive Periodontal Therapy, *J. Dent. Hyg., 63,* 214, June, 1989.

Echeverria, J.J., Manau, G.C., and Guerrero, A.: Supportive Care After Active Periodontal Treatment. A Review, *J. Clin. Periodontol., 23,* 898, October, 1996.

Mann, L.C.: Guidelines for Supportive Periodontal Therapy and When to Refer to a Periodontist, *Can. Dent. Hyg. Assoc. (Probe), 29,* 185, September, 1995.

McCullough, C.: Long-term Maintenance of the Treated Periodontal Patient, *Access, 8,* 45, March, 1994.

Merin, R.L.: Supportive Periodontal Treatment, in Carranza,

F.A. and Newman, M.G.: *Clinical Periodontology*, 8th ed. Philadelphia, W.B. Saunders Co., 1996, pp. 743–760.

Nevins, M.: Long-term Periodontal Maintenance in Private Practice, *J. Clin. Periodontol., 23*, 273, March, 1996.

Ogilvie, A.L.: Maintenance of the Periodontal Patient, in Schluger, S., Yuodelis, R., Page, R.C., and Johnson, R.H.: *Periodontal Diseases*, 2nd ed. Philadelphia, Lea & Febiger, 1990, pp. 732–746.

Parr, R.W.: *Periodontal Maintenance Therapy*. Berkeley, California, Praxis Publishing Co., 1974, 86 pp.

Parr, R.W., Green, E., and Miller, S.R.: *Hygienists in Periodontal Maintenance Therapy*. Berkeley, California, Praxis Publishing Co., 1978, 67 pp.

Ramfjord, S.P.: Maintenance Care and Supportive Periodontal Therapy, *Quintessence Int., 24*, 465, July, 1993.

Reiker, J., van der Velden, U., Barendregt, D.S., and Loos, B.G.: A Cross-sectional Study into the Prevalence of Root Caries in Periodontal Maintenance Patients, *J. Clin. Periodontol., 26*, 26, January, 1999.

Shiloah, J. and Patters, M.R.: Repopulation of Periodontal Pockets by Microbial Pathogens in the Absence of Supportive Therapy, *J. Periodontol., 67*, 130, February, 1996.

Somacarrera, M.L., Lucas, M., Cuervas-Mons, V., and Hernandez, G.: Oral Care Planning and Handling of Immunosuppressed Heart, Liver, and Kidney Transplant Patients, *Spec. Care Dent., 16*, 242, November/December, 1996.

Wang, N.J. and Holst, D.: Individualizing Recall Intervals in Child Dental Care, *Community Dent. Oral Epidemiol., 23*, 1, February, 1995.

Wang, N.J. and Riordan, P.J.: Recall Intervals, Dental Hygienists and Quality in Child Dental Care, *Community Dent. Oral Epidemiol., 23*, 8, February, 1995.

Wilson, T.G., ed.: Supportive Periodontal Treatment and Retreatment in Periodontics, *Periodontol. 2000, 12*, 1–140 (18 articles), 1996.

Von Troil-Lindén, B., Saarela, M., Matto, J., Alaluusua, S., Jousimies-Somer, H., and Asikainen, S.: Source of Suspected Periodontal Pathogens Re-emerging After Periodontal Treatment, *J. Clin. Periodontol., 23*, 601, June, 1996.

Treatment During Maintenance

Cattabriga, M., Pedrazzoli, V., Cattabriga, A., Pannuti, E., Trapani, M., and Verrocchi, G.C.: Tetracycline Fiber Used Alone or with Scaling and Root Planing in Periodontal Maintenance Patients: Clinical Results, *Quintessence Int., 27*, 395, June, 1996.

Drisko, C.H. and Lewis, L.H.: Ultrasonic Instruments and Antimicrobial Agents in Supportive Periodontal Treatment and Retreatment of Recurrent or Refractory Periodontitis, *Periodontology 2000, 12*, 90, 1996.

Greenstein, G.: Periodontal Response to Mechanical Nonsurgical Therapy: A Review, *J. Periodontol., 63*, 118, February, 1992.

Kaldahl, W.B., Kalkwarf, K.L., Patil, K.D., Molvar, M.P., and Dyer, J.K.: Long-term Evaluation of Periodontal Therapy: I. Response to 4 Therapeutic Modalities, *J. Periodontol., 67*, 93, February, 1996.

Pattison, A.M.: The Use of Hand Instruments in Supportive Periodontal Treatment, *Periodontology 2000, 12*, 71, 1996.

Compliance

Novaes, A.B., Novaes, Jr., A.B., Moraes, N., Campos, G.M., and Grisi, M.F.M.: Compliance with Supportive Periodontal Therapy, *J. Periodontol., 67*, 213, March, 1996.

Novaes, Jr., A.B., deLima, F.R., and Novaes, A.B.: Compliance with Supportive Periodontal Therapy and Its Relation to the Bleeding Index, *J. Periodontol., 67*, 976, October, 1996.

Wilson, T.G., Hale, S., and Temple, R.: The Results of Efforts to Improve Compliance with Supportive Periodontal Treatment in a Private Practice, *J. Periodontol., 64*, 311, April, 1993.

Wilson, T.G.: How Patient Compliance to Suggested Oral Hygiene and Maintenance Affect Periodontal Therapy, *Dent. Clin. North Am., 42*, 389, April, 1998.

VI

PATIENTS WITH SPECIAL NEEDS

INTRODUCTION

An understanding of each patient's general and/or oral health problems requires particular study. Actually, each patient is a "special" patient and must be considered according to individual needs. The patients with special needs who will be considered in the chapters following include patients with oral and general systemic conditions. Variations with respect to age and degree of physical and/or mental disability are considered.

Certain patients, however, have problems peculiar to their age group and/or unusual health factors that may complicate the plan for care generally provided. These special patients require more skillful application of dental hygiene knowledge and ability to accomplish a comparably favorable result than do what might be called "normal" patients.

The dental hygienist's obligation is to see that no patient needs special rehabilitative dental or periodontal services because of any condition that could have been prevented by dental hygiene care.

Consideration of the patient as a whole requires attention to general physical and emotional problems as well as oral problems. Basic psychologic needs for affection, belonging, independence, achievement, recognition, and self-esteem frequently influence the outcome of treatment, as does the patient's whole attitude toward dental and dental hygiene care.

Optimum oral health is frequently an important contributing factor in maintaining or restoring the patient's physical, emotional, vocational, economic, and social usefulness to the extent of individual capabilities.

With certain disabilities, oral health has assumed less importance in the mind of the patient because other health problems have demanded so much attention. For some of these patients, neglect has intensified the need for oral care.

SPECIAL ORAL PROBLEMS

In each specialty of dentistry, patients present with problems that can be helped by the services performed by the dental hygienist. Patients with dentofacial handicaps who have missing teeth or congenital malformations, patients requiring surgery, and patients afflicted with habits conducive to the initiation of dental caries are all examples of patients who need special adaptations of the preventive care and instruction the dental hygienist can provide.

PERIODONTAL RISK FACTORS

The new research that ties together periodontal infections with systemic conditions provides the basis for emphasis on periodontal health. Risk factors for peri-

odontal infections also may be risk factors for systemic conditions, for example, use of tobacco, certain nutritional deficiencies, and immune dysfunctions.

Periodontal infection is a risk factor for many systemic conditions, including diabetes mellitus, preterm low birth weight, osteoporosis, bacterial pneumonias, and cardiovascular diseases. Certain systemic conditions are risk factors for periodontal conditions including HIV/AIDS, diabetes mellitus, and medications with side effects of oral manifestations.

ORAL MANIFESTATIONS

The interrelationship between oral conditions and systemic diseases must be revealed through a patient's medical history and identified by clinical changes noted during the extra- and intra-oral examinations.

Oral manifestations may be evident in association with certain acute and chronic systemic diseases, particularly nutritional deficiencies, endocrine disturbances, blood diseases, and many chronic degenerative diseases. When an oral manifestation suggests the possibility of an undiagnosed systemic disease, dental personnel have a responsibility to refer the patient for medical evaluation.

DENTAL HYGIENE CARE

Patients with chronic conditions may or may not be able to go to a dental office or clinic for appointments. Certain conditions, particularly during the advanced stages of a disease, require the patient to remain confined and, in some instances, bedridden. Dental hygienists must understand the special procedures for care in these instances.

The basic approach to oral problems of the patient with a chronic disease or a physical or mental disability is through prevention. Individual initiative is vital if the impact of preventive measures is to be understood and necessary action taken. The public, including dental personnel, must incorporate into daily living fundamental health practices that contribute to optimum health and, hence, to the prevention of chronic disease. Dental hygiene care can improve the general health and influence the resistance to infection of the oral cavity.

INTEGRATION OF APPLICATIONS TO SPECIAL NEEDS

A patient may have more than one special need. For example, the patient who requires dental hygiene care prior to oral surgery may have a blood disorder. The pregnant patient may have diabetes. The use of the patient's medical history plays an important role when the total needs of the patient are outlined.

Part VI attempts to integrate learning from other areas of medical and social sciences into the dental and dental hygiene aspects. The dental hygienist is encouraged to supplement knowledge and apprecia-tion of the special needs of patients through the use of additional readings such as those suggested at the end of each chapter. By application of understanding of the patient's needs, clinical techniques and patient counseling may be directed more skillfully to provide *complete dental hygiene care*.

43

The Pregnant Patient and the Infant/Toddler

During pregnancy, attention is focused on good health practices for the mother. She is concerned for the health of her baby and for herself. This alertness to total health, of which oral health is an important part, provides an unusual opportunity to help the patient learn principles that may be applied to the future care of the child.

The term *prenatal care* refers to the supervised preparation for childbirth that helps the mother enjoy optimum health during and after pregnancy and provides the maximum chance for the baby to be born healthy. Such a program involves the combined efforts of the obstetrician and/or midwife, nurse practitioner, dentist, dental hygienist, nutritionist, and the expectant parents. Key words for study with this chapter are defined in Box 43-1.

Obstetricians, family practitioners, and nurses in private and public health settings should recommend dental and periodontal examination early in pregnancy. This brings to the dental office or clinic many women who previously would not have had a regular plan for obtaining professional service. Many of these

women have not known the advantages of personal habits of daily care and diet related to the health of the oral tissues. Numerous misconceptions must be counteracted when providing up-to-date information about the relationship of pregnancy and oral health.

Women who do not receive routine oral health care may appear for emergency dental services and may be receptive to a program of care and instruction to prevent further emergencies. The dental hygienist in public health, especially maternal and child health clinics, participates in community educational programs with public health nurses, whereby some less informed women may learn of the need for professional dental care and advice during pregnancy.

FETAL DEVELOPMENT

Pregnancy is arbitrarily divided into three periods of 3 months each called the first, second, and third trimesters. Normal pregnancy, or period of *gestation,* is

BOX 43-1 KEY WORDS: Pregnancy, Infants, and Toddlers

Amniocentesis: (am″nē-ō-sen-tē′sĭs): a testing procedure on fluid aspirated from the amniotic sac to detect chromosomal abnormalities and metabolic disorders.

Amniotic sac (am″nē-ot′ik): the innermost of the membranes enveloping the embryo *in utero*; **amniotic fluid** fills the sac in which the embryo is free to move and is protected against mechanical injury.

Cesarean section (sĕ-zar′ē-an): delivery of a fetus by incision through the abdominal wall and uterus.

Embryo: developing organism from conception to approximately the end of the second month.

Epulis: nonspecific term referring to a growth on the gingiva.

Estradiol: the most potent natural estrogen in humans; the circulating blood level of estradiol rises during the follicular phase of the reproductive cycle and drops when ovulation occurs (see Figure 45-1, page 679).

Fetus: developing organism from the second month after conception to birth.

Gestation: the period of pregnancy.

Granuloma: nonspecific term applied to a nodular inflammatory lesion containing macrophages and surrounded by lymphocytes.

   "Pyogenic" granuloma: a misnomer because it does not contain pus, but contains blood vessels and inflammatory cells.

In utero: within the womb; not yet born.

Infant: child younger than 1 year of age.

Intrapartum: occuring during childbirth.

Midwife: a person who attends a woman during delivery.

   Nurse-midwife: a registered nurse specializing in midwifery; requires additional education and special licensure in certain states and countries.

Neonate (ne′ōnāt): newborn.

   Neonatal: refers to the period immediately following birth and continuing through the first month of life.

Non-nutritive sucking: sucking fingers, pacifiers, or other objects.

Obstetrics: the branch of medicine that has to do with the care of the pregnant woman during pregnancy and parturition.

   Obstetrician: physician who practices obstetrics.

Parturition (pahr″tu-rĭ′shun) childbirth; labor; giving birth.

Postpartum: pertaining to the period following childbirth or delivery.

Premature birth: birth that occurs before the expected delivery date; denotes an infant born prior to 37 weeks of gestation.

Puerpera (pū-ĕr′pĕr-ah): woman who has just given birth to a child.

Pyogenic (pī″o-jĕn′ĭk): producing pus.

Teratogen (ter′ah-tō-jen): nongenetic factors that cause malformations and disease syndromes *in utero*.

Teratogenic agent: any drug, virus, or irradiation the exposure to which can cause malformation of the fetus.

Tippy cup: a special cup designed to teach a young child to drink.

Toddler: child from age 1 year to approximately 3 years of age.

Trimester: a period of 3 months; one third of a pregnancy.

Wean: to discontinue breast-feeding and bottle; to nourish the infant with other food.

---

approximately 40 weeks. *Premature birth* refers to a birth before 37 weeks' gestation.

Physiologic changes in the mother are related to nearly every bodily system. Early development of the embryo is greatly influenced by heredity and the overall health of the mother.

I. FIRST TRIMESTER

During the first trimester, the embryo is highly susceptible to injuries and malformations. Teratogenic effects can be produced by many sources, including maternal poor nutrition, infections, and drug intake.

All organ systems are formed (organogenesis) during the first trimester. By 12 weeks, the fetus moves and swallows. In the oral cavity, the following occurs:

A. Teeth
1. Tooth buds develop between the fifth and sixth week.
2. Initial mineralization occurs from the fourth to the fifth month.

B. Lips and Palate
1. Lips form during the fourth to the seventh week.

2. Palate forms between the eighth and the twelfth week.
3. Cleft lip is apparent by the eighth week; cleft palate, by the twelfth week (pages 665 to 668).

II. SECOND AND THIRD TRIMESTERS

The organs are completed, and growth and maturation continue. Fetal weight changes from 1 ounce at 3 months to an average of 7.5 pounds at birth.

III. FACTORS THAT CAN HARM THE FETUS

A. Periodontal Infection in the Mother
Severe periodontitis is a significant risk factor for preterm delivery with low birth weight. A pregnant mother with advanced periodontitis has a 7.5 to 7.9 fold increased risk for a preterm low birth weight infant.[1]

B. Other Infections
Protection from infectious diseases is necessary because damage to and infection of the fetus can result. Women of childbearing age should avail themselves of all available vaccines prior to conception.

Defects, deformities, and life-threatening infections can result from infection acquired during pregnancy or during delivery and after birth. Rubella (German measles), rubeola, varicella, herpes viruses, hepatitis B (page 25), human immunodeficiency virus (HIV) infection (page 32), syphilis (congenital syphilis), and gonorrhea all can have serious effects on the fetus.

C. Medications
Ideally no medications or other drugs should be used during pregnancy. Nearly all drugs can pass across the placenta to enter the circulation of the developing fetus. Many drugs have teratogenic effects. Table 43-1 lists selected drugs with examples of their possible effects on the fetus.
1. *Effect of Tetracycline.* Tetracycline is well known for intrinsic staining of tooth structure. The effect occurs during mineralization of the primary teeth beginning at about 4 months of gestation and of the permanent teeth near and after birth (page 289). When an antibiotic is required during pregnancy, a choice other than tetracycline can be made.
2. *Therapy for HIV Infection.*[2] Prevention of perinatal HIV transmission and health for the fetus and neonate are considered with the plan for optimal health care for the mother with HIV/AIDS infection. Antiretroviral medication is not withheld because of pregnancy and generally should be the same as for a nonpregnant adult.

With no long-term safety studies, whether antiretroviral agents are teratogenic is not known. Consideration by the mother can be given to withholding the antiretroviral treatment during the first 14 weeks of pregnancy. That is the period of maximal organogenesis and risk for teratogenicity.

D. Drugs of Abuse
Adverse effects of controlled substances, alcohol, and tobacco products are included in Table 43-1. There are many serious effects from their use. Additional information on the effects of smoking on pregnancy and smoking cessation can be found on page 429.

ORAL FINDINGS DURING PREGNANCY

Gingival inflammatory changes that occur during pregnancy are considered to be an exaggerated response of the tissues to bacterial plaque. When the periodontal tissues are in good health and the patient uses adequate personal oral care measures for plaque control, major adverse gingival changes are not expected.

The gingiva can show a reaction to the physiologic changes of pregnancy, as well as to the influence of the increased circulating levels of female sex hormones. Trauma, poor oral hygiene, and local irritation from calculus or prostheses may be contributory factors.

The gingival reaction in pregnancy is usually seen by the second month. When left untreated, the gingival inflammation continues as the hormone levels rise, to a maximum severity by the eighth month.

The symptoms abate after the birth of the child, but a completely healthy condition does not necessarily result. A patient with a gingival disturbance during pregnancy continues to have the disturbance, even if to a somewhat lessened degree, after the birth.

I. GINGIVITIS[3,4]

A. Clinical Appearance
The appearance varies and shows characteristics of inflamed tissues, including enlargement, redness, shiny surface, and bleeding on probing.

B. Predisposing Factors
1. Local irritation because of an unhygienic oral condition and bacterial plaque on the teeth and gingiva.
2. Hormonal changes during pregnancy that may alter the tissue reaction.

C. Microbiology[5,6]
Increased proportions of *Prevotella intermedia* have been found with an increase in gingivitis and elevated serum levels of the hormones of pregnancy (estrogen and progesterone).

II. GINGIVAL ENLARGEMENT[7]

An oral pyogenic granuloma may develop. It is a benign, inflammatory lesion. It has also been called an epulis gravidarum, a pregnancy granuloma, or a preg-

TABLE 43-1 Drugs Contraindicated During Pregnancy and Breast-Feeding

Classification	Drugs Prescribed for Treatment*	Possible Adverse Effects on Fetus and Infant
Anticoagulant	Warfarin (Coumadin) (D) Dicumarol (D)	Hemorrhagic; fetal death Birth Malformations
Anticonvulsant	Barbiturates (phenobarbital) (D) Phenytoin sodium (D) Trimethadione (D) Valproate sodium (D)	Congenital malformations Developmental delays Fetal phenobarbital syndrome Fetal hydantoin syndrome Fetal trimethadione syndrome Fetal valproate syndrome
Antimicrobial	Streptomycin (B) Tetracycline (D)	Toxic action on ear: 8th cranial nerve damage Bone growth inhibition; intrinsic dental stain
Antineoplastic	Cyclophosphamide (Cytoxan) (D) Mercaptopurine (D) Methotrexate (D)	Multiple anomalies; fetal death

Hormones	Clomiphene (Clomid) (X)
	 Estrogenic substances (X)
	    diethylstilbestrol (X)
	 Prednisone (C)
	 Progesterone (X)
		Increased anomalies; neural tube defects
		 Cancer of the vagina and cervix; genital tract anomalies; congenital
		    heart defects

Psychotrophic	Antianxiety
	    chlordiazepoxide (Librium) (D)
	    diazepam (Valium) (D)
	    meprobamate (Miltown) (D)
	 Antimanic
	    lithium carbonate (D)
		Low heart rate, muscle tone, respiration, poor sucking reflex
		
		 Taken near term may cause neonatal withdrawal syndrome or cardio-
		    respiratory instability
		
		 Lethargy, cyanosis, teratogenic (dose related)

Drugs of Abuse	Alcohol	Fetal alcohol syndrome (page 890) Spontaneous abortion; low birth rate Mental retardation

	Cocaine
	    prenatal exposure
	
	    inhale free-base vapors (postpartum)
		Decreased birth weight; prematurity
		 Fetal growth retardation; microcephaly
		 Teratogenic effects
		 Increased rate of seizures

	Narcotics
	    heroin
	    methadone
		Decreased birth weight
		 Withdrawal symptoms
		 Convulsions; sudden infant death

	Tobacco
	    cigarette smoking
	
	    involuntary smoking
	       Environmental
		Low birth weight; prematurity; miscarriage; still birth; infant mortality
		 Sudden infant death syndrome
		 Children: increased respiratory infections and symptoms
		 Deficiencies in physical growth, intellectual development
		 Higher incidence in mortality rate of infant and child

*United States Food and Drug Administration (FDA) categorizes drugs and their relation to pregnancy as: **A.** No risk demonstrated to fetus in any trimester. **B.** No adverse effects in animals; no human studies available. **C.** Only given after risks to fetus are considered; animal studies have shown no adverse reactions, no human studies available. **D.** Definite fetal risks; may be given in spite of risks if needed in life-threatening conditions. **X.** Absolute fetal abnormalities; not to be used at any time in pregnancy.

nancy tumor.[8,9] The use of the word tumor is misleading, because the lesion is not a tumor but a hyperplasia and also occurs in men and nonpregnant women. When the lesion is removed during pregnancy, there is some tendency for recurrence.

A. Clinical Appearance

The lesion appears as an isolated, discrete, soft, round enlargement near the gingival margin usually associated with an interdental area. It forms in a mushroomlike shape with a smooth, glistening surface. The pressure of the lip or cheek tends to make it flattened.

The color depends on the vascularity and may be purplish-red, magenta, or deep blue, sometimes dotted with red.

B. Symptoms

1. Bleeds readily with slight trauma.
2. Painless unless it becomes large enough to interfere with occlusion and mastication.

C. Significance

1. Interference during mastication: can contribute to inadequate nutritive intake for mother and baby because of discomfort when chewing.
2. Provides a site for bacterial growth: potential development of periodontal attachment loss and eventual bone destruction.
3. Results in bleeding and pain: may interfere with routine bacterial plaque removal using toothbrush and interdental aids.
4. Creates an undesirable cosmetic effect.

III. ENAMEL EROSION

Morning sickness with vomiting over an extended period can lead to demineralization and acid erosion primarily of the palatal surfaces. Nausea associated with early pregnancy can be relieved by frequent eating of small amounts of food. Careful selection of nutritious yet noncariogenic foods is necessary to avoid dental caries.

Advise patient to use a sodium bicarbonate rinse after vomiting to neutralize acid on the teeth. Vigorous toothbrushing should be avoided to prevent damage to tooth surface that has been slightly etched.

ASPECTS OF PATIENT CARE

The first few months may be challenging for the mother-to-be, because pregnancy provides an emotional experience with many adjustments that must be made. The second trimester is considered the safest for general dental treatment. However, dental hygiene care should start much earlier to keep the gingival tissues in optimum health and prevent oral infections.

I. ASSESSMENT

A. Early Appointment

The patient should be seen as early in her pregnancy as possible. Anticipatory guidance is mandatory relative to the effects of drugs, tobacco use, and periodontal infection on the development and subsequent health of the infant.

B. Medical History

1. Other health problems: conditions other than pregnancy may be present. For example, diabetes or cardiovascular diseases can involve serious complications.
2. Adolescent health: when the expectant mother is an adolescent, her own special needs differ from those of a mature woman. Aspects of adolescent development are described on pages 675 to 678.

C. Consultation

Contact with the patient's physician and/or obstetrician is necessary for integrating general and oral care. All reasonable treatment is acceptable unless the patient's obstetrician advises otherwise.

When a patient seeks dental and dental hygiene care and is not under the care of a physician, she should be urged and assisted to obtain medical supervision for her health and the health of her baby.

II. RADIOGRAPHY

A. Universal Safety Factors

Radiographs are not made for any patient unless necessary. When they are required during pregnancy, the patient is covered with a lead apron, a thyroid collar, and a second apron for the back to prevent secondary radiation from reaching the abdomen. As always, all current methods for radiation safety and protection are applied, including optimum filtration, collimation, use of the fastest film, and extended target film distance.

B. Exposures

Determine the minimum number of film exposures that will produce the required diagnostic information. The use of a paralleling technique does not require angulation directed toward the patient's abdomen. Careful and skillful film placement, angulation, processing, and all phases of technique prevent the need for remaking radiographs that are not acceptable for diagnosis.

III. PERIODONTAL TREATMENT

Areas of food impaction should be corrected and all overhanging restorations reshaped or replaced. All nonsurgical procedures should be carefully and thoroughly completed. Complicated elective periodontal treatment should be deferred until after delivery.

IV. OVERALL TREATMENT CONSIDERATIONS

A. Dental Hygiene Care Goal: Optimum periodontal health and hygiene.

B. Dental Care

1. *Elective Treatment:* Postpone until second trimester or early third trimester.
2. *Restorative:* Restorations should be completed with permanent restorative materials. One important contraindication for the use of temporary restorations is that, after the baby is born, the mother may be too busy to attend to appointments because of added family responsibilities and/or a return to career employment.

DENTAL HYGIENE CARE

The dental hygienist must be well informed about dental care to motivate the patient and alleviate fears related to certain services. The patient often consults with the dental hygienist for reassurance and interpretation of the dentist's recommendations and procedures.

Gingival disease need not be expected when the patient is motivated to practice conscientious self-care procedures for oral cleanliness and plaque control. This calls for a specific appointment plan for scaling and disease control instruction.

A concentrated plan for dental caries control is indicated. A multiple fluoride program and limitation of cariogenic foods are basic to the preventive efforts.

I. APPOINTMENT PLANNING

A. Frequency

Monthly appointments or appointments three times during the 9-month period may be required, depending on the patient's needs as well as ability and motivation to maintain a healthy oral environment.

B. Individual Appointments

An appointment should be short, for patient comfort. A series of appointments is indicated when calculus deposits are heavy.

C. Postpartum Maintenance Appointments

For the patient who has not been on a regular maintenance plan prior to pregnancy, emphasis must be placed on motivating the patient to continue regular appointments for dental hygiene and dental care after the baby is born.

II. CLINICAL CARE

It is not within the scope of this book to review all the physiologic changes that occur during pregnancy. Common physical changes should be identified because they can affect appointment procedures. Nearly every woman is bothered by one or more minor complaints at some time during her pregnancy.

Attention to details provides the patient with comfort and motivates her to continue oral care. Table 43-2 lists the more common physical changes of pregnancy and suggests a few appointment considerations.

A. Patient Positioning

1. *Effect of Supine Position.* The weight of the developing fetus in the uterus bears down directly on the major vessels, the aorta, and the inferior vena cava. The vessels are pressed between the spinal column and the uterus. During the third trimester, symptoms of circulatory insufficiency can appear when venous return is decreased.
2. *Alternate Positions* (Figure 43-1)[10]
   a. Patient lies on left side.
   b. Elevate the right hip to displace the uterus to the left. Use a pillow or rolled-up blanket.

B. Instrumentation

When a patient has gingival enlargement and inflammation, a good part of the first appointment should be spent on instruction in plaque control and other preventive measures. At the second appointment, evaluation is made and instruction continued.

Careful instrumentation for calculus removal is indicated. After consultation with the patient's physician, local anesthetics may be used in moderation. Nitrous oxide–oxygen sedation is contraindicated.[11] If stain removal is needed, the use of an abrasive cleaning paste should be postponed until the tissue has responded to the plaque control measures.

C. Fluoride Program

1. *Professional Topical Application.* All patients can benefit from a topical application of fluoride solution or gel after scaling and root planing. Applications can be indicated, especially for patients with a tendency toward rampant caries and who have numerous restorations. The fluoride agents and techniques are described in Chapter 29, pages 465 to 469.
2. *Self-Application.* A fluoride dentifrice is recommended for all patients. A daily non-alcohol-containing mouthrinse, gel tray, or other mode of application is essential, depending on the individual evaluation. A concentrated fluoride effort can be particularly important to the teeth of the adolescent mother-to-be.

PATIENT INSTRUCTION

The emphasis on general health during pregnancy provides the ideal setting for instruction relative to many aspects of oral health for the mother and her expected child, as well as for other members of the family. New developments in disease prevention and control should be explained.

TABLE 43-2 Appointment Adaptations for the Prenatal Patient

Characteristic	Dental Hygiene Implication
Fatigues easily, may even fall asleep	Short appointments; several in series, as needed Work with an assistant to accomplish more at each appointment
General awkwardness because of new shape and weight gain	Attend to details, such as gently lowering and straightening chair for patient Make sure rinsing facilities are convenient; or preferably, an assistant attends to evacuation
Frequent urination	Allow sufficient appointment time for interruptions Suggest at beginning of appointment that patient mention need for interruption
Discomfort of remaining in one position too long Backache	Position the patient on her left side and not in supine or Trendelenburg position (Figure 43-1) Interrupt in middle of appointment to allow patient to change position Assistance with evacuation during intra-oral instrumentation can shorten appointment time
Faintness and dizziness	Be prepared for emergency (Table 61-5, pages 910–911)
Adverse reaction to strong smells and flavors	Recommend less strong flavored dentifrice
Exaggerated reactions to odors and flavors of medicaments and other office materials	Determine particularly obnoxious odors for an individual patient and remove them; check office ventilation
Unpleasant taste in mouth	Advise: non-alcoholic mouthrinse; use a neutral sodium fluoride rinse Demonstrate tongue brushing
Nausea and vomiting (first trimester)	Explain why not to brush right after vomiting to prevent erosion (page 656)
Gagging	Recommend a small toothbrush Turn head down over sink while brushing; helps to relax throat and allow saliva to flow out Take care in instrument and radiographic film placement
Physician's recommendation for alleviation of nausea symptoms: frequent eating of small amounts of foods	Encourage use of noncariogenic foods
Unusual food cravings	If cravings are for sweets, clearly define relationship of frequent nibbling of cariogenic foods to dental caries Provide list of nutritious noncariogenic snacks

Printed materials concerning the prevention of periodontal infections and dental caries and the development and care of children's teeth are available from the American Dental Association.* Reading material that supplements personal discussions can contribute to patient understanding and cooperation.

*An American Dental Association catalog for the current year may be obtained by writing the Department of Salable Materials, 211 East Chicago Avenue, Chicago, IL 60611.

I. BACTERIAL PLAQUE CONTROL

A rigid schedule for self-care must be demonstrated and supervised. A series of instructional periods is usually needed.

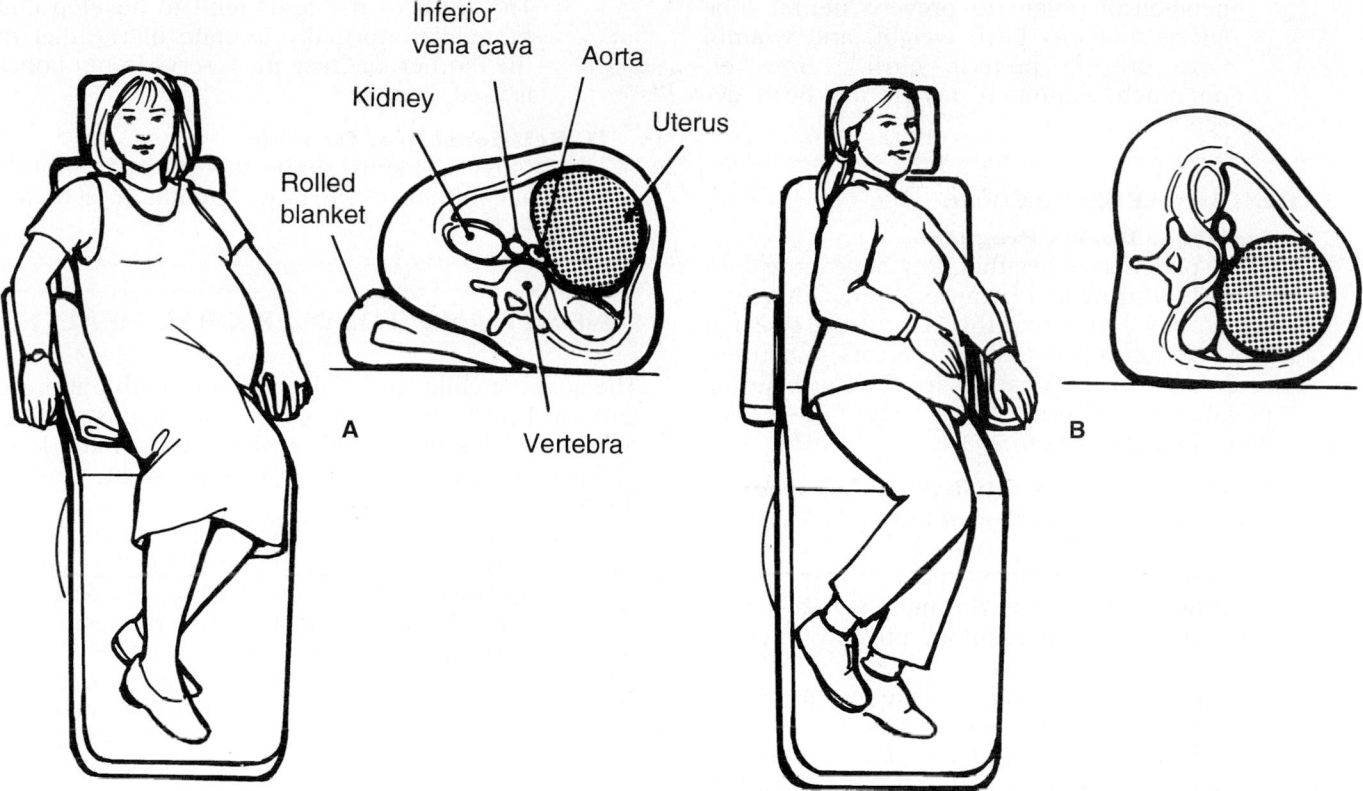

FIGURE 43-1 Positions During Pregnancy. The supine position allows the weight of the developing fetus to bear down directly on the major vessels. **(A)** Patient lies on left side with a pillow or blanket roll to elevate right hip. **(B)** Patient turned farther to left. Note position of fetus in cross sections of the abdomen.

II. PREVENTION OF PERIODONTAL DISEASE

A. Gingival changes during pregnancy (page 654) require continuing attention daily by the patient and periodically with professional appointments.

B. Severity of existing periodontal infection, or potential for the initiation of bone and attachment loss, can have serious effects on both mother and fetus.

C. Effect on preterm low birth weight: periodontal infection of the mother has a serious effect on the infant.[1]

III. SMOKING CESSATION

Use of tobacco, alcohol, and many substances of abuse during pregnancy has moderate to severe influences on the developing fetus as well as the child after birth. Pregnancy is an ideal time to motivate a patient to quit smoking. The mother's attention is captivated by doing her very best for a healthy child.

A. Explain increased risks for reduced birth weight, spontaneous abortions, perinatal deaths, and sudden infant death syndrome.

B. Present the steps in a cessation program (pages 436 to 438).

IV. DIET

Instruction must be provided in prevention of dental caries and maintenance of the health of the supporting structures of the teeth. The use of a varied diet containing the essential protective food groups, with a minimum of cariogenic foods, is necessary. The food guide pyramid is shown on page 445.

A. Purposes of Adequate Diet During Pregnancy

1. To maintain daily strength and feeling of well-being.
2. To provide the essential building materials for the developing fetus.
3. To protect and promote the health of the oral tissues of the mother.
4. To minimize postpartum problems.

B. Dietary Needs During Pregnancy

The mother's diet must be adequate to maintain her own nutritional status and to meet the needs of the fetus.

The particular needs of the fetus are:

1. Proteins, for general tissue construction.
2. Minerals, especially calcium and phosphorus, for bone and tooth mineralization; iron for blood corpuscles.
3. Vitamins, especially vitamin D for calcium

metabolism, folate to prevent neural tube defects and low birth weight, and vitamin A to prevent preterm birth.[12] However, too much vitamin A may cause birth defects.[13]

V. DENTAL CARIES CONTROL

A. Incidence During Pregnancy

Some patients believe that they have more dental caries during and because of pregnancy. Research has shown that this is not true, and that any relationship is indirect. Factors that result in dental caries formation are the same during pregnancy as at other times (Figure 28-1, page 443, and pages 272 to 273).

B. Factors That May Contribute to Apparent Increase in Dental Caries Rate

1. *Previous Neglect.* A patient may not have kept a regular appointment plan, so that the existing dental caries during pregnancy represents an accumulation, possibly even of years.
2. *Diet During Pregnancy.* Possible increase in intake of cariogenic foods:
   a. Unusual cravings may be for sweet foods.
   b. Frequency of eating: patient may be eating every few hours for prevention of nausea, and these foods may be cariogenic.
3. *Neglect of Personal Oral Care Procedures.* Patient may lack interest in daily bacterial plaque removal or be lax about rinsing immediately following intake of a cariogenic food.

C. Calcium and the Mother's Teeth

The misconception concerning the withdrawal of calcium from the mother's teeth and its relationship to dental caries is widespread. It is important to review the known facts, because the patient's beliefs may need clarification. In discussing the problem with the patient, a summary of the process of dental caries initiation can be helpful (pages 272 to 273).

1. Minerals contained in the erupted tooth enamel and dentin are not available, and no removal of minerals can occur by way of the pulp.
2. Minerals contained within the alveolar bone are available, as they are from other bones of the body. When the mother's diet does not contain sufficient calcium and phosphorus, her own reserve is utilized. The metabolism of calcium is complex.[12]
3. Most calcium and phosphorus of bones and teeth is added to the fetus during the third trimester. The incidence of dental caries in the mother is not different during that period, although the carious lesions may be larger if the teeth have been neglected throughout the pregnancy.

4. The teeth of the fetus tend to develop and mineralize normally in spite of the diet of the mother, because the reserve in her bones is used.

D. Relationship of Fluoride

No direct evidence shows that prenatal fluoride intake influences the rate of dental caries in the child.[14–16]

INFANT AND TODDLER ORAL HEALTH

The goal is a child free of dental caries with optimum gingival health. Parents need to understand the importance of the oral health of the newborn and how habits practiced during the early years of life can influence future health.

Counseling for parents starts before and continues after the birth of the baby. Before birth, the parents are looking ahead and planning for the very best care for their baby. They are most receptive to meaningful recommendations.

There are three primary areas for concern. Attention must be directed, first, to the parents' own oral hygiene for dental caries prevention and periodontal health; second, to the prevention of baby bottle tooth decay; and third, to the provision of adequate fluoride for the dental health of the entire family.

Through early guidance, parents can be aware of the infant's needs for oral health and anticipate the kind of attention that will be required. *Anticipatory guidance* is the term that has been applied to teaching ahead of time so that untoward, unfavorable conditions can be prevented.[17]

I. PRENATAL ANTICIPATORY GUIDANCE, BIRTH THROUGH 6 MONTHS (TABLE 43-3)

A. Help the parent understand that infants and toddlers can have dental caries and infections of the oral mucosa.
B. Suggest procedures for the parent's own oral health. The oral flora of the infant reflects the oral flora of the parents. *Streptococcus mutans* can be transmitted from the parents to the infant.
C. Plan for fluoride
   1. Determine the fluoride content of the water used at home (page 463).
   2. Analyze the need for prescription of fluoride supplements to start at 6 months of age (see Table 29-2, page 464).
D. Plan ahead for the infant's first dental hygiene visit.

II. FIRST DENTAL/DENTAL HYGIENE VISIT

A. Age

The first appointment should occur within 6 months of the eruption of the first primary tooth but no later than 12 months of age.[18]

TABLE 43-3 Anticipatory Guidance: Infants and Toddlers

Area of Concern	Birth to 6 Months	6 to 12 Months	18 Months
Developmental Milestone	Eruption of first tooth Pattern of eruption	Pattern of eruption Expected new teeth	Check tooth contacts Close contacts: teach to floss
Nutrition and Feeding	Cause and effects of baby bottle tooth decay Avoid use of nursing bottle If used: use only tap water Discourage parent sleeping with child Breast-feeding: passage of alcohol and drugs to infant	Discontinue bottle feeding Use regular cup Discuss sugar use, sugar retention, and caries initiation	Nutrition, snacking based on child's diet Snacking safety (aspiration) Reduce snacking frequency
Oral Hygiene and Caries Prevention	Oral health of parents; *Streptococcus mutans* transmission Clean teeth after each feeding (soft brush)	Use of brush Position of infant for brushing	Disclose for bacterial plaque Review brushing Parents are the role models
Fluoride Information	Explain the relation of F to teeth Anticipate need to supplement Check water supply for F content	When water supply is deficient, prescribe supplement (see Table 29-2, page 464) Discuss compliance Review manner of storage	Update fluoride status Use of small thin smear of fluoride dentifrice on brush
Trauma Prevention		Trauma-proofing Confirm emergency access to dental provider	Discuss oral electrical burns and child-proofing home Care of avulsed tooth
Habits/Function Behaviors	Discuss teething, non-nutritive sucking	Discuss oral signs of child abuse	Effects of continued thumb sucking
Environmental (Passive) Smoke	Detrimental at all ages Smoking parents must start tobacco cessation program	Provide smoke-free environment	Children need smoke-free environment
Dental/Dental Hygiene Visit	What happens at baby's first dental visit Parent's appointments for their dental care	First visit within 6 months of eruption of first tooth Parents make dental visit a happy event	Home preparation for dental hygiene visit Frequency depends on parent compliance with home preventive measures Parents build positive attitude toward dentist and dental hygienist

(Adapted from Casamassimo, P.S., Griffiths, P., and Nowak, A.: Anticipatory Guidance in Dentistry, *DentalHygienistNews, 5,* 19, Fall, 1992.)

B. Purposes

The early appointments are planned for prevention, introduction to dental hygiene, and oral assessment.

1. Discover, intercept, and change any practices applied by the parents that may be detrimental to the infant's oral health.
2. Initiate positive preventive measures, such as fluoride, feeding practices, and bacterial plaque removal.
3. Develop rapport with the baby and the family.
4. Provide anticipatory guidance (Table 43-3).

C. Record Medical, Dental, and Feeding History[19]

The forms for the histories may be best filled out before the appointment. They can be mailed to the parents prior to the first appointment.

D. Appointment Procedures

1. *Patient Position During Oral Examination.* Clinician and parent sit knee-to-knee with infant positioned on their laps. The clinician cradles the head; the parent gently holds the baby's

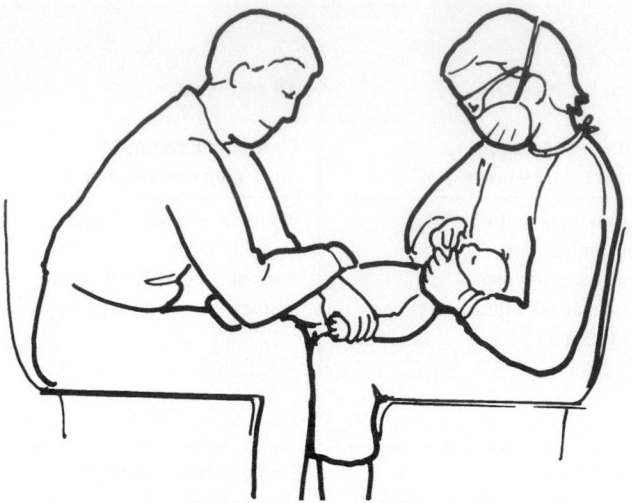

FIGURE 43-2 Infant's Dental/Dental Hygiene Visits. Clinician and parent sit knee-to-knee with the child across their laps. Parent stabilizes the infant's legs and holds the hands in a position that allows a good view of the patient's oral cavity for watching and learning. The clinician makes the oral examination, discusses any oral problems, and shows the parent oral care.

hands and may stabilize the legs with the elbows (Figure 43-2).

2. *Extra- and Intra-Oral Examination*
   a. Follow routine in Table 8-1 (page 119) and Table 11-1 (pages 194 and 195).
   b. Proceed calmly with soft talk. Anticipate that many infants will fuss and cry; reassure parent.
   c. Watch for physical signs of child abuse (page 128).
3. *Instruction for Bacterial Plaque Removal*
   a. Clinician demonstrates cleaning the teeth with a soft toothbrush; patient is held as described for the oral examination. Flossing is needed when teeth are in close contact.
   b. Parent demonstrates the cleaning procedure; the baby is turned around so that the clinician holds the hands and stabilizes the legs with the elbows.
4. *Counseling* (Table 43-3)
   All aspects of significance for the particular child are discussed with the parents: fluoride, diet and feeding, daily oral care. Reading materials are provided for review and discussion with the parents.

III. DAILY BACTERIAL PLAQUE REMOVAL

A. Planned Time

Parents need a routine for cleaning the infant's mouth. They must continue to care for the mouth until the child develops fine motor coordination, usually around 7 years of age.

1. Until the infant's first tooth erupts, place a clean damp cloth over finger and wipe over oral tissues and gingiva after each feeding.
2. After first tooth erupts, use a small, soft toothbrush with water only.

B. Position of Infant

Two family members can work together to make this experience pleasant and easy. Sit opposite each other with the infant between (Figure 43-2). For other positions, see Figure 50-11, page 754.

IV. DIETARY HABITS AND FEEDING[20]

A. Prevention of Baby Bottle Tooth Decay

1. Describe baby bottle tooth decay, how it is caused, and which teeth are most frequently involved (page 240).
2. Nap or nighttime bottle
   a. It is best never to start giving a bottle for bedtime use.
   b. If a bottle is used, do not use sweet juices or milk. Use only plain tap water.
   c. Do not use the bottle as a pacifier.
   d. Recommend discontinuance of bottle feeding at least by the age of 12 months and teaching the child to use a cup.[18]
3. Avoid "on-demand" breast-feeding practices. When the infant falls asleep, milk collects around the teeth. Demineralization begins, and dental caries can result.

B. Snacks

Noncariogenic snacks must be used. *Frequency* and *consistency* of snack foods are most significant (pages 450 and 451 and Figure 28-6).

C. Medications and Nutritional Supplements

Many medications and other products for child consumption are made with a sugar or syrupy base to disguise the bad flavor of the drug.[21,22] For counteractivity, rinse the child's mouth with clear water immediately after the medication is given.

V. MAINTENANCE

Certain risk factors need consideration when frequency of appointments is determined. The history and record of assessment contain most of the basic information needed. Infants with a high risk for dental caries need frequent preventive maintenance appointments. As the child grows older, attention must be paid to risks related to gingival conditions.

A. Low Risk

1. Family members oriented to oral health care; family with no history of needing extensive professional care.
2. Infant has received systemic fluoride through fluoridation or fluoride supplements in accord with the recommended schedule (see Table 29-2, page 464).

3. A normal general health history.

B. High Risk

1. Family members with history of irregular professional care in whom moderate to severe dental and periodontal treatment has been needed.
2. Residence in nonfluoridated community; private water supply not tested for fluoride level; systemic supplements not provided.
3. Presence of congenital or hereditary defect or developmental disability.
4. Administration of medications with potentially high sucrose base.
5. Dental examination that shows early eruption pattern, areas of demineralization, and notable bacterial plaque build-up.
6. Lack of parental supervision and reminders for maintenance of daily routine of oral hygiene.
7. Prolonged bottle/breast-feeding and feeding on demand.
8. Lack of general compliance with the plan for prevention.

REFERENCES

1. **Offenbacher, S.,** Katz, V., Fertik, G., Collins, J., Boyd, D., Maynor, G., McKaig, R., and Beck, J.: Periodontal Infection as a Possible Risk Factor for Preterm Low Birth Weight, *J. Periodontol., 67,* 1103, October, 1996, Supplement.
2. **International AIDS Society**—USA Panel: Antiretroviral Therapy for HIV Infection in 1997, *JAMA, 277,* 1962, June 25, 1997
3. **Loe,** H.: Periodontal Changes in Pregnancy, *J. Periodontol., 36,* 209, May–June, 1965.
4. **Carranza,** F.A. and Newman, M.G.: *Clinical Periodontology,* 8th ed. Philadelphia, W.B. Saunders, 1996, pp. 239–240, 193–194, 675–76.
5. **Kornman,** K.S. and Loesche, W.J.: The Subgingival Microbial Flora During Pregnancy, *J. Periodont. Res., 15,* 111, March, 1980.
6. **Jensen,** J., Liljemark, W., and Bloomquist, C.: The Effect of Female Sex Hormones on Subgingival Plaque, *J. Periodontol.,52,* 599, October, 1981.
7. **Fehrenbach,** M.J., Lemborn, U.E., and Phelan, J.A.: Inflammation and Repair, in Ibsen, O.A.C. and Phelan, J.A.: *Oral Pathology for the Dental Hygienist,* 2nd ed. Philadelphia, W.B. Saunders, 1996, pp. 96–98.
8. **Pindborg,** J.J.: *Atlas of Diseases of the Oral Mucosa,* 5th ed. Philadelphia, W.B. Saunders Co., 1992, p. 286–288.
9. **Shafer,** W.G., Hine, M.K., and Levy, B.M.: *A Textbook of Oral Pathology,* 4th ed. Philadelphia, W.B. Saunders Co., 1983, p. 359.
10. **Tarsitano,** B.F. and Rollings, R.E.: The Pregnant Dental Patient: Evaluation and Management, *Gen. Dent., 41,* 226, May–June, 1993.
11. **Little,** J.W., Falace, D.A., Miller, C., and Rhodus, N.L.: *Dental Management of the Medically Compromised Patient,* 5th ed. St. Louis, Mosby, 1997, pp. 437–440.
12. **Picciano,** M.F.: Pregnancy and Lactation, in Ziegler, E.E. and Filer, L.J., eds.: *Present Knowledge in Nutrition,* 7th ed. Washington, D.C., ILSI Press, 1996, pp. 384–395.
13. **Oakley,** G.P. and Erickson, J.D.: Vitamin A and Birth Defects, (Editorial), *N Engl. J. Med., 333,* 1414, November 23, 1995.
14. **Driscoll,** W.S.: A Review of Clinical Research on the Use of Prenatal Fluoride Administration for Prevention of Dental Caries, *ASDC J. Dent. Child., 48,* 109, March–April, 1981.
15. **Thylstrup,** A.: Is There a Biological Rationale for Prenatal Fluoride Administration? *ASDC J. Dent. Child., 48,* 103, March–April, 1981.
16. **Bawden,** J.W., ed.: Changing Patterns of Fluoride Intake, Workshop Report—Group III, *J. Dent. Res., 71,* 1224, Special Issue, May, 1992.
17. **Casamassimo,** P.S., Griffiths, P., and Nowak, A.: Anticipatory Guidance in Dentistry, *DentalHygienistNews, 5,* 19, Fall, 1992.
18. **American Academy of Pediatric Dentistry:** Oral Health Policies, Guidelines, and Quality Assurance Criteria, *Pediatr. Dent., 20,* 72, *Special Issue,* November, 1998.
19. **Goepferd,** S.: Examination of the Infant and Toddler, in Pinkham, J.R., ed.: *Pediatric Dentistry: Infancy Through Adolescence,* 2nd ed. Philadelphia, W.B. Saunders Co., 1994, pp. 181–191.
20. **Casamassimo,** P.: *Bright Futures in Practice: Oral Health.* Arlington, VA., National Center for Education in Maternal and Child Health, 1996, p. 107.
21. **Gehrke,** P.S. and Johnsen, D.S.: Bottle Caries Associated with Anti-HIV Therapy, *Pediatr. Dent., 13,* 73, January/February, 1991.
22. **Howell,** R.B. and Houpt, M.: More Than One Factor Can Influence Caries Development in HIV-Positive Children, *Pediatr. Dent., 13,* 247, July/August, 1991.

SUGGESTED READINGS

Casamassimo, P.: *Bright Futures in Practice: Oral Health,* Arlington, VA, National Center for Education in Maternal and Child Health, 1996. (Available from: National Maternal and Child Health Clearinghouse, 2070 Chain Bridge Road, Suite 450, Vienna, VA 22182-2536.)

Casamassimo, P.S.: Children's Oral Health. What's New and What's True, *DentalHygienistNews, 10,* 14, Number 1, 1997.

Lie, R.T., Wilcox, A.J., and Skjaerven, R.: A Population-based Study of the Risk of Recurrence of Birth Defects, *N. Engl. J. Med., 331,* 1, July 7, 1994.

Motulsky, A.G.: Screening for Genetic Diseases, (Editorial), *N. Engl. J. Med., 336,* 1314, May 1, 1997.

Nowak, A.J.: Rationale for the Timing of the first Oral Evaluation, *Pediatr. Dent., 19,* 8, January/February, 1997.

Nowak, A.J. and Casamassimo, P. S.: Using Anticipatory Guidance to Provide Early Dental Intervention, *J. Am. Dent. Assoc., 126,* 1157, August, 1995.

Shaw, G.M., Lammer, E.J., Wasserman, C.R., O'Malley, C.D., and Tolarova, M.M.: Risks of Orofacial Clefts in Children Born to Women Using Multivitamins Containing Folic Acid Periconceptionally, *Lancet, 346,* 393, August 12, 1995.

Sterling, E.S., Bauchmoyer, S.M., and Carr, M.P.: Infant Oral Health Care, *DentalHygienistNews, 7,* 18, Spring, 1994.

Pregnancy

Brown, Z.A., Selke, S., Zeh, J., Kopelman, J., Maslow, A., Ashley, R.L., Watts, H., Berry, S., Herd, M., and Corey, L.: The Acquisition of Herpes Simplex Virus During Pregnancy, *N. Engl. J. Med., 337,* 509, August 21, 1997.

D'Alton, M.E. and DeCherney, A.H.: Prenatal Diagnosis, *N. Engl. J. Med., 328,* 114, January 14, 1993.

Fraser, A.M., Brockett, J.E., and Ward, R.H.: Association of Young Maternal Age with Adverse Reproductive Outcomes, *N. Engl. J. Med., 332,* 1113, April 27, 1995.

Glick, M. and Goldman, H.: Viral Infections in the Dental Setting: Potential Effects on Pregnant HCWs, *J. Am. Dent. Assoc., 124,* 79, June, 1993.

Lawrenz, D.R., Whitley, B.D., and Helfrick, J.F.: Considerations in the Management of Maxillofacial Infections in the Pregnant Patient, *J. Oral Maxillofac. Surg., 54,* 474, April, 1996.

Robert, E.: Treating Depression in Pregnancy, *N. Engl. J. Med., 335,* 1056, October 3, 1996.

Serman, N.J. and Singer, S.: Exposure of the Pregnant Patient to Ionizing Radiation, *Ann. Dent., 53,* 13, Winter, 1994.

Sibai, B.M.: Treatment of Hypertension in Pregnant Women, *N. Engl. J. Med., 335,* 257, July 25, 1996.

Torres, H.O., Ehrlich, A., Bird, D., and Dietz, E.: The Special Patient (Part I), *Dent. Assist., 65,* 11, July/August, 1996.

Periodontal Aspects

Daley, T.D., Nartey, N.O., and Wysocki, G.P.: Pregnancy Tumor: An Analysis, *Oral Surg. Oral Med. Oral Pathol., 72,* 196, August, 1991.

Manus, D.A., Sherbert, D. and Jackson, I.T.: Management Considerations for the Granuloma of Pregnancy, *Plast. Reconstr. Surg., 95, 1045,* May, 1995.

Powell, J.L., Bailey, C.L., Coopland, A.T., Otis, C.N., Frank, J.L., and Meyer, I.: Nd: YAG Laser Excision of a Giant Gingival Pyogenic Granuloma of Pregnancy, *Lasers Surg. Med., 14,* 178, Number 2, 1994.

Raber-Durlacher, J.E., van Steenbergen, T.J.M., van der Velden, U., de Graaff, A.J., and Abraham-Inpijn, L.: Experimental Gingivitis During Pregnancy and Post-partum: Clinical, Endocrinological, and Microbiological Aspects, *J. Clin. Periodontol., 21,* 549, September, 1994.

Raber-Durlacher, J.E., Palmer-Bouva, C.C.R., Raber, J., and Abraham-Inpijn, L.: Experimental Gingivitis During Pregnancy and Post-partum: Immunohistochemical Aspects, *J. Periodontol., 64,* 211, March, 1993.

Sills, E.S., Zegarelli, D.J., Hoschander, M.M., and Strider, W.E.: Clinical Diagnosis and Management of Hormonally Responsive Oral Pregnancy Tumor (pyogenic granuloma), *J. Reprod. Med., 41,* 467, July, 1996.

Silverstein, L.H., Burton, C.H., Garnick, J.J., and Singh, B.B.: The Late Development of Oral Pyogenic Granuloma as a Complication of Pregnancy: A Case Report, *Compend. Cont. Educ. Dent., 17,* 192, February, 1996.

Soorlyamoorthy, M. and Gower, D.B.: Hormonal Influences on Gingival Tissue: Relationship to Periodontal Disease, *J. Clin. Periodontol., 16,* 201, April, 1989.

Whitaker, S.B., Bouquot, J. E., Alimario, A.E., and Whitaker, T.J.: Identification and Semiquantification of Estrogen and Progesterone Receptors in Pyogenic Granulomas of Pregnancy, *Oral Surg. Oral Med. Oral Pathol., 78,* 755, December, 1994.

Zachariasen, R.D.: The Effect of Elevated Ovarian Hormones on Periodontal Health: Oral Contraceptives and Pregnancy, *Women Health, 20,* 21, Number 2, 1993.

Drugs

Gleghorn, T. and Housholder, G.T.: Anti-infective Drug Therapy: Implications for the Lactating Mother and Nursing Infant, *J. Dent. Hyg., 69,* 130, May–June, 1995.

Howe, A.M. and Webster, W.S.: Vitamin K—Its Essential Role in Cranofacial Development. A Review of the Literature Regarding Vitamin K and Cranofacial Development, *Aust. Dent. J., 39,* 88, April, 1994.

Jacobson, J.L. and Jacobson, S.W.: Intellectual Impairment in Children Exposed to Polychlorinated Biphenyls in Utero, *N. Engl. J. Med., 335,* 783, September 12, 1996.

Mills, J.L.: Protecting the Embryo from X-rated Drugs, (Editorial), *N. Engl. J. Med., 333,* 124, July 13, 1995.

Rosenberg, N.M., Meert, K.L., Knazik, S.R., Yee, H., and Kauffman, R.E.: Occult Cocaine Exposure in Children, *Am. J. Dis. Child., 145,* 1430, December, 1991.

Slutsker, L.: Risks Associated with Cocaine Use During Pregnancy, *Obstet. Gynecol., 79,* 778, May, 1992.

Volpe, J.J.: Effect of Cocaine Use on the Fetus, *N. Engl. J. Med., 327,* 399, August 6, 1992.

Smoking

Cunningham, J., Dockery, D.W., and Speizer, F.E.: Maternal Smoking During Pregnancy as a Predictor of Lung Function in Children, *Am. J. Epidemiol., 139,* 1139, June 15, 1994.

DiFranza, J.R. and Lew, R.A.: Effect of Maternal Cigarette Smoking on Pregnancy Complications and Sudden Death Syndrome, *J. Fam. Practice, 40,* 385, April, 1995.

Fried, P.A.: Prenatal Exposure to Tobacco and Marijuana: Effects During Pregnancy, Infancy, and Early Childhood, *Clin. Obstet. Gynec., 36,* 319, June, 1993.

Schoendorf, K.C. and Kiely, J.L.: Relationship of Sudden Infant Death Syndrome to Maternal Smoking During and After Pregnancy, *Pediatrics, 90,* 905, December, 1992.

Waldman, H.B.: Do the Parent(s) of Your Pediatric Patients Smoke? *ASDC J. Dent. Child., 59,* 126, March–April, 1992.

Early Childhood Caries

Aaltonen, A.S. and Tenovuo, J.: Association Between Mother-infant Salivary Contacts and Caries Resistance in Children: A Cohort Study, *Pediatr. Dent., 16,* 110, March/April, 1994.

Berkowitz, R.J. and Jones, P.: Mouth-to-mouth Transmission of the Bacterium *Streptococcus mutans* between Mother and Child, *Arch. Oral Biol., 30,* 377, Number 4, 1985.

Bowen, W.H., Pearson, S.K., Rosalen, P.L., Miguel, J.C., and Shih, A.Y.: Assessing the Cariogenic Potential of Some Infant Formulas, Milk and Sugar Solutions, *J. Am. Dent. Assoc., 128,* 865, July, 1997.

Duggal, M.S., Toumba, K.J., Pollard, M.A., and Tahmassebi, J.F.: The Acidogenic Potential of Herbal Baby Drinks, *Br. Dent. J., 180,* 98, February 10, 1996.

Jones, S., Hussey, R., and Lennon, M.A.: Dental Health Related Behaviours in Toddlers in Low and High Caries Areas in St. Helens, North West England, *Br. Dent. J., 181,* 13, July 6, 1996.

Kanellis, M.J., Logan, H.L., and Jacobsen, J.: Changes in Maternal Attitudes Toward Baby Bottle Tooth Decay, *Pediatr. Dent., 19,* 56, January/February, 1997.

Kohler, B. and Andreen, I.: Influence of Caries-preventive Measures in Mothers on Cariogenic Bacteria and Caries Experience in Their Children, *Arch. Oral Biol., 39,* 907, October, 1994.

Matee, M.I., Mikx, F.H.M., Maselle, S.Y.M., and van Palenstein, W.H.: Mutans streptococci and Lactobacilli in Breast-fed Children with Rampant Caries, *Caries Res., 26,* 183, May–June, 1992.

Muller, M.: Nursing-bottle Syndrome: Risk Factors, *ASDC J. Dent. Child., 63,* 42, January–February, 1996.

Schwartz, S.S., Rosivack, R.G., and Michelotti, P.: A Child's Sleeping Habit as a Cause of Nursing Caries, *ASDC J. Dent. Child., 60,* 22, January–February, 1993.

Tinanoff, N. and O'Sullivan, D.M.: Early Childhood Caries: Overview and Recent Findings, *Pediatr. Dent., 19,* 12, January/February, 1997.

Wendt, L.-K., Koch, G., and Hallonsten, A.-L.: Parental Awareness of Dental Caries in Toddlers, *Swed. Dent. J., 20,* 161, Number 4, 1996.

The Patient With a Cleft Lip and/or Palate

44

Cleft lip and/or palate is the most common of the many types of congenital craniofacial anomalies. Cleft lip and/or palate frequently occurs as part of a syndrome with other birth defects.

The person with a cleft lip and/or palate can be dentally dysfunctional unless extensive habilitative care and supervision from birth is available. An interdisciplinary team of medical and dental specialists is required to provide adequate treatment and family counseling as needed. The dental hygienist is an important member of the team with responsibilities to coordinate dental and periodontal care.

Speaking ability and appearance are among the first factors considered when the long-range treatment program is planned, because the objective is to help the patient lead a normal life. Dental personnel need to maintain a current list of the health agencies, clinics, and other community resources where the patient and family can obtain assistance for the various phases of treatment and habilitation.

Key words relating to cleft lip and/or palate are defined in Box 44-1.

CLASSIFICATION OF CLEFTS

Classification is based on disturbances in the embryologic formation of the palate as it develops from the premaxillary region toward the uvula in a definite pattern. Interference with normal development of the palate may occur at one stage level of the embryo,

BOX 44-1 KEY WORDS: Cleft Lip and/or Palate

Autograft (aw'tō-graft): graft transferred from one part of the patient's body to another part.

Bifid uvula (bī'fĭd ū'vū-lah): cleft of the uvula of the soft palate that divides the uvula into two parts (Figure 44–1, Class 2).

Cheiloplasty (kī'lō -plăs" tē): surgical repair of a lip defect.

Cheilorhinoplasty (kī"lō -rī'nō-plăs" tē): plastic surgery of nose and lip.

Cleft lip: a unilateral or bilateral congenital fissure in the upper lip, usually lateral to the midline; can extend into one nostril or both and may involve the alveolar process; caused by defect in the fusion of the maxillary and globular processes.

Cleft palate: a congenital fissure in the palate caused by failure of the palatal shelves to fuse; may extend to connect with unilateral or bilateral cleft lip.

Congenital (kon-jen'ĭ-tal): present at and existing from the time of birth.

Craniofacial (krā"nē-ō-fā'shal): pertaining to the cranium, the part of the skull that encloses the brain, and the face.

Dentally dysfunctional: abnormal functioning of dental structures.

Graft: tissue that is transplanted and expected to become a part of the host tissue.

Heredity (hĕ-red'ĭ-tē): genetic transmission of traits from parents to offspring; the hereditary material, chromosomes, is contained within the ovum and the sperm (23 chromosomes each), which unite when the sperm penetrates the ovum.

Multifactorial (mul"ti-fak-tor'ē-al): pertaining to, or arising through the action of, many factors.

Obturator (ob'tuh-rā'tor): a prosthesis designed to close a congenital or acquired opening, such as a cleft of the hard palate.

Orthognathic surgery (or"thog-na'thick): surgical repositioning of all or parts of the maxilla or mandible.

Orthopedics (or"thō-pē'dĭks): branch of surgery dealing with the preservation and restoration of function of the skeletal system, its articulations, and associated structures.

Palatoplasty (pal'ah-tō-plas"tē): plastic reconstruction of the palate.

Premaxilla (prē-mak'sĭ-lah): anterior part of maxilla that contains the incisor teeth; bilateral cleft lips separate the premaxilla from its normal fusion with the entire maxilla.

Prosthesis (pros-thē'sĭs): an artificial replacement of an absent part of the human body; a therapeutic device to improve or alter function.

Rehabilitation (rē"hah-bil"ĭ-tā'shun): the process of restoring a person's ability to live and work as normally as possible after a disabling injury or illness; aims to help the individual to achieve maximum possible physical and psychologic fitness and to regain ability to carry out personal care.

Habilitation: the same goals and objectives as rehabilitation, but for a person with acquired disability for whom the ability to achieve maximum physical and psychologic fitness is acquired for the first time.

Rhinoplasty (rī'nō-plas" tē): plastic surgery of nose.

Speech aid prosthesis: a prosthetic device with a posterior section to assist with palatopharyngeal closure; also called bulb, speech bulb, or prosthetic speech appliance.

Pediatric speech aid prosthesis: a temporary or interim prosthesis used to close a defect in the hard and/or soft palate; may replace tissue lost as a result of developmental or surgical alterations; necessary for intelligible speech.

Adult speech aid prosthesis: a definitive prosthesis to improve speech by obturating (sealing off) a palatal cleft or occasionally assisting an incompetent soft palate.

Syndrome (sin'drōm): a combination of symptoms either resulting from a single cause or occurring so commonly together as to constitute a distinct clinical picture.

Tracheostomy (trā"kē-os'tuh-mē): creation of an opening into the trachea through the neck, with insertion of an indwelling tube to facilitate passage of air or evacuation of secretions.

Velopharyngeal insufficiency (vel'ō-fah-rin'jē-al): anatomic or functional deficiency in the soft palate or the muscle affecting closure of the opening between mouth and nose in speech; results in a nasal speech quality.

Velum (ve'lum): covering structure or veil.

Velum palatinum (ve'lum pal-ah-ti'num): soft palate.

and the normal pattern may be re-established at a later stage.

The first six classes are illustrated in Figure 44-1. All degrees are found, from an insignificant notch in the mucous membrane of the lip or uvula, which produces no functional disability, to the complete cleft defined by Class 6 of this classification.

Class 1. Cleft of the tip of the uvula.

Class 2. Cleft of the uvula (bifid uvula).

Class 3. Cleft of the soft palate.

Class 4. Cleft of the soft and hard palates.

Class 5. Cleft of the soft and hard palates that continues through the alveolar ridge on one side of the premaxilla; usually associated with cleft lip of the same side.

Class 6. Cleft of the soft and hard palates that continues through the alveolar ridge on both sides, leaving a free premaxilla; usually associated with bilateral cleft lip.

Class 7. Submucous cleft in which the muscle union is imperfect across the soft palate. The palate is short; the uvula is often bifid; a groove is situated at the midline of the soft palate; and the closure to the pharynx is incompetent.

ETIOLOGY

I. EMBRYOLOGY[1,2]

Cleft lip and palate represent a failure of normal fusion of embryonic processes during development in the first trimester of pregnancy. Figure 44-2 shows the locations of the globular process and the right and left maxillary processes. With normal fusion, no cleft of the lip results.

Formation of the lip occurs between the fourth and seventh week *in utero*. The development of the palate takes place during the eighth to twelfth week. Fusion begins in the premaxillary region and continues backward toward the uvula.

A cleft lip becomes apparent by the end of the second month *in utero*. A cleft palate is evident by the end of the third month.

II. RISK FACTORS[3,4]

Genetic and environmental factors can be significant. Rarely a single factor can be found as the specific cause. They are most often multifactorial. Early in the first trimester is the significant time for influences due to the environmental factors.

    A. Genetic

    B. Environmental

        1. Tobacco smoking.[5,6]

        2. Alcohol consumption.[7]

        3. Teratogenic agents: phenytoin, vitamin A (isotretinoin), corticosteroids, drugs of abuse (see Table 43-1, page 655).

        4. Inadequate diet: vitamins, especially folic acid deficiency.

        5. Lack of adequate prenatal care and instruc-

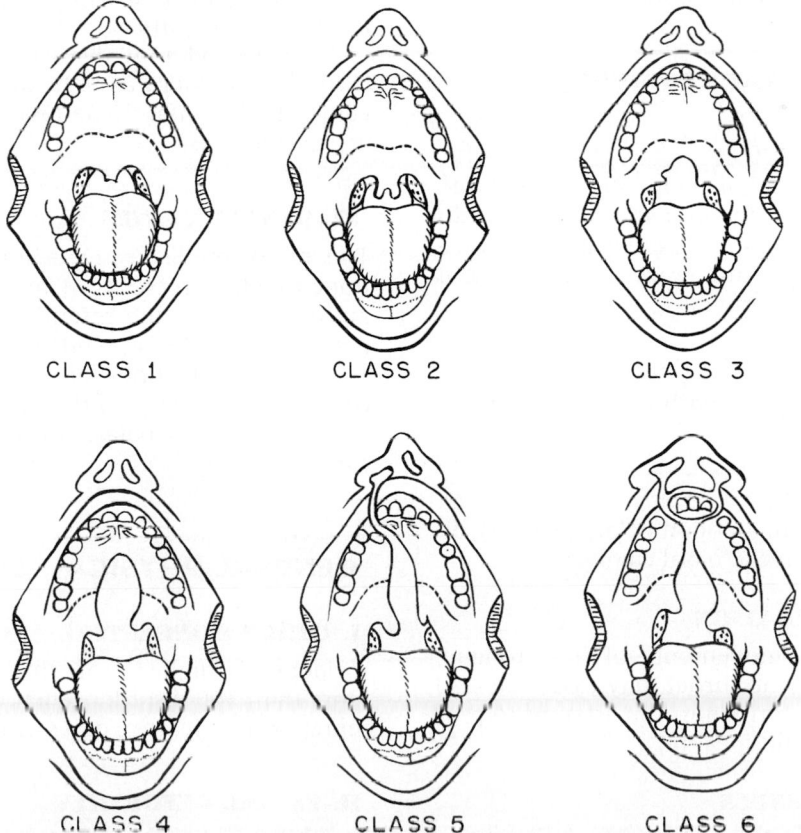

CLASS 1   CLASS 2   CLASS 3

CLASS 4   CLASS 5   CLASS 6

■ **FIGURE 44-1 Classification of Cleft Lip and Cleft Palate.** (Courtesy of O.E. Beder.)

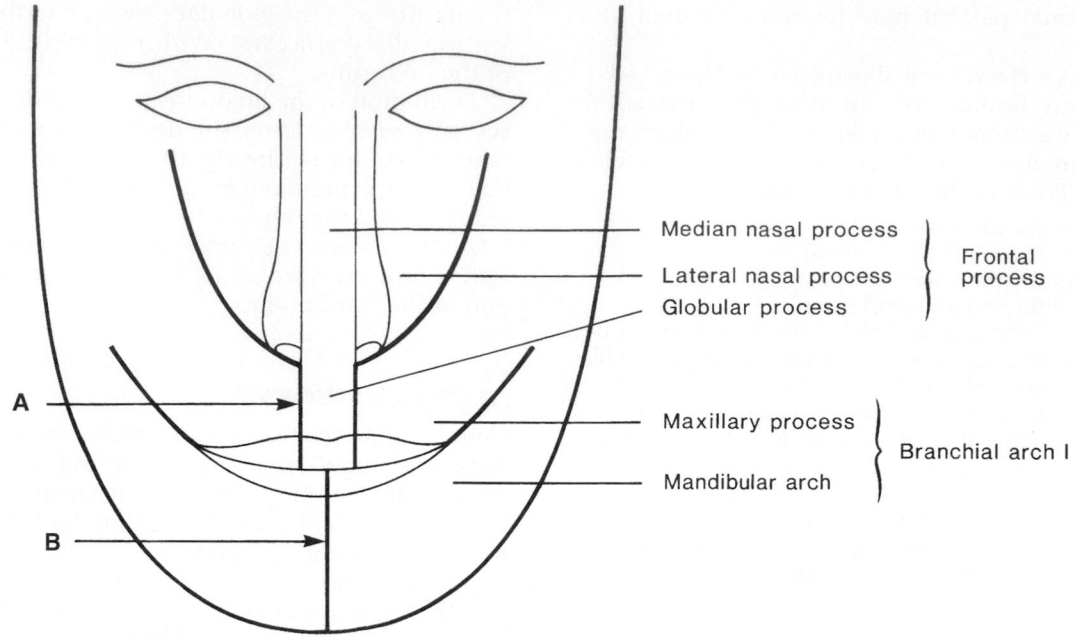

FIGURE 44-2 Developmental Processes of the Face. The derivations of parts of the face from the frontal process and the branchial arch. **A.** Location of cleft lip when fusion of the globular process and a maxillary process fails. **B.** Cleft of the mandible can occur at the midline. (Redrawn from Melfi, R.C.: *Permar's Oral Embryology and Microscopic Anatomy,* 8th ed. Philadelphia, Lea & Febiger, 1988.)

tion is a risk factor that has influence on all the environmental factors.

ORAL CHARACTERISTICS

I. TOOTH DEVELOPMENT

Disturbances in the normal development of the tooth buds occur more frequently in patients with clefts than in the general population. There is a higher incidence of missing and supernumerary teeth, as well as of abnormalities of tooth form.

II. MALOCCLUSION

A high percentage of patients with cleft lip and palate require orthodontic care.

III. OPEN PALATE

Before surgical correction, an open palate provides direct communication with the nasal cavity.

IV. MUSCLE COORDINATION

A lack of coordinated movements of lips, tongue, cheeks, floor of mouth, and throat may exist and lead to compensatory habits formed in the attempt to produce normal sounds while speaking.

V. PERIODONTAL TISSUES

Bacterial plaque accumulation is influenced by the irregularly positioned teeth; inability to keep lips closed; mouth breathing; and the difficulties in accomplishing adequate personal oral care, especially around the cleft areas.

Early periodontal disease with loss of bone and clinical attachment at cleft sites is common in adolescents.[8] Periodontal tissue loss in later years is greatest at the cleft sites.[9]

VI. DENTAL CARIES

The many predisposing factors relating to malpositioned teeth, problems of mastication, diet selection, and bacterial plaque retention are intensified for the person with a cleft lip and/or palate.

Feeding difficulties of infants and toddlers have contributed to baby bottle tooth decay. Children with a cleft lip and/or palate are at higher risk for dental caries.[10]

GENERAL PHYSICAL CHARACTERISTICS

I. OTHER CONGENITAL ANOMALIES

Incidence is higher than that in noncleft people. In more than 300 disorders, cleft lip, cleft palate, or both represent one feature of a syndrome.[11]

II. FACIAL DEFORMITY

Facial deformities may include depression of the nostril on the side with the cleft lip; deficiency of upper lip, which may be short or retroposed; and overprominent lower lip.

III. INFECTIONS

Predisposition to upper respiratory and middle ear infections is common.

IV. AIRWAY AND BREATHING

The craniofacial anomalies of the nose and throat area predispose the child with a cleft palate to airway obstruction and breathing problems.[12] Early treatment intervention is necessary for the infant to cope with feeding problems. Speech involves breathing and swallowing.

V. SPEECH[13]

Patients with cleft lip and/or cleft palate have difficulty in making certain sounds and may produce nasal tones. Anatomic structure, airway and breathing problems, and hearing difficulties all contribute to speech problems.

VI. HEARING LOSS

The incidence of hearing loss is significantly higher in individuals with cleft palate than in the noncleft population.

PERSONAL FACTORS

Most patients with a cleft lip or palate do not have more personality problems than people without clefts. Realization of the social effects of speech and appearance makes it possible to understand why some of these patients exhibit evidences of maladjustment. The ridicule of contemporaries soon leads even young children to think they are "different." Parental acceptance or rejection no doubt can be a strong influence. A few characteristics are suggested here.

I. SELF-CONSCIOUSNESS

Hypersensitivity to taunts or obvious pity.

II. FEELINGS OF INFERIORITY

The result may be a person who is quiet, unresponsive, and withdrawn, or one who is openly brash or rebellious until rapport is established.

TREATMENT

Treatment is coordinated by a team of specialists and is based on the patient's progress at each age period. Members of the interdisciplinary team are listed in Table 44-1.

The team is responsible for providing integrated case management. Quality and continuity of care are essential.[14] The need for attention to gingival health

---

TABLE 44-1 Members of an Interdisciplinary Team for Treatment of Patient With Cleft Lip or Palate

DENTAL PROFESSION

Dental Hygiene
Oral and Maxillofacial Surgery
Orthodontics
Pediatric Dentistry
Prosthodontics
Implantology
Periodontics

MEDICAL PROFESSION

Anesthesiology
Genetics/Dysmorphology
Imaging/Radiology
Neurology
Neurosurgery
Ophthalmology
Otolaryngology
Pediatrics
Physical Anthropology
Plastic Surgery
Psychiatry

ALLIED MEDICAL

Nursing
Nutrition
Genetic Counseling
Psychology
Social Work
Speech-Language Pathology
Vocational Counseling

---

throughout the years of treatment cannot be overemphasized.

I. CLEFT LIP

Surgical union of the cleft lip is made before 6 months. The infant's general health is a determining factor.

A. Purposes for Early Treatment
1. Aid in feeding.
2. Encourage development of the premaxilla.
3. Help partial closure of the palatal cleft.
4. Lessen concern of family about appearance of their infant.

B. Orthodontics and Dentofacial Orthopedics[15]
In preparation for cleft closure, orthodontic and orthopedic treatment may be needed to reduce the protrusion and stabilize the premaxilla.

II. CLEFT PALATE

Primary surgery to close the palate should be undertaken by age 18 months or earlier when possible.[14]

The combined efforts of many specialists are required (Table 44-1).

A. Goals for Treatment
1. Produce anatomic closure.
2. Maximize maxillary growth and development.
3. Achieve normal function, particularly normal speech.
4. Relieve problems of airway and breathing.
5. Establish good dental esthetics and functional occlusion.

B. Types of Secondary Surgical Procedures
Secondary surgical care refers to additional surgical procedures after primary closure of the clefts. Secondary surgery may involve the lips, nose, palate, and jaws. It may be to improve function, improve appearance, or both.

Treatment plans are individualized to fit the needs of the patient. Team evaluations on a periodic basis determine the effects of treatment to date and outline the next phase. Examples of what may be needed are:
1. Rhinoplasty and nasal septal surgery for an airway problem.
2. Velopharyngeal flap or other pharyngoplasty.
3. Closure of palatal fistulae.
4. Tonsillectomy and/or adenoidectomy.

C. Use of Bone Grafting[16,17]
Bone grafting is used to repair residual alveolar and hard palate clefts.
1. *Alveolar graft:* Placed before eruption of maxillary teeth at the cleft site, creates a normal architecture through which the teeth can erupt. A need for future prosthetic replacement of missing teeth is reduced. Support is provided for teeth adjacent to the cleft areas.
2. *Hard palate graft:* Provides closure of oronasal fistulae and helps to relieve a compromised airway.
3. *Sources for Autogenous Bone for Graft:* Rib, iliac crest, skull, or mandible.

D. Use of Osseointegrated Implant
After bone grafting, implants can be used to replace individual teeth or to support a complete prosthesis.[18,19]

III. PROSTHODONTICS

A. Types of Appliances
A removable prosthesis may be designed to provide closure of the palatal opening (obturator) and/or to complete the palatopharyngeal valving required for speech (speech aid prosthesis).

B. Purposes and Functions of a Prosthesis
The prosthesis may be designed to accomplish one or all of the following:
1. Closure of the palate.
2. Replacement of missing teeth.

3. Scaffolding to fill out the upper lip.
4. Masticatory function.
5. Restoration of vertical dimension.
6. Postorthodontic retainer.

IV. ORTHODONTICS

Treatment may be initiated as early as 3 years of age, depending on the problems of dentofacial development. Each stage of surgery and other treatment may require orthodontic intervention and follow-up.

Final formal orthodontic treatment for realigning the teeth and gaining a functional occlusion may start during the mixed dentition years or later. During that period, an intensive program for dental caries prevention and gingival health must be supervised.

V. SPEECH THERAPY

Training may be started with very young children and is particularly emphasized after the surgical or prosthodontic treatment has been accomplished.

VI. RESTORATIVE DENTISTRY (PEDIATRIC DENTIST OR GENERAL DENTAL PRACTITIONER)

A major problem can be dental caries, leading to tooth loss. With missing teeth, major difficulties arise related to all phases of treatment. Preservation of the primary teeth is very important.

DENTAL HYGIENE CARE

Preventive measures for preservation of the teeth and their supporting structures are essential to the success of the special care needed for the habilitation of the patient with a cleft palate.

Each phase of dental hygiene care and instruction, important for all patients, takes on even greater significance in the light of the magnified problems of the patient with a cleft lip and/or palate.

Every attempt should be made to avoid the need for removal of teeth, especially around the cleft area. In an area already weakened by lack of bone, the removal of teeth creates further complications. The presence of teeth encourages optimum arch growth.

Understanding by the patient and the parents of the value of preventive procedures is accomplished through explanation and instruction. When the patient has not had specialized care, the dental team has a responsibility to arrange referral to an available agency, clinic, or private practice specialist.

I. PARENTAL COUNSELING: ANTICIPATORY GUIDANCE
Items from Table 43-3 (page 661) pertain to the parents and infant with a cleft lip and/or palate. The primary concerns are daily bacterial plaque removal and prevention of baby bottle tooth decay.

II. OBJECTIVES FOR APPOINTMENT PLANNING

Frequent appointments, scheduled every 3 or 4 months, are usually needed during the maintenance phase of the patient's care.

A. To review plaque control measures and provide encouragement for the patient to maintain the health of the supporting structures and the cleanliness of the removable prostheses.

B. To remove all calculus and smooth the tooth surfaces as a supplement to the patient's personal daily care procedures.

C. To supervise a dental caries prevention program for both primary and permanent dentitions with fluorides and sealants.

III. APPOINTMENT CONSIDERATIONS

A. Patient Apprehension

A patient who has been seen often in hospital clinics may become "clinic tired" and be very apprehensive about dental and dental hygiene care.

B. Communication

1. *Speech.* Speech may be almost unintelligible, although with repeated contact, understanding can be developed. Referral for speech assessment, if not already done, is recommended.

2. *Hearing.* Depending on the severity of hearing loss, the approach is similar to that for speech difficulties. Suggestions for care of patients with hearing problems are described on pages 794 to 800.

C. Avoid Solicitousness or Undue Sympathy.
Approach as a normal patient.

D. Provide Motivations for Quiet, Unresponsive, or Bold Rebellious Types.
Use approach that helps them gain an objective attitude to the care of their mouths.

IV. DENTAL HYGIENE INTERVENTIONS

A. Infection Control
Although procedures for asepsis should be the same for all patients, one should remember that the open fistulae make the patient with a cleft palate particularly susceptible to infections.

B. Instrumentation
1. Adapt techniques to the oral characteristics. All objectives of scaling and other instrumentation have particular implications for the patient with a cleft palate.
2. Prevent debris or pieces of calculus from passing into or being retained in the clefts.
3. Remove an obturator or prosthesis for cleaning.

C. Topical Application of Fluoride
Short upper lip may complicate cotton-roll or tray placement.

V. PATIENT INSTRUCTION

A. Personal Oral Care Procedures
The self-conscious patient may actually fear or exhibit rejection toward the oral cavity. With a small child, the parents may be afraid of damaging the deformed areas or hurting the child if cleaning methods are employed. An empathetic approach and plan for continued instruction over a long period of time is needed.

1. *Teeth and Gingiva.* Select toothbrush, brushing method, and auxiliary aids according to the individual needs. A soft nylon brush with end-rounded filaments is indicated.

2. *Fluoride.* Instigate daily self-application of fluoride by way of mouthrinse, fluoride dentifrice, and diet supplements for a young child in a non-fluoridated community (pages 469 to 472).

3. *Rinsing Instruction.* Young children especially may need instruction in how to rinse when this procedure is new for them (page 384).

4. *Prosthesis or Speech Aid.* Halitosis may be a real problem when the prosthesis forms the soft palate and the floor of the nasal cavity. Mucus secreted in the nasal cavity accumulates on the prosthesis.
   a. Instruct patient in the need for frequent removal of prosthesis for cleaning, particularly following eating.
   b. Method for cleaning the prosthesis is the same as that for a removable partial denture (page 402).

B. Diet
1. *Need for a Varied Diet:* Should include adequate proportions of all essential food groups (see Figure 28-2, page 445).
2. *Need for Prevention of Dental Caries:* Limitation of cariogenic foods, particularly for between-meal snacks.

C. Smoking Cessation
Patients who smoke or use any form of smokeless tobacco should be informed about the effects of tobacco on all the oral tissues, with emphasis on the potential damage to the periodontal bone. Offer assistance with a smoking cessation program (pages 436 to 438).

VI. DENTAL HYGIENE CARE RELATED TO ORAL SURGERY

A. Presurgery (pages 709 to 711)
Objectives have particular significance because the patient with a cleft palate is unusually susceptible to infections of the upper respiratory area and middle ear. Every precaution should be taken to prevent complications.

B. Postsurgery Personal Oral Care
In certain of the palate operations, arm re-

straints are applied to prevent accidental damage to the repaired region. After each feeding (liquid diet for several days, soft diet for the next week), the mouth must be rinsed carefully.

Brushing must be accomplished with great care, usually by the parent or caregiver, to avoid damage to the healing suture lines. In some cases, a toothbrush with suction attachment may be useful (pages 764 to 765).

Water irrigation using low pressure can also be helpful where jaw repositioning surgery has been completed and wires have been used to stabilize the jaws for a period of time (pages 381 to 382).

REFERENCES

1. **Melfi**, R.C.: *Permar's Oral Embryology and Microscopic Anatomy,* 9th ed. Philadelphia, Lea & Febiger, 1994, pp. 25–41.
2. **Avery**, J.K. and Steele, P.F.: *Essentials of Oral Histology and Embryology.* St. Louis, Mosby, 1992, pp. 39–50.
3. **Slavkin**, H.C.: Meeting the Challenges of Craniofacial-oraldental Birth Defects, *J. Am. Dent. Assoc., 127,* 681, May, 1996.
4. **Berkowitz,** S.: *The Cleft Palate Story.* Chicago, Quintessence, 1994, pp. 45–49.
5. **Shaw**, G.M., Wasserman, C.R., Lammer, E.J., O'Malley, C.D., Murray, J.C., Basart, A.M., and Tolarova, M.M.: Orofacial Clefts, Parental Cigarette Smoking, and Transforming Growth Factor-Alpha Gene Variants, *Am. J. Hum. Genet., 58,* 551, March, 1996.
6. **Källén**, K.: Maternal Smoking and Orofacial Clefts, *Cleft Palate Craniofac. J., 34,* 11, January, 1997.
7. **Werler**, M.M., Lammer, E.J., Rosenberg, L., and Mitchell, A.A.: Maternal Alcohol Use in Relation to Selected Birth Defects, *Am. J. Epidemiol., 134,* 691, October 1, 1991.
8. **Brägger**, U., Schürch, E., Gusberti, F.A., and Lang, N.P.: Periodontal Conditions in Adolescents with Cleft Lip, Alveolus and Palate Following Treatment in a Coordinated Team Approach, *J. Clin. Periodontol., 12,* 494, July, 1985.
9. **Brägger**, U., Schürch, E., Salvi, G., von Wyttenbach, T., and Lang, N.P.: Periodontal Conditions in Adult Patients with Cleft Lip, Alveolus, and Palate, *Cleft Palate Craniofac. J., 29,* 179, March, 1992.
10. **Bokhout**, B., Hofman, F.X.W.M., van Limbeek, J., Kramer, G.J.C., and Prahl-Andersen, B.: Incidence of Dental Caries in the Primary Dentition in Children with a Cleft Lip and/or Palate, *Caries Res., 31,* 8, January, 1997.
11. **Cohen**, M.M., Jr. and Bankier, A.: Syndrome Delineation Involving Orofacial Clefting, *Cleft Palate Craniofac. J., 28,* 119, January, 1991.
12. **Perkins**, J.A., Sie, K.C.Y., Milczuk, H., and Richardson, M.A.: Airway Management in Children with Craniofacial Anomalies, *Cleft Palate Craniofac. J., 34,* 135, March, 1997.
13. **Berkowitz**: op cit., pp. 113–115.
14. **American Cleft Palate-Craniofacial Association**: Parameters for Evaluation and Treatment of Patients with Cleft Lip/Palate or Other Craniofacial Anomalies, *Cleft Palate Craniofac. J., 30,* Supplement 1, 1993.
15. **Figueroa**, A.A., Polley, J.W., and Cohen, M.: Orthodontic Management of the Cleft Lip and Palate Patient, *Clin. Plast. Surg., 20,* 733, October, 1993.
16. **Boyne**, P.J. and Sands, N.R.: Secondary Bone Grafting of Residual Alveolar and Palatal Clefts, *J. Oral Surg., 30,* 87, February, 1972.
17. **Kalaaji**, A., Lilja, J., Friede, H., and Elander, A.: Bone Grafting in the Mixed and Permanent Dentition in Cleft Lip and Palate Patients: Long-term Results and the Role of the Surgeon's Experience, *J. Craniomaxillofac. Surg., 24,* 29, February, 1996.

18. **Verdi**, F.J., Lanzi, G.L., Cohen, S.R., and Powell, R.: Use of the Branemark Implant in the Cleft Palate Patient, *Cleft Palate Craniofac. J., 28,* 301, July, 1991.
19. **Lund**, T.W. and Wade, M.: Use of Osseointegrated Implants to Support a Maxillary Denture for a Patient with Repaired Cleft Lip and Palate, *Cleft Palate Craniofac. J., 30,* 418, July, 1993.

SUGGESTED READINGS

Arcuri, M.R., LaVelle, W.E., Higuchi, K.W., and Svec, B.R.: Implant-supported Prostheses for Treatment of Adults With Cleft Palate, *J. Prosthet. Dent., 71,* 375, April, 1994.

Hudson, J.W. and Russell, R.: Contributions Within Dental Science to Cleft Lip/Palate Management: A Literature Review, *Compend. Cont. Educ. Dent., 15,* 116, January, 1994.

Kaufman, F.L.: Managing the Cleft Lip and Palate Patient, *Pediatr. Clin. North Am., 38,* 1127, October, 1991.

Pham, A.N.D., Seow, W.K., and Shusterman, S.: Developmental Dental Changes in Isolated Cleft Lip and Palate, *Pediatr. Dent., 19,* 109, March/April, 1997.

Ronchi, P., Chiapasco, M., and Frattini, D.: Endosseous Implants for Prosthetic Rehabilitation in Bone Grafted Alveolar Clefts, *J. Craniomaxillofac. Surg., 23,* 382, December, 1995.

Santi, E., Weinberg, M.A., and Abitol, T.E.: Periodontal and Prosthetic Treatment of a Cleft Lip and Palate Patient: A Case Report, *Cleft Palate Craniofac. J., 32,* 346, July, 1995.

So, L.Y.L. and Lui, W.W.K.: Alternative Donor Site for Alveolar Bone Grafting in Adults with Cleft Lip and Palate, *Angle Orthod., 66,* 9, Number 1, 1996.

Tolarova, M. and Harris, J.: Reduced Recurrence of Orofacial Clefts After Periconceptional Supplementation with High-dose Folic Acid and Multivitamins, *Teratology, 51,* 71, February, 1995.

Turvey, T.A. and Hegtvedt, A.K.: Surgical Correction of Craniofacial Malformations, *J. Oral Maxillofac. Surg., 51,* 69, January, 1993 (Supplement).

van der Velden, E.M. and van der Dussen, M.F.N.: Dermatography as an Adjunctive Treatment for Cleft Lip and Palate Patients, *J. Oral Maxillofac. Surg., 53,* 9, January, 1995.

Winters, J.C. and Hurwitz, D.J.: Presurgical Orthopedics in the Surgical Management of Unilateral Cleft Lip and Palate, *Plast. Reconstruct. Surg., 95,* 755, April, 1995.

Infants/Children

Copeland, M.: The Effects of Very Early Palatal Repair on Speech, *Br. J. Plast. Surg., 43,* 676, November, 1990.

Dahllöf, G., Ussisoo-Joandi, R., Ideberg, M., and Modeer, T.: Caries, Gingivitis, and Dental Abnormalities in Preschool Children with Cleft Lip and/or Palate, *Cleft Palate J., 26,* 233, July, 1989.

Fries, M.H., Kuller, J.A., Norton, M.E., Yankowitz, J., Kobori, J., Good, W.V., Ferriero, D., Cox, V., Donlin, S.S., and Golabi, M.: Facial Features of Infants Exposed Prenatally to Cocaine, *Teratology, 48,* 413, November, 1993.

Jocelyn, L.J., Penko, M.A., and Rode, H.L.: Cognition, Communication, and Hearing in Young Children with Cleft Lip and Palate and in Control Children: A Longitudinal Study, *Pediatrics, 97,* 529, April, 1996.

Osuji, O.O.: Preparation of Feeding Obturators for Infants with Cleft Lip and Palate, *J. Clin. Pediatr. Dent., 19,* 211, Spring, 1995.

Sierra, F.J. and Turner, C.: Maxillary Orthopedics in the Presurgical Management of Infants with Cleft Lip and Palate, *Pediatr. Dent., 17,* 419, November–December, 1995.

Strauss, R.P. and Broder, H.: Children with Cleft Lip/Palate and Mental Retardation: A Subpopulation of Cleft-craniofacial Team Patients, *Cleft Palate Craniofac. J., 30,* 548, November, 1993.

Wood, A.J. and Farrington, F.H.: Objective Evaluation of an Airway Management Appliance in Infants with Craniofacial Anomalies, *Spec. Care Dent., 10,* 30, January–February, 1990.

Zarrinnia, K., Hulnick, S., Athanasiou, A.E., and Zaghi, F.: Taking Dental Impressions in Infants with Cleft Lip and Palate, *Cleft Palate Craniofac. J., 30,* 248, March, 1993.

Adolescents

Kapp-Simon, K.A.: Psychological Interventions for the Adolescent with Cleft Lip and Palate, *Cleft Palate Craniofac. J., 32,* 104, March, 1995.

King, G.A., Shultz, I.Z., Steel, K., Gilpin, M., and Cathers, T.: Self-evaluation and Self-concept of Adolescents with Physical Disabilities, *Am. J. Occup. Ther., 47,* 132, February, 1993.

Leonard, B.J., Brust, J.D., Abrahams, G., and Sielaff, B.: Self-concept of Children and Adolescents with Cleft Lip and/or Palate, *Cleft Palate Craniofac. J., 28,* 347, October, 1991.

Peterson-Falzone, S.J.: Speech Outcomes in Adolescents with Cleft Lip and Palate, *Cleft Palate Craniofac. J., 32,* 125, March, 1995.

Richman, L.C.: Neuropsychological Development in Adolescents: Cognitive and Emotional Model for Considering Risk Factors for Adolescents with Cleft, *Cleft Palate Craniofac. J., 32,* 99, March, 1995.

45

Preadolescent to Postmenopausal Patients

The endocrine glands are glands of internal secretion. They secrete highly specialized substances—the hormones—that, with the nervous system, maintain body homeostasis.

Hormones are transported by the blood or lymph. They may act directly on body cells or indirectly to control the hormones of other glands. Their complex and unified action augments and regulates many vital functions, including growth and development, energy production, food metabolism, reproductive processes, and the responses of the body to stress.

The major endocrine glands are the pituitary, thyroid, parathyroids, pancreas, adrenals, and gonads. The anterior pituitary is called the master gland, because it regulates the output of hormones by other glands. In turn, the pituitary itself is regulated by the hormones of the other glands.

Both hyposecretion and hypersecretion of a hormone can cause physical and mental disturbances. Regulation of hormonal secretion is complex, and the mechanisms are not fully understood. Normally, hormones are secreted when needed. The external temperature, for example, can influence the production of thyroxine by the thyroid gland. The calcium level of the blood affects parathyroid activity.

Hormones of the reproductive system have an effect on the development and function of the individual. Some of the influences on oral health and patient care are described in this chapter. Key words are defined in Box 45-1.

PUBERTY AND ADOLESCENCE

I. PUBERTAL CHANGES

Puberty is a sign of growing up. Some individuals go through changes earlier and faster than others. Chronologic age is an unreliable indicator, because puberty may begin normally in either sex between 9 and

BOX 45-I KEY WORDS: Preadolescent to Postmenopausal Patients

Acne vulgaris (ak'nē vul-ga'rĭs): a chronic skin disorder with increased production of oil from the sebaceous glands and the formation of blackheads that plug the pores; may be inflammatory or noninflammatory; appears on the face, back, and chest, primarily in adolescents and young adults.

Adolescence: the period extending from the time the secondary sex characteristics appear to the end of somatic growth, when the individual is psychologically mature.

Amenorrhea: absence of spontaneous menstrual periods in a female of reproductive age.

Circumpubertal: on or around the age of puberty.

Climacteric: the phase in the aging of a woman that marks the transition from the reproductive to the nonreproductive stage.

Coitus: sexual union; copulation; intercourse.

Dysmenorrhea: difficult and painful menstruation.

Gynecologist (gī"nĕ-kol'ah-jist): physician who specializes in the conditions peculiar to women, particularly of the genital tract, female endocrinology, and reproductive physiology.

Homeostasis (hōmē-ō-sta'sĭs): the tendency of biologic systems to maintain constant internal stability while continually adjusting to external changes.

Hormonal replacement therapy: prescription of a purified or synthetic hormone to correct or prevent undesirable symptoms resulting from the surgical removal or degeneration of the hormone-producing organ.

Hormone: a chemical product of an organ or of certain cells within the organ that has a specific regulatory effect upon cells elsewhere in the body.

Mastalgia: fullness, soreness, or pain in the breast.

Maturity: state of complete growth.

Menarche: onset of menstruation; may occur from ages 9 to 17 years.

Menopause (men'ō-pawz): the time of life when a woman ceases menstruation; clinically defined as a period of 6 to 12 months of amenorrhea in a woman over 45 years of age.

Menses: menstruation.

Oligomenorrhea: menstrual intervals of greater than 45 days.

Premenstrual syndrome: a cluster of behavioral, somatic, affective, and cognitive disorders that appear in the premenstrual (luteal) phase of the menstrual cycle and that resolve rapidly with the onset of menses.

Puberty (pu'ber-tē): period in which the gonads mature and begin to function.

Pubescence (pu-bes'ens): coming to the age of puberty or sexual maturity.

---

17 years of age, depending on such factors as race, heredity, and nutritional status. Friends of the same age may look quite different from one another because there is a wide range of normal. Girls often begin puberty before boys. The secondary sex characteristics begin to appear between 10 and 13 years of age in girls, while changes in boys start at about 13 or 14 years. The major changes are usually complete in 3 to 4 years.

A. Hormonal Influences

Pituitary hormones control the hormones produced by the ovaries and the testes. The several hormones produced by the ovaries are known collectively as *estrogens,* and those produced by the testes are called *androgens.* They are responsible for the development of the sex organs, the accessory sex organs, and the secondary sex characteristics, and they have strong physical, mental, and emotional influences throughout the body.

B. Female Development
1. Accelerated growth spurt.

2. Development of the sex organs: fallopian tubes, uterus, vagina, and breasts.
3. Appearance of secondary sex characteristics:
   a. Growth of pubic and axillary hair.
   b. Skeletal development, increased height, enlargement of the pelvis.
   c. Fat deposition on the hips.
   d. Voice drops one or two tones.
4. Beginning of menstruation and ovulation. Menstruation may precede the first ovulation.

C. Male Development
1. Increase in size of testes and scrotum and beginning of spermatogenesis.
2. Development of the sex organs: vas deferens, seminal vesicles, prostate, and penis.
3. Appearance of secondary sex characteristics:
   a. Growth of facial, pubic, and axillary hair.
   b. Voice deepens.
4. Increased height, increased muscle volume and mass.

II. CHARACTERISTICS OF ADOLESCENCE

A. Growth Spurt

1. Varies in age of occurrence, extent, and duration; usually occurs in boys between 12 and 16 years, in girls between 11 and 14 years.
2. Marked by rapid, extensive growth in height, weight, and muscle mass.
3. Overeating with underexercise, along with psychological problems, makes obesity a difficult and serious problem.
4. Poor coordination and awkwardness in young adolescents may result from irregular, uneven stages of growth.

B. Nutritional Requirements

1. Highest of any time in life for boys; will be exceeded only during pregnancy for girls.
2. Undernutrition is common: in boys, because of overactivity and poor food selection; in girls, because of voluntary diet restrictions with poor food selection and fad diets in the attempt to be trim. Teens with a distorted image of their weight, size, or shape may take that dissatisfaction to extremes. Anorexia nervosa and/or bulimia may be a problem. Eating disorders can lead to severe health complications and even death. Successful treatment programs involve medical care, psychotherapy, and nutrition and family counseling (pages 830 to 833).
3. Iron-deficiency anemia is not uncommon among teenage girls, particularly after the onset of menstruation. It is usually treated with iron supplements, changes in diet, or both (page 870).

C. Skin Disorders

Acne vulgaris commonly results from overactivity of the sebaceous glands. Usually, relief occurs when adolescence is completed, although the condition may persist longer.

III. PERSONAL FACTORS

Adolescents are no longer children, and yet they have not reached adulthood. They may respond and wish to be treated as adults or as children at different times. They are learning to adapt to body changes, sexual impulses, secondary sex characteristics, and independence.

Causes of anxiety in adolescents include emotional health, violence, substance abuse, and sexuality. Peer pressures, family arguments, divorce, school performance, confusion over beliefs and values, and concern about their future can be troublesome. These issues can be addressed at the family, school, or individual level.[1] Younger, less healthy teenagers tend to show greater health concerns.

There is no fixed picture, but characteristics listed here are exhibited to one degree or another by many adolescents.

A. Increased Self-Interest

1. Adolescents have a great deal of concern for themselves and respond best to those who show concern for them.
2. They want attention and tend to reject those who do not listen.

B. Growing Independence

1. Adolescence is a period of rapidly growing independence of thought and action with conflicts between feelings of dependence and independence.
2. Childhood dependence on parents is gradually given up; the idea of infallibility of parents is lost; teachers and other authority figures are questioned.
3. Personal identity is sought; adolescents are uncertain about their place and role in society.
4. Independence from parents frequently means increased confidence in and respect for other adults outside the family.

C. Concern Over Physical Characteristics

1. Girls mature earlier than boys, and young female adolescents are usually taller than their male counterparts, which may present social problems.
2. Increased interest in personal appearance; adolescents want to dress and be like their peers.
3. Issues such as delayed growth, delayed sexual development, and obesity may be troublesome.

ORAL CONDITIONS

I. DENTAL CARIES

The incidence of dental caries is often higher during adolescence than in other age groups in communities without fluoridation. This is often related to the dietary and eating habits of the adolescent. Appetite becomes intensified by the demands of rapid growth, as well as by the emotional problems confronted, thus leading to frequent eating. Many cariogenic foods are chosen, particularly between meals and in social settings.

II. PERIODONTAL INFECTIONS

Adolescents are subject to all categories of periodontal infections (see Table 13-2, page 228). Gingivitis is common in this age group.

A. Gingivitis

1. *Contributing and Predisposing Factors.* Many of the factors described on pages 231 to 234 can be applied when considering the periodontal conditions of adolescents. Orthodontic appliances, dietary habits, and com-

pliance for bacterial plaque removal seem to be special problems for this age group.

Some teenagers have systemic conditions that may have affected the periodontal health, such as diabetes. Another example of contributing factors is the use of antiseizure medication, which could cause gingival enlargement.

2. *"Puberty" Gingivitis.* An exaggerated response to bacterial plaque and endotoxins can occur during puberty and may be related to hormonal changes. The gingiva enlarge, particularly the papillae; the tissue appears a bluish-red color and bulbous in shape.[2]

B. Early-Onset Periodontitis

Early-onset periodontitis (EOP) is the clinical classification term used to describe destructive periodontal infections that develop in children, adolescents, and young adults. When left untreated, EOP may progress rapidly and lead to early tooth loss.[3] Loss of periodontal attachment and supporting bone is evident in 5% to 47% of adolescents around the world.[4-6]

Careful probing and study of radiographs are indicated for each patient. Emphasis must be placed on preventive measures, early assessment, early treatment, and regular maintenance appointments.

C. Juvenile Periodontitis[7]

A specific category of EOP is juvenile periodontitis. The two distinct disease categories are localized (LJP) and generalized (GJP). Both types have a familial tendency.

1. *Localized Juvenile Periodontitis.* LJP is characterized by severe bone loss involving the first permanent molars and the incisors. It is usually first diagnosed during the circumpubertal years. The pathogenic microorganism of etiologic importance is the *Actinobacillus actinomycetemcomitans* (see Table 16-3, page 274). *A. actinomycetemcomitans* is a powerful microorganism that can invade tissue and destroy white blood cells. The patient usually has a neutrophil dysfunction with a compromised immune response.

2. *Generalized Juvenile Periodontitis.* GJP is characterized by generalized alveolar bone loss. It occurs in the older adolescent and young adult. The microflora found in pockets of GJP has similarities to the microflora of adult periodontitis. A neutrophil disturbance is also noted in this type of juvenile periodontitis.

D. Necrotizing Ulcerative Gingivitis/Periodontitis

Although found infrequently in children, necrotizing ulcerative gingivitis has its highest frequency in older adolescents and young adults. Stress, undernutrition, lack of bacterial plaque control, neglect of oral health, depressed immune reactions, and psychosomatic factors are predisposing influences in its development (pages 578 to 579).

DENTAL HYGIENE CARE

Dental and dental hygiene services during adolescence can impact oral health throughout the patient's lifetime. The knowledge, attitudes, and practices acquired and developed by adolescents can have wide-reaching significance as they become the parents and community participants of the future.

I. PATIENT APPROACH

Adolescence is a period of transition. Working with adolescents offers a challenge, and each situation requires its own approach. Some of the physical and psychological characteristics are listed in this chapter to provide a framework for what may be expected. A few basic suggestions for approach include the following:

A. Treat adolescents as adults. Physically, many of them are mature, although their emotional development varies.

B. Set the stage to let them know of your interest in them and their issues. Encourage them to talk, and then listen attentively.

C. Suggest and advise, but do not become impatient or take offense when they choose to make their own decisions.

D. Self-esteem plays a significant role in mediating changes in dental health behavior. High self-esteem has been positively correlated with oral hygiene self-care in adolescents.[8]

E. They are usually interested in health matters and details about their physical condition, although they may appear indifferent. Cleanliness and attractiveness are important to most teenage patients.

F. Health, including oral health, may be a real concern. Adolescents need to be well informed about their oral conditions, and explanations on a scientific basis are generally appreciated.

II. PATIENT HISTORY

Adolescents should provide their own information for the medical and dental histories. A consultation with the parent or guardian for additional details should be made, but not in the same interview with the patient and not without the patient's knowledge.

Adolescents need to take increasing responsibility for their own health. Although the initial dental visit may be at the insistence of the parents, every effort should be made to focus on the patient, not the parents.

The adolescent patient may have other health problems. The patient with diabetes; heart disease; a mental, physical, or sensory disability; or other systemic involvement requires special methods for approach as described in the various chapters of Part VI of this book. Medical clearance by parent or legal guardian is necessary for conditions requiring antibiotic coverage, local anesthesia, or other medication for a patient under legal age. Approval of the dental hygiene care plan by parent or legal guardian is necessary.

III. ORAL HEALTH PROBLEMS IN ADOLESCENCE[9]

Dental caries and periodontal infections of the adolescent years have been described. Some examples of other oral problems related to adolescent development and behavior characteristics are listed here.

A. Oral manifestations of sexually transmitted diseases (STD).
B. Effects of tobacco use, such as leukoplakia and periodontal damage from smokeless tobacco products. Effects of cocaine use and other drugs.
C. Potential effects of oral contraceptives on periodontal tissues (page 680).
D. Oral findings of anorexia nervosa or bulimia (pages 830 to 833).
E. Traumatic injury to teeth and oral structures from athletic activities and motorized vehicle accidents. Many adolescents participate in contact sports and other potentially dangerous activities such as the use of roller blades, jet skis, skateboards, and snowmobiles. Automobiles and motorcycles can also be dangerous.
F. Pregnancy and parenting may be issues for the adolescent. The dental hygienist has the opportunity to use anticipatory guidance in educating the patient on important dental health issues (see Table 43-3, page 661).
G. Oral piercings.

IV. BACTERIAL PLAQUE CONTROL

A clear explanation of the causes of dental caries and periodontal conditions, with the methods for their prevention, is basic. Adolescents need to understand the effects of the accumulation of bacterial plaque, the purposes of professional calculus removal, and the relation of the daily self-care plaque control program to the health status of the periodontal tissues.

For dental caries prevention, adolescents must appreciate the effects of fluoride and the need to restrict the intake of cariogenic foods. The program is outlined and conducted on the basis of these clear-cut preventive measures.

A. Instruction in self-care procedures.
B. Continuing reassessment over a series of appointments to develop daily practices that can be carried over into adult life.

V. INSTRUMENTATION

A series of appointments may be required, depending on probing depth and extent of calculus deposits.

Careful and complete scaling and root planing and removal of all local irregularities, such as inadequate margins of restorations, are the basic treatment procedures.

VI. FLUORIDE TREATMENT PROGRAM

A combined fluoride program is indicated for most adolescent patients, particularly for those who have not lived in a community with a fluoridated water supply. In addition to the topical applications made in conjunction with dental hygiene professional appointments, self-administered methods should include a fluoride dentifrice and a daily fluoride mouthrinse. A daily application of a fluoride gel in a custom-made tray may be necessary for remineralization in selected cases (pages 469 and 470).

VII. DIET CONTROL

A. **Dietary Assessment (pages 444 to 449)**
A study of the patient's diet and counseling relative to general nutrition and dental caries control can provide important learning experiences for many adolescents. The parent or other person who is in charge of shopping and food preparation must be included so that appropriate foods are available. As much responsibility as possible should be placed on the patient.

B. **Instruction Suggestions**
1. *Advise Foods From the Most Recent Food Guide Pyramid* (page 445). Emphasize foods for growth, energy, clear complexion, wellness, and prevention of illness.
2. *Emphasize a Good Breakfast.* Teenagers tend to slight or omit breakfast, particularly if they have to prepare it for themselves.
3. *Snack Selection.* Advise selecting from the nutritious foods, with recognition of cariogenic foods. Snacks suggested can include raw fruits and vegetables, nuts, nonsweetened milk, use of sugar-free foods when possible, and sugarless chewing gum if gum is used.

MENSTRUATION

The menstrual cycle refers to the cyclic structural changes in the uterus. These changes are instigated by hormones and represent periodic preparation of the lining of the uterus for pregnancy (Figure 45-1). When fertilization does not take place, changes in the mucous membrane lining the uterus (the endometrium) lead to the menstrual discharge. The fluid discharged is primarily blood combined with fragments of the disintegrated endometrium.

I. CHARACTERISTICS

A. **Occurrence**
The cyclic changes occur from puberty to menopause except during pregnancy and part

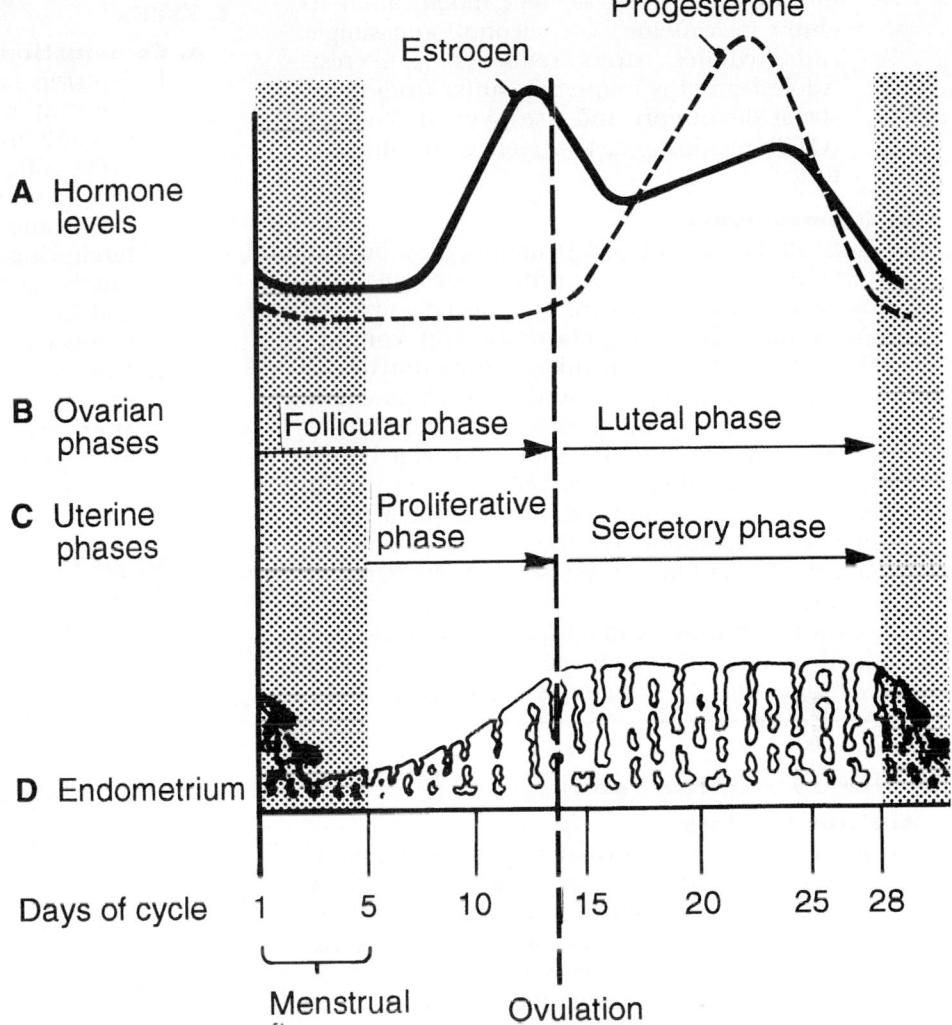

A Hormone levels

Estrogen

Progesterone

B Ovarian phases

Follicular phase | Luteal phase

C Uterine phases

Proliferative phase | Secretory phase

D Endometrium

Days of cycle   1   5   10   15   20   25   28

Menstrual flow   Ovulation

FIGURE 45-1 Changes During the Menstrual Cycle. The 28 days of a normal cycle are shown, with ovulation between days 12 and 15 and the menstrual flow between days 1 to 5 and again at day 28. *(A)* Hormonal levels show the estrogen peak shortly before ovulation during the follicular phase of the ovary *(B)* and the proliferative phase of the uterus *(C)*. *(D)* The endometrium builds up at the end of each menstrual flow. This prepares the area for possible implantation of a fertilized ovum.

of breast-feeding. Although the average cycle is complete in about 28 days, the normal range is from 22 to 34 days.

B. Menarche

Menstruation may begin at any time from ages 9 to 17 years. The mean age in the United States is between 12 and 13 years.

Menarche frequently occurs before the first ovulation, that is, before the pituitary and ovarian hormones are synchronized and ovulation becomes a part of the menstrual cycle. Timing and extent of flow may be irregular for several months or years after the onset of menstruation.

II. IRREGULARITIES

Although variations in the menstrual cycle are common, many females never have any problems or discomforts. The pattern of the cycle may be affected by factors such as changes in climate, changes in work

schedule, emotional trauma, acute or chronic illnesses, weight loss, or excessive exercise.

Menstruation may have strong emotional impact, and associated disturbances may have a psychologic basis. Intense emotional conflicts may be related to the inability to accept the feminine role and assume the responsibilities of womanhood. The symptoms of premenstrual tension and dysmenorrhea described in the following can continue beyond adolescence and even through menopause.

A. Premenstrual Syndrome

This condition is associated with fluid retention in the body and psychologic depression occurring within 10 days prior to menstruation.

1. *Physical Symptoms.* The most frequent symptoms are fatigue, headache, abdominal bloating, mastalgia, joint pain, increased appetite, and incoordination.
2. *Affective Symptoms.* Depression, anxiety, irritability, and hostility can be noted.
3. *Management.* Severe symptoms require medical care and supervision. Self-help methods

include daily exercise; diet modification to eliminate caffeine, salt, alcohol, and simple carbohydrates; stress reduction; and rest. Adolescent girls frequently suffer from menstrual discomfort and use over-the-counter (OTC) medications to manage the discomfort.[10]

B. Dysmenorrhea

Difficult or painful menstruation may be primary or secondary. With primary or functional dysmenorrhea, the organs are normal and there are symptoms of hyperactivity and contractions. Secondary or acquired dysmenorrhea is associated with organ disorders, such as endometriosis or pelvic inflammatory disease (PID).

Dysmenorrhea in the adolescent can be related to physiologic or psychologic factors. It may indicate emotional status, may be a result of poor preparation for the arrival of puberty and menstruation, or can result from parental example.

Although most women have little or no discomfort, a small percentage suffers severe pain with "cramps," sometimes accompanied by nausea and vomiting.

III. DENTAL HYGIENE CARE

A. Patient History

Menstruation is a normal process and should not be referred to as a "sick period" or a "monthly illness." When presenting questions for the patient history, use of terms such as the "period" or "monthly period" is preferable. A question about the regularity of menstruation should be included in each medical history review.

The menstrual history may provide indications of a woman's general health. Regularly excessive menstrual flow may be related to an anemic state, and medical examination and treatment are indicated.

B. Oral Findings[11]

No specific gingival changes are related to the menstrual cycle. An exaggerated response to local irritants or unusual gingival bleeding during or following scaling may be noted in an occasional patient. With control of local irritants through bacterial plaque control, self-care measures, and removal of calculus at regular maintenance appointments, bleeding usually can be controlled.

HORMONAL CONTRACEPTIVES

Birth control pills are recognized as the most effective method of contraception when they are taken as prescribed. Because of their convenience, they are used by millions of women worldwide.

I. TYPES[12]

A. Combination Preparations

1. *Estrogen and Progestin.* The combination of the synthetically produced hormones estrogen and progestin is nearly 100% effective in preventing ovulation. Estrogen inhibits the secretion of follicle-stimulating hormone (FSH) and progestin inhibits the release of luteinizing hormone (LH) by the anterior pituitary gland. Without the hormones FSH and LH, the ovum cannot be released from the ovary.
2. *Schedule of Administration.* One pill is taken each day for 20 or 21 days starting 5 days after the onset of the menstrual flow. Then, for a period of 7 days, no pill is taken. The routine is followed regardless of when menstruation starts or stops.

B. Single Preparations: Minipill

Progestin alone has been used when the effects of estrogen are contraindicated. Pregnancy prevention is slightly less effective with this pill. When this type of pill is used, menstrual cycles tend to be more irregular and side effects more frequent.

II. CONTRAINDICATIONS[12]

Contraceptives containing hormones should not be taken when the woman has a history of the following:

A. Thromboembolic disorders.
B. Cerebrovascular disease.
C. Severe hypertension.
D. Impaired liver function.
E. Known or suspected cancer of the breast or other estrogen-dependent neoplasia.
F. Undiagnosed uterine bleeding.
G. Smoking.
H. Pregnancy.

III. SIDE EFFECTS[12]

Side effects sometimes may be related more to incorrect use of the drug than to hormonal effects. Visual problems, mental depression, rashes, and bleeding irregularities occur in some women. The most significant effects are the following:

A. Cardiovascular (including increased blood pressure).
B. Weight gain.
C. Decreased effectiveness of the contraceptive when certain drugs are used, including the following:
   1. Antibiotics.[13,14]
   2. Anticonvulsants.
   3. Rifampin (used in treatment of tuberculosis).

IV. EFFECT ON THE GINGIVA

An exaggerated response to bacterial plaque and

other local irritants has been noted, especially when the personal oral hygiene is less than adequate. The gingivitis is similar to that described for pregnancy (page 654).

V. APPOINTMENT CONSIDERATIONS

A. Medical History
A record of the use of oral contraceptives should be updated with each history review.

B. Patient Information
1. Explain the need for exceptional personal oral care and regular professional maintenance appointments to prevent complications from gingivitis.
2. Explain the need for additional contraception when antibiotic premedication or other use of antibiotics is indicated.
3. Alert patient to side effects and advise medical evaluation if side effects become troublesome.
4. Smoking: quantity and frequency. There is an increased risk factor for cardiovascular disease when smoking is combined with the use of hormonal contraceptives. Risk increases with age.

MENOPAUSE AND CLIMACTERIC

Menopause is the cessation of menstruation. Menopause is one part of the natural cycle of a female's reproductive life. It is the end of menstruation, usually confirmed when a woman has no menstrual period for 12 consecutive months and there is no obvious biologic or physiologic cause. Menopause generally occurs between the ages of 45 and 55 years, with the average of approximately 51 years.

Menopause is not a disease or an illness, but a natural event, the end of fertility, resulting from the ovaries decreased production of two sex hormones: estrogen and progesterone. Menopause may be induced by surgical removal of the ovaries or by radiation therapy.

The female *climacteric* is that period of change during the gradual decline of ovarian efficiency when ovulation is less regular and finally ends, through the menopause, and including the period after menopause when the body is adjusting to endocrine and other changes. While adolescence is considered the transitional period from childhood into maturity, the climacteric has been described as the transitional period from maturity into senescence.

I. CHARACTERISTICS

Prior to menopause, menstruation decreases in frequency, duration, and amount of flow over a period of about 12 to 24 months. Menopause is accompanied by a number of characteristic changes. Although many women may experience minor symptoms, only a small percent have any pronounced effects from menopause.

A. General Symptoms
As ovarian function declines with diminishing estrogen, physiologic changes in body function take place.
1. *Vasomotor Reactions.* Vasomotor instability in the form of hot flashes, in which sudden, periodic surges of heat involving the whole body and accompanied by drenching sweats, may occur during the day or night. Although a strict distinction is not always made between flush and flash, the term hot flush may be used to mean a reaction of lesser degree in which a wave of warmth is felt over the face, neck, and upper thorax. Headaches, heart palpitations, and sleeplessness may occur.
2. *Emotional Disturbances.* Emotional problems are not caused specifically by estrogen deficiencies but are frequently related to personal and family circumstances and concern over growing old. Anxiety, tension, and irritability, with depression and feelings of uselessness, may appear in some women.

B. Postmenopausal Effects
1. Reproductive organs atrophy.
2. Changes in bones may lead to osteoporosis. This condition is less frequent among women who have used drinking water containing fluoride over the years, have met the daily requirement for calcium in the diet, and who have exercised regularly.
3. Skin and mucous membranes decrease in thickness and keratinization.
4. Predisposition to conditions including atherosclerosis, diabetes, and hypothyroidism.

II. ORAL FINDINGS
Oral changes can be related to the menopause.

A. Gingiva
Gingival changes associated with menopause usually represent an exaggerated response to bacterial plaque, which reflects the conditioning influence of the hormonal changes taking place. When local factors are controlled through preventive dental hygiene appointments for maintenance to supplement daily personal oral care, unusual gingival changes are uncommon.

Rarely, a condition that has been called menopausal gingivostomatitis may develop.[15] It may also occur after removal of, or radiation therapy to, the ovaries.

B. Mucous Membranes and Tongue
1. Dryness with burning sensations may be present. Altered salivary composition in some menopausal women may be due to psychologic stress.[16]

2. Epithelium may become thin and atrophic with decreased keratinization; tolerance for removable prostheses may lessen.
3. Altered taste perception.
4. Inadequate diet and eating habits may contribute to the adverse changes of the mucosal tissues. The appearance and symptoms frequently resemble those associated with vitamin deficiencies, particularly B vitamins.

C. Alveolar Bone Loss
As a result of systemic osteoporosis, ridge resorption and loss of teeth can occur.[17]

III. DENTAL HYGIENE CARE
In the approach to the patient, a specific relationship of oral conditions to menopause should not be made because the patient may tend to overemphasize such a relationship and de-emphasize the need for self-care measures. Because of the importance of local factors, attention should be directed to the need for regular and frequent professional care, as well as to increased efforts for daily plaque control.

A. Appointment Suggestions
The symptoms of physical and emotional changes should be kept in mind when planning and conducting the appointment. The patient's possible tenseness and irritability can be anticipated.
1. Rapport begins with the clinician's courtesy, personal attention, and friendly, unhurried manner.
2. Give particular attention to details, such as seating the patient promptly, handling materials and instruments efficiently and with calm assurance.
3. Maintain a conservativeness in conversation to prevent unnecessary annoyances to the patient.

B. Instruction of Patient
Preservation of oral health is particularly important to the woman who has her natural teeth. Because of the possible difficulties and discomforts of wearing prostheses, every effort should be made to prevent the need for tooth removal. If needed, a saliva substitute may provide a degree of relief from xerostomia and aid in the prevention of dental caries (pages 345 and 346).

Measures for the prevention of periodontal infections should be carefully explained, and emphasis should be placed on reasons for frequent calculus removal to supplement meticulous daily care. Because good general health practices are very important to this age group, the relationship of general and oral health can be emphasized.

C. Diet
A dietary survey may prove to be a helpful teaching–learning experience (pages 444 to 449) by helping the patient to identify and correct inadequately balanced food selection. Dietary supplementation with calcium and vitamin D can help to minimize bone loss. Dental caries prevention through selection of nutritious and noncariogenic foods is especially important for the patient who tends to indulge in between-meal eating.

D. Fluoride Therapy
A fluoride-containing dentifrice and a brush-on gel applied before retiring are necessary for nearly all patients in this age group (pages 471 to 472).

REFERENCES

1. **Resnick,** M.D., Bearman, P.S., Blum, R.W., Bauman, K.E., Harris, K.M., Jones, J., Tabor, J., Beuhring, T., Sieving, R.E., Shew, M., Ireland, M., Bearinger, L.H., and Udry, J.R.: Protecting Adolescents From Harm. Findings from the National Longitudinal Study on Adolescent Health, *JAMA, 278,* 823, September 10, 1997.
2. **Carranza,** F.A. and Newman, M.G.: *Clinical Periodontology,* 8th ed. Philadelphia, W.B. Saunders Co., 1996, pp. 192, 240.
3. **Albandar,** J.M., Brown, L.J., and Löe, H.: Clinical Features of Early-onset Periodontitis, *J. Am. Dent. Assoc., 128,* 1393, October, 1997.
4. **Bishop,** K., Dummer, P.M.H., Kingdon, A., Newcombe, R.G., and Addy, M.: Radiographic Alveolar Bone Loss from Posterior Teeth in Young Adults Over a 4-year Period, *J. Clin. Periodontol., 22,* 835, November, 1995.
5. **Hansen,** B.F., Gjermo, P., Bellini, H.T., Ihanamaki, K., and Saxén, L.: Prevalence of Radiographic Alveolar Bone Loss in Young Adults, A Multinational Study, *Internat. Dent. J., 45,* 54, February, 1995.
6. **Brown,** L.J., Albandar, J.M., Brunelle, J.A., and Löe, H.: Early-onset Periodontitis: Progression of Attachment Loss During 6 Years, *J. Periodontol., 67,* 969, October, 1996.
7. **Perry,** D.A., Beemsterboer, P.L., and Taggart, E.J.: *Periodontology for the Dental Hygienist.* Philadelphia, W.B. Saunders Co., 1996, pp. 103–109.
8. **Regis,** D., Macgregor, I.D.M., and Balding, J.W.: Differential Prediction of Dental Health Behaviour by Self-esteem and Health Locus of Control in Young Adolescents, *J. Clin. Periodontol., 21,* 7, January, 1994.
9. **American Academy of Pediatric Dentistry**: Oral Health Policies, Statement on Adolescent Oral Health, May, 1994, *Pediatr. Dent., 20,* 24, Special Issue, November, 1998.
10. **Campbell,** M.A. and McGrath, P.J.: Use of Medication by Adolescents for the Management of Menstrual Discomfort, *Arch. Pediatr. Adolesc. Med., 151,* 905, September, 1997.
11. **Carranza and Newman:** op. cit., p. 193.
12. **Greydanus,** D.E. and Patel, D.R.: Contraception, in McAnarney, E.R., Kreipe, R.E., Orr, D.P., and Comerci, G.D.: *Textbook of Adolescent Medicine.* Philadelphia, W.B. Saunders Co., 1992, pp. 676–685.
13. **Zachariasen,** R.D.: Effect of Antibiotics on Oral Contraceptive Efficacy, *J. Dent. Hyg., 65,* 334, September, 1991.
14. **American Dental Association,** Health Foundation Research Institute, Department of Toxicology: Antibiotic Interference with Oral Contraceptives, *J. Am. Dent. Assoc., 122,* 79, December, 1991.
15. **Carranza and Newman:** op. cit., p. 194.
16. **Ciberka,** R.M., Nelson, S.K., and Lefebvre, C.A.: Burning Mouth Syndrome; A Review of Etiologies, *J. Prosthet. Dent., 78,* 93, July, 1997.
17. **Jeffcoat,** M.K. and Chesnut, C.H.: Systemic Osteoporosis and Oral Bone Loss: Evidence Shows Increased Factors, *J. Am. Dent. Assoc., 124,* 49, November, 1993.

SUGGESTED READINGS

Bale, P., Doust, J., and Dawson, D.: Gymnasts, Distance Runners, Anorexics Body Composition and Menstrual Status, *J. Sports Med. Phys. Fitness, 36,* 49, March, 1996.

Folkers, S.A., Weine, F.S., and Weissman, D.P.: Periodontal Disease in the Life Stages of Women, *Compend. Cont. Educ. Dent., 13,* 52, October, 1992.

Miyajima, K., Nagahara, K., and Lizuka, T.: Orthodontic Treatment for a Patient After Menopause, *Angle Orthod., 66,* 173, Number 3, 1996.

Olson, L.: Answering the Challenges of Women's Oral Health, *Access, 11,* 15, May–June, 1997.

Schmidt, P.J., Nieman, L.K., Danaceau, M.A., Adams, L.F., and Rubinow, D. R.: Differential Behavioral Effects of Gonadal Steroids in Women With and in Those Without Premenstrual Syndrome, *N. Engl. J. Med., 338,* 209, January 22, 1998.

Zakrzewska, J.M.: Women As Dental Patients: Are There Any Gender Differences?, *Int. Dent. J., 46,* 548, December, 1996.

Adolescence

DuRant, R.H., Rickert, V.I., Ashworth, C.S., Newman, C., and Slavens, G.: Use of Multiple Drugs among Adolescents Who Use Anabolic Steroids, *N. Engl. J. Med., 328,* 922, April 1, 1993.

Dwyer, J.T.: Adolescence, in Ziegler, E.E. and Filer, L.J., eds.: *Present Knowledge in Nutrition,* 7th ed. Washington, D.C., ILSI Press, 1996, pp. 404–413.

Freeman, R. and Sheiham, A.: Understanding Decision-making Processes for Sugar Consumption in Adolescence, *Community Dent Oral Epidemiol., 25,* 228, June, 1997.

Macgregor, I.D., Regis, D., and Balding, J.: Self-concept and Dental Health Behaviours in Adolescents, *J. Clin. Periodontol., 24,* 335, May, 1997.

Macgregor, I.D., Balding, J., and Regis, D.: Toothbrushing Schedule, Motivation and "Lifestyle" Behaviours in 7,770 Young Adolescents, *Community Dent Health, 4,* 232, December, 1996.

Adolescents: Periodontitis

Aass, A.M., Tollefsen, T., and Gjermo, P.: A Cohort Study of Radiographic Alveolar Bone Loss During Adolescence, *J. Clin. Periodontol., 21,* 133, February, 1994.

Albandar, J.M., Brown, L.J., and Loe, H.: Dental Caries and Tooth Loss in Adolescents with Early-onset Periodontitis, *J. Periodontol., 67,* 960, October, 1996.

American Academy of Periodontology, Committee on Research, Science and Therapy: Position Paper: Periodontal Diseases of Children and Adolescents, *J. Periodontol., 67,* 57, January, 1996.

Clerehugh, V., Seymour, G.J., Bird, P.S., Cullinan, M.,

Drucker, D.B., and Worthington, H.V.: The Detection of Actinobacillus actinomycetemcomitans, Porphyromonas gingivalis and Prevotella intermedia Using an ELISA in an Adolescent Population with Early Periodontitis, *J. Clin. Periodontol., 24,* 57, January, 1997.

Ellwood, R., Worthington, H.V., Cullinan, M.P., Hamlet, S., Clerehugh, V., and Davies, R.: Prevalence of Suspected Periodontal Pathogens Identified Using ELISA in Adolescents of Differing Ethnic Origins, *J. Clin. Periodontol., 24,* 141, March, 1997.

Jenkins, S.M., Dummer, P.M.H., and Addy, M.: Radiographic Evaluation of Early Periodontal Bone Loss in Adolescents, an Overview, *J. Clin. Periodontol., 19,* 363, July, 1992.

Oral Contraceptives

Baird, D.T. and Glasier, A.F.: Hormonal Contraception, *N. Engl. J. Med., 328,* 1543, May 27, 1993.

Biron, C.: Questions Surface over Whether Antibiotics Neutralize "the pill," Resulting in Pregnancy, *RDH, 16,* 34, July, 1996.

Glasier, A.: Emergency Postcoital Contraception, *N. Engl. J. Med., 337,* 1058, October 9, 1997.

Menopause

Ben Aryeh, H., Gottlieb, I., Ish-Shalom, S., David, A., Szargel, H., and Laufer, D: Oral Complaints Related to Menopause, *Maturitas, 24,* 185, July, 1996.

Forabosco, A., Criscuolo, M., Coukos, G., Uccelli, E., Weinstein, R., Spinato, S., Botticelli, A., and Volpe, A.: Efficacy of Hormone Replacement Therapy in Postmenopausal Women with Oral Discomfort, *Oral Surg. Oral Med. Oral Pathol., 73,* 570, May, 1992.

Hormone Replacement

Covington, P.: Women's Oral Health Issues: An Exploration of the Literature, *Can. Dent. Hyg. (Probe), 30,* 173, September/October, 1996.

Ferris, G.M.: Alteration in Female Sex Hormones: Their Effect on Oral Tissues and Dental Treatment, *Compend. Cont. Educ. Dent., 14,* 1558, December, 1993.

Norderyd, O.M., Grossi, S.G., Machtei, E.E., Zambon, J.J., Hausmann, E., Dunford, R.G., and Genco, R.J.: Periodontal Status of Women Taking Postmenopausal Estrogen Supplementation, *J. Periodontol., 64,* 957, October, 1993.

Payne, J.B., Zachs, N.R., Reinhardt, R.A., Nummikoski, P.V., and Patil, K.: The Association Between Estrogen Status and Alveolar Bone Density Changes in Postmenopausal Women with a History of Periodontitis, *J. Periodontol., 68,* 24, January, 1997.

Taguchi, A., Tanimoto, K., Suei, Y., Otani, K., and Wada, T.: Oral Signs as Indicators of Possible Osteoporosis in Elderly Women, *Oral Surg. Oral Med. Oral Pathol., 80,* 612, November, 1995.

The Gerodontic Patient

CHAPTER OUTLINE

Preventive measures for the aging population through care and instruction require greater emphasis as the number of people involved in this group increases steadily. Members of the dental team are challenged by the need to help the aging population learn about personal care and seek professional care that will provide continuing oral comfort and function.

As the percentage of people in the older group has increased, the total number of older patients in a general or adult practice has grown. An increasing number of dental hygienists specialize in the care of the elderly and are employed in long-term care and resident facilities for the aged.

Tooth loss increases with age, but not because of age. Dental caries and periodontal diseases are the major causes of tooth loss. Periodontal diseases in the older population represent the cumulative effects of long-standing, undiagnosed, untreated, or neglected chronic infection.

With fluoridation and the application of current knowledge of preventive measures for oral diseases in younger age groups, it is anticipated that future generations of older people will not be subjected to the severe effects of uncontrolled and untreated oral diseases. Key words relating to older patients are defined in Box 46-1.

AGING

I. BIOLOGIC AND CHRONOLOGIC AGE

When aging is defined from a chronologic viewpoint, the aging population may be recognized as the "older population" (age 55 and over), the "elderly" (age 65 and over), the "aged" (75 years and older), and the "very old" (85 years and over).[1] Biologic age is not synonymous with chronologic age, and hence, signs of aging appear at different chronologic ages in different individuals. In other words, some people are old at 45 years, whereas others are not old at 75 years.

BOX 46-1 KEY WORDS: Gerodontic Patient

Aging: the continuous process (biologic, psychologic, social), beginning with conception and ending with death, by which organisms mature and decline.

Alzheimer's disease (awltz'hī-merz): a chronic brain syndrome, usually occuring in older adulthood, characterized by gradual deterioration of memory, disorientation, and other features of dementia.

Biologic age: the anatomic or physiologic age of a person as determined by changes in organismic structure and function; takes into account features such as posture, skin texture, strength, speed, and sensory acuity.

Chronologic age: the actual measure of time elapsed since a person's birth.

Dementia (de-men'shah): severe mental deterioration involving impairment of mental ability; organic loss of intellectual function.

Dysphagia (dĭs-fa'jē-ah): difficulty in swallowing.

Emphysema (em"fĭ-sē'mah): pathologic accumulation of air in tissues or organs; general use refers to **chronic pulmonary emphysema**, in which terminal bronchioles become plugged with mucus, the lung and tissue loses elasticity, and breathing difficulties ensue.

Geriatric dentistry: the branch of dentistry that deals with the special knowledge, attitudes, and technical skills required in the provision of oral health care for older adults.

Geriatrics: (jer"ē-at'rĭks): the branch of medicine that deals with the problems and illnesses of aging and their treatment.

Gerontology: study of the aging process; includes the biologic, psychologic, and sociologic sciences.

Hemostasis (hē"mō-stā'sis): arrest of the escape of blood by either natural (clot formation or vessel spasm) or artificial (compression or ligation) means, or by the interruption of blood flow to a part.

Life expectancy: average number of years that a person can be expected to live; expectancy from birth in 1900 averaged 47 years; in 1996 averaged 76.1 years; expectancy for the female population is about 6 years longer than that for the male population.*

Lifestyle: relatively permanent organization of activities, including work, leisure, and associated social activities, characterizing an individual.

Osteoid (os'tē-oid): young bone that has not undergone calcification.

Osteopenia (os"tē-ō-pē'nē-ah): decreased calcification or density of bone; inadequate osteoid synthesis.

Osteoporosis (os"tē-ō-pah-rō'sĭs): low bone mass resulting from an excess of bone resorption over bone formation, with resultant bone fragility and increased risk of fracture.

Presbyopia (pres"be-o'pe-ah): a condition of farsightedness resulting from a loss of elasticity of the lens of the eye due to aging.

Psychologic age: the age of a person as determined by his or her feelings, attitudes, and life perspective.

Senescence (se-nes'ens): the process of growing old.

Senility (sĕ-nĭl'ĭ-te): old age; loss of mental, physical, or emotional control; caused by physical and/or mental deterioration.

*****Centers for Disease Control and Prevention:** Mortality Patterns—Preliminary Data, United States, 1996, *MMWR, 46,* 941, October 10, 1997.

II. CLASSIFICATION BY FUNCTION

The degree of general health and physical activity provides a workable classification not based on age. Relative to the degree of impairment, older persons may be *functionally independent, frail,* or *functionally dependent.* Another term for the functionally independent is the *well elderly,* a more descriptive term for the many healthy, active, productive people who happen to be older than what is considered to be a reasonable retirement age.[2]

III. AGING AND DISEASE

Normal changes with aging should not be confused with the effects of pathologic influences that accelerate the aging process. Each age level brings changes in body metabolism, activity of the cells, endocrine balance, and mental processes.

An older person's health status is influenced by many factors. Both biologic and environmental factors influence longevity. Genetically, a person may belong to a family of healthy people who have exhibited great resistance to disease factors. Another person may have inherited a specific disease state. Even inherited diseases, for example, diabetes or sickle cell anemia, may be controllable through treatment or genetic counseling.

CHARACTERISTICS OF AGING

Changes with aging vary among individuals and among organs and tissues of the same individual. In a healthy person, free of chronic diseases and medications with their potential side effects, the tissue changes of aging are more subtle, appear at a later age, and definitely can be influenced by the person's lifestyle.

Over the years the risk factors of smoking, poor diet, lack of exercise, and obesity take their toll. Helping people to learn early in life the health maintenance procedures that prevent the development of chronic illnesses and disabilities is a responsibility of all health-care workers.

I. GENERAL PHYSIOLOGIC CHANGES

During aging, an overall gradual reduction in functional capacities occurs in most organs, with a decrease in cell metabolism and numbers of active cells. The tissues may show signs of dehydration, atrophy, fibrosis, reduced elasticity, and diminished reparative ability. Many of these characteristics cannot be separated from pathologic changes.

A. Increased Susceptibility to Infection[3]
With aging, an increased susceptibility to infection may be related to one or more of the following:
1. Lowered capacity in cell-mediated and humoral immunity and nonspecific host defenses.
2. Altered skin and mucosal barriers. In the oral cavity, the flora of the mucosa can be changed, especially when systemic conditions or medications lead to xerostomia.
3. Interaction of nutritional factors with underlying chronic conditions.
4. Decreased immunologic functioning of aging is a factor in increased susceptibility of both men and women to HIV infection and AIDS.[4]

B. Response to Disease
1. *Course and Severity:* Although the diseases that affect the elderly person also occur in younger persons, the course and effects of the diseases may differ. In the elderly person, disease may occur with greater severity and have a longer course, with slower recovery.
2. *Pain Sensitivity:* May be lessened.
3. *Temperature Response:* May be altered so that a patient may be very ill without the expected increase in body temperature.
4. *Healing*
   a. Decreased healing capacity.
   b. More prone to secondary infection.

II. COMMON CHANGES AND DISORDERS

A. Cardiovascular System (Chapter 58)
Effects of aging on the cardiovascular system include the following:
1. Tendency toward increased blood pressure usually secondary to disease.
2. Arteriosclerosis, with decreased circulation to the tissues.
3. Reduced cardiac output; increased heart size.
4. Postural hypotension, with dizziness or weakness when sitting up from recumbent position.

B. Pulmonary Disorders
1. Vital capacity is progressively diminished.
2. Decreased pulmonary efficiency may be related to lifestyle and lack of exercise.
3. Chronic obstructive pulmonary diseases (COPD): chronic bronchitis and emphysema are of particular concern for the longtime smoker.
4. Pneumonia and influenza.
5. Inactive tuberculosis (pages 21 to 22).

C. Musculoskeletal System
1. *Skeletal Integrity:* Significantly influenced by an insufficient intake of calcium, phosphorus, and fluoride.
2. *Bone Volume (Mass):* Decreases gradually after the age of 40, depending on diet, nutrition, and exercise.
3. *Osteoporosis:* Common in individuals older than age 60, and the incidence increases with age (page 687).
4. *Loss of Muscle Function:* Development of unsteadiness and tremor, diminishing of muscular strength, and decreased speed of response. Posture may become stooped; joints may stiffen as a result of loss of elasticity in the ligaments.
5. *Osteoarthritis:* A major cause of disability, it affects the weight-bearing joints. Also known as degenerative joint disease (pages 784 to 785).

D. Gastrointestinal System
1. Production of hydrochloric acid and other secretions gradually decreases.
2. Peristalsis is slowed.
3. Evaluation of digestive disorders is complicated by the general indiscriminate use of self-medications.

E. Skin
1. The skin may become thin, wrinkled, and dry, with pigmented spots, loss of tone, and atrophy of the sweat glands.
2. Reduced tolerance to temperature extremes and solar exposure is evident.

F. Special Senses (Chapter 53)
1. *Vision:* Decline in accommodation and color and depth perception, and difficulty in adapting from light to dark.
2. *Hearing:* Reduced hearing ability, with a loss of sensitivity to high tones.

G. Alcoholism[5,6]
1. *Early-Onset Drinkers:* May have lifetime pattern, with history of trauma, medical problems, hospitalizations, and detoxification.
2. *Late-Onset Drinkers:* Less likely to have chronic illnesses directly related to alcohol abuse; more likely to be living with family than early-onset drinkers.

3. *Related Factors:* Depression, loneliness, lack of social support, and loss of self-image.
4. *Effects of Aging:* Symptoms and effects are similar to younger people (Chapter 57); aging people are more vulnerable because of tissue changes and metabolism.

OSTEOPOROSIS

Osteoporosis is a bone disease involving loss of mineral content and bone mass. Although most prominent in postmenopausal women, the condition may also occur at other ages and in men.

I. CAUSES

A. Endocrine: hormonal disturbances; depletion of estrogen after menopause.
B. Calcium deficiency: defective absorption of calcium.
C. Steroid therapy.

II. RISK FACTORS

Several risk factors have been identified, some of which usually work together. From this list of risk factors, a list of methods for long-term prevention can be derived:

A. Female gender.
B. Caucasian or Asian ethnicity (worldwide, blacks are least affected).
C. Positive family history.
D. Low calcium and vitamin D intake (life-long).
E. Early menopause or early surgical removal of ovaries.
F. Sedentary lifestyle; lack of exercise.
G. Alcohol abuse.
H. Use of corticosteroids.
I. Cigarette smoking.
J. High caffeine intake.

III. RELATION TO PERIODONTAL DISEASE[7,8]

A. Relationship exists between the reduced bone mineral density of osteoporosis and oral bone loss in skeletal and mandibular bone; oral bone loss pertains to periodontal bone destruction and residual ridge loss in the edentulous person.
B. Osteoporosis and periodontal disease have mutual risk factors. Included are smoking, nutritional deficiencies, alcohol use, hormonal status, and others from the above list of risk factors for osteoporosis.
C. Osteoporotic bone is less dense and more readily absorbed; periodontal pathogenic microorganisms can provide the toxic products for increased periodontal breakdown.
D. Osteoporosis can be considered a risk factor for periodontal bone loss.

IV. SYMPTOMS

A. **Asymptomatic Period**
   Osteoporosis develops over many years; therefore a long asymptomatic period of bone change occurs with no clinical symptoms.

B. **Clinical Symptoms**
   1. Backache: stooping of the posture.
   2. Fractures: hip, spine, ends of long bones.
   3. Evidence of bone changes in the mandible: residual ridge resorption.

V. TREATMENT

A. **Medications**[9]
   1. Decrease bone resorption: estrogen; calcium.
   2. Increase bone formation: sodium fluoride.

B. **Activity**
   1. Activity and exercise require caution and preventive measures to avoid accidental falls.
   2. Severe involvement of the spine may require orthopedic support and medication for pain. Questions regarding the patient's medical history can elicit factors of importance.

C. **Behavioral**
   Avoid smoking and excessive alcoholic intake.

ALZHEIMER'S DISEASE

Alzheimer's disease is one of the non-reversible types of dementia. Dementia is severe impairment of the intellectual abilities, notably thinking, memory, and personality. At least one half of the patients with dementia have Alzheimer's disease.

I. SYMPTOMS

The common impairments of Alzheimer's disease may be divided into three or four overlapping stages that may extend over many years. In Table 46-1, characteristics are divided into early, middle, advanced, and terminal stages.

II. APPOINTMENT CONSIDERATIONS

During the early stages, perhaps even before a diagnosis of Alzheimer's disease has been made, the patient will be attending routine dental and dental hygiene appointments.

A. **Early Stages**
   An early sign of the disease may be a slow decline of interest in oral hygiene and personal care. Review of the patient's medical and dental history at each maintenance appointment may reveal lapses in memory and other items listed under the "Early Stage" in Table 46-1. An opportunity may be found to help a patient seek professional evaluation and care.

TABLE 46-1 Common Impairments Associated With Alzheimer's Disease

EARLY STAGE

Forgetfulness
Personality changes
Employment performance difficulty
Social withdrawal
Apathy
Errors in judgment
Inattentiveness
Personal hygiene neglect

MIDDLE STAGE

Disorientation
Loss of coordination
Restlessness/anxiety
Language difficulty
Sleep pattern disturbance
Progressive memory loss
Catastrophic reactions
Pacing

ADVANCED STAGE

Profound comprehension difficulty
Gait disturbances
Bladder and bowel incontinence
Hyperoralia
Inability to recognize family members
Seizures
Aggression
Lack of insight into deficits

TERMINAL STAGE

Physical immobility
Contractures
Dysphagia
Emaciation
Mutism
Pathologic reflexes
Unawareness of environment
Total helplessness

(From Fabiszewski, K.J.: Caring for the Alzheimer's Patient, *Gerodontology*, 6, 53, Summer, 1987, © Beech Hill Enterprises, Inc. Used by permission.)

B. Later Stages

Later stages may require that the patient reside in a long-term care facility. Dental hygienists in specialized facilities develop particular techniques for the variety of patients to be served.

ORAL FINDINGS IN AGING

As mentioned earlier in this chapter, changes related to aging must be separated from the long-term effects of chronic diseases.

I. SOFT TISSUES

A. Lips

1. *Tissue Changes.* Dry, purse-string opening results from dehydration and loss of elasticity within the tissues.
2. *Angular Cheilitis.*[10] Angular cheilitis is not specifically an age-related lesion, but it frequently is seen among elderly persons. It appears as skin folds with fissuring at the angles of the mouth and can be related to reduced vertical dimension or inadequate support of the lips. Primary etiologic factors are candidiasis and vitamin B deficiency. Contributing factors are summarized on page 702.

B. Oral Mucosa

Degenerative changes take several forms. The surface texture is affected by changes in lubrication of the tissue with decreased secretion of the salivary and mucous glands. Xerostomia is not a result of aging but is associated with certain diseases and medications.

1. *Atrophic Changes.* The tissue may become thinner and less vascular, with a loss of elasticity. Clinically, the smooth shiny appearance is related to thinning of the epithelium.
2. *Hyperkeratosis.* White, patchy areas may develop as a result of irritation from sharp edges of broken teeth, restorations, or dentures, and from use of tobacco.
3. *Capillary Fragility.* Facial bruises and petechiae of the mucosa are common.

C. Tongue

1. *Atrophic Glossitis (Burning Tongue).* The tongue appears smooth, shiny, and bald, with atrophied papillae. The condition is related to anemia that results from a deficiency of iron or combinations of deficiencies. Elderly people have deficiency anemias more frequently than do those in other age groups because of nutritional factors, but not because of aging specifically.
2. *Taste Sensations.* Taste buds are not reduced in number. Taste may be reduced or abnormal taste reactions may occur, primarily in people with a disease condition, but changes are not routinely observed in the healthy elderly person.
3. *Sublingual Varicosities*
   a. Clinical appearance: Deep, red or bluish nodular dilated vessels on either side of the midline on the ventral surface of the tongue.
   b. Significance: Although frequently occurring, these varicosities do not necessarily have a direct relation to systemic conditions.

D. Xerostomia

Dryness of the mouth is found frequently in

older people in conjunction with pathologic states, drug-induced changes, or radiation-induced degeneration of the salivary glands. Healthy people continue to have normal salivary flow.[11] Xerostomia is described in detail on pages 345 to 346.

II. TEETH

A. Color
The teeth may show color changes from long use of tobacco or foods with coloring agents, such as tea or coffee. Dark intrinsic stains from dental restorations may be evident.

B. Attrition
The teeth of elderly people frequently show signs of wear, which may be the long-term effects of diet, occupational factors, or bruxism. Figure 14-7, page 244, illustrates incisal wear. Attrition may be accompanied by chipping, and teeth may seem more brittle, particularly when compared with teeth of young people.

C. Abrasion
Abrasion at the neck of a tooth may be the result of extended use of a hard toothbrush in a horizontal direction with an abrasive dentifrice. With current preventive measures, use of soft-textured brushes, and attention to abrasiveness of dentifrices, future generations will be less likely to exhibit such tooth alterations.

D. Root Caries
1. *Occurrence.* With roots exposed by periodontal infections, an increase in caries of the cementum can result. Root caries is described on pages 240 to 242. An increase in caries with age is the result of root exposure, not of age. Risk factors for root caries are shown in Table 14-5 (page 243).
2. *Effect of Fluoride.* Adults with longtime residence in fluoridated community have substantially fewer root carious lesions than in a non-fluoridated community. This is especially true for lifelong residents where there has been natural fluoride in the water.[12]
3. *Rampant Caries.* Sometimes called "retirement caries." A noticeable increase in dental caries may occur after age 65. Factors influencing the development of dental caries include the following:
   a. Xerostomia. Tooth-protection factors of the saliva are missing (page 345).
   b. Masticatory abilities. Oral conditions and, possibly, tooth loss make mastication difficult. This leads to changes in food selections.
   c. Lifestyle. After retirement, without a daily work schedule, snacking and irregular mealtimes may lead to poor food selections and an excessively cariogenic diet.

E. Dental Pulp[13]
Whether pulpal changes can be considered results of aging is questionable. The pulpal changes develop as reactions to dental caries, restorations, bruxism, and other assaults during the elderly person's long life. The changes noted here may be observed at younger ages, but are seen more frequently in older people.
1. Narrowing of pulp chambers and root canals; increased deposition of secondary dentin.
2. Progressive deposition of calcified masses (pulp stones or denticles).

III. PERIODONTIUM

A. Clinical Findings
The periodontal tissues reflect the health and disease of the patient over the years. One of the following may apply to any patient.
1. *The Healthy Periodontium.* Healthy tissues that have been maintained over the years may have had a minimum of disease. The radiographs show little if any bone recession, the gingiva are firm, and the appearance is normal in every way. Probing reveals minimal sulcus depth with no bleeding. The teeth are not mobile.
2. *The Patient With Periodontal Infection.* Neglect or omission of preventive measures and therapy over the years may have resulted in a chronic periodontal infection with extension of tissue destruction into the bone, periodontal ligament, and cementum. Loss of attachment, deep periodontal pockets, tooth mobility, and radiographic signs of periodontitis may be present.
3. *The Treated Patient.* Although the patient was subject to periodontal infection, treatment was completed, and the tissues were maintained in health through personal care and professional supervision. The tissues may show the effects of the treated disease, such as scar tissue. Areas of recession with exposed cementum may also be evident. The teeth are not mobile.

B. Tissue Changes Related to Aging
1. *Bone*
   a. Osteoporosis may be present (page 687).[7,8]
   b. Depressed vascularity, a reduction in metabolism, and reduced healing power affect bone.
2. *Cementum.* Increased thickness has been demonstrated. In one series of measurements, the average overall thickness of the cementum at 20 years of age was 0.095 mm, whereas cementum from 60-year-old persons measured 0.215 mm.[14]
3. *Gingiva.* Most gingival changes can be traced to the effects of infection or to anatomic factors. For example, gingival recession is com-

mon in older individuals. Predisposing factors may be a lack of sufficient attached gingiva or malposition of the teeth.

PERSONAL FACTORS

The following list should not be considered typical of all elderly patients, because many are well adjusted. These characteristics are suggested to help the dental team members understand an older person's attitudes and actions.

I. INSECURITY

    A. Related to reduction in economic status, self-respect, and feeling of being needed.
    B. Inability to work.
    C. Reduced activity:
       1. Physical limitations.
       2. Overprotection by family.
    D. Rejection by family.
    E. Anxiety over health.

II. DEPRESSION

    A. Limited physical power; sensitivity about shortcomings of impaired vision, hearing, and lack of motor control.
    B. Changes in physical appearance.
    C. Loneliness:
       1. Loss of spouse and friends.
       2. Need for attention and concern from others; companionship.

III. INABILITY TO ADJUST TO CHANGES IN MODE OF LIFE

Tendency to develop fixed habits and ideas.

IV. SLOWING OF VOLUNTARY RESPONSES

Voluntary responses, association of thoughts, and speed of vocalization may all be slowed.

V. TENDENCY TO RETROSPECTION

Narrowing of interests; living in the past.

DENTAL HYGIENE CARE

When planning and conducting appointments for an older patient, many of the procedures included in Chapter 50 can be applied. Certain aging patients have physical and sensory limitations, and for those persons, adaptations are needed. It should be appreciated, however, that many members of the elderly population are independent, agile, and healthy people without systemic disease and who are not dependent on medications.

Care for the older patient should be planned in terms of comprehensive, not palliative, treatment.

Long-term maintenance for the prevention of oral disease must be the basic objective.

Many elderly people do not seek dental and dental hygiene care except when an emergency arises. A primary reason for the limited attention to professional care may be a lack of perceived need. Other reasons relate to physical and mental disabilities, chronic disease, and physical barriers such as transportation or accessibility of the dental office. Financial resources may be a reason for some people.

I. OFFICE OR CLINIC FACILITIES

Attention to dental office arrangement that eliminates physical barriers is important. An aged person's impaired vision, feebleness, or lack of motor control must be considered.

Hazards, such as small rugs, which can slide on polished floors; loose corners of rugs, which can be tripped over; and irregularities in floor levels, can be eliminated. Other considerations related to architectural barriers and how to assist an elderly person who may be disabled are described on pages 740 to 746.

II. ASSESSMENT

A. Patient History

Preparation of a careful and detailed medical and dental history takes on particular significance. Basic procedures for preparation of the history are described in Chapter 6.

Suggestions for good communication include the following:

1. Eliminate distracting background music or sounds.
2. Sit facing the patient, because hearing may be a problem. Other suggestions for the hearing-impaired patient are described on pages 794 to 800.
3. Do not shout; just increase volume and speak slowly and clearly.
4. Be courteous at all times; show respect for age. Do not call the patient by his/her first name unless the patient suggests doing so.
5. Present one idea at a time; be a good listener; older people do not like to be hurried.
6. Develop trust; reduce anxiety.

B. Medications

Older patients use more drugs and have more prescriptions, as well as more over-the-counter drugs, than does any other age group. Many have more than one chronic disease or disability requiring medication.

1. *Obtain the Correct List.* Ask the patient to bring in either the bottles that contain the various medications (over-the-counter as well as prescription items) or a written copy of the labels so that a list may be kept in the patient's record. The patient's physician may be the best source for an accurate list.

    The list of medications must be checked at

each maintenance appointment. Changes in health status can mean changes in prescriptions.

2. *References for Checking Drugs.* Each practice center or clinic needs current references, such as the *Physician's Desk Reference (PDR), Merck Manual,* and pharmacology textbooks.

3. Review patient's medication to determine:
   a. Potential adverse side effects.
   b. Possible drug interactions with products recommended or used during the appointment.
   c. A clear understanding of the patient's state of health to assure the clinician that the recommended procedure is right for the patient.

4. *Effects on Appointment.* Table 46-2 provides a partial list of effects of medications and the general classes of drugs that can produce each effect. Although the drug effects apply to all age groups, the elderly patient not only has more chronic disease and more prescriptions, but also can be more sensitive. Consultation with the patient's physician carries particular significance.

C. Need for Antibiotic Premedication
Many conditions that require prophylactic coverage are found fairly frequently in the elderly person.[15] Those with uncontrolled diabetes or those who receive chemotherapeutic or steroid treatments may have an increased susceptibility to infection. When the patient has a prosthetic joint replacement, pacemaker, or a history of other conditions listed on pages 101 to 104, consultation with the patient's physician is indicated.

D. Vital Signs
Blood pressure determination is recommended for each visit (pages 113 to 114).

E. Intra-Oral and Extra-Oral Examination
The need for careful, periodic examination of the oral mucosa from lips to throat cannot be overstressed at any age, but it is especially crucial for the elderly patient because oral cancer occurs with increasing frequency with advancing years. Many, in fact most, oral lesions exist without the patient being aware of them.

For some early surface lesions, biopsy is definitely indicated. For others, a cytologic smear can be prepared as directed by the dentist (pages 126 to 127).

III. PREVENTIVE CARE PLAN
Older patients need to have frequent appointments to maintain their oral health at a high level through supervision on a regular basis. The content of a care plan resembles that for other age groups, and emphasis on bacterial plaque control dominates. Appointment suggestions are summarized in Table 46-3.

TABLE 46-2 Effects of Medications

Effect of Medication Adjust Procedure	Drug Classes Involved
Abnormal hemostasis	Aspirin Warfarin (Coumadin) Dipyridamole
Need to minimize vaso-constrictor use	Antiarrhythmics Cardiac glycosides Sublingual and systemic nitrates Tricyclic antidepressants
Decreased tolerance for stress	Beta-blockers Calcium-channel blockers Cardiac glycosides Sublingual and systemic nitrates
Altered host resistance	Long-term antibiotics Insulin Oral hypoglycemics Systemic corticosteroids
Xerostomia	Antianxiety agents Anticholinergics Antidepressants Antihistamines/decongestants Antihypertensives Antiparkinsonism Antipsychotics Chemotherapy agents Diuretics
Movement disorders	Antipsychotics Levodopa Lithium
Gingival overgrowth	Phenytoin Nifedipine Cyclosporine

(Adapted from Levy, S.M., Baker, K.A., Semla, T.P., and Kohout, F.J.: Use of Medications with Dental Significance by a Noninstitutionalized Elderly Population, *Gerodontics, 4,* 119, June, 1988.)

A. Bacterial Plaque Control
Plaque control is described in detail in a subsequent section. Self-care provides the foundation for all preventive measures.

B. Periodontal Care
Treatment includes complete scaling, root planing, and follow-up to assess need for additional therapy.

C. Dental Caries Control
1. Diet record covering several days (pages 444 to 449).
2. Diet adjustment to eliminate cariogenic foods and make appropriate substitutions.

TABLE 46-3 Adaptations in Treatment Procedures for the Gerodontic Patient

Appointment Factors	Characteristic of the Gerodontic Patient	Dental Hygiene Implication
Medical history review	Many forms of chronic diseases Variety of medications used	Poor medical prognosis may limit extent of total treatment Need for antibiotic premedication for decreased immune response
Appointment planning	Low stress tolerance Tires more easily than does a younger patient	Morning appointments Shorter appointments Need for frequent maintenance appointments to provide high-level preventive care Appreciation of the real effort patient has made to get there
	Slower voluntary responses Sensitivity about shortcomings or lack of motor control	Do not rush Do not make the patient feel old by obvious physical assistance
	Lowered tolerance to extremes of heat and cold; less body cooling through perspiration	Adjust room temperature
	Impaired hearing; difficulty in hearing when there are distractions	Speak clearly and slowly; provide written memorandum of date and time of each appointment Eliminate background noises and music
Instrumentation	Loss of elasticity of lips and oral mucosa	Difficulty in retraction may provide patient discomfort
	Slowing of voluntary responses Cannot adjust to sudden muscular demands	Do not demand quick response to request for change of position of head, rinsing
	Pulp recession: variable pain threshold	Ask patient before administering anesthesia; the patient may not need
	Reduction in growth and repair processes Decreased resistance to infection Healing slowed	Provide as little trauma to gingiva as possible during instrumentation Suggest posttreatment care procedures to promote healing
	Inability to recover readily from stresses and strains Unsteadiness; tendency to postural hypotension	At completion of appointment, straighten chair back slowly and let patient sit up for short time before dismissing; assist out of chair

3. Emphasis on prevention of rampant root caries.
4. Fluoride therapy by use of daily self-applied preparations of dentifrice, rinse, or brush-on gel as needed (pages 469 to 472).

BACTERIAL PLAQUE CONTROL

I. OBJECTIVES

Basic objectives do not differ from those for younger people: infection must be eliminated and controlled.

Older individuals need to be as interested in their health and appearance as do people of any age. Esthetic deterioration may create emotional unhappiness, and when aging persons feel insecure or unwanted, they may lose their interest in personal oral care and diet.

Motivation through expression of sincere interest on the part of dental personnel can be an influencing factor in helping the patient to better health.

Certain people fear dentures because they associate them with "old" people. Patients with partial dentures may already have been impressed with the need for preserving the remaining teeth. Here, in the desire to save the teeth, lies the appeal for preventive measures for both the teeth and their supporting structures, and good use should be made of this very real motivating force.

II. APPROACH TO INSTRUCTION

A. New Habits With Old

In patient instruction, do not try to change all lifelong habits because doing so may create frustration and unhappiness.

B. Build Self-Confidence

Self-confidence, which has diminished because of lowering of physical capabilities and emotional satisfaction, must be built up. Major changes required because previous habits were detrimental must be brought about gradually if cooperation is to be expected. A more optimistic attitude is needed about the degree of oral health the elderly patient can be expected to achieve.

III. DENTAL PLAQUE FORMATION

The incidence and severity of periodontal diseases increase with age as an effect of disease accumulation. The extent of periodontal destruction reflects the length of time the tissues have been exposed to disease-producing factors, primarily plaque microorganisms.

A. Factors Contributing to Accumulation of Plaque

1. Gingival recession with wide embrasures that result from periodontal destruction provides a larger surface area for plaque retention.
2. Exposed cementum with areas of abrasion or dental caries at the neck of a tooth can create undercut areas where special adaptation of plaque removal devices is needed.

B. Plaque Retention and Removal

1. Exposed untreated cementum may hold plaque more readily than does enamel. A smooth root surface is less likely to hold plaque, and plaque removal efforts are more successful.
2. Decreased saliva production reduces or eliminates the cleansing and lubricating effects of saliva.
3. Restorations and prostheses provide a more complex dentition for personal care. Plaque removal requires more time, patience, and motivation.
4. Deficient restorations may have overhanging margins that provide areas of plaque retention.
5. Lack of dexterity related to disabling conditions resulting from chronic diseases, such as arthritis and parkinsonism, makes plaque removal more difficult.

IV. SPECIFIC RECOMMENDATIONS

A. Selection of Bacterial Plaque Removal Devices

1. Use of a power-assisted brush may help certain patients with impaired motor function.
2. Adaptations to alter the handle of a manual brush are described on pages 749 to 752.
3. Methods for the care of fixed and removable prostheses are described on pages 399 to 408.

B. Dentifrice Selection

1. Fluoride ingredient mandatory for root caries prevention.
2. Mild abrasive agent to prevent abrasion of root surfaces.
3. Desensitizing ingredient for exposed dentinal tubules.

C. Relief for Xerostomia

1. Recommendations are described on pages 345 to 346.
2. Provide specific instructions for use of a saliva substitute or other product.

D. Motivation and Instruction

Instruction and motivation techniques are applied gradually and regularly at frequent intervals for best results. Suggestions for adaptations of instruction to the physical and personal characteristics of the patient are listed in Table 46-4.

DIET AND NUTRITION

I. DIETARY HABITS

A. Nutritional Deficiencies

Dietary and resulting nutritional deficiencies are common in older people. For example, characteristic changes, such as burning tongue, angular cheilitis, and atrophic glossitis, may be related to vitamin B deficiencies. Unfortunately, many people believe that a diet rich in nutritive elements is important only for children.

B. Factors Contributing to Dietary and Nutritional Deficiencies

1. Limited budget.
2. Living alone or eating alone.
3. Not eating regular meals; frequently using nonnutritious snacks and foods for entertaining.
4. Alcoholism.
5. Lacking interest in shopping for or preparing food.
6. Acuteness of senses (taste, smell) lowered; may seek highly seasoned or sweetened foods.
7. Childish likes and dislikes; unusual cravings.
8. Tendency to follow food habits of lifetime; ignores newer knowledge of food preparation methods and dietary needs.
9. Inadequate masticatory efficiency because of tooth loss or dentures that no longer fit properly.
10. Adverse food selection may result from social embarrassment over inability to chew.
11. Adaptations in eating habits, made to compensate for deficiency, may interfere with adequate digestion and absorption of nutrients.

TABLE 46-4 Characteristics Affecting Instruction for the Gerodontic Patient

Characteristic of the Gerodontic Patient	Suggested Relation to Patient Instruction
Tendency for introspection; desire for attention	Patience needed in taking time to listen to complaints and accounts of past experiences
Feelings of insecurity Deprivation of physical capabilities Touchy sensitiveness, exaggerated imaginary or real pains, or attitudes of suspicion	Sympathetic understanding needed Build up self-confidence
Resistance to change; tendency to maintain fixed habits	Should not attempt to change all lifelong habits, only detrimental habits
Vision impaired	For the patient who wears prescription eyeglasses, make sure the glasses are worn while instruction is being given Recommend that eyeglasses be worn at home while performing plaque control procedures
Hearing impaired; loss of sensitivity to higher tones	Speak distinctly in normal voice Look directly at patient while speaking; many are lip readers
Slowing of voluntary responses Slowing of speed of thought associations Difficulty in timing sequential events; skills become separate movements, as by a child Least comfortable when must respond quickly to demanding sequential stimuli Rate of learning changed, ability to learn not changed Changes in speed of vocalization	Make suggestions gradually, over a series of appointments Do not demand learning a completely new procedure; adapt procedure already used Guide patient's demonstration of toothbrushing to prevent embarassment Do not expect perfection; go slowly, anticipate difficulties, give cues and clues Distinguish between slowness of learning and inability to learn
Memory shortened, mainly the result of lack of attention, lack of interest, or more selection of what patient wants to remember	Use motivating factors carefully. Provide written instructions; spoken instructions may be forgotten or misunderstood
Need for personal achievement	Help patient gain sense of accomplishment; commend for any success however minor Never compare the patient's condition with that of other patients

12. Following dietary fads that provide only a limited and unbalanced diet.
13. Loss of appetite, which may have physiologic, social, or economic causes.
14. Difficulty in swallowing.
15. Lack of self-discipline; feeling that aging brings privilege to eat only preferred foods.

II. DIETARY NEEDS OF THE AGED

The nutritional needs of older persons are not different from those of younger persons, except in quantity. Caloric intake must be decreased to control weight. Protein, vitamins, minerals, and water are particularly important for body function, repair, and resistance to disease.

A necessary objective in geriatric nutrition is to retard the progression of diet-induced chronic diseases. Examples of these are atherosclerosis related to high dietary cholesterol, anemias related to iron and folic acid deficiencies, and osteoporosis resulting from calcium and fluoride deficiency.

In addition to a better intake of calcium in the diet, fluoride intake over the years is beneficial in the prevention of osteoporosis and fractures of the bones. The relationship between fluoride in the drinking water and the decreased prevalence of root caries was described on page 461.

III. INSTRUCTION IN DIET AND ORAL HEALTH

A. Dietary Analysis

A 4- or 5-day record of the patient's diet can provide information to guide recommendations to be made. Difficulties in showing the procedure to the patient and obtaining accurate results may seem insurmountable. Inaccuracy of recent memory is a problem with some elderly people, so that even the 24-hour dietary record prepared during the appointment may not be complete.

The first consideration in making recommendations for aging patients is that a well-balanced diet be used with limited amounts of cariogenic foods for dental caries prevention. Food for an adequate diet is shown in Figure 28-2 on page 445.

B. Motivation

Appeal to the patient is made through personal

concerns for the relationships of dietary deficiencies to appearance, lowered resistance to disease, and premature aging, which may inspire the patient to improve daily habits. Educational materials are available to study with, and to give to, the patient.

TECHNICAL HINTS

Source of materials:

American Dental Association
Department of Salable Materials
211 E. Chicago Avenue
Chicago, IL 60611

REFERENCES

1. **World Health Organization:** *Planning and Organization of Geriatric Services.* Geneva, World Health Organization, Technical Report Series, Number 548, 1974, p. 11.
2. **Roddy,** J.A.: Dental Needs: The Well Elderly, *DentalHygienistNews, 3,* 13, Fall, 1990.
3. **Terpenning,** M.S. and Bradley, S.F.: Why Aging Leads to Increased Susceptibility to Infection, *Geriatrics, 46,* 77, February, 1991.
4. **Woolery,** W.A.: Occult HIV Infection: Diagnosis and Treatment of Older Patients, *Geriatrics, 52,* 51, November, 1997.
5. **Wartenberg,** A.A. and Nirenberg, T.D.: Alcohol and Other Drug Abuse in Older Patients, in Reichel, W., ed.: *Care of the Elderly. Clinical Aspects of Aging,* 4th ed. Baltimore, Williams & Wilkins, 1995, pp. 133–141.
6. **Gambert,** S.R.: Alcohol Abuse: Medical Effects of Heavy Drinking in Late Life, *Geriatrics, 52,* 30, June, 1997.
7. **von Wowern,** N., Klausen, B., and Kollerup, G.: Osteoporosis: A Risk Factor in Periodontal Disease, *J. Periodontol., 65,* 1134, December, 1994.
8. **Wactawski-Wende,** J., Grossi, S.G., Trevisan, M., Genco, R.J., Tezal, M., Dunford, R.G., Ho, A.W., Hausmann, E., and Hreshchyshyn, M.M.: The Role of Osteopenia in Oral Bone Loss and Periodontal Disease, *J. Periodontol., 67,* 1076, Supplement, October, 1996.
9. **Riggs,** B.L. and Melton, L.J.: The Prevention and Treatment of Osteoporosis, *N. Engl. J. Med., 327,* 620, August 27, 1992.
10. **Robinson,** H.B.G. and Miller, A.S.: *Colby, Kerr, and Robinson's Color Atlas of Oral Pathology,* 5th ed. Philadelphia, J.B. Lippincott Co., 1990, p. 141.
11. **Baum,** B.J.: Salivary Gland Fluid Secretion During Aging, *J. Am. Geriatr. Soc., 37,* 453, May, 1989.
12. **Stamm,** J.W., Banting, D.W., and Imrey, P.B.: Adult Root Caries Survey of Two Similar Communities With Contrasting Natural Water Fluoride Levels, *J. Am. Dent. Assoc., 120,* 143, February, 1990.
13. **Seltzer,** S. and Bender, I.B.: *The Dental Pulp. Biologic Considerations in Dental Procedures,* 3rd ed. St. Louis, Ishiyaku EuroAmerica, 1990, pp. 324–348.
14. **Zander,** H.A. and Hurzeler, B.: Continuous Cementum Apposition, *J. Dent. Res., 37,* 1035, November–December, 1958.
15. **Felder,** R.S., Nardone, D., and Palac, R.: Prevalence of Predisposing Factors for Endocarditis Among an Elderly Institutionalized Population, *Oral Surg. Oral Med. Oral Pathol., 73,* 30, January, 1992.

SUGGESTED READINGS

Berkey, D.B., Berg, R.G., Ettinger, R.L., and Mersel, A.: The Old-old Dental Patient. The Challenge of Clinical Decision-making, *J. Am. Dent. Assoc., 127,* 321, March, 1996.

Bryant, S.R., MacEntee, M.I., and Browne, A.: Ethical Issues Encountered by Dentists in the Care of Institutionalized Elders, *Spec. Care Dent., 15,* 79, March/April, 1995.

Friedlander, A.H. and Yoshikawa, T.T.: Pathogenesis, Management, and Prevention of Infective Endocarditis in the Elderly Dental Patient, *Oral Surg. Oral Med. Oral Pathol., 69,* 177, February, 1990.

Garcia, R.I.: Geriatric Dentistry, in Reichel, W., ed.: *Care of the Elderly. Clinical Aspects of Aging,* 4th ed. Baltimore, Williams & Wilkins, 1995, pp. 451–459.

Hoad-Reddick, G.: Organization, Appointment Planning, and Surgery Design in the Treatment of the Older Patient, *J. Prosthet. Dent., 74,* 364, October, 1995.

Kilmartin, C.M.: Managing the Medically Compromised Geriatric Patient, *J. Prosthet. Dent., 72,* 492, November, 1994.

Maddox, M.K. and Burns, T.: Positive Approaches to Dementia Care in the Home, *Geriatrics, 52,* S54, Supplement 2, September, 1997.

Reichel, W. and Rabins, P.V.: Evaluation and Management of the Confused, Disoriented, or Demented Elderly Patient, in Reichel, W., ed.: *Care of the Elderly. Clinical Aspects of Aging,* 4th ed. Baltimore, Williams & Wilkins, 1995, pp. 142–154.

van der Bijl, P.: Therapeutic Considerations in the Gerodontic Patient, *Compend. Cont. Educ. Dent., 15,* 478, April, 1994.

Yellowitz, J.A.: Alzheimer's Disease. An Oral Health Care Provider's Perspective, *DentalHygienistNews, 7,* 10, Fall, 1994.

Oral Health Problems

Loesche, W.J., Bretz, W.A., Grossman, N.S., and Lopatin, D.E.: Dental Findings in Geriatric Populations With Diverse Medical Backgrounds, *Oral Surg. Oral Med. Oral Pathol. Oral Radiol. Endod., 80,* 43, July, 1995.

MacEntee, M.I.: How Severe is the Threat of Caries to Old Teeth? *J. Prosthet. Dent., 71,* 473, May, 1991.

Niessen, L.C. and Gibson, G.: Aging and Oral Health: Implications for Women, *Compend. Cont. Educ. Dent., 14,* 1542, December, 1993.

Shay, K.: Identifying the Needs of the Elderly Dental Patient. The Geriatric Dental Assessment, *Dent. Clin. North Am., 38,* 499, July, 1994.

Soon, J.A.: Effects of Drug Therapy on Oral Health of Older Adults, *Can. Dent. Hyg. J. (Probe), 26,* 118, Autumn, 1992.

Vissink, A., Spijkervet, F.K.L., and Amerongen, A.V.N.: Aging and Saliva: A Review of the Literature, *Spec. Care Dent., 16,* 95, May/June, 1996.

Youngs, G.: Risk Factors for and the Prevention of Root Caries in Older Adults, *Spec. Care Dent., 14,* 68, March/April, 1994.

Periodontal Disease

Baelum, V., Luan, W.-M., Chen, X., and Fejerskov, O.: A 10-year Study of the Progression of Destructive Periodontal Disease in Adult and Elderly Chinese, *J. Periodontol., 68,* 1033, November, 1997.

Burt, B.A.: Periodontitis and Aging: Reviewing Recent Evidence, *J. Am. Dent. Assoc., 125,* 273, March, 1994.

Carranza, F.A. and Newman, M.G.: *Clinical Periodontology,* 8th ed. Philadelphia, W.B. Saunders Co., 1996, pp. 51–55, 423–426.

Fransson, C., Berglundh, T., and Lindhe, J.: The Effect of Age on the Development of Gingivitis. Clinical, Microbiological, and Histological Findings, *J. Clin. Periodontol., 23,* 379, April, 1996.

Klemetti, E., Collin, H.-L., Forss, H., Markkanen, H., and Lassita, V.: Mineral Status of Skeleton and Advanced Periodontal Disease, *J. Clin. Periodontol., 21,* 184, March, 1994.

McArthur, W.P., Bloom, C., Taylor, M., Smith, J., Wheeler, T., and Magnusson, N.I.: Antibody Responses to Suspected Periodontal Pathogens in Elderly Subjects With Periodontal Disease, *J. Clin. Periodontol., 22,* 842, November, 1995.

Persson, R.E., Persson, G.R., and Robinovitch, M.: Periodontal Conditions in Medically Compromised Elderly Subjects: Assessments of Treatment Needs, *Spec. Care Dent., 14,* 9, January/February, 1994.

Wheeler, T.T., McArthur, W.P., Magnusson, I., Marks, R.G., Smith, J., Sarrett, D.C., Bender, B.S., and Clark, W.B.: Modeling the Relationship Between Clinical, Microbiologic, and Immunologic Parameters and Alveolar Bone Levels in an Elderly Population, *J. Periodontol., 65,* 68, January, 1994.

Patient Instruction

Doherty, S.A., Ross, A., and Bennett, C.R.: The Oral Hygiene Performance Test: Development and Validation of Dental Dexterity Scale for the Elderly, *Spec. Care Dentist., 14,* 144, July/August, 1994.

Felder, R., James, K., Brown, C., Lemon, S., and Reveal, M.: Dexterity Testing as a Predictor of Oral Care Ability, *J. Am. Geriatr. Soc., 42,* 1081, October, 1994.

Felder, R., Reveal, M., Lemon, S., and Brown, C.,: Testing Toothbrushing Ability of Elderly Patients, *Spec. Care Dentist., 14,* 153, July/August, 1994.

Garry, P.J. and Vellas, B.J.: Aging and Nutrition, in Ziegler, E.E. and Filer, L.J., eds.: *Present Knowledge in Nutrition,* 7th ed. Washington, D.C., ILSI Press, 1996, pp. 414–419.

Ostuni, E. and Mohl, G.: Communicating More Effectively With the Confused or Demented Patient, *Gen. Dent., 43,* 264, May–June, 1995.

Shay, K. and Ship, J.A.: The Importance of Oral Health in the Older Patient, *J. Am. Geriatr. Soc., 43,* 1414, December, 1995.

Spencer, P.: The Dental Hygienist and the Senior Client, *Can. Dent. Hyg. J. (Probe), 31,* 89, May/June, 1997.

Osteoporosis

Dawson-Hughes, B., Harris, S.S., Krall, E.A., and Dallal, G.E.: Effect of Calcium and Vitamin D Supplementation on Bone Density in Men and Women 65 Years of Age or Older, *N. Eng. J. Med., 337,* 670, September 4, 1997.

Hillier, S., Inskip, H., Coggon, D., and Cooper, C.: Water Fluoridation and Osteoporotic Fracture, *Community Dent. Health, 13,* 63, September, 1996.

Jeffcoat, M.K. and Chesnut, C.H.: Systemic Osteoporosis and Oral Bone Loss: Evidence Shows Increased Risk Factors, *J. Am. Dent. Assoc., 124,* 49, November, 1993.

Kanis, J.A.: Treatment of Symptomatic Osteoporosis With Fluoride, *Am. J., Med., 95,* 53S, November 30, 1993.

Loza, J.C., Carpio, L.C., and Dziak, R.: Osteoporosis and Its Relationship to Oral Bone Loss, *Current Opinion in Periodontology, 3,* 27, 1996.

Pak, C.Y.C., Sakhaee, K., Rubin, C.D., and Zerwekh, J.E.: Sustained-release Sodium Fluoride in the Management of Established Postmenopausal Osteoporosis, *Am. J. Med. Sci., 313,* 23, January, 1997.

Talbot, L. and Craig, B.J.: Osteoporosis and Alveolar Bone Loss, *Canad. Dent. Hyg. Assoc. (Probe), 32,* 11, January–February, 1998.

Watson, E.L., Katz, R.V., Adelezzi, R., Gift, H.C., and Dunn, S.M.: The Measurement of Mandibular Cortical Bone Height in Osteoporotic vs. Non-osteoporotic Postmenopausal Women, *Spec. Care Dentist., 15,* 124, May/June, 1995.

47

The Edentulous Patient

The completely edentulous patient who wears a removable denture needs an appointment at least annually for careful observation of the oral tissues, as well as for supervision of bacterial plaque control for the dentures. The edentulous patient with an implant-supported denture requires more frequent appointments. Since the implants are surrounded and supported by gingival tissue and osseointegrated bone, professional care and supervision is more like that required by natural teeth.

For either type of denture, instruction for the patient who receives new dentures is a special concern. The patient must learn new personal oral health care and apply new bacterial plaque control measures to the new prosthesis. Information and procedures relating to implants and implant dentures are provided on pages 417 to 422. The present chapter will be concerned primarily with the traditional type of removable denture. Terminology related to dentures and the edentulous patient is defined in Box 47-1.

Various combinations are found among denture wearers. A patient may have a single complete denture and natural teeth in the opposing dental arch. There may be a complete denture for one arch and natural teeth and a partial fixed or removable denture in the other arch.

Of the completely edentulous population, particularly in the older age groups, some individuals have dentures they do not wear, others have full dentures but wear only one of them, and still others have no dentures. When there is a single denture, more frequently the maxillary denture is worn. It is not unusual to find that the same dentures have been worn for many years without having the dentures or the supporting oral tissues examined.

Dentures occasionally must be constructed to replace primary teeth. The teeth may be congenitally missing (anodontia) or may have required extraction because of rampant caries or trauma. Baby bottle tooth decay, which can result in severe breakdown

BOX 47-1 KEY WORDS: Edentulous Patient*

Anodontia (an'o-don"she-ah): congenital absence of all teeth, primary and permanent.

Complete denture prosthodontics: that body of knowledge and skills pertaining to the restoration of the edentulous arch with a removable prosthesis.

Denture: an artificial substitute for missing natural teeth and adjacent tissues.

> **Complete denture:** a removable dental prosthesis that replaces the entire dentition and associated structures of the maxilla or mandible.

Denture adhesive: a material used to adhere a denture to the oral mucosa; over-the-counter product that can be misused without professional instruction.

Denture characterization: modification of the form and color of the denture base and teeth to produce a more lifelike appearance.

Denture placement: the process of directing a prosthesis to a desired oral location; introduction of a prosthesis into a patient's mouth; other terms used are denture **delivery** or denture **insertion**.

Immediate denture: a complete denture fabricated for placement immediately following the removal of the natural teeth and/or other surgical preparation of the dental arches.

Implant prosthesis: any prosthesis that utilizes dental implants in part or whole for retention, support, and stability; the prosthesis may be a complete denture.

Overdenture: a removable denture that covers and is partially supported by one or more remaining natural teeth, roots, and/or dental implants and the soft tissue of the residual alveolar ridge; also called overlay denture.

Prosthesis (pros-thē'sĭs): an artificial replacement of an absent part of the human body.

> **Dental prosthesis:** artificial replacement of one or more teeth and/or associated structures.

Resection (rē-sĕk'shun): excision of a segment of any part; removal of articular ends of one or both bones forming a joint.

---

*Definitions are taken from or adapted from and in harmony with the *Glossary of Prosthodontic Terms*, 6th ed., 1993, from the Academy of Prosthodontics Foundation.

of the teeth soon after eruption, is described on page 240.

To provide esthetics and function, dentures can be constructed for the accepting child who is able to cooperate. As the permanent teeth begin to erupt, parts of the denture are cut away (Figure 47-1). A supervised caries prevention program is initiated for protection of the permanent dentition.

TYPES OF REMOVABLE COMPLETE DENTURES[1]

A. Tissue-Supported Complete Denture: a removable dental prosthesis that replaces the entire dentition and associated structures of the maxillae or the mandible and rests on the mucosal covered alveolar ridge.

B. Implant-Supported Complete Denture: a dental prosthesis supported by one or more dental implants.

C. Overdenture: a prosthesis that covers and is partially supported by remaining natural teeth, tooth roots, and/or dental implants (page 408 and Figure 25-15).

D. Provisional or Interim Prosthesis: a transitional prosthesis that provides protection, stabilization, and function prior to the fabrication of the definitive prosthesis. It may also

be used as a diagnostic device, for function during a healing process, or as a training prosthesis for an apprehensive patient. Originally serving as a transitional partial denture, artificial teeth may be added as natural teeth are removed. The definitive denture can be completed after postextraction tissue changes have occurred.

E. Immediate Denture: a denture fabricated

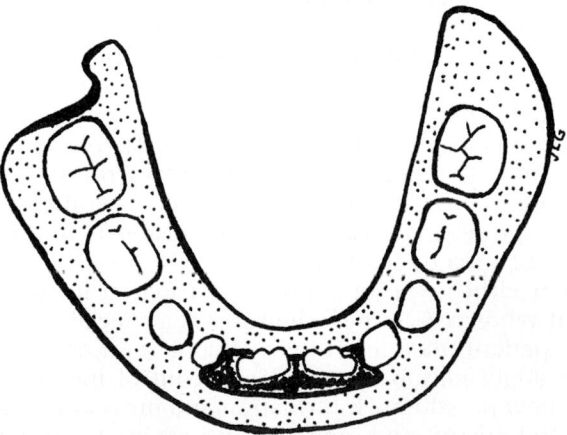

FIGURE 47-1 Denture for a Young Child. As permanent teeth erupt, parts of the denture are cut away. Shown are denture alterations for the mandibular right first permanent molar and the mandibular incisors.

for placement immediately following the removal of the natural teeth.

THE EDENTULOUS MOUTH

I. BONE

A. Residual Ridges

After the teeth are removed, the residual ridges enter into a continuing process of remodeling. The alveolar bone, which had supported the teeth, undergoes resorption. The rate and amount of bony resorption vary with each individual. The major bony changes occur during the first year after the teeth are removed, but changes continue throughout life. Mandibular bone loss is generally as much as four times greater than maxillary bone loss.[2] Because of the oral changes, it is usually necessary to have dentures rebased or remade at intervals.

B. Tori

The tori that interfere with dentures are benign bony outgrowths. Because of the size, shape, or location, a torus often must be removed surgically before a denture can be constructed.
1. *Torus Palatinus.* Bony enlargement located over the midline of the palate.
2. *Torus Mandibularis.* Bony mass(es) generally located on the lingual side of the mandibular arch in the premolar area; in a radiograph, a torus will appear as a radiopaque area in the region of the premolars.

II. MUCOUS MEMBRANE

As described on page 188, the oral mucosa is composed of masticatory, lining, and specialized mucosa. The edentulous ridges and the hard palate are covered with masticatory mucosa, which is continuous with the lining mucosa that covers the floor of the mouth, vestibules, and cheeks.

The mucous membrane covering the bony ridges is made up of two layers, the lamina propria and the surface stratified squamous epithelium which is keratinized in the healthy mouth. Underneath the mucous membrane is the submucosa, which is attached to the underlying bone.

The submucosa is composed of connective tissue with vessels, nerves, adipose tissue, and glands. The support or cushioning effect for the denture depends on the makeup of the submucosa, which varies in different parts of the mouth.

When an edentulous mouth is examined clinically and the lips and cheeks are retracted using a tension test technique (page 211), a line of demarcation similar to the mucogingival junction is apparent, separating the attached tissue over the bony ridge and the loose lining mucosa of the vestibule. Frenal attachments can be observed readily.

THE PATIENT WITH NEW DENTURES

I. PATIENT COUNSELING

The preparation for denture insertion has to begin well in advance of the day the dentures are delivered. Anticipatory guidance will help the patient gain a clear idea of what to expect and what procedures will be followed. Successful after-care and denture satisfaction depend to a large extent on conditioning the patient to the adjustments to be made and to the period of practice and learning with the new dentures that can be expected.

Many dental teams prepare their own printed educational materials, whereas others use those available from outside sources.

The preliminary counseling is followed through the initial postinsertion appointments, particularly to teach denture hygiene and to arrange for continuing maintenance appointments during the following years.

II. POSTINSERTION CARE

A. Immediate Denture

The patient receiving an immediate denture is instructed to leave the denture in place for 24 to 48 hours to aid in the control of bleeding and swelling. When the patient returns and the denture is removed, the mouth is rinsed and appropriate instructions are given. After initial healing, the denture care and other instructions are similar to those presented in Table 47-1.

B. New Dentures Over Healed Ridges
1. *Appointments.* Following insertion, adjustment appointments are scheduled routinely because adjustments can be expected. The first appointment is made within 48 hours of the time of insertion, and additional appointments are made in accord with individual needs.
2. *Instructions.*[3] Too many instructions given on the day of insertion may only confuse the patient. Basic denture care and other procedures of immediate concern can be reviewed. Slow repetition over several periods helps the patient to develop adequate denture management and hygiene habits.

   Basic information for the new denture wearer is provided in Table 47-1. Denture cleaning methods are described with other plaque control procedures for the care of dental prostheses on pages 403 to 408.

DENTURE-RELATED ORAL CHANGES

The condition of the mucous membranes, salivary glands, and alveolar bone is influenced by dietary and nutritional deficiencies, age, and various chronic dis-

TABLE 47-1 Patient Instruction for Complete Dentures

Item	Factors To Teach
Food selection	Use foods from the Food Guide Pyramid (page 445) Check each day's diet to fulfill needs for a balanced diet Older patients: use foods to prevent diet-induced chronic diseases (page 694) New denture wearer: Avoid foods that need incising Avoid raw vegetables, fibrous meats, and sticky foods until experience has been gained Cut food into small pieces Practiced denture wearer: Select a variety of foods, but do not expect the same efficiency as with the natural teeth
Incision or biting	Use the canine and premolar area. Insert for biting at the angle of the mouth. Push back as the food is incised; do not pull or tear the food in a forward direction
Chewing	Take small portions Try to chew with some food on each side at the same time to stabilize the denture Be patient and practice
Salivary flow	Anticipate an increased flow of saliva when a new denture is worn
Speaking	Speak slowly and quietly Practice by reading aloud at home, preferably in front of a mirror Repeat and practice words that seem the most difficult
Sneezing, coughing, yawning	Anticipate loss of denture retention Cover mouth with hand and handkerchief
Denture hygiene	Thoroughly clean dentures twice each day Immerse dentures in chemical solution and brush for plaque removal. Rinse thoroughly Complete denture care is described on pages 403–407 Devices to aid a disabled person are shown on pages 749–751
Mucosa	Tissues need to rest each day. Preferable to leave the dentures out while sleeping Brush and massage the mucosa to clean away plaque and debris and stimulate circulation
Storage of dentures	After careful cleaning to remove all bacterial plaque, store the denture in water (or cleaning solution) in a covered container Place in a safe place inaccessible to children or house pets Change water or cleaning solution daily and wash the container
Over-the-counter products	Never attempt to alter the denture for relief of discomfort Do not buy and use self-reline materials, adhesives, or other additives without consulting the dentist. They may be harmful to the dentures and/or the oral tissues Consult the dentist for advice about all denture problems
Maintenance	Understand the importance of the dentist's examination of the denture fit, occlusion, and wear, and the condition of the oral mucosa First year: expect reline, rebase, or remake of dentures because bone remodeling is greatest during the first year Subsequent appointment: an examination each year for most patients, provided the denture hygiene is ideal. Other patients in the cancer-susceptible category need an examination every 3 months

eases. Tissue alterations for an older patient are described on page 686. Some of the denture-related changes are listed here.

I. BONE CHANGES

A. Alveolar Ridge Remodeling
The continuing reduction in the size of the residual ridge may lead to loss of denture support, loss of facial height and lip support, increased prominence of the chin, possible temporomandibular joint manifestations, and occlusal disharmony.

B. Compensations by the Patient
1. Patients may adapt to the bone changes by making compensating adjustments in the way they wear and manage the dentures.

2. Other patients may resort to drugstore remedies, such as pads, adhesives, or self-reline
materials, which may be detrimental if used
improperly. Denture adhesives should never
be used to compensate for a poorly designed,
constructed, or ill-fitting denture.

C. Treatment by the Dentist

Dentures need relining, rebasing, or remaking
periodically.

II. ORAL MUCOSA

The tissue reaction under a denture varies considerably among individuals. Whereas one mouth may
have thinning of the mucosa, submucosa, and, particularly, the epithelium with an absence of keratinization, another may have normal keratinization or hy-
perkeratinization.

Factors that influence the mucosa include systemic
conditions that alter host response, aging, denture
and tissue hygiene, wearing the denture constantly,
xerostomia, and fit and occlusion of the denture itself.

III. EFFECT OF XEROSTOMIA

The causes of xerostomia are described on page 345.
Diminished salivary flow can influence denture retention and tissue lubrication, as well as reduce the resistance of the oral mucosa to trauma and infection.

A. Lubrication

The oral mucosa needs saliva for protection
against frictional irritation by the denture.

B. Retention

The film of saliva between the denture and the
mucosa contributes to retention of the denture.

IV. SENSORY CHANGES

A. Tactile Sense

With the dentures in place, sensitivity may be
diminished to small objects in the mouth, such
as small bones or bits of nut shells.

B. Taste

Occasionally, patients indicate that, since they
have been wearing dentures, food has a different taste for them. Although the taste buds that
are located in the tongue papillae are not affected by the dentures, the taste buds of the
palate are covered by the maxillary denture and
therefore are ineffective for taste perception.
Denture hygiene must be meticulous to ensure
that the denture does not develop thick odorif-
erous plaque, which may alter food flavors.

DENTURE-INDUCED ORAL LESIONS

When the mouth is examined extraorally and intraorally, the dentures are removed and the mucosa is
carefully and thoroughly examined. The patient may
tell of an area that has been sensitive and thus help-
fully call attention to a specific visible lesion. On the
other hand, a patient may be unaware of chronic mucosal lesions, which are often asymptomatic. Because
tissue changes may be important indicators of serious
disease, such as oral cancer, the intraoral examination
must be conducted thoroughly with good illumination.

I. PRINCIPAL CAUSES OF LESIONS UNDER DENTURES

The factors that singly or in combination cause most
oral lesions under dentures are infection, trauma, ill-
fit of the dentures, inadequate oral hygiene, and
wearing the dentures all the time, without relief for
the tissues.

A. Ill-Fitting Dentures

Because tissue changes under dentures occur
gradually over a long period, the patient may
not be aware of developing disease. The patient
may not realize or may not have been informed
of the importance of having regular professional examinations of the dentures and the
oral mucosa.

B. Lack of Oral Hygiene

The dentures and the oral mucosa need daily
care. Neglected dentures can accumulate heavy
plaque and calculus that may irritate the mucosa and cause infection.

C. Continuous Wearing of Dentures

Dentures need to be removed for a part of
every 24 hours so that the mucosa can have a
rest from the pressure of the hard acrylic during
occlusion, bruxism, and clenching. The rest period also allows the tissue to recover in its natural environment, where the tongue and saliva
provide a cleansing effect.

II. INFLAMMATORY LESIONS

A. Localized Inflammation (Sore Spots)

1. *Appearance.* Isolated red inflamed area, sometimes ulcerated.
2. *Contributing Factors.* Trauma from an ill-fitting denture, rough spot on a denture surface, tongue bite.

B. Generalized Inflammation

1. *Other Names.* "Denture sore mouth," "denture stomatitis."
2. *Appearance.* Generalized redness over the tissues that support the denture. The patient
may have pain and a burning sensation. This
occurs more frequently in the maxilla.
3. *Contributing Factors*
The following may occur singly or in combination.
   a. Denture trauma from the fit, occlusion,
   or parafunctional habits.

b. Inadequate denture hygiene and care of the mucosa.

c. Chemotoxic effect from residual cleansing paste or solution not thoroughly rinsed from the denture.

d. Allergy to the denture base (rare).

e. Continuous denture wearing without relief for the tissues.

f. Patient self-treatment with over-the-counter products for relining.

g. Systemic influence on the tolerance of the tissues to trauma and lowered resistance to infection; for example, vitamin and other nutritional deficiencies and immunosuppressant therapy, such as chemotherapy.

h. *Candida albicans* infection.[4] *C. albicans* is a customary member of the oral flora of people with or without teeth. In denture stomatitis, or in recognizable candidiasis or moniliasis, the numbers of the yeast-like fungus increase. Conditions that promote *C. albicans* overgrowth are depression of defense mechanisms by immunosuppressants, radiation therapy, and prolonged antibiotic therapy.

III. ULCERATIVE LESIONS

Localized ulcer-shaped lesions usually are related to an overextended denture border. The ulcer may resemble a cancerous lesion and should be biopsied if it persists longer than expected of a healing traumatic ulcer.

IV. PAPILLARY HYPERPLASIA[5]

A. Appearance

Papillary hyperplasia is located on the palatal vault, rarely outside the confines of the bony ridges (Figure 47-2). The overall lesion appears as a group of closely arranged, pebble-shaped, red, edematous projections.

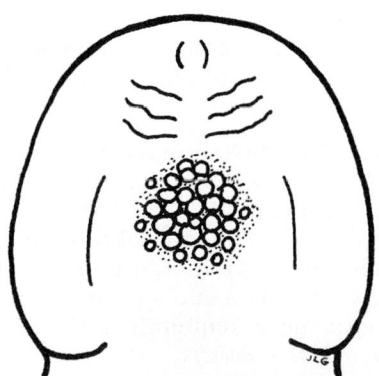

FIGURE 47-2 Papillary Hyperplasia. Outline of an edentulous palate shows the characteristic location of papillary hyperplasia within the bony ridges.

B. Contributing Factors

The cause is unknown but it is associated with poor denture hygiene, ill-fitting dentures, and possible *Candida albicans* infection.

V. DENTURE IRRITATION HYPERPLASIA[5] (EPULIS FISSURATUM)

Long-standing, chronic inflammatory tissue appears in single or multiple elongated folds related to the border of an ill-fitting denture.

VI. ANGULAR CHEILITIS[6]

A. Appearance

Angular cheilitis appears as fissuring at the angles of the mouth, with cracks, ulcerations, and erythema. Sometimes it is dry with a crust; other times, it is moist from saliva.

B. Contributing Factors

Angular cheilitis is usually initiated by lack of support of the commissure because of overclosure and by moistness from drooling. Secondarily, a riboflavin deficiency or an infection by *Candida albicans* or other organisms may be involved.

PREVENTION AND MAINTENANCE

I. DEVELOPMENT OF ATTITUDE AND UNDERSTANDING BY THE PATIENT

For continuing oral health and appropriate denture service, the patient needs to understand the following:

A. Purposes of regular maintenance appointments for finding early signs of disease, particularly chronic irritations and oral cancer.

B. Reasons why the dentist must supervise the function and fit of the dentures.

C. Damage that can result from wearing ill-fitting dentures for long periods of time (years) without tissue and denture examination.

D. Harmful effects to the oral tissue and damage to the dentures that can result from the unsupervised use of commercial products for denture retention or relief, or of home repair kits.

II. DAILY PREVENTIVE MEASURES

A. Denture Hygiene

Dentures must be cleaned after each meal. Details are explained on pages 403 to 408. Cleansing solutions must be changed daily.

B. Oral Mucosa

1. Brush to clean and massage.
2. Perform digital massage (page 407).

C. Rest for the Tissues

For most patients, having the dentures out while sleeping is the best procedure to provide rest for the oral tissues. When this is impossible, the patient should remove the denture for as long a daytime period as possible, such as while bathing. While the dentures are out of the mouth, they can be placed in a container with cleaning solution, and the mucosa can be cleaned and massaged.

D. Diet and Nutrition

The teaching of food selection cannot be overemphasized. For denture wearers, an emphasis on using foods from the basic food groups as shown in the pyramid (Figure 28-1, page 445) is necessary. Control of weight and avoidance of foods that are related to specific chronic conditions are important. A dietary analysis can provide a foundation for making specific recommendations.

The diet problems of the elderly patient have been described on pages 693 to 694. Factors that contribute to dietary deficiencies in patients of any age are magnified when dentures are ill-fitting and masticatory efficiency is decreased. The patient tends to overlook food value and to select foods that are within the limits of chewing ability or that can be swallowed without chewing.

E. Relief From Xerostomia

The use of a saliva substitute may be recommended (page 346).

F. Dental Caries Control for Overdenture Wearers

Meticulous denture hygiene and bacterial plaque control for the natural teeth are mandatory. Care of the overdenture is described on pages 408 to 409.

Sodium fluoride dentifrice is used while brushing the teeth. Daily fluoride application is made by placing gel drops inside the overdenture (page 409).

III. PROFESSIONAL SUPERVISION

A. Appointment Frequency

1. *First Year.* After the initial adjustments, the patient can expect the dentures to need reline, rebase, or remake in 6 months to 1 year.
2. *Subsequent Maintenance Period*
   a. For most patients, one appointment each year may be adequate.
   b. For patients who are careless with denture and tissue care, at least two appointments each year are recommended.
   c. For patients who are at high cancer risk because of age, tobacco use, and alcohol-drinking habits or have a previous history of cancer, examination three to four times per year should be scheduled.

B. Maintenance Appointment

Maintenance procedures as described on pages

644 to 645 are followed with necessary adaptations for the edentulous patient.

1. *Procedures*
   a. Review patient history; make necessary additions to the record.
   b. Determine blood pressure.
   c. Perform an extraoral and intraoral examination.
   d. Examine dentures for cleanliness and evidence of patient care.
      i. Ask patient to demonstrate the personal hygiene care procedures used routinely.
      ii. Supplement with additional demonstration and instruction when the care is less than adequate.
   e. Clean the dentures to remove calculus and stain. Procedures are described on pages 615 to 616.
2. *Procedures for the Dentist*
   a. Review the complete assessment.
   b. Examine the oral tissues and the fit and occlusion of the dentures.
   c. Treat as needed.
3. *Subsequent Appointment*
   Make necessary appointments for continuing current treatment or for maintenance.

DENTURE MARKING FOR IDENTIFICATION[7]

The need for denture marking is apparent in a variety of situations. A universal system for marking would be ideal. Marking is required by law in some countries and in most states of the United States. In forensic dentistry, or for identification of victims of war, such disasters as flood or fire, or transportation catastrophes, the dentition has been used increasingly as a means of identification.

Dentures provide a method for immediate identification. Prompt identification can be urgent when an individual is found unconscious from illness or injury or suffering from amnesia as a result of psychiatric or traumatic causes, as well as from senility.

The dentures of people in long-term residence or care facilities should be marked. Mislaid dentures can be returned and mix-ups by the direct care staff can be prevented. An important contribution to an oral health program is to introduce a plan for denture marking.

I. CRITERIA FOR AN ADEQUATE MARKING SYSTEM

Information on the denture must be specific so that rapid identification is possible.

A. Relative to the Denture

1. Must have no adverse effects on denture material.

2. Must not change the strength, surface texture, or fit of the denture.

3. Must be cosmetically acceptable; the label must be placed in an unobtrusive position.

B. Relative to the Procedure

1. Readily learned and simple to carry out.

2. Inexpensive.

3. Durable result. When the information is incorporated during denture processing, indefinite durability can be expected. A surface marker for a denture already in use should be able to withstand denture cleaning methods for a reasonable period of time.

C. Characteristics of the Material Used

1. *Fire and Humidity Resistant.* When the label is placed inside the posterior section of a denture, the surrounding tongue and maxillofacial parts offer protection except in the most severe conflagration.

2. *Radiopaque.* A metal marker can be of use as a means of identification by radiographic examination in the event the radiolucent acrylic denture is accidentally swallowed.

II. INCLUSION METHODS FOR MARKING

A. New Dentures

A typewritten or printed enclosure is inserted as a denture is being processed. Labels are positioned on the impression surfaces of the maxillary and mandibular dentures (Figure 47-3). They are covered, just before the final closure of the flask, with a clear acrylic material.

A label may be typewritten on onionskin paper or the tissue paper that separates sheets of packaged baseplate wax.[7,8] Another system

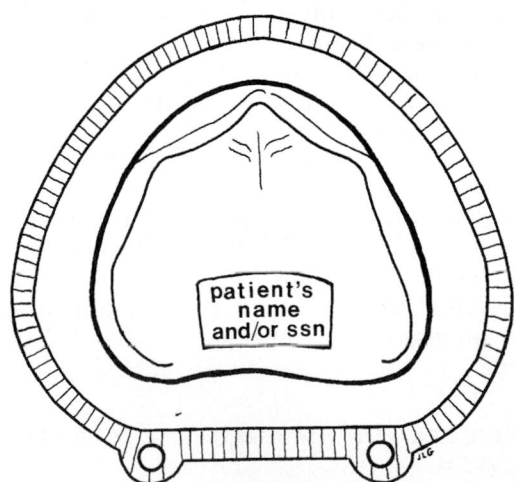

FIGURE 47-3 Inclusion Marker for New Denture. The label is inserted on the impression surface as the denture is being processed. In the flasked maxillary denture shown, the marker is positioned near the posterior border.

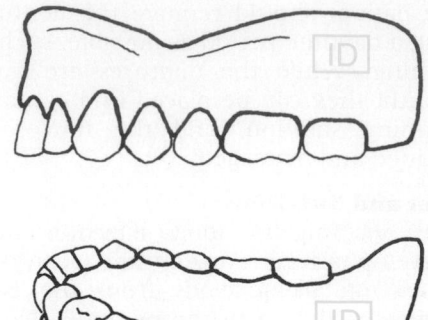
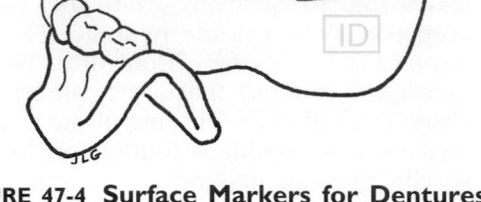

FIGURE 47-4 Surface Markers for Dentures. The labels are placed on the external denture surfaces for existing dentures. As shown, the markers are on the maxillary buccal flange and the mandibular lingual flange.

uses a thin metal strip for the insert. Stainless steel matrix bands, orthodontic bands, and thin metal strips (shim stock) have been used.[9]

B. Existing Dentures[10]

1. Clean the dentures thoroughly.

2. Use a No. 6 or 8 round bur and an inverted cone to cut small, shallow, box-like preparations in the posterior buccal flange of the maxillary denture and the lingual posterior flange of the mandibular denture (Figure 47-4). Do not go through to the impression surface.

3. Typewrite two copies of the patient's name (or other choice of identification) on onionskin paper, and trim the papers to fit the box-like preparations.

4. Cover the paper with cold-cure clear acrylic and fill to a slight excess; after the acrylic has cured, polish to a smooth finish.

III. SURFACE MARKERS

Surface markers are not as durable, but instruction can be provided for persons not trained in dental laboratory methods. In a skilled nursing facility or other long-term institution that has no resident dentist or dental hygienist, it may be important to teach a nurse or other staff member to mark dentures of residents as they are admitted. The methods described as follows have been used for this purpose.

A. Indelible Pen or Ballpoint

After cleaning and drying the denture, a small area near the posterior of the outer or polished denture surface is rubbed with an emery board until it is rough (Figure 47-4). The name, initials, or other identification is printed on the roughened area with an indelible pen and dried. Two or three coats of a fingernail acrylic (heavy nail protector) are painted over the area; each layer is dried before applying the next. Surface markings have been found to last at least 6 months.[11] Light-cured materials may also be used.[12,13]

B. Engraving Tool

An engraving tool is used to enter the name on the denture, and the grooves created are darkened with a special pencil before a sealing liquid is applied. Materials are available in a commercial kit.[14]

IV. INFORMATION TO INCLUDE ON A MARKER

For residents of a home or institution, using only the person's name and initials should suffice for temporary surface marking.

In a community, country, or international situation, the name alone would not provide enough identification, and the social security number, armed services serial number, or the equivalent in other countries should be included.

Other identification, such as blood type and vital drug or disease condition, has been suggested. In certain countries, the dentist's registration or hospital number has been used. In Sweden, the patient's date of birth and national registration number have been marked on the dentures. The markings that can provide *immediate* identification are the most significant.

FACTORS TO TEACH THE PATIENT

I. Dentures are not permanent prostheses.

II. Dentures and tissues must be examined at least once a year for care of the tissue-supported removable prosthesis; implant-supported, more frequently. Teach frequency of maintenance appointments for the individual, depending in part on that individual's ability to clean the dentures and maintain them free from plaque, stain, and calculus.

III. Dentures may need replacement periodically. Tissues under the denture change.

IV. Avoid use of drugstore remedies, reliners, and other home-applied materials unless the dentist has provided specific instruction.

V. Specific methods of care for dentures.

VI. Leaving the dentures out of the mouth overnight in accord with dentist's directions.

VII. Where to obtain and how to use a saliva substitute.

REFERENCES

1. **Academy of Prosthodontics Foundation**: The Glossary of Prosthodontic Terms, 6th ed. *J. Prosthet. Dent.*, 71, 41, January, 1994.
2. **Tallgren,** A.: The Continuing Reduction of the Residual Alveolar Ridges in Complete Denture Wearers: A Mixed-Longitudinal Study Covering 25 Years, *J. Prosthet. Dent.*, 27, 120, February, 1972.
3. **Gallagher,** J.B.: Insertion and Postinsertion Care, in Clark, J.W., ed.: *Clinical Dentistry,* Volume 5, Revised Edition—1984. Philadelphia, J.B. Lippincott Co., Chapter 14, pp. 1–27.
4. **Iacopino,** A.M. and Wathen, W.F.: Oral Candidal Infection and Denture Stomatitis: A Comprehensive Review, *J. Am. Dent. Assoc., 123,* 46, January, 1992.
5. **Robinson,** H.B.G. and Miller, A.S.: *Color Atlas of Oral Pathology,* 5th ed. Philadelphia, J.B. Lippincott, 1990, pp. 94-95.
6. **Robinson** and Miller: op. cit., p. 141.
7. **American Dental Association,** Council on Prosthetic Services and Dental Laboratory Relations: *Techniques for Denture Identification.* Chicago, American Dental Association, 1984, 12 pp.
8. **Dentsply International, Inc.:** *Method for Placing Permanent Record Data in Denture Base Without Affecting Tissue Adaptation,* Technical Bulletin, Dentsply International, Inc., York, PA 17404.
9. **Turner,** C.H., Fletcher, A.M., and Ritchie, G.M.: Denture Marking and Human Identification, *Br. Dent. J., 141,* 114, August 17, 1976.
10. **Bauer,** T.L.: Technique for Denture Identification, *J. Indiana Dent. Assoc., 58,* 28, Number 6, 1979.
11. **Deb,** A.K. and Heath, M.R.: Marking Dentures in Geriatric Institutions. The Relevance and Appropriate Methods, *Br. Dent. J., 146,* 282, May 1, 1979.
12. **Richards,** E.E., Williams, J.E., and Gauthier, G.: A Modified Light-cured Denture Identification Technique, *Spec. Care Dentist., 12,* 81, March/April, 1992.
13. **Lamb,** D.J.: A Simple Method for Permanent Identification of Dentures, *J. Prosthet. Dent., 67,* 894, June, 1992.
14. **Identure,** Geri, Inc., P.O. Box 9086, North St. Paul, MN 55109.

SUGGESTED READINGS

Cordioli, G., Majzoub, Z., and Castagna, S.: Mandibular Overdentures Anchored to Single Implants: A Five-year Prospective Study, *J. Prosthet. Dent., 78,* 159, August, 1997.

den Dunnen, A.C.L., Slagter, A.P., de Baat, C., and Kalk, W.: Professional Hygiene Care, Adjustments and Complications of Mandibular Implant-retained Overdentures: A Three-year Retrospective Study, *J. Prosthet. Dent., 78,* 387, October, 1997.

Fiske, J., Davis, D.M., and Horrocks, P.: A Self-help Group for Complete Denture Wearers, *Br. Dent. J., 178,* 18, January 7, 1995.

Hardy, D.L.: Dental Hygiene Care of the Denture Patient, *DentalHygienistNews, 5,* 22, Fall, 1992.

Joshipura, K.J., Willett, W.C., and Douglass, C.W.: The Impact of Edentulousness on Food and Nutrient Intake, *J. Am. Dent. Assoc., 127,* 459, April, 1996.

Kulak, Y., Arikan, A., and Delibalta, N.: Comparison of Three Different Treatment Methods for Generalized Denture Stomatitis, *J. Prosthet. Dent., 72,* 283, September, 1994.

Ramos, V., Giebink, D.L., Fisher, J.G., and Christensen, L.C.: Complete Dentures for a Child with Hypohidrotic Ectodermal Dysplasia: A Clinical Report, *J. Prosthet. Dent., 74,* 329, October, 1995.

Sebring, N.G., Guckes, A.D., Li, S.-H., and McCarthy, G.R.: Nutritional Adequacy of Reported Intake of Edentulous Subjects Treated with New Conventional or Implant-supported Mandibular Dentures, *J. Prosthet. Dent., 74,* 358, October, 1995.

Assessment

Allen, C.M.: Diagnosing and Managing Oral Candidiasis, *J. Am. Dent. Assoc., 123,* 77, January, 1992.

Ansari, I.H.: Panoramic Radiographic Examination of Edentulous Jaws, *Quintessence Int., 28,* 23, January, 1997.

Ettinger, R.L. and Jakobsen, J.R.: A Comparison of Patient Satisfaction and Dentist Evaluation of Overdenture Therapy, *Community Dent. Oral Epidemiol., 25,* 223, June, 1997.

Guggenheimer, J. and Hoffman, R.D.: The Importance of

Screening Edentulous Patients for Oral Cancer, *J. Prosthet. Dent., 72,* 141, August, 1994.

Kogon, S.L., Stephens, R.G., and Bohay, R.N.: An Analysis of the Scientific Basis for the Radiographic Guideline for New Edentulous Patients, *Oral Surg. Oral Med. Oral Pathol. Oral Radiol. Endod., 83,* 619, May, 1997.

Moltzer, G., van der Meulen, M.J., and Verheij, H.: Psychological Characteristics of Dissatisfied Denture Patients, *Community Dent. Oral Epidemiol., 24,* 52, February, 1996.

Denture Hygiene and Microbiology

Blair, Y., Bagg, J., MacFarlane, T.W., and Chestnutt, I.: Microbiological Assessment of Denture Hygiene Among Patients in Longstay and Daycare Community Places, *Community Dent. Oral Epidemiol., 23,* 100, April, 1995.

Danser, M.M., van Winkelhoff, A.J., and van der Velden, U.: Periodontal Bacteria Colonizing Oral Mucous Membranes in Edentulous Patients Wearing Dental Implants, *J. Periodontol., 68,* 209, March 1997.

Danser, M.M., Van Winkelhoff, A.J., De Graaff, J., and van der Velden, U.: Putative Periodontal Pathogens Colonizing Oral Mucous Membranes in Denture-wearing Subjects with a Past History of Periodontitis, *J. Clin. Periodontol., 22,* 854, November, 1995.

DePaola, L.G. and Minah, G.E.: Isolation of Pathogenic Microorganisms from Dentures and Denture-soaking Containers of Myelosuppressed Cancer Patients, *J. Prosthet. Dent., 49,* 20, January, 1983.

Jeganathan, S., Thean, H.P.Y., Thong, K.T., Chan, Y.C., and Singh, M.: A Clinically Viable Index for Quantifying Denture Plaque, *Quintessence Int., 27,* 569, August, 1996.

Kulak, Y., Arikan, A., and Kazazoglu, E.: Existence of *Candida albicans* and Microorganisms in Denture Stomatitis Patients, *J. Oral Rehabil., 24,* 788, October, 1997.

Marsh, P.D., Percival, R.S., and Challacombe, S.J.: The Influence of Denture-wearing and Age on the Oral Microflora, *J. Dent. Res., 71,* 1374, July, 1992.

Radford, D.R. and Radford, J.R.: A SEM Study of Denture Plaque and Oral Mucosa of Denture-related Stomatitis, *J. Dent., 21,* 87, April, 1993.

Adhesives, Materials

Granström, G.: Upper Airway Obstruction Caused by a Do-it-yourself Denture Reliner, *J. Prosthet. Dent., 63,* 495, May, 1990.

Grasso, J.E.: Denture Adhesives: Changing Attitudes, *J. Am. Dent. Assoc., 127,* 90, January, 1996.

Jagger, D.C. and Harrison, A.: Denture Fixatives—An Update for General Dental Practice, *Br. Dent. J., 180,* 311, April 20, 1996.

Jagger, D.C. and Harrison, A.: Complete Dentures—the Soft Option. An Update for General Dental Practice, *Br. Dent. J., 182,* 313, April 26, 1997.

Kelsey, C.C., Lang, B.R., and Wang, R.-F.: Examining Patients' Responses about the Effectiveness of Five Denture Adhesive Pastes, *J. Am. Dent. Assoc., 128,* 1532, November, 1997.

Shay, K.: Denture Adhesives. Choosing the Right Powders and Pastes, *J. Am. Dent. Assoc., 122,* 70, January, 1991.

Waters, M.G.J., Williams, D.W., Jagger, R.G., and Lewis, M.A.O.: Adherence of *Candida albicans* to Experimental Denture Soft Lining Materials, *J. Prosthet. Dent., 77,* 306, March, 1997.

Denture Identification

Berry, F.A., Logan, G.I., Plata, R., and Riegel, R.: A Postfabrication Technique for Identification of Prosthetic Devices, *J. Prosthet. Dent., 73,* 341, April, 1995.

Coss, P. and Wolfaardt, J.F.: Denture Identification System, *J. Prosthet. Dent., 74,* 551, November, 1995.

Cunningham, M. and Hoad-Reddick, G.: Attitudes to Identification of Dentures: The Patients' Perspective, *Quintessence Int., 24,* 267, April, 1993.

Frese, P: Denture Identification. A Valuable Clinical Service, *DentalHygienistNews, 9,* 4, Number 3, 1996.

Goshima, T., Gettleman, L., Goshima, Y., and Yamamoto, A.: Evaluation of Radiopaque Denture Liner, *Oral Surg. Oral Med. Oral Pathol., 74,* 379, September, 1992.

Milward, P.J., Shepherd, J.P., and Brickley, M.R.: Automatic Identification of Dental Appliances, *Br. Dent. J., 182,* 171, March 8, 1997.

48

The Oral and Maxillofacial Surgery Patient

Oral and maxillofacial surgery is the specialty of dentistry that includes the diagnostic, surgical, and adjunctive treatment of diseases, injuries, and defects involving both the functional and the esthetic aspects of the hard and soft tissues of the oral and maxillofacial regions.[1] Table 48-1 lists types of treatment included in this specialty with examples.

The practice of an oral surgeon may be primarily in a group clinical setting, in a hospital, or in a private office with outpatient hospital facilities available. With the oral surgeon is a team of specially trained individuals that might include surgical assistants, anesthetists, registered nurses, and dental hygienists.

The surgeon is involved with various dental practitioners, including general dentists and specialists. Maxillofacial surgery can be programmed, for example, with prosthodontists, orthodontists, implantologists, and specialists caring for any of the patients suggested by the list in Table 48-1. Terminology that relates to maxillofacial surgery is defined in Box 48-1.

Surgery for treatment of diseases and correction of defects of the periodontal tissues is categorized specifically as *periodontal surgery*. Within the scope of periodontal surgery are procedures for pocket elimination, gingivoplasty, treatment of furcation involvements, correction of mucogingival defects, and treatment for bony defects about the teeth. Preparation for periodontal surgery is not specifically described in this chapter.

PATIENT PREPARATION

I. OBJECTIVES

Dental hygiene care and instruction prior to oral and

TABLE 48-1 Categories of Oral and Maxillofacial Treatments

DENTOALVEOLAR SURGERY

Exodontics
    Impacted tooth removal
    Alveolar bone surgery: alveoloplasty

INFECTIONS

Abscesses
Osteomyelitis

TRAUMATIC INJURY

Fractures of jaws, zygoma
Fracture of teeth, alveolar bone

NEOPLASMS

Cysts
Tumors

DENTAL IMPLANT PLACEMENT

PREPROSTHETIC RECONSTRUCTION

Maxillofacial prosthetics
Immediate denture

ORTHOGNATHIC SURGERY

Prognathism correction
Facial esthetics

CLEFT LIP/PALATE

TEMPOROMANDIBULAR DISORDERS (TMD)

SALIVARY GLAND OBSTRUCTION

---

maxillofacial surgery may contribute to the patient's health and well-being by one or more of the following:

A. Reduce Oral Bacterial Count
1. Aid in the preparation of an aseptic field for the surgery.
2. Make postsurgical infection less likely or less severe.

B. Reduce Inflammation of the Gingiva and Improve Tissue Tone
1. Lessen local bleeding at the time of the surgery.
2. Promote postsurgical healing.

C. Remove Calculus Deposits
1. Remove a source of plaque retention and thus improve gingival tissue tone.
2. Prevent interference with placement of surgical instruments.
3. Prevent pieces of calculus from breaking away.

    a. Danger of inhalation, particularly when a general anesthetic is used.
    b. Possibility of calculus falling into a socket or other surgical area and acting as a foreign body to inhibit healing.

D. Instruct in Presurgical Personal Oral Care Procedures
Such instruction contributes to reducing inflammation and thus improves tissue tone and helps to prepare the patient for postsurgical care.

E. Instruct in the Use of Foods
The patient should be instructed about foods that provide the elements essential to tissue building and repair during pre- and postsurgical periods.

For the patient who will have teeth removed and immediate complete or partial dentures inserted, the importance of a diet containing all essential food groups should be emphasized.

F. Interpret the Dentist's Directions
Explanation should be given for the immediate presurgical preparation with respect to rest and dietary limitations, particularly when a general anesthetic is to be administered.

G. Motivate the Patient Who Will Have Teeth Remaining
The patient who will have teeth remaining after surgery should be motivated to prevent further tooth loss through routine dental and dental hygiene professional care and personal oral care procedures.

II. PERSONAL FACTORS

The extent of the surgery to be performed and previous experiences affect the patient's attitude. Many patients who are in the greatest need of presurgical dental hygiene care and instruction may be people who have neglected their mouths for many years. They have been indifferent to or unaware of the importance of obtaining adequate care. Their only visits to a dentist may have been to have a toothache relieved by extraction. Their knowledge of preventive measures may be limited. A few of the characteristics are suggested here.

A. Apprehensive and Fearful
1. Apprehensive and indifferent toward need for personal care of teeth.
2. Fearful of all dental procedures, particularly oral surgery and anesthesia.
3. Fearful of cancer or other disease.
4. Fearful of personal appearance after surgery.

B. Impatient
When teeth have caused discomfort and pain, the patient may have difficulty understanding the need for delay while oral hygiene procedures are accomplished.

BOX 48-1 KEY WORDS: Oral and Maxillofacial Surgery

Ecchymosis (ek-i-mō'sis): a hemorrhagic spot, larger than a petechia, in the skin or mucous membrane caused by extravasation of blood; forms a nonelevated, rounded, or irregular purplish patch.

Exodontics (ek"sō-don'tiks): branch of dentistry dealing with the surgical removal of teeth.

Exostosis (ek"sos-tō'sis): benign new growth projecting from the surface of bone.

Intermaxillary fixation (in"ter-mak'sĭ-lār'ē): fixation of the maxilla in occlusion with the mandible held in place by means of wires and elastic bands; the healing parts are stabilized following fracture or surgery.

Maxillofacial (mak'sĭl-ō-fā'shal): pertaining to the jaws and the face.

Maxillofacial prosthetics: the branch of prosthodontics concerned with the restoration of the mouth and jaws and associated facial structures that have been affected by disease, injury, surgery, or a congenital defect.

Miniplate osteosynthesis: a method of internal fixation of mandibular fractures utilizing miniaturized metal plates and screws made of titanium or stainless steel.

Orthognathic surgery: surgery to alter relationships of the dental arches and/or supporting bone; usually coordinated with orthodontic therapy.

Orthognathics (or'thog-na'thiks): science dealing with the causes and treatment of malposition of the bones of the jaws.

Trismus (triz'mus): motor disturbance of the trigeminal nerve with spasm of masticatory muscles and difficulty in opening the mouth (lockjaw).

C. Ashamed

Of appearance or of having neglected the teeth.

D. Resigned

Feeling of inevitableness of the situation; lack of appreciation for natural teeth.

E. Discouraged

Over tooth loss or development of soft tissue lesions.

F. Resentful

1. Toward time lost from work.
2. Toward the financial aspects of dental care.
3. Toward inconvenience and discomfort.

DENTAL HYGIENE CARE

A review of the patient's record shows preliminary procedures that need to be completed. For example, a thorough intraoral and extraoral examination, a recording of vital signs, photographs, and additional radiographs may be required. The patient's medical and dental history reveals essential information relative to the need for prophylactic antibiotics or other precautions.

I. PRESURGERY TREATMENT PLANNING

The pending date for the surgery and the patient's attitude may limit the time to be spent.

A. First Appointment

1. Develop rapport; explain purposes of presurgical appointments.

2. Explain and demonstrate bacterial plaque control principles.
3. Present dietary record form for completion before the next appointment (pages 444 to 449).
4. Perform scaling to prepare for tissue healing.
5. Give postappointment instruction for rinsing with basic saline or with chlorhexidine 0.12% for tissue conditioning.

B. Second Appointment

1. Observe gingival tissue response; apply disclosing agent. Review disease control procedures. Introduce the use of dental floss or other interdental aids when applicable.
2. Receive the dietary record and review it with the patient. Present diet recommendations.
3. Complete or continue the scaling. More than two appointments may be needed for patients who will have surgery for oral cancer or who have a cardiovascular or other condition for which all periodontal and dental treatment must be completed. When radiation or chemotherapy will be used following surgery for oral cancer, or when a prosthetic heart valve or total joint replacement will be involved, complete oral care is necessary as described on page 725.

II. PATIENT INSTRUCTION

A. Bacterial Plaque Control

1. *Brush.* Soft.
2. *Technique.* For a patient who may not have practiced careful brushing on a regular plan, a simple brushing technique is preferred.

Time for establishing habits may be limited until postsurgical healing is complete. Use of disclosing agent for the patient's own evaluation is important.

B. Auxiliary Procedures

Interdental plaque removal and care of fixed and removable prostheses are included in instruction. The patient who is to have multiple extractions for the placement of an immediate denture or other prosthesis, such as an obturator following cleft palate, tumor, or other surgery, needs postsurgical instruction for the specific care of the prosthesis.

III. INSTRUMENTATION

A. Scaling

1. *Problems*
   a. Teeth with large carious lesions.
   b. Mobile teeth.
   c. Edentulous areas.
   d. Sensitive, enlarged gingival tissue that bleeds readily.
2. *Suggestions for Procedure*
   a. Provide preprocedural antimicrobial rinse to lessen bacteremia and aerosol contamination.
   b. Use local anesthetic.
   c. Maintain a clear field, using evacuation techniques.
   d. Use alternate finger rests to adapt to mobile teeth or edentulous areas: stabilize mobile teeth during scaling strokes.
   e. Ultrasonic scaling may be the technique of choice; high power evacuation is essential.

B. Stain Removal

1. *Contraindications*
   a. Enlarged, inflamed, sensitive gingiva.
   b. Deep pockets.
   c. Profuse hemorrhage.
2. *Effects*
   a. Irritation to tissue by polishing abrasive and action of rubber polishing cup.
   b. Abrasive particles forced into the gingival tissues by movement of rubber cup.

C. Rinsing Instruction

1. *Objectives.* To promote tissue healing following scaling and to remove debris; to initiate the habit of rinsing for postsurgical care later.
2. *Rinsing Solution.* Warm, mild, hypertonic salt solution.
3. *Frequency.* Recommended for several times each day after the surgical procedure.

D. Follow-up Evaluation

Scaling and planing should be planned for a few weeks after oral surgery. Emphasis must be placed on review and redemonstration of personal daily care.

IV. PATIENT INSTRUCTION: DIET SELECTION

The nutritional state can influence the resistance to infection and wound healing, as well as general recovery powers. Nutritional deficiencies can occur because of the inability to ingest adequate nutrients orally.

Specific recommendations of what to include and not to include in the diet should be given to the patient. Postsurgical suggestions may differ from presurgical; for example, when difficulty in chewing is a postsurgical problem, a liquid or soft diet may be required. When major oral surgery requires hospitalization, tube feeding may be used during the initial healing period. Tube feeding is described on page 717.

A. Nutritional and Dietary Needs

Diets outlined are designed to include the essential foods from the Food Guide Pyramid (Figure 28-2, page 445).
1. *Essential for Promotion of Healing.* Protein and vitamins, particularly vitamin A, vitamin C, and riboflavin.
2. *Essential for Building Gingival Tissue Resistance.* A varied diet that includes adequate portions of all essential food groups.
3. *Essential for Dental Caries Prevention.* Noncariogenic foods. When a patient has not been able to masticate properly, the diet employed frequently may have included many soft and cariogenic foods.

B. Suggestions for Instruction

1. Provide instruction sheets that show specific pre- and postsurgery meal plans. Foods for liquid and soft diets are listed on pages 717 to 718.
2. Express nutritional needs in terms of quantity or servings of foods so that the patient clearly understands.
3. For the patient who will receive dentures, careful instruction must be provided over a period of time. At the presurgical appointment, only an introduction can be given, particularly because the patient is probably more concerned about the surgery than about the aftereffects.

   When the patient loses the teeth because of dental caries, the diet has likely been highly cariogenic. Emphasis should be placed on helping the patient include nutritious foods for the general health of the body and, more specifically, the health of the alveolar processes, which will support the dentures.

V. PRESURGICAL INSTRUCTIONS[2]

At the appointment just prior to the oral surgery appointment, instructions relative to the surgical procedure should be discussed with the patient. The objective is to let the patient know what to expect so that full cooperation is possible. The patient may have concerns about the anesthesia, the surgical procedure, and the outcome.

A. Explain the general procedures for anesthesia and surgery.

B. Provide printed instructions. Information in the printed instructions should include the following:

1. *Food and Liquid Intake.* Specify the number of hours before the time of the surgery when the patient should stop further intake of food and fluids.

2. *Alcohol and Medications Restrictions.* Certain proprietary self-medications are not compatible with the anesthetic and drugs to be used during and following the surgical procedure. The patient should be instructed to discontinue use.

3. *Transport to and from the Appointment.* When a general anesthetic or light sedation is used, the patient should not drive. Plans for someone to accompany and assist the patient should be made.

4. *The Night Before the Appointment.* In addition to food and alcohol restrictions, a good night's rest is advocated.

5. *Personal Items*
   a. Clothing. The clothing worn should be loose and comfortable. The sleeves should be easily drawn up over the elbows.
   b. Care of contact lenses and prostheses. The patient will be asked to remove contact lenses and prostheses, and should bring containers for their safe keeping.

VI. POSTSURGICAL CARE

A. Immediate Instructions

Printed postsurgical instructions are provided following all oral procedures. The prepared material is reviewed with the patient after surgery. Specific details vary, but basic information for postsurgical instruction sheets includes the following:

1. *Control Bleeding.* Keep the sponge in the mouth over the surgical area for ½ hour; then discard it. When bleeding persists at home, place a gauze pad or cold wet teabag over the area and bite firmly for 30 minutes.

2. *Rinsing.* Do not rinse for 24 hours after the surgical appointment. Then use warm salt water (½ teaspoonful salt in ½ cup [4 ounces] of warm water) after toothbrushing and every 2 hours.

3. *Bacterial Plaque Control.* Brush the teeth even more thoroughly than usual. Avoid the surgery site.

4. *Rest.* Get plenty of rest; at least 8 to 10 hours

of sleep each night. Avoid strenuous exercise during the first 24 hours, and keep the mouth from excessive movement.

5. *Diet.* Use a liquid or soft diet high in protein. Drink water and fruit juices freely. Avoid foods that require excessive chewing.

6. *Pain.* If needed, use a pain-relieving preparation prescribed by the dentist. Adhere to directions.

7. *Icepack.* Following a flap procedure or when swelling is likely to occur, apply icepack (ice cubes in a plastic bag) for 15 minutes followed by 15 minutes off, or apply for 15 minutes after 30 minutes off, as directed by the dentist. Heat is not used for swelling.

8. *Complications.* Instructions should include the telephone number to call after office hours, should complications arise; complications may include uncontrollable pain, marked bleeding, temperature rise, difficulty in opening the mouth, or unusual swelling a few days after the surgery.

B. Follow-up Care

The dental hygienist may participate in suture removal, irrigation of sockets, and other postsurgical procedures when the patient returns. Appropriately, instruction concerning plaque control, rinsing, oral irrigation, and other personal care, as well as diet supervision, can be continued.

PATIENT WITH INTERMAXILLARY FIXATION

The limited access for personal oral care procedures and the effect of the liquid diet required for most cases define the need for special dental hygiene care for the patient with intermaxillary fixation. Attention to rehabilitation of the oral tissues during the period following the removal of appliances takes on particular significance lest permanent tissue damage result or inadequate oral care habits be continued indefinitely.

Descriptions in this section are related to a fractured jaw, but intermaxillary fixation is required for a variety of corrective surgeries and other conditions, including temporomandibular joint treatment and reconstructive and orthognathic surgeries. Regardless of the reason for intermaxillary fixation, instructions for dental hygiene care (page 716) are similar, and the patient's problems are much the same.

The patient with a fractured jaw may be hospitalized. A dental hygienist employed in a hospital would be called upon to assume a part of the responsibility for patient care or to give oral hygiene instruction to direct-care personnel. After dismissal from the hospital, the patient may require special attention in the private dental office for a long period of time.

Treatment of a fractured jaw may be complex, and the patient may suffer considerably, both physically and mentally. Some basic knowledge of the nature of fractures and their treatment is helpful in understanding the patient's needs.

I. CAUSES OF FRACTURED JAWS

A. Traumatic

From automobile, bicycle, and sports injuries, industrial accidents, and physical violence (blows, fistfights).

B. Predisposing

Pathologic conditions, such as tumors, cysts, osteoporosis, or osteomyelitis, weaken the bone; thus, slight trauma or even tooth removal can cause fracture.

II. EMERGENCY CARE

Immediate attention must be paid to measures for care of the patient's general condition. Emergency care is given for airway, breathing, and circulation ("A-B-C," page 900). Hemorrhage, shock, and skull or internal head injuries are next in the sequence of concern.

Almost any category of emergency care may be required (Tables 61-5 and 61-6, pages 910 to 916). Although treatment for the fractured jaw must not be postponed for any great length of time, its immediate care takes second place to the vital aspects of patient care.

Tetanus prophylaxis may be indicated as soon as medical treatment is available.

III. RECOGNITION

A. History

Except for a pathologic fracture, a history of trauma should be available.

B. Clinical Signs

The patient has pain, especially on movement, and tenderness on slight pressure over the area of the fracture. Teeth may be displaced, fractured, or mobile. Because of muscle pull or contraction, segments of the bones may be displaced, and the occlusion of the teeth may be irregular.

Muscle spasm is a common finding, particularly when the fracture is at the angle or ramus of the mandible. Crepitation can be heard if the parts of bone are moved.

The soft tissue in the area of the fracture may show laceration and bleeding, discoloration (ecchymosis), and enlargement.

IV. TYPES

A fracture is classified by using a combination of descriptive words for its *location, direction, nature,* and *severity.* Fractures may be single or multiple, bilateral or unilateral, complete or incomplete.

A. Classification by Nature of the Fracture (Figure 48-1)

1. *Simple.* Has no communication with outside.
2. *Compound.* Has communication with outside.
3. *Comminuted.* Shattered.
4. *Incomplete.* "Greenstick" fracture has one side of a bone broken and the other side bent. It occurs in incompletely calcified bones (young children, usually). The fibers tend to bend rather than break.

B. Mandibular (described by location)

1. Alveolar process.
2. Condyle.
3. Angle.
4. Body.
5. Symphysis.

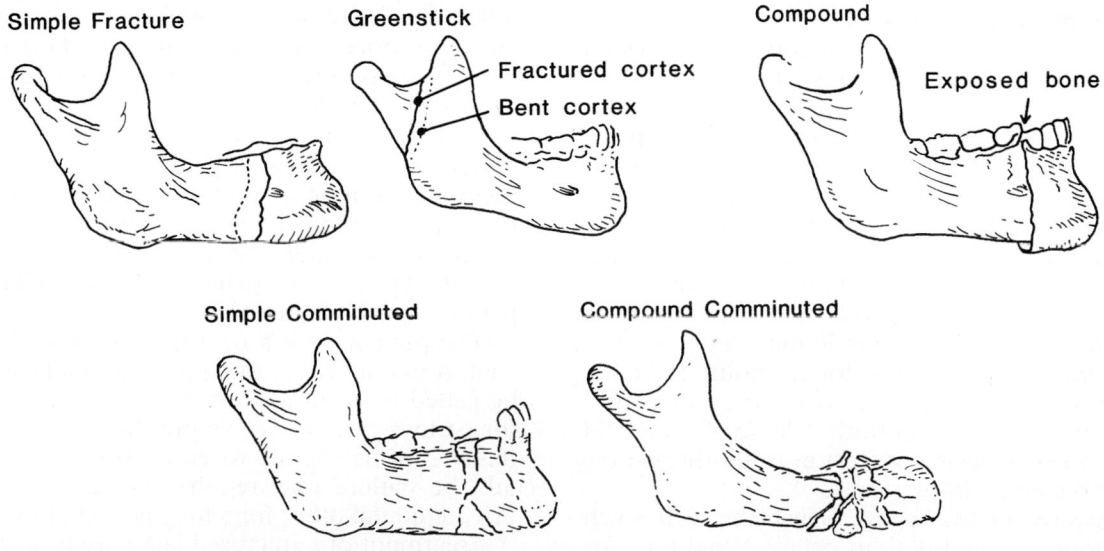

FIGURE 48-1 Types of Fractures. (From Kruger, G.O.: *Textbook of Oral and Maxillofacial Surgery,* 6th ed. St. Louis, Mosby, 1984.)

C. Maxillary

1. *Alveolar Process.* The alveolar process fracture does not extend to the midline of the palate.
2. *Le Fort I.*[3] The Le Fort classification is used widely to identify the three general levels of maxillary fractures, as shown in Figure 48-2.

   Le Fort I is a horizontal fracture line above the roots of the teeth, above the palate, across the maxillary sinus, below the zygomatic process, and across the pterygoid plates.
3. *Le Fort II.* The midface fracture extends over the middle of the nose, down the medial wall of the orbits, across the infraorbital rims, and posteriorly, across the pterygoid plates.
4. *Le Fort III.* The high-level craniofacial fracture extends transversely across the bridge of the nose, across the orbits and the zygomatic arches, and across the pterygoid plates

TREATMENT OF FRACTURES[4,5]

Each fracture differs from the next, and the methods used in treatment vary with the individual case. Many factors are involved when the oral surgeon selects the methods to be used, particularly the location of the fracture or fractures, the presence or absence of teeth, existing injuries to the teeth, other head injuries, and the general health and condition of the patient.

Treatment of a fracture consists of *reduction* of the fracture, *fixation* of the fragments, and *immobilization* of the jaw. A temporary, removable splint may be necessary when a patient must be transported to another location for specialized treatment. An accident or war casualty may occur many miles from a professional treatment facility.

I. REDUCTION

Reduction means the positioning of the parts on either side of the fracture so they are in apposition for healing and restoration of function. The closure of the teeth is the guide for position in the dentulous patient.

A. Closed Reduction

1. Manual manipulation of the parts.
2. Elastic traction. The most common traction is applied with elastic bands hooked to arch bars, which are also part of the method for fixation. The method is described under the topic "intermaxillary fixation" (page 714).

B. Open Reduction

The bone fracture ends are exposed surgically by a flap procedure, and the two ends are brought together. They are then fixed as described under "transosseous wires or metal plate."

II. FIXATION

The fracture is first reduced or positioned, and then is

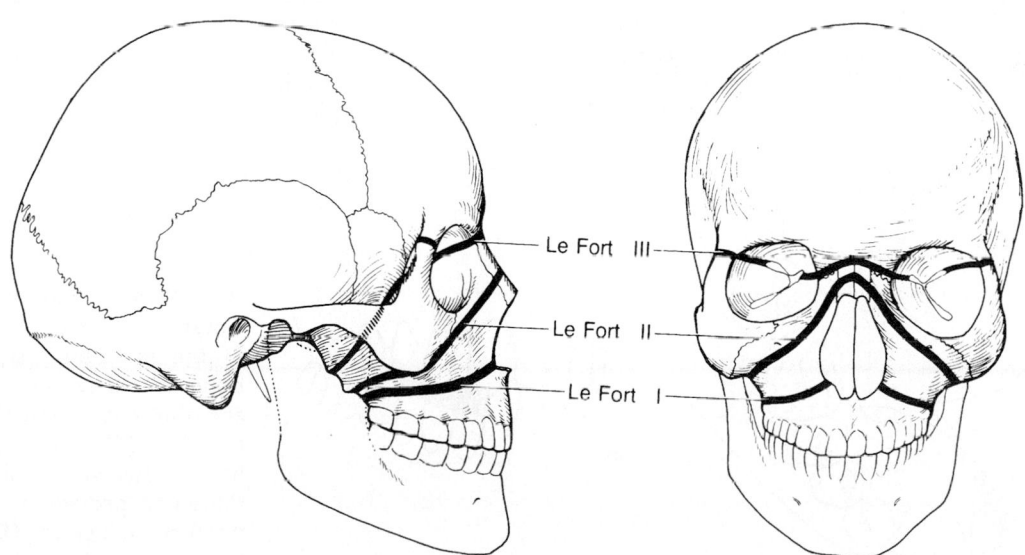

FIGURE 48-2 Le Fort Classification of Facial Fractures. *Le Fort I,* horizontal fracture above the roots of the teeth, below the zygomatic process, and across the pterygoid plates. *Le Fort II,* midface fracture over the middle of the nose and across the intraorbital rims. *Le Fort III,* transversely across the bridge of the nose, across the orbits and the zygomatic bone. (From Archer, W.H.: *Oral and Maxillofacial Surgery,* 5th ed. Philadelphia, W.B. Saunders Co., 1975; from Committee on Trauma, American College of Surgeons: Early Care of the Injured Patient. Philadelphia, W.B. Saunders Co., 1972.)

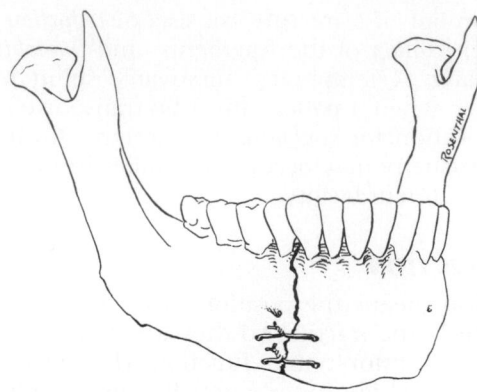

FIGURE 48-3 Open Reduction for Mandibular Fracture. Transosseous wiring is shown to hold bony parts in position for healing at the fracture line. (From Waite, D.E.: *Practical Oral Surgery*, 2nd ed. Philadelphia, Lea & Febiger, 1978.)

fixed or stabilized in that position. Fractures take several weeks to heal, and fixation apparatus is left in place long enough to ensure union of the bony parts.

A. Transosseous Wires or Metal Plate

When the bony parts are reduced by open reduction, they are fastened together either by a wire suture threaded through holes drilled on either side of the fracture line (Figure 48-3) or by a metal plate. The metal plate is designed to cross over the fracture line and is held in place by screws on either side.

B. Intermaxillary Fixation

Intermaxillary fixation is fixation obtained by applying wires or elastic bands between the maxillary and mandibular arches. This treatment is sufficient for many fractures. More complicated types of fractures may require additional or supplemental types of therapy.

Ready-made, contoured, metal arch bars are available, or wires may be custom made with loops on which to hook wires or elastics to connect the mandible and maxilla in occlusion. The arch bars are adapted carefully to fit accurately to each tooth, and then are wired into place so that the hooks project up in the maxilla and down in the mandible.

Elastics are positioned to provide a steady, gradual pull to aid in reducing the fracture (Figure 48-4C). A small horizontal elastic may be positioned across the fracture to reduce the lateral displacement (Figure 48-4D).

C. External Skeletal Fixation (Figure 48-5)

1. *Indications.* Management of a fracture cannot always be accomplished satisfactorily by intermaxillary wiring alone. The following are indications for external skeletal fixation:

   a. Insufficient number of teeth in good condition for intermaxillary fixation.

   b. As a supplement to intermaxillary fixation when no teeth are present in the fractured portion of the mandible.

   c. Loss of bone substance. When bone substance is lost because of an accident, a gunshot wound, or a pathologic condition, a bone graft may be indicated.[6]

   The extraoral fixation is used first to hold the fractured parts in a normal relationship, and then to immobilize the area during healing following the bone graft surgery.

   d. Certain patients may be unable to have the jaws closed for a long period. Examples of these are

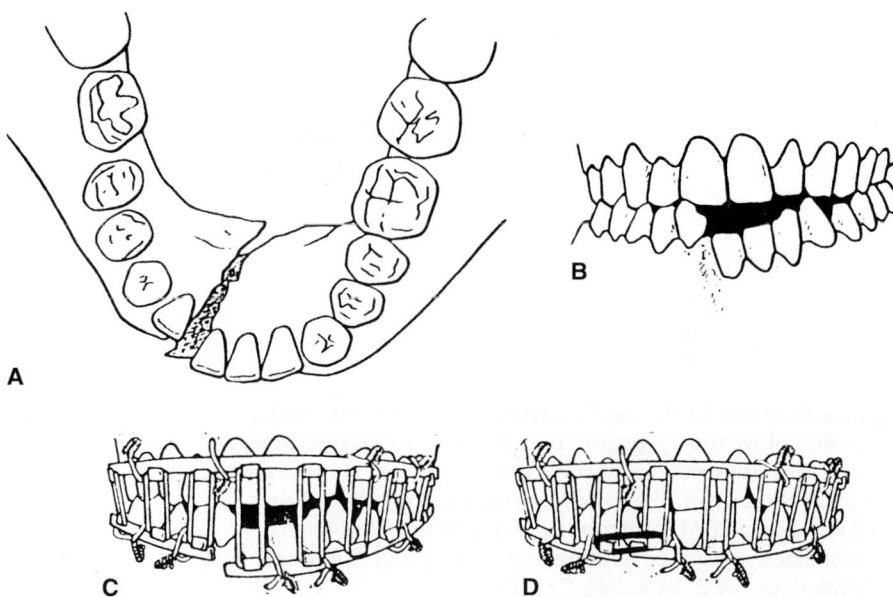

FIGURE 48-4 Intermaxillary Fixation. (A) Location of fracture of the mandible. **(B)** Segments of bone on either side of the fracture are displaced by muscle pull or contraction. **(C)** Metal arch bars are held in place with rubber bands positioned to provide a steady pull for fracture reduction. **(D)** Note small horizontal rubber band extending from the hook at the mandibular right central incisor to the mandibular right canine to reduce the lateral displacement. (From Archer, W.H.: *Oral and Maxillofacial Surgery*, 5th ed. Philadelphia, W.B. Saunders Co., 1975.)

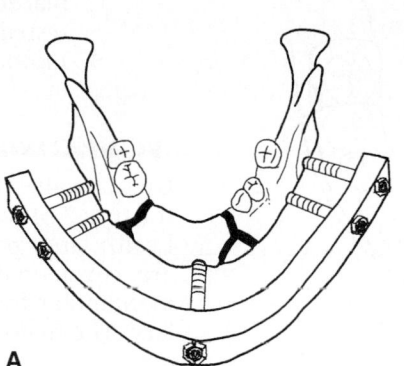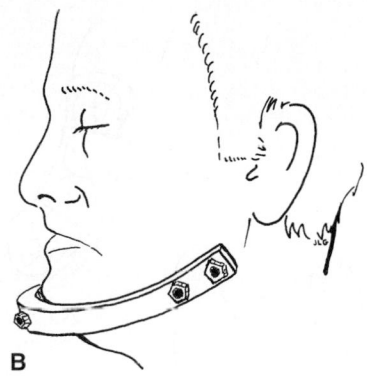

■FIGURE 48-5 External Skeletal Fixation. (A) Precision bone screws placed on either side of the fractures shown by heavy black lines. (B) Molded acrylic bar positioned over the bone screws and locked into position with nuts.

A   **B**

i. Patient with a vomiting problem, such as during pregnancy.
ii. Patient with a mental or physical disability, such as cerebral palsy, epilepsy, or mental retardation.
e. Edentulous mandible when the fracture fragments are greatly displaced, when the fracture is at the angle of the mandible, or when the mandible is atrophic or thinned.

2. *Description.* Two special bone screws are placed via skin incisions on either side of the fracture. An acrylic bar is molded and, while still pliable, is pressed over the threads of the bone screws and locked into position with the screw nuts (Figure 48-5).

III. EDENTULOUS PATIENT

The use of external skeletal fixation for an edentulous mandible was described earlier. Other procedures are included here.

A. Open Reduction Using Transosseous Wiring

Transosseous wiring for an edentulous mandible is similar to that described for the dentulous mandible. The bony parts are brought together and held in place by wire sutures (Figure 48-6).

B. Circumferential Wiring

The patient's denture can be used for a splint. If the denture was broken when the mandible was fractured, it may be repaired immediately or a temporary edentulous splint may be fabricated. Wires are placed around the denture and the arch together by threading the wire, using surgical procedures (Figure 48-7). When the line of fracture is not under the denture-covered area, additional procedures are needed for the uncovered portion.

Because considerable trauma may be associated with the fracture, swelling may occur that prevents denture placement. In addition, the insertion of circumferential wires may cause

more trauma to the soft tissues. An external skeletal fixation may be a preferred treatment.

C. Intermaxillary Fixation

The mandibular denture may be wired to the maxillary complete denture for additional mobilization. Mandibular anterior denture teeth may be cut away to allow the patient to feed by straw or glass feeding tube.

IV. MAXILLARY FRACTURE

Maxillary fractures are more difficult to handle because of the number of bones, the associated anatomy, and the complications of basal skull fractures.

A. Intermaxillary Fixation

Whether the fracture is Le Fort I, II, or III (Figure 48-2), intermaxillary fixation is completed first to establish the occlusal relationship (Figure 48-4). The next step is to accomplish craniomaxillary immobilization.

B. Craniomaxillary Immobilization

A rigid craniomaxillary fixation is necessary. A

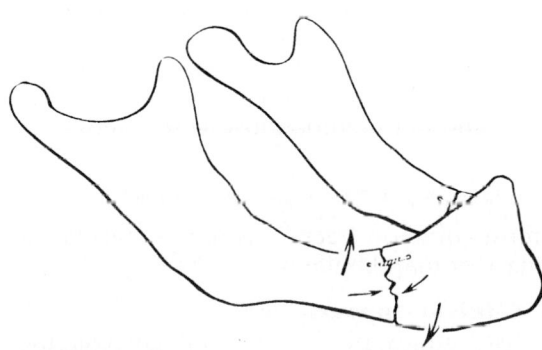

■FIGURE 48-6 Edentulous Mandible to Show the Use of Open Reduction. Transosseous wiring placed. (From Archer, W.H.: *Oral and Maxillofacial Surgery*, 5th ed. Philadelphia, W.B. Saunders Co., 1975; from Dingman, R.A. Natvig, P.: *Surgery of Facial Fractures*, Philadelphia, W.B. Saunders Co., 1964.)

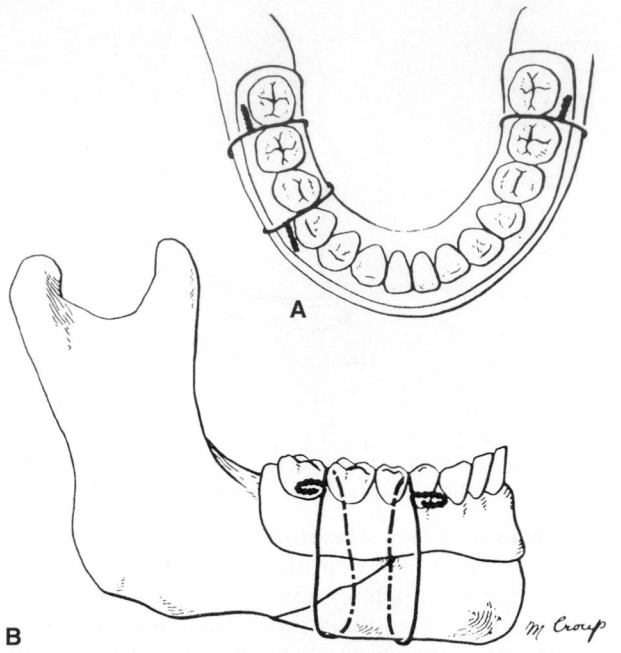

FIGURE 48-7 Removable Denture Used as Splint.
(A) Wires are placed around the denture and the edentulous arch and twisted together to stabilize the reduction. **(B)** Note the line of fracture with the denture positioned to cover it. (From Archer, W.H.: *Oral and Maxillofacial Surgery*, 5th ed. Philadelphia, W.B. Saunders Co., 1975.)

variety of methods has been used, some internal and others external.

1. *Cranial Suspension to the Nearest Superior Unfractured Bone.* Pins are used to provide a connection for the attachment of wires from a stable bone, such as the supraorbital area, to the mandibular arch bar.
2. *Headcap.* A plaster headcap can provide a means for extraoral traction. This method is used infrequently.
3. *Internal Suspension Wires.* A maxilla with a Le Fort I fracture may be suspended by internal wires over the zygoma. In the oral cavity, the wires are connected to the mandibular arch bar. When the zygoma is also fractured, another method must be selected.

V. ALVEOLAR PROCESS FRACTURE

The most common fracture is of the alveolar process, maxillary or mandibular.

A. Clinical Appearance
Lacerations of the lips and gingiva; mobility, fracture, or displacement of teeth; swelling; bruising; and hemorrhage are usual signs.

B. Treatment
1. Replantation of displaced teeth.
2. Immobilization with interdental wiring. A temporary fixed splint of acrylic may be placed over the wires. The teeth must be tested periodically for vitality.
3. Endodontic therapy may be required later.

VI. HEALING

Union is affected by the location and character of the fracture. Much depends on the patient's general health and resistance and cooperation. Six weeks are considered the average for the uncomplicated mandibular fracture and 4 to 6 weeks for the maxillary. The major cause of complication is infection.

DENTAL HYGIENE CARE

I. PROBLEMS

Fixation apparatus, however carefully placed to prevent tissue irritation, interferes with normal function. The length of time the appliances must be in place is sufficient for considerable disturbance of tissue metabolism. Identification of possible effects of treatment provides the basis for planning dental hygiene care.

A. Development of Gingivitis or Periodontal Complications
1. Thick plaque formation and food debris accumulation provide sources of irritation to the gingiva.
2. Gingivitis can develop in 9 to 19 days.[7]
3. Lack of normal stimulation to the circulation of the periodontium and of cleansing effects usually provided by the action of the tongue, lips, and facial muscles contributes to stagnation of saliva and to bacterial plaque accumulation.
4. Tender, sensitive gingiva make plaque control more difficult, even on available surfaces.

B. Dental Caries Initiation
An appetizing soft or liquid diet is difficult to plan using limited cariogenic foods for dental caries prevention.

C. Loss of Appetite
Loss of appetite related to monotonous liquid or soft diet may lead to weight loss and lowered physical resistance. Secondary infections, including those of the oral tissues, may result.

D. Difficulty in Opening the Mouth
1. When the temporomandibular joint has been injured, the patient wearing fixation appliances that involve only the mandible has difficulty in applying a toothbrush to the lingual surfaces of teeth.
2. After removal of appliances, all patients have a degree of muscular trismus that hinders toothbrushing and mastication.

II. INSTRUMENTATION

A. Presurgical

Gross calculus is removed, insofar as possible, before wiring or the placement of metal or acrylic splints. Trauma to surrounding soft tissues of lip, tongue, and cheeks limits accessibility.

B. During Treatment

Periodic scaling in conjunction with plaque control contributes to oral health. Although access is only from the facial aspect for a patient with intermaxillary wiring, some benefit can be obtained. An assistant must provide continual suction during treatment.

C. After Removal of Appliances

A few weeks after removal of appliances, when the patient can open the mouth normally and plaque control procedures have been initiated, complete scaling and planing can be performed.

III. DIET

Many patients with fractured jaws tend to lose weight, which is generally related to an inadequate nutrient and caloric intake. Objectives in planning the diet are to help the patient maintain an adequate nutritional state, to promote healing, to increase resistance to infection, and to prevent new carious lesions.

Attention must be given to the patient's willingness and ability to follow the recommendations made. The patient may be in the hospital for a few days to a few weeks, depending on the severity of other injuries. A greater length of time is spent as an outpatient, when the diet is much more difficult to supervise. The patient's understanding of dietary instructions and what is expected appears to be much more significant than the specific components of the diet recommended.

A. Nutritional Needs

After a surgical fixation procedure, the diet must be planned to promote tissue building and repair.

1. All essential food elements.
2. Emphasis on protein, vitamins, particularly A and C, and minerals, particularly calcium and phosphorus.
3. Usual caloric requirements for patient's age, taking into consideration lack of physical exercise and loss of appetite while ill.

B. Methods of Feeding

1. *Plastic Straw.* Liquid is sucked through the teeth or through an edentulous area. Straw can be bent to accommodate a patient who cannot sit up.
2. *Spoon Feeding.* When a patient's arms are not functional, direct assistance is needed. The mouth may have injuries that prevent sucking food through a straw.

3. *Tube Feeding.* Tube feeding may be indicated following various types of extensive oral surgery, facial trauma, burns, immobilized fractured jaw, and other conditions that prevent ingesting sufficient calories and nutritional foods by way of the mouth.

A nasogastric tube is used (Figure 48-8). Blenderized food can be prepared, or special tube formulas are available commercially. When commercial preparations are used, contents can be selected to meet the specific nutritional and caloric requirements of an individual patient.

C. Liquid Diet

A *clear liquid* diet to help prevent dehydration may be prescribed initially, but it is nutritionally inadequate. A *full liquid* diet to provide high protein and other healing elements is of a consistency to be taken by a cup. A *blenderized liquid* diet can be passed through a straw.

1. *Indications*
   a. All patients with jaws wired together.
   b. All patients with no appliance or single-jaw appliance who have difficulty in opening the mouth because of a condition, such as temporomandibular joint involvement or tongue or lip injury, that hinders insertion of food or manipulation of food in the mouth.
2. *Examples of Foods.* Fruit juices, milk, eggnog, meat juices and soups, cooked thin cereals, and canned baby foods. Strained vegetables and meats (baby foods) may be added to meat juices and soups.
3. *Use of a Blender.* Regular table foods can be

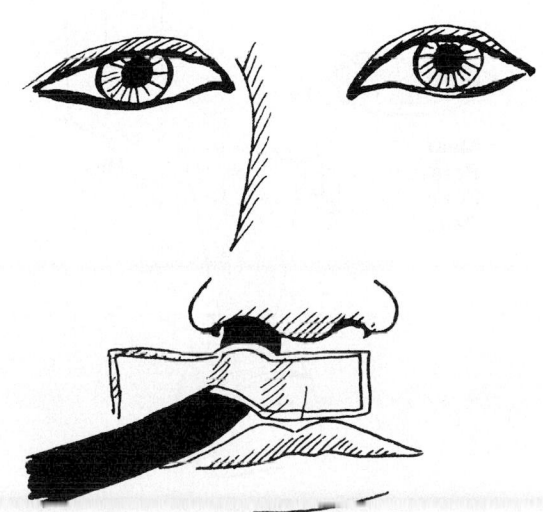

▪ **FIGURE 48-8 Nasogastric Feeding Tube.** To prevent injury to the nasopharyngeal passages, the tube is taped securely between the upper lip and the nares. (From Lewis, C.M.: *Nursing Considerations in Tube-fed Patients.* Philadelphia, F.A. Davis Co., 1976.)

mixed in a food blender. With liquid, such as clear soup or milk, added, a fluid consistency can be obtained that will pass through a straw (Figure 48-9).

D. Soft Diet
1. *Indications*
   a. Patient with no appliance or with single-jaw appliance without complications in opening the mouth or in movement of the lips and tongue.
   b. Patient who has been maintained on liquid diet throughout treatment period. After appliances are removed, the soft diet is recommended for several days to 1 week to provide the stomach with foods that are readily digestible rather than making a drastic change to a regular diet. A soft diet can also aid by protecting tender oral tissues from the rough textures of a regular diet until the tissues have had a chance to respond to softer foods and a regular bacterial plaque control routine.
2. *Examples of Foods.* Soft-poached, scrambled, or boiled eggs; cooked cereals; mashed soft-cooked vegetables, including potato; mashed fresh or canned fruits; soft, finely divided meats; custards; plain ice cream.

E. Hints for Diet Planning With the Nonhospitalized Patient
1. Provide instruction sheets that show specific meal plans.
2. Express nutritional needs in quantities or servings of foods.

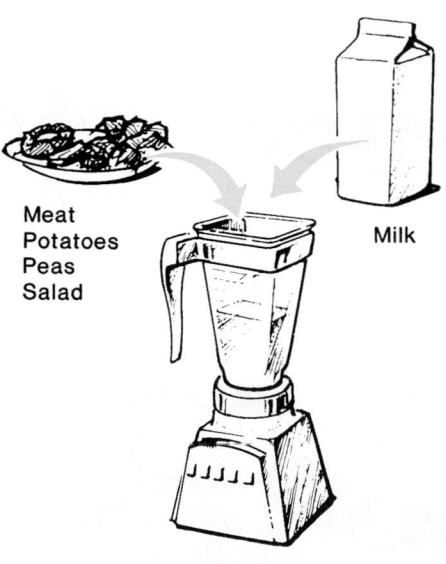

Meat
Potatoes
Peas
Salad

Milk

Blender

▪ **FIGURE 48-9 Preparation of a Liquid or Soft Diet.** Regular table foods can be blenderized with milk or other nutritious liquid. (From Schultz, R.C.: *Facial Injuries,* 2nd ed. Copyright © 1977 by Yearbook Medical Publishers, Inc., Chicago.)

3. Show methods of varying the diet. A liquid or soft diet is at best monotonous because of the sameness of texture.
4. Suggest limitation of cariogenic foods as an aid to prevention of dental caries.

IV. PERSONAL ORAL CARE PROCEDURES

Every attempt to keep the patient's mouth as clean as possible for comfort and sanitation, and as plaque-free as possible for disease prevention, should be made. The extent of possible care depends on the appliances; the condition of the lips, tongue, and other oral tissues; and the cooperation of the patient.

Encouragement must be given to the patient to begin toothbrushing as soon as possible after the surgical procedure, but until the patient is able, a plan for care is outlined for a caregiver.

A. Irrigation
1. *Indications.* During the first few days after the surgical procedure, while the mouth may be too tender for brushing, frequent irrigations are required; irrigation also serves as an adjunct to toothbrushing.
2. *Method.* In a hospital, irrigations with suction are possible. At home, the patient irrigates with the head lowered over a sink (pages 381 to 382).
3. *Mouthrinse Selection.* The oral surgeon should be consulted for specific instructions.
   a. Physiologic saline.
   b. Chlorhexidine gluconate (page 386).
   c. Fluoride rinse after toothbrushing, after each meal, and before going to sleep (page 470).

B. Early Mouth Cleansing
Before a toothbrush can be used effectively, a premoistened swab or toothette may be necessary to clean and lubricate the lips, mucosa, and gingiva. Because plaque removal should be attempted as soon as possible, a very soft toothbrush with suction can be applied. The toothbrush with suction is described on pages 764 to 765.

C. Personal Care by the Patient
As soon as possible, the patient is instructed in personal care. A toothbrushing method and other aids, such as those used for orthodontic appliances, are recommended and demonstrated (pages 396 to 397).

Because interdental and proximal tooth-surface care is limited to access only from the facial approach, the choice of devices is limited.[8] Some spaces permit insertion of an interdental brush. With instruction, most patients can use a toothpick in a holder (page 379).

The patient must be shown why care must be taken not to entangle the toothbrush filaments in the wires. When the tongue is not injured, the patient can be instructed to use the tongue as an aid in cleaning the lingual surfaces of the teeth and massaging the gingiva.

The ambulatory patient can use a water irrigator. A low-pressure setting is used, and the spray is directed carefully to prevent tissue injury (pages 381 to 382).

D. After Appliances Are Removed

A step-by-step series of lessons is usually necessary before the patient can carry out adequate plaque control.

A method for daily self-applied fluoride, such as a mouthrinse, brush-on gel, or customized fluoride trays, should be introduced along with the use of a fluoride dentifrice. Demineralization and dental caries can result from plaque retention about the appliances.

DENTAL HYGIENE CARE PRIOR TO GENERAL SURGERY

Completing dental and dental hygiene treatment and bringing the oral cavity to a state of health have special significance for certain patients who will have surgical procedures other than oral. When emergency surgery is performed, preparation of the mouth is not possible, and postsurgical examination and care may be complicated by various limitations.

When surgery is elective, or planned well in advance, the patient can be encouraged to have complete dental and periodontal treatment. Protection against complications related to broken appliances or restorations can be very meaningful to the hospitalized patient. Types of patients are described briefly here. Other examples are found in the various special patient chapters throughout this section of the book.

I. PATIENTS IN WHOM SURGICAL PROCEDURES AFFECT THEIR RISK STATUS

Susceptibility to infection is greatly increased in certain patients, for example, those with prosthetic heart valves, prostheses for joint replacement, and transplanted organs. Patients who receive chemotherapeutic agents as partial treatment after surgery for various types of cancer, and others who use immunosuppressant drugs, require special management to prevent complications during dental and dental hygiene appointments. Antibiotic premedication to prevent infective endocarditis and other infections is mandatory for certain patients (pages 101 to 104).

Prior to surgery for prostheses, transplants, cancer, and other serious conditions, patients can be informed of the need for completing oral care treatments and practicing preventive daily personal care.

II. PREPARATION OF THE MOUTH PRIOR TO GENERAL INHALATION ANESTHESIA

Plaque control and professional instrumentation aid in reducing the oral bacterial count. Because the mouth is an entrance to the respiratory chamber, the possibility always exists that debris and fluids may be inhaled from the mouth. Inhalation could occur during the administration of an anesthetic or when the patient coughs.

III. PATIENT WITH A LONG CONVALESCENCE

Patients whose surgery requires a long convalescence are unable to keep a regular maintenance appointment. When the patient has a healthy mouth before the hospitalization and convalescence, the problems of postsurgical oral care are lessened but not eliminated.

Instruction for the caregiver may be needed. A home visit by the dental hygienist may be possible.

TECHNICAL HINTS

I. WRITTEN CONSENT

Surgical treatment is not provided to minors without consent of parent or guardian. Written consent is mandatory.

II. ACCIDENT PREVENTION

A. Seat Belts

Encourage patients to use the seat belts in their cars. Professional people should set the example by using their own seat belts.

B. Bicycle Helmet

Bicycle accidents are frequent, and serious trauma can result.

REFERENCES

1. **American Dental Association,** Council on Dental Education, Chicago, 1990.
2. **Chuong,** R.: Perioperative Management of the Surgical Patient, in Peterson, L.J., ed.: *Oral and Maxillofacial Surgery.* Philadelphia, J.B. Lippincott Co., 1992, pp. 63–85.
3. **Haskell,** R.: Applied Surgical Anatomy, in Rowe, N.L. and Williams, J.L.: *Maxillofacial Injuries.* London, Churchill Livingstone, 1985, pp. 21–24.
4. **Kruger,** G.O., ed.: *Textbook of Oral and Maxillofacial Surgery,* 6th ed. St. Louis, Mosby, 1984, pp. 364–435.
5. **Luyk,** N.H.: Principles of Management of Fractures of the Mandible, in Peterson, L.J., ed.: *Oral and Maxillofacial Surgery.* Philadelphia, J.B. Lippincott Co., 1992, pp. 407–434.
6. **Boyne**, P.J.: *Osseous Reconstruction of the Maxilla and the Mandible.* Chicago, Quintessence, 1997, pp. 64–74.
7. **Löe,** H., Theilade, E., and Jensen, S.B.: Experimental Gingivitis in Man, *J. Periodontol., 36,* 177, May–June, 1965.
8. **Phelps-Sandall,** B.A. and Oxford, S.J.: Effectiveness of Oral Hygiene Techniques on Plaque and Gingivitis in Patients Placed in Intermaxillary Fixation, *Oral Surg., 56,* 487, November, 1983.

SUGGESTED READINGS

Acton, C.H., Nixon, J.W., and Clark, R.C.: Bicycle Riding and Oral/Maxillofacial Trauma in Young Children, *Med. J. Aust., 165,* 249, September 2, 1996.

Bunn-Minsky, K.C., Hunt, V., Mona, R.A., and Tal, K.: Nutrition of the Hospitalized Patient, in Zambito, R.F., Black, H.A., and

Tesch, L.B., eds.: *Hospital Dentistry. Practice and Education.* St. Louis, Mosby, 1997, pp. 243–282.

Costello, B.J., Betts, N.J., Barber, H.D., and Fonseca, R.J.: Preprosthetic Surgery for the Edentulous Patient, *Dent. Clin. North Am., 40,* 19, January, 1996.

Ehrlich, A. and Torres, H.O.: *Essentials of Dental Assisting.* Philadelphia, W.B. Saunders Co., 1992, pp. 505–578.

Fun-Chee, L. and Shanmuhasuntharam, P.: A Simple Method to Enable Feeding During Maxillomandibular Fixation of the Jaws, *Oral Surg. Oral Med. Oral Pathol., 75,* 549, May, 1993.

Hollinger, J. and Wong, M.E.K.: The Integrated Processes of Hard Tissue Regeneration with Special Emphasis on Fracture Healing, *Oral Surg. Oral Med. Oral Pathol. Oral Radiol. Endod., 82,* 594, December, 1996.

Holman, A.R., Brumer, S., Ware, W.H., and Pasta, D.J.: The Impact of Interpersonal Support on Patient Satisfaction with Orthognathic Surgery, *J. Oral Maxillofac. Surg., 53,* 1289, November, 1995.

Kaban, L.B.: Diagnosis and Treatment of Fractures of the Facial Bones in Children 1943–1993, *J. Oral Maxillofac. Surg., 51,* 722, July, 1993.

Ramsey, W.O.: Valved Feeding Devices: Adjuncts in Rehabilitation of the Oral Phase of Swallowing, *Int. J. Periodontics Restorative Dent., 10,* 321, No. 4, 1990.

Schmidt, B., Kearns, G., Perrott, D., and Kaban, L.B.: Infection Following Treatment of Mandibular Fractures in Human Immunodeficiency Virus Seropositive Patients, *J. Oral Maxillofac. Surg., 53,* 1134, October, 1995.

Shetty, V. and Freymiller, E.: Teeth in the Line of Fracture: A Review, *J. Oral Maxillofac. Surg., 47,* 1303, December, 1989.

Mandibular Fracture

Bavitz, J.B. and Collicott, P.E.: Bilateral Mandibular Subcondylar Fractures Contributing to Airway Obstruction, *Int. J. Oral Maxillofac. Surg., 24,* 273, August, 1995.

Eyrich, G.K.H., Grätz, K.W., and Sailer, H.F.: Surgical Treatment of Fractures of the Edentulous Mandible, *J. Oral Maxillofac. Surg., 55,* 1081, October, 1997.

Iannetti, G. and Cascone, P.: Use of Rigid External Fixation in Fractures of the Mandibular Condyle, *Oral Surg. Oral Med. Oral Pathol. Oral Radiol. Endod., 80,* 394, October, 1995.

Shonberg, D.C., Stith, H.D., Jameson, L.M., and Chai, J.Y.: Mandibular Fracture Through an Endosseous Implant, *Int. J. Oral Maxillofac. Implants, 7,* 401, Fall, 1992.

Thorén, H., Iizuka, T., Hallikainen, D., and Lindqvist, C.: Different Patterns of Mandibular Fractures in Children. An Analysis of 220 Fractures in 157 Patients, *J. Craniomaxillofac. Surg., 20,* 292, October, 1992.

Tolman, D.E. and Keller, E.E.: Management of Mandibular Fractures in Patients with Endosseous Implants, *Int. J. Oral Maxillofac. Implants, 6,* 427, Winter, 1991.

Tuovinen, V., van Steenis, K., and Sindet-Pedersen, S.: Internal Fixation of a Mandibular Fracture in a 6-month-old Girl—A Case Report, *Int. J. Oral Maxillofac. Surg., 24,* 210, June, 1995.

The Patient With Cancer

Care of the cancer patient before, during, and after therapy has as its main purposes attaining and maintaining oral health at the highest possible level and contributing to the patient's general and mental health. The patient may be under the care of a team of specialists, including the dentist, oral surgeon, dental hygienist, oncologist, nurse, dietitian, and pharmacist. Special rehabilitation personnel, such as a plastic surgeon, psychiatrist, speech therapist, physical therapist, maxillofacial prosthodontist, and social worker are frequently involved.

Oral cancers (pages 124 to 126) and leukemias (pages 874 to 876) are forms of cancer that have par-

ticular relevance, because the cancers themselves and their treatment modalities (radiation, chemotherapy, surgery, and transplantation) have significant effects on the oral tissues. In Box 49-1, terminology relating to cancer is defined.

DESCRIPTION

Cancer refers to a group of neoplastic diseases in which there is transformation of normal body cells into malignant ones. As cancer cells proliferate, the

BOX 49-1 KEY WORDS: Cancer

Alopecia (al-ō-pē′shē-ah): a loss of hair.

Anaplasia (an″ah-plā′zē-ah): an irreversible alteration in adult cells toward more primitive (embryonic) cell types; characteristic of tumor cells.

Benign (bē-nīn′): not malignant; not recurrent; remains localized; favorable for recovery (Table 49-1).

Carcinogen (kar″-sin′ō-jen): an agent that may cause cancer; may be chemical, physical (ionizing radiation), or biologic; biologic carcinogens may be external (for example, viruses) or internal (genetic defects).

Carcinoma (kar″sĭ-nō′mah): a malignant tumor of epithelial origin.

Chemotherapy (kē-mō-ther′ah-pē): treatment of illness by chemical means, that is, by medication or drugs.

Dysgeusia (dis-gū′zē-ah): distortion of the sense of taste.

Dysplasia (dis-pla′ze-ah): an abnormality of development; in pathology, alteration in size, shape, and organization of adult cells.

Endoscopy (en-dos′kō-pē): visual examination of interior structures of the body with an endoscope.

Hematologic profile (hē-mah-tō-loj′ĭk): an analysis of the blood and blood-forming tissues (for normal blood values see Table 59-2, page 868).

Hematopoiesis (hē-mah-tō-poi-ē′sĭs): formation and development of blood cells.

Hyperbaric oxygen (hī-per-bar′ĭk): the patient is placed in a sealed chamber and given pure oxygen through a face mask. At the same time, compressed air is introduced into the chamber to raise the atmospheric pressure to several times normal. This equalizes the pressure inside and outside of the body, thereby flooding the tissues with oxygen. An increase in oxygen to the irradiated tissues can temporarily compensate for the reduction in circulation.

Imaging (im′ah-jing): the production of diagnostic images, including radiography, ultrasonography, or scintigraphy.

Infiltration (in-fil-trā′shun): the diffusion or accumulation in a tissue of cells or substances not normal to it or in amounts in excess of normal; in leukemia, for example, white blood cells infiltrate body tissues.

Infusion (in-fū′zhun): slow therapeutic introduction of fluid other than blood into a vein; infusion flows by gravity.

In situ (in si′tū): in its normal place; confined to the site of origin.

Interstitial (in″ter-stish′al): pertaining to, or situated in, the interstices (small spaces) of a tissue.

Intrathecal (in″trah-thē′kal): within a sheath; through the theca of the spinal cord into the subarachnoid space; in leukemia, for example, the location for the delivery of various chemotherapeutic drugs.

Isogenic (ī″sō-jen′ik): having the same genetic constitution; syngeneic.

Leukemia (loo-kē′mē-ah): an acute or chronic progressive malignant neoplasm of the blood-forming organs, marked by diffuse proliferation of immature white blood cells (leukocytes); subsequent reduction in erythrocytes and platelets results.

Lymphadenectomy (lĭmfad″e-něk′tō-mē): excision of one or more lymph nodes.

Malignant (mah-lig′nant): tending to become progressively worse and to result in death; having the properties of anaplasia, invasiveness, and metastasis; said of tumors (Table 49-1).

Metastasis (mě-tas′tah-sis): transfer of disease from one organ or part to another not directly connected with it; for example, regional or distant spread of cancer cells from the site primarily involved.

Neoplasm (nē′ō-plazm): any new and abnormal growth, specifically one in which cell multiplication is controlled and progressive; may be benign or malignant.

Oncology (ong-kol′ō-jē): the sum of knowledge regarding tumors: the study of tumors.

Palliative (păl′ē-ā″tiv): affording relief; but does not cure.

Pancytopenia (pan″sī-tō-pē′nē-ah): abnormal depression of all cellular elements of the blood.

Pleomorphism (plē″ō-mor′fism): occurrence in more than one form; the assumption of various distinct morphologic types by a single organism or cell.

Radiotherapy (radiation therapy): the treatment of disease by ionizing radiation; may be external megavoltage or internal by use of interstitial implantation of an isotope (radium).

Radium (rā′dē-um): a highly radioactive chemical element found in uranium minerals; used in the treatment of malignant tumors in the form of needles or pellets for interstitial implantation.

(continued)

BOX 49-I KEY WORDS: Cancer (Continued)

Radon (rā'don): radioactive element produced by the disintegration of radium and is used in radiotherapy; referred to as **radium emanation.**

Relapse (rē'-laps): the return of a disease weeks or months after its apparent cessation.

Remission (rē-mish'un): diminution or abatement of the symptoms of a disease; the period during which such diminution occurs.

Sarcoma (sar-kō'mah): a tumor, often highly malignant, composed of cells derived from connective tissue such as bone and cartilage, muscle, blood vessel, or lymphoid tissue.

Staging (stāj'ing): the succinct, standardized description of a tumor with regard to origin and spread. This clinical classification is based on physical assessments, biopsy, imaging, endoscopy. Each stage (I–IV) consists of three components: T (size of tumor); N (lymph node involvement); and M (presence or absence of distant metastasis).

Trismus (triz'mus): limitations of opening because of spasm and/or fibrosis of the muscles of mastication and/or temporomandibular joint located in the field of radiation.

---

mass of abnormal tissue that is formed enlarges and sheds cells that spread the disease locally or to distant sites (metastasis). Characteristics of benign and malignant neoplasms are compared in Table 49-1.

There are numerous types of cancers. They are classified on the basis of the (1) origin of the tissue involved, that is, carcinomas from epithelial tissue, and sarcomas from connective tissue; and (2) type of cell from which they arise, namely, an epithelial or connective tissue cell.[1]

I. INCIDENCE

Cancer is the second leading cause of death in the

TABLE 49-1 Characteristics of Benign and Malignant Neoplasms

Characteristic	Benign	Malignant
Cell Characteristics	Cells resemble normal cells of the tissue from which the tumor originated	Cells often bear little resemblance to the normal cells of the tissue from which they arose; there is both anaplasia and pleomorphism
Mode of Growth	Tumor grows by expansion and does not infiltrate the surrounding tissues; encapsulated	Tumor grows at the periphery and sends out processes that infiltrate and destroy the surrounding tissues
Rate of Growth	Rate of growth is usually slow	Rate of growth is usually relatively rapid and is dependent on level of differentiation; the more anaplastic the tumor, the more rapid the rate of growth
Metastasis	Does not spread by metastasis	Gains access to the blood and lymph channels and metastasizes to other areas of the body
Recurrence	Does not recur when removed	Tends to recur when removed
General Effects	Is usually a localized phenomenon that does not cause generalized effects unless by location it interferes with vital functions	Often causes generalized effects, such as anemia, weakness, and weight loss
Destruction of Tissue	Does not usually cause tissue damage unless location interferes with blood flow	Often causes extensive tissue damage as the tumor outgrows its blood supply or encroaches on blood flow to the area; may also produce substances that cause cell damage
Ability to Cause Death	Does not usually cause death unless its location interferes with vital functions	Usually causes death unless growth can be controlled

(From Porth, C., *Pathophysiology: Concepts of Altered Health States,* 2nd ed. Philadelphia, J.B. Lippincott Co., 1986.)

United States. The three most commonly diagnosed cancers among women involve the breast, lung and bronchus, and colon and rectum. Among men, the most common cancers are of the prostate, lung and bronchus, and colon and rectum.[2]

A. Survival Rates

A cured patient is one that shows no evidence of disease and has the same life expectancy as a person who has never had cancer. Most forms of cancer are considered cured after survival for 5 years without symptoms following treatment.

B. Oral Cancer

Oral/pharyngeal cancers annually account for 3.3% of cancers in men and 1.6% in females.[2] The incidence rate for oral/pharyngeal cancer is about 1.5 times higher in African Americans than in whites. The overall mortality rate has declined slightly over the past 15 years. The 5-year survival rate for posterior oral structures such as the pharynx is lower than that for anterior oral structures, namely the lip.[3] Approximately 90% of all oral carcinomas are of the squamous cell type. They spread by local extension and the lymphatic system.

C. Leukemia

Many new cases of leukemia occur annually. Slightly more than half of the cases occur in males. An equal number of leukemia cases are chronic as are acute in type. Cancer is the leading cause of death in children aged 1 to 14; approximately one third of the deaths occur from leukemia.[3]

II. ETIOLOGY AND PREDISPOSING FACTORS

Although the etiologic factors of cancer are not known, extensive research is being conducted. Several factors predispose an individual to cancer formation. Implicated have been weakened immunity, a history of syphilis and other infections, diet, and tobacco. Table 49-2 lists the sites of cancer and their risk factors.

A. Risk Factors For Oral Cancer[3]

1. Excessive use of alcohol and tobacco in combination. Chronic alcoholic persons have more lesions of the tongue and floor of the mouth than of other locations of the oral cavity.
2. Long-term exposure to the chemical carcinogens of tobacco (smoking or smokeless).
3. Poor oral hygiene, particularly in chronic alcohol and tobacco users.
4. Overexposure to sunlight. Persons with occupations requiring outdoor activity in the sun and weather have a higher risk for developing lip cancer.

TABLE 49-2 Risk Factors for Cancer

Agent	Sites of Cancer
Tobacco related	Lung, bladder, kidney, renal pelvis, pancreas, cervix
Tobacco and alcohol related	Oral cavity, esophagus
Diet related	High fat, low fiber, low in vegetables & fruits—large bowel, breast, pancreas, prostate, ovary, endometrium Pickled, salted foods, low in vegetables & fruits—stomach Alcohol, certain mushrooms—liver, esophagus
Bacterial	*Helicobacter pylori*—stomach
Sunlight	Skin (melanoma)
Occupational	Various carcinogens—bladder, liver, other organs
Lifestyle and Occupation	Tobacco and asbestos; tobacco and mining; tobacco and uranium and radium—lung, respiratory tract
Iatrogenic	Radiation, drugs—diverse organs, leukemia
Genetic	Retinoblastoma, soft-tissue sarcomas
Viral	Human T-cell lymphotropic virus type I (HTLV-1); adult T-cell lymphoma; human papillomavirus—cervix, penis, anus
Origin Uncertain	Lymphomas, leukemias, sarcomas, cervical cancer

(Adapted from the *American Cancer Society Cancer Statistics*, 1998[2], and the *Textbook of Clinical Oncology*, 1995, p. 18.[3])

B. **Risk Factors For Leukemia[3]**
1. Radiation.
2. Toxic exposure to chemicals, namely benzene.
3. Previous bone marrow disorders.
4. Congenital disorders such as Down's syndrome (pages 814 to 816).

PREPARATION FOR TREATMENT

Time may be a factor for the patient with advanced malignancy. Once the extent and severity of the cancer has been ascertained, or staging has been completed, as is the case with tumors of the head and neck, the type and length of therapy can be determined and initiated. Basic preparation follows the same general outline as described on pages 709 to 711 for a patient undergoing oral surgery.

I. OBJECTIVES

The aim in preparation of a patient for the treatment of cancer is to restore the mouth to optimal health prior to radiation, chemotherapy, surgery, or bone marrow transplantation. The objectives of preparing a patient for treatment include steps to:
A. Assess the oral cavity.
B. Eliminate sources of infection.
C. Motivate the patient in preventive oral care measures.
D. Reduce the oral microbial count.
E. Provide a better environment for therapeutic procedures.
F. Improve the conditions for healing.

II. ORAL FINDINGS

The extent and severity of the oral side effects of cancer therapy are related to the condition of the teeth and soft tissues before therapy and the patient's hematologic profile. If some or all of the following oral findings are encountered they must be corrected prior to therapy:
A. Extensive carious lesions.
B. Retained root tips.
C. Periodontal involvement.
D. Ill-fitting prostheses (partial or complete dentures).
E. Orthodontic appliances that cause excessive irritation may require removal or wax coverage to protect soft tissues.
F. Poor oral hygiene.

DENTAL/DENTAL HYGIENE TREATMENT PLAN[4,3]

Dental procedures, such as tooth removal, periodontal surgery, and endodontic treatment, that could open a channel for infection to reach the bone or systemic circulation are contraindicated during cancer therapy and, in the case of radiation, after therapy as well. When consideration is given to proper preparation of the oral cavity prior to cancer therapy and supervision of preventive measures continues during and after therapy, the incidence of harmful effects can be minimized.

The patient's total treatment plan prior to the initiation of therapy should include at least the following:

I. ASSESSMENT

A complete oral and dental assessment must be performed to establish a baseline for measuring changes and evaluating the effectiveness of oral care. Areas of assessment should include:
A. Oral–facial soft tissue.
B. Hard tissues for dental caries, impacted teeth, ill-fitting prostheses.
C. Periodontium for presence of deposits on the teeth, probing depths, bone loss.
D. Amount and consistency of saliva.
E. Previous history of oral complications associated with cancer therapy.
F. Cultures performed before and throughout treatment when it is suspected that a patient is exhibiting an oral mucosal infection, such as *Candidiasis*.

II. PREVENTION PROGRAM

A. Bacterial Plaque Control
1. Start oral hygiene instruction at first appointment.
2. Emphasize preventive infection control procedures and potential oral side effects associated with cancer therapy.

B. Daily Fluoride Therapy
1. Indicated for patients about to undergo head and neck radiation therapy, if the salivary glands are in the field of radiation.
2. Make impressions and fabricate custom fluoride trays.
3. Advise patient to apply custom trays lined with 1.1% neutral sodium fluoride gel to the teeth for 4 minutes once daily or use brush-on method, if trays are not feasible.
4. Advise patient to refrain from eating, drinking, or rinsing for 30 minutes following tray removal.

C. Dietary Instructions
1. Instruct patient or caregiver in the preparation of foods in a blender.
2. Avoid highly cariogenic or spicy foods.

D. Avoid Alcohol and Smoking

III. PERIODONTAL THERAPY

A. Complete scaling and root debridement.
B. Perform surgical procedures when time permits follow-up for healing.
C. Adjust occlusion when necessary.

IV. RESTORATION OF CARIOUS LESIONS

A. Restore all clinically and radiographically detected caries.

B. Remove all overhanging margins.

C. Finish and polish all restorations.

D. Seal newly erupted teeth.

V. PROSTHODONTIC THERAPY

A. Correct ill-fitting prostheses.

B. Instruct patient to leave prostheses out of the mouth as much as possible once therapy has begun.

C. Fabricate new prostheses 3 to 6 months after radiation.

D. Motivate patient to maintain meticulous denture hygiene.[6]

1. Dentures should be cleansed and soaked in an antimicrobial solution overnight.

2. Disposable cups should be used to soak the denture.

3. Denture adhesives should be avoided.

VI. REMOVAL OF NONRESTORABLE TEETH

A. Indications

Extensively involved teeth may need extraction because of severe bone loss, mobility, and other signs of advanced periodontal infection, large carious lesions with pulpal exposures not conducive to endodontic therapy, or periapical radiographic findings.

B. Rationale

In the past, treatment frequently called for complete extraction of all teeth that would be in the pathway of radiation whether or not they were broken down or diseased. Now, only teeth that are definitely beyond saving or loose primary teeth are removed.

C. Healing

Alveoloplasty to remove bone spicules is necessary. A healing period of at least 10 to 14 days should be allowed before starting radiation therapy, because when bone is irradiated, healing and remodeling cease.

VII. SURGICAL PROCEDURES

Removal of residual root tips, gingival opercula which have the potential to trap food debris and become infected, and other subsurface pathologic areas that are found in radiographs of edentulous areas is advised.

VIII. ENDODONTIC THERAPY

Endodontic therapy for essential abutment teeth may be necessary. Treatment planning for prosthetic replacements must be done in advance so that abutment teeth can receive proper treatment before radiation therapy.

RADIATION THERAPY[7,8]

Therapeutic radiation may be the only treatment for oral cancer or it may be used in conjunction with surgery.

I. OBJECTIVES

A. As a Total Treatment

Exposures are usually given as daily doses, made in fractions of the total dose.

B. In Conjunction With Surgery

1. *Preoperatively.* To reduce the size of the neoplasm as an aid to surgery by limiting the surgical area.

2. *Postoperatively.* To control residual disease.

II. TYPES

A. External Beam

1. *Orthovoltage.* Low-yield radiation may be used for superficial lesions, such as lip lesions or small lesions in the oral cavity, where radiation is applied by an intraoral cone.

2. *Mega- or Supervoltage.* High-yield radiation includes cobalt-60 and the linear accelerator. It has a spraying effect on skull and bone and less scatter radiation to surrounding tissues than does orthovoltage. Divided doses are given over 6 to 8 weeks on an outpatient appointment plan.

3. *Field of Radiation.* Areas of application. Figure 49-1 illustrates exposure areas for external irradiation. The neoplasms and regional lymph nodes cannot be exposed without radiation also going to the oral cavity, salivary glands, maxilla, and mandible. The side effects to the exposed normal tissues are induced by the unwanted radiation.

B. Internal: Interstitial Implant

The source of radiation is placed within the body. Less radiation is delivered to surrounding tissues than when an external source is utilized. Radium needles and radioactive radon and gold seeds are used.

III. DOSAGE AND DURATION

A. Dosage

The dosage of radiation therapy may range from 3,000 to > 7,000 centigray (cGy) for a 3- to 8-week period.

B. Factors Affecting Duration

1. Tumor type and location.

2. Single or combination therapy.

3. Patient's ability to tolerate therapy.

4. Infiltration of cancer cells into CNS.

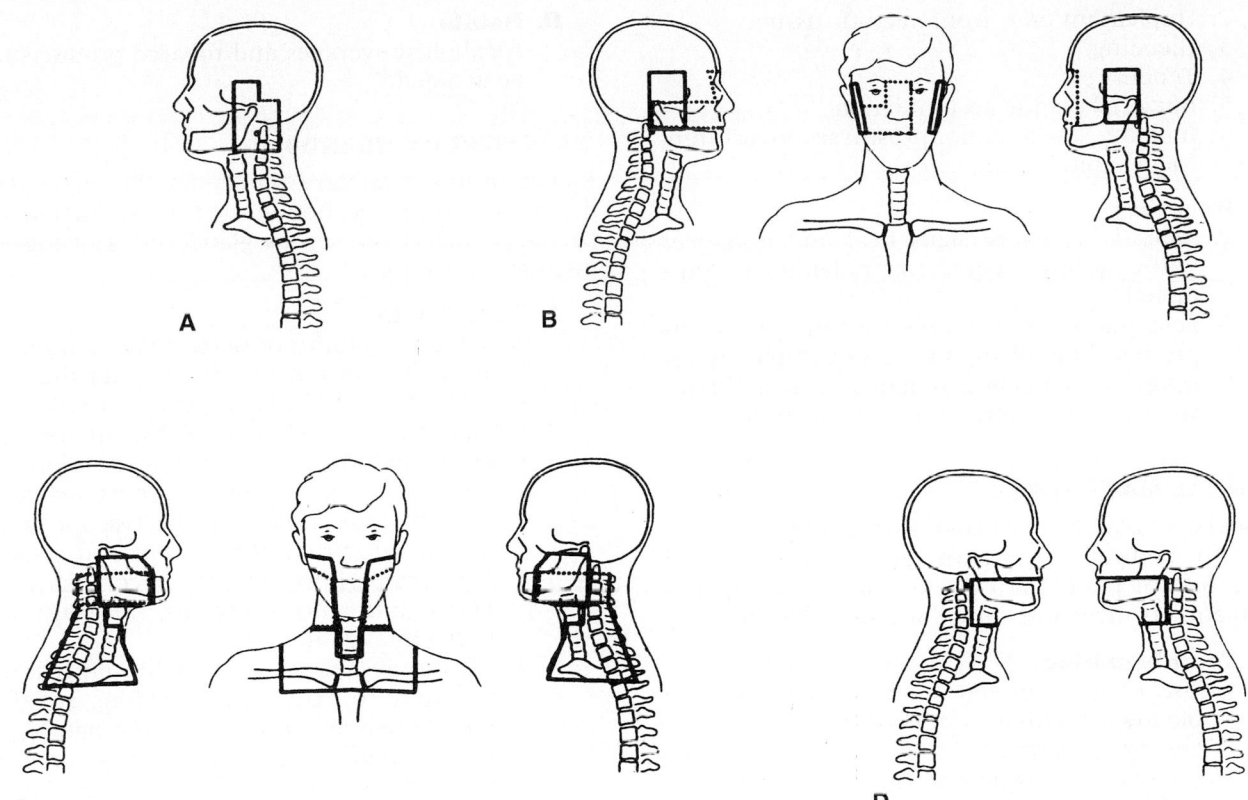

FIGURE 49-1 Common Fields of Radiation for Head and Neck Tumors. Dotted lines show fields when increased dosages are needed. **(A)** Parotid field. **(B)** Antrum field. **(C)** Oropharynx field. **(D)** Floor of mouth field. (From Jansma, J.: *Oral Sequelae Resulting from Head and Neck Radiotherapy.* Groningen, Drukkerij van Denderen B.V., 1991.)

ORAL EFFECTS OF RADIATION THERAPY AND MANAGEMENT[4,9–14]

Irradiation is the exposure of tissues to electromagnetic radiation (e.g., heat, light, x rays). The purpose is to destroy cancerous cells. Damage to surrounding normal tissue cannot be avoided, but the severity of damage can be minimized.

I. TISSUE CHANGES

Ionizing radiation induces tissue changes, some of which are apparent during the treatment period and may continue for a few weeks or months after cessation of irradiation. Other changes may not be evident until after treatment and may have long-term significance. Therefore, the patient should be seen often during therapy (at least once weekly), and indefinitely following therapy.

A. Onset: Early Changes (damage to exposed tissues in the field of radiation with rapid cell turnover rates)
1. Dermatitis.
2. Mucositis.
3. Alopecia.
4. Reduced salivary flow.

B. Late Changes (damage to exposed tissues in the field of radiation with slow turnover rates)
1. Xerostomia.
2. "Radiation Caries."
3. Osteoradionecrosis.
4. Trismus.

II. MUCOSA

A. Inflammatory Changes
1. *Time Sequence.* Inflammation of the mucosa usually occurs 1 to 2 weeks after the onset of radiation therapy.
2. *Severity.* Effects of radiation are more severe in patients with susceptible oral tissues secondary to alcoholism and/or heavy smoking.

B. Cellular Changes
1. *Initial Inflammatory Response.* Edema of the tissues is noted first, followed by ulcerations and necrosis with sloughing.
2. *Latent Response.* Fibrosis develops as a result of chronic inflammation.

C. Clinical Signs
1. Sensitivity to pressure and temperature extremes.

2. Unpleasant odor from necrotic tissue.
3. Bleeding.
4. Tenderness.
5. Bacterial plaque accumulation.
6. Inability to tolerate prostheses over thin, fragile epithelium.

D. Recovery

1. *Immediate.* Severe signs heal and disappear within a few weeks after radiation is completed.
2. *Long Range.* Thin, fragile mucosa with compromised blood supply never completely recovers and healing remains difficult in response to exposure to future infections.

III. ORAL MANAGEMENT

Personal care may be neglected because of preoccupation with medical concerns or sensitivity of the oral tissues, but the patient must be urged to be compliant with plaque control and daily fluoride application.

A. Toothbrushing

1. Use of a super-soft toothbrush to remove plaque is highly recommended.
2. Lemon-glycerine swabs are ineffective in the removal of plaque and may further dry the oral mucosa.
3. A flavored dentifrice may not be tolerated, but a dentifrice containing fluoride is essential.

B. Mouthrinses

1. Rinsing with a baking soda/saline solution throughout the day followed by a plain water rinse is suggested. Salt may be eliminated.
2. Chlorhexidine rinsing may also be recommended to reduce inflammation, particularly when mechanical plaque control methods are compromised owing to mucositis pain.
3. Commercial mouthwashes with high alcohol content should be avoided owing to their drying and irritating effects.
4. Hydrogen peroxide should be diluted with water to a 1:4 concentration. Use of hydrogen peroxide 3% should be limited to short-term use to prevent disruption of the normal oral flora.
5. Gauze or a tooth sponge may be employed as a vehicle for applying rinsing agents to the teeth and sensitive oral soft tissues.

C. Diet

1. Topical anesthetic or anti-inflammatory rinses, ointments, or gels may be applied as needed or before eating to alleviate mucositis pain.
2. Liquids are needed with meals to moisten food for swallowing.
3. A soft, bland, noncariogenic diet eaten at a low temperature is recommended.

D. Habits

Alcoholic beverages and tobacco products must be avoided.[15]

IV. SALIVARY GLANDS

Radiation to the salivary glands may be unavoidable, depending on the location of the tumor. The radiation primarily affects the serous gland cells causing a reduction in secretion.

A. Xerostomia

A reduced quantity of saliva may be noticed as early as the third or fourth day after the beginning of radiation, thus decreasing the self-cleansing ability of the oral cavity. Subsequent candidiasis or periodontal infections may develop.

1. *Changes in Saliva.* Saliva is more acidic and viscous, thus increasing the risk for enamel demineralization. Mastication and swallowing become impaired by the combination of xerostomia and mucositis, making nutritional intake difficult.
2. *Changes in Mucosa.* Dry friable mucosa may be prone to cracks and bleeding, creating a portal of entry for infection. The patient who wears a denture may be unable to tolerate it because of a reduced surface tension between the dry mucosa and the prosthesis.

B. Management

1. *Pilocarpine Therapy.* This parasympathomimetic drug has been shown to be effective in relieving symptoms of xerostomia and improving salivary flow when given in a dosage of 5–10 mg 3 to 4 times daily.[16-19]
2. *Saliva Substitutes.* Adjunctive artificial salivas with fluoride may be used as often as needed to provide temporary relief from xerostomia. The only contraindication is if the patient is on a low sodium diet. The patient should be instructed to spray directly on the tissues, or if in gel form, place a drop or two in the mouth and spread around with the tongue.
3. *Water and Ice Chips.* Frequent sips of water or sucking on ice chips help to alleviate xerostomia on a short-term basis.
4. *Diet.* The patient should be advised to eat moist foods, chew sugarless gum, and avoid sucking on lozenges or candy with sugar to moisten the mouth.
5. *Humidify Air.* Humidifiers can be used to manage dry air at home, particularly during the winter months when the house is heated.

V. TEETH

A. Radiation Caries

1. *Description.* Teeth with exposed root surfaces are especially susceptible. The lesions develop in the gingival third and gradually encircle the necks of the teeth (Figure 14-4,

page 242). The carious lesions appear black or dark brown.

2. *Predisposing Factors.* Xerostomia, neglect of plaque control measures, soft cariogenic diet, sore mouth, and changes in oral flora are responsible, not radiation directly.

3. *Prevention.* Intensified preventive measures involving daily fluoride application, bacterial plaque control, and noncariogenic diet are warranted. The use of a saliva substitute containing fluoride is also indicated (page 728).

B. Tooth Development

Radiation in children can affect the odontogenic cells. A tooth bud may be completely destroyed if irradiated before mineralization has started.[20]

C. Sensitivity of Teeth

Teeth with dental caries are particularly sensitive, but all teeth may react to temperature extremes. Daily fluoride therapy and tooth sensitivity dentifrices with fluoride will also lessen tooth sensitivity. Extreme hot or cold foods should be avoided.

VI. INFECTIONS

A. Fungal

Candidiasis is the most common oral infection during or after radiation therapy. The increase in *Candida* infection is related to hyposalivation and the changed composition of the saliva. Fungal infections should be treated with an antifungal agent, ideally one that does not contain sugar.

B. Bacterial

Radiation leaves the patient with susceptible oral tissues. Gram-negative bacilli increase and are often related to the secondary infections occurring in the later stages of ulcerative mucositis.

VII. BONE: OSTEORADIONECROSIS

Radiation damages bone cells and blood vessels within the bone. Changes in the endothelial cells lead to sclerosis of the vessels. The result is change in the growth potential of the bone and lowered resistance to infection.

A. Portals of Entry for Infection

1. Mucosal ulceration.
2. Bacterial plaque.
3. Deep periodontal pockets.
4. Periapical lesion.
5. Open socket from tooth extraction.

B. Signs

1. Pain.
2. Trismus.
3. Exposed bone, sequestration, pathologic fracture.
4. Suppuration.
5. Halitosis.

C. Management

Administration of a series of hyperbaric oxygen treatments to facilitate healing of the compromised bone is the treatment for osteoradionecrosis. Advanced cases may involve extended antibiotic therapy and surgery for the removal of the sequestra, or even part of the mandible.[21-24]

D. Prevention

Correct pre- and postradiation procedures have had a definite effect on lowering the incidence of osteoradionecrosis. Maintenance of oral cleanliness and health are contributing preventive factors.

E. Development

Children who receive radiation to the developing facial bones may experience altered craniofacial growth.[20]

VIII. DYSGEUSIA

A. Changes

Taste can be altered or lost by degeneration of taste buds or by changes in the quantity of saliva.

B. Duration

Altered taste may begin as early as the first 200–400 cGy. Taste acuity is usually regained in 2 to 4 months after therapy, if saliva flow is adequate.

C. Management

Taste aversions should be considered if a person other than the patient is responsible for preparing meals. Meats, for example may, elicit a metallic taste. Dietary supplements of zinc have been recommended to alleviate taste disturbances.[21]

IX. LOSS OF APPETITE

A. Factors

1. Sore mouth; alteration in taste.
2. Diminished saliva; inability to wear prostheses.
3. Depression.

B. Sequelae

1. Dehydration; weight loss.
2. Impaired healing.
3. Fatigue.

X. TRISMUS

A. Duration

Trismus may occur 3 to 6 months after therapy has stopped. Opening of the mouth is difficult and often painful. Oral care, eating, and speaking may be adversely affected.

B. Management

Exercises and stretching appliances have been used for treatment.

POSTRADIATION THERAPY[4,5,13]

When radiation therapy has been completed and the acute oral side effects have resolved, dental hygiene care must continue on a routine basis to eliminate the risk of infection. The risk of osteoradionecrosis in the patient who has undergone radiation therapy persists throughout life. The dental hygienist's contribution to the oral health success after radiation therapy is as significant as the care and supervision required before and during therapy.

I. DENTAL HYGIENE ASSESSMENT AND CARE PLAN

A. Evaluate Periodontal Health
1. Complete periodontal examination with charting
2. Assess bacterial plaque control and provide additional motivation and instruction
3. Perform scaling and root debridement

B. Examine and Chart Dental Caries
1. Review home fluoride program
2. Administer topical application

C. Assess Salivary Flow
Review care plan for xerostomia.

D. Counsel in Dietary Practices

E. Manage Additional Effects of the Radiation Therapy

F. Make Referrals for Dental Treatment

G. Arrange Frequent Maintenance Appointments

II. DENTAL TREATMENT FOLLOW-UP

A. New or Routine Adjustment of Prostheses

B. Restoration of Carious Lesions

C. Extractions
If extraction is the only option to manage extensive dental or periodontal disease, hyperbaric oxygen therapy before and after tooth removal, antibiotic prophylaxis, and meticulous surgical technique are warranted.

D. Extraction Alternative: Endodontic therapy

E. Implants Preceded by Hyperbaric Oxygen Therapy[25,26]

CHEMOTHERAPY[13,14,27-30]

Chemotherapeutic agents destroy or deactivate rapidly dividing cancer cells with as little destruction of normal cells as possible. Side effects from the drugs are significant and frequently involve the oral tissues.

I. OBJECTIVES
A. Control widely scattered neoplasms.
B. Supplement surgery and/or radiation.
C. Palliative care for patients with advanced squamous cell carcinomas of the head and neck.[21]

II. TYPES OF CHEMOTHERAPEUTIC AGENTS[31]

A. Categories (Table 49-3)

B. Use: Single or combination therapy

III. SYSTEMIC SIDE EFFECTS OF CHEMOTHERAPY

Rapidly proliferating normal cells are susceptible to the suppression action of chemotherapeutic agents. The most common side effects include:
A. Alopecia.
B. Myelosuppression (bone marrow suppression causing a reduction in blood counts leading to anemia, leukopenia, and thrombocytopenia).
C. Immunosuppression (inhibition of antibody responses resultant from leukopenia).
D. Nausea and vomiting, diarrhea.
E. Loss of appetite.

IV. ORAL EFFECTS OF CHEMOTHERAPY AND MANAGEMENT[32]

For chemotherapy-induced oral complications identical to those encountered in the patient undergoing head and neck radiation, follow the management recommendations outlined on page 728, and Table 49-4.

A. Factors Affecting Severity of Oral Effects
1. Dosage and duration of drugs administered.
2. Patient's age.
3. Patient's oral health status and dietary habits.
4. Patient's systemic condition/hematologic profile.

B. Direct Cytotoxic Effects
Chemotherapy drugs act on the oral structures.
1. Ulcerative mucositis.
2. Transient xerostomia.
3. Jaw pain.
4. Abnormal enamel and root development.[20]
5. Delayed eruption.[20]

C. Indirect Cytotoxic Effects
Chemotherapy drugs act indirectly on the oral tissues; caused by myelosuppression.

TABLE 49-3 Categories of Cancer Chemotherapy Drugs
Alkylating Agents
Antibiotics
Antimetabolites
Plant Alkaloids
Steroids/Hormones
Miscellaneous

TABLE 49-4 Oral Complications of Cancer Therapy and Their Management

Oral Side Effects	Source	Management
Fungal Infections	Prescription	Amphotericin B Nystatin Clotrimazole Ketoconazole Fluconazole
Viral Infections	Prescription	Acyclovir Penciclovir
Bacterial Infections	Prescription	Peridex® Procter & Gamble Periogard® Colgate

Ulcerations/Mucositis	Prescription	Dyclonine HCl
		Clark's solution
		   Maalox
		   Bonodryl
		   Lidocaine
		Topical Steroids
		   Sucralfate

	OTC	Kank-A®—Blistex Orabase-B®—Colgate Orajel®—Del Pharmaceuticals Tanac®—Del Pharmaceuticals Zilactin®—Zila Pharmaceuticals
Xerostomia	Prescription	Pilocarpine, Fluorides
	OTC	Biotene®—Laclede Optimoist®—Colgate Moi-stir®—Kingswood Labs Glandosane®—Kenwood Labs Salivart®—Gebauer Co.
Bleeding	Prescription	Collacote®—Calcitek, Inc. Gelfoam®—Pharmacia & Upjohn, Inc. Instat®—Johnson & Johnson Surgicel®—Johnson & Johnson Thrombogen®—Johnson & Johnson

1. Hemorrhage
   a. Gingival bleeding.
   b. Oral petechiae and ecchymoses.
2. Infection
   a. Bacterial (gram-negative, *Pseudomonas, Klebsiella, Proteus, E. coli, Serratia,* or *Enterobacter*).
   b. Viral (herpes simplex).
   c. Fungal (*Candida*).

V. ORAL CARE

A. Scheduling
Appoint patient and determine need for antibiotic prophylaxis in consultation with the oncologist. The best time to schedule treatment is after the patient's blood counts have recovered, usually just prior to the next course of chemotherapy.

B. Blood Counts
Request blood values the day before or the day of the dental appointment to confirm the patient can be treated. For normal blood values see Tables 59-1 and 59-2 (pages 867 and 868).

C. Platelet Transfusions[4]
Platelet replacement may be necessary prior to any dental procedures if the platelet count is less than 40,000/mm³.

D. Antibiotic Prophylaxis
The granulocyte count and the presence of an

indwelling catheter may suggest the need for antibiotic coverage prior to dental procedures.

VI. PREVENTION

A. Recommend use of super-soft toothbrush and frequent rinsing.
B. Disinfect brush with chlorhexidine; change toothbrush often.
C. Prevent mucosal lacerations with subsequent bacteremia during periods of profound neutropenia and thrombocytopenia: avoid using toothpicks, irrigating devices, floss, and eating crunchy or sharp foods.

VII. REMISSION

A. Characteristics of Remission
1. Neoplastic cells diminish.
2. Blood counts return to normal.
3. Oral complications subside.

B. Place on Routine Dental Hygiene Maintenance (pages 642 to 645)

C. Relapse
The cycle of therapy begins again, and the need for bone marrow transplantation is evaluated.

SURGICAL TREATMENT

Surgery may be required to remove a tumor located in the head and neck area. Pre- and postoperative care of the surgery patient is described on pages 709 to 711.

I. INDICATIONS FOR SURGERY[7]

A. Neoplasms that are not radiosensitive and could not be treated by radiotherapy alone.
B. Neoplasms recurring in an area that had already undergone radiotherapy.
C. Situations where side effects of radiation could be more severe than healed surgical defects.
D. Neoplasms involving bone, lymph nodes, and salivary glands.

II. TYPES OF SURGERY

A. Primary Lesion
Surgical treatment is to remove the primary lesion and the regional lymph nodes. Some small lesions are totally removed when a biopsy is used for diagnosis.

B. Cervical Lymphadenectomy ("Neck Dissection")
1. *Area.* The neck dissection includes wide removal of tissues around a tumor.
2. *Purposes.* To ensure removal of as many neoplastic cells as possible from the oropharynx and neck and to prevent the spread of the cancer to the lymph nodes.

BONE MARROW TRANSPLANTATION (BMT)[33,34]

Bone marrow transplantation is used to treat a variety of neoplasms and blood diseases. The purpose is to substitute bone marrow from a healthy, compatible donor to restore or reconstitute the blood–cell-producing capacity of the bone marrow of the patient.

I. TYPES OF TRANSPLANTS

The five basic types of transplants are shown in Table 49-5.

II. STAGES OF THE TRANSPLANTATION PROCESS[33]

A. Patient Selection
1. Indications: patient not responsive to chemotherapy alone; relapse occurs after one or more remissions.
2. Evaluation: medical and dental assessments are completed to ensure patient is free of infection and physically stable to undergo preparative regimen.

B. Donor Regimen
1. Histocompatibility matching.
2. Bone marrow aspirated from iliac crest, ribs, or sternum.

C. Conditioning of Patient to Receive Bone Marrow Graft
1. Preparative high-dose immunosuppressive regimen: chemotherapy alone or with total body irradiation.
2. Purposes
   a. Kill malignant cells.
   b. Suppress immune system so new marrow can engraft.

D. Transplantation: Intravenous infusion of donor's marrow

E. Pancytopenic Period: All cellular elements of the blood are depressed
1. Protective isolation for patient is required; patient highly susceptible to infection.
2. Function of new marrow (to produce peripheral blood elements) begins after 10 to 20 days.

F. Recovery: Immune recovery 3 to 12 months; long-term recovery 1 to 3 years.

III. PRIMARY COMPLICATIONS

A. Oral Effects
1. Mucositis, candidiasis, and xerostomia are similar in signs and symptoms to those resulting from chemotherapy and radiotherapy (pages 727 to 728).

TABLE 49-5 Types of Bone Marrow Transplants

Type of Transplant	Donor Source	Frequency
Autologous	Self	30–50%
Unrelated	Any matched donor (complete or partial)	25–30%
Allogeneic	Sibling	15–25%
Haploidentical	Parent	< 5%
Syngeneic	Identical twin	< 5%

(Adapted from Rhodus, N.L. and Little, J.W.: Dental Management of the Bone Marrow Transplant Patient, *Compend. Cont. Educ. Dent.*, 13, 1040, November, 1992.)

2. Daily oral care supervision is similar to management for chemotherapy- and radiotherapy-induced oral effects (pages 728 and 731).
3. Team supervision is essential.

B. Opportunistic Infection: Interstitial pneumonia

C. Graft Versus Host Disease[33,35]
  1. *Description*. Bone marrow recipient adversely reacts to the donated marrow and rejects it, or when the donor's immunologically competent cells react against the host.
  2. *Symptoms*
    a. Acute. Skin rash on palms and soles; persistent anorexia and/or diarrhea; liver disease during first 3 months after transplant.
    b. Chronic. Facial rash, arthritis, and obstructive lung and liver disease occur or persist beyond 3 months after the transplantation.
  3. *Prevention and Treatment*
    a. Antirejection drugs.
    b. Steroids.
  4. *Oral Care*
    a. Meticulous oral hygiene.
    b. Only consider emergency dental needs for treatment.
    c. Consult physician regarding blood counts and need for antibiotic prophylaxis.

PERSONAL FACTORS[36]

Patient attitudes and feelings may be similar to those of any patient with a major chronic disease or disability. As with other diseases with limited hope for cure, strong feelings of hopelessness and despair predominate.

The very word *cancer* brings fear and anxiety to the patient. The concerns of a patient may differ at different stages of treatment.

I. PATIENT PROBLEMS

A. Early Fears and Anxieties
  1. Outcome.
  2. Imminent surgery, radiation, chemotherapy, or other treatment.
  3. Disfigurement, changes in appearance, and pain.
  4. Extended hospitalization.
  5. Financial stress.

B. During and Following Therapy
  1. Preoccupation with details of examinations, treatments, symptoms, or medications.
  2. Depression and grief, which may lead to withdrawal and isolation.
  3. Major concerns may include obvious facial deformity, speech difficulty, swallowing difficulty, drooling, hair loss, weight loss, nausea, and odors from debris collection and tissue changes.

II. SUGGESTIONS FOR APPROACH TO PATIENT

A. Provide explanations before and after therapy to prevent misconceptions and apprehensions and to attempt to allay fears.
B. Provide paper and pencil for patient with a speech difficulty to write questions and requests.
C. Show acceptance. Acknowledge the appropriateness of the patient's concerns.
D. Express empathy, but avoid oversolicitousness.
E. Help to direct thoughts and efforts toward restoration of functional activity.
F. Instill trust and security by demonstrating genuine interest.
G. Assist the patient who is alcoholic, uses tobacco products excessively, or has other habits that have to be eliminated. The patient may need the help of psychiatry, Alcoholics Anonymous, counseling for a tobacco cessation program, or other type of support.

TECHNICAL HINTS

I. PREPARATION OF HISTORY

Preparation of a medical and dental history for all patients should include questions relative to a cancer diagnosis and the type(s) of therapy received. Therapy during childhood should be recorded as well as that during adulthood.

II. PATIENT REFERRAL

When a patient is referred to a specialist or specialty clinic, a check must be made to ascertain that the patient arrives for the appointment. Frightened patients may become confused or may postpone the visit if they do not realize the urgency of the condition.

III. SOURCES OF MATERIALS

American Cancer Society
1599 Clifton Road N.E.
Atlanta, GA 30329
Local cancer society addresses can be obtained from the Atlanta office or local telephone book.

National Cancer Institute
31 Center Drive
MSC 2590
Bethesda, Maryland 20892

FACTORS TO TEACH THE PATIENT

I. The importance of oral soft tissue screening and complete oral examination at regular frequent intervals.
II. Bacterial plaque control methods, gel-tray application, use of saliva substitute, and all other details of personal care to reduce oral side effects induced by the disease and/or therapy.
III. Encourage adherence to daily oral care regimen.
IV. Why use of alcohol and tobacco must be stopped.
V. Instruction for family members in oral health care for the sick and dependent patient.

REFERENCES

1. **Miller**, B.F. and Keane, C.B.: *Encyclopedia and Dictionary of Medicine, Nursing, and Allied Health*, 6th ed. Philadelphia, W.B. Saunders Co., 1997.
2. **Cancer Statistics, 1997**, *CA., 48*, 1, January/February, 1998.
3. **Murphy**, G.P., Lawrence, W., and Lenhard, R.E., eds.: *Clinical Oncology*, 2nd ed. Atlanta, GA, American Cancer Society, 1995, pp. 1–39.
4. **Little**, J.W., Falace, D.A., Miller, C.S., and Rhodus, N.L.: *Dental Management of the Medically Compromised Patient*, 5th ed. St. Louis, Mosby–Year Book, 1997, pp. 532–542.
5. **Stevenson-Moore**, P.: Essential Aspects of Pretreatment Oral Examination, *NCI Monogr., 9*, 33, 1990.
6. **DePaola**, L.G. and Minah, G.E.: Isolation of Pathogenic Microorganisms from Dentures and Denture Soaking Containers of Myelosuppressed Cancer Patients, *J. Prosthet. Dent., 49*, 20, January, 1983.
7. **Kraus**, D.H. and Pfister, D.G.: Head and Neck Oncology, in Noble, J., ed.: *Textbook of Primary Care Medicine*, 2nd ed. St. Louis, Mosby, 1996, pp. 467–475.
8. **Harrison**, L.B. and Fass, D.E.: Radiation Therapy for Oral Cavity Cancer, *Dent. Clin. North Am., 34*, 205, April, 1990.
9. **Whitmyer**, C.C., Waskowski, J.C., and Iffland, H.A.: Radiotherapy and Oral Sequelae: Preventive and Management Protocols, *J. Dent. Hyg., 71*, 23, January–February, 1997.
10. **Semba**, S.E., Mealey, B.L., and Hallmon, W.W.: The Head and Neck Radiotherapy Patient: Part I—Oral Manifestations of Radiation Therapy, *Compend. Cont. Educ. Dent., 15*, 250, February, 1994.
11. **Madeya**, M.L.: Oral Complications from Cancer Therapy: Part 1—Pathophysiology and Secondary Complications, *Oncol. Nurs. Forum, 23*, 801, June, 1996.
12. **Madeya**, M.L.: Oral Complications from Cancer Therapy: Part 2—Nursing Implications for Assessment and Treatment, *Oncol. Nurs. Forum, 23*, 808, June, 1996.
13. **Barker**, G.J., Barker, B.F., and Gier, R.E.: *Oral Management of the Cancer Patient. A Guide for the Health Care Professional*, 5th ed. Kansas City, MO, Biomedical Communications, University of Missouri-Kansas City, School of Dentistry, January, 1996, 19 pp.
14. **American Academy of Periodontology**, Committee on Research, Science, and Therapy: Position Paper: *Periodontal Considerations in the Management of the Cancer Patient, J. Periodontol., 68*, 791, August, 1997.
15. **Browman**, G.P., Wong, G., Hodson, I., Sathya, J., Russell, R., McAlpine, L., Skingley, P., and Levine, M.N.: Influence of Cigarette Smoking on the Efficacy of Radiation Therapy in Head and Neck Cancer, *N. Engl. J. Med., 328*, 159, January 21, 1993.
16. **Wiseman**, L.R. and Faulds, D.: Oral Pilocarpine: A Review of Its Pharmacological Properties and Clinical Potential in Xerostomia, *Drugs, 49*, 143, January, 1995.
17. **Zimmerman**, R.P., Mark, R.J., Tran, L.M., and Juillard, G.F.: Concomitant Pilocarpine During Head and Neck Irradiation Is Associated with Decreased Posttreatment Xerostomia, *Int. J. Radiat. Oncol. Biol. Phys., 37*, 571, February 1, 1997.
18. **Garg**, A.K. and Malo, M.: Manifestations and Treatment of Xerostomia and Associated Oral Effects Secondary to Head and Neck Radiation Therapy, *J. Am. Dent. Assoc., 128*, 1128, August, 1997.
19. **Guchelaar**, H.J., Vermes, A., and Meerwaldt, J.H.: Radiation-Induced Xerostomia: Pathophysiology, Clinical Course and Supportive Treatment, *Support Care Cancer, 5*, 281, July, 1997.
20. **Ried**, H., Zietz, H., and Jaffe, N.: Late Effects of Cancer Treatment in Children, *Pediatr. Dent., 17*, 273, July/August, 1995.
21. **Peterson**, D.E. and D'Ambrosio, J.A.: Nonsurgical Management of Head and Neck Cancer Patients, *Dent. Clin. North Am., 38*, 425, July, 1994.
22. **Ashamalia**, H.L., Thom, S.R., and Goldwein, J.W.: Hyperbaric Oxygen Therapy for the Treatment of Radiation-Induced Sequelae in Children. The University of Pennsylvania Experience, *Cancer, 77*, 2407, June 1, 1996.
23. **Neovius**, E.B., Lind, M.G., and Lind, F.G.: Hyperbaric Oxygen Therapy for Wound Complications After Surgery in the Irradiated Head and Neck: A Review of the Literature and a Report of 15 Consecutive Patients, *Head Neck, 19*, 315, July, 1997.
24. **Wong**, J.K., Wood, R.E., and McLean, M.: Conservative Management of Osteoradionecrosis, *Oral Surg., Oral Med., Oral Pathol., Oral Radiol., Endod., 84*, 16, July, 1997.
25. **Granström**, G., Jacobsson, M., and Tjellström, A.: Titanium Implants in Irradiated Tissue: Benefits from Hyperbaric Oxygen, *Int. J. Oral Maxillofac. Implants, 7*, 15, Spring, 1992.
26. **Esser**, E. and Wagner, W.: Dental Implants Following Radical Oral Cancer Surgery and Adjuvant Radiotherapy, *Int. J. Oral Maxillofac. Implants, 12*, 552, July, 1997.
27. **Savarese**, D.: Principles of Cancer Therapy, in Noble, J., ed.: *Textbook of Primary Care Medicine*, 2nd ed. St. Louis, Mosby, 1996, pp. 777–788.
28. **NIH Consensus Development Conference Statements**:

Oral Complications of Cancer Therapies: Diagnosis, Prevention, and Treatment, *NCI Monogr., 9,* 3, 1990.

29. **DeBiase**, C.B.: *Dental Health Education: Theory and Practice,* Philadelphia, Lea & Febiger, 1991, pp. 228–239.

30. **Krywulak**, M.L., Hsu, E., Vietti, T., and DeBiase, C.B.: Mouth and Dental Care, in Ritchey, K., ed.: *Pediatric Oncology Group Supportive Care Manual,* Smith Kline Beecham, 1996, pp. 1–14.

31. **Terezhalmy**, G.T., Whitmyer, C.C., and Markman, M.: Cancer Chemotherapeutic Agents, *Dent. Clin. North Am., 40,* 709, July, 1996.

32. **Little**, Falace, Miller, and Rhodus: op. cit., pp. 543–544.

33. **Rhodus**, N.L. and Little, J.W.: Dental Management of the Bone Marrow Transplant Patient, *Compend. Cont. Educ. Dent., 13,* 1040, November, 1992.

34. **DeBiase**, C.B.: Oral Care for the Bone Marrow Transplant Patient, *Case Studies in Periodont. Mgmt., 2,* 1, November, 1996.

35. **Appelbaum**, F.R.: The Use of Bone Marrow and Peripheral Blood Stem Cell Transplantation in the Treatment of Cancer, *CA, 46,* 142, May/June, 1996.

36. **Allen**, J.: The Psychosocial Effects of Cancer and Its Treatment in the Elderly, *Spec. Care Dentist., 4,* 13, January/February, 1984.

SUGGESTED READINGS

Barasch, A. and Safford, M.M.: Management of Oral Pain in Patients with Malignant Diseases, *Compend. Cont. Educ. Dent., 14,* 1376, November, 1993.

Joyston-Bechal, S: Prevention of Dental Diseases Following Radiotherapy and Chemotherapy, *Int. Dent. J., 42,* 47, February, 1992.

Lunn, R.: Oral Management of the Cancer Patient. Part I: Overview of Cancer and Oral Cancer, *Can. Dent. Hyg. Assoc. (PROBE), 31,* 137, July/August, 1997.

Schein, J.: The Many Faces of Cancer: Sifting Through the Facts, *RDH, 15,* 24, October, 1995.

Souliman, S.K. and Christie, J.: Pacemaker Failure Induced by Radiotherapy, *PACE, 17,* 270, March, 1994, Part I.

Toth, B.B., Martin, J.W., and Fleming, T.J.: Oral Complications Associated with Cancer Therapy. An M.D. Anderson Cancer Center Experience, *J. Clin. Periodontol., 17,* 508, August, 1990 (Part II).

Yellowitz, J.A., Goodman, H.S., and Farooq, N.S.: Knowledge, Opinions, and Practices Related to Oral Cancer: Results of Three Elderly Racial Groups, *Spec. Care Dentist., 17,* 100, May/June, 1997.

Children

Berg, J. and Bleyer, A.: Pediatric Dentistry in Care of the Cancer Patient, *Pediatr. Dent., 17,* 257, July/August, 1995.

Chan, K.W.: Pediatric Bone Marrow Transplantation, *Pediatr. Dent., 17,* 291, July/August, 1995.

Kennedy, L. and Diamond, J.: Assessment and Management of Chemotherapy-Induced Mucositis in Children, *J. Pediatr. Oncol. Nurs., 14,* 164, July, 1997.

Chemotherapy

Peterson, D.E. and Sonis, S.T., eds.: *Oral Complications of Cancer Chemotherapy.* The Hague/Boston/London, Martinus Nijhoff Publishers, 1983, pp. 1–12.

Rosenberg, S.W.: Oral Care of Chemotherapy Patients, *Dent. Clin. North Am., 34,* 239, April, 1990.

Semba, S.E., Mealey, B.L., and Hallmon, W.W.: Dentistry and the Cancer Patient: Part 2—Oral Health Management of the Chemotherapy Patient, *Compend. Cont. Educ. Dent., 15,* 1378, November, 1994.

Radiation

Epstein, J.B. and van der Meij, E.H.: Complicating Mucosal Reactions in Patients Receiving Radiation Therapy for Head and Neck Cancer, *Spec. Care Dentist., 17,* 88, May/June, 1997.

Epstein, J.B., Corbett, T., Galler, C., and Stevenson-Moore, P.: Surgical Periodontal Treatment in the Radiotherapy-treated Head and Neck Cancer Patient, *Spec. Care Dent., 14,* 182, September/October, 1994.

Meraw, S.J. and Reeve, C.M.: Dental Considerations and Treatment of the Oncology Patient Receiving Radiation Therapy, *J. Am. Dent. Assoc., 129,* 201, February, 1998.

Wang, R.R., Pillai, K., and Jones, P.K.: In vitro Backscattering from Implant Materials During Radiotherapy, *J. Prosthet. Dent., 75,* 626, June, 1996.

Whitmeyer, C.C., Esposito, S.J., and Terezhalmy, G.T.: Radiotherapy for Head and Neck Neoplasms, *Gen. Dent., 45,* 363, July/August, 1997.

Patient Health and Oral Hygiene

Addems, A., Epstein, J.B., Damji, S., and Spinelli, J.: The Lack of Efficacy of a Foam Brush in Maintaining Gingival Health: A Controlled Study, *Spec. Care Dentist., 12,* 103, May/June, 1992.

American Cancer Society 1996 Advisory Committee on Diet, Nutrition, and Cancer Prevention: Guidelines on Diet, Nutrition, and Cancer Prevention: Reducing the Risk of Cancer with Healthy Food Choices and Physical Activity, *CA, 46,* 325, November/December, 1996.

Bland, K.I.: Quality-of-Life Management for Cancer Patients, *CA, 47,* 194, July/August, 1997.

Epstein, J.B., van der Meij, E.H., Lunn, R., Le, N.D., and Stevenson-Moore, P.: Effects of Compliance with Fluoride Gel Application on Caries and Caries Risk in Patients After Radiation Therapy for Head and Neck Cancer, *Oral Surg. Oral Med. Oral Pathol. Oral Radiol. Endod., 82,* 268, September, 1996.

Ghalichebaf, M., DeBiase, C.B., and Stookey, G.K.: A New Technique for the Fabrication of Fluoride Carriers in Patients Receiving Radiotherapy to the Head and Neck, *Compend. Cont. Educ. Dent., 15,* 470, April, 1994.

Care of Patients With Disabilities

Many types of disabilities require special attention and adaptations during dental and dental hygiene appointments. The general term *disability* refers to any reduction of a person's activity that has resulted from an acute or chronic health condition and affects motor, sensory, or mental functions.

A disability may be permanent or temporary. A temporary impairment may be physical, such as a fracture of a leg, or physiologic with physical limitations, such as during pregnancy. Chronic systemic diseases may result in crippling disabilities. The causes of disabilities may be factors of heredity, systemic disease, trauma, or combinations of these. Box 50-1 supplies key words and definitions pertaining to impairments, disabilities, and handicaps.

I. DEFINITION AND CLASSIFICATION

As defined by the *United States Americans with Disabilities Act (ADA)*, an individual with a disability is a per-

son who *"has a physical or mental impairment that substantially limits one or more major life activities, has a record of such impairment, or is regarded as having such impairment."*[1]

The *International Classification of the World Health Organization* clarifies the meaning of impairment, disability, and handicap.[2] An *impairment* is an abnormality of structure or function of a limb or body organ, whereas the *disability* is the inability to perform a task or activity as a result of the impairment. The *handicap* is the disadvantage or limitation that an individual has when compared to others of the same age, sex, and background that has resulted from the impairment and the disability. Table 50-1 lists categories and examples of each.

II. REHABILITATION TRENDS

Current trends toward deinstitutionalization have brought alternative living, educational, and work

---

BOX 50-1 KEY WORDS: Impairment, Disability, Handicap

Accessibility standards: the ADA prohibits discrimination on the basis of a disability and requires places of public accommodation and commercial facilities to meet requirements of accessibility by removing architectural, transportation, and communication barriers.

AwDA: Americans with Disabilities Act; abbreviation sometimes used to prevent confusion with the ADA (American Dental Association).

Barrier-free: area that is freely accessible to all without discrimination on the basis of a disability; obstacles to passage or communication have been removed.

Behavior modification: an approach to correction of undesirable conduct that focuses on changing observable actions; modification of behavior is accomplished through systematic manipulation of the environmental and behavioral variables related to the specific behavior to be changed.

Behavior therapy: an approach in which the focus is on the patient's observable behavior, rather than on conflicts and unconscious processes presumed to underlie the maladaptive behavior; accomplished through systematic manipulation of the environmental and behavioral variables related to specific behavior to be modified.

Deinstitutionalization: returning patients to home and community as quickly as possible after treatment rather than housing them permanently or for long periods in custodial institutions, the elimination of mental health institutions, for example, has been made possible by (1) the use of new medications that control the symptoms of illness, and (2) community health centers that serve as support.

Desensitization: the treatment of phobias and related disorders by intentionally exposing the patient, in imagination or real life, to emotionally distressing stimuli; desensitization of a fearful patient to accept dental treatment might consist, for example, of short exposures to the dental chair, instruments, air syringe, and the sound of a handpiece along with building trust in the dental team members.

Developmental disability: a substantial handicap of indefinite duration with onset before the age of 18 years, attributable to mental retardation, autism, cerebral palsy, epilepsy, or other incurable neuropathy.

Disability: any restriction or lack of ability (resulting from an impairment) to perform an activity in the manner or within the range considered normal for a human being of the same age, sex, and background.

Handicap: a disadvantage for an individual, resulting from an impairment or a disability, that limits or prevents fulfillment of a role that is within the normal range for a human of the same age, sex, and social and cultural factors as the affected individual.

Impairment: any loss or abnormality of psychologic, physiologic, or anatomic structure or function.

Mainstreaming: integration of people with disabilities into their community through programs of rehabilitation; process by which persons with special needs (educational, physical, psychologic) are included within the mainstream of society rather than segregated.

Normalization: making available to all individuals patterns and conditions of everyday life that are as close as possible to the norms and patterns of the mainstream of society.

TABLE 50-1 Impairments, Disabilities, and Handicaps

Impairments	Disabilities	Handicaps
Intellectual impairments	Behavior disabilities	Orientation handicap
Mental retardation	Awareness	To surroundings
Memory, thinking	Motivation	Relates to behavior and communication disability
Psychologic impairments	Communication disabilities	Physical independence handicap
Consciousness	Speaking	Dependence on others
Perception	Listening	Mobility handicap
Language impairments	Personal care disabilities	Reduced mobility
Communication	Personal hygiene	Dwelling restriction
Voice function	Dressing	Occupation handicap
Aural impairments	Locomotor disabilities	Adjusted occupation
Hearing impairment	Ambulation	Restricted because of disability
Auditory sensitivity	Transport	Social integration handicap
Ocular impairments	Body disposition disabilities	Restricted participation
Visual acuity	Subsistence	Socially isolated
Blindness	Dexterity disabilities	Economic self-sufficiency handicap
Visceral impairments	Daily activity	Fully self-sufficient
Internal organs	Grasping	Impoverished
Impaired mastication, swallowing	Situational disabilities	
Skeletal impairments	Environmental temperature	
Mechanical and motor	Dependence	
Deficiency of parts	Endurance	
Paralysis	Particular skill disability	
Disfiguring impairments	Task fulfillment	
Structural deformity	Learning ability	
Generalized, sensory impairment	Dexterity	
Susceptible to trauma		

(From World Health Organization: *International Classification of Impairments, Disabilities and Handicaps,* Geneva, 1980.)

arrangements to many individuals with physical and mental disabilities. Children taken out of institutional life and trained for community living in transitional homes are being integrated or "mainstreamed" into regular school and health programs.

Through a program of rehabilitation, persons with disabilities may receive vocational, educational, placement, medical, and dental services as needed. Specially staffed community housing for group living has been made available.

DENTAL AND DENTAL HYGIENE CARE

Oral health for the individual with a disability takes on more than usual significance and presents a challenge to dental personnel. For the patient, the disability provides enough of a burden without additional oral problems, which can reduce an already lowered potential for normal living. Preventive measures, particularly fluoridation and other means for protecting the teeth with fluoride, must be encouraged and promoted through community effort and personal instruction to minimize oral problems.

Imagination, ingenuity, and flexibility are neces-

sary for those involved in treating people with disabilities. Individualization and modification of usual procedures are necessary in addition to the material described in this chapter. Patience, calmness, and kindness are keys to approaching the special patient.

I. OBJECTIVES

The dental team can make a significant contribution to the well-being, independent mobility, and sense of personal value of a patient with a disability. Whether employed in private practice, working in an institutional or community clinical and educational setting, or contributing on a volunteer basis, the dental team must have as its objectives to:

A. Motivate the patient and the caregiver. Personal oral care practices conducive to maintaining healthy oral tissue with freedom from infection must be developed.

B. Contribute to the patient's general health, of which oral health is an integral part. Prevention of tooth loss increases the ability to masticate food, which, in turn, is essential to prevent malnutrition and to increase resistance to infection.

C. Prevent the need for extensive dental and periodontal treatment that the patient may not be able to undergo because of lowered physical stamina or the inability to cooperate. Dentures or other removable prostheses can be hazardous for certain patients or impossible for others.

D. Aid in the improvement of appearance, thereby contributing to social acceptance. An untidy person with unclean teeth and halitosis (from local causes) is much less acceptable socially than is one with a clean mouth.

E. Make appointments pleasant and comfortable experiences.

II. TYPES OF CONDITIONS

A variety of impairments are found among persons with disabilities. An individual may have more than one type of crippling or limiting problem. The lists in Table 50-1 are representative. Many of the diseases and syndromes with symptoms of impairments are described in the various chapters throughout Part VI of this book.

III. PRETREATMENT PLANNING

Most patients with disabilities can be treated in the private dental office setting. Only a relatively small number need hospitalization because of marked difficulties in management or because of a systemic condition that would require special medical supervision.

A. Preliminary Information

Information about the younger and/or dependent, mentally retarded, or elderly senile patient is obtained from a parent, relative, advocate, or other person responsible for the patient. The essential information can be obtained in advance by telephone or interview.

Medical and other record forms can be mailed to the home for completion. Advance information permits the dental team to be prepared for the patient so that valuable appointment time is not used up and complete attention can be devoted to the patient's needs.

B. Records and Forms

1. *Medical History.* In addition to the usual topics covered by questions (Table 6-3, pages 96–100), information relative to the disabling condition is needed. At least the following should be included:
   a. Specific disabling condition. When diagnosed, history of treatments, hospitalizations, current medications and other therapy, names and addresses of specialists involved.
   b. Record of institutionalization.
   c. History of communicable diseases; most recent blood tests; immunizations.
   d. Seizures. History, frequency, treatment.
   e. Muscular coordination. Mobility, dexterity.
   f. Communication. Speech, vision, hearing.
   g. Mental capacities. Schooling, special classes.
   h. Degree of independence. Self-care, ability to dress and feed self and to perform own oral care with brush, floss, other aids.
   i. Dietary restrictions.

2. *Dental History*
   a. Previous dental experiences. Patient's attitude, ability to cooperate.
   b. Difficulties in obtaining appointments in other locations.
   c. Most recent care. Scaling, restorations, extractions, other.
   d. Oral infections and oral habits.
   e. Fluoride history. Fluoridation, dietary supplements, self- or professionally applied topical methods, including years, ages, and frequency.
   f. Current home care methods. Aids and special devices, frequency, degree of self-care.
   g. Patient/parent. Concepts of perceived needs, attitudes, and apparent emphasis on dental care.

3. *Consent Forms.* Consent forms for minor, dependent, and/or incompetent patient must be signed by parent or legal guardian.

C. Consultations With Physicians and Other Specialists

Medical aspects of the patient's care are integrated into treatment planning for oral care. The physician can supply information the dentist can apply in the selection of antibiotic, sedative, or other necessary pharmaceutical agents. Additional pertinent information may be obtained from other medical specialists and the social worker.

D. Discussion With Parent or Other Caregiver

1. Determine familial interrelationships. Many parents devote their lives to the care of their disabled child. Dental personnel must make every effort to learn from the parents or other caregivers the capabilities of the patient and the methods most effective for gaining cooperation. The names, ages, and interrelationships of other family members can prove helpful.

   Families may overindulge the special child. Sweets may be used as rewards or bribes to pacify. Poor behavior may be condoned.

2. Describe to the parent the cooperation and assistance needed. Special help may be needed during the appointment and for supervision of oral care on a daily basis in the total preventive care program.

3. Solicit parental help in preparing the patient for the appointments. Ask that procedures and facilities be described in advance in a

pleasant and positive manner to reassure the patient.

4. Invite the patient to the office or clinic before the appointment to see the facility and become familiar with the surroundings and staff.

5. List special aids the patient must bring to the appointment, such as a transfer board for transfer into the dental chair, hearing aid, dental prostheses and bacterial plaque control devices currently in use.

APPOINTMENT SCHEDULING

I. DETERMINE SPECIAL REQUIREMENTS

Determine whether special requirements of the patient's daily schedule influence time selection. The cooperation of the patient may be decreased if basic routines are disturbed. Some examples follow:

A. Appointment for the patient with diabetes must not interfere with medication, meal, or between-meal eating schedules.

B. Elderly person who rises early may feel better during a morning appointment.

C. Patients with arthritis may have greater mobility late in the morning or in the afternoon.

D. Child's nap schedule should be respected.

E. Early morning appointment may be difficult for a patient who requires a long time for morning preparation, such as a patient with a spinal cord injury or colostomy.

II. EFFECT OF TRANSPORTATION REQUIREMENTS

A. A family member who accompanies the patient should not be expected to lose a day's work if the dental appointment can be accommodated otherwise. Families may have limited financial resources because of expenses related to treatment of the person with the disability.

B. Wheelchair patient may need to reserve a public wheelchair transport vehicle and, thus, may be limited by the schedule.

III. TIME OF APPOINTMENT

A. Arrange a time when the patient will not have to wait a long time after arrival. If daily appointments tend to run increasingly off schedule by late morning or afternoon, the patient with a disability should be scheduled for the appointment at the start of the day or for the first appointment in the afternoon.

B. Schedule a difficult patient when the clinician is at optimum energy and patience.

C. Allow sufficient time so that the patient does not feel rushed; many persons with disabilities cannot hurry.

IV. FOLLOW-UP

The frequency of maintenance appointments must be individualized. The time depends on the patient's oral problems and general disabilities. Frequent appointments are encouraged for the following reasons:

A. To decrease length of single appointment by keeping the oral tissues at an optimum level of health.

B. To assist the patient whose disability limits the ability to perform personal oral hygiene adequately.

C. To provide motivation through monitoring of plaque and review of procedures for the patient and the parent or other caregiver involved.

BARRIER-FREE ENVIRONMENT

A variety of factors can explain the general lack of dental and dental hygiene care of the elderly patient or of individuals of any age who are disabled. One of the more significant reasons is the existence of physical barriers confronting patients who may attempt to keep appointments. Fear of not being able to cope with architectural barriers, fear of falling, or fear of attracting attention in an embarrassing way all can be hindrances to seeking oral care.

In general, a facility that is barrier-free for a patient in a wheelchair is accessible to all other individuals. The patient in a wheelchair requires more space for turning and positioning than does a patient with crutches or a walker, or than a patient accompanied by another person walking at the side to guide or provide support.

In addition to space requirements, special features are needed for other specific disabilities. For example, braille floor indicators can be installed beside the numbers on elevators. For people with limited vision, doorways, steps, and stairways can be outlined with bright colors that contrast with the background.

Guidelines and specifications for a barrier-free environment are available. The descriptions that follow represent general features based on governmental regulations for accessibility standards, along with suggested applications for a dental clinic or office.[3]

I. EXTERNAL FEATURES

A. Parking

A reserved area, clearly marked, should be close to the building entrance and 13 feet wide (8-foot car space with 5-foot access aisle) to permit a person with a disability to open car doors for exiting and reboarding.

B. Walkways

A 3-foot-wide walkway is needed for wheelchair accommodation. The surface must be solid and nonslip without irregularities. Curb ramps (cuts) from the street and from the parking area are necessary.

C. Entrance

At least one entrance to the building should be on ground level or be accessible by a gently sloping ramp (rise of 1 inch for every 12 inches). An easily grasped handrail (height 30 to 34 inches) is needed on at least one side, and preferably both sides, to accommodate left- and right-handed cane and one-crutch users.

D. Door

The lightweight door with a lever type of handle must open at least 32 inches for a wheelchair and a person using a tall crutch (Figure 50-1).

II. INTERNAL FEATURES

Official regulations specify dimensions for accessibility of all aspects, including passageways, floors, drinking fountains, and restrooms. A few are described here.

A. Passageways

The passageways should be at least 3 feet wide with handrails along the sides. They should be free from obstructions, such as hanging signs with which a tall blind person could collide.

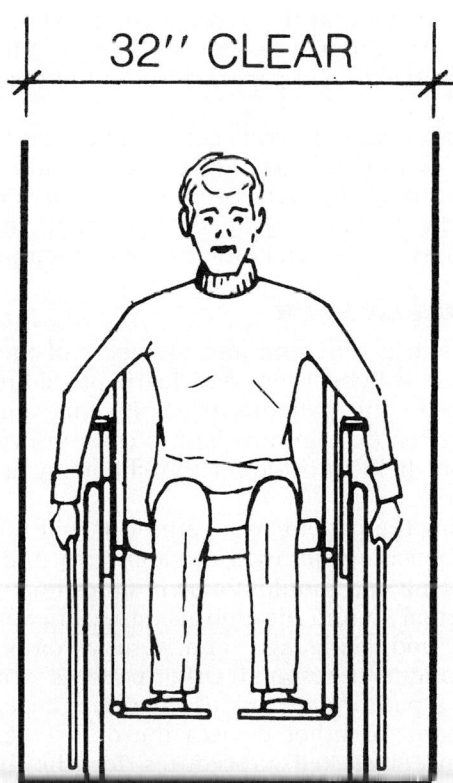

FIGURE 50-1 Wheelchair Accessibility. Wheelchairs designed for adults vary in width from 2 feet 3 inches to 2 feet 8 inches. A clear door width of 32 inches to accommodate these wheelchairs has been accepted as the official regulation.

B. Floors

Level floors with nonslip surfaces are important. Thick or small unattached movable rugs or carpets present obstacles for wheelchairs or walkers and hazards for a patient with crutches, cane, or leg brace.

C. Reception Area

At least part of the furniture should permit easy access during seating and rising. Preferred are chairs with 18-inch-high, flat, firm seats and arms for support when pushing oneself up by the arms. Chairs must not slide or tip as the person rises.

III. THE TREATMENT ROOM

In a group of several treatment rooms in which a limited number of patients in wheelchairs is served, only one room needs to be made accessible. Dental personnel should be versatile in exchanging rooms to serve special patients.

A. Dimensions

Space is needed for both the dental chair and related dental equipment, as well as for the wheelchair. The doorway must be at least 32 inches wide. The wheelchair is placed beside and parallel to the dental chair for patient transfer. In a small facility, the dental chair can be rotated to give room for turning the wheelchair.

When planning or redesigning for wheelchair accessibility, the dental chair selected should be able to be lowered to 19 inches from the floor, and be accessible from both sides for wheelchair transfer. An x-ray machine in the same treatment room can simplify the problems of moving the patient into a separate radiography room.

B. Wheelchair Used During Treatment

The wheelchair of a patient who is unable to transfer easily, if at all, is positioned for direct utilization.

1. *Portable Headrest.* A portable headrest may be attached to the wheelchair handles.
2. *Position of Dental Chair.* The dental chair can be swiveled to permit the wheelchair to be backed up to place the patient's head in a usual treatment position. The dental light can then be directed into the patient's oral cavity and adjusted for access to the equipment.
3. *Wheelchair Lift.* An automatic wheelchair lift that tilts the chair back to a usual working position can be obtained for a clinical facility where wheelchair patients are treated frequently.

IV. PATIENT INSTRUCTION

When a teaching area is planned for patient instruction, attention must be given to ensure accessibility for a patient in a wheelchair. The same facility can be used by a seated nondisabled patient.

A. Dimensions

The usual 32-inch doorway and turnabout space for a wheelchair are indicated. The tabletop and washbasin built at a height of 32 to 34 inches permit clearance underneath for knees and wheelchair arms (Figure 50-2). The same regulations are used for a lavatory sink.

B. Washbasin

Lever- or blade-type handles on faucets are usable by patients who cannot grip round handles or who have no hands. Hot pipes under the sink must be covered or insulated, because patients who have no sensation in their legs could be burned. The hot water temperature should be regulated, if possible.

C. Mirror

Mirrors and dispensers are positioned low. A tilt mirror could provide better viewing of the teeth during instruction. A tilt mirror with a hinge has more adaptability for tall and short patients and for patients with bifocal eyeglasses.

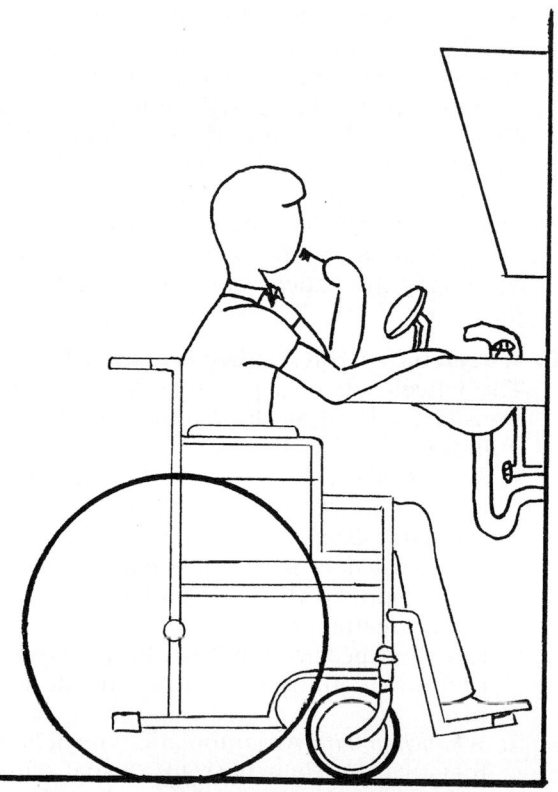

FIGURE 50-2 Plaque Control Facility. The tabletop and washbasin in a patient instruction area or lavatory should be built at a height of 32 to 34 inches to provide clearance underneath for knees of the patient and arms of the wheelchair. Hot pipes under a sink must be covered or insulated because patients with no sensation could be burned.

An unattached hand mirror, preferably on a pedestal that tilts, is a necessary supplement to the wall mirror. A magnifying mirror can provide an excellent aid for viewing the disclosed plaque and the devices for plaque removal.

PATIENT RECEPTION: THE INITIAL APPOINTMENT

The orientation of a patient with a disability paves the way for long-term dental and dental hygiene supervision and care. When a patient is passive, follows instructions, and possibly has received sedative medication, the situation is different from that of a patient who is apprehensive and fearful, perhaps because of past medical and dental experiences. Other patients have difficulties of communication or have limitations of body movement and control. The problems of management and care become greatly intensified for such patients.

I. ORIENTATION

The first appointment includes and, when necessary, may be devoted entirely to a basic orientation to the facilities, the dental chair, and the personnel. The examination of the oral cavity is started, and dependent on the degree of patient cooperation, various steps in the assessment may be completed. Preventive personal care procedures to alleviate gingival inflammation are initiated, and participation of the caregiver is solicited.

Several orientation visits may be necessary because hurrying or forcing a patient may cause more severe problems. In a long-term care facility where patients live on the premises, daily short visits to the clinic may be possible to condition or desensitize a patient.

II. COMMUNICATION

Each patient is different, and members of the dental team must watch, listen, and learn procedures that will develop the patient's trust. Parents and other caregivers can explain how best to communicate. The parent can help to interpret the changing moods of the patient.

Even for the patient who cannot or will not speak or may appear withdrawn, the ability to understand what is being said should not be underestimated.

Nonverbal communication using facial expression, pointing, body language, and demonstration helps certain patients to respond. Other patients write messages on a pad of paper or use sign language, a language board, or other devices the dental personnel can learn. Suggested procedures for the hearing-impaired patient are described on pages 795 to 800.

III. PREVENTIVE CARE INTRODUCTION

Whether or not the assessment and treatment plan are completed at the initial visit, the personal oral daily care program should be introduced. After finding out what the current daily care has been, instruction for the parent or other caregiver is presented along with that for the patient.

The first step in treatment is the control of gingival infection. This goal can be accomplished primarily by daily plaque removal. When dental caries is present, or in keeping with routine practice policy, a food record form is explained in preparation for daily recording at home. The completed form can be brought in or mailed in so that it can be ready for review at the next appointment.

The complete instruction and prevention program is described on pages 444 to 449.

WHEELCHAIR TRANSFERS[4,5]

Three basic transfer techniques are described here. The size, weight, and mobility of the patient, along with any special physical conditions, influence the choice. The patient may prefer to transfer from the left or the right side of the dental chair depending on which side of the body is stronger.

When the patient is in a total support wheelchair, transfer to the dental chair may not be advisable. Dental and dental hygiene care may be hampered, however, unless a portable headrest and possibly a wheelchair lift, as described on page 741, are available.

I. PREPARATION FOR WHEELCHAIR TRANSFER

A. Clear the Area
Before starting a transfer, clear the area by moving the clinician's stool, bracket tray, portable unit, and dental light. After the trans-

fer, release the wheelchair brake to move it aside. In a small treatment room, the wheelchair may be folded and set aside.

B. Special Needs of Patient
1. *Chair Padding.* Special padding is usually used in a wheelchair as a protection from pressure sores. Depending on the length of the appointment, the patient will decide whether the padding should be moved to the dental chair. Pressure sores are described on page 770.
2. *Bags and Catheters.* Patients who do not have control of urine discharge, such as those with paraplegia or quadriplegia, have a bag with tubing for collection. The bag may be attached to the leg of the patient or to the wheelchair. After transfer, the tubing must be checked to be sure it is not bent or twisted.
3. *Spasms.* Ask the patient about susceptibility to spasms, and what procedures to follow for prevention.
4. *Advice Concerning Transfer.* Ask the patient, family member, or caregiver how best the clinician can help during the transfer. The patient must be allowed to do as much as possible.

II. MOBILE PATIENT TRANSFER
When a patient can support his or her own weight, the "stand and pivot" technique can be used (Figure 50-3).

A. Position the Wheelchair
Face the wheelchair in the same direction as

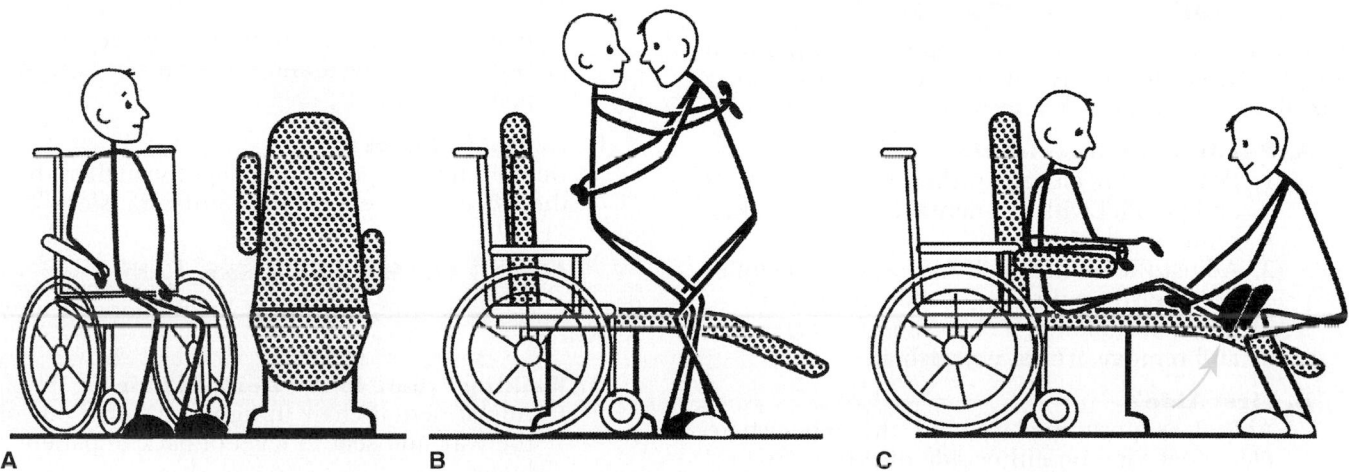

A   **B**   **C**

FIGURE 50-3 Wheelchair Transfer for a Mobile Patient. (A) Position wheelchair at level of or lower than the dental chair; set wheel locks, remove footrests and arm rest, and raise the dental chair arm. **(B)** Clinician places feet outside of patient; grasps patient around waist under arms, locks hands or grasps belt in back; patient holds clinician around shoulders or neck; patient is lifted up and pivoted to dental chair side. **(C)** Patient is gently lowered to sitting position; dental chair arm is lowered; clinician grasps legs together to lift on to dental chair.

the dental chair at approximately an angle of 30°; set brakes; remove footrests and wheelchair armrests. The patient will adjust a power-driven chair and set the brakes before turning it off.

B. Prepare Dental Chair
1. Adjust dental chair to same height as or lower than the wheelchair.
2. Clear path for transfer by uplifting the dental chair arm.

C. Approach to Patient
1. Detach patient's safety belt.
2. Face the patient and place feet outside the patient's feet for pivoting. Clinician's knees should be close to or against the patient's knees to prevent buckling.
3. Place hands under the patient's arms and grasp the waist belt in back. Patient places arms around clinician's neck or places hands on wheelchair arms to push up. Clinician lifts patient to standing position (Figure 50-3B).

D. Pivot to Dental Chair
1. Pivot together slowly until the patient is backed up to the side of the dental chair with the backs of the legs touching. The patient is gently lowered to sitting position. Reposition the arm of dental chair.
2. Grasp patient's legs together between the ankles and knees, and lift them onto the dental chair (Figure 50-3C).

E. Repeat in Reverse
After the appointment, the patient is returned to the wheelchair in the reverse order of procedure.

III. IMMOBILE PATIENT TRANSFER

When the patient is unable to support his or her own weight, two aides are required. The parent or other caregiver may serve as the second person.

A. Position the Wheelchair
1. Position wheelchair in the same direction as and parallel with the dental chair; set brakes; remove footrests.
2. Adjust the dental chair to the same height as or lower than the seat of the wheelchair.
3. Move arm of dental chair out of transfer area and remove arm of wheelchair.

B. First Aide
Aide I is positioned behind the wheelchair. Place feet, one on either side of the rear wheel nearest the dental chair; place hands under the patient's arms below the elbows, pressing forearms against the patient's lower thorax area. Clasp hands or wrists under patient's rib cage.

C. Second Aide
Aide II may do either of the following, depending on the size and weight of the patient.

1. Face patient and grasp hands under the patient's knees.
2. Face dental chair and place one arm under the thighs and the other under the calves of the lower legs.

D. Transfer
On a prearranged signal, with a steady motion, the patient is lifted and gently transferred to the dental chair.

E. Repeat in Reverse
After the appointment, the patient is returned to the wheelchair in the reverse order of procedure.

IV. SLIDING BOARD TRANSFER

A patient may bring a sliding board or one may be kept in the office or clinic. Two persons are needed when the patient is heavy or less mobile.

A. Position the Wheelchair
1. Position the wheelchair in the same direction as and parallel with the dental chair; set the brakes; remove the footrests.
2. Adjust the seat of the dental chair to slightly lower than the wheelchair seat.
3. Move the arm of the dental chair out of transfer area and remove the arm of the wheelchair.

B. Adjust the Sliding Board
Patient or clinician places the sliding board well under the hip of the patient. The board is extended across the dental chair.

C. Transfer
1. Patient slides by shifting weight, balancing on hands, and walking the buttocks across the board. The clinician who faces the patient can assist or even do the transfer by holding the patient under the axillae.
2. Board is removed and replaced after the appointment.

D. Repeat in Reverse
Dental chair is positioned slightly higher than the wheelchair seat for the return transfer.

V. WALKING FRAME, CRUTCHES, CANE

The clinician asks the patient for instructions in how to assist.

A. Walking Frame to the Dental Chair
1. Adjust dental chair upright with arm out of the way and seat to level of back of patient's knees.
2. Patient backs up to dental chair until back of legs touch, then lowers into the chair. Clinician stabilizes the walking frame.
3. Clinician takes patient by the ankles to lift legs and turn patient onto the dental chair.
4. Remove walker to a place out of the way of dental personnel.

B. Walking Frame From the Dental Chair

1. Raise dental chair to upright and ask patient to wait while the walker is positioned. Allow ample time for patient to adjust to upright position to prevent effects of postural hypotension.
2. Move arm of dental chair; position chair to approximate height of patient's knees.
3. Grasp ankles, gently turn patient, and swing legs down.
4. Reposition walker.
5. Patient uses one hand to push up and other to grasp walker. When walker is used for balance, one hand must be in the middle to prevent tipping.
6. If patient wants assistance when rising, clinician can hook an arm under the patient's arm on left side if patient is right-handed. The patient's dominant hand is used to grasp the walker.

C. Crutches

1. Dental chair is positioned upright at a level with patient's knees. Some patients need the chair higher so seating does not require knees to be bent.
2. Clinician assists, as directed by patient, while patient lowers into the chair; the legs are lifted onto the dental chair.
3. After the appointment, with patient seated on the side of the dental chair, pass the crutches together to one hand. The patient usually uses the other hand to push up. If assistance in rising is requested, the clinician can hook an arm under the patient's arm as directed.

D. Cane

1. Dental chair is positioned at the level of the patient's knees or higher if the patient may have difficulty in bending the knees.
2. Patient may need assistance in lifting the legs onto the dental chair.
3. After the appointment, when the patient is seated on the side of the dental chair, the clinician passes the cane to the patient and assists patient to rise only as directed.

PATIENT POSITION AND STABILIZATION

The objectives in patient positioning and stabilization are to let the patient feel comfortable and secure while the professional person performs in a position that provides adequate illumination, visibility, and accessibility. A hyperactive patient or a patient with involuntary muscle movements can wear a special stabilizing device to enable the clinician to work and to prevent damage to the oral tissues by accidental movement of instruments.

I. CHAIR POSITION

A. Tip Chair Back Slowly

Immediately after a patient with cerebral palsy or other condition that involves a lack of muscle control is in the dental chair, start to tip the chair back feet up first to provide balance so that the patient cannot fall. While tipping back the chair, place one hand on the patient's shoulder to offer assurance and support. Never place the chair back quickly. Advance in steps to allow the patient to adjust.

B. Chair Up

A patient with a respiratory complication must have the chair back up. A patient with a cardiac disease or a patient wearing a pacemaker should be asked "How many pillows do you use at night?" The chair can be adjusted accordingly.

II. BODY ADJUSTMENTS

During the appointment, patients with a spinal cord injury must do a "push up" and patients with quadriplegia must shift their weight every 20 minutes for 10 to 15 seconds. By doing so, the patient can maintain good circulation and healthy tissue of the buttocks, where there is no sensation. The procedure is a preventive measure for decubitus ulcers and should be a consideration during long dental procedures (page 770).

III. BODY STABILIZATION

Body movement can be limited by providing support for paralyzed limbs. When a support of any type is to be used, it should be explained to the patient. The patient must understand that the devices are used to help the clinician and to make the patient more comfortable, and are by no means a form of punishment.

A. Body Enclosure

Although a small patient may be held by a parent, such positioning can be tiring and insecure and not recommended. Better cooperation is usually obtained by the use of aids, such as commercial wraps, which are available, or improvised wraps.

1. *Pediwrap.* The *Pediwrap* is made of nylon mesh and encloses the patient from neck to ankles. It is available in 3 sizes to fit infants and children through 10 years of age. It is frequently used with support straps about the patient's legs and arms.
2. *Papoose Board.* A *papoose board* is a board with padded wraps to enclose a patient (Figure 50-4). It is available in three sizes, from a small child size to an adult size.
3. *Bedsheet or Blanket.* The parent can bring from home a blanket or sheet that is familiar to the patient. The sheet or blanket is folded firmly around the patient twice and held se-

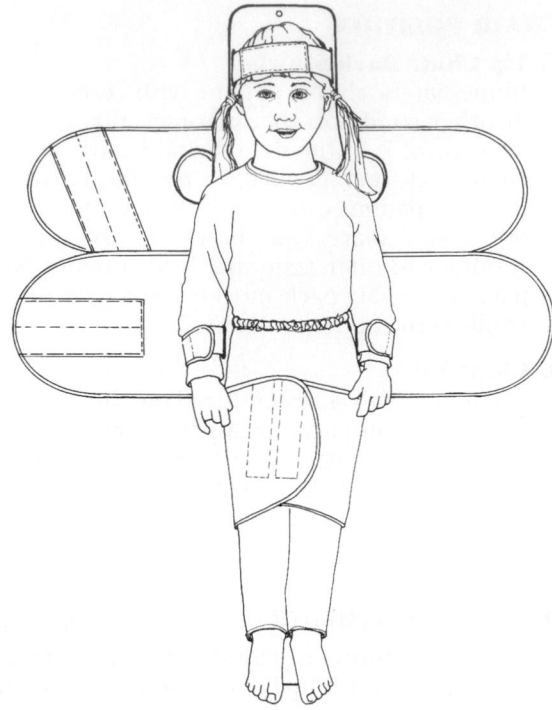

FIGURE 50-4 Papoose Board. Stabilization is accomplished by three body wraps and a head restrainer. The arms are secured at the wrists, as shown, before the large center wrap is closed. (From King, E.M., Wieck, L., and Dyer, M.: *Illustrated Manual of Nursing Techniques.* Philadelphia, J.B. Lippincott Co., 1977, page 311.)

curely by a Velcro strap around the body. Support straps about the legs and body provide the patient with additional control.

B. Support Straps

Adhesive tape (2 or 3 inches wide), canvas, or Velcro straps may be used with or without body enclosure. A soft strap may be made from a soft material, such as flannel, with a padded section to place over the wrists, ankles, or where needed. Ties 4 to 6 inches wide may be passed around the dental chair or may be tied to the arms of the chair.

C. Head Stabilization

1. *Arm of Clinician.* From a working position at 12 o'clock (top of patient's head), the non-dominant arm is placed around the patient's head to hold it in position.
2. *Mouth Prop* (page 758).

ASSESSMENT OF PATIENT

As many as possible of the procedures for assessment are accomplished at the first appointment. The goals should be the same for all patients, namely, to prepare the assessment material to be reviewed and analyzed for care planning. Suggestions for preparing the medical history are on page 739.

The patient may not be able to complete all the steps in the assessment, and extra time may be needed for orientation. Each clinic procedure is prefaced by an explanation and demonstration. Several trials may be needed.

ORAL MANIFESTATIONS

Oral diseases of disabled individuals are not different in kind from those of nondisabled persons. The two principal diseases found are dental caries and periodontal infections. Other oral findings include congenital malformations, oral injuries, and malocclusions. In the chapters devoted to describing specific individuals with disabilities, oral characteristics of each are included.

For a majority of patients with disabilities, dental and dental hygiene treatment is not different once the patient is in the dental chair, sedated if needed, and stabilized physically. For a few other patients, an oral manifestation can be caused by, or be a result of, the patient's disabling condition or the treatment for it. Examples are included here.

I. CONGENITAL MALFORMATIONS

A. Cleft Lip or Palate (Pages 665 to 668)

B. Other Craniofacial Anomalies

C. Tooth Defects

An increased incidence of malformations has been observed with developmental disabilities, for example:

1. Variations in number and structure of teeth.
2. Dentinogenesis imperfecta, amelogenesis imperfecta, enamel hyperplasia, and other abnormalities of tooth structure.

II. ORAL INJURIES

A. Attrition

Attrition caused by bruxism is particularly common among individuals with cerebral palsy and mental retardation.

B. Trauma to Teeth and Soft Tissues

Trauma to teeth and soft tissues may result from accidents (instability, falling), self-abuse, or seizures. The individual with epilepsy is particularly susceptible to accidents. Chipped and fractured teeth, as well as residual scars in the tongue and lips, may be seen frequently.

Because of personal limitations and living a protected life, many patients with disabilities are not exposed to contact sports, traffic accidents, and other accident-prone situations. The incidence of facial trauma may be expected to be less.

III. FACIAL WEAKNESS OR PARALYSIS

When a patient has muscle weakness or paralysis of one side of the face, bilateral mastication is not possible. Plaque usually collects more heavily, and food debris is retained on the involved side. Certain patients may have bilateral weakness.

IV. MALOCCLUSION

Malocclusion is frequently found among persons with developmental disabilities. Factors contributing to problems of occlusion include skeletal and muscular deformities, macroglossia, congenitally missing teeth, and such oral habits as tongue thrust and mouth breathing.

V. THERAPY-RELATED ORAL FINDINGS

A. Phenytoin-Induced Gingival Overgrowth

Patients whose treatment for seizures requires phenytoin (Dilantin) may be susceptible to a slight to severe gingival enlargement. The severity of the enlargement usually depends on the maintenance of healthy gingival tissue associated with adequate daily plaque control. A description of phenytoin-induced gingival overgrowth is included in Chapter 54, page 805.

B. Chemotherapy

Oral ulcerations, mucositis, and susceptibility to infection are frequent manifestations following cancer chemotherapy. Patients with leukemia have a high incidence of oral manifestations, including lymphadenopathy, gingival changes with bleeding, and petechiae, that are more severe following chemotherapy.

C. Radiation Therapy

When radiation therapy of the head and neck area involves the cells of the salivary glands, xerostomia can result and contribute to an increased incidence of dental caries. The symptoms and treatment aspects of radiation therapy are described on pages 727 to 730.

DENTAL HYGIENE CARE PLAN

Parts of the total care plan can be identified under preventive, educational, and therapeutic services.

I. PREVENTIVE THERAPY

A. Bacterial Plaque Control

B. Fluoride Program

1. Supervision of self-applied daily fluoride.
2. Periodic professionally applied topical fluoride.

C. Pit and Fissure Sealants

II. EDUCATIONAL

A. Orientation

Patient orientation to each dental hygiene and dental procedure.

B. Counseling

Parental counseling starting as early as possible after an infant is known to have a disability.

C. Instruction in Disease Control

1. Plaque control for natural teeth and prostheses.
2. Daily fluoride, systemic and/or topical.
3. Dietary and nutritional effects.

III. THERAPEUTIC

A. Patient's plaque control for therapeutic purposes until tissue health is attained, followed by planned maintenance.
B. Complete scaling and root debridement.
C. Removal of overhanging fillings.
D. Re-evaluation for additional periodontal therapy.
E. Restorative phase; finishing restorations.

DISEASE PREVENTION AND CONTROL

I. PREVENTIVE PROGRAM COMPONENTS

A. Bacterial plaque control.
B. Fluorides.
C. Pit and fissure sealants.
D. Diet counseling.
E. Smoking cessation.
F. Regular professional examinations and treatment at intervals as recommended by the dentist and dental hygienist.

II. FUNCTIONING LEVELS

For a patient who does not have a mental or physical disability, neglect of personal oral hygiene usually can be explained by either a lack of knowledge and understanding about the need for plaque removal and how it is accomplished or a lack of motivation to carry out the necessary daily routines. For certain patients with disabilities, the problem of disease control becomes greatly magnified because of a lack of the necessary mental and/or physical coordination to carry out even the simplest of oral hygiene measures.

Depending on the severity of the disability, many patients need either complete or partial assistance. Assistance must be provided by parents and other family members when living at home, or by an aide or other caregiver responsible for the patient's care in a residence or institutional setting. There is a twofold responsibility to teach and supervise the patient and the patient's caregivers. Suggestions for in-service education are on page 756.

A *high, moderate,* or *low* functioning level refers to the daily living skills (bathing, toothbrushing, dressing, for example) an individual can do alone, what range or degree of assistance is needed, or whether the person depends on others for complete care. The functioning levels have also been called *self-care, partial care,* or *total care.* In another concept, the terms *supervised, supervised/assistance,* and *maintenance (by others)* have been used.[6]

A. High Functioning Level

The high functioning, self-care group includes those capable of flossing and brushing their own teeth. Many patients, particularly children and those of all ages who are mentally retarded, need varying degrees of encouragement, motivation, and supervision.

B. Moderate Functioning Level

The moderate functioning, partial-care group includes those capable of carrying out at least part of their oral hygiene needs, but who require considerable training, assistance, and direct supervision. The assistance may be verbal, gestural, or hand-over-hand.

C. Low Functioning Level

The low functioning, total-care group includes those who are unable to attend to their own care and are therefore dependent. Patients in this group may be bedridden and nonambulatory, although others may be confined to wheelchairs. With training, some may be able to attempt a part of their own care.

III. PREPARATION FOR INSTRUCTION

A. Basic Planning Questions

1. What is the patient's functioning level?
2. Will the patient do all or part of the plaque removal personally or require partial or total care?
3. Is the patient involved in any community dental health programs (home, school, or day activity), and can the dentist and/or dental hygienist in such a program be contacted to coordinate the instruction given?
4. Will the parent or caregiver do part or all of the oral care?
5. What disabilities have the greatest influence on the extent of self-care possible and anticipated success of the overall preventive program? Mental? Physical? Sensory? Learning? Oral?
6. Which techniques and procedures will best fit the situation of the particular patient and the parent or caregiver?
7. How can the patient be helped to be as independent as possible?

B. Introduction

For the answers to these questions, an initial plan is made, with the realization that the system is on a trial-and-error basis. As the skills of the patient and parent improve and less plaque is observed and recorded on succeeding appointments, adaptations can be made. In the meantime, communication improves and the patient's trust develops as the sincere concern of the dental team is realized.

For all patients, with or without a disability, the aim is complete daily plaque control. Such an ideal result may seem far from reality with a moderate or low functioning person, but with continuing reinforcement and inspiration, progress can be made. Patient and parental attitudes, willingness to participate, and acceptance of the recommended procedures must be taken into consideration.

BACTERIAL PLAQUE REMOVAL

I. COMPONENTS

General procedures for instruction and methods for toothbrushing, interdental plaque removal, and care of fixed and removable prostheses are described in Chapters 23 through 26. Individualization for each patient's needs and abilities is necessary. Each step must be explained slowly and carefully.

A. Provide Basic Information

Plaque formation and disease development are described on a level at which the patient and parent can learn and be motivated.

B. Disclose and Show Plaque

An ongoing record of the extent of plaque in graphic form by which the patient and parent can watch progress may help to motivate many patients.

C. Toothbrushing

1. Provide a soft toothbrush and ask the patient to remove the disclosed plaque from the teeth. For the completely dependent patient, the parent will demonstrate. Alternative positions for the parent are described on pages 753 and 754 and in Figure 50-11.
2. Plaque removal is more important than the specific technique used, as long as damage is not done to the gingiva or teeth. A scrub-brush or circular Fones method may be appropriate and within the capability of certain patients (page 361).
3. Explain each step and demonstrate slowly.
4. Adaptations for brush handles and other devices to promote or make possible a patient's independent performance are described on pages 749 to 752.

D. Dentifrice

A dentifrice containing fluoride is recommended for patients who can use a dentifrice. An ingestible dentifrice may prove useful. The factors to consider when deciding whether a standard noningestible dentifrice should be used include the following:

1. When a patient cannot rinse or expectorate, a dentifrice should not be used. The person who is institutionalized and severely disabled may be treated with a suction brush as described on pages 764 to 765.
2. When a parent or other caregiver is performing the brushing, the paste may limit visibility for thorough plaque removal. When a paste is used, only a small amount should be

placed on the brush (pea size, Figure 29-8, page 472).

3. Dentifrice may increase a gag reflex for certain patients.

4. For the patient whose problem is brush manipulation, and for whom special adaptations of the brush are recommended, management of the dentifrice may be awkward and messy.

5. Dentifrice is not essential to plaque removal, and other means for daily fluoride application may prove easier for certain patients. A brush-on gel may be recommended.

E. Dental Floss

With time and repeated instruction, many patients with disabilities can learn to use dental floss, and some can learn to use other interdental aids. The use of a floss holder can make flossing possible for certain patients, such as those with limited digital dexterity or the use of only one hand (Figure 50-8 and 50-9).

The holder may also be useful for the parent or other caregiver. Methods for increasing the size of a toothbrush handle may be adapted for the handle of a floss holder.

II. EVALUATION

Many patients, parents, and other caregivers can learn with demonstration and practice how to examine the teeth and gingiva. The signs of healthy gingiva, especially color and absence of bleeding on brushing, can be noted.

For selected patients, the thoroughness of brushing can be improved if a disclosing agent is used at the start. The visible objective then is to remove all the color. Another system is to apply a disclosing agent after brushing to determine completion of plaque removal. Then, any additional plaque noted is brushed and removed.

When a patient brushes first, followed by the caregiver, the disclosing agent might be applied by the caregiver so the task of removal can be completed. Because the patient is encouraged to do as much as possible and is praised for whatever successes are accomplished, the plaque disclosed for the caregiver to remove may be a factor of discouragement to the patient who really had done the very best to the extent of individual capability. A better plan could be for the patient to do all the brushing and flossing once a day, and for the caregiver to do all the brushing and flossing at a different time.

SELF-CARE AIDS

Although a caregiver may be willing to brush the patient's teeth, as much as possible should be carried out by the patient. Psychologic benefits to the patient result in feelings of self-esteem and accomplishment when able to manage the important and worthwhile task of brushing.

For patients of all ages whose main deterrent to personal self-care is related to grasp, manipulation, or control of a toothbrush, adaptations of the brush have been devised.[7-9] Modifications to accommodate specific needs include enlarged handles, hand attachments, and elongated handles.

I. GENERAL PREREQUISITES FOR A SELF-CARE AID

A. Cleanable.

B. Durable. Can withstand exposure to water and saliva.

C. Resistant to absorption of oral fluids.

II. TOOTHBRUSHING

A. For Patient With Fingers Permanently Fixed in a Fist

Insert the brush handle into the grasp.

B. For Patient Who Cannot Grasp and Hold

1. *Objective.* To fasten the brush handle to the open hand.

2. *Methods*

   a. Velcro strap around hand has a slit on the palm side into which the brush handle can be inserted. A vinyl pocket with an adjustable Velcro strap is commercially available. The toothbrush handle fits into the pocket (Figure 50-5A). The device can be used to hold other utensils for the patient, such as eating utensils.

   b. Handle of fingernail brush attached to toothbrush by adhesive water-resistant tape (Figure 50-5B).

   c. Wide rubber strap or a length of small-diameter rubber tubing attached through the hole in the toothbrush handle and tied adjacent to the brush head so the patient's hand can be slipped under the rubber and the brush can be held firmly (Figure 50-5C).

C. For Patient With Limited Hand Closure (unable to manipulate usual toothbrush handle or floss holder)

1. *Objective.* Enlarge the diameter of the handle.

2. *Methods*

   a. Bicycle handle grip. Insert toothbrush handle (Figure 50-6A).

   b. Soft rubber ball or a styrofoam ball. Push brush handle in (Figure 50-6B). Styrofoam balls are available in various sizes from craft shops.

   c. Juice or soda pop can. Place the rubber ball with toothbrush inside the can (Figure 50-6C).

   d. Foam rubber hair roller. Insert brush handle.

   e. Quick-cure acrylic. Obtain an impression of the hand grasp by having the patient grasp a cylinder of base plate wax. Then, fill the wax cylinder with quick-cure

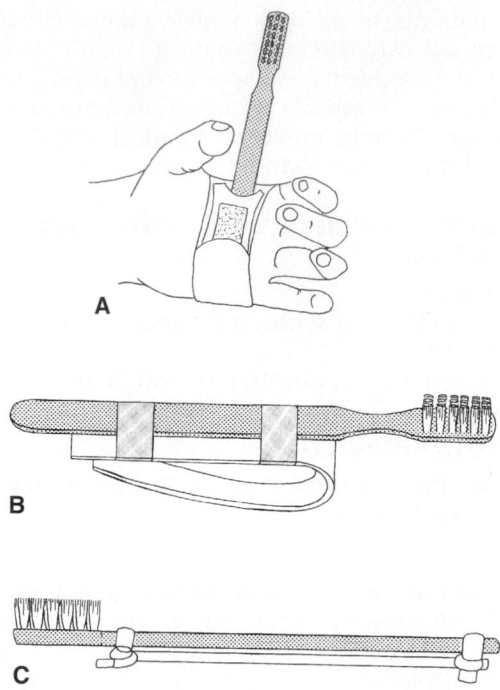

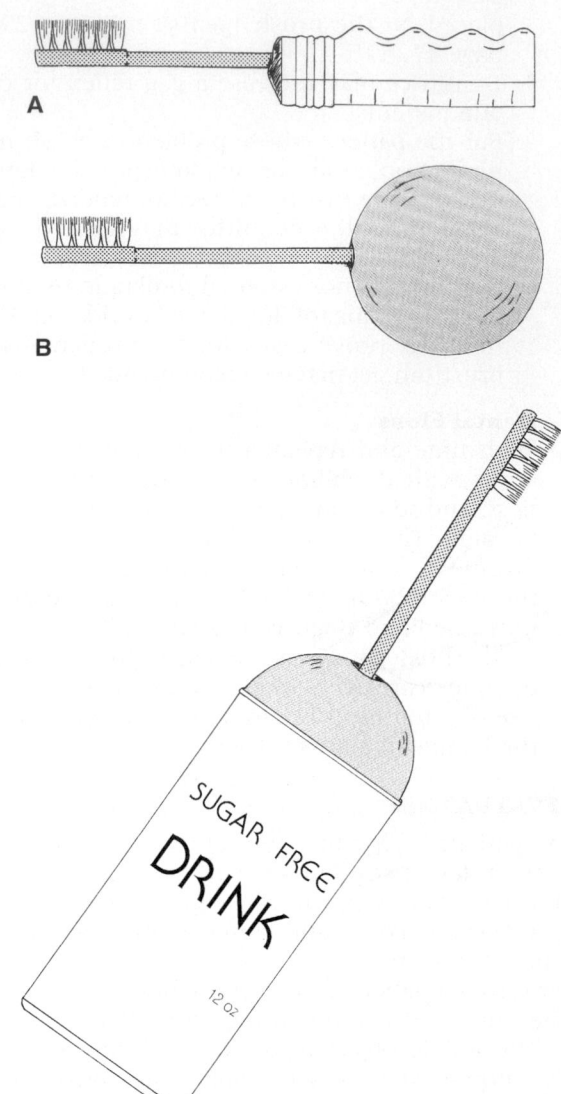

■ **FIGURE 50-5 Aids for Patient Who Cannot Grasp and Hold. (A)** Adjustable Velcro strap around hand has a pocket designed to hold the toothbrush handle. **(B)** Handle of a fingernail brush attached to toothbrush by adhesive tape. **(C)** Rubber tubing attached firmly to toothbrush handle enables patient to hold brush across the palm of the hand. A floss holder also may be held by these methods.

acrylic. Insert the toothbrush handle before the acrylic sets. The angle may be adjusted to set the brush head for the patient's convenient use. Polish the acrylic.

D. For Patient Unable to Lift Hand or Arm (with limited shoulder or elbow movement)

1. *Objective.* Lengthen the handle of the brush.
2. *Prerequisite.* The material must be strong or rigid enough to maintain the brush contact with sufficient lateral pressure to remove plaque from the tooth surfaces.
3. *Methods*
   a. Cylinder of wood with brush handle cemented inside.[7]
   b. Two brushes. Cut the head from an old brush and fasten the handle to the end of the new brush handle (glue, tape, heat).
   c. Tongue depressors taped to the brush handle, then one or two other tongue depressors taped to overlap and provide an extension.
   d. Bicycle spoke, coat hanger, or other means for elongation fixed with a handle of acrylic resin. The metal tip may be

■ **FIGURE 50-6 Aids for Patient with Limited Grasp. (A)** Toothbrush inserted into a bicycle handle grip. **(B)** Toothbrush inserted into a soft rubber ball. **(C)** Toothbrush in soft rubber ball inserted into a juice or soda pop can can provide a handle of appropriate diameter for patients with limited hand closure.

heated and pushed into the toothbrush handle.[10,11] Use double or triple thickness to avoid flexibility.

E. For Patient Who Can Hold and Position the Toothbrush but Cannot Manipulate to Make Strokes for Plaque Removal

1. *Specially Designed Toothbrush.* A manual brush that brushes exposed tooth surfaces simultaneously (Figure 50-7). With curved outer filaments and a short stiff center row of filaments, the brush requires only a back-and-forth stroke. Research showed a similar reduction in debris and bacterial plaque with

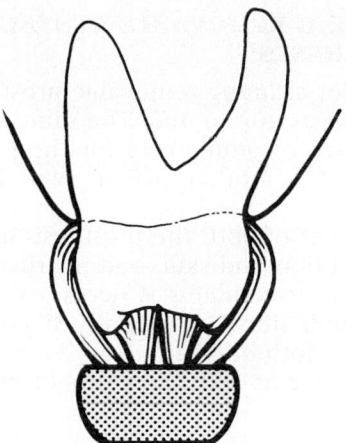

■FIGURE 50-7 **Aid for Patient with a Brushing Problem.** A specially designed toothbrush *(Collis Curve)* is shown on the mesial of a maxillary second primary molar. Used with a back-and-forth motion, the filaments remove debris and bacterial plaque simultaneously from the facial, lingual (palatal), and occlusal tooth surfaces.

this brush when compared with such reduction with a conventional brush.[12]

2. *Patient Moves Head Instead of Hand.* Guide patient to learn to move the head up and down and from side to side while a conventional soft brush is held against the teeth.[11]

F. Use of a Power-Assisted Toothbrush

A power-assisted brush can serve as a motivational adjunct for selected patients (pages 362 to 363). For an uncoordinated patient, a power-assisted brush could be harmful. The various models present different characteristics.

1. *Advantages and Disadvantages*[13]
   a. The extra weight of the handle may prove advantageous for some patients, but disadvantageous for others with limited arm strength.
   b. The on/off mechanism may require more strength and finger coordination to operate than certain patients can manage.
   c. The brush handle is thick and therefore helpful for a patient with grasping problems.
   d. The vibration created during use cannot be tolerated by certain patients.
2. *Suggestions for Use*
   a. For use without hands, attach the brush handle by means of a clamp in a stationary upright position lower than the patient's mouth when bending down. An alert, controlled patient can insert the brush and apply to the teeth, moving the head for application to all surfaces. The use of a dentifrice probably would be contraindicated because splashing might be uncontrollable.

b. A Velcro cuff around the hand and the brush can aid in brush control.

3. *Institutional Use.* Although not possible for most institutionalized patients to use for themselves, power-assisted brushes have been found effective by caregivers in certain situations. Handles must be disinfected between uses and replaced promptly when out of order, which may present problems in some institutions.

Cross-contamination is a problem even when individual brush tips are labeled, washed, and kept apart. Special instruction for the caregivers is needed, and repeated motivation for any toothbrushing program is essential. Using a power-assisted brush is not encouraged by many dental hygienists associated with long-term care institutions.

III. USE OF FLOSS HOLDER

A. Types

Several types of plastic floss holders are available (Figure 50-8).

B. Use

Careful instruction should be provided and supervision given periodically to prevent tissue

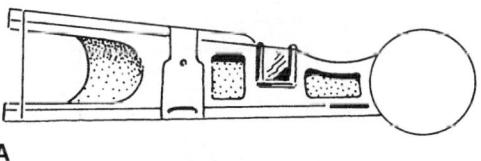

A

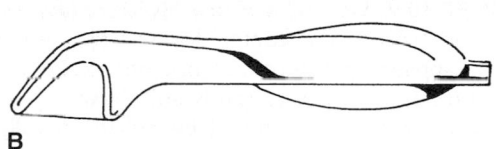

B

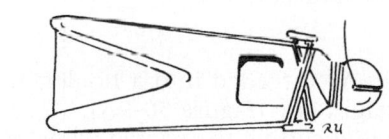

C

■FIGURE 50-8 **Floss Holders.** A variety of floss holders are available. **(A)** A holder with a replaceable floss container. **(B)** A holder with a replaceable floss cartridge and a thin edge for cleaning the tongue. **(C)** A holder with a threading mechanism for a 24-inch length of floss applied at each use. A fourth type, shown in Figure 50-9, is operated in a manner similar to that shown in **C.**

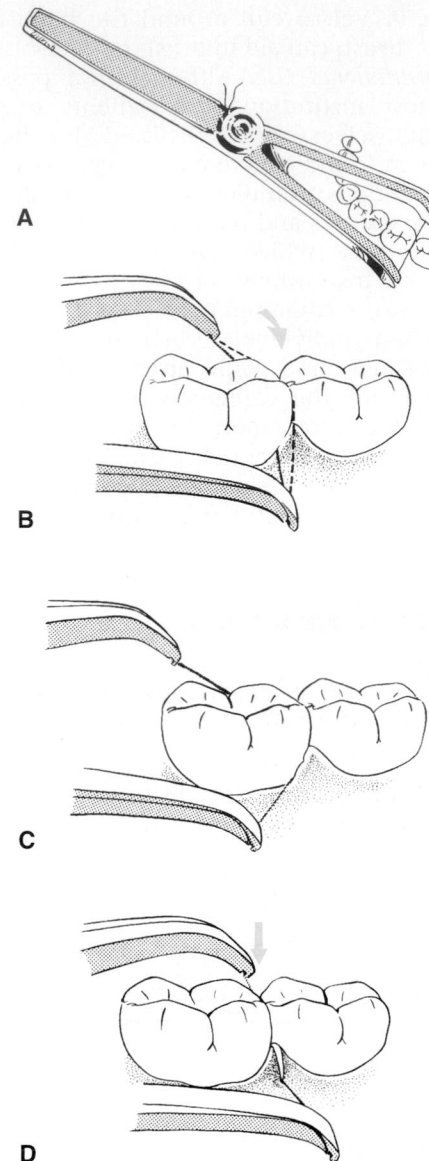

FIGURE 50-9 Use of a Floss Holder. (A) The floss is held over the proximal contact for insertion. A hand rest should be applied on the chin to prevent excess pressure. **(B)** As the floss is lowered gently and drawn through the contact area, the holder should be pulled mesially when the floss is applied to the distal surface and pushed distally when the floss is applied to the mesial surface. **(C)** Floss is lowered slightly below the gingival margin. **(D)** Floss cut in the papilla when used incorrectly.

damage. As threaded into a holder, the floss is in a straight line (Figure 50-9A).

To avoid cutting the papilla when applied interproximally:

1. Use a rest or fulcrum to prevent snapping through the contact.
2. Pull the floss mesially (to clean the distal surface of a tooth) or push distally (to clean mesial surface) to allow floss to be positioned on the side of the papilla (Figure 50-9C).

IV. CLEANING REMOVABLE DENTAL PROSTHESES[7,14]

The details for cleaning removable prostheses are described on pages 402 to 408. The same materials and procedures are recommended for the patient with a disability or for another person who cares for the prosthesis.

Management of both the prosthesis and the brush requires attention and skill, and instruction in methods that prevent accidents is necessary. In all procedures, the sink must be partially filled with water, and/or a face cloth or small towel should be placed in the sink to serve as a cushion should the denture be dropped.

A. Grasp Problem

For the patient with difficulty grasping or holding the brush, a denture brush handle may be adapted by any of the methods described for the regular toothbrush (Figure 50-6). A fingernail brush may be used instead of a standard denture brush, provided all denture surfaces can be reached for plaque removal.

B. One Hand

For the patient handicapped by hemiplegia or for the patient with use of two hands but who needs to grasp the denture with two hands to prevent accidents, the following are recommended:

1. Fingernail brush with suction cups.
2. Denture brush in mounting that has suction cups. These are available commercially (Figure 50-10A).
3. Denture brush with suction cups to attach low inside the sink bowl (Figure 50-10B).

INSTRUCTION FOR CAREGIVER

Individuals who need partial or total care present with varying degrees of ability to cooperate, depending on the nature of the disability. The size of the patient and whether the patient is ambulatory, bedridden, or in a wheelchair are among the factors that influence the technique for management.

The instruction for the parents or the other caregiver should be given where the specific techniques can actually be demonstrated as they will be done at home. When the patient lies down with the head in the parent's lap, for example, a suitable couch should be used, or chairs can be placed together. Time and repeated practice sessions are needed for successful plaque removal for a difficult patient.

I. SELF-CARE AND ATTITUDE

Whenever possible, instruction for the parents, family members, or other caregivers begins with their own personal oral care. The most success comes when those who care for the patient have knowledge and

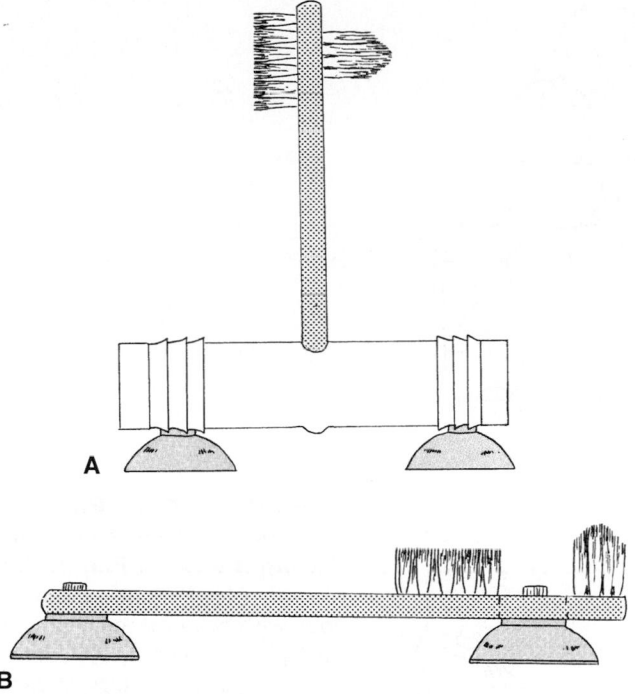

FIGURE 50-10 Denture Brushes with Suction Cups. (A) Denture brush in a commercially available mounting. **(B)** Suction cups attached directly to a denture brush. Either brush may be positioned in a sink to aid the person who has one hand or who needs to grasp the denture with two hands to prevent accidental dropping and breakage.

understanding of the purposes and techniques and can demonstrate their own bacterial plaque removal.

An appreciation for the need for preventive care and for why the health of the teeth and gingiva are of great importance to the well-being and overall health of the patient can help those responsible to develop the patience and take the necessary time from their own busy schedules.

II. GENERAL SUGGESTIONS

A. Place

The plaque removal procedures must be performed where both the patient and the caregiver can be comfortable and relaxed. A small bathroom may be the least desirable place because positioning the patient may be awkward except when a standing position can be used.

Good light, easy visibility of the teeth, and control of the head of the person with the disability are prerequisites.

B. Teaching Techniques for Plaque Removal

1. *Use of Finger and Hand Rests.* The person performing the plaque removal must learn how to balance the toothbrush, dental floss, floss aid, or any other implement with a finger or hand rest on the side of the patient's face or chin. Such contact contributes to total patient control and to effective use of the plaque removal device.

2. *Use of a Mouth Prop.* For certain patients, plaque removal is impossible without a mouth prop, and demonstration for insertion on both sides is needed. For home use, a washable, rubber prop is practical.

III. POSITIONS

General positions that involve one or two people are suggested here.[15] When the patient is young, hyperactive, and unable to cooperate, and the assistance of a second person is not available, the use of a blanket or sheet wrap may be necessary (page 745).

In the following description, the term "parent" is used to mean the family member or other caregiver who may be performing the plaque removal.

A. Parent Standing

With the parent standing from behind, the arm is brought around the patient's head and the chin is cupped while using the thumb and index finger to retract the lips and cheeks. The other hand applies the toothbrush, floss aid, or other device. This technique requires that the patient be able to bend the head back far enough for the parent to see the maxillary teeth. The procedure may be applicable for the following.

1. Short patient standing in front of and backed up to the parent.
2. Tall patient seated in a chair with the head tipped back to lean against the parent, or seated in a large chair or sofa with the head stabilized against the top of chair back.
3. Patient in a wheelchair leaning back against the parent. Wheelchair brakes are set.

B. Parent Seated

1. Patient seated on pillow on floor in front of parent, with back close to the chair and head turned back into parent's lap (Figure 50-11A). The parent may place his/her legs over the shoulders of the patient to restrain arms and body movements (Figure 50-11B).
2. Parent is seated at the end of a sofa or couch, and patient is lying down with the head in parent's lap (Figure 50-11C).
3. For a bedridden patient, the parent may sit at the patient's head and place the head in the lap. When body and arm movements must be controlled, the parent can sit beside the patient, lean across the patient's chest, and hold the patient's arm against the body with the elbow. The hand of the restraining arm can hold the mouth prop, retract, or do whatever is necessary. If the patient is particularly difficult, a sheet or blanket wrap is indicated.

C. Two People

In any of the positions previously mentioned, the parent may need the assistance of a second

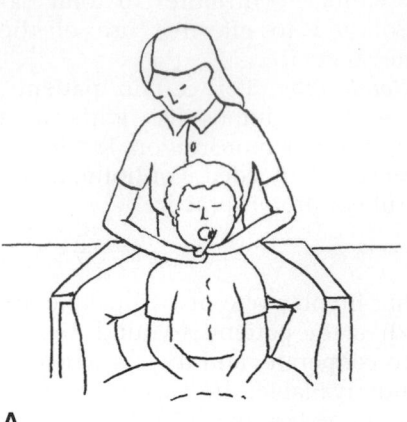

A

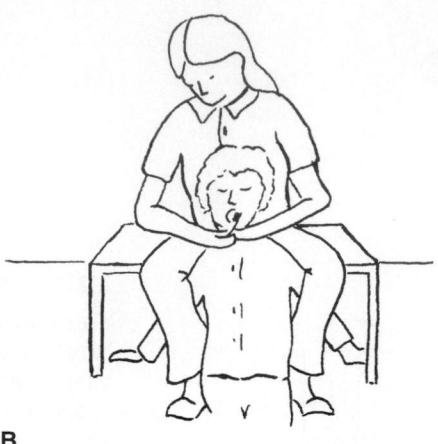

B

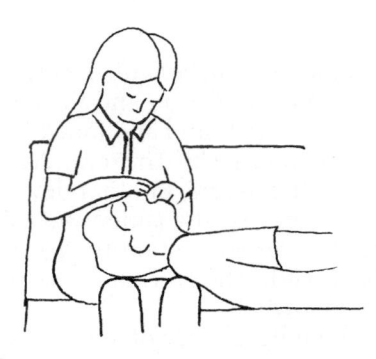

C

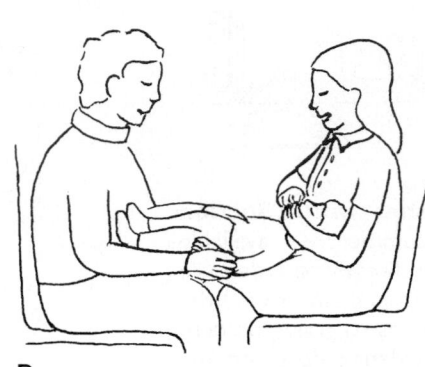

D

■ FIGURE 50-11 **Positions for Child or Disabled Patient During Bacterial Plaque Removal. (A)** Patient seated on floor with head turned back into the lap of caregiver. **(B)** Patient's arms restrained by legs of caregiver. **(C)** Patient reclining on couch with head in lap of caregiver. **(D)** Two people participating with small child between. One holds patient for stabilization while other holds the head for toothbrushing and flossing.

person to hold the hands and arms or otherwise restrain the patient.

A small child may be placed across the laps of two persons seated facing each other. One stabilizes the head and brushes and flosses while the other person holds hands, arms, and legs, as needed (Figure 50-11D).

FLUORIDES

Selection of a multiple fluoride program for an individual patient depends on the age, the caries status, and the concentration of fluoride in the water supply. In addition, for a patient with a disability, the abilities to cooperate, to accept the vehicle and mode of application, and to master the technique required for a self-administered preparation dictate the final recommendation.

I. FLUORIDATION

A. Community Water Fluoridation

As more communities begin to fluoridate the water supplies, more of the total population, including persons with disabilities, will benefit.

B. Institutional Water Fluoridation

Research has shown the benefits derived from fluoridation of a school water supply when the community in which the school was located could not or did not have fluoridation. These programs were summarized in Chapter 29, page 462.

Institutions where individuals with disabilities reside may have a water supply that could be fluoridated. Installation is a relatively inexpensive procedure when the health benefits and the decreased need for professional care are realized.

II. DIETARY SUPPLEMENTS

When the community water supply is deficient in fluoride content, the fluoride level is below optimum, or the water intake by a child is low, a supplement is recommended, as shown in Table 29-2, page 464. Depending on the masticatory function of the child, that is, whether chewing or rinsing is possible, the fluoride can be prescribed in the form of a chewable tablet, lozenge, drops, or mouthwash to swallow after swishing.

III. PROFESSIONALLY APPLIED TOPICAL FLUORIDE

When water fluoridation is not available or when the benefits of water fluoridation must be supplemented, at least two topical applications per year are indicated, and more frequently if the dental caries rate is high. the method for application and system for isolation of the teeth depend on the patient's ability to cooperate.

IV. SELF-APPLIED PROCEDURES

Whether the individual with a disability is a child or an adult, a home fluoride program is indicated.

After disease control techniques for flossing and toothbrushing have been completed before the patient retires, a mouthrinse, for the patient who can rinse; a gel applied by tray or toothbrush; or a chewable tablet, for the patient who can chew and who needs a fluoride supplement, may be advised. For a young, dependent, low-functioning person, brushing with a gel or swabbing with a fluoride rinse might be most applicable.

Parental supervision and cooperation are essential. Motivation of the parent or caregiver needs regular reinforcement by the dental team.

PIT AND FISSURE SEALANTS

Pit and fissure sealants have been used for children with developmental disabilities with satisfactory results.[16,17] The principles for application are the same as those described for all patients (pages 482 to 485) The use of a rubber dam is especially important for patients with excess saliva, hyperactivity of the tongue, or other management difficulties.

When a severely disabled patient will be administered general anesthesia for restorative procedures, pit and fissure sealants should be placed in all noncarious occlusal surfaces while the patient is under control. For all young patients, the sealant can be placed as soon after eruption as the tooth will hold a rubber dam.[15]

DIET INSTRUCTION

Efforts to help adults who are disabled and the parents, family members, advocates, and other caregivers responsible to understand the general dietary requirements for oral health and how to put the principles into daily practice are a distinct part of the total preventive program. Information from Chapter 28 is applicable to patients with special needs as well as to all patients.

A careful assessment of current eating habits, extent of knowledge, family customs, and economic factors as they relate to a patient's condition is necessary before specific recommendations can be made. In an institutional setting, efforts can be directed to contact and work with the administrative personnel, teachers, dietitians, and aides. Coordination of plaque control, snack selection, and snack availability, together with the fluoride program, opens the way to caries control.

I. FACTORS THAT INFLUENCE DIET HABITS

For certain patients, diet selection and utilization center around problems of mastication, whereas for others, the transport of food to the mouth is a major undertaking. The problems of the elderly patient are described on pages 693 to 695.

The following partial list of problems is suggested to help during dietary analysis and counseling. Many of the problems are directly related to increases in plaque accumulation and resultant dental caries and periodontal infections.

A. Masticatory or Feeding Problems
Problems in eating can lead to the use of a soft diet, often composed mainly of carbohydrates.

B. Overindulgence in Sucrose-Containing Foods
Sweets are sometimes used as rewards or bribes by unsuspecting family members or teachers involved in behavior modification procedures in training programs.

Nonambulatory or otherwise confined patients may have less access to between-meal foods and, therefore, may eat more regularly, as served. On the other hand, the confined person may have snacks and sweets readily available, which can lead to dental destruction.

C. Inability to Accomplish Personal Plaque Control Measures
Problems of daily bacterial plaque removal can be related to a physical disability or lack of assistance from a parent or aide, combined with a diet high in cariogenic foods, which leads to dental caries development.

D. Lack of Professional Care and Instruction
Many patients do not receive adequate professional care because of unavailability, inability to obtain care because of physical barriers, inadequate financial support, lack of knowledge of the importance of oral health, or preoccupation with other major health problems.

E. Medications
1. Medications with a side effect of xerostomia contribute to dental caries.
2. Medications that diminish appetite as a side effect influence diet habits.
3. Medications contained within a sucrose base designed to mask the flavor of the agent or to pacify the patient contribute to dental caries incidence.[18]

F. Obesity
Obesity is a problem with certain patients who suffer from inactivity, overeating, boredom, or lack of knowledge of proper food selection.

G. Food Preparation
Difficulty of food preparation can be a major limitation to diet selection for adults with neu-

romuscular disorders. Wheelchair confinement, lack of muscular coordination, hemiplegia or paraplegia, and dependence on others for grocery shopping are examples of problems encountered.

II. DIET ASSESSMENT AND COUNSELING

A. Food Record
A high-functioning patient, except the very young, may be able to keep a food record, and participation should be encouraged. The parent, advocate, or other caregiver can assist or, in the case of a low- or moderate-functioning person, may complete the entire record. With the aid of the record and the information from the medical and dental histories, items for counseling can be selected.

B. Recommendations
General procedures for assessment and counseling are described on pages 444 to 449. Adaptations involve long-range planning for gradual modification of each patient's diet.

The person who selects and prepares the food must be involved in the planning. Sugarless snacks and sugarless rewards during behavior modification training are especially important to control.

Parents need instruction as early as possible after a newborn is known to be developmentally disabled, so that fluoride, diet, early personal hygiene, and the prevention of baby bottle caries can be coordinated into the daily program. As described on pages 660 to 662, the infant's early care should include an oral examination by the dentist and dental hygienist within 6 months of the eruption of the first tooth and no later than 12 months of age.

GROUP IN-SERVICE EDUCATION

In-service programs may be provided for teachers, registered nurses, other health professionals, parents, and volunteers in school and community preventive programs. For example, all persons mentioned could be involved in the preparation for a program of classroom weekly rinsing with a fluoride mouthrinse. When a program is citywide and many dental hygienists are involved, in-service preparation for the dental hygienists themselves is necessary.

A special need exists for in-service instruction in oral health measures for the caregivers in extended care institutions. Many patients in such facilities are unable to care for their own needs and may require total care, partial assistance, supervision, or regular reminders. The dental hygienist is able to work with the caregivers to teach them appropriate techniques and to motivate them to incorporate oral care into the daily routine for each resident or patient.

The general suggestions outlined in the following sections pertain to preparation and content for in-service workshops for the oral care of long-term patients.

I. PREPARATION FOR AN IN-SERVICE PROGRAM

A. Planning
An in-service program needs careful planning. For many groups, time for an in-service is taken from an already busy work schedule. Nonmotivated participants require special considerations. A leading factor contributing to the success of a program is the genuine concern and enthusiasm of the program leader in motivating the participants.

The material must be clear and to the point, interestingly presented with appropriate visual aids, and stimulating for learning. Objectives should be defined in writing and serve as a guide to preparation and evaluation.

Problems of the staff must be recognized. Some members may have negative oral health attitudes, minimal educational background, and poor personal oral health.

Initially, basic preparation includes learning about the functioning levels of the clients and assessing the procedures used for their oral care. A survey of the plaque control materials and devices available and in current use, methods for labeling or storing individual brushes, and the frequency of use is important.

B. Use of Clinic Records
Clinic records for each patient should be examined for information relative to the dental status and to those who wear dentures. Medical histories must be reviewed so that special general or oral health problems can be considered and necessary precautions taken.

When a dental hygienist is employed regularly within an institution, a much more complete assessment can be made. The dental hygienist invited to the institution for the specific purpose of presenting the workshop must arrange a preworkshop visit for observing the caregivers and the clients.

C. Gingival/Plaque Index
The use of a gingival or plaque index (pages 298 to 302, 307) can provide a baseline of information from which progress can be evaluated. The caregivers could carry out the daily plaque program and see the changes that take place by comparing survey results at a later date. Such continuing participation could provide a real motivation to the group.

II. PROGRAM CONTENT

A. The Participants' Own Plaque Control
Based on the premise that persons who are motivated to care for their own mouths have a

clearer understanding of the effects and importance of oral care and give a higher priority to the time spent daily, an in-service education group needs to participate in a personal plaque control program. A plaque-free score (pages 299 to 302) or other evaluation device can be used. A group may be willing to work in pairs and learn to evaluate and score each other, thereby learning the techniques to be applied to their clients.

B. Facts About Cause and Prevention

Basic information about plaque, its formation, and how gingivitis and dental caries develop are important to most groups. The progress of disease from reversible gingivitis to severe periodontitis can be explained, as can the process of dental caries, which begins with a small cavity and progresses to a diseased pulp. Prevention through bacterial plaque control, fluoride, dietary controls, sealants, and early treatment for restorations must be carefully presented. Handout materials and colorful visual aids promote learning.

C. Oral Examination

1. *Oral Mucosa.* Techniques demonstrated and practiced by the participants on each other should include the use of a tongue depressor to retract and a disposable mouth mirror and a light source to see the oral mucosa.
2. *Tongue.* How to hold the tongue, using a sponge to lift and inspect all parts, can be shown.
3. *Gingiva.* Color, size, and bleeding that occurs spontaneously or while brushing can be explained and demonstrated. When projection is possible, slides can be included for all aspects of the instructional material. When a camera is available for intraoral photography, "before" and "after" pictures of the patients can be shown. Changes effected by the plaque control supervised by the caregivers are more meaningful than are pictures of strangers.
4. *Bacterial Plaque.* Inspection for plaque can be demonstrated when the disclosing agent is used prior to plaque scoring and removal.
5. *Denture-Supporting Mucosa.* Patients with dentures need the supporting tissues examined periodically by the dentist, but caregivers can notice changes that should be called to the dentist's attention as a result of their daily cleaning and massaging of the mucosa while the denture is out of the mouth for cleaning.
6. *Dentures.* Sample dentures may be used to help the participants learn to examine each denture for cracks or sharp edges. Examination for deposits can be made by the patient and the caregivers and compared with the denture after it has been cleaned.

D. Techniques of Mouth Care and Disease Control

Staff members can be trained to work in pairs.[19] Working in pairs is more efficient, particularly in the care of difficult patients.

A plan for each patient can be worked out with the caregivers so that individual problems relative to dental caries prevention, gingival disease control, or complete or partial denture care can be solved. Teaching some or all of the following may be included, depending on the needs of the clients.

1. *Plaque Control.* Instruction includes positioning of the patient (Figure 50-11), application of disclosing agent, examination for plaque on the teeth, toothbrush selection and technique, use of a mouth prop, and flossing with or without a floss aid. The use of a portable or bedside suction unit for removing debris from a patient's mouth can be practiced by a paired team.[19]
2. *Fluoride Application.* The objectives and techniques for brushing with a gel, swabbing with a mouthrinse, assisting the patient with a chewable tablet, or applying a gel tray can be included.
3. *Denture Care.* Procedures for care of dentures and of the mucosa under the denture are shown.
4. *Saliva Substitute.* Use of saliva substitute for dry mouth is demonstrated; instruction includes how to use a swab with saliva substitute to provide relief for certain patients (page 346).

E. Denture Marking Procedure

Not all members of the staff need to learn the technique for marking dentures for personal identification. Because dentures should be marked soon after arrival, personnel involved with admissions of new clients are most in need of the instruction.

In a large hospital or rehabilitation center, new dentures made in the dental clinic are marked during processing. The techniques for denture marking are outlined in Chapter 47, pages 703 to 705.

III. RECORDS

A record form to be completed for each client is essential to follow-up and evaluation. During the instruction periods, the staff can learn how to complete the record and where to file the copies.

The form can be designed with spaces to record information obtained during the oral examination, the functioning level and degree of cooperation, the procedures needed for dental caries control, periodontal health, and/or denture care. In addition, the instruction provided, the implements and materials used, the planned future instruction, the prognosis, and any other personal notes can be included.

IV. FOLLOW-UP

After caregivers have tried their newly learned procedures, an opportunity to have questions answered should be provided. Direct observation by the dental hygienist of techniques performed with and for the clients, advice concerning oral problems of particular patients, and corrections when necessary can motivate and encourage both client and caregiver.

Disclosing and recording the plaque for comparison of scores before and after the program can show the progress being made.

V. CONTINUING EDUCATION

A. Individual instruction must be provided for each new employee during the orientation period for that employee.

B. Periodic updating for all employees can be accomplished at regular intervals. Questions and problems can be discussed, and plans can be introduced for changing a certain procedure based on new research evidence.

C. A specific plan for scheduled oral health programs may be a requirement for licensure of a health-care facility.

INSTRUMENTATION

Customary procedures must be adapted. With basic knowledge of methods for maintaining patient stability, adequate visibility of working area, secure instrument grasps and finger rests, and well-controlled strokes, instrumentation for calculus removal and root planing can be effectively accomplished.

Patients who are hyperactive, lack muscular control, or have a mental impairment provide many challenges. With some patients, the tasks of keeping the head and mouth positioned, the profuse saliva controlled, and the oversized or hyperactive tongue held back may seem insurmountable. Patience, a gentle but firm touch, and continuing experience are essential.

I. PREPARATION FOR INSTRUMENTATION

A. Premedication

1. Antibiotic coverage as indicated for susceptible patients (pages 101 to 104).
2. Sedative for control of selected patients.

B. Plaque Control Instruction Precedes Scaling

1. Provide a clean mouth for professional instrumentation (conditioning).
2. Disclose and present or review information on plaque.
3. Continue practice on plaque removal methods that were selected for the particular patient. The patient and caregiver demonstrate.

II. STABILIZATION

For certain patients, opening the mouth is difficult and maintaining the mouth in an open position is impossible. A mouth prop can be used to assist the patient. Verbal encouragement of the patient must continue throughout the appointment.

A. Ratchet Type (Molt's Mouth Gag)

The most stable mouth prop is a sterilized prop that can be nearly closed for insertion between the teeth. It can be opened gradually to hold the jaws to the necessary position. The tips are covered with rubber tubing and are positioned over the maxillary and mandibular teeth on one side while the clinician treats the opposite side.

B. Rubber Bite Block

A long piece of dental floss should be tied through the holes in a commercially available rubber mouth prop so that, in case of a sudden respiratory change, the prop can be quickly pulled out and breathing normalized.

C. Tongue Depressors

A practical, disposable mouth prop can be made from three to six tongue depressors taped together. A folded sponge should be placed under the tape to provide a cushion.

D. Precautions for the Use of a Mouth Prop

1. Mobile teeth could be knocked out and aspirated.
   a. Loose primary teeth in young patient.
   b. Mobile teeth in advanced periodontal infection.
2. Fatigue of the patient's facial and masticatory muscles and temporomandibular joint.
3. Patient must know that all stabilization devices are for comfort and to make the work easier and that they are in no way meant to hurt or punish.

III. TREATMENT BY QUADRANTS

For many patients, particularly those with generalized heavy supra- and subgingival calculus, treatment by quadrants under local anesthesia is the procedure of choice. Removal of calculus and overhanging fillings can be completed more efficiently.

A. Scaling Requirements

The occurrence of generalized heavy calculus deposits in disabled patients is not unusual. The reason may be inadequate personal and professional care or factors related to the disabling condition.

The objective of the clinical procedures is the complete removal of calculus and periodontal pocket debridement. The compromising or rationalization of complete treatment neglects the patient's needs and permits advanced periodontal disease to develop.

B. Need for Assistance

Four-handed dental hygiene procedures (page 79) are needed while treating many types of patients with disabilities. Many patients have excess saliva, whereas others have uncontrollable tongue and general body movements, all of which can hinder instrumentation.

1. *Stabilization and Visibility.* With assistance for stabilization, visibility, and maintenance of a clear field, the procedure is less traumatic for the patient and less time-consuming for all.
2. *Precaution During Evacuation.* Patients with chronic lung disorders, asthma, or cystic fibrosis and patients with cerebral palsy are considered "aspiration risks." For example, a sudden spasm in the facial, neck, or throat areas could cause a patient with cerebral palsy to aspirate foreign matter from the mouth into the airway.

C. Instruments

1. Unbreakable mirrors are recommended for use with a patient subject to spasm or sudden closure.
2. Use single-end sharp instruments to prevent accidents. When an unrestrained patient moves involuntarily, the nonworking end of an instrument can be a hazard.
3. Use of an ultrasonic scaler is contraindicated for an aspiration-risk patient. It also should not be used for patients who overreact to sensory stimuli, such as a patient with autism (pages 816 to 817).

D. Technique Suggestions

1. *Introduce Each Procedure and Sound to Prevent Startling a Patient.* Follow the basic instruction rule to "show, tell, then do." When a patient is blind or deaf, the rule has double significance.
2. *Finger Rests.* Firm, dependable finger rests are needed. Supplemental or reinforced rests can contribute to instrument stability. With certain patients, external finger and hand rests may be safer for the clinician.[20]

REFERENCES

1. **United States Equal Employment Opportunity Commission and the U.S. Department of Justice:** *Americans with Disabilities Act Handbook.* EEOC-BK-19, October, 1991, Appendix N. Title II Highlights.
2. **World Health Organization:** *International Classification of Impairments, Disabilities, and Handicaps.* Geneva, World Health Organization, 1980.
3. **United States Equal Employment Opportunity Commission and the U.S. Department of Justice:** *Americans with Disabilities Act Handbook.* EEOC-BK-19, October, 1991, Appendix B. ADA Accessibility Guidelines.
4. **Posnick,** W.R. and Martin, H.H.: Wheel Chair Transfer Techniques for the Dental Office, *J. Am. Dent. Assoc., 94,* 719, April, 1977.
5. **Stiefel,** D.J.: Wheelchair Transfers in the Dental Office, *DentalHygienistNews, 8,* 21, Number 4, 1995.
6. **Meador,** H.G.: Toothbrushing: A Sensible Approach for the Mentally Retarded, *Dent. Hyg., 53,* 462, October, 1979.
7. **Duncan,** J.L.: Incorporating Oral Hygiene Procedures in Geriatric Nursing Homes, *Dent. Hyg., 53,* 519, November, 1979.
8. **Price,** V.E.: Toothbrush Modifications for the Handicapped, *Dent. Hyg., 54,* 467, October, 1980.
9. **Sroda,** R. and Plezia, R.A.: Oral Hygiene Devices for Special Patients, *Spec. Care Dentist., 4,* 264, November–December, 1984.
10. **Albertson,** D.: Prevention and the Handicapped Child, *Dent. Clin. North Am., 18,* 595, July, 1974.
11. **Ettinger,** R.L. and Pinkham, J.R.: Oral Hygiene and the Handicapped Child, *J. Int. Assoc. Dent. Child., 9,* 3, July, 1978.
12. **Williams,** N.J. and Schuman, N.J.: The Curved-bristle Toothbrush: An Aid for the Handicapped Population, *ASDC J. Dent. Child., 55,* 291, July–August, 1988.
13. **Mulligan,** R.A.: Design Characteristics of Electric Toothbrushes Important to Physically Compromised Patients, *J. Dent. Res., 59,* 450, Abstract 731, Special Issue A, March, 1980.
14. **Ettinger,** R.L. and Pinkham, J.R.: Dental Care for the Homebound—Assessment and Hygiene, *Aust. Dent. J., 22,* 77, April, 1977.
15. **Nowak,** A.J.: *Dentistry for the Handicapped Patient.* St. Louis, Mosby, 1976, pp. 167–192.
16. **Ripa,** L.W. and Cole, W.W.: Occlusal Sealing and Caries Prevention: Results 12 Months After a Single Application of Adhesive Resin, *J. Dent. Res., 49,* 171, January, 1970.
17. **Richardson,** B.A., Smith, D.C., and Hargreaves, J.A.: A 5-Year Clinical Evaluation of the Effectiveness of a Fissure Sealant in Mentally Retarded Canadian Children, *Community Dent. Oral Epidemiol., 9,* 170, August, 1981.
18. **Feigal,** R.J. and Jensen, M.E.: The Cariogenic Potential of Liquid Medications: A Concern for the Handicapped Patient, *Spec. Care Dentist., 2,* 20, January–February, 1982.
19. **Gertenrich,** R.L. and Hart, R.W.: Utilization of the Oral Hygiene Team in a Mental Health Institution, *ASDC J. Dent. Child., 39,* 174, May–June, 1972.
20. **Pattison,** A.M. and Pattison, G.L.: *Periodontal Instrumentation.* 2nd ed. Norwalk, CT, Appleton & Lange, 1992, pp. 355–408.

SUGGESTED READINGS

Alty, C.T.: Finding a Place in Your Heart for Special Smiles, *RDH, 16,* 19, February, 1996.

Belles, M.T.: Long-Term Care Facilities: An In-service Education Program, *DentalHygienistNews, 6,* 14, Spring, 1993.

Boj, J.R. and Davila, J.M.: Differences Between Normal and Developmentally Disabled Children in a First Dental Visit, *ASDC J. Dent. Child., 62,* 52, January–February, 1995.

Brandes, D.A., Wilson, S., Preisch, J.W., and Cassamassimo, P.S.: A Comparison of Opinions from Parents of Disabled and Nondisabled Children on Behavior Management Techniques Used in Dentistry, *Spec. Care Dentist., 15,* 119, May–June, 1995.

Carr, M.P.: Ensuring Treatment for the Special Needs Population, *Access, 8,* 33, February, 1994.

Finger, S.T. and Jedrychowski, J.R.: Parents' Perception of Access to Dental Care for Children with Handicapping Conditions, *Spec. Care Dentist., 9,* 195, November–December, 1989.

Glassman, P., Miller, C., Wozniak, T., and Jones, C.: A Preventive Dentistry Training Program for Caretakers of Persons with Disabilities Residing in Community Residential Facilities, *Spec. Care Dentist., 14,* 137, July/August, 1994.

Lange, B.M., Entwistle, B.M., and Lipson, L.F.: *Dental Management of the Handicapped: Approaches for Dental Auxiliaries.* Philadelphia, Lea & Febiger, 1983, 169 pp.

Ogasawara, T., Watanabe, T., Hosaka, K., and Kasahara, H.: Hypoxemia Due to Inserting a Bite Block in Severely Handicapped Patients, *Spec. Care Dentist., 15,* 70, March/April, 1995.

Perlman, S.P. and Miller, C.: Preventive Oral Health Care for Patients with Disabilities, *Compend. Cont. Educ. Oral Hyg., 4,* 3, Number 2, 1997.

Ramsey, W.O.: Valved Feeding Devices: Adjuncts in Rehabilitation of the Oral Phase of Swallowing, *Int. J. Periodontics Restorative Dent., 10,* 321, Number 4, 1990.

Raynak, S.: Dental Hygiene Care for Individuals with Special Needs, *Can. Dent. Hyg. Assoc./Probe, 29,* 184, September, 1995.

Saunders, R.H., Davila, C.E., Hayes, A.L., Fu, J., and Zero, D.T.: The Effectiveness of Sponge-Type Intraoral Applicators for Applying Topical Fluorides in Institutionalized Older Adults, *Spec. Care Dentist., 14,* 224, November/December, 1994.

Sfikas, P.M.: What's a "Disability" under the Americans with Disabilities Act? *J. Am. Dent. Assoc., 127,* 1406, September, 1996.

Tesini, D.A. and Fenton, S.J.: Oral Health Needs of Persons with Physical or Mental Disabilities, *Dent. Clin. North Am., 38,* 483, July, 1994.

Waldman, H.B.: Respite Care: A New Social Program for Children at Risk, *ASDC J. Dent. Child., 58,* 241, May–June, 1991.

Wyatt, C.C.L. and MacEntee, M.I.: Dental Caries in Chronically Disabled Elders, *Spec. Care Dentist., 17,* 196, November/December, 1997.

Patient Management

American Academy of Pediatric Dentistry: Oral Health Policies. Guidelines for Behavior Management, *Pediatr. Dent., 18,* 40, Number 6, Special Issue, December, 1996.

Burtner, A.P. and Dieks, J.L.: Providing Oral Health Care to Individuals with Severe Disabilities Residing in the Community: Alternative Care Delivery Systems, *Spec. Care Dentist., 14,* 188, September/October, 1994.

Carroll, B.: Dental Hygiene and Preventive Care for People with Disabilities, *Access, 11,* 35, April, 1997.

Casamassimo, P.S.: A Primer in Management of Movement in the Patient with a Handicapping Condition, *J. Mass. Dent. Soc., 40,* 23, Winter, 1991.

Chalmers, J.M., Levy, S.M., Buckwalter, K.C., Ettinger, R.L., and Kambhu, P.P.: Factors Influencing Nurses' Aides' Provision of Oral Care for Nursing Facility Residents, *Spec. Care Dentist., 16,* 71, March/April, 1996.

Frankel, R.I.: The Papoose Board® and Mothers' Attitudes Following Its Use, *Pediatr. Dent., 13,* 284, September/October, 1991.

Gordon, S.M., Dionne, R.A., and Snyder, J.: Dental Fear and Anxiety as a Barrier to Accessing Oral Health Care Among Patients with Special Health Care Needs, *Spec. Care Dentist., 18,* 88, March/April, 1998.

Kayser-Jones, J., Bird, W.F., Redford, M., Schell, E.S., and Einhorn, S.H.: Strategies for Conducting Dental Examinations Among Cognitively Impaired Nursing Home Residents, *Spec. Care Dentist., 16,* 46, March/April, 1996.

Malamed, S.F., Gottschalk, H.W., Mulligan, R., and Quinn, C.L.: Intravenous Sedation for Conservative Dentistry for Disabled Patients, *Anesth. Prog., 36,* 140, July–October, 1989.

Nunn, J.H., Davidson, G., Gordon, P.H., and Storrs, J.: A Retrospective Review of a Service to Provide Comprehensive Dental Care Under General Anesthesia, *Spec. Care Dentist., 15,* 97, May/June, 1995.

Williams, E.O. and Seals, R.R.: Treating Patients in Wheelchairs, *J. Prosthet. Dent., 67,* 431, March, 1992.

Bacterial Plaque Control

Brownstone, E.: Handicapped Dental Patients: Mechanical Methods and Modifications for Oral Hygiene Care, *Can. Dent. Hyg./Probe, 24,* 32, Spring, 1990.

Carr, M.P., Sterling, E.S., and Bauchmoyer, S.M.: Comparison of the Interplak® and Manual Toothbrushes in a Population with Mental Retardation/Developmental Disabilities (MR/DD), *Spec. Care Dentist., 17,* 133, July/August, 1997.

Finizio, J.M., Fox, D.W., and Yasser, D.S.: Power-Assisted Toothbrushes Simplify Hygiene for Those Who Need Extra Help, *RDH, 16,* 42, January, 1996.

Stiefel, D.J., Truelove, E.L., Chin, M.M., and Mandel, L.S.: Efficacy of Chlorhexidine Swabbing in Oral Health Care for People with Severe Disabilities, *Spec. Care Dentist., 12,* 57, March/April, 1992.

Stiefel, D.J., Truelove, E.L., Chin, M.M., Zhu, X.C., and Leroux, B.G.: Chlorhexidine Swabbing Applications Under Various Conditions of Use in Preventive Oral Care for Persons with Disabilities, *Spec. Care Dentist., 15,* 159, July/August, 1995.

The Patient Who Is Homebound, Bedridden, or Helpless

51

HOMEBOUND PATIENTS

Within recent years, efforts have been made through research and organized programming to devote more attention to the oral health needs of people with a chronic illness and a disability. Patients of all age groups who are confined to hospitals, hospices, institutions, nursing homes, skilled nursing facilities, or private homes need special adaptations for oral care. Portable equipment is available, and special training for dental personnel is encouraged.

Dental care for the chronically ill must be completed in a variety of surroundings. For the hospitalized person, dental clinics frequently are available to provide care for in-patients. Those who are not hospitalized may be confined to their homes or may be able to be transported to the dental office or clinic in a wheelchair, depending on the severity and extent of disability.

Private practice clinicians have occasion to attend to patients confined to their homes. Dental hygiene procedures lend themselves to care for the bedridden because nearly the entire treatment can be completed with manual instruments. Instruction in personal oral preventive procedures has particular significance for the comfort, as well as the health, of the patient. Sug-

gestions relative to planning and conducting a home visit are included in this chapter. Key words and definitions are included in Box 51-1.

I. OBJECTIVES

  A. Aid in preventing dental caries and periodontal infections that require extensive treatment.
  B. Assist in preventing further complication of the patient's state of health by lessening oral care problems.
  C. Contribute to the patient's comfort, mental ease, general well-being, and quality of life.
  D. Encourage adequate personal care procedures, whether performed by the patient or a caregiver.
  E. Contribute to general rehabilitation or habilitation of the patient.
  F. Provide palliative care for the individual with a shortened life span.

II. PREPARATION FOR THE HOME VISIT

  A. Understanding the Patient
    1. Consider the characteristics associated with the particular chronic illness or disease and the effect oral infection may have on the severity of the illness.

BOX 51-1 KEY WORDS: Homebound and Helpless Patients

Coma (kō′mah): state of unconsciousness from which the patient cannot be aroused.

Irreversible coma: brain death.

Comatose (kō′mah-tōs): pertaining to or affected with a coma.

Hospice (hos′pĭs): a medically directed, nurse-coordinated program providing a continuum of home and inpatient care for the terminally ill patient and family; employs an interdisciplinary team acting under the direction of an autonomous hospice administration; the program provides palliative and supportive care to meet the special needs arising out of the physical, emotional, spiritual, social, and economic stresses that are experienced during the final stages of illness and during dying and bereavement.[1]

Interdisciplinary team: consists of specialists of many fields; combines expertise and resources to provide insight into all aspects of a given special area.

Palliative (pal′ē-ā″tiv): affording relief but not cure.

Sordes (sor′dēz): foul matter that collects on the lips, teeth, and oral mucosa in low fevers; consists of debris, microorganisms, epithelial elements, and food particles; forms a crust.

Terminally ill patient: a person who is experiencing the end stages of a life-threatening disease, for whom there is no longer hope of a cure.

---

2. Consider special problems related to age. (For example, for the gerodontic patient, see Chapter 46.)
3. Review patient's medical history (by telephone, if preliminary visit is not practical) to determine unusual precautions that must be taken. Arrange with physician and dentist when premedication is indicated (pages 101 to 104).

B. Instruments and Equipment
1. *Protective Barriers.* Mask, protective eyewear, gloves, and gown.
2. *Instruction Materials.* Toothbrush, interdental aids (several types, until needs of patient are known).
3. *Sterile Equipment.* Sterile instruments and other items are transported in the sealed packages in which they were sterilized.
4. *Disposable Items.* Gauze sponges, cotton rolls and pellets, wood points, fluoride application trays, and other essential disposable items are prepared in packages that are convenient to open and use at the bedside.
5. *Pharmaceuticals.* Such substances as the pretreatment mouthrinse, disclosing agent, and topical fluoride preparation are carried in small, tightly closed bottles.
6. *Coverall.* A large plastic drape is of particular importance, because in certain types of illness the patient's coordination during rinsing may be limited.
7. *Emesis Basin for Patient Rinsing.* Although a small basin undoubtedly would be available at the home, the kidney-shaped emesis basin facilitates the rinsing process.
8. *Lighting.* Adaptation of available possibilities.
   a. Headlight or reflector. Dentist may have as part of the office equipment; with

practice, the dental hygienist can learn to use with ease.
   b. Photography spot light. Might be available either from the dentist or from the patient's home; need a type with a narrow, concentrated beam.
   c. Gooseneck lamp. Might be available in patient's home; need bulb of adequate wattage.
9. *Miscellaneous Items Usually Available at the Home.* Arrangements must be made (by telephone) in advance of appointment.
   a. Large towels. For covering pillows.
   b. Pillows. Types of pillows available that may be firm enough to assist in maintaining patient's head in reasonably stationary position.
   c. Hospital bed. Can be adjusted most effectively for patient's position.
   d. Container for prosthesis.
   e. Hand mirror for patient instruction.

C. Appointment Time
Arrange during the patient's usual waking hours at as convenient a time as possible in relation to nursing care and mealtime schedule.

III. APPROACH TO PATIENT
Because a majority of patients who come to the dental office are active people with good general health, the adjustment to the relatively helpless, chronically ill person is sometimes difficult. One may tend to be oversolicitous, an attitude that may not contribute to the development of a cooperative patient.

Usually, a direct approach with gentle firmness is most successful. Establishment of rapport with the patient depends in part on whether the patient has requested and anticipated the appointment or whether those caring for the patient have insisted on and arranged for the visit.

A. Personal Factors

Frequently, the well-adjusted chronically ill person may show more appreciation for the care provided than does the healthy patient who comes to the dental office. The ill patient may also be well aware of the difficulties under which the clinician is working. The cooperation obtained frequently depends on the patient's attitude toward the illness or disability.

A prolonged illness that may have been accompanied by suffering is not conducive to a healthy outlook on life. Monotonous confinement contributes to the development of characteristics such as those that follow.

1. Unable to maintain a cheerful attitude.
2. Bored or dissatisfied with sameness of daily routine.
3. Easily depressed.
4. Discouraged about recovery; leads to mental state that may retard recovery.
5. Sensitive and easily offended.
6. Demanding; enjoys being waited on if used to having prompt attention to each request.
7. Indifferent to personal appearance and general rules of personal hygiene.
8. Preoccupied with details of medical examinations, tests, treatment, medications, and symptoms.

B. Suggestions for General Procedure

1. Request the caregiver to be present to assist as needed and to learn method for care of the patient's mouth on a daily basis. Other visitors should be asked to remain out of the room during the appointment to prevent distraction of patient.
2. Introduce each step slowly to be sure patient knows what is being done.
3. Do not make the patient feel rushed. Listen attentively: socializing is one of the best ways to establish rapport.
4. Regardless of inconvenience of arrangements, plan two or more appointments when extensive scaling is required.
   a. Need to avoid tiring the patient.
   b. Need for observing tissue response.
   c. Need to give encouragement in plaque control procedures.

IV. DENTAL HYGIENE CARE AND INSTRUCTION

A. The Working Situation

Because many patients can sit up in a chair or wheelchair for at least 1 or 2 hours each day, only rarely must procedures be performed while the patient is in bed. For the patient in a chair, a kitchen or large bathroom may be most satisfactory for working. In either situation, ingenuity is needed to arrange patient position, head stabilization, and proper lighting to maintain patient comfort and yet provide access for the clinician.

1. *Patient in Bed*
   a. Hospital bed. Adjust to lift patient's head to desirable height.
   b. Ordinary bed. Use firm pillows to support patient.
2. *Patient in Wheelchair.*
   a. Portable headrest may be attached to back of plain chair or wheelchair.
   b. Although the chair can be backed against a wall and a pillow inserted for the head, the patient preferably should be moved to a davenport or chair where a more stable headrest could be provided.
3. *Small Patient.* Positions for plaque control described on page 753 and shown in Figure 50-11 may be applicable during treatment.
4. *Suggestions for Lighting*
   a. Overhead lighting. Turn off to reduce shadows in the mouth.
   b. Headlight. Usually the most convenient and efficient form of lighting because of concentrated beam.
   c. Head reflector. Reflect light from bed lamp attached to bed behind patient's head.
   d. Gooseneck or photographer's light. Care must be taken not to direct the light into patient's eyes.
5. *Instrument Arrangement.* Use instruments directly from a sterile package or cassette.

B. Assessment Treatment Plan

1. Vital signs.
2. Extraoral/intraoral examination.
3. Periodontal assessment.
4. Dental examination.

C. Personal Oral Care

1. Provide specific instruction for caregiver of helpless or uncoordinated patient. Demonstrate in patient's mouth. A power-assisted toothbrush may prove valuable for certain patients (pages 362 to 363).
2. Specific instruction for cleaning and care of prostheses is needed.
3. Xerostomia can be a serious problem with patients using certain medication. Avoiding cariogenic candies and beverages is mandatory. Instruction for use of a saliva substitute is included.

D. Instrumentation

Scaling is complicated by instability of the head. A mouth prop may be needed when patient has difficulty holding the mouth open.

E. Fluoride Application

Selection of method for fluoride application varies with the patient and the home situation. The use of self-care techniques depends on the patient's disability and the cooperation of the caregiver. The greatest benefit is obtained from a daily mouthrinse, chewable tablet, or gel applied in a mouthguard tray or brushed on (pages 469 to 472).

F. Dietary Suggestions

1. Consultation with physician concerning a prescribed diet is necessary. When significant relationships of diet to oral health are suspected, they should be reported to the physician. The patient's problem then can be discussed with the physician and dietary adjustments made.
2. Cariogenic foods should be avoided as snacks. The patient and those who provide the patient's food need specific suggestions for food substitutes that are noncariogenic.
3. Factors influencing suggestions for diet
   a. Patient's appetite may be poor, particularly if the patient is discouraged about the state of health.
   b. The patient who is finicky in food selection may have affected the general nutritional state or may have used cariogenic foods in excess.
   c. Monotony of meals may have lessened the desire to eat.

G. Appointment Plan for Maintenance

THE HELPLESS OR UNCONSCIOUS PATIENT

Personal oral care procedures for the unconscious patient are accomplished by the caregiver because self-care by the patient is impossible. Planning and conducting an oral health in-service program for a nursing staff and other caregivers are described on pages 756 to 758.

Understanding the possible procedures for oral care of hospitalized patients is important to all dental hygienists, whether or not they are employed in a hospital, if they are to appreciate ramifications of dental hygiene care for the many types of patients with special needs.

Skill is required to carry out routine methods of toothbrushing, rinsing, and cleaning of removable dentures for the conscious patient who is able to cooperate. Methods must be adapted when the patient's head cannot be elevated. When the patient's illness or injury involves the oral cavity, the advice and recommendations of the attending oral surgeon are followed.

Maintenance of oral cleanliness for the acutely ill or unconscious patient requires special procedures because of the complete helplessness of the patient. Objectives and methods described in the following sections have application for patients with other special needs, for example, the patient with a fractured jaw (pages 716 to 719) or severe mental retardation (page 811).

I. OBJECTIVES OF CARE

A. Prevent debris in the mouth from being aspirated and clogging air passages.
B. Minimize the possibility of oral infection.
C. Clean the mouth and provide comfort for the patient.
D. Relieve mouth dryness.

II. CARE OF REMOVABLE DENTURES

A. Remove dentures from the patient's mouth. Usual hospital policy requires removal of dentures when a patient is unconscious.
B. Procedure for removal is described on page 615.
C. Clean the dentures (pages 403 to 407) and store in water in a covered container by the patient's bedside. Fresh water or denture cleanser must be provided daily to prevent bacterial growth.[2]

III. GENERAL MOUTH CLEANING

A. Edentulous and Dentulous

1. Clean the mouth at least three times each day to prevent dryness and sordes. Sordes is a crust-like material that collects on the lips, teeth, and gingiva of a patient with a fever or dehydration in a chronic debilitating disease.
2. Toothbrushing and flossing are essential for mechanical plaque removal. Other devices, such as swabs or gauze sponges, are much less effective and more time consuming.[3]

B. Brushing and Flossing

1. *Patient Who Can Rinse.* When unable to manipulate brush or floss but able to rinse and expectorate, a patient can be propped upright and an emesis basin used.
2. *Patient Who Cannot Participate.* Suction is a necessity. When suction is used, an assistant is needed, except for the suction toothbrush described in the following section.
3. *Brush.* A power-assisted brush may be more efficient and thorough than a manual brush when a caregiver must brush a helpless patient's teeth. A mouth prop can be placed in one side while the other side is retracted.

IV. TOOTHBRUSH WITH SUCTION ATTACHMENT

The toothbrush with attached suction provides an efficient and safe method for patient care.

A. Description of the Brush[4,5]

1. Soft-textured nylon brush with the hole drilled between the filaments in the middle of the head of the brush.
2. Small plastic tubing inserted into hole; end

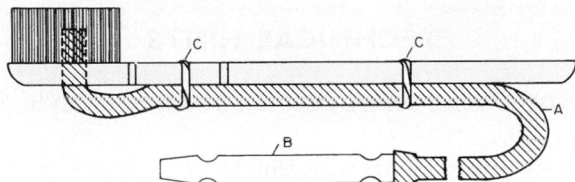

FIGURE 51-1 Suction Toothbrush. (A) Plastic tubing. **(B)** Adapter for attachment of the tubing to an aspirator or suction outlet. **(C)** Small rubber bands attach the tubing to the brush handle. The plastic tube is inserted through a hole in the head of the brush and extended to a level slightly below the brushing plane.

adjusted slightly below level of brushing plane.

3. Other end of tubing passed across back of brush handle and attached to handle by small rubber bands (Figure 51-1).
4. Tubing is connected by an adapter to aspirator or suction outlet.
5. Suction brushes are also manufactured commercially (see "Technical Hints" at the end of chapter).

B. Procedure for Use of Brush
The detailed procedure should be outlined for hospital personnel and included in the nursing procedures manual. An abbreviated outline of the basic steps is included here.

1. Prepare patient
   a. Although not able to respond in a usual manner, the patient may be aware of what is going on.
   b. Tell patient that the teeth are going to be brushed, and thereafter maintain a one-way conversation despite patient's inability to respond verbally.
   c. Turn patient on a side and place a pillow at the back for support.
   d. Place a face towel under patient's chin and over bedding.
2. Attach toothbrush to suction outlet and lay brush on towel near patient's mouth.
3. Place a rubber bite block on one side of the patient's mouth between the teeth. Floss tied to bite block is fastened to the patient's gown with a safety pin.
4. Dip brush in fluoride mouthrinse; turn on suction.
5. Gently retract lip and carefully apply the appropriate toothbrushing procedures; apply suction over each tooth surface with particular care at each interproximal area. Moisten brush frequently.
6. Move bite block to opposite side of mouth and continue brushing procedure.
7. Place brush in cup of clear water to allow water to be sucked through to clear the tub-

ing during the procedure if there is clogging and to clean the tube after brushing.
8. Remove bite block; wipe patient's lips with paper wipe and apply a water-based lubricant, such as plain hydrous lanolin.
9. Wash brush and bite block; prepare materials for next use.

V. RELIEF FOR XEROSTOMIA
A. Use Saliva Substitute
Swab the oral mucosa using a saliva substitute containing fluoride. Lemon and glycerin swabs formerly were used by hospital personnel, but the acidic effect of the lemon led to demineralization of enamel, and the drying effect of the glycerin was contradictory to the intended outcome.[6,7] Swabs prepared with saliva substitute are available to relieve xerostomia and can be used as frequently as needed throughout the day and night.[8]

B. Composition of Saliva Substitutes
1. *Remineralizing Effect.* Products containing fluoride (F), calcium (Ca), and phosphorus (P) ions have remineralizing capacity. Without F, Ca, and P, demineralization can occur.
2. *Alcohol and Glycerin.* Avoid products that contain alcohol or glycerin, which are drying to the oral tissues.

THE TERMINALLY ILL PATIENT

The role of the dental hygienist in the care of the terminally ill patient is to provide comfort care. The emphasis is on symptom relief and a clean environment, which may enhance the patient's sense of dignity and improve quality of life, no matter how brief the life is to be.

Although complicated dental procedures are not usually indicated for terminally ill patients, there is no excuse for neglect of oral cleanliness. Daily oral hygiene must be provided.

While hospice program caregivers are becoming more aware of the oral care needs of their patients, standardized oral health protocols are not followed in many programs.[9] The major difference in caring for a terminally ill patient is that the focus is on short-term palliative care rather than long-term preventive care.

I. OBJECTIVES OF CARE
A. Provide oral care that emphasizes patient comfort rather than only preventive or restorative aspects of care.
B. Provide relief of painful or aggravating symptoms of oral disease or lesions.
C. Provide a "clean mouth" environment to reduce malodor and improve appearance, which

may enhance personal interaction with care-givers and family members.

II. GENERAL MOUTHCARE CONSIDERATIONS

A. Cleanliness
Gentle but thorough daily cleaning of teeth, tongue, and oral mucosa is necessary. It is important to provide cleansing in any way the patient will allow. Dentifrice or other oral products are not necessary, but they can add a refreshing flavor that the patient may like.

B. Visual Inspection
Regular visual inspection of the patient's mouth is necessary to identify oral lesions that can cause discomfort or lead to serious infection.

C. Oral Lesions
Mucosal soreness and ulceration, candidiasis, glossitis, and xerostomia are frequently found on clinical examination.

1. *Candidiasis Infection.* Oral cultures of *Candida albicans* have been found in as many as 79% of terminally ill patients.[10] The infection may become life threatening in immunocompromised individuals. It is easily treated with antifungal medication.

2. *Xerostomia.* Xerostomia is common among terminally ill individuals owing to medications, dehydration, or mouthbreathing.[9,10] Intraoral tissues and lips should be moistened constantly using water, ice chips, or appropriate over-the-counter products as mentioned earlier in this chapter.

3. *Oral Mucosa.* Approximately 75% of hospice patients in one study had evidence of pathologic changes in the oral mucosa and 42% reported soreness of the oral mucosa.[10] Active oral lesions in the terminally ill may cause extreme discomfort when eating or talking as well as present an opportunity for development of secondary infections. Daily examination of tissues and immediate care of developing lesions is recommended.

4. *Denture Problems.* Because of severe weight loss, many terminally ill patients find that dentures no longer fit. More than 70% of hospice patients who wore dentures reported having some kind of difficulty wearing their dentures.[10]

   Individuals who continue to wear ill-fitting prostheses may find chewing and talking difficult. A more serious concern would be development of active intraoral lesions secondary to denture movement along with the collection of denture plaque microorganisms due to lack of daily cleaning of the denture. Denture-induced lesions are described in Chapter 47, pages 701 to 702. Several soft reline materials are available that may solve the problem for the duration of the patient's life.

TECHNICAL HINTS

I. SOURCES FOR SUCTION TOOTHBRUSHES
Ora Genics
5699 S.E. International Way, Unit D
Milwaukee, OR 97222
Vac-U-Brush

Trademark Corp.
1053 Headquarters Park
Fenton, MO 63026-2033
Plak-Vac

II. INSURANCE
Check practice liability insurance for alternate practice settings, such as a private home or nursing care facility.

REFERENCES

1. **National Hospice Organization (NHO),** 1978, in Zimmerman, J.M.: *Hospice Complete Care for the Terminally Ill,* 2nd ed. Baltimore-Munich, Urban & Schwarzenberg, 1986, p. 17.
2. **DePaola,** L.G. and Minah, G.E.: Isolation of Pathogenic Microorganisms from Dentures and Denture-Soaking Containers of Myelosuppressed Cancer Patients. *J. Prosthet. Dent., 49,* 20, January, 1983.
3. **Seto,** B.G., Wolinsky, L.E., Tsutsui, P., and Avera, C.: Comparison of the Plaque-Removing Efficacy of Four Nonbrushing Oral Hygiene Devices, *Clin. Prev. Dent., 9,* 9, March–April, 1987.
4. **Capps,** J.S.: New Device for Oral Hygiene, *Am. J. Nurs., 58,* 1532, November, 1958.
5. **Tronquet,** A.A.: Oral Hygiene for Hospital Patients, *J. Am. Dent. Assoc., 63,* 215, August, 1961.
6. **Daeffler,** R.J.: Oral Care, *Hospice J., 2,* 81, Spring, 1986.
7. **Poland,** J.M.: Xerostomia in the Oncologic Patient. Combating Complications of Treatment, *Am. J. Hospice Care, 4,* 31, May/June, 1987.
8. **Moi-stir Oral Swabsticks,** Kingswood Laboratories, Inc., 10375 Hague Road, Indianapolis, IN 46256.
9. **Wyche,** C.J. and Kerschbaum, W.E.: Michigan Hospice Oral Healthcare Needs Survey, *J. Dent. Hyg., 68,* 35, January/February, 1994.
10. **Aldred,** M.J., Addy, M., Bagg, J., and Finlay, I.: Oral Health in the Terminally Ill: A Cross-sectional Pilot Survey, *Spec. Care Dentist., 11,* 59, March/April, 1991.

SUGGESTED READINGS

Allman, R.M.: Pressure Ulcers Among the Elderly, *N. Engl. J. Med., 320,* 850, March 30, 1989.

Baker, K.A., Levy, S.M., and Chrischilles, E.A.: Medications with Dental Significance: Usage in a Nursing Home Population, *Spec. Care Dentist., 11,* 19, January/February, 1991.

Bowes, D. and Murray, K.: The Palliative Care Team and the Dental Hygienist, *Can. Dent. Hyg. Assoc./Probe, 31,* 127, July/August, 1997.

Casamassimo, P.S., Coffee, L.M., and Leviton, F.J.: A Comparison of Two Mobile Treatment Programs for the Homebound and Nursing Home Patient, *Spec. Care Dentist., 8,* 77, March–April, 1988.

Crosson, B.: Mobile Oral Hygiene Services, *Can. Dent. Hyg. Assoc./Probe, 30,* 72, March/April, 1996.

Epstein, J., Ransier, A., Lunn, R., and Spinelli, J.: Enhancing the Effect of Oral Hygiene with the Use of a Foam Brush with Chlorhexidine, *Oral Surg. Oral Med. Oral Pathol., 77,* 242, March, 1994.

Kambhu, P.P. and Levy, S.M.: An Evaluation of the Effectiveness of Four Mechanical Plaque-Removal Devices When Used by a Trained Care-Provider, *Spec. Care Dentist., 13,* 9, January/February, 1993.

Krust, K.S. and Schuchman, L.: Out-of-Office Dentistry: An Alternative Delivery System, *Spec. Care Dentist., 11,* 189, September/October, 1991.

Lugo, R.I., Braun, R.J., and Gray, S.A.: Homebound Dental Care of the HIV+ Individual, *J. Dent. Educ., 60,* 189, Abstract no. 58, February, 1996.

McFall, D.B.: Choosing a Portable Delivery System, *Dental-HygienistNews,* 5, 14, Spring, 1992.

Paunovich, E.: Assessment of the Oral Health Status of the Medically Compromised Homebound Geriatric Patient: A Descriptive Pilot Study, *Spec. Care Dentist., 14,* 80, March/April, 1994.

Practice Profile: Bruce Coyle: Dental Hygienist Provides Mobile Dental Hygiene Services, *Can. Dent. Hyg. Assoc./Probe, 32,* 15, January/February, 1998.

Rotty, R.W.: Oral Healthcare for the Homebound Patient, *Access,* 10, 22, February, 1996.

Shaver, R.D.: Portable Dentistry Benefits Homebound and Providers, *N.Y. State Dent. J.,* 57, 30, October, 1991.

Smith, D.M.: Are We Missing an Important Segment of the Population? *RDH, 12,* 30, March, 1992.

Strayer, M.S.: Perceived Barriers to Oral Health Care Among the Homebound, *Spec. Care Dentist., 15,* 113, May/June, 1995.

Williams, J.N. and Butters, J.M.: Sociodemographics of Homebound People in Kentucky, *Spec. Care Dentist., 12,* 74, March/April, 1992.

Terminally Ill

Aldred, M.J., Addy, M., Bagg, J., and Finlay, I.: Oral Health in the Terminally Ill: A Cross-sectional Pilot Survey, *Spec. Care Dentist., 11,* 59, March/April, 1991.

Bennett, L.: Hospice Care, *Can. Dent. Hyg. Assoc./Probe, 31,* 92, May/June, 1997.

Brown, J.O. and Hoffman, L.A.: The Dental Hygienist as a Hospice Care Provider, *Am. J. Hosp. Palliat. Care,* 7, 31, March–April, 1990.

Brown, J.: Community Hospices: Their Role in Palliative Care, *Can. Dent. Hyg. Assoc./Probe, 31,* 50, March/April, 1997.

Buckingham, R.W.: Dental Care Policies for Treating the Terminal Cancer Patient, *Dent. Hyg.,* 55, 23, April, 1981.

Cassel, C.K. and Vladeck, B.C.: ICD-9 Code for Palliative or Terminal Care, *N. Engl. J. Med., 335,* 1232, October 17, 1996.

Gordon, S.R., Berkeley, D.B., and Call, R.L.: Dental Needs Among Hospice Patients in Colorado: A Pilot Study, *Gerodontics, 1,* 125, June, 1985.

Jobbins, J., Bagg, J., Finlay, I.G., Addy, M., and Newcombe, R.G.: Oral and Dental Disease in Terminally Ill Cancer Patients, *Br. Med. J., 304,* 1612, June 20, 1992.

Kutscher, A.H., Schoenberg, B., and Carr, A.C.: *The Terminal Patient: Oral Care.* New York, Foundation of Thanology, 1973, 273 pp.

Kutscher, A.H. and Goldberg, I.K.: *Oral Care of the Aging and Dying Patient.* Springfield, Charles C Thomas, 1973, 209 pp.

Kutscher, A.H., Schoenberg, B., Carr, A.C., Rappaport, S., De-

Bellis, R., and Blitzner, A.: *Oral Care: The Mouth in Critical and Terminal Illness.* New York, Arno Press, 1980, 216 pp.

Rhymes, J.A.: Clinical Management of the Terminally Ill, *Geriatrics, 46,* 57, February, 1991.

Nursing Homes and Hospitals

Anderson, J.L.: Dental Treatment for Homebound and Institutionalized Patients, in Nowak, A.J.: *Dentistry for the Handicapped Patient.* St. Louis, Mosby, 1976, pp. 211–224.

Hardy, D.L., Brangan, P.P., Darby, M.L., Leinbach, R.M., and Welliver, M.R.: Self-Report of Oral Health Services Provided by Nurses' Aides in Nursing Homes, *J. Dent. Hyg.,* 69, 75, March–April, 1995.

Helgeson, M.J. and Smith, B.J.: Dental Care in Nursing Homes: Guidelines for Mobile and On-site Care, *Spec. Care Dentist., 16,* 153, July/August, 1996.

Henry, R.G. and Ceridan, B.: Delivering Dental Care to Nursing Home and Homebound Patients, *Dent. Clin. North Am., 38,* 537, July, 1994.

Hoyen-Chung, D.J.: Oral Hygiene Training Programmes in Long-stay Hospitals, *Br. Dent. J., 167,* 178, September 9, 1989.

Kambhu, P.P. and Levy, S.M.: Oral Hygiene Care Levels in Iowa Intermediate Care Facilities, *Spec. Care Dentist., 13,* 209, September/October, 1993.

Kambhu, P.P., Warren, J.J., Hand, J.S., Levy, S.M., and Cowen, H.J.: Medical and Functional Changes Among Nursing Facility Residents: Implications for Dentistry, *Spec. Care Dentist., 16,* 22, January/February, 1996.

Kemper, P. and Murtaugh, C.M.: Lifetime Use of Nursing Home Care, *N. Engl. J. Med., 324,* 595, February 28, 1991.

Libow, L.S. and Starer, P.: Care of the Nursing Home Patient, *N. Engl. J. Med., 321,* 93, July 13, 1989.

MacEntee, M.I., Weiss, R.T., Waxler-Morrison, N.E., and Morrison, B.J.: Opinions of Dentists on the Treatment of Elderly Patients in Long-term Care Facilities, *J. Public Health Dent., 52,* 239, Summer, 1992.

Meurman, J.H., Sorvari, R., Peittari, A., Rytömaa, I., Franssila, S., and Kroon, L.: Hospital Mouth-cleaning Aids May Cause Dental Erosion, *Spec. Care Dentist., 16,* 247, November/December, 1996.

Montgomery, M.T. and Christen, A.G.: Primary Preventive Dentistry in a Hospital-Based Setting, in Harris, N.O. and Christen, A.G.: *Primary Preventive Dentistry,* 4th ed. Norwalk, CT, Appleton & Lange, 1995, pp. 509–549.

Pellegrini, J.M., Fitch, J.A., Munro, C.L., and Glass, C.A.: Oral Hygiene in the Intensive Care Unit: An Interdisciplinary Approach to Oral Health, *J. Pract. Hyg.,* 6, 15, July/August, 1997.

Strayer, M.S. and Ibrahim, M.F.: Dental Treatment Needs of Homebound and Nursing Home Patients, *Community Dent. Oral Epidemiol., 19,* 176, June, 1991.

Thai, P.H., Shuman, S.K., and Davidson, G.B.: Nurses' Dental Assessments and Subsequent Care in Minnesota Nursing Homes, *Spec. Care Dentist., 17,* 13, January/February, 1997.

Warren, J.J., Kambhu, P.P., and Hand, J.S.: Factors Related to Acceptance of Dental Treatment Services in a Nursing Home Population, *Spec. Care Dentist., 14,* 15, January/February, 1994.

The Patient With a Physical Impairment

CHAPTER OUTLINE

Many diseases of the locomotor system and nervous system have as a symptom or leave as a chronic after-effect loss of function in the form of a physical impairment.

This chapter contains brief descriptions of selected diseases or conditions to illustrate the types of care necessary and the adaptations that must be made by the patient, as well as by the professional person, during treatment appointments. Box 52-1 lists key words and their definitions relating to physical impairments and disabilities.

General suggestions that may be adapted to a variety of patients with disabilities were described in Chapter 50. From those descriptions, methods and materials can be selected as they apply in the situations created by the different disorders included in this chapter and encountered in practice.

SPINAL CORD DYSFUNCTIONS

There are many causes of disruption of spinal cord function. Major causes are listed here with examples provided in parentheses.

BOX 52-1 KEY WORDS: Physical Impairments

Akinesia (ah"-kĭ-nē'zē-ah): absence or loss of power of voluntary motion.

Ankylosis (ang"kĭ-lō'sĭs): immobility due to direct union between parts.

Bony ankylosis: union of bone with bone or bone with tooth resulting in complete immobility; the periodontal ligament of an ankylosed tooth is completely obliterated.

Aphasia (ah-fā'zē-ah): defect in, or loss of power of, expression by speech, writing, or signs, or of comprehension of spoken or written language.

Ataxia (ah-tak'sē-ah): failure of muscular coordination; irregularity of muscle action.

Atrophy (at'rō-fē): wasting; decrease in size; occurs when muscle fibers are not used or are deprived of their blood supply, or when the nerve connection is interrupted.

Bradykinesia (brād'ē-kĭn-nē'sē-ah): abnormal slowness of movements.

Cerebrovascular accident (CVA): a focal neurologic disorder caused by destruction of brain substance as a result of intracerebral hemorrhage, thrombosis, embolism, or vascular insufficiency; also called stroke.

Decubitus ulcer (dē-ku'bĭ-tus): ulcer that usually occurs over a bony prominence as a result of prolonged, excessive pressure from body weight; also called pressure sore or bed sore.

Demyelinate (dē-mī'ĕ-lin-āt): destruction/removal of the myelin sheath of a nerve.

Diplopia (dī-plo'pe-ah): double vision; perception of two images of a single object.

Dysphagia (dĭs-fa'je-ah): difficulty in swallowing.

Hypercholesterolemia (hī"per-kō-les"ter-ol-ē'mē-ah): excess of cholesterol in the blood.

Ischemia (is-kē'mē-ah): deficiency of blood caused by functional constriction or actual obstruction of a blood vessel.

Kyphosis (kī-fō'sĭs): abnormally increased convexity in the curvature of the thoracic spine (viewed from the side).

Microcephaly (mī"krō-sef'ah-lē): head that is small in relation to the rest of the body; contrast with **macrocephaly**, head that is large in relation to the rest of the body.

Myopathy (mī-op'ah-thē): any disease of muscle.

Orthosis (or-thō'sĭs): orthopedic appliance or apparatus used to support, align, prevent, or correct deformities or to improve the function of a movable part of the body.

Pallidotomy (pal"i-dot'o-me): surgical excision or destruction of part of the globus pallidus in the basal ganglia to prevent symptoms of Parkinsonism including tremor, muscular rigidity, and bradykinesia.

Paralysis (pah-ral'ĭ-sis): a symptom of the loss or impairment of motor function in a body part caused by a lesion of the neural or muscular mechanism.

Diplegia (dī-ple'jē-ah): paralysis of like parts on either side of the body.

Hemiplegia (hem"e-ple'je-ah): paralysis of one side of the body; usually caused by CVA or a brain lesion.

Paraplegia (par"ah-ple'jē-ah): paralysis of the legs and in some cases the lower part of the body.

Quadriplogia (kwod"rĭ-ple'jē-ah): paralysis of all four limbs from neck down; tetraplegia.

Triplegia (trī-ple'jē-ah): paralysis of three limbs; hemiplegia with additional paralysis of one limb on the opposite side.

Paresis (pah-rē'sis): slight or incomplete paralysis.

Paresthesia (par"es-the'ze-ah): abnormal sensation as burning, prickling, tingling.

Parkinsonism (par'kin-sun-izm): a symptom complex comprising any combination of tremor, akinesia or bradykinesia, rigidity, loss of postural reflexes, and flexed posture. There are many causes of parkinsonism, one of which is Parkinson's disease.

Sclerosis (sklĕ-rō'sĭs): induration or hardening; especially hardening from inflammation and in disease of the interstitial substance.

Shunt: passage between two natural channels; to bypass or drain an area.

Ventriculoatrial shunt: surgical creation of a communication between a cerebral ventricle and a cardiac atrium by means of a plastic tube; for relief of hydrocephalus.

Ventriculoperitoneal shunt: communication between a cerebral ventrical and the peritoneum by means of a plastic tube; for relief of hydrocephalus.

Tia: transient ischemic attack; brief episode of cerebral ischemia that results in no permanent neurologic damage; symptoms are warning signals of impending CVA (stroke).

Visceral (vĭs'er-al): pertaining to internal organs (digestive, respiratory, urogenital, endocrine, spleen, heart, and great vessels).

I. Trauma (spinal cord injury).
II. Neoplasms (within the cord or extradural).
III. Viral or bacterial infections (poliomyelitis).
IV. Progressive degenerative disorders (multiple sclerosis).
V. Vascular accidents (hemorrhage, thrombus, embolus, hematoma).
VI. Compression from an arthritic spur (spondylitic osteoarthritis).
VII. Congenital anomalies or deformities (myelomeningocele, meningocele, spina bifida).

SPINAL CORD INJURY

Spinal cord injury is the impairment of spinal cord function resulting from the application of an external traumatic force. The effect is partial or complete paralysis to a degree related to the spinal cord level and the extent of the injury.

I. OCCURRENCE

At least one half of the trauma cases result from motor vehicle accidents; other causes are falls, diving accidents, and violence, such as from gunshot or stabbing wounds. Most patients are teenage or young adult men.

II. THE INITIAL INJURY

Total or partial loss of sensory, motor, and autonomic function occurs below the level of injury. The injury may be diagonal and leave one side with better function than the other at that particular level.

A. Types of Injury
Damage to the spinal cord may result from one or more of the following:
1. Fracture, dislocation, or both, of one or more vertebrae.
2. Compression, stretching, bending, or severing of the spinal cord.

B. Emergency Patient Care[1,2]
At the scene of an accident, severe damage can be done by inexpert care. The patient should be placed in a supine position, but when back injury is suspected, the arms and legs should be straightened with caution. Any twisting motion may produce irreversible injury to the spinal cord by bony fragments cutting into or severing the cord. When transfer is made, the patient must be moved by at least four persons and placed on a board for transport.

C. Spinal Shock
Immediately after the injury, spinal shock causes a complete loss of reflex activity. The result is a flaccid paralysis below the level of injury. The state of spinal shock may last from several hours to 3 months.

III. CHARACTERISTICS OF SPINAL CORD INJURY

The pattern of signs and symptoms depends on the nature and level of injury to the spinal cord. There are 7 cervical (C), 12 thoracic (T), and 5 lumbar (L) vertebrae, with paired spinal nerves extending from each.

The areas of the body that are controlled at the different levels are illustrated in Figure 52-1. The patient's condition is referred to by the letter C, T, or L, followed by the specific vertebra number where the injury occurred. The most severely disabled patients have a lesion level above C6, which refers to the sixth cervical vertebral level.

A. Sensorimotor Effects
1. *Complete Lesion.* A complete transection or compression of the spinal cord leaves no sensation or motor function below the level of the lesion.
2. *Incomplete Lesion.* Partial transection or injury of the spinal cord leaves some evidence of sensation or motor function below the level of the lesion. The sensation and motor function may return within a few hours after injury, and maximum return may occur in 6 months to 1 year.

B. Other Possible Effects
1. Impairment of voluntary bladder and bowel control.
2. Impairment of sexual function.
3. Impairment of vasomotor and body temperature regulatory mechanisms.

IV. SECONDARY COMPLICATIONS THAT MAY OCCUR[3,4]

Most of the complications described here do not occur in patients with lesions below the T6 level.

A. Respiratory Function
Respiratory difficulties may occur. During dental hygiene therapy, attention to patient position and continuous suction to keep passageways clear are vital. Some quadriplegic patients are unable to elicit a functional cough and need assistance. By placing manual pressure over the abdomen, below the diaphragm, after the patient has inhaled, the patient may be assisted while an attempt to cough is made.[3]

B. Tendency for Pressure Sores
A pressure sore (decubitus ulcer) is caused by pressure exerted on the skin and subcutaneous tissues by bony prominences and the object on which they rest, such as a mattress. The result is tissue anoxia or ischemia. The cutaneous tissue becomes broken or destroyed, thereby leading to destruction in the subcutaneous tissue. The ulcer that forms may be very slow to heal and may become infected by secondary bacterial invasion. Anemia and poor nutrition may also contribute.

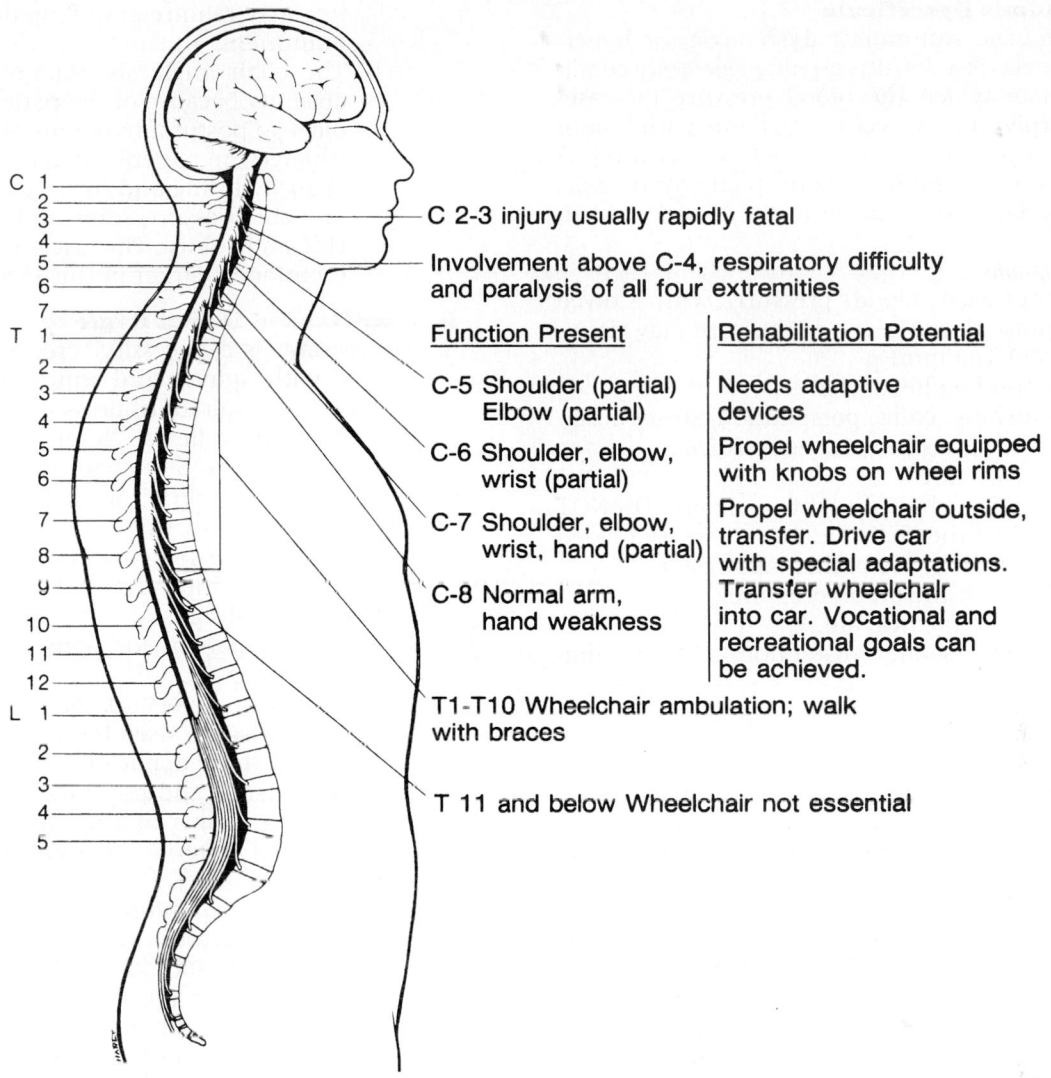

C 2-3 injury usually rapidly fatal

Involvement above C-4, respiratory difficulty
and paralysis of all four extremities

Function Present	Rehabilitation Potential
C-5 Shoulder (partial) Elbow (partial)	Needs adaptive devices
C-6 Shoulder, elbow, wrist (partial)	Propel wheelchair equipped with knobs on wheel rims
C-7 Shoulder, elbow, wrist, hand (partial)	Propel wheelchair outside, transfer. Drive car with special adaptations. Transfer wheelchair into car. Vocational and recreational goals can be achieved.
C-8 Normal arm, hand weakness	

T1-T10 Wheelchair ambulation; walk
with braces

T 11 and below Wheelchair not essential

■ FIGURE 52-1 Levels of Spinal Cord Injury. On the left, the vertebrae are designated as C (cervical), T (thoracic), and L (lumbar). The effects of spinal cord injury depend
on the level of injury, as shown by the information under Function Present at the specific
level. The most severely disabled patient has a lesion above level C6. (From Smeltzer, S.C.
and Bare, B.G.: *Brunner and Suddarth's Textbook of Medical-Surgical Nursing,* 7th ed. Philadelphia, J.B. Lippincott Co., 1992, page 1739.)

Prevention of pressure can be accomplished
by the use of padding and by regular turning of
the patient. The dental chair can be positioned
to prevent pressure. The patient may be asked
to bring special padding to be used during the
appointment, and also may be asked to provide
instruction for the dental personnel so correct
procedures can be followed.

C. Spasticity
As spinal shock subsides, muscle-reflex spasticity develops from a slight to a severe degree.
Stimuli, such as pressure sores, infections, and
sensory irritation, may bring on a spasm. Before
dental hygiene treatment, the patient should be
asked about susceptibility to spasms and to de-

scribe the procedure to follow should one
occur.

D. Body Temperature
High-level quadriplegic patients are unable to
regulate body temperature. A blanket may be
needed in colder weather and air cooling during summer. When air conditioning is not
available, the patient's temperature should be
monitored. In the event of a rise in temperature, treatment should be postponed.

E. Vulnerability to Infection
Infections related to elimination, decubitus
ulcer, and respiratory problems are the most
common.

F. Autonomic Dysreflexia

1. *Definition.* Autonomic dysreflexia, or hyper-reflexia, is a life-threatening *emergency* condition in which the blood pressure increases sharply. It may occur in patients with lesions at T6 or above, but not below that level. A variety of stimuli may precipitate dysreflexia, especially an irritation to the bowel or bladder.

2. *Symptoms*
   a. Increased blood pressure with slowed pulse rate. The blood pressure may rise to 300/160 mmHg.
   b. Pounding headache.
   c. Flushing, chills, perspiration, stuffy nose.
   d. Restlessness; increased spasticity.

3. *Emergency Care*[3]
   a. Position chair upright gradually. Do NOT recline the chair, because increased blood pressure in the brain could result.
   b. Monitor the blood pressure.
   c. Call for medical aid.
   d. Check bladder distention and unclamp catheter.

V. PERSONAL FACTORS

The typical patient is a young man, possibly a former athlete. Depression and discouragement along with the pain and pressure of treatment and rehabilitation make psychiatric therapy necessary for many patients.

Physical and occupational therapists provide self-care training and preparation for discharge from the rehabilitation hospital. As much responsibility as possible is given the patient for personal care. Daily oral care, which at first may have been carried out by the nursing care staff, gradually should become a part of the daily hygiene routine accomplished by the patient, depending on the cord level of injury.

VI. DENTAL HYGIENE CARE

Emergency dental care may be needed during the patient's hospital period of recovery and treatment.

By the time the patient is able to be transported to a dental office or clinic, physical and psychologic preparation for daily living is at a stage where the patient has developed a stable routine.

Most of the information necessary for patient management and instruction is presented in Chapter 50. A few special considerations are described here.

A. Dental Chair Position

1. Wheelchair transfers (pages 743 to 744).
2. Chair angle[3]
   a. For the patient with a gravity-drained urinary appliance, the chair may be adjusted to accommodate the drainage, or the patient should be uprighted at intervals to allow drainage to take place. The bag may require emptying during the appointment.
   b. The chair angle should not be changed abruptly because of the patient's susceptibility to postural hypotension.
   c. Change the patient's body position in the chair by lifting and turning at intervals to prevent pressure sores and pain in muscles and joints. The use of padding was mentioned earlier in this section.

B. Four-Handed Dental Hygiene

An assistant is a necessity. Precautions for the patient with spinal cord injury relate to the problems of respiration, pressure sores, spasms, autonomic dysreflexia, temperature control, and other factors that were described earlier. Assistance is definitely needed in many ways, including the following:

1. Assist in wheelchair transfer and in turning the patient at intervals.
2. Monitor vital signs.
3. Watch the patient for signs of body needs, emergencies.
4. Assist with rubber dam. A rubber dam should always be used for appropriate procedures, such as application of topical fluorides, sealants, and polishing of restorations, because of danger of a respiratory complication should materials be inhaled.
5. Suction
   a. Prevent aspiration of foreign materials, such as calculus.
   b. Use ultrasonic instruments with great caution, if at all. When use of such instruments is unavoidable, care must be taken to prevent aspiration of water, to avoid spraying the throat and stimulating a gag reflex or cough, and to watch for patient sensitivity.
6. Assist with all procedures to make the total treatment time as brief and efficiently used as possible without sacrificing patient comfort.

C. Disease Control

A complete preventive program with bacterial plaque control, fluorides, and diet counseling is essential. Frequent appointments usually are necessary to motivate, follow up with additional instruction, and assist the patient in carrying out the recommended procedures. Instruction for the caregiver for the severely injured patient must be provided.

Care of removable appliances includes cleaning of mouth-held implements.

VII. MOUTH-HELD IMPLEMENTS

The patient without hands or without the use of hands may utilize the mouth for performing many tasks and the teeth for holding objects. The maintenance of optimum oral health has special significance for these individuals because many of these functions could not be accomplished in an edentulous mouth.

A. Uses

Mouth-held appliances have been fabricated that are effective in carrying out a variety of basic procedures and that contribute to increased independence for a person without the use of hands. A device makes possible such activities as pressing light switches, writing, typewriting, dialing a telephone, pushing an elevator button, or turning the pages of a book.

B. Criteria

Criteria for an adequate oral orthosis include the following.[5]
1. Does not harm the oral tissues.
   a. Stabilization of occlusion with contact for all fully erupted teeth and the biting forces distributed to as many teeth as possible.
   b. Is not traumatic to the periodontal supporting structures.
   c. Does not prevent eruption of teeth.
2. Is comfortable, and does not cause fatigue.
   a. Patient can talk, swallow, and moisten the lips.
   b. Orthosis can be inserted and removed by the patient.
   c. Orthosis is adaptable for the various needs of the quadriplegic patient.
3. Can be cleaned and cared for easily.
   a. Taste is pleasant; no odors.
   b. Surface texture is smooth.
4. Is relatively easy to construct; inexpensive.

C. Limitations

The formerly used plain mouthsticks required gripping the stick with the teeth. The teeth could be damaged from chipping and undue and uneven pressures that led to periodontal trauma. When the appliance was adapted to anterior teeth only, tipping and extrusion of the incisors resulted.

A minimum requirement for the preparation of an orthosis is that it cannot damage soft or hard oral tissues. One prerequisite is the use of a sanitary material that can be cleaned easily.

D. Oral Care

Before making impressions for constructing a mouthpiece, periodontal and restorative therapy should be completed and the occlusion adjusted. Plaque control procedures must be effective, and the patient must be instructed carefully in the importance and methods of oral hygiene and appliance care.

MYELOMENINGOCELE[6]

Spina bifida is a congenital defect or opening in the spinal column. A portion of the spinal membranes may protrude through the opening with or without spinal cord tissue. When the spinal cord protrudes through the spina bifida, the condition is called *myelomeningocele.*

Embryologically, a neural tube forms during the first month of pregnancy. From the neural tube, the brain, brain stem, and spinal cord arise, and eventually, the vertebrae form and enclose the spinal cord. When a place in the spinal column fails to close, the result is an open defect in the spinal canal, which is called a spina bifida. Anticipatory guidance prior to conception must include the use of multivitamins containing folic acid. A reduced risk of offspring with spina bifida and other neural tube defects has been shown when mothers received folic acid.[7]

I. TYPES OF DEFORMITIES

A. Myelomeningocele

A myelomeningocele is a protrusion or outpouching of the spinal cord and its covering (meninges) through an opening in the bony spinal column. Because part of the spinal cord and nerve roots protrude, flaccid paralysis of the legs and part of the trunk results, depending on the level of the protrusion (herniation).

B. Meningocele

A meningocele is a protrusion of the meninges through a defect in the skull or spinal column. Because no neural elements are contained in the protrusion, paralysis is uncommon.

C. Spina Bifida

Spina bifida is a congenital cleft in the bony encasement of the spinal cord. When no outpouching of the meninges or spinal cord exists, the condition is called *spina bifida occulta.* Usually, spina bifida occulta has no symptoms.

II. PHYSICAL CHARACTERISTICS

Depending on the level of the myelomeningocele, some or all of the signs and physical characteristics listed here may be found.

A. Bony Deformities

Muscle imbalance from paralysis can cause dislocation of the hip, club foot, and spinal curvatures, such as humpback (kyphosis), curvature (scoliosis), or swayback (lordosis).

B. Loss of Sensation

Lack of skin sensitivity to pain, temperature, and other sensations can lead to problems of inadvertent burn or trauma unrecognized by the patient or caregiver, or to pressure sores, described on page 770. Frequent position changes are necessary.

C. Bladder and Bowel Paralysis

The nerve supplies to bladder and bowel are usually affected. Lack of bowel and bladder control requires continual attention. Kidney infection with loss of kidney function is one cause of shorter life expectancy.

D. Hydrocephalus

Hydrocephalus is a condition characterized by an excessive accumulation of fluid in the brain. The fluid dilates the cerebral ventricles, causes compression of brain tissues, and separates the cranial bones as the head enlarges (Figure 52-2). Development is slowed, and mental retardation is present. Many of these patients have seizures.

A high percentage of children with myelomeningocele have hydrocephalus.

III. MEDICAL TREATMENT

Surgical, orthopedic, medical, urologic, and physical and occupational therapy may constitute a minimum of specialties involved in the care of a patient with myelomeningocele.

A. Neurosurgery

1. *Closure of the Myelomeningocele.* Surgical closure helps to prevent infections that may otherwise enter into the spinal cord. Paralysis is not lessened by the surgery.

2. *Treatment of the Hydrocephalus.* Permanent drainage systems may be accomplished in the form of a ventriculoatrial shunt between the cerebral ventricle and the atrium of the heart (Figure 52-3). Sometimes, drainage by

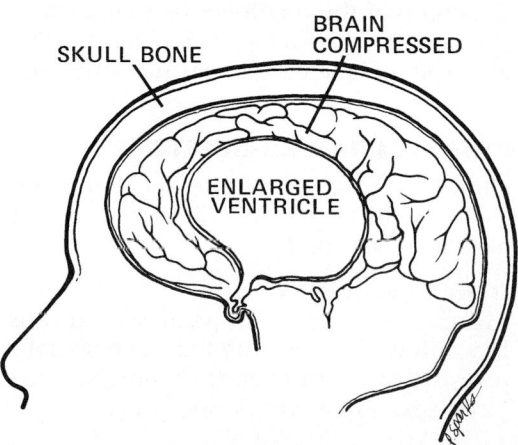

FIGURE 52-2 Hydrocephalus. The ventricle is enlarged because of the accumulation of fluid. Brain tissues are compressed. (From Bleck, E.E. and Nagel, D.A.: *Physically Handicapped Children. A Medical Atlas for Teachers.* New York, Grune & Stratton, 1975.)

Labels in figure: SKULL BONE, BRAIN COMPRESSED, ENLARGED VENTRICLE

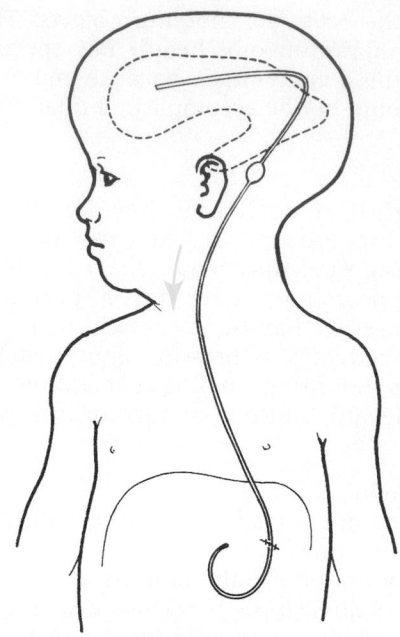

FIGURE 52-3 Shunt for Hydrocephalus Treatment. Fluid is drained by way of a ventriculoatrial or ventriculoperitoneal shunt. (Adapted from Bleck, E.E. and Nagel, D.A.: *Physically Handicapped Children. A Medical Atlas for Teachers.* New York, Grune & Stratton, 1975.)

way of the abdomen in the form of a ventriculoperitoneal shunt is used.

B. Orthopedic Surgery

Bracing to support the trunk and lower limbs is used in accord with the extent of the individual's paralysis. Ambulation varies from dependency on a wheelchair, walker, or use of crutches or cane to near normal with only foot problems. Orthopedic surgical procedures can assist by reducing or correcting deformities.

IV. DENTAL HYGIENE CARE

A. General Management

Management for the physical impairments of the patient with myelomeningocele can be adapted from the information in Chapter 50. Wheelchair transfers and assistance for patients with crutches are described on pages 743 to 744.

B. Need for Premedication

Ventriculoatrial shunts, but not ventriculoperitoneal shunts, need antibiotic premedication for dental and dental hygiene instrumentation.[8]

C. Latex Allergy

Patients with spina bifida appear to be specifically at risk for latex allergy. Proper precautions must be taken (page 51).

D. Gingival Care

Special adaptations for plaque control techniques are needed when the cervical or thoracic body level is involved, and the assistance of an attendant may be required.

Patients with seizures treated with phenytoin may need gingival treatment for phenytoin-induced gingival overgrowth. The condition is described on pages 805 to 806.

CEREBROVASCULAR ACCIDENT (STROKE)

Cerebrovascular accident (CVA) or stroke is a sudden loss of brain function resulting from interference with the blood supply to a part of the brain. CVA is the clinical manifestation of cerebrovascular disease. As a result, the patient is frequently disabled by changes in motor, communication, and perception functions. Hemiplegia or hemiparesis is common.

I. ETIOLOGIC FACTORS[11]

The stroke may be severe and followed by death within minutes. The less severe attack leaves the patient with the symptoms and signs described below. Strokes are usually brought on by one of the following:

A. Thrombosis

A clot within a blood vessel of the brain or neck closes or occludes the vessel and shuts off the oxygen supply to the portion of the brain supplied by that vessel, thus resulting in cerebral infarction.

B. Intracerebral Embolism

A blood vessel is blocked by a clot or other material carried through the circulation from another part of the body.

C. Ischemia

The blood flow decreases to an area of the brain, usually as the result of an atheromatous constriction of the arteries supplying the area.

Transient ischemic attack (TIA) is the most common manifestation.

D. Cerebral Hemorrhage

A cerebral blood vessel may rupture and bleed into the brain tissues.

E. Predisposing Factors

Patients with certain conditions may be considered "risk" patients, or persons more susceptible to having strokes. Early diagnosis and treatment for control of the following predisposing factors are necessary in the prevention of stroke and its devastating effects. Risk factors related to atherosclerosis are described on page 855, and to hypertension on page 852.

1. Atherosclerosis.
2. Hypertension, the greatest risk factor that leads to stroke.
3. Hypercholesterolemia.

4. Cigarette smoking.
5. Cardiovascular disease (rheumatic heart disease, congestive heart failure, history of TIAs).
6. Diabetes mellitus.
7. Use of oral contraceptives (enhanced by hypertension, cigarette smoking, age over 35, and high estrogen levels).
8. Drug abuse (especially in adolescents and young adults).

II. OCCURRENCE

A. Cerebral thrombosis is the most common cause of stroke.
B. Stroke is the third leading cause of death in the United States.

III. SIGNS AND SYMPTOMS

The effects of a stroke depend on the location of the damage to the brain, as well as to the degree or extent of involvement.

A. Transient Ischemic Attack (TIA)

"Little strokes" may last a few minutes to an hour, and may leave no damage. A history of transient attacks is a possible risk factor or warning.

B. Acute Symptoms of a Stroke

Acute symptoms and emergency procedures are included in Table 61-5, page 912.

C. Residual or Chronic Effects

Approximately two thirds of those who survive have some degree of permanent disability. Temporary or permanent loss of thought, memory, speech, sensation, or motion results. The side of the brain affected influences the symptoms.

The side of the face and body affected is opposite to that of the brain injury (Figure 52-4). Persons with right hemiplegia have more difficulty with verbal communication and are more apt to be cautious, anxious, and disorganized. Patients with left hemiplegia have difficulty with action requiring physical coordination and may respond impulsively with overconfidence.

Common signs and symptoms are described briefly here for application during clinical patient care.

1. *Paralysis.* Hemiplegia (one side of the body) or portions, such as an arm, leg, or the face.
2. *Articulation.* Difficulty of speech, which may be caused by involvement of the tongue, mouth, or throat, as well as by brain damage related to the speech centers.
3. *Salivation.* Difficulty in control of saliva complicated by difficulty in swallowing.
4. *Sensory.* Loss in affected parts may result in superficial anesthesia, or the opposite may

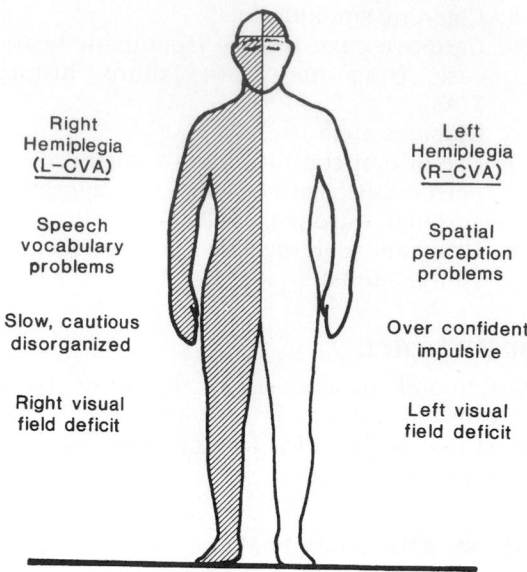

FIGURE 52-4 Cerebrovascular Accident (Stroke). Right hemiplegia is the result of left-side brain damage; left hemiplegia results from right-side brain damage.

occur with resultant increased sensitivity to pain and touch.

5. *Visual Impairment.* Blurred vision, or diminished visual acuity.

6. *Mental Function.* May be unaffected, but slowness, poor memory, and loss of initiative are common. Brain deterioration may occur over a period of time.

7. *Personal Factors.* Personality changes relate to emotional trauma, fear, discouragement, and dependency. Anxiety neuroses and periods of depression, which are common, may require assistance from a psychiatrist, psychologist, or social worker.

IV. MEDICAL TREATMENT

A. Surgical
Treatment may include surgical correction of aneurysms, clots, or malformations. Newer developments include surgery in the intracranial arteries using an operating microscope to remove very small clots or to perform minute grafting to bypass blocked vessels and provide collateral circulation.

B. Physical and Occupational Therapy
Rehabilitation techniques are vital to the patient's functioning.

C. Drugs
Careful recording of the medical history includes the listing of medications. The patient may be taking a variety of drugs for some or all of the following purposes:
1. Anticoagulant (to thin the blood).
2. Antihypertensive (to lower the blood pressure).
3. Thrombolytic (to dissolve clots).
4. Vasodilator (to relax the blood vessels of the brain).
5. Steroid (to control brain swelling).
6. Anticonvulsant (to help to control seizures).

V. DENTAL HYGIENE CARE

Elective dental treatment is not usually advisable until 6 months or more after a stroke, but when possible, preventive measures and plaque control procedures should be introduced or reinstated early. Regular appointments for preventive care should be initiated as soon as a release can be obtained from the physician.

Patients may be homebound or brought to the clinic or office by wheelchair or walker. Factors described in Chapter 50 apply for the patient who has had a stroke. Every attempt should be made to provide complete care, because temporary care may increase the severity of needs at a later time. Complete scaling and root planing to control the periodontal status are especially important.

A. Appointment Procedures
Because of weakness, treatment may best be accomplished in shorter appointments and small increments of instrumentation. The application of four-handed dental hygiene during instrumentation is necessary for all the same reasons described on page 772 for the patient with a spinal cord injury.

B. Disease Control
Techniques for plaque control may need special adaptations. When the right-handed person is paralyzed on the right side (or the left-handed on the left), development of dexterity for the manipulation of plaque removal implements with the nondominant hand takes time and patience. The patient must be as self-sufficient as possible, but should be encouraged to have the paralyzed side deplaqued daily (brush, floss, and supplementary aids) by a family member or other caregiver for whom instruction has been provided.

The paralyzed side of the face tends to sag or droop, and because of inactivity of the tongue on the same side, self-cleansing is ineffective. Lack of sensation hinders the patient from realizing that collection of food debris and tooth deposits may be extensive.

Rinsing is difficult or impossible. Thus, one method for daily fluoride application can be the use of a gel tray by the caregiver or the brushing of the teeth with a fluoride gel. When xerostomia is present, substitute saliva can be recommended (page 346).

Modified handles for toothbrushes and floss holders are shown on pages 749 to 751. The patient who wears dentures requires a suction cup brush to clean the denture with one hand (Figure 50-10, page 753).

MUSCULAR DYSTROPHIES[12]

The muscular dystrophies are genetic myopathies characterized by progressive severe weakness and loss of use of groups of muscles. The term *dystrophy* means degeneration and is associated with atrophy and dysfunction.

The syndromes of muscular dystrophy have been separated by clinical and genetic means, and range from mild types (Becker) with a later onset to more severe types (Duchenne, facioscapulohumeral). The cause of each type is not known, but the underlying pathologic processes do not differ. Generally, the diseases are limited to skeletal muscles, with cardiac muscle only rarely involved.

All muscular dystrophies are rare. The two types described are the more common.

I. DUCHENNE MUSCULAR DYSTROPHY (PSEUDOHYPERTROPHIC)

A. Occurrence
The Duchenne type is primarily limited to males and transmitted by female carriers.

B. Age of Onset
The condition is present at birth and becomes apparent during early childhood, usually between 2 and 5 years, but before 10 years.

C. Characteristics
1. *Musculature.* Enlargement (pseudohypertrophy) of certain muscles, particularly the calves, is present in early years.
2. *Weakness of Hips.* Child falls frequently, has increasing difficulty in standing erect.
3. *Lordosis.* With an abdominal protuberance.
4. *Gait*
   a. Waddling. Either walks on toes or flatfoot as a result of muscle contracture.
   b. Balance. Precarious; patient arches back in attempt to find center of gravity; gait is slow because balance must be attained with each step.
5. *Progressive Muscular Wasting.* Eventual involvement of thighs, shoulders, trunk; weakness of respiratory muscles; inactivity is detrimental and increases the individual's helplessness and dependency.
6. *Intellectual Impairment.* Average IQ in the range of 80 to 90; some patients have normal intelligence and others have a moderate to severe level of retardation.

D. Prognosis
Disablement severe by puberty; child is confined to a wheelchair. Patients rarely live to reach their third decade.

II. FACIOSCAPULOHUMERAL MUSCULAR DYSTROPHY

A. Occurrence
Males and females are equally affected.

B. Age of Onset
Between 10 and 18 years, with an average at 13 years, after puberty. Mild symptoms may appear at later ages.

C. Characteristics
1. Facial muscles involved, particularly the obicularis oris.
2. Scapulae prominent; shoulder muscles weak; difficulty in raising the arms.
3. Difficulty in closing eyes completely.

D. Prognosis
Progression is slower than that of the Duchenne type. Most patients live a normal life span and become incapacitated late in life.

III. MEDICAL TREATMENT

A specific treatment is not known. Symptoms may be relieved. The patient is encouraged to lead as full a life as possible and to keep active.

Preventive treatment consists of prenatal diagnosis, carrier detection, and genetic counseling.

IV. DENTAL HYGIENE CARE

Adaptations depend on the patient's disability. Patients may have slight muscular involvement, may be ambulatory but have balancing difficulties, may be in a wheelchair, or may be bedridden. Factors described for general consideration of patients with disabilities have application (Chapter 50). Suggestions that follow are useful for certain patients.

A. Patient Reception and Seating
1. *Assistance for the Walking Patient*
   a. Certain patients do better without assistance, because they have developed their own method of balancing and the slightest touch may upset them.
   b. Many patients gain balance by holding both hands on the partially flexed forearm of person walking beside them.
2. *Seating Preparation.* Raise chair and chair arm. Allow patient to sit directly. Lift patient's legs onto dental chair if such assistance is needed.
3. *Seated Patient.* Tilt chair back gently; balance is precarious while sitting as well as standing; patient may fall forward.
4. *Assistance for Patient While Rising From Chair*
   a. Stand directly in front of patient. Lock arms around lower back and pull forward near hips.
   b. Allow patient to sway upper trunk back while rising to standing position.

c. Provide support until balance is obtained for walking.

B. Patient Instruction
1. *Problems of Oral Cleanliness*
   a. Facial muscle weakness may interfere with self-cleansing mechanisms and prevent adequate rinsing by the patient with facioscapulohumeral dystrophy.
   b. Effect of gaping lips on oral tissues is similar to that of mouth breathing.
   c. Weakness of arm and shoulder causes difficulty in applying toothbrush. A power-assisted brush under supervision or an adapted handle for a regular brush (pages 749 to 751) may have advantages.
2. *Oral Disease Control*
   a. Instruct parent or other caregiver.
   b. When patient is receiving therapy, solicit assistance and advice from the occupational and physical therapists.

MYASTHENIA GRAVIS

Myasthenia gravis is an autoimmune neuromuscular disease characterized by weakness and fatigability of symmetrical voluntary muscles. It is caused by an autoimmune process that results in a defect in nerve impulse transmission at the neuromuscular junctions. In myasthenia gravis, the numbers of acetylcholine receptors in each neuromuscular junction are reduced markedly when compared to the normal number of receptors.[13]

The patient with myasthenia gravis has a special significance for dental professionals because the facial and oral parts served by certain cranial nerves are involved early. Muscles of the eyes, facial expression, mastication, and swallowing are affected. In advanced severe forms of the disease, muscle involvement may be extensive and result in total paralysis.

I. OCCURRENCE
The onset of myasthenia gravis may occur at any age. The early peak at about age 20 affects women twice as frequently as men. In late adult life, more men than women are affected.

II. SIGNS AND SYMPTOMS
A. Early Signs
Weakness of eye movements with double vision (diplopia) and drooping eyelids (ptosis) may be the initial indicators. In certain patients, the disease may not progress further.

B. Oral and Facial Problems
Involvement of muscles of the face, mastication, and tongue lead to swallowing difficulties (dysphagia) and a lack of facial expression. Disturbed speech and expression, with a weak voice that sounds tired and muffled, are typical. A patient may support the chin with one hand to help during talking.

C. Progressive Involvement
When the muscles that are used during breathing become involved, serious respiratory complications can result. Because of the lack of facial expression, distress may be difficult for the patient to convey.

Generalized fatigue is usually not so evident in the morning or immediately after rest. Weakness may increase as the day goes by, a factor pertinent to the time selected for dental and dental hygiene appointments.

D. Precipitating Factors
Individual reactions vary, but the more common predisposing, aggravating factors affecting the severity of muscular involvement include emotional excitement, surgical procedures, loss of sleep, alcoholic intake, and, especially, infections. Prevention of oral infections and of the need for dental or periodontal surgery contributes to patient stability. Myasthenic crisis is best avoided by elimination and prevention of infection and all precipitating factors.

E. Types of Crises
1. *Myasthenic Crisis*[14]
   a. Cause. A myasthenic crisis may result from undermedication or increased severity of the disease, or it may be precipitated by one of the aggravating factors previously mentioned. The relative deficiency of acetylcholine, which leads to the crisis symptoms, can usually be corrected by the administration of anticholinesterase by the physician.
   b. Symptoms and signs. The inability to swallow, speak, or maintain a patent airway is sudden. Marked weakness of respiratory and pharyngeal muscles leads to depression of respiration and obstruction. The patient may also have double vision and drooping eyelids.
   c. Emergency care.
      i. Suction.
      ii. Provide a patent airway.
      iii. Obtain medical assistance; transport to hospital emergency facility.
2. *Cholinergic Crisis*
   a. Cause. The cholinergic crisis results from overmedication with anticholinesterase.
   b. Symptoms and signs. Increased muscle weakness occurs within 30 to 60 minutes of taking the medication. Excessive pulmonary secretion, cramps, and diarrhea also are characteristic.
   c. Treatment. No further medication should be taken at that time. Medical assistance is needed promptly. When respiratory

symptoms develop, ventilation is urgent (pages 910 to 911).

III. MEDICAL TREATMENT[13]

Medical treatment may have two purposes: (1) to influence the course of the disease, and (2) to induce disease remission. Anticholinesterase agents are used for most patients at intervals during the day. A sustained-release preparation may be used at bedtime, particularly for the patient who awakens with severe weakness.

Current therapy for attempting to induce remission includes surgical removal of the thymus gland, particularly if a tumor of the gland develops, and drug therapy. Immunosuppressive medications include corticosteroids, azathioprine (when corticosteroids are contraindicated), and cyclosporine. Among the side effects of cyclosporine is gingival enlargement (page 234).

IV. DENTAL HYGIENE CARE

Dental hygiene care takes on special significance because the presence of infection can worsen the myasthenic weakness. Treatment with immunosupressive drugs makes the patient vulnerable to infection. The health of the oral cavity with minimal inflammation of the periodontal tissues contributes to the overall health of the patient.

A. Appointment Factors

1. *Time and Length.* Short appointments planned early in the day and in conjunction with the patient's medication schedule. Weakness worsens with activity.
2. *Maintenance.* Frequent appointments to aid the patient in obtaining and maintaining freedom from oral infection.
3. *Preparation for the Appointment.* Office emergency equipment for a possible respiratory emergency must be checked and in order. Stress-reduction procedures should be followed.

   At the outset, the patient should be asked about medication and whether it has been taken on schedule prior to the appointment.

B. Four-Handed Dental Hygiene

For any patient who is a potential respiratory risk, an assistant is needed to aid in observing the patient and to monitor vital signs. Because the patient with myasthenia gravis may have difficulty in providing a warning of distress, the need for supervision is indicated.

1. *Suction.* An assistant is needed to maintain the airway, to ensure no problem of aspiration, and to provide a clean field for efficient instrumentation to minimize appointment time. A side effect of the anticholinesterase medication is increased salivation.
2. *Rubber Dam.* Apply for appropriate proce-

dures to prevent aspiration of harmful substances.

C. Patient Instruction for Disease Control

1. *Diet Evaluation.* A dietary survey and instruction are recommended. The patient with myasthenia gravis may have difficulty in masticating and swallowing, and adequate food selection for oral health and dental caries prevention may be difficult.
2. *Plaque Control.* Weakness and fatigue may have discouraged the patient's routine daily plaque control efforts. A power-assisted brush or other aids can be recommended. Instruction for a family member or other caregiver may be needed to provide the severely disabled patient with assistance.

MULTIPLE SCLEROSIS[15,16]

Multiple sclerosis is a chronic demyelinating disease of the central nervous system characterized by progressive disability. It is a genetically linked disease of adults with motor, sensory, cognitive, and emotional (depression, mania) changes. Women are affected twice as frequently as men.

Pathologically, the myelin sheath is destroyed within the white matter of the central nervous system. The sheath degenerates in patches called *MS plaques* and is replaced by sclerotic tissue. There is interference with the transmission of nerve impulses and frequent involvement of the spinal cord and optic nerves.

I. OCCURRENCE

A. Onset
Usually, the onset is between 20 and 40 years of age, rarely before 15 or after 55 years.

B. Geographic
The disease is more prevalent in temperate climates.

II. CHARACTERISTICS

A. Initial Symptoms
1. May be visual impairment, diplopia, difficulty in coordination, tremor, fatigue, or weakness.
2. Transient tingling paresthesia of the hands or feet.
3. May have a sudden onset of severe illness with paralysis or marked weakness.

B. Course of Disease
1. *Relapses and Remissions.* An attack may last several days or weeks and be followed by a symptom-free period. Physical impairment varies, but the condition worsens with each attack.
2. *Risk Factors for Exacerbations*
   a. Infection. Various types of infection, systemic or local, can stimulate a relapse. Oral infections are no exception.

b. Pregnancy. For certain patients, pregnancy may appear to increase the risk and bring on an attack. Because the effect is more likely to be noticed during the first several months after delivery, fatigue and stress may be the direct precipitating effects.

Effects of multiple sclerosis on the pregnancy should also be recognized. Possible side effects of medications on the developing fetus should be considered, because certain medications used may have to be discontinued if they are teratogenic.

3. *Longevity.* People with multiple sclerosis may live many years. Fewer than half of those afflicted may eventually become nonambulatory.

C. Physical Symptoms

A wide distribution of areas is affected. Symptoms fluctuate, and several years may elapse between attacks. With extended rest, symptoms usually subside.

1. Fatigue
2. Involuntary motion of eyes (nystagmus); may later become partially or completely blind.
3. Speech disorders; possible loss of speech in advanced stages.
4. Changes in muscular coordination and gait; loss of balance; spasms.
5. Paralysis of one or more extremities; occasionally, facial paralysis.
6. Autonomic derangements, such as urinary frequency and urgency; later urinary incontinence.
7. Susceptibility to infection, particularly upper respiratory.

III. CATEGORIES

A. Relapsing-Remitting: acute episodes worsening with recovery and a stable course between relapses.

B. Secondary Progressive: gradual neurologic deterioration with or without superimposed acute relapses in a patient who previously had relapsing-remitting multiple sclerosis.

C. Primary Progressive: gradual, nearly continuous neurologic deterioration from the onset of symptoms.

D. Progressive Relapsing: gradual neurologic deterioration from the onset of symptoms but with subsequent superimposed relapses (very uncommon).

IV. TREATMENT

A. Objectives of Treatment

Since the direct cause of multiple sclerosis is not known, the first objective is to prevent relapses and progressive worsening of the disease. Prompt diagnosis and early treatment by 6 months is crucial to prevent neurologic damage. Treatments are based on the following:

1. *Psychologic Support.* The ramifications of having an incurable disease can be devastating. Understanding dental personnel can contribute in this area.
2. *Disease Course Modification.* Patients with relapsing-remitting multiple sclerosis have the best responses to treatment.
3. *Symptom Relief.*

B. General Treatment Procedures

1. General hygienic care; adequate nutrition, rest, avoidance of strain, prevention of infections, and prevention of injury.
2. Physical and occupational therapy; exercise, but not strenuous exertion, is important.
3. Patient should continue in a usual occupation as long as possible; activity should be encouraged.
4. Psychotherapy for personality problems and morale building is frequently necessary.

C. Medications

1. *Corticosteroids.* Antiinflammatory and immunomodulatory effects.
2. *Interferon Beta (1a and 1b).* Reduce or prevent severity and frequency of future exacerbations.
3. *Glatiramer Acetate.* Reduce or prevent relapse. Useful for patients who become resistant to interferon-beta.
4. *Methotrexate.* Used for progressive multiple sclerosis to slow the disease process.

V. DENTAL HYGIENE CARE

Because relapses may be precipitated by infections, dental hygiene care for the prevention of periodontal infection assumes particular significance.

Many factors described in Chapter 50 have direct application for the patient with a disability associated with multiple sclerosis. For the patient with paraplegia or quadriplegia, items from the section on patients with spinal cord injuries can be used (page 772).

A. Appointment Considerations

1. Provide a warm, quiet, comfortable atmosphere. The patient needs to remain relaxed mentally and physically; people nearby cannot be tense, restless, or noisy.
2. Frequent short appointments contribute to the prevention of fatigue, emotional stress, and advanced dental or periodontal conditions.

B. Patient Instruction

1. *Problems of Personal Oral Care*
   a. Involvements of the tongue and facial

muscles interfere with the self-cleansing mechanisms.

  b. Paralysis may make grasping and manipulating a toothbrush difficult or impossible. Adaptive aids are described on pages 749 to 751.

 2. *Factors Affecting Teaching*

  a. Slow response of patient; give instruction slowly and simply.

  b. Visual disturbances (pages 792 to 794).

CEREBRAL PALSY

Palsy means impairment of the ability to control movement, and cerebral palsy means a condition in which injury to parts of the brain has occurred prenatally, natally, or postnatally and has resulted in paralysis or disruption of motor parts. Such a condition can occur at any age as a result of brain injury from a variety of causes.

Cerebral palsy can be caused by anoxia during pregnancy or delivery, maternal infection during pregnancy (for example, rubella), blood type incompatibility, severe nutritional lack during pregnancy, or maternal diabetes endocrine imbalance. Later in infancy, infectious diseases, such as meningitis or encephalitis, lead poisoning, direct trauma from accidents, or battering (nonaccidental injury) may be implicated.

Symptoms usually can be observed during the first year after birth but may not appear for several years. General symptoms that may occur are tense, contracted muscles; uncontrolled movements of limbs, eyes, or head; poor coordination; muscle spasms; problems with hearing and/or seeing; and a lack of manual dexterity.

I. TYPES OF CHARACTERISTICS[17,18]

Classified by motor activity, six types have been named. In each type, different parts of the brain are damaged, and the symptoms vary respectively. More than 50% of those with cerebral palsy are in the spasticity group, 15% to 20% are athetoid, and the remainder are divided among the other four types or have mixed types.

A. Spasticity (could bite; deep reflex)

 1. Muscles have increased tone, tension, and activity.

 2. Condition characterized by spasms, which are sudden, involuntary contractions of single muscles or groups of muscles.

 3. Patient has complete or partial loss of ability to control muscular movement; therefore, movements are awkward and stiff.

 4. Lack of control causes patient to fall easily; patient tends to avoid activity and thus may gain weight, particularly during teenage years; caloric requirement is therefore low.

 5. Brain damage to motor area of cerebral cortex (Figure 52-5).

B. Athetosis

 1. Condition characterized by constant, involuntary, unorganized muscular movement.

 2. Patient lacks ability to direct muscles in the motions desired; probably the most difficult dental patient.

 3. Grimacing, drooling, and speech defects are common.

 4. Factors influencing movements

  a. Effort by patient to control muscle activity results in exaggerated muscle movement.

  b. May be initiated and aggravated by stimuli outside body, such as sudden noises, bright lights, or quick movements by people or things in the area.

  c. Intensity influenced by emotional factors. Patient is least in control in an emotionally charged environment, such as the dental office.

 5. Patient constantly in motion; burns up energy; usually very thin; caloric requirement of diet is therefore high.

 6. Brain damage to basal ganglia (Figure 52-5).

C. Ataxia 10%

 1. Loss of equilibrium; balance and orientation difficult; walk uncertain; has difficulty in sitting straight.

 2. Lack of coordination; needs time to execute changes.

 3. Patient inactive because of balance disturbance; tends to put on weight; caloric requirement in diet is therefore low.

 4. Brain damage to cerebellum (Figure 52-5).

D. Rigidity

 1. Muscles may be rigid and stiff, with resistance to movement and hypertonicity.

 2. Tendency to lack of activity.

E. Tremor

Involuntary muscle quivering may affect part or all of the body.

F. Flaccidity

 1. Hypotonia or atonia of muscles that are flabby and weak.

 2. Unable to stand or raise head.

 3. Drooling; difficulty in swallowing and chewing; speech problems.

G. Mixed

Various combinations of the six types occur.

II. CONDITIONS ACCOMPANYING MOTOR ACTIVITY

In addition to impaired movement, weakness, and lack of coordination, the following disabling conditions may also occur.

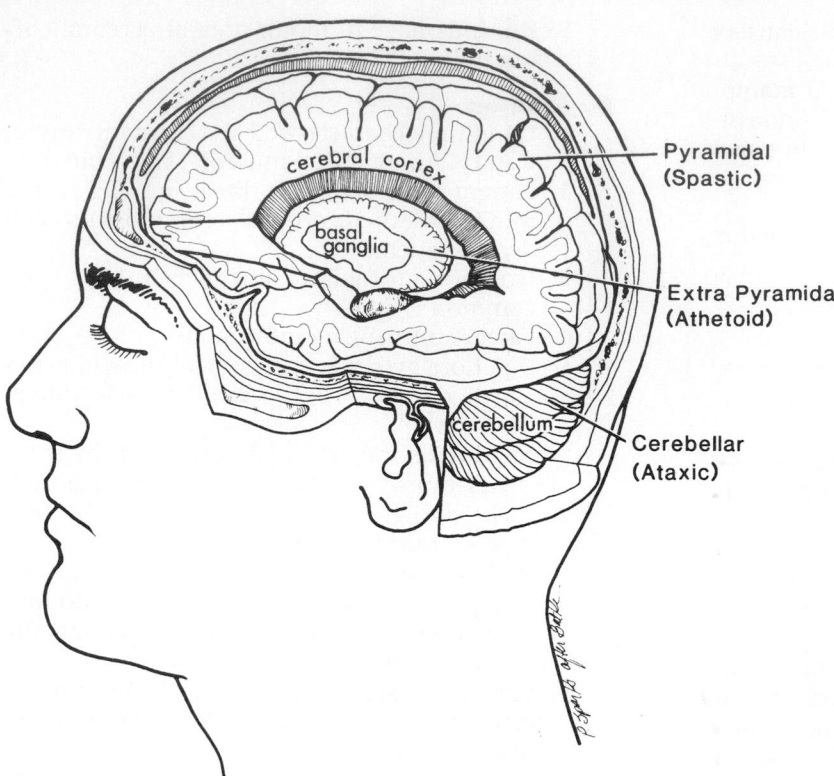

cerebral cortex

basal ganglia

cerebellum

Pyramidal (Spastic)

Extra Pyramidal (Athetoid)

Cerebellar (Ataxic)

■ **FIGURE 52-5 Cerebral Palsy.** Shown are the major parts of the brain involved in each of the three major types of cerebral palsy—spastic, athetoid, and ataxic. (From Bleck, E.E. and Nagel, D.A.: *Physically Handicapped Children. A Medical Atlas for Teachers.* New York, Grune & Stratton, 1975.)

A. Mental Retardation

Fewer than 50% of individuals with cerebral palsy also have mental retardation.

B. Learning Disabilities

Of the 50% who are not mentally retarded, many have problems of learning because of sensory defects, especially hearing and seeing, and perceptive-cognitive deficiencies. Speech difficulties and inability to move about freely can also contribute to learning problems.

C. Seizures

Between 25% and 30% have seizures and undergo related drug therapy.

D. Sensory Disorders

Seeing and hearing problems are common.

III. MEDICAL TREATMENT

Surgical, orthopedic, and medical care, as well as speech, physical, and occupational therapy, may constitute a minimum of specialties involved in the care of a patient with cerebral palsy. Bracing to support the lower limbs and the use of canes, crutches, walkers, or wheelchairs help to increase function. Surgery may be needed for orthopedic deformities or for correcting eye or ear difficulties.

Patients may use tranquilizers to reduce tension or aid in limiting problems associated with nerve damage. Other medication may include drugs for seizure control. Cerebral palsy has no cure.

IV. ORAL CHARACTERISTICS

A. Disturbances of Musculature

Facial grimacing, abnormal muscle function, facial asymmetry, and problems of mastication and swallowing are common. Opening of the mouth may present problems during dental and dental hygiene therapy, as well as during plaque control at home.

B. Malocclusion

The incidence of malocclusion is high. Oral habits of mouth breathing, tongue thrusting, and faulty swallowing contribute to orthodontic needs.

C. Attrition

Severe, constant, involuntary grinding of teeth wears down tooth structure and restorations. Bruxism is most extensive in the athetoid group.

D. Fractured Teeth

Patients fall frequently; accidents to anterior teeth result.

E. Dental Caries

The rate of dental caries may be slightly higher, but the factors that operate for the patient with cerebral palsy are the same as those for the physically normal population. Difficulties in maintaining plaque control and problems of mastication, which lead to the use of a soft diet, may predispose to an environment for bacterial plaque formation.

F. Periodontal Infections
Periodontal or gingival infections are found in a high percentage of patients with cerebral palsy.
1. *Phenytoin-Induced Gingival Overgrowth.* When phenytoin is used for the prevention of seizures, the patient is susceptible to gingival enlargement. The condition and its prevention are described on pages 805 to 807.
2. *Predisposing Factors to Periodontal Involvement.* Mechanical difficulties related to plaque control, mouth breathing, and increased food retention because of ineffective self-cleansing all lead to increased periodontal involvement and plaque collection. Many patients with cerebral palsy have heavy calculus deposits.

V. DENTAL HYGIENE CARE

Procedures described in Chapter 50 apply in the management of the patient with cerebral palsy. Many special adaptations are needed, and experience contributes to developing the necessary patience and confidence.

Dental hygiene care is complicated by the difficulties the patient has in cooperating and by the oral manifestations previously listed. Understanding the physical characteristics is particularly necessary to the success of the appointments. Athetoid movements should not be interpreted as lack of cooperation, and a patient's inability to communicate does not mean lack of comprehension.

Dentists occasionally must use general anesthesia in a hospital situation for the unmanageable patient.

Dangers for both the patient and dental personnel may result from the uncontrolled movement of the patient. The sudden forceful closure of the mouth on the finger of the clinician or on a mouth mirror is an example.

Assistance throughout appointments is important. Suggestions for management should be solicited from family or caregivers. Sedation through premedication may be possible, and various stabilizing procedures may be used (pages 745 to 746).

Selected patients with cerebral palsy may use a mouth-held instrument as described on pages 772 to 773. Oral care and preventive measures are vital to this group of patients.

BELL'S PALSY

Bell's palsy is paralysis of the facial muscles innervated by the facial or seventh cranial nerve. Although the cause is not known, various possible agents have been implicated, including bacterial and viral infections, particularly herpes simplex, trauma from tooth removal, or surgery of the parotid gland area, such as the removal of a tumor.

I. OCCURRENCE
Although relatively rare, the incidence increases with each decade of life. Women are more frequently affected than men in younger age groups, but after age 50, the disorder is more common in men.

II. CHARACTERISTICS[19]
A. Signs and Symptoms
Abrupt weakness or paralysis of facial muscles, usually without preceding pain, occurs on one side of the face.
1. *Mouth.* The corner of the mouth droops, and salivation with drooling is uncontrollable.
2. *Eye.* Eyelids cannot be closed. Watering and drooping of the lower lid invite infection.

B. Functional Problems
Speech and mastication are difficult.

C. Prognosis
A majority of patients experience a return to normal within a month; many have a spontaneous recovery. Others may have lasting residual effects or permanent paralysis.

III. MEDICAL TREATMENT
Without knowledge of the specific cause, treatment has not been definitive. Temporary palliative measures, such as protecting the eye during sleep and massaging the involved muscles, provide some relief.

A. Drugs
Steroids have been used to improve the prognosis.

B. Surgical
The objectives for surgical procedures have been to improve the appearance, provide facial symmetry with voluntary motion, and provide control of the eye and the mouth. Surgery has included repair of the facial nerve, nerve transplantation and grafting, crossover nerve grafts from the uninvolved side of the face, muscle transfers, and free muscle grafts. Prosthetic rehabilitation has been combined with surgical treatment.

IV. DENTAL HYGIENE CARE
Instruction and frequent appointments to supplement the patient's efforts usually are needed. A removable prosthesis needs daily care because debris and plaque collect readily. The involved side needs meticulous bacterial plaque removal because self-cleansing ability has been lost.

When only the seventh nerve is affected, sensory responses are still intact. When anesthesia is used on the opposite side, special precautions should be provided for posttreatment care until the anesthesia has worn off.

Protective eyewear should be worn by the patient. Care is necessary to ensure that calculus, polishing paste, or other foreign material does not enter the eye because the eyelid lacks its natural ability to close for protection.

PARKINSON'S DISEASE

Parkinson's disease is a progressive disorder of the central nervous system characterized by loss of postural stability, slowness of spontaneous movement, resting tremor, and muscular rigidity. It is also known as *paralysis agitans* and *Parkinson's syndrome*.

Although the cause is not known, the basis for the specific group of symptoms is degeneration of certain neurons in the substantia nigra of the basal ganglia, where posture, support, and voluntary motion are controlled. In addition, a severe deficiency of dopamine, one of the substances that participates in nerve transmission, occurs.

I. OCCURRENCE

Parkinson's disease affects middle-aged and older persons primarily, with a higher incidence in men than in women.

II. CHARACTERISTICS

The signs and symptoms center around tremor, rigidity, and loss or impairment of motor function (akinesia). These three factors also occur in other conditions, which must be differentiated by a physician when a diagnosis is made.

A. General Manifestations
1. Body posture bent, with bent head and general stiffness.
2. Motion and responses slowed; difficulty in keeping balance.
3. Gait slow and shuffling.
4. Speech monotonous and slow.
5. Tremor of one or both hands; the fingers may be involved in a pill-rolling motion in which the thumb and index finger are rubbed together in a circular movement. The tremor can be reduced or stopped when the person engages in purposeful action.
6. Intellect is seldom affected except in the advanced stages.
7. Eventually, after 10 to 20 years, the person may become incapacitated and may require complete care.

B. Face and Oral Cavity
1. Expression is fixed and masklike with diminished eye blinking.
2. Tremor in lips, tongue, and neck, and difficulty in swallowing.
3. Excess salivation and drooling.

III. TREATMENT
Maintenance of good general health, with plenty of rest and nutritious meals, is encouraged. Professional physical therapy and occupational therapy have particular significance for a patient's well-being.

Although no known cure exists for Parkinson's disease, symptomatic control can be accomplished, at least in part, by replenishing the dopamine shortage with levodopa. Side effects are common, and may indicate an overdose. Orthostatic hypotension and dizziness may be expected and should be considered when adjusting the dental chair.

Surgical relief for symptoms has been accomplished using pallidotomy. The surgery alters the globus pallidus in the basal ganglia. The location of the basal ganglia in the brain is shown in Figure 52-5.

IV. DENTAL HYGIENE CARE

Various adaptations of procedures can be anticipated from knowledge of the physical characteristics previously noted. Personal interest, attention, and encouragement contribute to help the patient to bear the stresses of the disability.

General suggestions for the gerodontic patient in Chapter 46 (pages 690 to 693) may prove useful, as well as suggestions related to physical disabilities in Chapter 50. Special adaptations for plaque control may be needed.

ARTHRITIS

Diseases of the joints, including arthritis, are among the most common causes of chronic illness in the United States. In addition to arthritis as a disease entity, arthritic manifestations are produced as part of various other chronic diseases. The disability may be temporary or permanent, partial or complete. A person may suffer from more than one type at a time.

Arthritis means inflammation in a joint. It may occur in an acute or chronic form and may be localized or generalized. When many joints are involved, the term *polyarthritis* may be applied.

Factors that have been implicated in the cause of rheumatic and arthritic diseases include infectious agents, traumatic disorders, endocrine abnormalities, tumors, allergy and drug reactions, and inherited or congenital conditions. When the cause is known, specific medical, physical, and surgical therapies may be available to alleviate pain and disability.

I. RHEUMATOID ARTHRITIS
Rheumatoid arthritis is a chronic, immunologic systemic disease in which inflammation of the joints occurs in exacerbations and remissions. The cause is unknown, and the means by which the inflammation in the joints is initiated remains a question.

A. Occurrence
The onset usually occurs between ages 20 and 40, although it may occur at any age. More women than men are affected. It is rare in tropical countries.

B. Signs and Symptoms

1. Joint pain and swelling. Rheumatoid arthritis is a polyarthritis with migratory pain, swelling, tenderness, and warmth in symmetrical joints. Fingers, hands, and knees are usually affected first.
2. Morning stiffness and stiffness after periods of inactivity.
3. Weakness, fatigue, loss of appetite and weight, anemia, low-grade fever.
4. Subcutaneous nodules in elbows, wrists, or fingers in approximately 20% of the patients; nodules may appear in other body organs.
5. Possible temporomandibular joint involvement. There may be pain with jaw movements and difficulty in chewing. Ankylosis may develop but is not a common finding.
6. Progressive deformity, with limited motion in the more severely involved joints and muscle atrophy adjacent to the joints.

C. Medical Treatment

Without a specifically known cause, therapy is limited to an individualized program involving pain relief, physical and occupational therapy, and overall health maintenance with adequate nutrition.

Drugs used in treatment include nonsteroidal anti-inflammatory drugs (NSAIDS) and drugs to aid in controlling the disease including methotrexate, gold compounds, azathioprine, and cyclosporine.[20] Selected patients have been treated by joint replacement surgery.

II. JUVENILE RHEUMATOID ARTHRITIS

Rheumatoid arthritis occurring in children under 16 years of age differs from the disease in adults. The onset is usually more acute, with prolonged fever and enlargement of the spleen and lymph nodes. The inflammation of many joints, particularly knees, wrists, and spine, may appear after a few weeks. Figure 52-6 shows the shape of affected fingers. The temporomandibular joint may be involved, with pain and limited oral opening.

Many patients have complete remissions, some have increasing disability, and others may have mild arthritic symptoms that continue for years. Children are encouraged to lead as normal a life as possible. The long-term treatment program includes activity to maintain function and drugs to relieve pain.

III. DEGENERATIVE JOINT DISEASE[21]

Degenerative joint disease (DJD), or osteoarthritis as it is frequently called, affects the weight-bearing joints particularly. Because inflammation is not the basic joint problem, degenerative joint disease is a more accurate term.

No specific cause is known, but predisposing factors may include repeated trauma, obesity, age-related

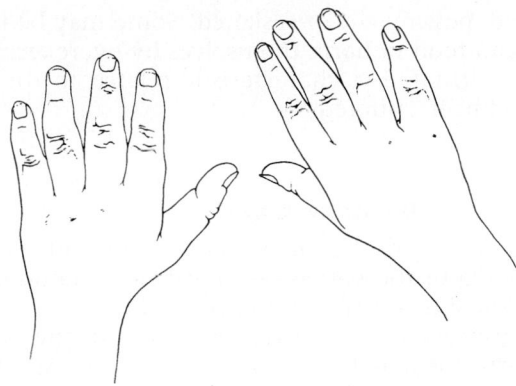

FIGURE 52-6 Child with Rheumatoid Arthritis. The fingers are tapered from fat central areas. The joint nearest the tip of the finger is the least involved. (From Bleck, E.E. and Nagel, D.A.: *Physically Handicapped Children. A Medical Atlas for Teachers.* New York, Grune & Stratton, 1975.)

changes in the joint tissues, mechanical stresses to the weight-bearing joints, and genetic predisposition.

A. Occurrence

The onset occurs between 50 and 70 years of age, with the average onset 20 years later than that of rheumatoid arthritis. As many as 85% of people over age 70 have evidence of degenerative joint disease.

B. Symptoms

At first insidious, with slight stiffness of a single joint, the eventual condition leads to much pain, deformity, and limitation of movement.

1. Hips, knees, fingers, and vertebrae affected most frequently.
2. Swelling rare; ankylosis does not occur.
3. Stiffness in the morning on rising and after periods of inactivity; diminishes with exercise.
4. Pain aggravated by temperature changes and bearing body weight.
5. Temporomandibular joint usually without pain or other clinical symptoms, although crepitation, clicking, or snapping may occur when the joints are exercised.

C. Medical Treatment

Moderate exercise, pain-relieving drug therapy, weight reduction for obese patients, physical therapy, and selected orthopedic surgical procedures comprise the general treatments available. Total hip or knee joint replacement has proved satisfactory for many patients, and has been used more widely for DJD than for rheumatoid arthritis.

IV. PERSONAL FACTORS

With long-term illnesses, patients are frequently discouraged or apprehensive. Certain patients may be worried, pessimistic, or resigned. Some may be impatient and tend to harm themselves by overexercise. A few are irritable, a characteristic related to the pain that has been suffered.

V. DENTAL HYGIENE CARE

A high standard of general health contributes to the well-being of the patient with arthritis. Maintenance of oral health contributes to general health.

Adjustments for physical disabilities of the patient with arthritis may be found in Chapter 50. Assistance with ambulation, chair positioning, and other special adaptations are needed.

A. Patient History

Questions to determine whether the patient has a joint prosthesis should be included in the patient history. Because of the susceptibility to infection at the interface of the bone and the prosthesis, prophylactic antibiotic premedication to prevent bacteremia is recommended.[22] A patient who is anticipating surgery for a joint replacement should be counseled to complete all needed periodontal and restorative therapy before the surgery to prevent the need for repeated antibiotic premedication.

B. Instrumentation

For the patient with arthritis of the temporomandibular joint, instrumentation may need adaptations to accommodate a minimal opening of the mouth. Fatigue in the joint may be reduced by rest periods, by minimizing the pressure on the mandible, and by overall efficiency to shorten the necessary appointment time. More frequent appointments can contribute to keeping the oral health at a maximum and thus preventing long, difficult scaling sessions.

C. Bacterial Plaque Control

Because of hand and arm involvement, a patient may have difficulty grasping a toothbrush or lifting the arm for sufficient periods to clean the mouth completely. Adapted brushing procedures may be applied (pages 749 to 751).

D. Diet and Nutrition

1. No special nutritional factors are known to be associated with the course or treatment of arthritis. Physicians generally recommend a normal, well-balanced diet with a controlled caloric intake for weight control. Encouragement of restriction of sweets and selection of noncariogenic between-meal snacks can help to improve oral health.
2. Obtaining a food diary for several days to a week can be important for dietary analysis and counseling, especially for the gerodontic arthritic patient.

SCLERODERMA (PROGRESSIVE SYSTEMIC SCLEROSIS)

Scleroderma is an autoimmune disease of connective tissue characterized by an overproduction of collagen. The most striking physical symptom is the immobility and rigidity of the skin, but inflammation and sclerosis occur throughout the body. Thus, the disease has the full title of *progressive systemic sclerosis.*

The cause is not known, but collagen synthesis irregularities, associated immunologic disorders, and microvascular abnormalities have been implicated. Hereditary factors are not involved.

I. OCCURRENCE

Scleroderma usually has its onset between ages 30 and 50, but may affect persons of any age, even infants. It may develop over months or years and is 2 to 5 times more common in females.

II. CHARACTERISTICS

Scleroderma may be localized and involve only the skin, or it may be generalized and involve all body organs. The most notable changes are in the skin, gastrointestinal tract, kidneys, heart, muscles, and lungs. Eventual death results from renal failure, cardiac failure, pulmonary insufficiency, or intestinal malabsorption. Symptoms vary, and all individuals do not have all the symptoms and signs that follow.

A. General Manifestations

1. *Joints.* Pain, swelling, and stiffness of the fingers and knee joints.
2. *Polyarthritis.* Symmetrical polyarthritis, similar to rheumatoid arthritis.
3. *Skin.* Hard and fixed; ivory-white, yellow, or gray, sometimes with brown pigmentation in the late stages.
4. *Face.* When affected, the face becomes masklike and expressionless.

B. Oral Characteristics

1. *Lips.* Thin, rigid, with oral stricture and difficulty in opening and closing.
2. *Mucosa.* Thin, pale, tender, rigid, with poor healing capacity.
3. *Gingiva.* Pale and unusually firm.
4. *Teeth.* Mobility is common.
5. *Radiographic Findings.* Marked widening of the periodontal ligament spaces. This finding is sometimes considered pathognomonic for scleroderma.
6. *Mastication.* Difficult; temporomandibular joint movement is limited.
7. *Tongue.* May be immobile; speech difficult.

III. MEDICAL TREATMENT

Specific therapy is not known. Medications that retard collagen deposition have not yet been effective for scleroderma. Treatment, therefore, has been directed at specific system complications, physical therapy, and attempts to maintain normal activities.

IV. DENTAL HYGIENE CARE

The tightening of the skin and lips limits opening of the mouth and complicates all dental and dental hygiene procedures, as well as daily self-care by the patient. Every effort for preservation of the teeth and gingiva in health should be made to prevent the need for extensive treatment. With oral stricture, the preparation and wearing of dentures are difficult or impossible as the disease becomes more severe.

Patients with scleroderma are sensitive to cold and dampness, stress, undue emotional tension, and fatigue. All these factors can be considered for the dental hygiene appointment.

REFERENCES

1. **Smeltzer,** S.C. and Bare, B.G.: *Brunner and Suddarth's Textbook of Medical-Surgical Nursing,* 7th ed. Philadelphia, J.B. Lippincott Co., 1992, pp. 1737–1744.
2. **Chiles,** B.W. and Cooper, P.R.: Acute Spinal Injury, *N. Engl. J. Med., 334,* 514, February 22, 1996.
3. **Schubert,** M.M., Snow, M., and Stiefel, D.J.: *Dental Treatment of the Spinal Cord Injured Patient.* Disability Dental Instruction, 4919 NE 86th Street, Seattle, WA 98115, 34 pp.
4. **Thornton,** J.B., Sneed, R.C., Tomaselli, C.E., and Boraz, R.A.: Dental Management of Patients with Spinal Cord Injury, *Compend. Cont. Educ. Dent., 13,* 122, February, 1992.
5. **Ruff,** J.C.: Selection Criteria for Static and Dynamic Mouthsticks, *Gen. Dent., 38,* 414, November–December, 1990.
6. **Akar,** Z.: Myelomeningocele, *Surg. Neurol., 43,* 113, February, 1995.
7. **United States Centers for Disease Control:** Recommendations for the Use of Folic Acid to Reduce the Number of Cases of Spina Bifida and Other Neural Tube Defects, *MMWR, 41,* RR-14, September 11, 1992.
8. **Little,** J.W., Falace, D.A., Miller, C.S., and Rhodus, N.L.: *Dental Management of the Medically Compromised Patient,* 5th ed. St. Louis, Mosby, 1997, pp. 74, 607.
9. **Engibous,** P.J., Kittle, P.E., Jones, H.L., and Vance, B.J.: Latex Allergy in Patients with Spina Bifida, *Pediatr. Dent., 15,* 364, September/October, 1993.
10. **Nelson,** L.P., Soporowski, N.J., and Shusterman, S.: Latex Allergies in Children with Spina Bifida: Relevance for the Pediatric Dentist, *Pediatr. Dent., 16,* 18, January/February, 1994.
11. **Malamed,** S.F.: *Medical Emergencies in the Dental Office,* 4th ed. St. Louis, Mosby, 1993, pp. 262–275.
12. **Bennett,** J.C. and Plum, F., eds.: *Cecil Textbook of Medicine,* 20th ed. Philadelphia, W.B. Saunders Co., 1996, p. 2161.
13. **Drachman,** D.B.: Myasthenia Gravis, *N. Engl. J. Med., 330,* 1797, June 23, 1994.
14. **Appel,** S.H.: Myasthenia Gravis, in Rakel, R.E., ed.: *Conn's Current Therapy, 1998.* Philadelphia, W.B. Saunders Co., 1998, p. 929.
15. **Silberberg,** D.H.: Multiple Sclerosis, in Rakel, R.E., ed.: *Conn's Current Therapy, 1998.* Philadelphia, W.B. Saunders Co., 1998, p. 922.
16. **Rudick,** R.A., Cohen, J.A., Weinstock-Guttman, B., Kinkel, R.P., and Ransohoff, R.M.: Management of Multiple Sclerosis, *N. Engl. J. Med., 337,* 1604, November 27, 1997.
17. **Sorenson,** H.W.: Physically Handicapped, in Nowak, A.J.: *Dentistry for the Handicapped Patient.* St. Louis, Mosby, 1976, pp. 23–38.
18. **Danforth,** H.A., Snow, M., and Stiefel, D.J.: *Dental Manage-*

ment of the Cerebral Palsied Patient. Disability Dental Instruction, 4919 NE 86th Street, Seattle, WA 98115, 30 pp.
19. **Regezi,** J.A. and Sciubba, J.: *Oral Pathology. Clinical-Pathologic Correlations,* 2nd ed. Philadelphia, W.B. Saunders Co., 1993, pp. 581–582.
20. **Cash,** J.M. and Klippel, J.H.: Second-Line Drug Therapy for Rheumatoid Arthritis, *N. Engl. J. Med., 330,* 1368, May 12, 1994.
21. **Neustadt,** D.H.: Osteoarthritis, in Rakel, R.E., ed.: *Conn's Current Therapy, 1998.* Philadelphia, W.B. Saunders Co., 1998, p. 995.
22. **American Dental Association and American Academy of Orthopaedic Surgeons:** Advisory Statement: Antibiotic Prophylaxis for Dental Patients with Total Joint Replacements, in *ADA Guide to Dental Therapeutics.* Chicago, ADA Publishing Co., 1998, Appendix E., pp. 547–550.

SUGGESTED READINGS

Anderson, R.A. and Ewell-Jackson, T.: Scleroderma in Pediatric Patients, *ASDC J. Dent. Child., 57,* 462, November–December, 1990.

Ertürk, N. and Dogan, S.: The Effect of Neuromuscular Diseases on the Development of Dental and Occlusal Characteristics, *Quintessence Int., 22,* 317, April, 1991.

Hughes, G.B.: Acute Peripheral Facial Paralysis (Bell's Palsy), in Rakel, R.E., ed.: *Conn's Current Therapy, 1998.* Philadelphia, W.B. Saunders Co., 1998, p. 943.

Kellman, R.: The Cervical Spine in Maxillofacial Trauma. Assessment and Airway Management, *Otolaryngol. Clin. North Am., 24,* 1, February, 1991.

Munsat, T.L.: Poliomyelitis—New Problems with an Old Disease, *N. Engl. J. Med., 324,* 1206, April 25, 1991.

Sonies, B.C. and Dalakas, M.C.: Dysphagia in Patients with Post-polio Syndrome, *N. Engl. J. Med., 324,* 1162, April 25, 1991.

Vita, A.J., Terry, R.B., Hubert, H.B., and Fries, J.F.: Aging, Health Risks, and Cumulative Disability, *N. Engl. J. Med., 338,* 1035, April 9, 1998.

Zuckerman, J.D.: Hip Fracture, *N. Engl. J. Med., 334,* 1519, June 6, 1996.

Arthritis

Akerman, S., Jonsson, K., Kopp, S., Petersson, A., and Rohlin, M.: Radiologic Changes in Temporomandibular, Hand, and Foot Joints of Patients with Rheumatoid Arthritis, *Oral Surg. Oral Med. Oral Pathol., 72,* 245, August, 1991.

Carpenter, E.H., Plant, M.J., Hassell, A.B., Shadforth, M.F., Fisher, J., Clarke, S., Hothersall, T.E., and Dawes, P.T.: Management of Oral Complications of Disease-Modifying Drugs in Rheumatoid Arthritis, *Br. J. Rheumatol., 36,* 473, April, 1997.

Gynther, G.W., Holmlund, A.B., Reinholt, F.P., and Lindblad, S.: Temporomandibular Joint Involvement in Generalized Osteoarthritis and Rheumatoid Arthritis: A Clinical Arthroscopic, Histologic, and Immunohistochemical Study, *Int. J. Oral Maxillofac. Surg., 26,* 10, February, 1997.

Harris, E.D: Rheumatoid Arthritis. Pathophysiology and Implications for Treatment, *N. Engl. J. Med., 322,* 1277, May 3, 1990.

Liang, M.H. and Fortin, P.: Management of Osteoarthritis of the Hip and Knee, *N. Engl. J. Med., 325,* 125, July 11, 1991.

Pinals, R.S.: Polyarthritis and Fever, *N. Engl. J. Med., 330,* 769, March 17, 1994.

Risheim, H., Kjaerheim, V., and Arneberg, P.: Improvement of Oral Hygiene in Patients with Rheumatoid Arthritis, *Scand. J. Dent. Res., 100,* 172, June, 1992.

Russell, S.L. and Reisine, S.: Investigation of Xerostomia in Patients with Rheumatoid Arthritis, *J. Am. Dent. Assoc., 129,* 733, June, 1998.

Tanchyk, A.P.: Dental Considerations for the Patient with Juvenile Rheumatoid Arthritis, *Gen. Dent., 39,* 330, September–October, 1991.

Wright, E.F., DesRosier, K.F., Clark, M.K., and Bifano, S.L.:

Identifying Undiagnosed Rheumatic Disorders Among Patients with TMD, *J. Am. Dent. Assoc., 128*, 738, June, 1997.

Zifer, S.A., Sams, D.R., Potter, B.J., and Jerath, R.: Clinical and Radiographic Evaluation of Juvenile Rheumatoid Arthritis: Report of a Case, *Spec. Care Dentist., 14*, 208, September/October, 1994.

Spinal Cord Injury

Ditunno, J.F. and Formal, C.S.: Chronic Spinal Cord Injury, *N. Engl. J. Med., 330*, 550, February 24, 1994.

Lancashire, P., Janzen, J., Zach, G.A., and Addy, M.: The Oral Hygiene and Gingival Health of Paraplegic Inpatients—A Cross-sectional Survey, *J. Clin. Periodontol., 24*, 198, March, 1997.

Laskowski-Jones, L.: Acute SCI. How to Minimize the Damage, *Am. J. Nursing, 93*, 22, December, 1993.

Rosenblatt, R.: New Hopes, New Dreams. Christopher Reeve is Preparing to Walk Again, *TIME, 148*, 40, August 26, 1996.

Stiefel, D.J., Truelove, E.L., Persson, R.S., Chin, M.M., and Mandel, L.S.: A Comparison of Oral Health in Spinal Cord Injury and Other Disability Groups, *Spec. Care Dentist., 13*, 229, November/December, 1993.

Taniguchi, M.H. and Schlosser, G.A.: Adolescent Spinal Cord Injury: Considerations for Post-acute Management, *Adolescent Medicine, 5*, 327, June, 1994.

Mouth-Held Orthosis

Blaine, H.H. and Nelson, E.P.: A Mouthstick for Quadriplegic Patients, *J. Prosthet. Dent., 29*, 317, March, 1973.

Budning, B.C. and Hall, M.: A Practical Mouthstick for Early Intervention with Quadriparetic Patients, *J. Can. Dent. Assoc., 56*, 243, March, 1990.

DiPietro, G.J., Warfield, D.K., and Bradshaw, A.J.: A Jaw-Operated Proximity Switch for a Paraplegic Patient, *J. Prosthet. Dent., 56*, 711, December, 1986.

Drago, C.J.: Design Considerations for Construction of a Mouthstick Prosthesis, *Quintessence Dent. Technol., 10*, 451, July–August, 1986.

Hock, D.A.: The Use of the Maxillary Interocclusal Splint as a Mouthpiece for the Mouthstick Prosthesis, *J. Prosthet. Dent., 62*, 56, July, 1989.

Nunn, J.H. and Wood, I.: The Use of a Vacuum-Molded Polyvinyl Acetate-Polyethylene Copolymer (PVAC.PE) for a Handicapped Patient, *Spec. Care Dentist., 12*, 122, May/June, 1992.

Rodeghero, P., Claman, L., Cellier, S., and Lotz, J.W.: The Long-term Effect of Mouthsticks on Periodontal Support, *Spec. Care Dentist., 5*, 251, November–December, 1985.

Stroke

Bronner, L.L., Kanter, D.S., and Manson, J.E.: Primary Prevention of Stroke, *N. Engl. J. Med., 333*, 1392, November 23, 1995.

Carter, L.C., Haller, A.D., Nadarajah, V., Calamel, A.D., and Aguirre, A.: Use of Panoramic Radiography Among an Ambulatory Dental Population to Detect Patients at Risk of Stroke, *J. Am. Dent. Assoc., 128*, 977, July, 1997.

Cieslak, S.: Stroke Dental Care for Stroke Survivors, *DentalHygienistNews*, 11, 14, No. 1, 1998.

Ostuni, E.: Stroke and the Dental Patient, *J. Am. Dent. Assoc., 125*, 721, June, 1994.

Reddy, M.P. and Reddy, V.: After a Stroke: Strategies to Restore Function and Prevent Complications, *Geriatrics, 52*, 59, September, 1997.

Roth, E.J.: Rehabilitation of the Stroke Patient, in Rakel, R.E., ed.: *Conn's Current Therapy, 1998*. Philadelphia, W.B. Saunders, 1998, p. 868.

Wright, S.M.: Denture Treatment for the Stroke Patient, *Br. Dent. J., 183*, 179, September 13, 1997.

Muscular Dystrophy

Darras, B.T., Harper, J.F., and Francke, U.: Prenatal Diagnosis and Detection of Carriers with DNA Probes in Duchenne's Muscular Dystrophy, *N. Engl. J. Med., 316*, 985, April 16, 1987.

Dubowitz, V.: The Muscular Dystrophies—Clarity or Chaos? (Editorial), *N. Engl. J. Med., 336*, 650, February 27, 1997.

Duggan, D.J., Gorospe, J.R., Fanin, M., Hoffman, E.P., and Angelini, C.: Mutations in the Sarcoglycan Genes in Patients with Myopathy, *N. Engl. J. Med., 336*, 618, February 27, 1997.

Eckhardt, L. and Harzer, W.: Facial Structure and Functional Findings in Patients with Progressive Muscular Dystrophy, *Am. J. Orthod. Dentofacial Orthop., 110*, 185, August, 1996.

Shapiro, F., Specht, L., and Korf, B.R.: Locomotor Problems in Infantile Facioscapulohumeral Muscular Dystrophy. Retrospective Study of 9 Patients, *Acta Orthop. Scand., 62*, 367, August, 1991.

Smith, P.E.M., Calverley, P.M.A., Edwards, R.H.T., Evans, G.A., and Campbell, E.J.M.: Practical Problems in the Respiratory Care of Patients with Muscular Dystrophy, *N. Engl. J. Med., 316*, 1197, May 7, 1987.

Myasthenia Gravis

Linton, D.M. and Philcox, D.: Myasthenia Gravis, *Disease-a-Month, 36*, 595, November, 1990.

Lloyd, J.M. and Mitchell, R.G.: Myasthenia Gravis as a Cause of Facial Pain, *Oral Surg. Oral Med. Oral Pathol., 66*, 45, July, 1988.

Patton, L.L. and Howard, J.F.: Myasthenia Gravis: Dental Treatment Considerations, *Spec. Care. Dentist., 17*, 25, January/February, 1997.

Multiple Sclerosis

Confavreux, C., Hutchinson, M., Hours, M.M., Cortinovis-Tourniaire, P., Moreau, T., and The Pregnancy in Multiple Sclerosis Group: Rate of Pregnancy-Related Relapse in Multiple Sclerosis, *N. Engl. J. Med., 339*, 285, July 30, 1998.

Robinson-Akande, D.A.: Trigeminal Neuralgia as a Complication of Multiple Sclerosis, *Gen. Dent., 43*, 436, September–October, 1995.

Symons, A.L., Bortolanza, M., Godden, S., and Seymour, G.: A Preliminary Study into the Dental Health Status of Multiple Sclerosis Patients, *Spec. Care Dentist., 13*, 96, May/June, 1993.

Trapp, B.D., Peterson, J., Ransohoff, R.M., Rudick, R., Mörk, S., and Bö, L.: Axonal Transection in the Lesions of Multiple Sclerosis, *N. Engl. J. Med., 338*, 278, January 29, 1998.

Waxman, S.G.: Demyelinating Diseases—New Pathological Insights, New Therapeutic Targets (Editorial), *N. Engl. J. Med., 338*, 323, January 29, 1998.

Cerebral Palsy

Bhat, M., Nelson, K.B., Cummins, S.K., and Grether, J.K.: Prevalence of Developmental Enamel Defects in Children with Cerebral Palsy, *J. Oral Pathol. Med., 21*, 241, July, 1992.

Croft, R.D.: What Consistency of Food Is Best for Children with Cerebral Palsy Who Cannot Chew? *Arch. Dis. Child., 67*, 269, March, 1992.

DeBiase, C.B.: Treating the Patient with Cerebral Palsy, *DentalHygienistNews, 5*, 13, Summer, 1992.

Hallet, K.B., Lucas, J.O., Johnston, T., Reddihough, D.S., and Hall, R.K.: Dental Health of Children with Cerebral Palsy Following Sialodocho-plasty, *Spec. Care Dentist., 15*, 234, November/December, 1995.

Kaufman, E., Meyer, S., Wolnerman, J.S., and Gilai, A.N.: Transient Suppression of Involuntary Movements in Cerebral Palsy Patients During Dental Treatment, *Anesth. Prog., 38*, 200, November–December, 1991.

Kuban, K.C.K. and Leviton, A.: Cerebral Palsy, *N. Engl. J. Med., 330*, 188, January 20, 1994.

Loiacono, C.: Dental Hygiene Care for the Patient with Cerebral Palsy, *Access, 10*, 34, July, 1995.

MacDonald, D.: Cerebral Palsy and Intrapartum Fetal Monitoring (Editorial), *N. Engl. J. Med., 334*, 659, March 7, 1996.

Nelson, K.B., Dambrosia, J.M., Ting, T.Y., and Grether, J.K.: Uncertain Value of Electronic Fetal Monitoring in Predicting Cerebral Palsy, *N. Engl. J. Med., 334*, 613, March 7, 1996.

Nielsen, L.A.: Caries Among Children with Cerebral Palsy: Relation to CP-Diagnosis, Mental and Motor Handicap, *ASDC J. Dent. Child., 57,* 267, July–August, 1990.

Oliver, R.G.: Theoretical Aspects and Clinical Experience with the Palatal Training Appliance for Saliva Control in Persons with Cerebral Palsy, *Spec. Care Dentist., 7,* 271, November–December, 1987.

Parkinson's Disease

Agid, Y.: Parkinson's Disease: Pathophysiology, *Lancet, 337,* 1321, June, 1, 1991.

Clough, C.G.: Parkinson's Disease: Management, *Lancet, 337,* 1324, June 1, 1991.

Grandinetti, A., Morens, D.M., Reed, D., and MacEachern, D.: Prospective Study of Cigarette Smoking and the Risk of Developing Idiopathic Parkinson's Disease, *Am. J. Epidemiology, 139,* 1129, June 15, 1994.

Kennedy, M.A., Rosen, S., Paulson, G.W., Jolly, D.E., and Beck, F.M.: Relationship of Oral Microflora with Oral Health Status in Parkinson's Disease, *Spec. Care Dentist., 14,* 164, July/August, 1994.

Persson, M., Osterberg, T., Granérus, A.-K., and Karlsson, S.: Influence of Parkinson's Disease on Oral Health, *Acta Odontol. Scand., 50,* 37, February, 1992.

Salzman, E.W.: Living with Parkinson's Disease (Editorial), *N. Engl. J. Med., 334,* 114, January 11, 1996.

The Patient With a Sensory Disability

Successful management and treatment of any patient depend to a large extent on the interpersonal communication between the patient and the clinician. When a patient has a vision or hearing impairment, communication assumes a different dimension. Suggestions for adaptations for patients with hearing or visual problems are described in this chapter. Box 53-1 contains key words and definitions pertaining to sensory impairments.

The Americans with Disabilities Act defines an individual with a disability as a person who has a physical or mental impairment that substantially limits a major life activity. The examples of physical and mental impairments provided with the Act include visual and hearing impairments. For the visually impaired, certain qualifications related to physical facilities are specified, such as the removal of physical barriers and the use of braille markers for elevators.

In the section on communications, the Act specifies that communications with individuals with hearing and vision impairments must be as effective as communications with nondisabled people, and appropriate auxiliary aids must be provided. Examples of auxiliary aids are such services and devices as qualified interpreters, assistive listening headsets, text telephone devices for deaf persons (TTYs), readers, taped texts, brailled materials, and large-print materials.

Special skills used to counsel, motivate, and educate a patient with a sensory disability must be developed and practiced. Although visual channels provide a primary method of communication with the deaf person, audible and "touch" channels are essential for the person with visual disability.

VISUAL IMPAIRMENT

Limitations of sight cover a broad spectrum from the slightly affected to the completely blind with no perception of light. Loss of sight is a major physical deprivation. In many persons, blindness is secondary to a primary condition that may have been the cause of the blindness and in itself may be disabling.

In the United States, "legal blindness" is defined as follows: having central vision (or acuity) of not more than 20/200 in the better eye with correction (glasses), or having peripheral fields (side vision) of no more than 20 degrees diameter or 10 degrees radius. Only approximately 3% of legally blind persons are totally blind. The term "legal blindness" is a legal term, not a medical one, but certification of the degree of severity of blindness is obtained from an ophthalmologist.

BOX 53-1 KEY WORDS AND ABBREVIATIONS: Sensory Disabilities

VISION

Astigmatism (ah-stig′mah-tizm): impaired vision caused by irregularities in the curvature of the cornea or lens.

Blind spot: the area on the retina that marks the site of entrance of the optic nerve.

Blindness: no perception of visual stimuli; lack or loss of ability to see.

  Legal blindness: less than 20/200 vision with corrective eyeglasses (see text).

Braille (brāl): a system of writing and printing by means of raised points representing letters; enables people with a visual disability to read by touch.

Cataract (kat′ah-rakt): clouding or opacity of the lens of an eye.

Color blindness: inability to distinguish between certain colors; most common is red/green confusion; color vision is a function of the cones of the retina.

Diplopia (dĭ-plō′pē-ah): double vision; perception of two images of a single object.

Glaucoma (glaw-kō′mah): group of diseases of the eye characterized by intraocular pressure from pathologic changes in the optic disc; person has visual-field defects.

Hyperopia (hi″per-ō′pē-ah): farsightedness; eyeball is shorter behind the retina; vision is better for distant objects than for near objects.

Myopia (mī-ō′pē-ah): nearsightedness; longer eyeball from front to back so the image is focused in front of the retina.

Nyctalopia (nik″tah-lo′pe-ah): night blindness; may be hereditary or related to vitamin deficiency.

Ocular (ok′ū-lar): pertaining to the eye.

Ophthalmologist (of″thal-mol′ō-jist): physician who specializes in diagnosing and prescribing treatment for defects, injuries, and diseases of the eye (obsolete term: oculist).

Ophthalmology (of″thal-mol′ō-je): the branch of medicine that deals with the anatomy, diagnosis, pathology, and treatment of the eye.

Optician (op-tish′an): technician who prepares and adapts lenses; fills prescriptions from an ophthalmologist.

Optometrist (op-tom′ĕ-trist): a specialist in **optometry**, the measurement of visual acuity and the adaptation of lenses for correction of visual defects.

Retinitis (ret″i-ni′tis): inflammation of the retina.

Retinopathy (ret′ĭ-nop′ah-thē): noninflammatory disease of the retina; identified by the chronic disease of which it is a symptom; for example, **diabetic retinopathy** reflects the retinal manifestations of diabetes mellitus, including microaneurysms.

Retinopathy of prematurity: a condition peculiar to premature infants; characterized by opaque tissue behind the lens resulting from a high concentration of oxygen, which causes spasm of the retinal vessels, leads to retinal detachment, and arrests eye growth and development; prevented by keeping oxygen administration as low as possible and discontinuing the oxygen as soon as possible.

HEARING

Audiogram (aw′dē-ō-gram): graphic record of the findings of an audiometer.

Audiologist (aw′dē-ol′ō-jist): certified allied health worker, often with advanced degrees; trained in the identification, diagnosis, measurement, and rehabilitation of hearing impairment.

Audiometer (aw″dē-om′ĕ-ter): instrument used to determine degree and type of hearing ability.

Aural (aw′ral): pertaining to the ear.

Decibel (des′ĭ-bel): unit for expressing the relative loudness of a sound; abbreviation, **dB.**

Hearing: the sense by which sounds are perceived; conversion of sound waves into nerve impulses, which are then interpreted by the brain.

Otitis (ō-tī′tis): inflammation of the ear.

  Otitis media: inflammation of the middle ear.

Otologist (ō-tol′ō-jist): physician specialist in **otology,** branch of medicine dealing with the anatomy, physiology, pathology, and treatment of the ear.

Speechreading: recognizing spoken words by watching the speaker's lips, face, and gestures.

TDD: Telecommunication Device for the Deaf.

Tinnitus (tĭ-nī′tus): noise in the ears, as ringing, buzzing, or roaring.

TTY: Text telephone device.

(continued)

BOX 53-1 KEY WORDS AND ABBREVIATIONS: Sensory Disabilities (Continued)

Tuning fork: instrument used to test for hearing loss; vibrations of the fork produce sound waves that can be heard in both ears by a person with normal hearing when the stem is placed on top of the head; sound is heard louder in an ear affected by conductive loss and softer in an ear affected by sensorineural loss.

Tympanic membrane: ear drum; vibrates when sound waves strike; transmits waves to nerve endings by way of ossicles in middle ear and to cochlea in the inner ear.

Vertigo (ver-tĭ-gō): sensation of rotation or movement of one's self (subjective vertigo) or of one's surroundings (objective vertigo); a subtype of dizziness, but not a synonym.

I. CAUSES OF BLINDNESS

The leading causes of blindness are diabetic retinopathy, age-related macular degeneration, senile cataracts, glaucoma, vascular disease, trauma, and infections. At least one half of the blindness in children is of prenatal origin, particularly resulting from maternal infections (rubella, syphilis, toxoplasmosis). Other causes are injuries, neoplasms, and retinopathy of prematurity (formerly called retrolental fibroplasia). The incidence of retinopathy of prematurity has increased as more premature babies survive.

II. PERSONAL FACTORS

Each person with visual impairment must be considered in relation to individual aptitudes, interests, abilities, and potentialities, with sight as one factor involved. No pattern of patient attitudes and personality characteristics can be described. The only common characteristic this group of patients has is difficulty in seeing. A few suggestions of factors involved are mentioned here.

A. Patient History

Assistance in completing the personal questionnaire may be needed. Specific details of the patient's limitations must be recorded so that adaptations can be made during the appointment.

B. Child

1. *Learning Ability*
   a. Sensory defects often mask a child's intellectual capacity because responses cannot be the same as in other children.
   b. Blind children may learn to speak later than sighted children and may start school when they are a year or two older.
   c. A blind child takes longer than does the sighted child to cover the same amount of material; therefore, the educational level for the blind child may be different from that for the sighted child of the same chronologic age.
   d. Blind children are deprived of the opportunity to learn by imitation.

2. *Personal Factors.* Environment influences the child's adjustment, and parental attitude affects the blind child as it does the sighted child. When the parent is overindulgent and protective, the child may be self-centered, dependent, and emotionally less stable.

C. Adult

The adult who has always been blind or has been so since childhood has made adjustments and may be employed in a limited but useful occupation. The greater number of those who become blind after adulthood experience an immediate natural reaction of depression and feeling of helplessness.

When loss of vision is incipient, the reactions of shock and upheaval usually are less, but dread, worry, and anxiety may be experienced for years in anticipation. When the patient begins to accept the disability, efforts for rehabilitation are made easier. Independence and self-confidence should be developed, and the patient must be helped to avoid helplessness.

III. DENTAL HYGIENE CARE: TOTALLY BLIND

A. Factors in Patient Care

1. A blind person can perceive a new experience readily if told about it in detail.
2. Because of the visual disability, the patient must rely more on other senses and cultivate them.
3. A blind person must be neat and orderly. If something is put down, it must be located readily again.
4. A blind person does things deliberately and slowly to gain perception and prevent accidents.
5. A blind person learns to interpret and rely on tone of voice more than do persons with sight who can watch facial expressions.

B. Patient Reception and Seating

1. Lower dental chair prior to receiving patient; move other dental equipment, such as the

bracket tray and clinician's stool, from pathway.

2. Guide to dental chair. Patient holds arm and is led without being pushed or pulled (Figure 53-1).

3. Provide forewarnings of potential hazards in the pathway.

4. The patient who has become familiar with office arrangement from previous appointments should be informed of changes to prevent embarrassment.

5. Protective eyewear. The patient usually will prefer to wear the personal glasses regularly worn. Many wear dark glasses.

6. When leaving the treatment room during the appointment, explain absence; prevent embarrassment of patient speaking to someone who is not there; speak when re-entering the room.

C. The Dog Guide

1. Do not distract a dog guide on duty by speaking to or touching it.

2. Ask the patient where the best place would be for the dog to stay during the appointment. The dogs are gentle, carefully trained animals, and may lie quietly in a corner of the treatment room as directed by the patient.

D. Introduce Clinical Procedures

1. Describe each step in detail before proceeding. Explain instruments and materials, and how each will be applied. Mention flavors.

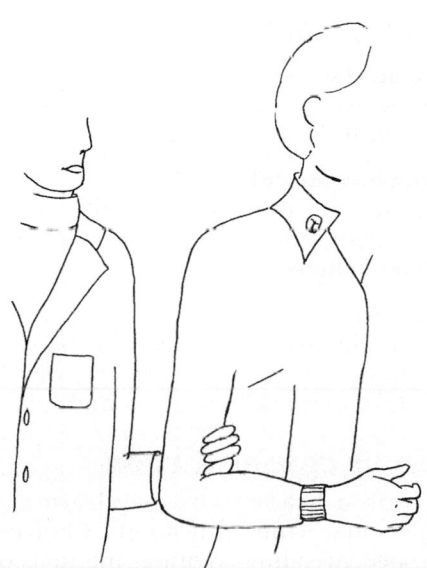

■ **FIGURE 53-1 Escorting a Blind Person.** The blind person holds the arm of the guide just above the elbow and walks beside and slightly behind. The guide verbally gives advance notice of approaching changes. The blind person can sense the body motion of the guide and anticipate changes.

2. Permit patient to handle dull instruments, such as a mouth mirror. This applies particularly to a child patient who is not familiar with dental procedures.

3. Use other instruments of a similar size and shape when describing scalers or explorers because handling sharp instruments would be dangerous for the patient.

4. Prepare patient for power-driven instruments.
   a. Avoid surprise applications of compressed air, water from syringe, or power-driven instruments.
   b. Apply moving rubber cup to child's finger. When power-driven instruments disturb the patient, a porte polisher may be used when stain removal is considered necessary.

5. Speak before touching the patient. By maintaining contact of a finger on a tooth or through retraction while changing instruments, repeated orientation can be avoided.

6. Rinsing
   a. Use evacuator when possible.
   b. Without evacuation, explain the water syringe and place rinsing cup in the patient's hand each time. Do not expect the patient to pick it up from unit.
   c. Help the patient avoid embarrassment if water is spilled.

E. Instructions for Patient

1. Give instructions clearly and concisely.

2. Demonstrate toothbrushing in patient's mouth. Help learning by the feeling of the filament tips on and under the gingival margin and the feeling of clean teeth.

IV. DENTAL HYGIENE CARE: PARTIALLY SIGHTED

Persons with sight often underestimate how useful a little vision can be. Patience is needed for helping a patient to make full use of available vision, without oversolicitousness. Although many of the procedures described for the totally blind person can be applied to the partially sighted person, a few additional hints are suggested here.

Elderly patients with failing sight rarely admit such an impairment. Sight failure in the older individual or lowered vision in a person of any age may be suspected from the patient's unusual squinting, blinking, or lack of continued attention. Procedures can be adapted without mention of sight to the patient.

A. Patient Position

Adjust for patient comfort. Tilting back a patient with glaucoma may increase pain and pressure in the eyes.

B. Light

Avoid glare of the dental light in the patient's

eyes. Sensitivity to light is characteristic of many eye conditions.

C. Patient Instruction

1. Position patient for best vision. For example, a patient with glaucoma has no peripheral vision; thus instruction should be given directly from the front.
2. Do not expect patient to see fine detail, such as that in a radiograph or on a small model.
3. Work patiently and give instruction slowly. Patient may have slow visual accommodation.

HEARING IMPAIRMENT

When hearing is impaired to the extent that it has no practical value for the purpose of spoken communication, a person is considered deaf. When hearing is defective but functional with or without a hearing aid, the terms "a person who is hard of hearing" or "a person with hearing loss" are used. Terminology is changing and reflects the ways in which people prefer to identify themselves.

I. CAUSES OF HEARING IMPAIRMENT

The auditory system includes the anatomic parts from the outer ear to the termination of the auditory nerve in the brain. The cause of hearing loss may be associated with the outer, middle, or inner ear mechanisms, singly or in combinations.

Many factors may contribute to deafness. Heredity, prenatal infection in the mother, especially rubella, and birth trauma are significant in the earliest years. Chronic inner ear infections, infectious diseases (meningitis), trauma, and toxic effects of drugs have all been implicated.

II. TYPES OF HEARING LOSS

A. Conductive Hearing Loss
Outer or middle ear involvement of the conduction pathways to the inner ear.

B. Sensorineural Hearing Loss
Damage to the sensory hair cells of the inner ear or the nerves that supply the inner ear.

C. Mixed Hearing Loss
Combination of conductive and sensorineural.

D. Central Hearing Loss
Damage of the nerves or nuclei of the central nervous system in the brain or the pathways to the brain.

III. CHARACTERISTICS SUGGESTING HEARING LOSS

Partial deafness may not have been diagnosed, or certain patients, particularly an elderly person, may not admit hearing limitation. Clues to the identification of a hearing problem are listed as follows.

A. Lack of attention; fails to respond to conversation.
B. Intentness; strained facial expression; stares at others.
C. Turns head to one side; hearing may be good on one side only.
D. Gives unexpected answer unrelated to question; does one thing when told to do another.
E. Frequently asks others to repeat what was said.
F. Unusual speech quality.

IV. HEARING AIDS

A hearing aid is an electronic device that amplifies and shapes sound waves that enter the external auditory canal. Current hearing aids are more technically advanced, more esthetic in their invisibility, and more commonly used. Standards for the manufacture and distribution of hearing aids are set by the U.S. Food and Drug Administration. A medical evaluation is required along with extensive audiologic testing.

Figure 53-2 shows five types of hearing aids that are available. The body aid and the eyeglass models are used less frequently as the newer types are more electronically sophisticated and powerful. The small units may be difficult to operate for people without finger dexterity. The aids are delicate and require special instruction for care.

A. Body Aid Model
The unit is in a case for carrying in a pocket or attaching to clothing.

B. Eyeglass Model
A thickened temple bar of the eyeglasses holds the essential parts, and the earmold is connected by a small tube.

C. Behind-the-Ear Model
The device hooks over the ear and contains tone controls.

D. In-the-Ear Model
Because the unit is practically invisible and lightweight, the in-the-ear model has been a frequent choice.

E. Canal Aid
This model fits entirely within the canal and is the most cosmetically acceptable of all types. It may take extra skill to adjust and remove.

V. MODES OF COMMUNICATION

A person with a hearing loss may learn a particular way of personal communication. Choices include speaking, speechreading, writing, manual, or a combination. Manual communication includes using sign language or "signing" and fingerspelling. *Always ask your patient which means of communication is preferred and how you can improve communication.*

A. American Sign Language (ASL)
The American manual alphabet is shown in

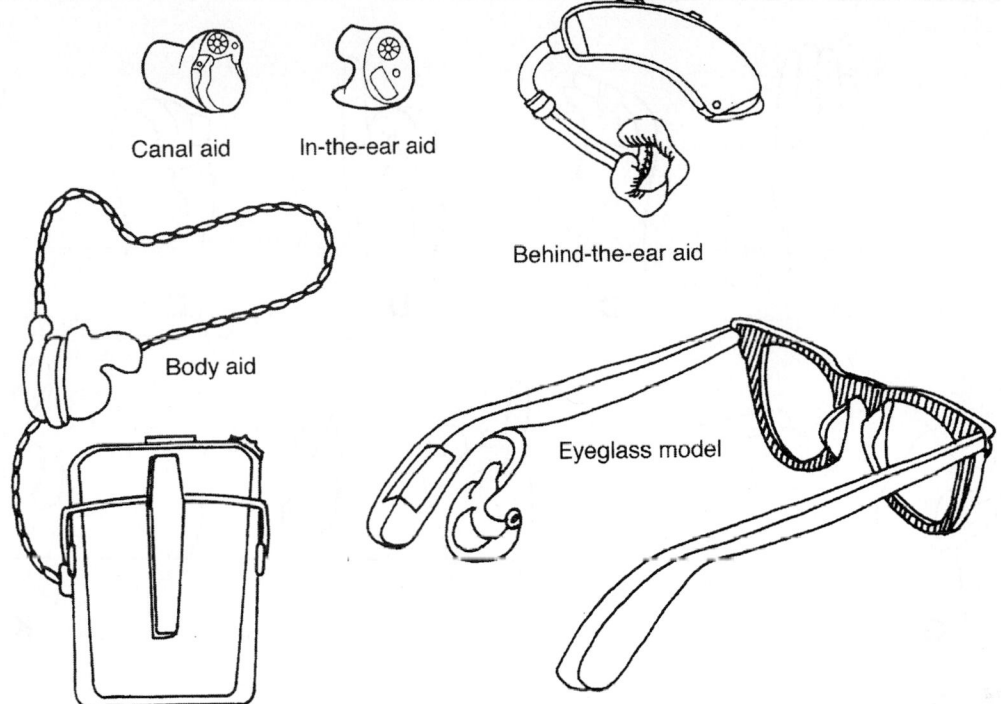

Canal aid · In-the-ear aid · Behind-the-ear aid · Body aid · Eyeglass model

□FIGURE 53-2 Types of Hearing Aids. Hearing aids are electronic devices made with tiny controls to amplify sounds. The hearing aids may be able to fit over or inside the ear, connect to eyeglasses, or be fastened to clothing. None of the illustrations are drawn to scale. (From Series 2: *The Ear and Hearing.* Gallaudet University, 1986. Used with permission.)

Figure 53-3.[1] A few examples of signs are shown in Figure 53-4 A,B,C.

American Sign Language is a visual/gestural language with a unique grammar and syntax. Many deaf people who prefer this mode of communication grew up using ASL and consider themselves part of a cultural group. Other individuals who have become deaf in later years may learn sign language and use the signs in English word order.

Some deaf people prefer to communicate using ASL in medical or dental situations. They can request the services of an ASL interpreter.

Although a universal sign language has not been recognized, many countries have their own.

B. Fingerspelling

Spelling "in the air" is often combined with sign language. When making an introduction, for example, the name is fingerspelled. New words that enter the scientific language often do not have signs and are fingerspelled.

C. Oral Communication

Oral communication by a deaf person means a combination of some speech, residual hearing, and speechreading.

D. Speechreading

Speechreading consists of recognizing spoken words by watching the lips, face, and gestures. Because many of the mouth movements for spoken words have the same appearance as one or more other words, speechreading may need to be combined with another method of communication. Speechreading is not a reliable means of communication for extended, complex discussions for most people with hearing loss.

E. Writing

Writing may be an alternative when other methods are not satisfactory.

VI. DENTAL HYGIENE CARE

Patients with hearing problems are of all ages; some have been deaf all their lives, and others lost their hearing later in life. Each has special problems. Determination of the mode of communication is an important step at the outset. Always ask the patient.

When the patient's preferred mode of communication is sign language and the clinician does not know sign language, or when the patient lipreads but cannot read the clinician's lips because the clinician is wearing a mask, writing on a pad of paper may be the first choice. Some deaf individuals may not be fluent

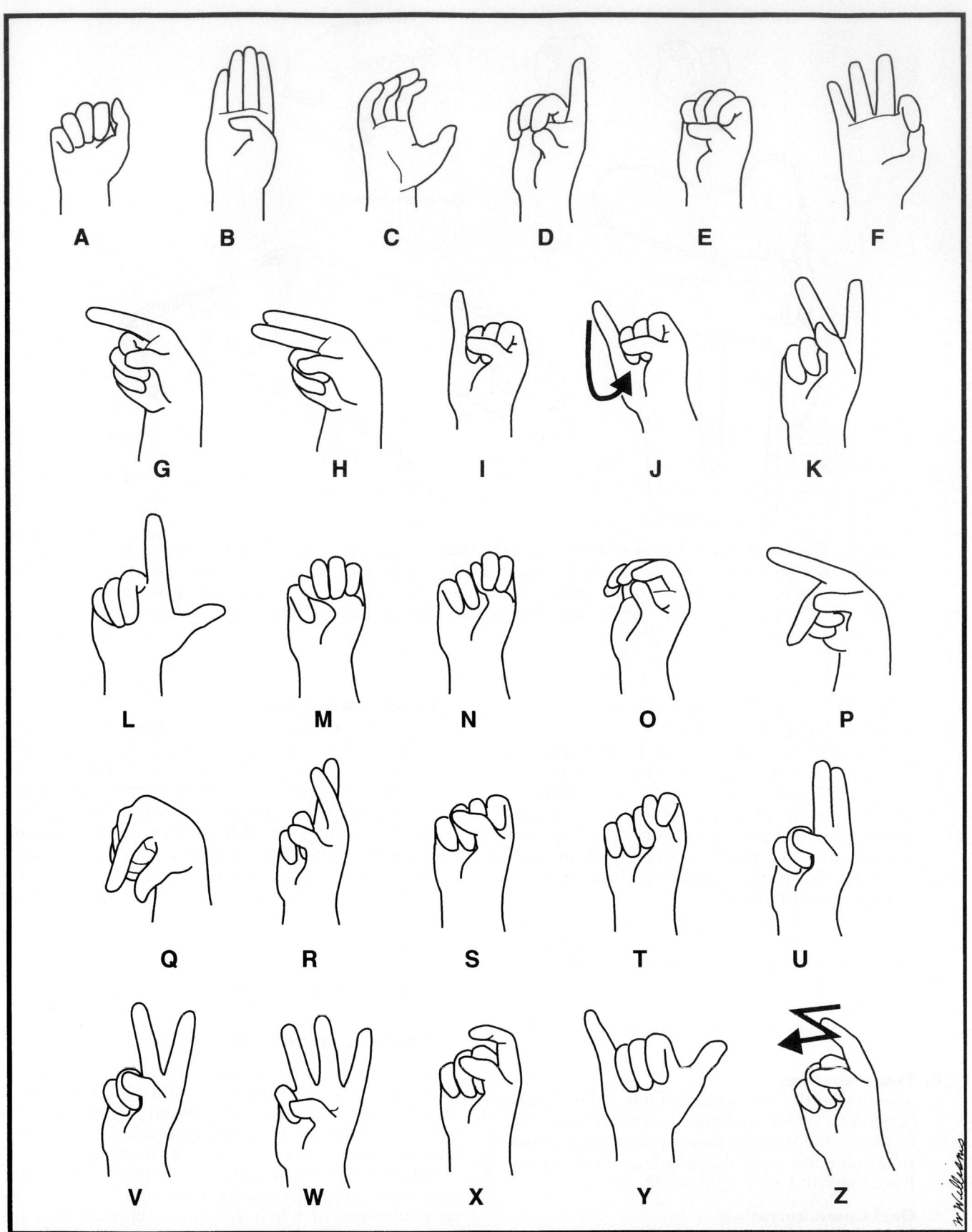

■**FIGURE 53-3 American Manual Alphabet.** Fingerspelling is used in combination with signs and lip reading. (From Lane, L.G.: *The Gallaudet Survival Guide to Signing.* Washington, D.C., Gallaudet University Press, 1990. Reproduced by permission.)

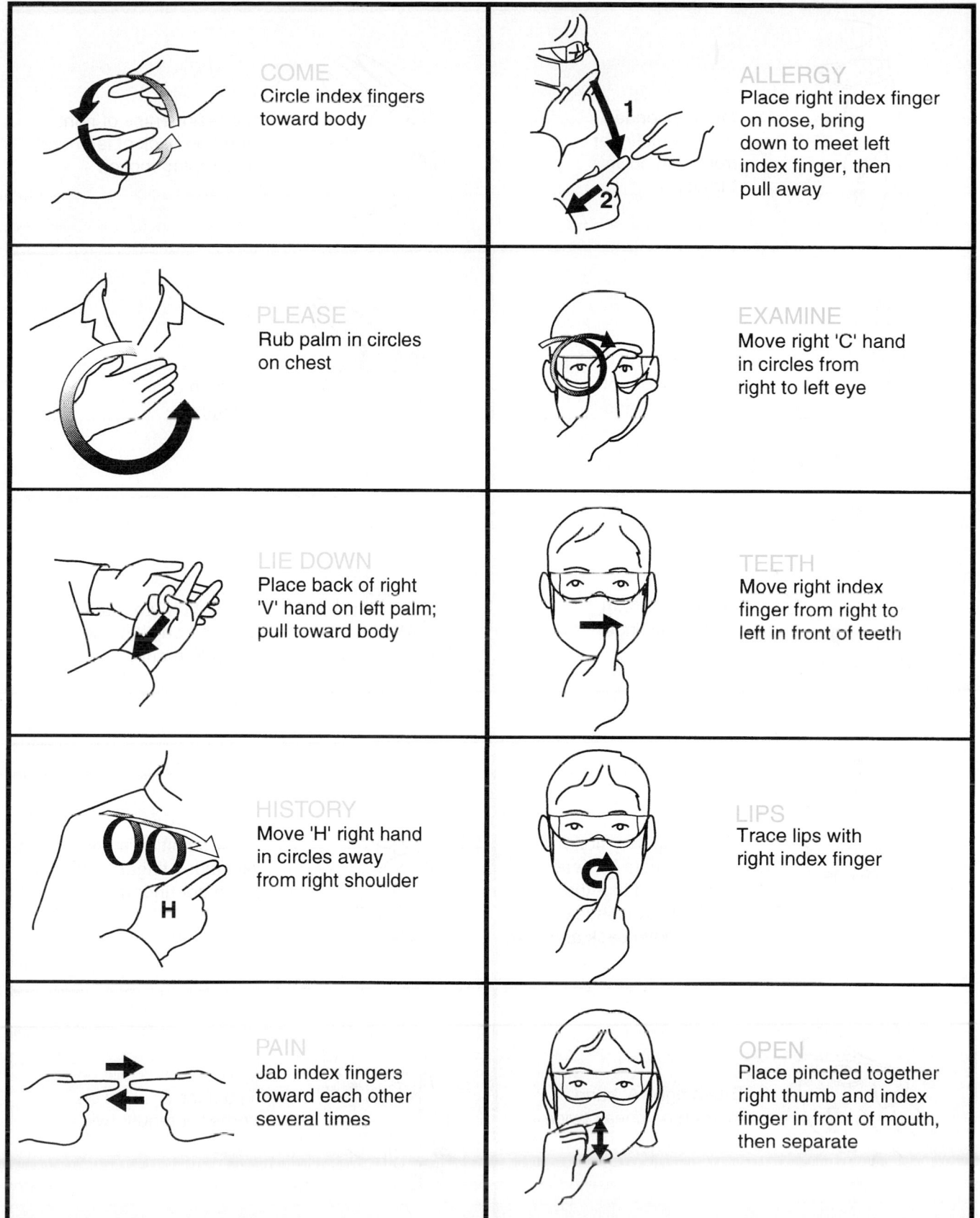

COME
Circle index fingers toward body

ALLERGY
Place right index finger on nose, bring down to meet left index finger, then pull away

PLEASE
Rub palm in circles on chest

EXAMINE
Move right 'C' hand in circles from right to left eye

LIE DOWN
Place back of right 'V' hand on left palm; pull toward body

TEETH
Move right index finger from right to left in front of teeth

HISTORY
Move 'H' right hand in circles away from right shoulder

LIPS
Trace lips with right index finger

PAIN
Jab index fingers toward each other several times

OPEN
Place pinched together right thumb and index finger in front of mouth, then separate

■ **FIGURE 53-4 Examples of Signing.** Selected words that may be used during a patient's dental appointment. (From Lane, L.G.: *The Gallaudet Survival Guide to Signing.* Washington, D.C., Gallaudet University Press, 1990. Reproduced by permission.)

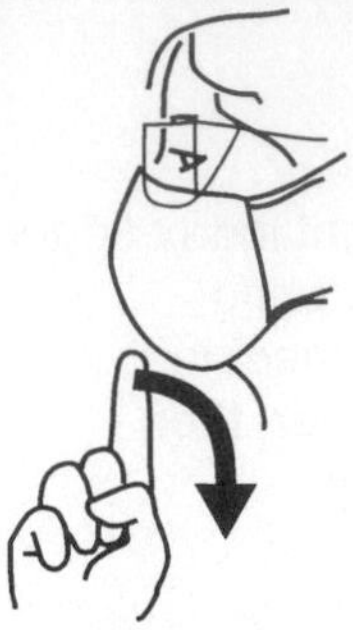

SWALLOW
Move extended right index finger from chin down throat

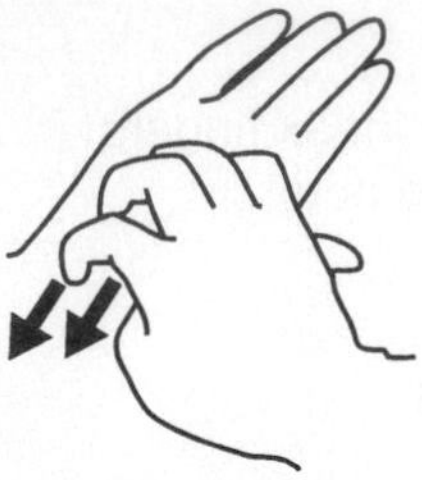

SCRAPE
Move fingertips of right hand on back of left hand in scraping motion

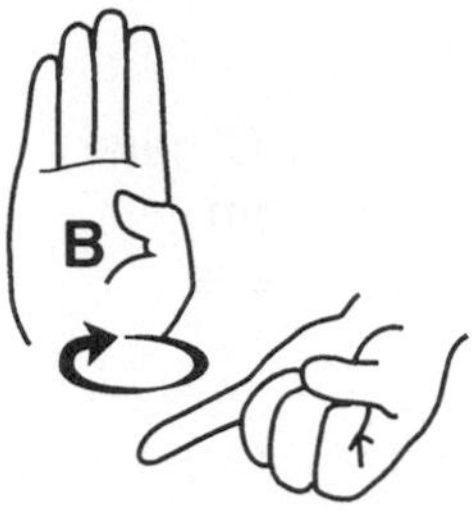

BACTERIA
Right 'B' hand circles on little finger of palm up 'I' hand

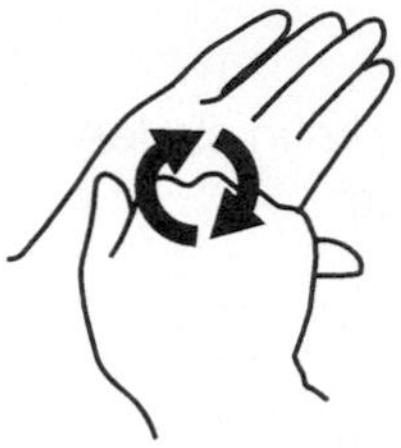

POLISH
Rub knuckles of right hand on back of left hand

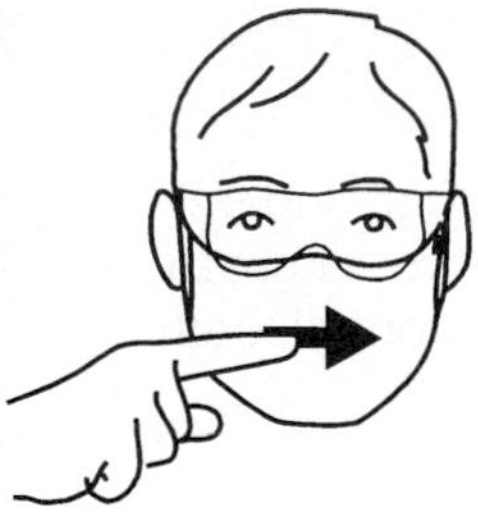

TOOTHBRUSH
Brush teeth with right index finger

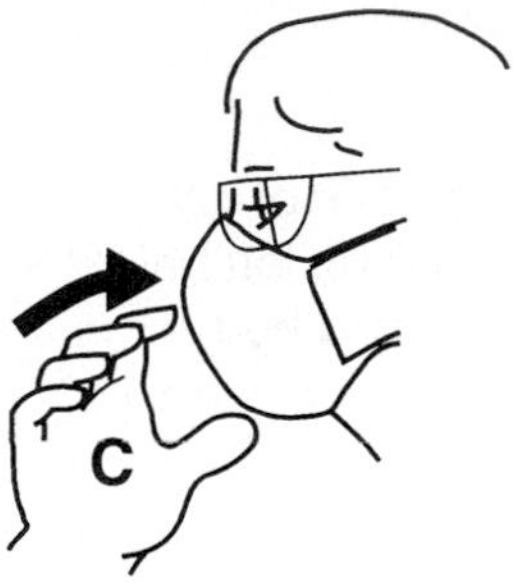

DRINK
Place thumb of right 'C' hand on chin and tip up to mouth

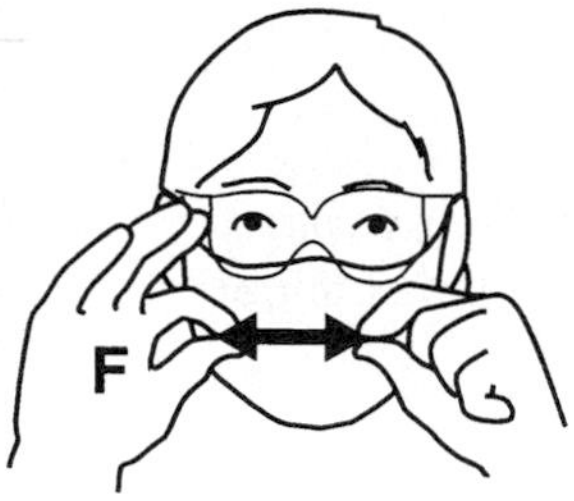

FLOSS
Hold imaginary floss between right 'F' hand and pinched together left thumb and index finger; move back and forth

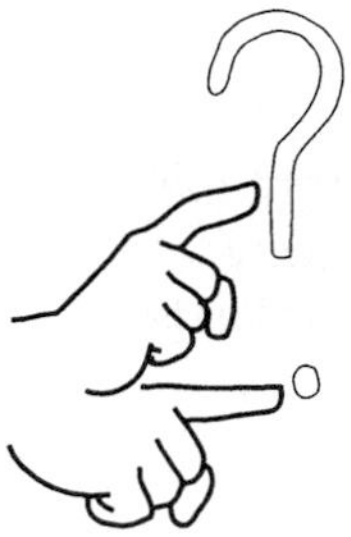

QUESTION
Draw question mark with index finger; place dot underneath

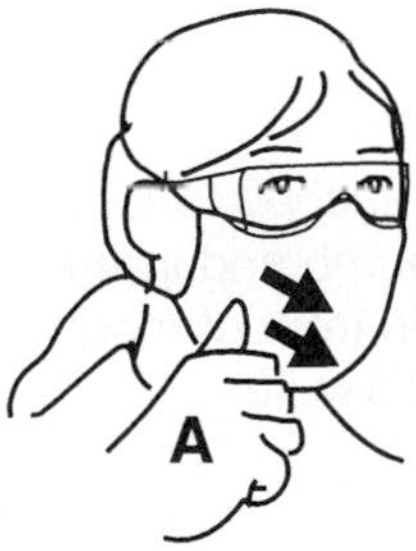

DAILY
Brush right 'A' hand forward on cheek twice

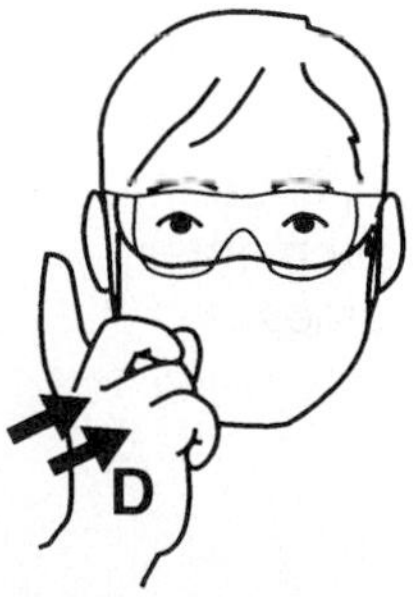

DENTIST
Tap right 'D' hand on corner of mouth twice

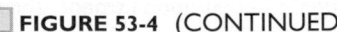

■ **FIGURE 53-4** (CONTINUED)

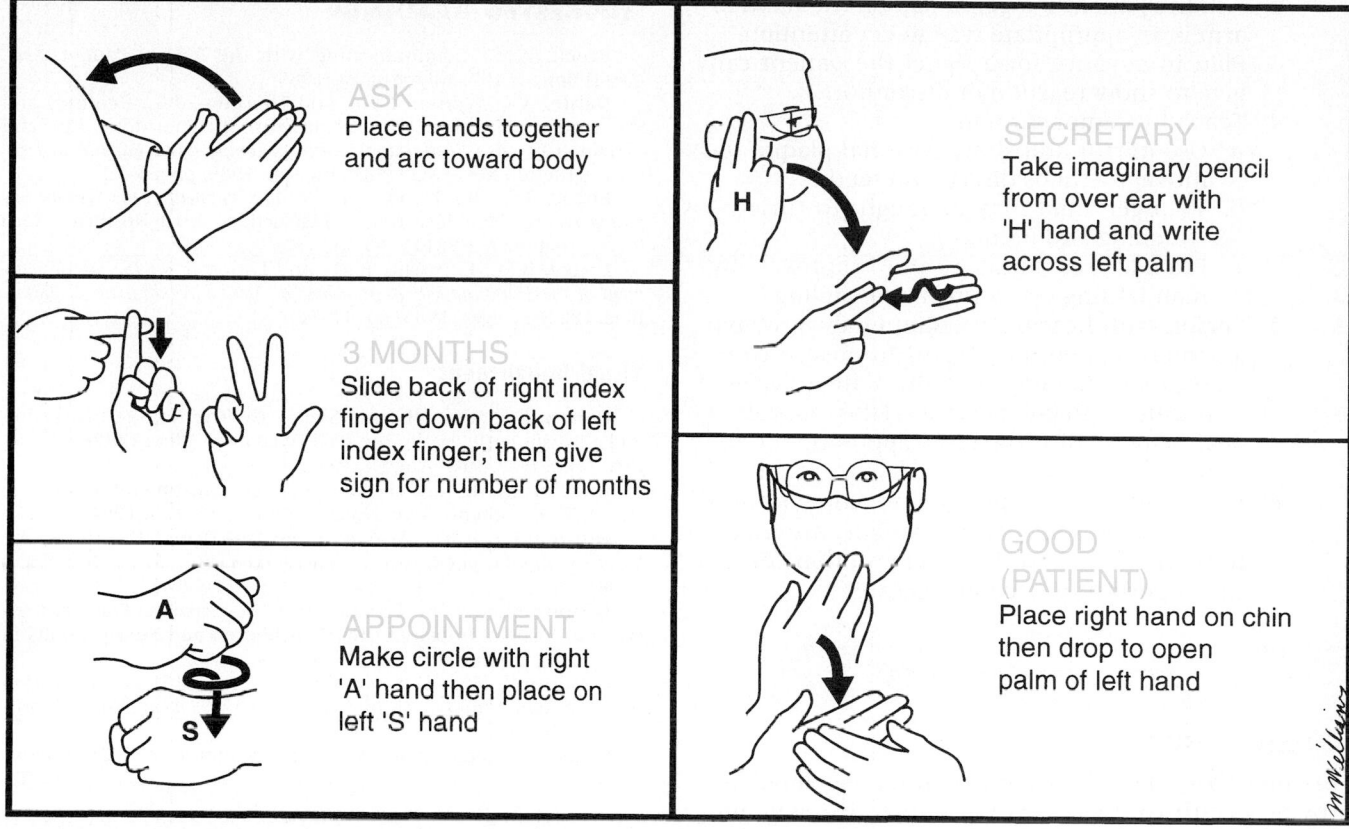

ASK
Place hands together and arc toward body

3 MONTHS
Slide back of right index finger down back of left index finger; then give sign for number of months

APPOINTMENT
Make circle with right 'A' hand then place on left 'S' hand

SECRETARY
Take imaginary pencil from over ear with 'H' hand and write across left palm

GOOD (PATIENT)
Place right hand on chin then drop to open palm of left hand

■ **FIGURE 53-4** (CONTINUED)

in the English language and will need the services of an interpreter for extensive communication such as review of an involved treatment plan.

A. Patient With Hearing Aid
1. Be careful not to touch a hearing aid when it is turned on.
2. Ask patient to turn off or remove a hearing aid when a power-driven dental instrument, particularly a power-driven scaler, will be used. The noise can be amplified many times, much to the discomfort of the patient.

B. Patient With Partial Hearing Ability
1. Speak clearly and distinctly. If you must talk, be sure the patient can see your face. With the dental light directed toward the patient's mouth, the clinician's face may be in the background.
2. Eliminate interfering noises from street outside or from saliva ejector suction.

C. Speechreader
1. Be sure patient is looking; do not turn to side; speak directly.
2. Speaker's face must be clearly visible so patient can read lips easily; difficult when dental light is directed to patient's face or the clinician has back to window.
3. Speak in normal tone; do not exaggerate

words; slow the pace of speech; pause more frequently than usual.
4. Do not raise voice; raising voice can distort lip movements and make lipreading more difficult.
5. When patient cannot understand, use alternate words to express the same thought; many letters and combinations of letters look the same on the lips; others are not visible at all.
6. Keep calm; display of irritation or annoyance over difficulties in conversing discourages or upsets the patient.
7. Write proper names or unusual words the patient fails to understand.
8. When wearing a mask, certain gestures may be agreed upon in advance.

D. Sign Language
All the points previously mentioned for the speechreader apply to patients who use sign language because lips are read along with signs. When a dental hygienist knows a few signs to use, a deaf patient will greatly appreciate them.

E. General Suggestions
1. For written messages, use a clipboard with a marker-type pen attached and large paper, at least 8½ × 11 inches. Write clearly.

2. Ask the patient if a gentle tap on the hand or arm is an appropriate way to get attention.
3. Plan in advance for a signal the patient can give to show reaction or discomfort.
4. Teach by demonstration
   a. Use mirror and show bacterial plaque removal methods directly on teeth.
   b. Younger child may be taught to rinse by watching and imitating.
   c. Provide reassurance and approval by maintaining eye contact and smiling.
5. Person with hearing loss should always have a written appointment card to ensure complete understanding. Use the state Telecommunication Relay Service (TRS) to call a deaf patient directly with appointment reminders.
6. Use judgment in prolonging conversation with deaf person. Certain patients are under tension and tire easily, whereas others enjoy the opportunity to communicate.

TECHNICAL HINTS

I. BASIC SKILLS

Learning basic sign language and finger spelling can provide health-care workers with an added skill and reduce stress for the deaf patient.

II. SOURCES OF MATERIALS AND INFORMATION

American Foundation for the Blind
15 East 16th Street
New York, NY 10011
National Society to Prevent Blindness and Its Affiliates
79 Madison Avenue
New York, NY 10016
National Information Center on Deafness, Gallaudet University
800 Florida Avenue, N.E.
Washington, D.C. 20002-3695
Local State Office or Community Service Center for Deaf Persons

REFERENCE

1. **Lane,** L.G.: *The Gallaudet Survival Guide to Signing.* Washington, DC, Gallaudet University Press, 1990.

SUGGESTED READINGS

Brock, A.M.: Communicating with the Elderly Patient, *Spec. Care Dentist., 5,* 157, July–August, 1985.

Dahle, A.J., Wesson, M.D., and Thornton, J.B.: Dentistry and the Patient with Sensory Impairment, in Thornton, J.B. and Wright, J.T., eds.: *Special and Medically Compromised Patients in Dentistry.* Littleton, MA, PSG Publishing Co., 1989, pp. 63–72.

Engar, R.C. and Stiefel, D.J.: *Dental Treatment of the Sensory Impaired Patient.* Disability Dental Instruction, 4919 Northeast 86th Street, Seattle, WA 98115, 65 pp.

Lange, B.M., Entwistle, B.M., and Lipson, L.F.: *Dental Management of the Handicapped: Approaches for Dental Auxiliaries.* Philadelphia, Lea & Febiger, 1983, pp. 11–38.

Visual Impairment

Cohen, S., Sarnat, H., and Shalgi, G.: The Role of Instruction and a Brushing Device on the Oral Hygiene of Blind Children, *Clin. Prev. Dent., 13,* 8, July–August, 1991.

Geurink, K.M.: The Visually Impaired. Creating a Comfortable Dental Environment, *DentalHygienistNews, 7,* 15, Fall, 1994.

Hunter, L.H.: "The Way We See It"—Dental Health for the Visually Handicapped, *Dental Health (London), 27,* 3, June/July, 1988.

O'Donnell, D.: The Prevalence of Nonrepaired Fractured Incisors in Visually Impaired Chinese Children and Young Adults in Hong Kong, *Quintessence Int., 23,* 363, May, 1992.

O'Donnell, D. and Crosswaite, M.A.: Dental Health Education for the Visually Impaired Child, *Dent. Health (London), 30,* 8, February/March, 1991.

Schein, J.: Keeping an Eye on Your Vision, *RDH, 9,* 28, August, 1989.

Hearing Impairment

Arnos, K.S.: Hereditary Hearing Loss, (Editorial) *N. Engl. J. Med., 331,* 469, August 18, 1994.

Busch, L.: Communication: The Key to Treatment of the Hearing Impaired, *Spec. Care Dentist., 2,* 150, July–August, 1982.

Clark, C.A., Cangelosi-Williams, P., Lee, M.A., and Morgan, L.: Dental Treatment for Deaf Patients, *Spec. Care Dentist., 6,* 102, May–June, 1986.

Glicken, S.R.: Health Care for Deaf Adolescents, *Adolescent Medicine, 5,* 345, June, 1994.

Graves, C.E. and Portnoy, E.J.: Identifying Hearing Impairment among Older Adults, *J. Dent. Hyg., 65,* 138, March–April, 1991.

Hollingsworth, R.A.: Sign for the Times, *RDH, 12,* 40, June, 1992.

Merrell, H.B. and Claggett, K.: Noise Pollution and Hearing Loss in the Dental Office, *Dent. Assist., 61,* 6, Third Quarter, 1992.

Nadol, J.B.: Hearing Loss, *N. Engl. J. Med., 329,* 1092, October 7, 1993.

O'Brien, S.: A Special Challenge, *RDH, 9,* 18, March, 1989.

Smela, D.-M.: Interacting With the Hearing Impaired, *DentalHygienistNews, 7,* 11, Summer, 1994.

Zazove, P. and Kileny, P.R.: Devices for the Hearing Impaired, *Am. Fam. Physician, 46,* 851, September, 1992.

54

The Patient With a Seizure Disorder

Epilepsy is not a disease entity but is, rather, a term used to describe a syndrome or group of symptoms of disordered function of the central nervous system. A person with epilepsy may be susceptible to recurrent involuntary loss of consciousness or awareness with or without convulsive movements or spasms. Some patients may have seizures without loss of consciousness.

The patient's medical history should reveal a susceptibility to seizures, and the physician must be consulted when additional information other than that provided by the patient is required. The well-controlled patient who is under anticonvulsant medication usually presents no specific problems. An uncontrolled patient may require special treatment. A knowledge of symptoms is important in all

cases, and dental personnel should know and be able to apply emergency measures in or out of the dental office.

Care of the oral cavity of a person with epilepsy becomes important for its relationship both to general health and to oral accidents that may occur during a severe attack. All patients are advised by their physicians to live a moderate lifestyle and pay strict attention to general health rules.

Occupation may be limited because the person with epilepsy cannot participate in activities that may precipitate a seizure or that provide hazards in the event of a seizure. Such limitation is particularly depressing to adults who acquire epilepsy after reaching the working age and thus may be required to change their vocation.

EPILEPTIC SYNDROMES

I. CLASSIFICATION

The epileptic syndromes are complex. Diagnosis is made from clinical symptoms, the history, electroencephalography (EEG), and functional neuroimaging. The syndromes have been classified by the following:

A. Age-related onset

B. Symptoms (particularly the type of seizure)

C. Anatomic localization in the brain (temporal, frontal, parietal, or occipital lobes)

II. TYPES OF SEIZURES[1,2]

A seizure is a convulsive disorder that results from a transient, uncontrolled alteration in brain function. It is a sudden paroxysmal electrical discharge of neurons in the brain. The effect is an abrupt onset of symptoms that may be of a motor, sensory, or psychic nature, depending on which brain cells are involved.

The two basic types of seizures are *generalized* and *partial*. The international classification of seizures is outlined in Table 54-1.

A seizure that is focal in origin and involves only a part of the brain is called a partial seizure. A generalized seizure, on the other hand, is not specific in area of origin and affects the entire brain at the same time. Terminology used in Table 54-1 and in the study of epilepsy is defined in Box 54-1.

III. ETIOLOGY

In addition to epilepsy, seizures can be a symptom of many different conditions from birth throughout life. During infancy, seizures can be related to maternal infection (rubella), birth injury, or congenital abnormalities, whereas in older children, additional causes include trauma, infections, toxins, and cerebral degenerative diseases. In middle age and older, vascular disease and tumors are added to the list.

The causes can be divided into primary and secondary.

A. Primary (Idiopathic) Epilepsy

Genetic predisposition to seizures or to other neurologic abnormalities for which seizure may be a symptom.

B. Secondary (Symptomatic) Epilepsy

Seizures can arise during many neurologic and non-neurologic medical conditions. A few are listed here.

1. Congenital conditions, such as maternal infection (rubella); toxemia of pregnancy.
2. Perinatal injuries.
3. Brain tumor.
4. Cerebrovascular disease (stroke).
5. Trauma (head injury).
6. Infection (meningitis, encephalitis, opportunistic infections of AIDS).
7. Degenerative brain disease.
8. Metabolic and toxic disorders, including alcoholism and drug addiction; seizures are common during drug withdrawal.

TABLE 54-1 International Classification of Seizures

PARTIAL SEIZURES (SEIZURES BEGINNING LOCALLY)

A. Simple Partial Seizures (without loss of consciousness)
1. With motor signs
2. With somatosensory or special sensory symptoms
3. With autonomic symptoms
4. With psychic symptoms

B. Complex Partial Seizures
1. Simple partial onset followed by impairment of consciousness
2. With impairment of consciousness at onset

C. Partial Seizures Evolving to Generalized Tonic-Clonic Convulsions (secondarily generalized)

GENERALIZED SEIZURES (BILATERALLY SYMMETRICAL, WITHOUT LOCAL ONSET)

A. Nonconvulsive Seizures
1. Absence seizures
2. Atypical absence seizures
3. Myoclonic seizures
4. Atonic seizures

B. Convulsive Seizures
1. Tonic-clonic seizures
2. Tonic seizures
3. Clonic seizures

UNCLASSIFIED EPILEPTIC SEIZURES

(From International League Against Epilepsy, Commission on Classification andTerminology: Proposal for Revised Clinical and Electroencephalographic Classification of Epileptic Seizures, *Epilepsia, 22,* 489, August, 1981.)

CLINICAL MANIFESTATIONS[3]

I. PRECIPITATING FACTORS

For the patient with epilepsy or predisposed to seizures, various factors may be involved. The patient or a caregiver may provide helpful information to prepare health care workers to handle an emergency. Possible precipitating factors include the following:

A. Psychologic stress; apprehension.

B. Fatigue; sleep deprivation.

C. Sensory stimuli, such as flashing lights, noises, peculiar odors.

D. Alcohol use; withdrawal from alcohol or other substances.

II. AURA

Not all patients have a warning, or aura, before a seizure. A patient with a warning may seek a safe place to sit or lie down in privacy. In the dental environment, the patient can inform the personnel, so that procedures can be terminated and brief preparations made.

BOX 54-I KEY WORDS: Seizures

Absence: a generalized seizure of sudden onset characterized by a brief period of unconsciousness. Formerly called **petit mal.**

Anticonvulsant (an"ti-kon-vul'sant): a drug that inhibits or suppresses convulsions.

Antiepileptic (an"te-ep"i-lep'tik): a remedy for epilepsy.

Ataxia (ah-tak'sē-ah): failure of muscular coordination; irregularity of muscular action.

Atonic: relaxed; without normal tone or tension.

Aura (aw'rah): warning sensation felt by some people immediately preceding a seizure; may be flashes of light, dizziness, peculiar taste, or a sensation of prickling or tingling.

Automatism (aw-tōm'ah-tizm): involuntary motor activity, such as lip smacking or repeated swallowing.

Autonomic symptoms: pallor, flushing, sweating, pupillary dilation, cardiac arrhythmia, incontinence.

Clonic: alternate contraction and relaxation of muscle; **clonic phase** is the convulsion phase of a seizure.

Consciousness: degree of awareness and/or responsiveness of a person to externally applied stimuli.

Convulsion: violent spasm.

Cryptogenic (krĭp'tō-jen'ik): a disorder for which the cause is hidden or occult.

Diplopia (di-plō'pē-ah): perception of two images of a single object; double vision.

Dyspepsia (dis-pep'sē-ah): impairment of the power or function of digestion.

Electroencephalography (e-lek'-trō-en-sef'-ah-log'rah-fē): the recording of changes in electric potentials in various areas of the brain by means of electrodes placed on the scalp or on/in the brain itself and connected to a vacuum-tube radio amplifier that amplifies the impulses more than a million times; the impulses move an electromagnetic pen that records the brain waves; a clinical test used for partial diagnosis of epilepsy.

Facies (fā'shē-ēz): expression or appearance of the face.

Grand mal (grahn-mahl): former name for a generalized or major seizure as contrasted with **petit mal** (pĕ-tē' mahl), a minor or relatively mild seizure.

Hirsutism (her'soot-izm): abnormal hairiness.

Ictal (ik'tal): pertaining to or resulting from a stroke or an acute epileptic seizure.

Myoclonus (mi'ōk-lō'nus): isolated or repetitive shock-like contractions of a muscle or group of muscles; adj., myoclonic.

Paresthesia (par'es-thē'zē-ah): an abnormal sensation, such as burning, prickling, or tingling.

Paroxysm (par'ok-sizm): sharp spasm or convulsion; sudden recurrence or intensification of symptoms.

Petit mal (pe-tē' mahl): attack or brief impairment of consciousness often associated with flickering of the eyelids and mild twitching of the mouth.

Prodrome (prō'drōm): a premonitory symptom; a symptom indicating the onset of a disease or condition; adj., prodromal.

Psychic (sī'kik): pertaining to the mind or psyche.

Refractory epilepsy: not readily yielding to basic treatment; usually with a single antiepileptic drug.

Seizure (sē'zhur): paroxysmal spell of transitory alteration in consciousness, motor activity, or sensory phenomenon; convulsion.

Spasm (spazm): sudden involuntary contraction of a muscle or group of muscles; may be tonic or clonic; may vary from small twitches to severe convulsions.

Status epilepticus (sta'tus ĕp'ĭ-lĕp'tĭ-cus): rapid succession of epileptic spasms without intervals of consciousness; life threatening; emergency care urgent.

Teratogenesis (ter"ah-tō-jen' e-sis): production of deformity in the developing embryo.

Tonic (ton'ik): state of continuous, unremitting action of muscular contraction; patient appears stiff.

Tonic-clonic: in a seizure, a sudden sharp tonic contraction of muscles followed by clonic convulsive movements.

The aura may be a special sensory stimulus, a sensation of numbness, tingling, or a twitching or stiffness of certain muscles.

III. PARTIAL SEIZURES

A. Simple
1. Cessation of ongoing activity.
2. Staring spell; dizziness.

3. Jerking of muscles around the mouth.
4. No loss of consciousness.

B. Complex
1. Trance-like state with confusion lasts usually for a few minutes, sometimes for hours.
2. Consciousness is impaired to varying degrees.
3. Patient may manifest purposeless move-

ments or actions followed by confusion, incoherent speech, ill humor, bad temper; does not remember what happened during the attack.

IV. GENERALIZED ABSENCE

A. Loss of consciousness for 5 to 30 seconds.
B. Patient usually does not fall; posture becomes fixed; may drop whatever is being held.
C. May become pale.
D. May have rhythmic twitching of eyelids, eyebrows, or head.
E. Attack ends as abruptly as it begins. Patient resumes activities; may or may not be aware of attack.

V. GENERALIZED TONIC-CLONIC

A. Loss of Consciousness: sudden and complete; the patient falls. A patient may slide out of the dental chair.

B. Voluntary Musculature Contraction
1. Tonic phase: tension with rigidity.
2. Clonic movements follow: with intermittent muscular contraction and relaxation.

C. Air Forced Out
1. Muscles of the chest and pharynx may contract at the same time, thus forcing air out.
2. Sound emitted is known as the "epileptic cry."

D. Color
1. Pale at first; then superficial veins become engorged.
2. Chest becomes fixed and aeration of blood ceases; face becomes cyanotic.

E. Eyes: Pupils dilate.

F. Muscular Contractions
1. Intermittent contractions rapid at first, then less frequently.
2. Tongue: may be bitten if between teeth.

G. Time
1. Incident lasts from 1 to 3 minutes.
2. Bladder, and rarely the rectum, may be emptied.

H. Respiration
1. Respiration returns.
2. Saliva, which previously could not be swallowed, may become mixed with air and appear as foam.

I. Postconvulsive Coma
1. Characterized by fixed or sluggish pupils; noisy breathing; profuse perspiration.
2. Cyanosed lips; complete relaxation of the body muscles.

J. Postconvulsive Phase
1. Drowsiness, headache, muscle aches.
2. Falls into a deep sleep.

TREATMENT

I. MEDICATIONS[4]

Anticonvulsant drugs are used to prevent seizures. Frequently prescribed medications are carbamazepine, phenytoin, valproic acid, phenobarbitol, primidone, and succinimides. Each has its own side effects.[5] Side effects such as drowsiness, depression, nausea, and gingival overgrowth are important when planning dental hygiene care.

The goal of treatment is to control all seizures with the lowest possible dose of a drug. The expectancy is that side effects will be lowered with lower doses.

II. SURGERY

A variety of surgical interventions are available and especially indicated when epilepsy is refractory to traditional therapy. New treatments have been made possible through the advances in EEG monitoring and neuroimaging, improvements in surgical techniques, and greater understanding of the symptomatic epilepsies.[6]

ORAL FINDINGS

Epilepsy in itself produces no oral changes. Specific effects relate to side effects of anticonvulsant therapy and to the results of oral accidents during seizures.

I. GINGIVAL OVERGROWTH

Gingival overgrowth occurs in 25% to 50% of persons using phenytoin for treatment.[7] Other anticonvulsant drugs also induce gingival overgrowth less frequently, some only rarely.[8]

Phenytoin and the other anticonvulsant drugs have been used in the treatment of many conditions other than epilepsy. These include behavior problems, stuttering, headaches, neuromuscular disturbances, and cardiac conditions. The presence of gingival enlargement and a history of use of a particular drug should not lead to the assumption that the patient has epilepsy.

II. EFFECTS OF ACCIDENTS DURING SEIZURES

A. Scars of Lips and Tongue
During generalized tonic-clonic seizures, the oral tissues, particularly tongue, cheek, or lip, may be bitten. Scars may be observed during the extraoral/intraoral examination, and the cause may be differentiated from other types of healed wounds.

B. Fractured Teeth
During the tonic and clonic movements, the teeth may be clamped and bruxing may be forceful enough to fracture teeth.

PHENYTOIN-INDUCED GINGIVAL OVERGROWTH

Gingival overgrowth is one of several side effects from treatment with phenytoin. The condition also has been called Dilantin hyperplasia, Dilantin-induced hyperplasia, diphenylhydantoin-induced hyperplasia, diphenylhydantoin gingival hyperplasia, Dilantin-induced gingival fibrosis, and phenytoin-induced hyperplasia.

I. SIDE EFFECTS OF PHENYTOIN

In addition to gingival overgrowth, other long-term side effects may influence dental hygiene appointments. During history preparation and the extraoral/intraoral examination, the effects described as follows can aid in understanding the patient and planning treatment.

A. General Effects That May Occur[5]
Drowsiness, gastric distress, skin rash, ataxia, and restlessness are not uncommon. Increased growth of body and facial hair may occur in women.

B. Nutritional Influences[9]
Vitamins K, D, and folic acid are affected by anticonvulsant drugs. A megaloblastic anemia can result from a low folic acid blood level, which is described on page 871.

C. Fetal Hydantoin Syndrome[10]
Children of women receiving anticonvulsant therapy during pregnancy are more susceptible to malformations (Table 43-1, page 655). They may have craniofacial abnormalities, growth retardation, mental deficiency, congenital heart defects, and cleft lip and/or palate.

II. OCCURRENCE[11]

A. Age
Incidence is greater in younger patients than in older patients just beginning therapy.

B. Initial Enlargement
The gingiva may start to enlarge within a few weeks or even after a few years following the initial administration of the drug.

C. Dosage and Length of Treatment
The size of the dose and the length of treatment are not necessarily factors in the incidence or nature of the gingival enlargement.

D. Sites
The anterior gingiva are usually more affected than are the posterior, and the maxillary more than the mandibular. Facial and proximal areas are usually larger than lingual and palatal areas.

E. Edentulous Areas
Although rare, an overgrowth of tissue may occur in an edentulous area. A source of trauma, irritation from a denture, the presence of retained roots, or unerupted teeth usually have been associated with the overgrowth.[12,13]

F. Dental Implants
Overgrowth of tissue surrounding titanium implants can occur.[14]

III. TISSUE CHARACTERISTICS

A. Early Clinical Features
The overgrowth appears as a painless enlargement of interdental papillae with signs of inflammation. Eventually, the tissue becomes fibrotic, pink, and stippled, with a mulberry- or cauliflower-like appearance (Figure 54-1B).

B. Advanced Lesion
With time, the tissue increases in size, extends to include the marginal gingiva, and covers a large portion of the anatomic crown. Often, cleftlike grooves occur between the lobules (Figure 54-1A).

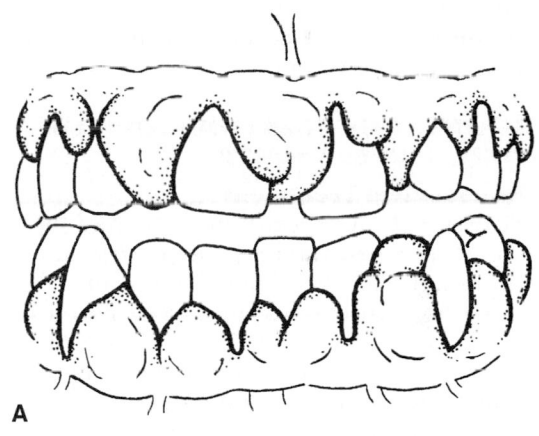

A

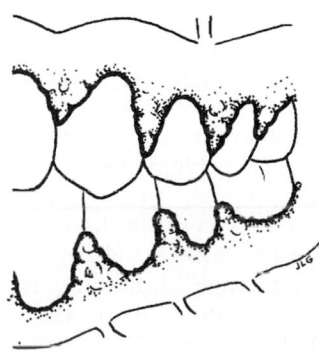

B

☐ FIGURE 54-1 Phenytoin-induced Gingival Enlargement. (A) Papillary enlargement with cleft-like grooves. Note the effect of the pressure of the fibrotic tissue on the position of teeth. Maxillary incisors and the mandibular left canine have been wedged away from normal positions. (B) Mulberry-like shape of interdental papillae.

C. Severe Lesion
Large, bulbous gingiva may cover the enamel, tend to wedge the teeth apart, and interfere with mastication. Note the severe growth about the mandibular left canine in Figure 54-1A.

D. Microscopic Appearance
During therapy, phenytoin is present in the saliva, blood, gingival sulcus fluid, and bacterial plaque. The number of fibroblasts and the amount of collagen in the connective tissue increases. The stratified squamous epithelium is thick, with long rete ridges. Inflammatory cells are in greatest abundance near the base of the pockets.

IV. COMPLICATING FACTORS

A. Bacterial Plaque and Gingivitis
Adequate plaque control, particularly if started before the administration of phenytoin, helps to control the extent of gingival overgrowth.

B. Contributing Factors
Mouth breathing, overhanging and other defective restorations, large carious lesions, calculus, and other plaque-retaining factors encourage gingival overgrowth. Treatment must include removal of overhangs and calculus and restoration of carious lesions.

V. TREATMENT OF PHENYTOIN-INDUCED GINGIVAL OVERGROWTH

A. Nonsurgical Treatment
Scaling with a concentrated program of bacterial plaque control may help early lesions to regress. Once the tissue has become fibrotic, however, shrinkage cannot be expected.

A program of prevention and control should be started prior to, or simultaneously with, the initial administration of phenytoin.

B. Change in Drug Prescription
Phenytoin alone or with phenobarbital has been a drug of choice for use with patients subject to generalized seizures since the drug was introduced in 1938. When the patient has a severe problem and is faced with embarrassment and social problems because of the appearance of the gingiva, the physician could be approached concerning the possibility of changing the prescription to a different drug. If possible, such a change should be made just prior to a surgical removal procedure that may be planned.

C. Surgical Removal
Assuming a sufficient band of attached gingiva exists, one surgical procedure that has been used for tissue removal has been gingivectomy. A flap procedure may be the choice for healing and esthetics.[15] Prior to surgery, a regulated program of plaque control should be introduced and continued as soon as surgical dressings have been removed.

DENTAL HYGIENE CARE

For the patient with epilepsy, general health has special significance, and oral health contributes to general health. For the patient with drug-induced gingival enlargement, emphasis in appointments is on a rigid oral hygiene program if the gingival overgrowth is to be kept to a minimum.

I. PATIENT HISTORY
Except in an unusual situation, most patients with epilepsy have had a thorough medical examination prior to the dental appointment. In preparing the patient history, however, all patients should be asked whether they ever had a seizure or currently have recurrent or occasional seizures. When the answer is positive, additional questioning is indicated.

A. History of Seizures
Questioning includes type, frequency, severity, and duration of episodes. The precipitating factors, need for any special premedication, and all information that may have application during the dental and dental hygiene appointments must be carefully documented.

B. Medications
The type, dosage, effectiveness in seizure control, and known side effects of medication are recorded. Patients using valproic acid may be subject to blood coagulation defects and should be questioned concerning bleeding and ease of bruising.[16] Prior to deep scaling or surgical procedures, when bleeding can be expected, blood testing for platelet count and bleeding time provides important information for the prevention of an emergency situation.

II. PATIENT APPROACH
A. Provide a calm, reassuring atmosphere.
B. Treat with patience and empathy; avoid over-solicitousness.
C. Encourage self-expression, particularly if the patient tends to be quiet and withdrawn and has narrowed interests.
D. Recognize possible impairment of memory when reviewing personal oral care procedures.
E. Help patient to develop interest in caring for the mouth; commend all little successes.
F. Drugs used in treatment tend to make patient drowsy.
   1. Be understanding when patient is late or misses an appointment.
   2. Plan telephone reminder at opportune time if patient is chronically late.
   3. Do not mistake drowsiness (effect of drugs) for inattentiveness.

III. CARE PLAN: INSTRUMENTATION

The treatment needs of a patient with drug-induced gingival overgrowth were described earlier. The dental hygiene care, planned within the total treatment plan, is determined by whether the patient is just starting phenytoin therapy or, if already receiving phenytoin, the severity of the gingival overgrowth.

A. Prior to and at the Start of Phenytoin Therapy

A rigorous plaque control program and complete scaling are introduced in preparation for phenytoin therapy. The patient (and parents) must understand that, with controlled oral hygiene and emphasis on all phases of prevention, gingival overgrowth can be prevented to a large degree.

B. Initial Appointment Series for Patient Treated With Phenytoin

Weekly appointments for complete plaque control instruction and scaling are planned with the following objectives:

1. *Slight or Mild Gingival Overgrowth.* Nonsurgical treatment, including frequent thorough scalings, can be expected to lead to tissue reduction, provided the patient cooperates in daily plaque control. Frequent maintenance appointments can contribute to function and comfort with minimum periodontal involvement.

2. *Moderate Gingival Overgrowth.* After the initial series of weekly plaque instruction and scalings, re-evaluation of the tissue can determine whether further procedures are needed. An optimum level of oral health may be attained by changing the medication to another anticonvulsant drug, using surgical pocket removal, and continuing frequent maintenance appointments.

3. *Severe Fibrotic Overgrowth.* Initial scaling and plaque control are carried out to prepare the mouth for surgical pocket removal. Plans for changing the drug or altering the dose should be discussed with the patient's physician.

C. Maintenance Appointment Intervals

Frequent appointments on a 1-, 2-, or 3-month plan are indicated, depending on the severity of the gingival enlargement and the ability and motivation of the patient to maintain the oral health. Most patients need continuing assistance and supervision, and their response is influenced by the instruction and devotion of the dental personnel.

IV. CARE PLAN: PREVENTION

Daily plaque removal and fluoride therapy, the use of pit and fissure sealants, and dietary control all have a vital part in the care of the patient with a seizure disorder. Initiation of preventive measures as soon as possible after the disorder has been diagnosed can contribute to the total health and well-being of the patient.

EMERGENCY CARE[3]

When a seizure occurs, no attempt should be made to stop the convulsion or to restrain the patient.

I. OBJECTIVES

A. To prevent body injury.
B. To prevent accidents related to the oral structures, such as:
1. Tongue bite.
2. Broken or dislocated teeth.
3. Dislocated or fractured jaw.
4. Broken fixed or removable dentures.
C. To ensure adequate ventilation.

II. PREPARATION FOR APPOINTMENT

When the patient's medical history indicates epilepsy, precautions may prevent complications should a seizure occur.

A. Put emergency materials in a convenient place.
B. Have patient remove dentures for duration of appointment.
C. Provide a calm and reassuring atmosphere.
D. Have other dental personnel available in case of an emergency.

III. EMERGENCY PROCEDURE (FIGURE 54-2)

The dental clinic or office team has assigned responsibilities during any emergency as described in Chapter 61 (pages 897 to 900). Initiation of procedures for seizure emergency follows the usual practice.

A. Terminate procedure; call for assistance; place medical emergency call.
B. Position patient; lower chair and tilt to supine; raise feet.
C. Push aside movable equipment and instrument trays.
D. Loosen tight belt, collar, necktie.
E. DO NOT place (or force) anything between the teeth.
F. Establish airway; check for breathing obstruction; provide basic life support when indicated.
G. Monitor vital signs.
H. Stay beside patient to prevent personal injury.

IV. POSTICTAL PHASE

A. Complete the record of emergency (Figure 61-1, page 898).
B. Allow patient to rest.
C. Talk to patient in a low, reassuring tone. Ask onlookers to leave the patient in privacy.

MANAGEMENT OF GENERALIZED TONIC-CLONIC SEIZURES (GRAND MAL)

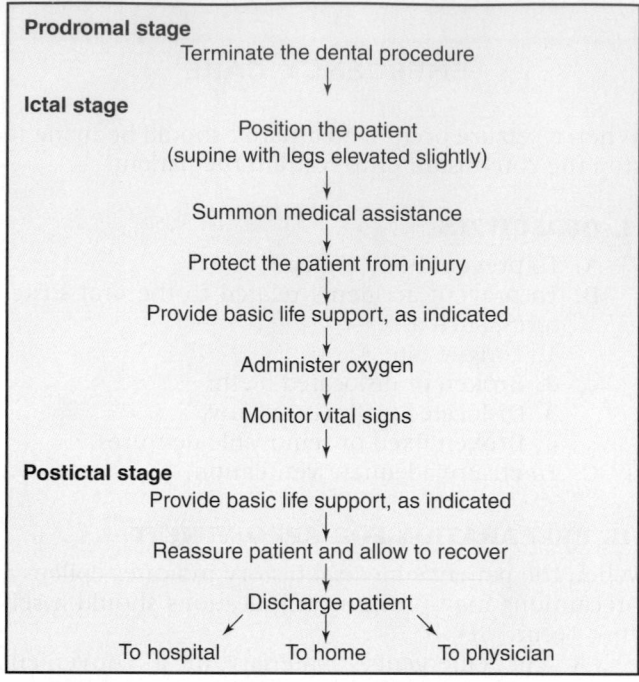

Prodromal stage

Terminate the dental procedure
↓

Ictal stage

Position the patient
(supine with legs elevated slightly)
↓
Summon medical assistance
↓
Protect the patient from injury
↓
Provide basic life support, as indicated
↓
Administer oxygen
↓
Monitor vital signs
↓

Postictal stage

Provide basic life support, as indicated
↓
Reassure patient and allow to recover
↓
Discharge patient
↓
To hospital   To home   To physician

■ **FIGURE 54-2 Emergency Procedure During a Seizure.** (From Malamed, S.F.: *Medical Emergencies in the Dental Office*, 4th ed. St. Louis, Mosby, 1993, page 295.)

D. Check oral cavity for trauma to teeth or tissues. Palliative care can be administered. When a tooth is broken, the piece must be located so that aspiration can be prevented.

TECHNICAL HINTS

I. Never use a glass syringe or other breakable instrument when a seizure could occur.

II. When a patient vomits during a seizure, use high-power evacuator with wide tip to remove material from the mouth as a first aid measure against aspiration of vomitus into the airway.

III. Be sensitive to the self-consciousness or embarrassment a patient may experience after a seizure.

FACTORS TO TEACH THE PATIENT

I. Always give full information for the medical history.

II. Take medication on schedule. Noncompliance with medications is a major factor in the recurrence of seizures.

III. Personal bacterial plaque control is important at all times, but an extra effort is needed when a drug is prescribed that can cause gingival en-

largement. Excellent personal bacterial control is vital to minimize gingival overgrowth.

IV. When seizure prone, a person should wear the Medic Alert jewelry.

REFERENCES

1. **International League Against Epilepsy,** Commission on Classification and Terminology: Proposal for Revised Clinical and Electroencephalographic Classification of Epileptic Seizures, *Epilepsia, 22,* 489, August, 1981.

2. **International League Against Epilepsy,** Commission on Classification and Terminology: Proposal for Revised Classification of Epilepsies and Epileptic Syndromes, *Epilepsia, 30,* 389, July/August, 1989.

3. **Malamed**, S.F.: *Handbook of Medical Emergencies in the Dental Office,* 4th ed. St. Louis, Mosby, 1993, pp. 279–297.

4. **Wyllie,** E.: *The Treatment of Epilepsy: Principles and Practice,* 2nd ed. Baltimore, Williams & Wilkins, 1997, pp. 808–855.

5. **Brodie,** M.J. and Dichter, M.A.: Antiepileptic Drugs, *N. Engl. J. Med., 334,* 168, January 18, 1996.

6. **Engel,** J.: Surgery for Seizures, *N. Engl. J. Med., 334,* 647, March 7, 1996.

7. **Angelopolous,** A.P. and Goaz, P.W.: Incidence of Diphenylhydantoin Gingival Hyperplasia, *Oral Surg., Oral Med., Oral Pathol., 34,* 898, December, 1972.

8. **Rees,** T.D. and Levine, R.A.: Systemic Drugs as a Risk Factor for Periodontal Disease Initiation and Progression, *Compend. Cont. Educ. Dent., 16,* 20, January, 1995.

9. **Poppell,** T.D., Keeling, S.D., Collins, J.F., and Hassell, T.M.: Effect of Folic Acid on Recurrence of Phenytoin-Induced Gingival Overgrowth Following Gingivectomy, *J. Clin. Periodontol., 18,* 134, February, 1991.

10. **Delgado-Escueta,** A.V. and Janz, D.: Consensus Guidelines: Preconception Counseling, Management, and Care of the Pregnant Woman With Epilepsy, *Neurology, 42,* 149, Supplement 5, April, 1992.

11. **Hassell,** T.M.: *Epilepsy and the Oral Manifestations of Phenytoin Therapy.* Monographs in Oral Science, Volume 9. London, S. Karger, 1981, pp. 116–127.

12. **Bredfeldt,** G.W.: Phenytoin-Induced Hyperplasia Found in Edentulous Patients, *J. Am. Dent. Assoc., 123,* 61, June, 1992.

13. **McCord,** J.F., Sloan, P., and Hussey, D.J.: Phenytoin Hyperplasia Occurring Under Complete Dentures: A Clinical Report, *J. Prosthet. Dent., 68,* 569, October, 1992.

14. **Chee,** W.W.L. and Jansen, C.E.: Phenytoin Hyperplasia Occurring in Relation to Titanium Implants: A Clinical Report, *Int. J. Oral Maxillofac. Implants, 9,* 107, No. 1, 1994.

15. **Carranza,** F.A.: Treatment of Gingival Enlargement, in Carranza, F.A. and Newman, M.G.: *Clinical Periodontology,* 8th ed. Philadelphia, W.B. Saunders Co., 1996, pp. 674–675.

16. **Hassell,** T.M., White, G.C., Jewson, L.G., and Peele, L.C.: Valproic Acid: A New Antiepileptic Drug With Potential Side Effects of Dental Concern, *J. Am. Dent. Assoc., 99,* 983, December, 1979.

SUGGESTED READINGS

Biron, C.R.: Anticonvulsants, *RDH, 14,* 34, September, 1994.

Devinsky, O.: Quality of Life with Epilepsy, in Wyllie, E.: *The Treatment of Epilepsy: Principles and Practice,* 2nd ed. Baltimore, Williams & Wilkins, 1997, pp. 1145–1150.

Dichter, M.A. and Brodie, M.J.: New Antiepileptic Drugs, *N. Engl. J. Med., 334,* 1583, June 13, 1996.

Hassell, T.M., Burtner, A.P., McNeal, D., and Smith, R.G.: Oral Problems and Genetic Aspects of Individuals with Epilepsy, *Periodontology 2000, 6,* 68, 1994.

Henskens, Y.M.C., Strooker, H., van den Keijbus, P.A.M., Veerman, E.C.I., and Nieuw Amerongen, A.V.: Salivary Protein Composition in Epileptic Patients on Different Medications, *J. Oral Pathol. Med., 25,* 360, August, 1996.

Rosa, F.W.: Spina Bifida in Infants of Women Treated With Carbamazepine During Pregnancy, *N. Engl. J. Med., 324,* 674, March 7, 1991.

Sanders, B.J., Weddell, J.A., and Dodge, N.N.: Managing Patients Who Have Seizure Disorders: Dental and Medical Issues, *J. Am. Dent. Assoc., 126,* 1641, December, 1995.

Schuh, L.A. and Drury, I.: Epilepsy in Adolescents and Adults, in Rakel, R.E., ed.: *Conn's Current Therapy,* 1997. Philadelphia, W.B. Saunders Co., 1997, p. 889.

Tennison, M., Greenwood, R., Lewis, D., and Thorn, M.: Discontinuing Antiepileptic Drugs in Children With Epilepsy, A Comparison of a Six-Week and a Nine-Month Taper Period, *N. Engl. J. Med., 330,* 1407, May 19, 1994.

Vining, E.P.G.: Epilepsy in Infants and Children, in Rakel, R.E., ed.: *Conn's Current Therapy, 1997.* Philadelphia, W.B. Saunders Co., 1997, p. 897.

Drug-Induced Gingival Overgrowth

Ball, D.E., McLaughlin, W.S., Seymour, R.A., and Kamali, F.: Plasma and Saliva Concentrations of Phenytoin and 5-(4-hydroxyphenyl)-5-Phenylhydantoin in Relation to the Incidence and Severity of Phenytoin-Induced Gingival Overgrowth in Epileptic Patients, *J. Periodontol., 67,* 597, June, 1996.

Brown, R.S., Beaver, W.T., and Bottomley, W.K.: On the Mechanism of Drug-Induced Gingival Hyperplasia, *J. Oral Pathol. Med., 20,* 201, May, 1991.

Brown, R.S., DiStanislao, P.T., Beaver, W.T., and Bottomley, W.K.: The Administration of Folic Acid to Institutionalized Epileptic Adults With Phenytoin-Induced Gingival Hyperplasia. A Double-Blind, Randomized, Placebo-Controlled, Parallel Study, *Oral Surg., Oral Med., Oral Pathol., 71,* 565, May, 1991.

Dahllöf, G., Axiö, E., and Modéer, T.: Regression of Phenytoin-Induced Gingival Overgrowth After Withdrawal of Medication, *Swed. Dent. J., 15,* 139, Number 3, 1991.

Hall, W.B.: Dilantin Hyperplasia: A Preventable Lesion? *Compend. Cont. Educ. Dent., 11,* S502, Supplement 14, 1990.

Hassell, T.M., Harris, E.L., Boughman, J.A., and Cockey, G.C.: Gingival Overgrowth: Hereditary Considerations, *Compend. Cont. Educ. Dent., 11,* S511, Supplement 14, 1990.

Katz, J., Givol, N., Chawshu, G., Taicher, S., and Shemer, J.: Vigabatrin-Induced Gingival Overgrowth, *J. Clin. Periodontol., 24,* 180, March, 1997.

McLaughlin, W.S., Ball, D.E., Seymour, R.A., Kamali, F., and White, K.: The Pharmokinetics of Phenytoin in Gingival Crevicular Fluid and Plasma in Relation to Gingival Overgrowth, *J. Clin. Periodontol., 22,* 942, December, 1995.

Mealey, B.L.: Periodontal Implications: Medically Compromised Patients. Medications Associated With Gingival Overgrowth, *Annals Periodontol., 1,* 303, November, 1996.

Thomason, J.M., Seymour, R.A., and Rawlins, M.D.: Incidence and Severity of Phenytoin-Induced Gingival Overgrowth In Epileptic Patients in General Medical Practice, *Community Dent. Oral Epidemiol., 20,* 288, October, 1992.

55

The Patient With Mental Retardation

With trends toward deinstitutionalization and emphasis on special training and education in local agencies and schools, more people with mild and moderate mental retardation have appeared in private dental offices and clinics, as well as in school and community dental facilities. Opportunities are available in all settings to contribute to the health and well-being of this special group.

MENTAL RETARDATION

Mental retardation refers to significantly subaverage general intellectual functioning with onset before 18 years that exists concurrently with deficits in adaptive behavior. Mental retardation is one of several developmental disorders that usually is first diagnosed in infancy, childhood, or adolescence. Table 55-1 lists the major categories of developmental disorders, and Box 55-1 provides descriptive terminology and other key words.

The levels of intellectual functioning are designated *mild, moderate, severe,* and *profound.* Standardized intelligence tests are used to determine individual levels. The Intelligence Quotient (IQ) expresses the test results. A category of *Unspecified Mental Retardation* is used when standard tests cannot be performed because of lack of cooperation, severe impairment, or infancy.

Adaptive functioning refers to the person's effectiveness in social skills, communication, and daily living skills, as well as to how standards of personal independence and social responsibility characteristic of the age and cultural group are met. Adaptive functioning is influenced by such factors as motivation, education, and social and vocational opportunities and has more chance for improvement by remedial efforts than does IQ, which tends to be more fixed.[1]

Adaptive functioning is described briefly for each of the categories listed in the following sections. An understanding of expected capabilities can help to provide necessary background information for teaching basic oral care procedures.

TABLE 55-1 Disorders Usually First Diagnosed in Infancy, Childhood, or Adolescence

MENTAL RETARDATION

Mild, moderate, severe, profound

LEARNING DISORDERS

Reading
Mathematics
Written expression

MOTOR SKILLS DISORDERS

Coordination

PERVASIVE DEVELOPMENTAL DISORDER

Autistic disorder

DISRUPTIVE BEHAVIOR DISORDERS

Overaggressiveness, hostility, hyperactivity, inattention,
    impulsiveness
Poor attention span
Conduct disorder; delinquency
Use of alcohol; stealing; destructive acts

ANXIETY DISORDERS

Unrealistic fears of the unfamiliar
Fear of separation

FEEDING DISORDERS

Failure to eat adequately
Pica
Rumination disorder

TIC DISORDERS

Tourette's syndrome
Chronic motor or vocal tic disorder

COMMUNICATION DISORDERS

Expressive language
Stuttering

(Adapted from American Psychiatric Association: DSM-IV, 1994, pp. 37–38.)

I. MILD RETARDATION

A. IQ
50–55 to approximately 70.

B. Adaptive Functioning
1. *Child.* In special classes for the educable, the child advances to a level of third to sixth grade. Practical skills can be learned.
2. *Adult.* At adult level, the individual cares for personal hygiene and other necessities, with reminders. Communication is good, although the attention span and memory are less than average. Activities that do not require involved planning or rapid implementation can be carried out satisfactorily. Most

educable individuals can engage in semi-skilled or simple skilled work with guidance, and so maintain themselves.

II. MODERATE RETARDATION

A. IQ
35–40 to 50–55.

B. Adaptive Functioning
1. *Child.* A marked developmental lag occurs in the early years, but the child can be trained in personal care and hygiene with help. These children attend classes and learn simple habits and skills, but they do not learn to read and write. They speak in short sentences, and understand best when single-thought, short sentences are used. They participate well in group activities.
2. *Adult.* As adults, these individuals attend to personal care, with reminders, and have a relatively short attention span and memory. Although they may have problems of coordination, they perform simple tasks and are conscientious about taking responsibility for errands and helpful duties. Although not completely capable of self-maintenance, many do unskilled work with direct supervision.

III. SEVERE RETARDATION

A. IQ
20–25 to 35–40.

B. Adaptive Functioning
1. *Child.* Children at this level can benefit from systematic habit training and may make attempts at personal care and dressing with assistance. They usually walk, use some speech, and respond to directions.
2. *Adult.* Adults conform to a daily routine and may help with household and other small tasks, in spite of a limited attention span. Many adapt to life in the community in group homes or with their families.

IV. PROFOUND RETARDATION

A. IQ
Below 20 or 25.

B. Adaptive Functioning
1. *Child.* Delays occur in all phases of development, and close supervision and care are necessary.
2. *Adult.* Many remain inert and placid throughout the early years and never learn to sit up. In a highly structured setting and with constant supervision, self-care and communication skills may improve. Some perform simple tasks in a sheltered, supervised setting.

BOX 55-1 KEY WORDS: Mental Retardation

Autism (aw'tizm): a syndrome beginning in infancy characterized by extreme withdrawal and an obsessive desire to maintain the status quo.

Brachycephalic (brak-ē-se-fal'ik): having a short, wide head.

Dysmorphism (dis-mor'fizm): abnormality in morphologic development.

Echolalia (ek"ō-lā'li-ah): echo reaction; the involuntary repetition of a word or sentence just spoken by another person.

Epicanthus (ep"i-kan' thus): a vertical fold of skin on either side of the nose, sometimes covering the inner canthus; a normal characteristic in persons of certain races.

Hyperactivity (hi"per-ak-tiv'ĭtē): abnormally increased activity.

  Development hyperactivity (hyperkinesis): characterized by constant motion, fidgetiness, excitability, impulsiveness, and a short attention span.

Intelligence quotient (IQ): numeric rating determined through psychologic testing that indicates the approximate relationship of a person's mental age (MA) to chronologic age (CA).

Macroglossia (mak"rō-glos'ē-ah): very large tongue.

Microcephaly (mī"krō-sef'ah-lee): small size of head in relation to the rest of the body.

Mutism (mu'tĭzm): inability or refusal to speak; deafness may prevent learning to speak.

Elective mutism: persistent refusal to talk in children with demonstrated ability to speak.

Pathognomonic (pa-thog-nō-mon'ĭk): characteristic or indicative of a particular disease or syndrome; especially one or more typical symptoms.

Pervasive: throughout entire individual, entire development is severely and markedly impaired, as in autism.

Pica (pi'kah): persistent craving/eating of nonnutritive substances or unnatural articles of food.

Rumination (roo"mĭ-na-shun): repeated regurgitation of food in the absence of any associated gastrointestinal illness.

Self-injury: act of deliberate harm to one's own body. Also called self-abuse, self-directed aggression, self-harm, self-inflicted injury, self-mutilation.

Tic: an involuntary, sudden, rapid, recurrent, nonrhythmic, stereotyped motor movement or vocal sound.

  Tourette's syndrome: multiple motor and one or more vocal tics; may involve squatting, twirling, grunts, barks, sniffs, and coprolalia.

  Coprolalia (kop'rō-lā'lē-ah): involuntary utterance of vulgar or obscene words.

Ultrasonography (ul'trah-so-nog'ra-fee): the location, measurement, or delineation of deep structures by measuring the reflection or transmission of ultrasonic waves. Used in examination of fetus to determine birth defects.

ETIOLOGY OF MENTAL RETARDATION[1]

Mental retardation represents a more or less important symptom in well over 200 different conditions. Many of these are rare. A variety of means of classification is found in the literature. It has been convenient to divide the causes into factors operating before birth, at birth, and after birth.

A majority of cases of mental retardation results from prenatal influences; a small number is effected as injuries at birth. Diagnosis may be complicated and difficult, and many cases can only be classified as of unknown origin.

I. PREDISPOSING FACTORS[1]
  A. Heredity.
  B. Early alterations of embryonic development.
  C. Pregnancy and perinatal problems.
  D. General medical disorders acquired in childhood.
  E. Environmental influences.
  F. Unknown.

II. EXAMPLES DURING PRENATAL PERIOD
  A. Infections
  Brain damage can result from maternal infection during pregnancy. Serious infections during the first trimester are most likely to cause physical malformations.
  1. *Congenital Rubella Syndrome.* German measles virus infection during the first trimester may cause abnormalities, including mental retardation. The rubella syndrome also may include cataracts, cardiac anomalies, deafness, and microcephaly.
    Immunization with rubella vaccine has reduced the incidence of the disease and retardation related to the virus infection has been reduced.
  2. *Congenital Syphilis.* Transfer of syphilis from the mother leads to numerous symptoms.

When the central nervous system is involved, hydrocephalus, convulsions, and mental retardation can result. Hutchinson's triad, which is associated with the late stage of congenital syphilis, includes deafness, interstitial keratitis, and dental defects. Hutchinsonian incisors, which are notched and tapered, mulberry molars, and microdontia are typical (Figure 14-6, page 244).

3. *Neonatal Congenital Toxoplasmosis.* Infection of the fetus transplacentally may lead to miscarriage, stillbirth, or a living baby with severe clinical disease. The effects may include hydrocephalus or microcephalus, blindness, and mental retardation.

B. Drugs Used During Pregnancy

1. *Contraindicated Drugs.* Table 43-1 (page 655) lists drugs contraindicated during pregnancy and the possible adverse effects the drugs can have on the fetus. Birth malformations and syndromes that include mental retardation are identified.

2. *Fetal Alcohol Syndrome (FAS).* The signs and symptoms of FAS are described on page 840, and the facial features are shown in Figure 57-1.

C. Metabolic Disorders

1. *Phenylketonuria (PKU).* Phenylketonuria results from an error of metabolism in which the enzyme necessary for digestion of the amino acid phenylalanine is missing. Severe mental retardation is a consequence. Early recognition of the missing enzyme with early dietary control lessens the severity of retardation. Many states require blood and urine screening tests soon after an infant is born. A diet free from animal and vegetable protein is necessary.

2. *Congenital Hypothyroidism.* Cretinism results from partial or complete absence of the thyroid gland at birth. Symptoms of defective development include mental retardation.

D. Chromosomal Abnormality

Down's syndrome is described in a separate section on pages 814 to 816.

III. EXAMPLES DURING BIRTH

A. Mechanical Injury at Birth

Damage leading to mental retardation may have a variety of causes, including difficulties of labor and delivery.

B. Hypoxia

Asphyxiation from prolonged oxygen deficiency may result from labor complications.

IV. EXAMPLES DURING POSTNATAL PERIOD

A. Infections

Cerebral infection may be caused by a wide variety of diseases, including encephalitis and meningitis.

B. Postnatal Trauma

Accidents may result in a fractured skull or prolonged unconsciousness.

GENERAL CHARACTERISTICS

I. PHYSICAL FEATURES

Because most individuals with mental retardation are in the borderline and mild categories, no unusual physical characteristics should be expected. There may be delayed growth and development.

Facial or other characteristics may be pathognomonic for a particular condition or syndrome; for example, Down's syndrome, described later in this chapter.

Skull anomalies include microcephaly (smaller), hydrocephalus (larger, contains fluid), spherical, conical, or otherwise asymmetrical shapes. Other dysmorphic features, such as asymmetries of the face, malformations of the outer ear, anomalies of the eyes, or unusual shape of the nose, may become apparent as the child develops.

II. ORAL FINDINGS

A higher incidence of oral developmental malformations has been observed, some specifically associated with particular syndromes or conditions. Oral findings that have been observed to occur more frequently in individuals with mental retardation than in those with normal intelligence include the following:

A. Lips

Thickness of the lips is common. Lip biting is one of the self-injurious habits.

B. Tooth Anomalies

Teeth may be imperfectly formed; eruption patterns may be delayed or irregular.

C. Periodontal Conditions

Gingivitis and periodontitis are common in individuals with mental retardation. Patients with Down's syndrome have more severe disease than do those from other groups with mental retardation. The incidence is greater among the institutionalized patients when compared with those living in the community.[2]

D. Habits

Incidence of clenching, bruxing, mouthbreathing, and tongue thrusting is increased.

E. Dental Caries[2]

The factors that are effective in the control of dental caries in the special group are the same as those in a population of normal intelligence. These factors include exposure to fluoridation and other forms of fluoride, form and frequency of cariogenic foods in the diet, and the control of bacterial plaque.

Studies have shown that, when all degrees of retardation are grouped together, dental caries incidence is generally higher for noninstitutionalized than for institutionalized patients, particularly among the profoundly retarded group. Institutionalized individuals have a controlled diet with less food available between meals. They also may have less accessibility to snacks containing refined carbohydrates, except those brought by visitors.

The private water supply for many institutions has been fluoridated. This may also be true of the community water supply where noninstitutionalized individuals reside.

When the figures for dental caries incidence are separated according to degree of retardation, the severely and profoundly retarded patients have been shown to have significantly more dental caries.[2] Mild and moderate retarded people can be trained in self-care.

DENTAL AND DENTAL HYGIENE CARE AND INSTRUCTION

Procedures for management and care of a patient with a disability are described in Chapter 50 with suggestions for various types of adaptations. The patient with mental retardation may have physical and sensory disabilities or systemic disease problems; therefore, information from various chapters can be applied during treatment. Patients with any type of mental retardation need basic periodontal therapy consisting of intensive daily plaque control, scaling, and frequent maintenance supervision. Patience and repetition are needed to learn and develop motor skills.

In the following pages, the special characteristics and problems of patients with Down's syndrome and autistic disorder are described.

DOWN'S SYNDROME

A special and unique group of individuals with mental retardation has a chromosomal abnormality manifested in Down's syndrome or trisomy 21 syndrome. Prenatal serum testing and genetic counseling have contributed to lowering the incidence of Down's syndrome.

Formerly, the incidence of births of babies with Down's syndrome increased with advancing maternal age. In recent years, however, the average age of mothers of infants with Down's syndrome has decreased.[3] Also, statistical evidence shows that the father can be the source of the chromosomal abnormality.[4]

Patients with Down's syndrome have a combination of characteristic abnormalities that is relatively constant. They tend to resemble one another.

I. PHYSICAL CHARACTERISTICS

A. Stature
Small, with a short neck; awkward, waddling gait; general growth retardation.

B. Head
Microcephaly; flat on facial and occipital sides; short, underdeveloped nose with depressed bridge; scanty hair.

C. Eyes
Oblique slant laterally with narrow opening between eyelids; fold of skin continues from upper eyelid over the inner angle of the eye (epicanthic fold) (Figure 55-1). Nearsightedness, eyes crossing inward, and cataracts are common.

D. Hands
Broad, with short stubby fingers. The little fingers are curved inward. A single transverse palmar crease may also be present (Figure 55-2).

II. LEVEL OF MENTAL RETARDATION

Generally, the IQ of patients with Down's syndrome is under 70. Those who have been institutionalized for a long period of time may show lower IQ scores.

Socially, many of the children are more advanced, and may appear to have more intelligence than actu-

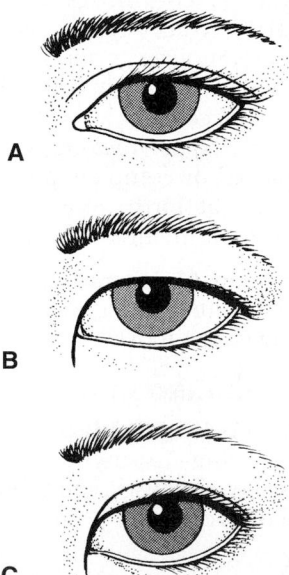

FIGURE 55-1 Down's Syndrome: Eye Characteristics. (A) Absence of an epicanthic fold. **(B)** Epicanthic fold in Oriental populations. **(C)** Epicanthic fold of person with Down's syndrome. (Redrawn from Smith, G.F. and Berg, J.M.: *Down's Anomaly*, 2nd ed. Edinburgh, Churchill Livingstone, 1976.)

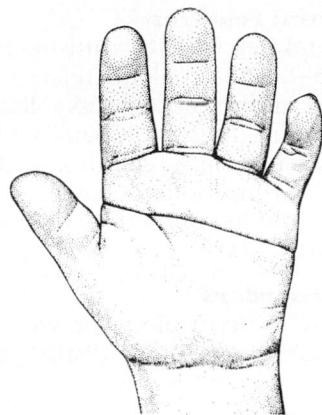

FIGURE 55-2 Down's Syndrome: Hand. Short, stubby fingers with little finger curved inward are characteristic. An identifying feature is the single transverse palmar crease. (From Smith, G.F. and Berg, J.M.: *Down's Anomaly*, 2nd ed. Edinburgh, Churchill Livingstone, 1976.)

ally exists. The characteristics of friendliness and personal interaction are described later.

Many people with Down's syndrome are fond of music and have a good sense of rhythm. They enjoy singing, playing an instrument, and listening to music. Background music in the dental office or clinic may be helpful in gaining rapport with these special patients.

III. PERSONAL CHARACTERISTICS

The newborn baby with Down's syndrome is considered a "good" baby by the parents. Later, many of the small children are cheerful, happy, and responsive to learning. Individual differences can be noted, and personality disturbances may occur.

Typical characteristics listed here may suggest management approaches for dental and dental hygiene appointments.

    A. Like attention; require affection for feeling of security.

    B. Cheerful disposition; rarely irritable; easily amused.

    C. Sociable, observant; take initiative.

    D. Tendency to imitate; mischievous.

    E. Periods of stubbornness; obstinate and determined to have their own way. Parental discipline is necessary. In the dental hygiene appointment, the initial approach can be important to continued control and cooperation.

IV. ORAL FINDINGS

A. Lips

Habitually, the young person with Down's syndrome holds the mouth open with the tongue protruded. The lips are often thickened, cracked, and dry, a result of excessive bathing in saliva while the mouth is open.

Mouth breathing is common. Because respiratory infections frequently exist, and the tonsils and adenoids are often enlarged, breathing through the nose may not be easy.

B. Tongue and Palate

The tongue is generally deeply fissured and appears large. The narrow jaws and short, narrow palate tend to force the tongue into protrusion. It appears larger than it actually may be.

The incidence of cleft lip, cleft palate, or cleft uvula is greater than that in the general population.[5]

C. Teeth

Eruption is delayed and irregular in sequence. There may be microdontia and congenitally missing teeth. Such anomalies as fused teeth and peg lateral incisors occur frequently.

D. Occlusion

Angle's Class III and posterior crossbite are common and relate to the flat face and underdevelopment of the midfacial region. Frequently, the teeth are spaced because certain anomalous teeth are narrow and require less space.

E. Periodontal Disease[6,7]

Periodontal conditions are more severe in people with Down's syndrome. Even at early ages, bone loss and other effects of periodontal infection are present. Leukocyte function is altered by impaired chemotaxis and phagocytosis, and the altered immune system contributes to the increased severity of periodontal infection.

Necrotizing ulcerative gingivitis (NUG), superimposed over gingivitis or periodontitis, has been found more in patients with Down's syndrome than in those with other types of mental retardation.

V. HEALTH PROBLEMS SIGNIFICANT TO DENTAL HYGIENE CARE

The mortality rate has been high during the early years because of high susceptibility to respiratory infections, leukemia, and congenital heart lesions. More recent improvements in child health care and immunizations have brought a longer life expectancy.

A. Susceptibility to Infection

Defects in the body's immune defense mechanisms lead to greater susceptibility to various infections.

B. Obstructive Airway Problems[8]

    1. Contributing factors: macroglossia, increased secretions, frequent respiratory infections, obesity, enlarged tonsils and adenoids.

    2. Dental hygiene adaptations: chair position, fluid suctioning, gag reflex.

C. Congenital Heart Lesions

Antibiotic premedication will be needed for many patients. There is a high incidence of mitral valve prolapse.[9]

D. Relation to Alzheimer's Disease

Adults with Down's syndrome age prematurely. Many over the age of 40 develop an Alzheimer's-like dementia with pathologic brain changes similar to those of Alzheimer's disease.[10] Changes occur in memory, speech, gait, personality, and other characteristics. Alzheimer's disease is described on pages 687 to 688.

AUTISTIC DISORDER

Autism is a pervasive behavioral developmental disability manifested by limited ability to understand and communicate. Autistic disorder appears during the first years of life.[11]

Other names that have been used for the condition are Kanner's syndrome, early infantile autism, primary autism, infantile or childhood autism, and childhood psychosis. Because autism is a life-long disability and autistic people can live a normal life span, names that refer to infancy or childhood are less accurate.

Children all over the world have autism, and no factor of race, ethnic background, parental intelligence, social class, or parental personality has been shown to be related. Approximately three fourths are mentally retarded, with an IQ below 70. Autism is found in males three to four times more frequently than in females.

I. CHARACTERISTICS

Autism is a severely incapacitating condition. It is present at birth, but may not be identified specifically for months or years.

A. Behavioral Features

Behavioral features of autism are shown in Table 55-2. The problems relate to social interaction, communication, and a limited range of activities and interests. Cognitive abnormalities are apparent. Many children with autism engage in self-injurious behaviors, such as head banging or biting of their own fingers, wrists, or other parts.

B. Other Disorders

Autism may occur alone or with other conditions such as metabolic disturbances and seizures.

C. Prognosis

Individuals with autism may live a normal life span. A few become relatively self-sufficient with regular employment.

II. INTERVENTIONS[12,13]

No drug or other treatment cures autism. Many patients do not require medications.

A. Education

Special education classes that address behavioral and communication disorders are of primary importance. In addition to a structured school environment, families need training to provide support and consistent treatment.

B. Parental Counseling

Parents of an autistic child are under such stress that emotional disorders of the parents may emerge. Along with supportive counseling, the need for psychotherapy may become evident.

TABLE 55-2 Characteristics of Autism

A. Impairment in Social Interaction
1. Impairment in use of nonverbal behaviors (e.g., eye-to-eye gaze, facial expression, gestures)
2. Failure to develop peer relationships appropriate to developmental level
3. Lack of spontaneous seeking to share enjoyment, interests, or achievements with others
4. Lack of social or emotional reciprocity

B. Impairment in Communication
1. Delay or total lack of spoken language
2. Individuals with adequate speech: impairment in conversational abilities
3. Stereotyped and repetitive use of language
4. Lack of spontaneous make-believe play

C. Restricted Repetitive and Stereotyped Patterns of Behavior
1. Preoccupation with stereotyped and restricted patterns of interest
2. Inflexible adherence to routines or rituals
3. Stereotyped, repetitive body movements and mannerisms
4. Persistent preoccupation with parts of objects

D. Delays or Abnormal Functioning Prior to Age 3 Years
1. Social interaction
2. Language as used in social communication
3. Symbolic or imaginative play

(Adapted from American Psychiatric Association, DSM-IV, 1994, pp. 70–71.)

C. Pharmacotherapy[13]

Various psychotropic drugs, hormones, megavitamins, and other pharmaceutical agents have been tried. Drug therapy depends on the individual needs. The main objective is to make the child more receptive to education and other therapies.

Patients may have other drugs in their complete treatment regimen that need consideration during dental and dental hygiene appointments. The patient with seizures may receive an anticonvulsant. Drug-induced gingival overgrowth may be a problem (pages 804 to 806).

III. PERSONAL FACTORS AND DENTAL HYGIENE CARE

For many patients with autism, appointments for health care, medical or dental, are frightening, difficult experiences. Because of language disability, lack of communication, anxiety, and limited social contact, dental care may have been neglected.

Although not all autistic patients are difficult to treat, a few are impossible to treat without sedation, general anesthesia, or immobilization.

A. Oral Health Problems

Except when autism is combined with a developmental disability of a different nature, no specific oral manifestation exists. The general health and factors that must be considered for preappointment planning, such as antibiotic premedication, are also not manifestations specifically related to autism. Several factors can contribute to a condition of poor oral health.

1. *Previous Dental Care.* The parent may not have taken the child to obtain care because of fear of the child being hurt or fear of embarrassment that would result from the behavior of the difficult child. Frustration at home over continuous management of the disabled child could lead a parent to place dental care at a low priority level.

   For the child who had been taken to a dental office or clinic, previous dentists and dental hygienists may not have succeeded in accomplishing treatment of a satisfactory quality.

2. *Dental Caries.* Problems of feeding may have led the parent to lines of least resistance in the serving of foods the child would accept, without regard for nutritive content or dental caries prevention.

   The child's need for sameness may have been applied to dietary selection. A minimal, limited diet may or may not have included excess cariogenic foods.

   A second factor is the possibility that the rewards used in behavior modification therapy may be sweets. Frequent repetition of cariogenic rewards over long periods could have a major effect on dental caries development.

3. *Oral Hygiene.* Even a parent or caregiver who is well informed about current plaque control procedures may have had such difficulty in coping with an uncooperative autistic child that daily oral care procedures have never been carried out adequately.

B. Dental Staff Preparation

Advanced review and discussion of the patient's medical, dental, and personal histories and information from the physician, psychiatrist, teacher, or other persons associated with the patient may be necessary as the dental team members begin to learn how to work with the patient. Several short orientation appointments may be planned initially.

The same members of the dental team should be involved at each appointment so that the patient is not disturbed by changes and time is not lost in reorientation.

C. Dental Hygiene Care Plan

1. Plan four-handed dental hygiene for the difficult patient.
2. Frequent appointments to include all phases of prevention:
   a. Bacterial plaque control for the patient and the caregiver.
   b. Scaling, fluoride therapy, sealants.

D. Appointment Interventions[14]

1. Provide the child with predictable and consistent experiences.
2. Create a quiet environment free from sensory stimuli. Avoid use of loud, inconsistent background music, noisy dental apparatus, and irrelevant conversations. Avoid touching as this may be disturbing to the patient.
3. Desensitization
   a. Begin with orientation to the setting and to each part of the equipment. The first appointment may not include any instruments, as the patient may not be ready. Patience and firmness are necessary elements. Instruction takes the form of "show-tell-do" repeated many times.
   b. Use the parent to help to condition the patient. Give the parent a plastic mouth mirror and a few dental films to take home for practice in the mouth each day.
4. Apply behavior modification procedures when the child is trained by that method. Use the parent or therapist-teacher to assist in presenting in a simple step-by-step manner the preventive measures. Reinforcers or rewards are given immediately following each success. By using noncariogenic or, better still, nonedible rewards, the parent or teacher can be educated.
5. Physical immobilization: various procedures

were described in Chapter 50. A papoose board (pages 745 to 746, Figure 50-4) may provide a safe environment for a severely autistic patient unable to respond to desensitization.

TECHNICAL HINTS

I. INFORMED CONSENT
Written approval of the care plan is obtained from the parent or legal guardian.[15]

II. BEHAVIOR MODIFICATION
Encourage caregivers to include oral care procedures in patient behavior modification.

III. TOBACCO USE
Residences and institutions for individuals with mental retardation should be designated tobacco free for the health of those incapable of understanding the health risks of use of smoke and smokeless tobacco products.

When the employees are permitted to use tobacco products while on duty, rules must be enforced to control disposal of unused portions. The residents are known to collect and chew or smoke discarded cigarette butts left by institutional employees.[16]

REFERENCES

1. **American Psychiatric Association:** *Diagnostic and Statistical Manual of Mental Disorders* (DSM-IV). Washington, DC, American Psychiatric Association, 1994, pp. 37–43.
2. **Tesini,** D.A.: An Annotated Review of the Literature of Dental Caries and Periodontal Disease in Mentally Retarded Individuals, *Spec. Care Dentist., 1,* 75, March/April, 1981.
3. **Holmes,** L.B.: Decreasing Age of Mothers of Infants with the Down's syndrome, *N. Engl. J. Med., 298,* 1419, June 22, 1978.
4. **Cohen,** F.L.: Paternal Contributions to Birth Defects, *Nurs. Clin. North Am., 21,* 49, March, 1986.
5. **Schendel,** S.A. and Gorlin, R.J.: Frequency of Cleft Uvula and Submucous Cleft Palate in Patients with Down's Syndrome, *J. Dent. Res., 53,* 840, July–August, 1974.
6. **Izumi,** Y., Sugiyama, S., Shinozuka, O., Yamazaki, T., Ohyama, T., and Ishikawa, I.: Defective Neutrophil Chemotaxis in Down's Syndrome Patients and Its Relationship to Periodontal Destruction, *J. Periodontol., 60,* 238, May, 1989.
7. **Modéer,** T., Barr, M., and Dahllöf, G.: Periodontal Disease in Children with Down's Syndrome, *Scand. J. Dent. Res., 98,* 228, June, 1990.
8. **Jacobs,** I.N., Gray, R.F., and Todd, N.W.: Upper Airway Obstruction in Children with Down syndrome, *Arch. Otolaryngol. Head Neck Surg., 122,* 945, September, 1996.
9. **Barnett,** M.L., Friedman, D., and Kastner, T.: The Prevalence of Mitral Valve Prolapse in Patients With Down's Syndrome: Implications for Dental Management, *Oral Surg., Oral Med., Oral Pathol., 66,* 445, October, 1988.
10. **Sigal,** M.J. and Levine, N.: Down's Syndrome and Alzheimer's Disease, *J. Can. Dent. Assoc., 59,* 823, October, 1993.
11. **American Psychiatric Association:** op. cit., pp. 66–71.
12. **Edwards,** D.R. and Bristol, M.M.: Autism: Early Identification and Management in Family Practice, *Am. Fam. Physician, 44,* 1755, November, 1991.
13. **Rapin,** I.: Autism, *N. Engl. J. Med., 337,* 97, July 10, 1997.
14. **Loiacono,** C.: Care of the Autistic Patient, *DentalHygienistNews,* 7, 19, Summer, 1994.
15. **Snow,** M.K. and Stiefel, D.J.: *Dental Treatment of the Mentally Retarded.* Disability Dental Instruction, 4919 NE 86th Street, Seattle, WA 98115, 1978, p.7.
16. **Burtner,** A.P., Wakham, M.D., McNeal, D.R., and Garvey, T.P.: Tobacco and the Institutionalized Mentally Retarded: Usage Choices and Ethical Considerations, *Spec. Care Dentist., 15,* 56, March/April, 1995.

SUGGESTED READINGS

Asher, R.S. and Winquist, H.: Appliance Therapy for Chronic Drooling in a Patient With Mental Retardation, *Spec. Care Dentist., 14,* 30, January/February, 1994.

Becking, A.G. and Tuinzing, D.B.: Orthognathic Surgery for Mentally Retarded Patients, *Oral Surg. Oral Med. Oral Pathol., 72,* 162, August, 1991.

Davila, J.M. and Menendez, J.: Relaxing Effects of Music in Dentistry for Mentally Handicapped Patients, *Spec. Care Dentist., 6,* 18, January/February, 1986.

Dicks, J.L. and Banning, J.S.: Evaluation of Calculus Accumulation in Tube-Fed, Mentally Handicapped Patients: The Effects of Oral Hygiene Status, *Spec. Care Dentist., 11,* 104, May/June, 1991.

Drews, C.D., Yeargin-Allsopp, M., Decoufle, P., and Murphy, C.C.: Variation in the Influence of Selected Sociodemographic Risk Factors for Mental Retardation, *Am. J. Public Health, 85,* 329, March, 1995.

Eyman, R.K., Grossman, H.J., Chaney, R.H., and Call, T.L.: The Life Expectancy of Profoundly Handicapped People with Mental Retardation, *N. Engl. J. Med., 323,* 584, August 30, 1990.

Gabre, P. and Gahnberg, L.: Dental Health Status of Mentally Retarded Adults With Various Living Arrangements, *Spec. Care Dentist., 14,* 203, September/October, 1994.

Gabre, P. and Gahnberg, L.: Inter-relationship Among Degree of Mental Retardation, Living Arrangements, and Dental Health in Adults With Mental Retardation, *Spec. Care Dentist., 17,* 7, January/February, 1997.

Kendall, N.P.: Oral Health of a Group of Non-institutionalized Mentally Handicapped Adults in the UK, *Community Dent. Oral Epidemiol., 19,* 357, December, 1991.

Kulkarni, G. V. and Levine, N.: Fragile X (Martin-Bell) Syndrome, *Spec. Care Dentist., 14,* 21, January/February, 1994.

Loiacono, C., Jenkins, J., and Campbell, P.R.: Management of the Patient With Mental Retardation: A Case Report, *Can. Dent. Hyg. Assoc.* (PROBE), *32,* 18, January/February, 1998.

Lovell, R.W. and Reiss, A.L.: Dual Diagnoses. Psychiatric Disorders in Developmental Disabilities, *Pediatr. Clin. North Am., 40,* 579, June, 1993.

Oilo, G., Hatle, G., Gad, A.-L., and Dahl, B.L.: Wear of Teeth in a Mentally Retarded Population, *J. Oral Rehabil., 17,* 173, March, 1990.

Vittek, J., Winik, S., Winik, A., Sioris, C., Tarangelo, A.M., and Chou, M.: Analysis of Orthodontic Anomalies in Mentally Retarded Developmentally Disabled (MRDD) Persons, *Spec. Care Dentist., 14,* 198, September/October, 1994.

Wakham, M.D., Burtner, A.P., McNeal, D.R., Garvey, T.P., and Bedinger, S.: Pica: A Peculiar Behavior with Oral Involvement, *Spec. Care Dentist., 12,* 207, September/October, 1992.

Willette, J.C.: Lip-chewing: Another Treatment Option, *Spec. Care Dentist., 12,* 174, July/August, 1992.

Down's Syndrome

Cooley, W.C. and Graham, J.M.: Common Syndromes and Management Issues for Primary Care Physicians. Down Syndrome—An Update and Review for the Primary Pediatrician, *Clin. Pediatr., 30,* 233, April, 1991.

Desai, S.S.: Down Syndrome. A Review of the Literature, *Oral Surg. Oral Med. Oral Pathol. Oral Radiol. Endod., 84,* 279, September, 1997.

Evenhuis, H.M.: The Natural History of Dementia in Down Syndrome, *Arch. Neurol., 47,* 263, March, 1990.

Hunt, N.: *The World of Nigel Hunt: The Diary of a Mongoloid Youth.* New York, Garrett, 1967, 126 pp.

Klaiman, P. and Arndt, E.: Facial Reconstruction in Down Syndrome: Perceptions of the Results by Parents and Normal Adolescents, *Cleft Palate J., 26,* 186, July, 1989.

Klaiman, P., Witzel, M.A., Margar-Bacal, F., and Munro, I.R.: Changes in Aesthetic Appearance and Intelligibility of Speech after Partial Glossectomy in Patients with Down Syndrome, *Plast. Reconstr. Surg., 82,* 403, September, 1988.

Kumasaka, S., Miyagi, A., Sakai, N., Shindo, J., and Kashima, I.: Oligodontia: A Radiographic Comparison of Subjects With Down Syndrome and Normal Subjects, *Spec. Care Dentist., 17,* 137, July/August, 1997.

Morinushi, T., Lopatin, D.E., and Tanaka, H.: The Relationship Between Dental Caries in the Primary Dentition and Anti *S. mutans* Serum Antibodies in Children With Down's Syndrome, *J. Clin. Pediatr. Dent., 19,* 279, Summer, 1993.

Navazesh, M., Mulligan, R., and Sobel, S.: Toxic Shock and Down Syndromes in a Dental Patient: A Case Report and Review of the Literature, *Spec. Care Dentist., 14,* 246, November/December, 1994.

Randell, D.M., Harth, S., and Seow, W.K.: Preventive Dental Health Practices of Non-institutionalized Down Syndrome Children: A Controlled Study, *J. Clin. Pediatr. Dent., 16,* 225, Spring, 1992.

Shapira, J. and Stabholz, A.: A Comprehensive 30-Month Preventive Dental Health Program in a Pre-adolescent Population With Down's Syndrome: A Longitudinal Study, *Spec. Care Dentist., 16,* 33, January/February, 1996.

Down's Syndrome: Periodontal

Barr-Agholme, M., Dahllof, G., Linder, L., and Modéer, T.: *Actinobacillus actinomycetemcomitans, Capnocytophaga* and *Porphyromonas gingivalis* in Subgingival Plaque of Adolescents with Down's Syndrome, *Oral Microbiol. Immunol., 7,* 244, August, 1992.

Morinushi, T., Lopatin, D.E., and Poperin, N.V.: The Relationship Between Gingivitis and Serum Antibodies to the Microbiota Associated With Periodontal Disease in Children With Down's Syndrome, *J. Periodontol., 68,* 626, July, 1997.

Reuland-Bosma, W. and van Dijk, J.: Periodontal Disease in Down's Syndrome: A Review, *J. Clin Periodontol., 13,* 64, January, 1986.

Reuland-Bosma, W., van Dijk, L.J., and van der Weele, L.: Experimental Gingivitis Around Deciduous Teeth in Children with Down's Syndrome, *J. Clin. Periodontol., 13,* 294, April, 1986.

Reuland-Bosma, W., Liem, R.S.B., Jansen, H.W.B., van Dijk, L.J., and van der Weele, L.T.: Cellular Aspects of and Effects on the Gingiva in Children with Down's Syndrome During Experimental Gingivitis, *J. Clin. Periodontol., 15,* 303, May, 1988.

Santos, R., Shanfeld, J., and Casamassimo, P.: Serum Antibody Response to *Actinobacillus actinomycetemcomitans* in Down's Syndrome, *Spec. Care Dentist., 16,* 80, March/April, 1996.

Shapira, J., Stabholz, A., Schurr, D., Sela, M.N., and Mann, J.: Caries Levels, *Streptococcus mutans* Counts, Salivary pH, and Periodontal Treatment Needs of Adult Down Syndrome Patients, *Spec. Care Dentist., 11,* 248, November/December, 1991.

Sohoel, P.D.C., Johannessen, A.C., Kristoffersen, T., Haugstvedt, Y., and Nilsen, R.: In situ Characterization of Mononuclear Cells in Marginal Periodontitis of Patients With Down's Syndrome, *Acta Odontol. Scand., 50,* 141, June, 1997.

Stabholz, A., Mann, J., Sela, M., Schurr, D., Steinberg, D., Dori, S., and Shapira, J.: Caries Experience, Periodontal Treatment Needs, Salivary pH, and *Streptococcus mutans* Counts in a Preadolescent Down Syndrome Population, *Spec. Care Dentist., 11,* 203, September/October, 1991.

Ulseth, J.O., Hestnes, A., Stovner, L.J., and Storhaug, K.: Dental Caries and Periodontitis in Persons with Down Syndrome, *Spec. Care Dentist., 11,* 71, March/April, 1991.

Yavuzyilmaz, E., Ersoy, F., Sanal, O., Tezcan, I., and Ercal, D.: Neutrophil Chemotaxis and Periodontal Status in Down's Syndrome Patients, *J. Nihon Univ. Sch. Dent., 35,* 91, June, 1993.

Autism

Davila, J.M. and Jensen, O.E.: Behavioral and Pharmacological Dental Management of a Patient with Autism, *Spec. Care Dentist., 8,* 58, March/April, 1988.

Johnson, C.D., Matt, M.K., Dennison, D., Brown, R.S., and Koh, S.: A Case Report Preventing Factitious Gingival Injury in an Autistic Patient, *J. Am. Dent. Assoc., 127,* 244, February, 1996.

Kamen, S. and Skier, J.: Dental Management of the Autistic Child, *Spec. Care Dentist., 5,* 20, January/February, 1985.

Lowe, O. and Lindemann, R.: Assessment of the Autistic Patient's Dental Needs and Ability to Undergo Dental Examination, *ASDC J. Dent. Child., 52,* 29, January–February, 1985.

Shapira, J., Mann, J., Tamari, I., Mester, R., Knobler, H., Yoeli, Y., and Newbrun, E.: Oral Health Status and Dental Needs of an Autistic Population of Children and Young Adults, *Spec. Care Dentist., 9,* 38, March/April, 1989.

Bacterial Plaque Control and Chlorhexidine

Bratel, J. and Berggren, U.: Long-term Oral Effects of Manual or Electric Toothbrushes Used by Mentally Handicapped Adults, *Clin. Prev. Dent., 13,* 5, July/August, 1991.

Burtner, A.P., Low, D.W., McNeal, D.R., Hassell, T.M., and Smith, R.G.: Effects of Chlorhexidine Spray on Plaque and Gingival Health in Institutionalized Persons with Mental Retardation, *Spec. Care Dentist., 11,* 97, May/June, 1991.

Burtner, A.P., Smith, R.G., Tiefenbach, S., and Walker, C.: Administration of Chlorhexidine to Persons With Mental Retardation Residing in an Institution: Patient Acceptance and Staff Compliance, *Spec. Care Dentist., 16,* 53, March/April, 1996.

Chan, J.C. and O'Donnell, D.: Ingestion of Fluoride Dentifrice by a Group of Mentally Handicapped Children During Toothbrushing, *Quintessence Int., 27,* 409, June, 1996.

Chikte, U.M., Pochee, E., Rudolph, M.J., and Reinach, S.G.: Evaluation of Stannous Fluoride and Chlorhexidine Sprays on Plaque and Gingivitis in Handicapped Children, *J. Clin. Periodontol., 18,* 281, May, 1991.

McKenzie, W.T., Forgas, L., Vernino, A.R., Parker, D., and Limestall, J.D.: Comparison of a 0.12% Chlorhexidine Mouthrinse and an Essential Oil Mouthrinse on Oral Health in Institutionalized Mentally Handicapped Adults: One-year Results, *J. Periodontol., 63,* 187, March, 1992.

Ozeki, M., Zinda, K., Matsumoto, S., Ohkouchi, K., Kobayashi, Y., and Moriyama, T.: Bacteriological Examination of Fissure Plaques from Seriously Mentally Retarded Adults, *Caries Res., 24,* 318, Number 5, 1990.

Shapira, J., Sgan-Cohen, H.D., Stabholz, A., Sela, M.N., Schurr, D., and Goultschin, J.: Clinical and Microbiological Effects of Chlorhexidine and Arginine Sustained-release Varnishes in the Mentally Retarded, *Spec. Care Dentist., 14,* 158, July/August, 1994.

Shaw, L., Shaw, M.J., and Foster, T.D.: Correlation of Manual Dexterity and Comprehension with Oral Hygiene and Periodontal Status in Mentally Handicapped Adults, *Community Dent. Oral Epidemiol., 17,* 187, August, 1989.

Stabholz, A., Shapira, J., Shur, D., Friedman, M., Guberman, R., and Sela, M.N.: Local Application of Sustained-release Delivery System of Chlorhexidine in Down's Syndrome Population, *Clin. Prev. Dent., 13,* 9, September/October, 1991.

Stiefel, D.J., Truelove, E.L., Chin, M.M., and Mandel, L.S.: Efficacy of Chlorhexidine Swabbing in Oral Health Care for People with Severe Disabilities, *Spec. Care Dentist., 12,* 57, March/April, 1992.

56

The Patient With a Mental Disorder

A mental disorder is a complex, clinically significant behavioral or psychological syndrome or pattern that is associated with present distress or disability. The causes may be related to behavioral, psychologic, or biologic dysfunction in the individual.[1]

A classification of mental disorders does not classify people, but rather it is the disorders that people have that are classified. For example, the patient should be referred to as "an individual with schizophrenia," not as "a schizophrenic."[1]

With the discovery and official approval of new psychotropic drugs for more effective therapy, and with the current policies of deinstitutionalization, more individuals with mental disorders are seeking dental and dental hygiene care in dental offices and clinics. Care for a person with a psychiatric illness, or

for one who may be undergoing an emotional crisis, presents increased challenges for health professionals.

The American Psychiatric Association has classified more than 200 types of mental disorders in the document *Diagnostic and Statistical Manual of Mental Disorders* (DSM-IV). The DSM is in accord with the International Classification of Diseases (ICD) published by the World Health Organization.[2] A partial list of the classified primary mental disorders is shown in Table 56-1. Each disorder has characteristic signs and symptoms. Terminology related to the disorders is listed and defined in Box 56-1.

This chapter includes descriptions of frequently encountered psychiatric disorders, namely, schizophrenia, mood disorders, anxiety disorders, and eating disorders. Other disorders are described elsewhere in the

TABLE 56-1 Primary Mental Disorders: Classification

COGNITIVE IMPAIRMENT DISORDERS

Delirium
Dementia (HIV, p. 35; Alzheimer's, pp. 687 to 688; Parkinson's,
   p. 784; Alcoholism, p. 836)
   Amnestic Disorders

SUBSTANCE-RELATED DISORDERS

Drugs of abuse, pp. 129 to 131
Nicotine-related disorders, p. 425
Alcohol-related disorders, p. 839

SCHIZOPHRENIA AND OTHER PSYCHOTIC DISORDERS (P. 821)

MOOD DISORDERS

Major Depressive disorder (p. 825)
Bipolar disorder I and II (p. 826)

ANXIETY DISORDERS (P. 828)

Panic disorder with and without agoraphobia
Phobias
Obsessive-compulsive disorder
Post-traumatic stress disorder
Generalized anxiety disorder

SOMATOFORM DISORDERS

Conversion disorder
Hypochondriasis
Body dysmorphic disorder
Pain disorder

FACTITIOUS DISORDERS

Physical symptoms
Psychologic symptoms

DISSOCIATIVE DISORDERS

Dissociative amnesia
Depersonalization disorder

SEXUAL AND GENDER IDENTITY DISORDERS

Sexual dysfunctions
Paraphilias

EATING DISORDERS (P. 830)

Anorexia nervosa
Bulimia nervosa

SLEEP DISORDERS

IMPULSE CONTROL DISORDERS

Kleptomania
Pyromania
Pathologic gambling

PERSONALITY DISORDERS

Paranoid personality disorder
Narcissistic personality disorder

(Adapted from *American Psychiatric Association*, DSM-IV, 1994, pp.
13–24.)

text, for example, alcoholism (Chapter 57), other substance abuse (Chapter 8), Alzheimer's disease (Chapter 46), dementia due to acquired immunodeficiency syndrome (Chapter 2), and dementia due to Parkinson's disease (Chapter 52).

Knowledge of the types of mental disorders and their signs and symptoms can help the clinician to recognize a patient's needs and to understand the patient's behaviors. Confidence and trust by the patient are essential for communication and the patient's acceptance of clinical care.

Principles of informed consent are applied for patients of all ages with mental disorders. Many patients with mental disorders are capable of signing their own consent form. Information for obtaining informed consent is described on page 328.

SCHIZOPHRENIA

Schizophrenia is a complex, chronic mental disorder. Disturbances in feeling, thinking, and behavior significantly impair function to a level below normal for the individual. Schizophrenia is a major psychotic illness in which the individual may be out of touch with reality. Symptoms include delusions, hallucinations, disorganized thinking, and incoherence.

The onset is usually between the ages of 17 and 25 in females, slightly older than for males. Although the cause is not fully understood, genetic factors can make an individual more vulnerable. Periods of remission and recurrence may occur.

I. SYMPTOMS OF SCHIZOPHRENIA

The disturbance progresses from subchronic to remission with acute exacerbations of varying frequencies. Symptoms may be triggered by social, psychologic, or environmental stresses.

The three phases are described as *prodromal, active,* and *residual.* Prodromal symptoms may appear as signs of deterioration for as long as 1 year before the active phase. Table 56-2 shows the symptoms of each phase.

Active-phase symptoms are *positive,* those that reflect unusual, profound behavior, or *negative,* those that show the absence of behavior that might be expected normally.

Rates of alcohol and drug abuse are high among patients with schizophrenia. Many patients diagnosed with schizophrenia also qualify for a diagnosis of alcohol abuse. Drug and alcohol abuse can aggravate psychiatric symptoms and lead to poor treatment compliance, increased hospitalization, homelessness, and suicide.[3]

II. TREATMENT OF SCHIZOPHRENIA

The response to initial treatment is a critical predictor of the long-term prognosis. The prognosis has generally been considered guarded to poor. Evidence shows that, although deterioration may occur during the

BOX 56-1 KEY WORDS: Mental Disorders

Affect (af'ekt): emotion or feeling; tone of reaction to persons and events.

Agitation: excessive motor activity, usually nonpurposeful and associated with internal tension.

Amnestic disorder (am-nes'tik): impaired short- and long-term memory attributed to a specific organic cause.

Anxiolytic medication: ability to relieve anxiety or emotional tension, also called antianxiety agent.

Bradykinesia (brad'e-kin-ne'ze-ah): abnormal slowness of movement; sluggish physical and mental responses.

Catatonia (kat"ah-tō'ne-ah): no voluntary movement; physical rigidity; fixed position may be maintained for hours.

Cognitive (kog'nĭ-tiv): mental process of comprehension, judgment, memory.

Conversion disorder: involuntary alteration or limitation of physical function as a result of psychologic conflict or need, not physical.

Decompensate: appearance or exacerbation of a mental disorder.

Delusion: false belief firmly held though contradicted by social reality.

Dementia (de-men'shē-ah): loss of cognitive and intellectual functions sufficiently severe to interfere with social and occupational functioning.

Dissociation (di-sō"sē-ā'shun): separation; psychologically induced loss of memory, consciousness, or identity.

   Dissociative fugue: unexpected wandering from home or one's customary place of work with inability to recall one's past.

Dysmorphic disorder (dis-mor'fik): imagined belief in a defect in appearance of all or a part of the body.

Euphoria (u-for're-ah): feeling of well-being; in psychiatry, abnormal or exaggerated sense of well-being.

Factitious (fak-tish'us): artificial, self-induced; production of psychologic or physical symptoms to assume a sick role.

Hallucination (hah-lu-sĭ-nā'shun): false sensory perception in the absence of an actual external stimulus.

Hypochondriasis (hī"pō-kon-dri'ah-sĭs): morbid fear or belief that one has a serious disease even though none exists.

Kleptomania (klep-tō-mā'nē-ah): compulsive stealing, without apparent need for the stolen objects.

Insomnia (in-som'ne-ah): wakefulness; inability to sleep in the absence of noise or other disturbance.

Melancholia (mel"an-ko'li-ah): mental state characterized by extreme sadness or depression.

Narcolepsy (nar'ko-lep"se): recurrent attacks of uncontrollable desire to sleep.

Narcissistic personality disorder (nar"sĭ-sis'tik): pervasive pattern of grandiosity and overconcern with issues of self-esteem.

   Narcissism (nar'sĭ-sizm): self-love.

Neurosis (nu-rō'sis): a mental disorder that usually involves the use of unconscious defense mechanisms as a means of coping; individual is not out of touch with reality.

Noncompliance: failure to carry out prescribed health-care plan, for example, failure to take medications as prescribed.

Paranoia (par"ah-noi'ah): mental disorder characterized by delusions of persecution, illusions of grandeur, or combination of both.

Paraphilia (par"ah-fil'ē-ah): sexual interests, impulses, fantasies, or practices that are unusual, deviant, or bizarre.

Perimylolysis (per"ĭ-my-lol'ē-sis): erosion of enamel and dentin as a result of chemical and mechanical effects.

Phobia (fo'be-ah): persistent, unrealistic pathologic fear or dread out of proportion to the stimulus from a particular object or situation.

Prodrome (pro'drom): a premonitory symptom; a symptom indicating the onset of disease.

Psychosis (sī-kō'sis): a significant major mental disorder that so greatly impairs perception, thinking, emotional response, and/or personal orientation that the individual loses touch with reality.

Psychotherapy (sī"kō-ther'ah-pē): treatment of emotional, behavioral, personality, and psychiatric disorders by means of individual or group verbal or nonverbal communication with the patient.

Psychotrophic medication (sī"kō-trop'ik): a medication that alters the mind; the major categories are antipsychotic, antianxiety, antidepressant, an antimanic agents.

Pyromania (pi"ro-ma'ni-ah): obsessive preoccupation with fire; morbid compulsion to set fires.

Somatoform disorder: physical symptoms without organic impairment.

Tardive dyskinesia (tar'div dĭs-kĭ-nē'zē-ah): involuntary movements of the mouth, lips, tongue, and jaws, usually associated with long-term use of antipsychotic medication.

TABLE 56-2 Symptoms of Schizophrenia

Prodromal and Residual Symptoms	Active-Phase Symptoms

Marked social isolation or withdrawal
Marked impairment in role functioning (as wage earner, student, homemaker)
Markedly peculiar behavior
Marked impairment in personal hygiene
Blunted or inappropriate affect
Digressive, vague speech or lack of speech
Odd beliefs or magical thinking
Unusual perceptual experiences
Marked lack of initiative, interests, or energy
	Positive Symptoms
	  Delusions
	  Hallucinations
	  Disorganized speech
	  Catatonia
	  Disorganized or bizarre behavior
	Negative Symptoms
	  Flat affect
	  Lack of voluntary action
	  Speechlessness
	  No pleasure from events that usually give pleasure

(Adapted from *American Psychiatric Association*, DSM-IV, 1994, pp. 285, 290)

early years, the condition may stabilize with treatment during middle age.

A. Pharmacotherapy[4]

The objectives of treatment are to reduce or alleviate the delusions, hallucinations, and other positive symptoms (Table 56-2) and to enable the patient to function in daily living. The use of antipsychotic medications has improved the outcomes of treatment and led to the process of deinstitutionalization.

Schizophrenia is associated with an excess of dopamine at specific synapses in the brain. Medications are used to block dopamine receptors.

1. *Typical Antipsychotic Drugs*[4,5]
   a. Phenothiazines (chlorpromazine [Thorazine])
   b. Butyrophenones (haloperidol [Haldol])
   c. Thioxanthenes (thiothixene [Navane])
2. *Atypical Drugs*
   a. Dibenzodiazepines (clozapine)
   b. Benzisoxazoles (risperidone)

B. Adverse Effects of Medications

Careful monitoring is essential because side effects can be severe. For example, weekly white blood cell counts are needed during clozapine therapy because of the high risk of agranulocytosis.[5] Table 56-3 lists a few of the many side effects of antipsychotic medication with suggestions for appointment adaptations.

C. Maintenance

After an acute episode, the dosage is adjusted for the remission period. A minimal effective dose is important because of the risk of tardive dyskinesia. Noncompliance in continuing medication is a common cause of psychotic relapse and rehospitalization.[4]

D. Psychosocial Therapy

Psychosocial therapy is integrated with pharmacotherapy. Objectives include to ensure compliance with the use of prescribed medications and to give support in the effort to cope with stress.

Long-term treatment for psychosocial and vocational recovery after an acute psychotic episode must include family and all those close to the patient. Psychotherapy may include a variety of vocational rehabilitation efforts and training in social skills.

III. DENTAL HYGIENE CARE

A. Oral Implications[6,7]

1. Overall degeneration of health factors may have occurred because of neglect of diet, exercise, sleep, general cleanliness, personal grooming, and oral care.
2. Concurrent alcohol and/or drug abuse, as well as smoking, can influence dental and periodontal health.
3. Xerostomia leads to an increase in rampant dental caries. Candy used for stimulating saliva can have devastating effects.

B. Appointment Planning

Elective dental and dental hygiene treatment is not carried out during an acute exacerbation. Treatment is undertaken when the patient's symptoms are reasonably controlled by medications.

If the patient decompensates during a dental or dental hygiene appointment, immediate referral is needed. Because schizophrenia can be a lifelong disorder, planning for future oral health is essential.

C. Appointment Interventions

1. Review medical and medications history; study possible drug side effects for necessary appointment modifications (Table 56-3).

TABLE 56-3 Effects of Antipsychotic Medication

Side Effects	Implications for Appointment
Dystonia Muscle contractions	Laryngeal spasm; coughing Unable to turn head
Dysarthria Difficult speech	Communication problem

Parkinson-like syndrome
   Shuffling gait
   Muscular rigidity
   Resting tremor (pill rolling)
   Facial grimacing
   Bradykinesia
	Difficult to gain cooperation
	Patient positioninhg
	Instrument positioning;
	   retraction

Akathisia
   Restlessness
   Pacing
	Plan short appointments

Akinesia
   Loss of voluntary
      movement
   Lethargy, fatigue feelings
	Adjust patient position

Tardive dyskinesia
   Involuntary mouth and
      jaw movements
	Difficulty in instrumentation
	Wearing dentures difficult or
	   impossible
	Muscle fatigue; may need
	   mouth prop

Anticholinergic effects
   Xerostomia
   Blurred vision
	Dental caries prevention
	Fluoride dentifrice; saliva
	   substitute
	Seeing visual aids

Cardiovascular
   Postural hypotension
   Tachycardia, palpitations
	Have patient sit up slowly and
	   wait before standing
	Monitor vital signs

Sedation
   Drowsiness
	Interfere with patient's daily
	   routine
	Patient may be late; needs
	   reminders

Blood
   Reduced leukocytes
   Agranulocytosis
	Increased susceptibility to
	   infection
	Oral candidiasis may be
	   present

2. Review consultation notes from mental health physician (psychiatrist) relative to medications, alcohol or other substance use, and medical-legal competence for informed consent.
3. Plan a simple routine. For a series of appointments and maintenance, use a familiar, organized routine that is comfortable for the patient.
4. Decrease stimulation; create a restful atmos-

phere; if background music is present, keep it low and soft.
   a. Never contradict or argue. Listen with the realization that an answer is not always needed.
   b. Avoid unnecessary physical contact.
5. Provide instruction in oral care.
   a. Help the patient to improve the level of personal oral care on a daily basis.
   b. When applicable, evaluate the patient's personal caregiver for attitude and knowledge and provide information and instruction.
6. Use a mouth prop to assist the patient with tardive dyskinesia. Remember the patient does not have control of mouth movements and can appreciate stability.

MOOD DISORDERS

The primary mood disorders are *major depressive disorder* and *bipolar disorder*. A major depressive disorder is unipolar, whereas a bipolar disorder is marked by severe mood swings from depression to elation (mania). Both unipolar and bipolar disorders are characterized by periods of remission and recurrence.

Depression is among the most common of the many psychiatric illnesses, yet it may not always be recognized and treated. Bipolar disorder may begin by ages 25 to 30, whereas major depression is more often first evident in middle age. All ages may be affected, but middle-aged women and elderly persons of both sexes are particularly vulnerable to severe depression. Risk factors for depression are listed in Table 56-4.

Transient depressed moods occur in the lives of most people. Sadness over unforeseen tragic events, illnesses, death, or disappointments in career or other life plans causes depressed feelings.

Depression is a disturbance marked by apathy, fear, sadness, and loss of mobility and energy. Transient depressed moods usually can be overcome in

TABLE 56-4 Risk Factors for Depression

Prior episodes of depression
Family history of depression
Prior suicide attempts
Female gender
Age of onset <40 years
Postpartum period
Lack of social support
Stressful life events
Personal history of sexual abuse
Current substance abuse

(Adapted from Stuart, G.W. & Sundeen, S.J.: *Principles & Practice of Psychiatric Nursing,* 5th ed., St Louis, Mosby, 1995 p. 431.)

time and need to be differentiated from depression as a major depressive illness.

MAJOR DEPRESSIVE DISORDER

I. CHARACTERISTICS OF A MAJOR DEPRESSIVE EPISODE

Characteristics of a major depressive episode are listed in Table 56-5. Both thought disorders and physical signs are involved. Depression increases the risk of suicide.

The manifestations of depression can vary considerably among patients and between age groups. Some individuals experience only one episode of major depression in their entire lives.

For children, depression interferes with interrelations with other children and with motivations to learn and play. The adolescent may demonstrate with substance abuse, antisocial behavior, school difficulties, and/or poor hygiene.[8]

Depressed adults lack motivation and initiative and may find interactions with people at work or in social settings difficult. Elderly depressed individuals can feel isolated because many friends and family members have passed away. In addition, their lives may be influenced by physical and mental changes associated with aging (pages 686, 690)

II. TREATMENT OF DEPRESSION

Treatment may include lifestyle changes, correction of sleep disorders, new diet and eating patterns, and exercise, along with counseling and practical psychotherapy. Severe depression requires antidepressant medication.

Hospitalization may be indicated when potential danger of suicide or harm to others exists. Severe health problems can be related to self-neglect with excessive weight loss.

A. Psychotherapy

Patients with lesser degrees of depression may benefit from psychotherapy alone. Psychotherapy and pharmacotherapy lend support to each other. Improvement in work performance and social adjustment with increased compliance in carrying out basic personal health needs, including oral hygiene, can be noted.

B. Psychopharmacotherapy[9,10]

Antidepressive medications are indicated for major depression and the depressive stage of bipolar disorder. For a patient with a substance-induced mood disorder, antidepressant or mood-stabilizing therapy is withheld for at least 30 days to confirm medical diagnosis of primary mood disorder.

Antidepressants are also used for other depressive spectrum disorders, premenstrual accentuation of mood problems, panic disorder, social phobia, obsessive-compulsive disorder, bulimia, and migraine.

Each drug has characteristic adverse reactions. Xerostomia is the major oral problem. Although nonaddictive, the tricyclics are toxic in excess amounts and therefore must be prescribed in small quantities, especially for the suicidal patient.

1. SSRIs (Selective Serotonin Re-uptake Inhibitors)
   a. Advantages: tolerability better than earlier drugs; better compliance; safety in overdose.
   b. Specific products: fluoxetine (Prozac); sertraline (Zoloft); paroxetine (Paxil); fluvoxamine (Luvox).
2. Tricyclic Antidepressants: less used than in past; risk of overdose.
3. MAOIs (monoamine oxidase inhibitors): certain foods and other drugs must be avoided to prevent hypertensive crisis.

C. Electroconvulsive Therapy: Indications[10]

1. Patient for whom antidepressant medications are contraindicated.
2. Patient who is nonresponsive to optimal pharmacotherapy.
3. Patient with major depression who also has delusions.
4. Patient with overwhelming suicidal preoccupation or substantially diminished food intake.
5. The need for an immediate response (such as for a catatonic patient).

III. DENTAL HYGIENE CARE

The patient with a major depressive disorder and the patient with the depressive phase of bipolar disorder have the same general characteristics as those described in this section.

A. Personal Factors

The symptoms of the depressed individual not controlled by medication are listed in Table 56-5

TABLE 56-5 Characteristics of a Major Depressive Episode

- Depressed mood
- Markedly diminished interest or pleasure in all or almost all activities
- Significant weight loss or gain
- Insomnia or hypersomnia
- Psychomotor agitation or retardation
- Fatigue or loss of energy
- Feelings of worthlessness or excessive guilt
- Diminished ability to concentrate; indecisiveness
- Recurrent thoughts of death or suicide
- Feelings of hopelessness

(Adapted from *American Psychiatric Association: DSM-IV*, 1994, p. 327.)

and can be considered in preparation for dental hygiene care. By appearance and facial expression the patient may appear to be pessimistic and show feelings of sadness and gloom. Inattentiveness, memory impairment, and diminished motivation are typical. On the other hand, the medicated patient may demonstrate symptoms of the side effects of medication.

When food and alcoholic beverages are used as coping mechanisms, weight gain may be considerable. Food choices frequently include many sweets, which contribute to dental and periodontal breakdown. Oral problems related to alcohol abuse are described on pages 842 to 843.

B. Oral Health Implications[11]
1. Side effects of medications: xerostomia, which leads to high risk of enamel and root caries and to problems of denture retention.
2. Omission of general health habits and neglect of oral care make the person susceptible to various infections and illnesses.
3. Loss of taste perception can contribute to a diet high in cariogenic foods with high levels of sucrose.

C. Appointment Interventions[11,12]
1. *Assessment*
   a. Monitor the medical and medications histories closely; review consultation with medical/psychiatric specialists caring for the patient.
   b. Intraoral/extraoral examination: check for signs of xerostomia.
2. *Approach*
   a. Provide positive reinforcement and reassurance. Avoid negative guilt-inducing words. Depressed patients already blame themselves for all bad things.
   b. Show genuine interest, but avoid attempts to cheer the patient by joking or laughing or making such remarks as, "Let's see you smile now."
3. *Preventive Instruction*
   a. Bacterial plaque control: Teach patient and caregivers the need for daily measures to preserve the teeth and periodontal tissues.
   b. Xerostomia
      i. Home fluoride custom tray daily
      ii. Saliva substitute containing fluoride
      iii. Alcohol-free, over-the-counter fluoride rinse or brush-on gel
4. *Scaling and Debridement*
   a. Adjust dental light carefully and provide tinted protective eyewear for the patient with photosensitivity, a side effect of certain medications.
   b. Use local anesthesia. Anxious and depressed patients can be sensitive and may need profound anesthesia.

c. For a patient with a history of being suicidal, keep sharp instruments out of view of the patient.
d. Provide fluoride treatment after scaling.
e. Use care to prevent postural hypotension. Sit the patient up slowly from a reclined position and have the patient remain seated a few moments before standing.

BIPOLAR DISORDER

Bipolar disorder is the major mood disorder in which episodes of mania (elation) and depression occur. It was formerly called "manic-depressive" disorder. When untreated, periods of elation can average 6 months in duration, whereas periods of depression may last longer. A return to normal behavior between episodes is usual.

I. PHASES AND SYMPTOMS
A. Depressive Phase
The characteristics for a major depressive episode (Table 56-5) and for a depressed episode of bipolar disorder are similar.

B. Manic Phase
Mania is characterized by excessive elation, hyperactivity, and accelerated thinking and speaking. A severe manic episode causes marked impairment in occupational and social functioning. Characteristics of a manic episode are listed in Table 56-6.

C. Mixed
The "mixed" category is used when symptoms of depression and mania are concurrent or when rapid changes between the two states occur within days or weeks.

II. TREATMENT OF BIPOLAR DEPRESSION
Three distinct treatment strategies apply, one for the manic phase, one for the depressive phase, and one

---

TABLE 56-6 Characteristics of Manic Episode

- Inflated self-esteem or grandiosity
- Decreased need for sleep
- More talkative than usual or pressure to keep talking
- Flight of ideas
- Distractibility (that is, attention easily drawn to unimportant or irrelevant external stimuli)
- Increase in goal-directed activity (socially, at work or school, or sexually) or psychomotor agitation
- Excessive involvement in pleasurable activities that have a high potential for painful consequences (for example, engages in unrestrained buying sprees, sexual indiscretions, or foolish business investments)

(Adapted from *American Psychiatric Association: DSM-IV*, 1994, p. 332.)

for the normal phase, which requires maintenance therapy. Treatment for the depressive phase is described under major depression on page 825.

Both pharmacotherapy and psychotherapy are used for the manic phase. Initially, hospitalization may be needed to protect the individual from harm to self or others.

A. Pharmacotherapy[9,13,14]

1. Sedation may be needed for the acute stage of mania when the patient is severely agitated.
2. Mood stablizer: lithium carbonate.[9,13]
   a. Prevents recurrence of bipolar disorder when given on a maintenance drug level.
   b. Possible side effects include gastrointestinal irritation, fine hand tremor, thirst, polyuria, and muscular weakness. Prolonged use may lead to renal tube damage and hypothyroidism.
   c. Frequent monitoring is important to guard against lithium toxicity, which can occur with long-term drug use.
3. Antidepressant therapy may be needed for the patient with moderate to severe bipolar depression to protect against a drug-induced switch to mania.

B. Psychotherapy

Psychotherapy can help to lower stress factors and uncover early warning signs of an approaching high or low mood. Psychosocial support is important to prevent relapse.

III. DENTAL HYGIENE CARE

A. Personal Factors

Characteristics of an individual during a manic episode can be studied in Table 56-6. During the manic phase, the patient is overactive, restless, and in constant motion, and behaves in an aggressive, fearless manner.

Many patients talk quickly, jump from thought to thought, and have a short attention span. A tendency to argue and become irritable may be apparent if pressured in any way.

B. Oral Health Implications

1. Oral hygiene needs are often unmet.
2. Patient unlikely to report injury or illness; a complete oral assessment can be especially significant.
3. Gingival tissues may appear abraded and lacerated because of over-eager grandiose brushing motions.
4. Xerostomia from long-term use of medications will require use of a saliva substitute. A complete preventive program with daily fluoride therapy and an anticariogenic diet is important.
5. Lithium may impart a metallic taste in the mouth.

C. Appointment Interventions

Lithium medication and other treatments usually provide control for the nonhospitalized patient. The need for protecting the patient and others from overactive behavior may not be experienced in the private clinical setting because elective dental and dental hygiene appointments usually are postponed until the patient is under medical control.

1. Simplify the surroundings; provide a comfortable uncluttered environment.
2. Do not rush the patient, as doing so can lead to anger and hostility.
3. Use quiet persuasion; keep the voice firm and low-pitched with a coaxing quality.
4. When applicable, help the patient's caregiver to learn procedures for dental caries prevention and periodontal health.
5. Patient instruction is difficult because the patient has a short attention span and may not like fine detail. Avoid long descriptions.

POSTPARTUM MOOD DISTURBANCES[15]

The puerperium is the 6-week period after childbirth when the body undergoes physical and physiologic changes. During the entire postpartum period, many physiologic and psychologic stresses are related to the changes taking place in the mother's life. Degrees of emotional reactions are evident and range from postpartum blues to psychosis. Postpartum psychosis is considered a major psychiatric emergency.

I. POSTPARTUM BLUES

A period of nonpsychotic depression for a few days after giving birth is not uncommon. There may be crying, irritability, and mood shifts.

II. POSTPARTUM DEPRESSION

A moderate to severe depression may begin by the second to third week postpartum. Symptoms include excessive fatigue, insomnia, loss of appetite, and loss of interest and enthusiasm.

III. POSTPARTUM PSYCHOSIS

Postpartum or puerperal psychosis is a mood disorder. It may be of a depressive or manic type.

A. Underlying Causes

1. Secondary to pre-existing mental illness, such as bipolar disorder or schizophrenia.
2. Stress.
3. Conflicts about motherhood, such as unwanted pregnancy, fears about mothering, and marital problems.

B. Symptoms

1. *Early.* Complaints of insomnia, restlessness,

tearfulness, fatigue, and emotional unsteadiness.

2. *Progressive.* Confusion, irrationality, delirium,
   and obsessive concerns about the baby.
   Thoughts of bringing harm to the baby or
   oneself are not unusual.

C. Treatment

Without treatment, risk of suicide, infanticide,
or both exists. A favorable outcome can be expected with appropriate treatment, family support, and no pre-existing illness.

1. *Medical Care.* Treat for other (organic) illnesses.
2. *Suicidal Precautions.* Baby should not be left
   alone with mother.
3. *Pharmacotherapy.* In accord with symptoms of
   depression.
4. *Psychotherapy.* Individual and marital. Arrangements for assistance at home must be
   made before hospital release.
5. *Extended Treatment.* Counseling in infant care
   with observation for emergence of major
   mood disorder.

ANXIETY DISORDERS

Anxiety is experienced as apprehension, tension, or
dread that results from the anticipation of danger, the
source of which is unknown or unrecognized. Anxiety is the result of feeling a threat to the person's
being, self-esteem, or identity. Fear, on the other
hand, is an emotional or physiologic response to a
recognized source of danger.

In normal life, some mild anxiety provides an effective stimulus to improved performance. As a psychiatric symptom, anxiety can be excessive, irrational,
and beyond the control of the individual.

I. TYPES AND SYMPTOMS OF ANXIETY DISORDERS[16]

The types of anxiety disorders are listed in Table 56-7.
The disorders have symptoms of fear, excess worry,

TABLE 56-7 Anxiety Disorders

- Panic disorder without agoraphobia
- Panic disorder with agoraphobia
- Agoraphobia without history of panic disorder
- Specific phobia
- Social phobia
- Obsessive-compulsive disorder
- Post-traumatic stress disorder
- Acute stress disorder
- Generalized anxiety disorder
- Anxiety disorder due to a general medical condition
- Substance-induced (intoxication/withdrawal) anxiety disorder

(Adapted from *American Psychiatric Association: DSM-IV*, 1994, p. 393.)

TABLE 56-8 Symptoms of Panic Attack

- Shortness of breath
- Dizziness, unsteady feelings, or faintness
- Palpitations or accelerated heart rate
- Trembling or shaking
- Sweating (clammy hands)
- Choking
- Nausea or abdominal stress
- Numbness or tingling sensations
- Flushes (hot flashes) or chills
- Chest pain or discomfort
- Fear of dying
- Fear of going crazy or losing control

(Adapted from *American Psychiatric Association: DSM-IV*, 1994, p. 395.)

---

and avoidance behavior that are revealed in a variety
of ways and degrees of severity. The anxiety disorders
also can produce varying degrees of occupational and
social dysfunction. Certain patients may have secondary problems of alcohol and other substance
abuse. The abuse may be the result of an attempt at
self-medication.

A. Panic Attack

The symptoms that may occur in a panic attack
are listed in Table 56-8. The panic attack itself is
a symptom in several of the anxiety disorders.
*An overwhelming sense of impending doom is the
cardinal symptom of the attack.*

A panic attack may be unexpected (uncued)
or "situationally bound" (cued). A situationally
bound panic attack invariably results from exposure to a specific trigger. Such triggers are
characteristic of social and specific phobias that
are described in this section.

B. Panic Disorder

Panic disorder is characterized by recurrent
panic attacks that are usually unexpected.
Panic disorder may occur alone or with agoraphobia.

Agoraphobia is the fear of being in places or
situations from which escape might be difficult
or embarrassing or in which help might not be
available in the event of a panic attack. The fear
is of open spaces, of crowds, or of going outside
the home alone and away from a safe place.

C. Agoraphobia Without History of Panic Disorder

Agoraphobic fear may be related to a genuine
medical concern. An example is a nonpsychi-
atric medical condition, such as a heart attack
after which the patient avoids leaving home,
especially alone.

D. Phobic Disorder

1. *Specific Phobic Stimulus.* Examples include fear
   of heights, such as riding in an elevator or

airplane, certain animals, fire, or the sight of blood.

2. *Social Phobia.* Examples include the inability to speak in public or to be in a situation in which the individual can be exposed to possible scrutiny and thus fears that he or she may show humiliating anxiety symptoms.

3. *Reaction.* The individual must avoid the phobic stimulus, endure it with marked stress, or have an anxiety reaction, perhaps in the form of a panic attack (Table 56-8).

E. Obsessive-Compulsive Disorder[17]

Obsessive thoughts and compulsive actions characterize this disorder. The disorder may begin in early childhood or early adulthood, and unless specific treatment is introduced, the condition may last throughout life.

1. *Obsessions.* An obsession is a repetitive intrusive thought or impulse. Preoccupation with a single idea can result in neglect of daily work and other responsibilities.

2. *Compulsions.* Compulsions are repetitive, ritualistic behaviors or mental acts that the individual is compelled to perform against the person's conscious wishes or standards. Examples are counting, frequent handwashing, and checking and rechecking.

F. Posttraumatic Stress Disorder

An initiating traumatic event has occurred outside the range of usual human experience. It may be destruction to the home or family, or may result from a manmade disaster, such as war, imprisonment, torture, rape, or other exposure associated with intense horror, fear, or serious threat to life. A child may have stress disorder brought on by physical or sexual abuse.

Flashbacks of the traumatic experience and the attendant terror may be precipitated by a stimulus that can be readily associated with the original event. Through dreams or recollections, the patient may have the feeling of reliving the event. Symptoms of depression or panic attacks may be evident in an acute episode.

G. Generalized Anxiety Disorder

There is persistent, pervasive anxiety and excessive worry but not associated with life-threatening fears or "attacks." It may be complicated by depression, alcohol abuse, or anxiety related to a general medical condition.

II. TREATMENT OF ANXIETY DISORDERS[18,19]

A. Basic Therapeutic Approach

1. Eliminate the intake of caffeine, alcohol, and drugs of abuse. Anxiety disorders are frequently complicated by alcohol abuse.

2. Diagnose and treat other medical and psychiatric problems. Anxiety disorders may emerge with depression, which should be treated first or at least simultaneously.

3. Exercise. Participation in vigorous aerobics or an active sport helps to eliminate physical and psychologic symptoms and enhances the patient's sense of control. Working and keeping busy are important.

B. Cognitive-Behavioral Therapy

For phobic disorders, compulsive actions, and the event associated with a posttraumatic stress disorder, repeated exposure to a feared object, act, or situation may help to overcome the problem. The support of family and friends can be significant.

A skilled behavioral therapist is needed. Relaxation, biofeedback, and other behavioral therapies have shown selective successes.

C. Pharmacotherapy

As few medications as possible should be used. Treatment can best be focused on the patient's sleeping habits, physical activity, and attainment of personal control in general. Determination of a patient's specific problem is essential because treatment for each disorder is different. When treatment is indicated, antianxiety and antidepressant medications are the drugs of choice.

1. *Antianxiety Medications.*[18,19] Benzodiazepines.
   a. Objectives. Reduce tension and relieve anxiety; induce sleep.
   b. Prescription. Short-term basis for immediate need only; gradual discontinuance to prevent withdrawal symptoms.
   c. Possible side effects. Confusion, dizziness, muscle weakness, difficulty in speaking, skin rash.
   d. Adverse effects. Potential for addiction, withdrawal symptoms, diminished alertness (drowsiness), impaired eye-hand coordination, xerostomia.

2. *Antidepressant Medication.* Antidepressants may be used in the treatment of panic attack (page 825).

III. DENTAL HYGIENE CARE

A. Personal Factors

Each anxiety disorder has its own specific characteristics. Individuals suffering from an anxiety disorder maintain contact with reality and may be aware of the type of their disorder. Relationships with other people are often strained.

Physical complaints, such as rapid heart beat, hyperventilation, tightness in the throat, and constant fatigue, are common. Such symptoms may lead to an anxiety about the anxiety.

B. Oral Implications

1. Hypersensitivity of the teeth, related to patient's general tenseness and irritability, may be present.

2. Xerostomia related to medications can cause severe problems for dental caries. Candy or cariogenic beverages used to allay dry mouth lead to enamel and root caries.

3. Oral cleanliness may not be present, even in a patient with an obsession for cleanliness. The opposite may be true, however, and a patient may perform such excessive, vigorous tooth brushing that gingival and dental abrasion result.

C. Appointment Interventions[17]

1. Help the patient to feel in control. Patient may appear very nervous, jumpy, and tense. Accept the patient without judgment or criticism. Attempting to change behavior could cause symptoms of panic attack.

2. Explain each step to the patient and keep communication as open as possible. When the patient must remain still, such as during sealant placement, explain and then distract with trivial chatter.

3. Effective pain control is needed for these highly nervous, anxious patients. Use local anesthesia for subgingival scaling. Provide gentle, painless injections.

4. Appointments are best scheduled in the morning; patient should not have to wait in the reception area unnecessarily; length of appointment can be minimized and planned to prevent stress.

5. Be alert to symptoms of panic attack (Table 56-8), such as sweating or hyperventilation. Allow the patient to sit up and enjoy short breaks.

EATING DISORDERS

Anorexia nervosa, bulimia nervosa, and bulimarexia (a combination of the two) are examples of serious eating disorders. They occur primarily in adolescent girls and young adult women, but men and people of other age groups may be involved. The incidence and awareness of the conditions have increased possibly because of better recognition and diagnosis.

Recognition of the oral manifestations can lead to detection of the patient's problem. Referral and medical evaluation may be life saving because serious medical problems may exist and psychiatric therapy may be indicated. Because of patient resistance and denial, however, referral for help may be difficult or impossible.

An interdisciplinary team approach for successful rehabilitation of an individual with an eating disorder involves, at the least, medical, psychiatric, nutritional, dental, and dental hygiene professionals. Sometimes dental and dental hygiene care must be postponed until the eating disorder is under control. For other patients, definitive dental care can provide the patient

with confidence and encouragement through improved esthetics and relief from tooth sensitivity.

ANOREXIA NERVOSA[20,21,22]

The syndrome anorexia nervosa is characterized by a refusal of the individual to maintain body weight over the minimal normal weight for age and height. The aversion to eating results in life-threatening weight loss.

Anorexia involves self-imposed starvation that results from an obsessive desire to be thin and a marked fear of gaining weight. Perceptual disturbances relative to body image are present (Figure 56-1). The course of the disease may continue until hospitalization is necessary to prevent death.

I. SIGNS AND SYMPTOMS

The characteristics of anorexia nervosa are listed in Table 56-9. The two types are defined in the table. Many anorectic persons have major depression or a family history of major depression or bipolar disorder.

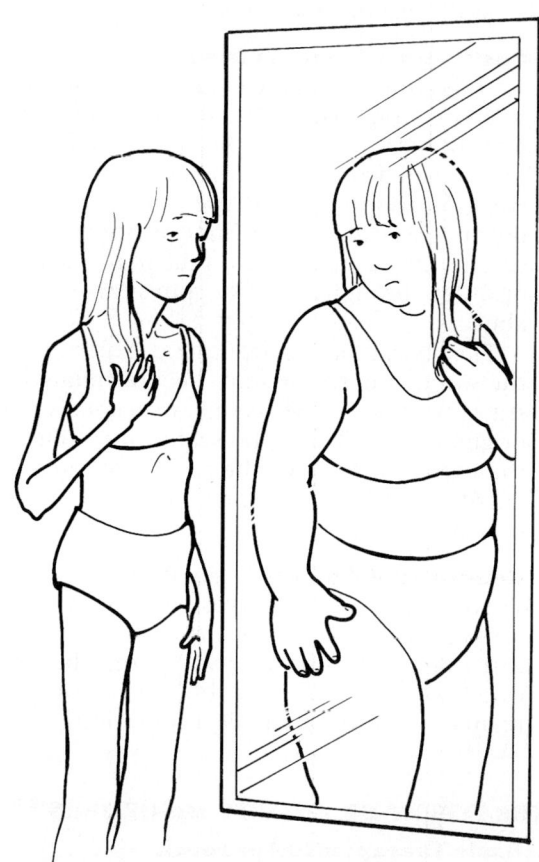

■ **FIGURE 56-1 Anorexia Nervosa.** The person with anorexia typically has a distorted body self-image. Although small and waif-like in real life, the mirror image appears as an overweight individual.

TABLE 56-9 Characteristics of Anorexia Nervosa
• Refusal to maintain body weight over a minimally normal weight for age and height.
• Intense fear of gaining weight or becoming fat, even though underweight.
• Disturbance in the way in which one's body weight or shape is experienced.
• Denies the seriousness of the current low body weight
• In females, absence of menstrual cycles when otherwise expected to occur.
TYPES
Restricting Type: does not regularly engage in binge-eating or purging behavior (i.e., self-induced vomiting or misuse of laxatives, diuretics, or enemas)
Binge-Eating/Purging Type: regularly engages in binge-eating or purging behavior (i.e., self-induced vomiting or the misuse of laxatives, diuretics, or enemas)
(Adapted from *American Psychiatric Association: DSM-IV,* 1994, pp. 544–545.)

A. General Characteristics

1. Severe weight loss with emaciation; "waif-like" appearance.
2. Refusal to eat, yet a preoccupation with food; strange habits, such as hoarding but not eating food (except in the binge-eating/purging type, when recurrent episodes of binge eating do occur).
3. Hyperactivity and excessive exercising.
4. Abuse of diuretics and laxatives.
5. Dry, flaky skin, brittle fingernails; hair growth on the arms and face.

B. Medical Complications

1. *Malnutrition and Dehydration.*
2. *Vital Signs.* Low pulse rate, hypotension, decreased respiratory rate, and low body temperature.
3. *Metabolic Changes.* Gastrointestinal, cardiovascular, hematologic, and renal system disturbances.
4. *Amenorrhea.*

II. TREATMENT OF ANOREXIA[20,21]

Medical and psychiatric therapies are necessary, with hospitalization for the severely ill patient. The primary objectives are to promote weight gain and restore the nutritional status. Treatment may require months or even years.

Pharmacotherapeutic agents are not usually involved, although the patient may be taking antidepressants, tranquilizers, antipsychotics, or antianxiety medication. Vitamin supplements may have been prescribed.

Psychotherapy varies and involves individual behavior modification, as well as group and family therapies. Professional therapists can help the individual to discover the underlying causes of the problems and the sources of the anorectic and bulimic behaviors.

III. DENTAL HYGIENE CARE

A. Personal Factors

The individual with anorexia is frequently engaged in excessive exercise and preoccupied with food and weight loss. Depression may be apparent and shown by crying spells, sleep disturbances, and even thoughts of suicide. The person frequently is a high achiever and highly motivated scholastically, but is socially isolated, withdrawn, and shy.

B. Oral Implications

1. Xerostomia from medications, leading to enamel and cervical root caries.
2. Perimylolysis and other findings of bulimia can be noted in the binge-eating/purging–type of anorexia.

C. Appointment Interventions

1. Respect the patient's shy, anxious manner. Gently encourage the patient to talk to develop rapport.
2. Recognize that denial of anorexia is common.
3. Be aware that answers to medical and personal history questions concerning diet, medications, use of laxatives and diuretics, and weight and weight loss may provide strong suspicions of anorexia or bulimarexia.
4. Assess the nutritional status through use of a dietary assessment.
5. Record vital signs.
6. Introduce a concentrated preventive program. Apply significant points itemized for bulimia.

BULIMIA NERVOSA[21,22,23]

Bulimia nervosa is a psychiatric compulsive disorder marked by recurrent episodes of uncontrollable binge eating. The two types of bulimic individuals are known as the purging type and the nonpurging type (Table 56-10). Because of the fear of becoming overweight, self-induced vomiting after eating or the use of laxatives or diuretics is characteristic of the purging type, whereas the nonpurging type uses strict dieting, fasting, and/or vigorous exercise.

The individual with bulimarexia has bulimic-type anorexia and shows symptoms of both anorexia and bulimia. All of these individuals are concerned with body weight and shape.

I. SIGNS AND SYMPTOMS

The characteristics of a person with bulimia nervosa are listed in Table 56-10. The illness may last over

TABLE 56-10 Characteristics of Bulimia Nervosa

- Recurrent episodes of binge eating. An episode of binge eating is characterized by both the following:

    Eating, within any 2-hour period, an amount of food that is definitely larger than most people would eat in a similar period of time.

    A sense of lack of control over eating during the episode, for example, a feeling that one cannot stop eating or control what or how much one is eating.

- Recurrent inappropriate behavior to prevent weight gain, such as self-induced vomiting; misuse of laxatives, diuretics, enemas; fasting; or excessive exercise.

- Self-evaluation is unduly influenced by body shape and weight.

TYPES

Purging Type: regularly engages in self-induced vomiting or the misuse of laxatives, diuretics, or enemas.

Nonpurging Type: uses inappropriate compensatory behaviors such as fasting or excessive exercise, but does not engage in self-induced vomiting or the misuse of laxatives, diuretics, or enemas.

(Adapted from *American Psychiatric Association, DSM-IV*, 1994, pp. 549–550.)

many years, and may alternate with periods of normal eating or periods of fasting.

A. General Characteristics

1. Normal body weight or slightly overweight is typical in contrast to the thin anorectic person.
2. Food consumed during a binge may include cariogenic items with a high caloric content, sweet taste, and a texture that allows rapid eating. Often, favorite foods are selected.
3. Drug and/or alcohol abuse by the patient or in the family history is not uncommon.

B. Medical Complications

1. Problems include dehydration, electrolyte imbalance, protein malnutrition, and cardiac arrhythmia.
2. Self-medications include abuse of laxatives and diuretics, which contribute to gastrointestinal disturbances.
3. Amenorrhea when the person also has a history of anorexia nervosa.
4. Complications of drug and alcohol abuse.

II. TREATMENT OF BULIMIA

Electrolyte imbalance and metabolic disturbances may necessitate hospitalization. Antidepressants may be prescribed because anxiety and depressive symptoms are common.

Treatment is focused on the psychologic aspects with individual psychotherapy and family group ther-

apy. Behavior modification is particularly important in the attempt to help the patient practice a normal eating pattern.

III. DENTAL HYGIENE CARE

A. Personal Factors

The individual with bulimia nervosa tends to be socially extroverted and outgoing in contrast to the shy, introverted person with anorexia. Like the anorectic person, perfectionism in life is sought, especially physical perfection through body shape and weight. The patient is well aware that the eating habits are abnormal, and may suffer low self-esteem and guilt feelings.

B. Oral Findings[24,25]

1. *Perimylolysis.* Perimylolysis is the chemical erosion of the tooth surfaces by acid from the regurgitation of stomach contents. After vomiting, acid is retained by the tongue papillae and provides longer contact with the palatal surfaces of maxillary teeth.

    The earliest evidence of bulimia may be on the smooth palatal surfaces of the teeth. With time, the erosion extends over the occlusal and incisal surfaces. The mandibular teeth are protected in part by the tongue, lips, and cheeks.

2. *Restorations.* Restorations may appear raised because of erosion of the enamel around the margins.

3. *Dental Caries.* An increase in caries incidence is found, particularly in cervical caries. Demineralization results from the pH changes in the saliva, from xerostomia, and from the large quantities of cariogenic foods ingested during binges.

4. *Saliva.* The decrease in quantity, quality, and pH of the saliva limits its buffering and lubricating properties. Dehydration of the oral soft tissues occurs.

5. *Xerostomia.* Body fluid is lost from vomiting and the use of diuretics. Xerostomia is also a side effect of antidepressant medication prescribed for certain patients with bulimia and anorexia.

6. *Hypersensitive Teeth.* The loss of enamel and the exposure of dentin results in sensitivity, which can be especially noticeable for the maxillary anterior teeth.

7. *Oral Trauma*

    a. The soft palate can be traumatized by fingers, comb, pencils, or toothbrush used to induce vomiting. The same implement may injure the mouth at the commissures.

    b. Pharyngeal trauma is caused by a large food bolus that is swallowed or regurgitated.

    c. Callous formation or scars on fingers or

knuckles used for self-induced vomiting may be seen.

8. *Parotid Gland.* Enlargement may occur for 2 to 6 days after a binge. A cause for the enlargement is not known, but it has been related to malnutrition.

9. *Bruxism.* Tooth wear related to stress and tension.

10. *Taste.* Impairment of taste perception.

C. Appointment Interventions

1. Patient instruction in cause and prevention of perimylolysis and dental caries.
   a. Reduce use of cariogenic foods; provide list of suggestions for substituting sugar-free products.
   b. Improve personal oral care. Show use of appropriate brushing and flossing with additional interdental aids if required for plaque removal. Clean the tongue (page 365).
   c. Do not brush after vomiting. Demineralization of the tooth surface by the acid from the stomach starts immediately on contact. Brushing may abrade the demineralized areas. Remineralization can be helped by an alkaline rinse of sodium bicarbonate or magnesium hydroxide solution to neutralize the acid. A 0.05% neutral sodium fluoride rinse should also be used.

2. Fluoride therapy to reduce dental hypersensitivity and build resistance of teeth to acid demineralization.
   a. Use fluoride dentifrice with several brushings daily.
   b. Use neutral pH sodium fluoride mouthrinse (0.05%) daily.
   c. Custom-fitted tray for daily home application (1.1 neutral sodium fluoride gel) (pages 469 to 472).

3. Reduction in problems caused by xerostomia.
   a. Advise sugar-free mints or chewing gum if patient uses them to stimulate saliva flow.
   b. Recommend saliva substitutes containing fluoride (page 346).

4. Reduction in problems caused by hypersensitive teeth.
   a. Use sugar-free foods and other products.
   b. Use fluoride dentifrice, mouthrinse, and gel tray to ease the sensitivity. (Additional suggestions can be found in Chapter 37, page 600.)

PSYCHIATRIC EMERGENCIES

I. PSYCHIATRIC EMERGENCY

A psychiatric emergency in a dental clinic or private dental practice would be rare. The most common causes of emergency include panic attack, atypical drug reaction, and schizophrenic or manic decompensation.[26]

II. RISK PATIENTS FOR EMERGENCIES

A. Patient with a significant psychiatric history.
B. Patient with a known substance abuse history.
C. Patient new to the clinic or office; not known by the practitioners.

III. PREVENTION OF EMERGENCIES

A. Prepare a complete history: collect as much information as possible; consult with the patient's physician and psychiatrist.
B. Be alert to risks and characteristic symptoms of each disorder.
C. Learn and apply all the principles of stress management.
D. Know the patient's medications and when they are taken. Request that patient (or caregiver if accompanied) have readily available any necessary medication that may be effective in an emergency.
E. Develop rapport with each patient; do not confront or threaten a patient who may react.

IV. PREPARATION FOR AN EMERGENCY

A. Attend to surroundings, such as door access, objects in the room.
B. Arrange for colleagues to be aware of the possible needs of a special patient appointment; plan for an assistant to participate in clinical procedures.
C. Review characteristics of specific emergencies; have necessary equipment ready.
D. Keep names of the patient's case worker, psychiatrist, and responsible family member in the record in a prominent position for ready reference.

V. INTERVENTION

A. Panicked Patient

1. Stay with the patient; request colleague to contact patient's case worker, psychiatrist, or other responsible person.
2. Maintain a calm, serene manner; talk quietly but firmly.
3. Move the patient to a quiet, less stimulating environment. The dental equipment and environment may have contributed to the patient's disturbance.
4. Assist with medication when indicated.

B. Other General Emergencies

See Chapter 61, Table 61-5, page 910, and 61-6, page 915.

REFERENCES

1. **American Psychiatric Association:** *Diagnostic and Statistical Manual of Mental Disorders, DSM-IV,* 4th ed. Washington, DC, American Psychiatric Association, 1994, p. xxi.
2. **World Health Organization:** *International Classification of Diseases (ICD-10).* Geneva, World Health Organization, 1993.
3. **Selzer,** J.A. and Lieberman, J.A.: Schizophrenia and Substance Abuse, *Psych. Clin. North Am., 16,* 401, June, 1993.
4. **Kane,** J.M.: Drug Therapy: Schizophrenia, *N. Engl. J. Med., 334,* 34, January 4, 1996.
5. **Meltzer,** H.Y. and Fatemi, S.H.: Schizophrenia, in Rakel, R.E., ed.: *Conn's Current Therapy, 1997.* Philadelphia, W.B. Saunders Co., 1997, pp. 1161–1166.
6. **Steifel,** D.J., Truelove, E.L., Menard, T.W., Anderson, V.K., Doyle, P.E., and Mandel, L.S.: A Comparison of the Oral Health of Persons With and Without Chronic Mental Illness in Community Settings, *Spec. Care Dentist., 10,* 6, January/February, 1990.
7. **Friedlander,** A.H. and Liberman, R.P.: Oral Health Care for the Patient with Schizophrenia, *Spec. Care Dentist., 11,* 179, September/October, 1991.
8. **Friedlander,** A.H., Friedlander, I.K., Yagiela, J.A., and Eth, S.: Dental Management of the Child and Adolescent With a Major Depression, *ASDC J. Dent. Child., 60,* 125, March–April, 1993.
9. **Berlow,** R. and Akiskal, H.S.: Mood (Affective) Disorders, in Rakel, R.E., ed.: *Conn's Current Therapy, 1997.* Philadelphia, W.B. Saunders Co., 1997, pp. 1154–1161.
10. **Potter,** W.Z., Rudorfer, M.V., and Manji, H.: The Pharmacologic Treatment of Depression, *N. Engl. J. Med., 325,* 633, August 29, 1991.
11. **Friedlander,** A.H. and West, L.J.: Dental Management of the Patient With Major Depression, *Oral Surg. Oral Med. Oral Pathol., 71,* 573, May, 1991.
12. **Friedlander,** A.H., Kawakami, K.K., Ganzell, S., and Fitten, L.J.: Dental Management of the Geriatric Patient With Major Depression, *Spec. Care Dentist., 13,* 249, November/December, 1993.
13. **Price,** L.H. and Heninger, G.R.: Lithium in the Treatment of Mood Disorders, *N. Engl. J. Med., 331,* 591, September 1, 1994.
14. **Stuart,** G.W. and Sundeen, S.J.: *Principles & Practice of Psychiatric Nursing,* 5th ed. St. Louis, Mosby–Year Book, 1995, pp. 680–683.
15. **Parry,** B.L.: Postpartum Psychiatric Syndromes, in Kaplan, H.I. and Sadock, B.J., eds.: *Comprehensive Textbook of Psychiatry/VI.* Baltimore, Williams & Wilkins, 1995, pp. 1059–1066.
16. **Tancer,** M.E. and Uhde, T.W.: Anxiety Disorders, in Rakel, R.E., ed.: *Conn's Current Therapy, 1997.* Philadelphia, W.B. Saunders Co., 1997, pp. 1147–1151.
17. **Friedlander,** A.H. and Serafetinides, E.A.: Dental Management of the Patient with Obsessive-Compulsive Disorder, *Spec. Care Dentist., 11,* 238, November/December, 1991.
18. **Woods,** S.W. and Goddard, A.W.: Panic Disorder, in Rakel, R.E., ed.: *Conn's Current Therapy, 1997.* Philadelphia, W.B. Saunders Co., 1997, pp. 1166–1168.
19. **Stuart** and Sundeen: op. cit., pp. 669–673.
20. **American Psychiatric Association:** op. cit., pp. 539–544.
21. **Brown,** S. and Bonifazi, D.Z.: An Overview of Anorexia and Bulimia Nervosa, and the Impact of Eating Disorders on the Oral Cavity, *Compend. Cont. Educ. Dent., 14,* 1594, December, 1993.
22. **Robb,** N.D. and Smith, B.G.N.: Anorexia and Bulimia Nervosa (the Eating Disorders): Conditions of Interest to the Dental Practitioner, *J. Dent., 24,* 7, January/March, 1996.
23. **American Psychiatric Association:** op. cit., pp. 545–550.
24. **Mueller,** J.A.: Eating Disorders. Identification and Intervention, *DentalHygienistNews, 8,* 3, Winter, 1995.
25. **Burke,** F.J.T., Bell, T.J., Ismail, N., and Hartley, P.: Bulimia: Implications for the Practising Dentist, *Br. Dent. J., 180,* 421, June 8, 1996.
26. **Storrie-Lombardi,** M.C., Storrie-Lombardi, I.J., Margon, C., and Stiefel, D.J., eds.: *Dental Treatment of the Patient with a Major Psychiatric Disorder.* A Self-instructional Series in Rehabilitation Dentistry. Seattle, University of Washington School of Dentistry, 1987, p. 36.

SUGGESTED READINGS

Asher, R.S., McDowell, J.D., and Winquist, H.: HIV-related Neuropsychiatric Changes: Concerns for Dental Professionals, *J. Am. Dent. Assoc., 124,* 80, August, 1993.

Avorn, J., Soumerai, S.B., Everitt, D.E., Ross-Degnan, D., Beers, M.H., Sherman, D., Salem-Schatz, S.R., and Fields, D.: A Randomized Trial of a Program to Reduce the Use of Psychoactive Drugs in Nursing Homes, *N. Engl. J. Med., 327,* 168, July 16, 1992.

Bickley, S.R.: Dental Hygienists' Attitudes Towards Dental Care for People With a Mental Handicap and Their Perceptions of the Adequacy of Their Training, *Br. Dent. J., 168,* 361, May 5, 1990.

Canning, E.H., Hanser, S.B., Shade, K.A., and Boyce, W.T.: Mental Disorders in Chronically Ill Children: Parent-Child Discrepancy and Physician Identification, *Pediatrics, 90,* 692, November, 1992.

Chiodo, G.T. and Rosenstein, D.I.: Tardive Dyskinesia, *Gen. Dent., 38,* 289, July–August, 1990.

Friedlander, A.H., Mills, M.J., and Cummings, J.L.: Consent for Dental Therapy in Severely Ill Patients, *Oral Surg. Oral Med. Oral Pathol., 65,* 179, February, 1988.

Hede, B.: Dental Health Behavior and Self-reported Dental Health Problems Among Hospitalized Psychiatric Patients in Denmark, *Acta Odontol. Scand., 53,* 35, February, 1995.

Hede, B. and Petersen, P.E.: Self-assessment of Dental Health Among Danish Noninstitutionalized Psychiatric Patients, *Spec. Care Dentist., 12,* 33, January/February, 1992.

Kessler, R.C., Frank, R.G., Edlund, M., Katz, S.J., Lin, E., and Leaf, P.: Differences in the Use of Psychiatric Outpatient Services Between the United States and Ontario, *N. Engl. J. Med., 336,* 551, February 20, 1997.

Kinney, R.K., Gatchel, R.J., Ellis, E., and Holt, C.: Major Psychological Disorders in Chronic TMD Patients: Implications for Successful Management, *J. Am. Dent. Assoc., 123,* 49, October, 1992.

Milgrom, P., Weinstein, P., Roy-Byrne, P., and Tay, K.-M.: Dental Fear Treatment Outcomes for Substance Use Disorder Patients, *Spec. Care Dentist., 13,* 139, July/August, 1993.

Reveal, M. and Lemon, S.: Survey of Dental Hygienists Perceptions of Their Educational Preparation Regarding Oral Care for the Mentally Ill, *J. Dent. Hyg., 65,* 20, January, 1991.

Schizophrenia

Baldessarini, R.J. and Frankenburg, F.R.: Clozapine. A Novel Antipsychotic Agent, *N. Engl. J. Med., 324,* 746, March 14, 1991.

Carpenter, W.T. and Buchanan, R.W.: Schizophrenia, *N. Engl. J. Med., 330,* 681, March 10, 1994.

Clark, D.B.: Dental Care for the Psychiatric Patient: Chronic Schizophrenia, *J. Can. Dent. Assoc., 58,* 912, November, 1992.

Friedlander, A.H.: The Dental Management of Patients with Schizophrenia, *Spec. Care Dentist., 6,* 217, September/October, 1986.

Friedlander, A.H., Friedlander, I.K., Eth, S., and Freymiller, E.G.: Dental Management of Child and Adolescent Patients with Schizophrenia, *ASDC J. Dent. Child., 60,* 281, July–October, 1993.

Meltzer, H.Y.: New Drugs for the Treatment of Schizophrenia, *Psychiatr. Clin. North Am., 16,* 365, June, 1993.

Shaner, A., Eckman, T.A., Roberts, L.J., Wilkins, J.N., Tucker, D.E., Tsung, J.W., and Mintz, J.: Disability Income, Cocaine Use, and Repeated Hospitalization Among Schizophrenic Cocaine Abusers. A Government-sponsored Revolving Door? *N. Engl. J. Med., 333,* 777, September 21, 1995.

Thomas, A., Lavrentzou, E., Karouzos, C., and Kontis, C.: Factors Which Influence the Oral Condition of Chronic Schizophrenia Patients, *Spec. Care Dentist., 16,* 84, March/April, 1996.

Depression

Biron, C.R.: Antidepressants, *RDH, 15,* 34, January, 1995.

Chambers, C.D., Johnson, K.A., Dick, L.M., Felix, R.J., and Jones, K.L.: Birth Outcomes in Pregnant Women Taking Fluoxetine, *N. Engl. J. Med., 335,* 1010, October 3, 1996.

Eisenberg, L.: Treating Depression and Anxiety in Primary Care. Closing the Gap Between Knowledge and Practice, *N. Engl. J. Med., 326,* 1080, April 16, 1992.

Friedlander, A.H.: The Dental Management of Depressed Patients, *Spec. Care Dentist.,* 7, 65, March/April, 1987.

Friedlander, A.H. and Brill, N.Q.: The Dental Management of Patients with Bipolar Disorder, *Oral Surg. Oral Med. Oral Pathol.,* 61, 579, June, 1986.

Haddad, L.M.: Managing Tricyclic Antidepressant Overdose, *Am. Fam. Phys.,* 46, 153, July, 1992.

Nulman, I., Rovet, J., Stewart, D.E., Wolpin, J., Gardner, H.A., Theis, J.G.W., Kulin, N., and Koren, G.: Neurodevelopment of Children Exposed in Utero to Antidepressant Drugs, *N. Engl. J. Med.,* 336, 258, January 23, 1997.

Ramsey, R.D.: Clinical Depression: A Debilitating Disease, *RDH,* 14, 44, October, 1994.

Robert, E.: Treating Depression in Pregnancy (Editorial), *N. Engl. J. Med.,* 335, 1056, October 3, 1996.

Wolfe, F.: Soul-deep Blues, *RDH,* 17, 28, March, 1997.

Anxiety

Biron, C.R.: Antianxiety Drugs, *RDH,* 14, 24, March, 1994.

Enneking, B.A., Milgrom, P., Weinstein, P., and Getz, T.: Treatment Outcomes for Specific Subtypes of Dental Fear: Preliminary Clinical Findings, *Spec. Care Dentist.,* 12, 214, September/October, 1992.

Friedlander, A.H., Freymiller, E.G., Yagiela, J.A., and Eth, S.: Dental Management of the Adolescent With Panic Disorder, *ASDC J. Dent. Child.,* 60, 365, November–December, 1993.

Friedlander, A.H. and Eth, S.: Dental Management Considerations in Children with Obsessive-Compulsive Disorder, *ASDC J. Dent. Child.,* 58, 217, May–June, 1991.

Jonas, B.S., Franks, P., and Ingram, D.D.: Are Symptoms of Anxiety and Depression Risk Factors for Hypertension? *Arch. Fam. Med.,* 6, 43, January/February, 1997.

Schmaling, K.B. and Bell, J.: Asthma and Panic Disorder, *Arch. Fam. Med.,* 6, 20, January/February, 1997.

Eating Disorders

Altshuler, B.D.: Eating Disorder Patients. Recognition and Intervention, *J. Dent. Hyg.,* 64, 119, March–April, 1990.

Ediger, M.: Do the Eating Habits of Anorexics and Bulimics Have an Effect on Their Oral Health? *J. Canad. Dent. Hyg. Assoc./ Probe,* 28, 139, July/August, 1994.

Kneisl, C.R., ed.: Eating Disorders (12 articles), *Nurs. Clin. North Am.,* 26, 665–800, September, 1991.

Liew, V.P., Frisken, K.W., Touyz, S.W., Beumont, P.J.V., and Williams, H.: Clinical and Microbiological Investigations of Anorexia Nervosa, *Aust. Dent J.,* 36, 435, December, 1991.

Milosevic, A. and Dawson, L.J.: Salivary Factors in Vomiting Bulimics With and Without Pathological Tooth Wear, *Caries Res.,* 30, 361, September–October, 1996.

Robb, N.D., Smith, B.G., and Geidrys-Leeper, E.: The Distribution of Erosion in the Dentitions of Patients With Eating Disorders, *Br. Dent. J.,* 178, 171, March 11, 1995.

Ruff, J.C., Koch, M.O., and Perkins, S.: Bulimia: Dentomedical Complications, *Gen. Dent.,* 40, 22, January–February, 1992.

Tylenda, C.A., Roberts, M.W., Elin, R.J., Li, S.-H., and Altemus, M.: Bulimia Nervosa. Its Effect on Salivary Chemistry, *J. Am. Dent. Assoc.,* 122, 37, June, 1991.

The Patient With an Alcohol-Related Disorder

The use of alcohol is common in a large percentage of the population of all ages from teenage through the elderly. Some people are considered light drinkers; some moderate; and others heavy or problem drinkers. A small percent are dependent on alcohol and suffer from *alcoholism.* Alcohol dependence is a chronic, progressive disease that is treatable and can be arrested. Treatment for this illness implies control, not complete cure. The *recovering alcoholic* must be dedicated to life-long abstinence.

People from each category of alcohol use appear as patients needing dental and dental hygiene care. Knowledge of their social and physical health histories and of the effect alcohol use may have on oral health is essential to dental hygiene care planning.

Other substance abuse drugs are described in Chapter 8 (pages 129 to 131).

DESCRIPTION

Key words and terminology to describe the use and abuse of alcohol are defined in Box 57-1. Alcohol used for drinking purposes is ethyl alcohol or ethanol. Other alcohols are methyl, an industrial solvent, and isopropyl, used for rubbing alcohol.

I. CLINICAL PATTERN OF ALCOHOL USE

Alcohol dependency develops after periods of use of

BOX 57-1 KEY WORDS AND ABBREVIATIONS: Alcoholism

Abstinence (ab'stĭ-nens): refrain from use; complete abstinence from alcohol is the objective of a recovering alcoholic.

Abuse: substance abuse with respect to alcohol abuse involves persistent patterns of heavy alcohol intake associated with health consequences and/or impairment in social functioning.

Acne rosacea (ak'ne rō-sa'cē-ah): facial skin condition usually characterized by a flushed appearance; often accompanied by puffiness and a "spider-web" effect of broken capillaries.

Addiction (ah-dik'shun): physiologic and/or psychologic dependence.

> **Drug addiction:** state of periodic or chronic intoxication produced by repeated consumption of a drug; characterized by an overwhelming desire to continue the use of the drug and a tendency to increase the dosage.

Alcoholism (al'kō-hol-izm): alcohol dependence; progressive chronic disease with physiologic, psychologic, and behavioral implications.

Amnesia (am"nē'zē-ah): impairment of long- and/or short-term memory.

Analgesia (an"al-jē'ze-ah): loss of sensibility to pain without loss of consciousness.

Antabuse (an'tah-bus): brand name of the generic drug **disulfiram;** used to deter consumption of alcohol by persons being treated for alcohol dependency by inducing vomiting.

Blackout: temporary amnesia occurring during periods of intensive drinking; person in not unconscious.

Chemical dependence: a primary chronic disease with genetic, psychosocial, and environmental factors influencing its development and manifestations.

Delirium (dě-lēr'e-um): extreme mental and usually motor excitement marked by a rapid succession of confused and unconnected ideas; often with illusions and hallucinations; may be accompanied by tremors.

Delirium tremens: "DTs"; a serious, acute condition associated with the last stages of alcohol withdrawal.

Dementia (de-men'shē-ah): condition of deteriorated mentality characterized by a marked decline of intellectual functioning.

Dependence: drug or substance dependence; with respect to alcohol refers to a physical and psychologic dependence on alcohol that results in impaired ability to control drinking behavior; dependence is differentiated from abuse by manifestations of craving, tolerance, and physical dependence, as well as by an inability to exercise restraint over drinking.

Detoxification (de"tok-sĭ-fĭ-kā'shun): treatment designed to assist in recovery from the toxic effects of a drug; involves withdrawal, and may include pharmacologic and/or non-pharmacologic treatment with psychotherapy and counseling.

DSM-IV: *Diagnostic and Statistical Manual of Mental Disorders,* 4th ed., published by the American Psychiatric Association.

Euphoria (ū-for'rē-ah): feeling of well-being, elation; without fear or worry.

Fetal alcohol effects (FAE): offspring of alcoholic mother who does not have all of the criteria of FAS.

Fetal alcohol syndrome (FAS): an abnormal pattern of growth and development in some children born to chronically alcoholic mothers.

Hallucination (hah-lu"sĭ-nā'shun): a sensory impression (sight, touch, sound, smell, or taste) that has no basis in external stimulation; may have psychologic causes, or may result from use of drugs (including alcohol), brain tumor, senility, or exhaustion.

Hyperthermia (hi"per-ther'-me-ah): greatly increased temperature.

Illicit: illegal; not authorized; not sanctioned by law.

Micrognathia (mi-kro-nath' e-ah): abnormal smallness of the jaws, especially of the mandible.

Nystagmus (nĭs-tag'mus): involuntary, rapid, rhythmic movement of the eyeball.

Polysubstance dependence: addiction to at least three categories of psychoactive substances (not including nicotine or caffeine) but in which no single psychoactive substance predominates.

Psychotropic drug (si"kō-trop'ik): a drug capable of modifying mental activity; used in the treatment of mental illness.

Recovering alcoholic: a person afflicted with the disease of alcoholism who is abstaining from the use of alcohol; recovering alcoholics prefer the term "recovering" to reformed, cured, "ex," or recovered, because recovering implies an ongoing process.

Tolerance: ability to endure without effect or injury.

> **Drug tolerance:** the need for higher and higher doses of a drug to achieve the same effects.

alcohol followed by pathologic abuse. In the early period, the person functions appropriately in work, family, and social situations.

As drinking continues in the alcoholic person, episodes may occur of alcohol intoxication with amnesia and blackouts. Early evidences of withdrawal symptoms require more alcohol for self-treatment, thus creating a vicious circle leading to dependency.

A. Signs of Alcohol Abuse[1]
1. *Adult*
   a. Health problems.
   b. Arrest, accident involvement.
   c. Impairment of job performance.
   d. Difficulties in personal relationships.
2. *Adolescent*
   a. Poor school performance.
   b. Trouble with parents.
   c. Involvement with law enforcement personnel.

B. Signs of Alcohol Intoxication[1]
Intoxication results from recent ingestion of excessive amounts of alcohol. It is characterized by behavioral changes that tend to alter the usual behavior of the individual.
1. *Behavioral Changes.* Aggressiveness, mood instability, impaired judgment, impaired social or occupational functioning, and impaired attention and memory.
2. *Physical Characteristics.* Slurred speech, incoordination, unsteady gait, nystagmus, and flushed face.
3. *Complications*
   a. Irresponsible actions in work and family settings.
   b. Accidents with resultant bruises, fractures, or brain trauma.
   c. Suicide.

C. Signs of Alcohol Dependence
1. Impaired control: inability to stop drinking before intoxication occurs; inability to cut down or limit drinking in spite of repeated attempts; binge drinking.
2. Amnesia for events happening during a period of intoxication.
3. Continuation of drinking in spite of other serious physical or mental disorder that is aggravated by alcohol use.
4. Tolerance; increased amount of alcohol needed to achieve intoxication.
5. Preoccupation with drinking: spending excess time on activities related to drinking.
6. Withdrawal leads to withdrawal symptoms, such as morning-after "shakes"; relief obtained by use of more alcohol.

II. ETIOLOGY[2]
Genetic, psychosocial, and environmental factors influence the development of alcoholism. Children of alcohol-dependent parents have a significantly higher incidence of alcoholism than do children of nonalcoholics.

Various precipitating factors may be involved when considering environmental influences. Included are psychologic stress, social contacts, being raised in a setting where heavy drinking is encouraged or tolerated as acceptable, and current lifestyle.

METABOLISM OF ALCOHOL[3]

I. INGESTION AND ABSORPTION
A. Upon intake, alcohol is promptly absorbed from the stomach and small intestine; less rapidly in the presence of food.
B. Transported to liver for metabolism; it is also partly metabolized in the stomach.

II. LIVER METABOLISM
More than 90% of ingested alcohol is converted into acetaldehyde, then into acetone, and finally into carbon dioxide and water, by action of various liver enzymes. High acetaldehyde levels and chronic alcohol consumption impair liver function and lead to liver damage.

III. DIFFUSION
A. Alcohol is quickly diffused into all cells and intercellular fluid of the body.
B. Less than 10% is excreted directly through the lungs, skin, and kidney (breath, sweat, and urine).

IV. BLOOD ALCOHOL CONCENTRATION (BAC)[4]
A. Within 5 minutes after ingestion, alcohol can be detected in the blood. BAC is measured in milligrams per deciliter (mg/dL).
B. BAC is used in the legal testing of automobile drivers. In most states in the United States, 100 mg/dL (0.1%) or less is the maximum legal driving level. The blood level usually is not measured; it is estimated from the amount present in the expired air and is expressed as a percentage.

C. Effects of BAC at Various Levels
1. The tolerance level varies among individuals. Whereas the inexperienced drinker may lose self control and become nauseated with low levels of alcohol, the experienced drinker tolerates a higher level of alcohol without nausea.
2. Ethanol is a powerful depressant of the central nervous system. In low doses, alcohol can act as a disinhibitor and as a relaxant. Euphoria may be produced. In high doses, alcohol can produce analgesic effects, with reduction of anxiety generally accompanied by reduced alertness and reduced judgment.

3. BACs at various levels produce the following characteristic effects.

50 mg/dL	sedation, tranquility
	fine motor coordination reduced
	unsteadiness on standing
50–100 mg/dL	reduced anxiety
	enhanced self-esteem
	reduced critical judgment
	reduced alertness; slowed reaction time
	impulsive risk-taking behavior
100–200 mg/dL	slowed reaction time
	slurred speech
	staggering
	mood swings
	memory deficits (blackouts)
	increased aggressive behavior
300–400 mg/dL	labored breathing
	nystagmus
	lowered blood pressure
	lowered body temperature
	loss of consciousness
400–500 mg/dL	depressed respiration
	alcoholic coma
	possibly fatal

HEALTH HAZARDS

Prolonged alcohol use causes many serious medical disorders. The alcohol-dependent person is most seriously afflicted, but even less heavy drinkers may have complications. Alcohol-related illnesses may involve any body system. A few are mentioned here.

I. LIVER DISEASE

A. Of all the body organs, the liver is the most severely affected. Chronic alcohol abuse is the most outstanding cause of morbidity and mortality from liver diseases.

B. Injurious effects of alcohol lead to fatty liver, early fibrosis, alcoholic hepatitis, and cirrhosis.

II. IMMUNITY AND INFECTION

A. Alcoholic persons have diminished immune response: suppression of immune system defense and disturbed function of neutrophils.

B. Risk for many bacterial infections is increased, particularly pulmonary diseases (pneumonia, tuberculosis) and viral infections (hepatitis B).

III. DIGESTIVE SYSTEM

A. Alcohol ingestion alters the stomach mucosa, stimulates gastric acid secretion, and affects gastric function.

B. Bleeding lesions may develop with desquamation of the stomach lining (acute gastritis).

C. Injury to small intestines can lead to diarrhea, weight loss, and vitamin deficiencies.

IV. NUTRITIONAL DEFICIENCIES

A. The diet of a person who consumes large quantities of alcohol regularly may be limited because the person loses interest in food. The alcohol provides an excess of caloric intake.

B. Marked deficiencies can result from malabsorption of vitamins and other essential nutrients.

C. Secondary malnutrition develops because of the direct effects of alcohol on the gastrointestinal tract. Malabsorption and maldigestion occur following cellular changes in the intestinal wall.

V. CARDIOVASCULAR DISEASES

A. Risk for cardiomyopathy, hypertension, sudden death, and hemorrhagic stroke is greater for chronic alcohol abusers; decreased risk for heart attack and stroke is associated with light to moderate alcohol use.[5]

B. Heavy alcohol consumption increases the death rate from cardiovascular disease.

VI. NEOPLASMS

A. Alcohol use increases the risk for many types of cancers, notably of the alimentary and respiratory tracts.[6]

B. Alcohol combined with tobacco use has long been associated with increased neoplasms of the oral cavity, pharynx, and larynx (page 724).

VII. NERVOUS SYSTEM

A. Central and Peripheral
Long-term alcohol abuse combined with malnutrition can lead to damage of both central and peripheral nervous systems. Other factors may be involved including alcohol-related head injuries and psychiatric status.

Early changes affect intellectual actions, such as judgment and learning ability. With prolonged and heavy alcohol consumption, chronic brain damage results.

B. Wernicke-Korsakoff's Syndrome
This disorder involves ocular and gait disturbances, confusion, and psychosis. It is a result of nutritional deficiency, specifically thiamine deficiency, in conjunction with chronic alcoholism and liver damage.

VIII. REPRODUCTIVE SYSTEM
Alcohol affects every branch of the endocrine system, directly and indirectly, through the body's organization of the endocrine hormones. Possible effects of chronic alcohol abuse are listed here.

A. Female
Menstrual disturbances, failure to ovulate, and

early menopause. Fetal alcohol syndrome is described in the next section.

B. Male
Testicular atrophy, suppression of testosterone, loss of mature sperm cells, feminization, and failure of gonadal function.

FETAL ALCOHOL SYNDROME (FAS)

I. ALCOHOL USE DURING PREGNANCY

A. No Safe Amount
The use of alcohol during the prenatal period can be seriously threatening to the health of the baby. Even children born to mothers who have been occasional drinkers, but not alcoholics, may have alcohol-related developmental or behavioral problems. The amount of alcohol, if any, that might be considered "safe" to consume during pregnancy has not been established. Complete abstinence is safest.

B. Other Factors
Many women who abuse alcohol have poor health habits and inadequate nutritional intake, use tobacco regularly, and abuse other substances. These other factors also may influence the health of the baby.

C. No Placental Barrier
Alcohol passes freely across the placenta. Increased incidence of spontaneous abortions and stillbirths has been related to alcohol intake. The most severe effects result in fetal alcohol syndrome (FAS).

D. Fetal Growth Pattern
A characteristically abnormal pattern of growth and development can be found in children with fetal alcohol syndrome. Individually, the signs or symptoms of alcohol-related birth defects cannot be considered specific for alcohol because they appear in other conditions; but grouped together, they form the syndrome.

II. CHARACTERISTICS OF FETAL ALCOHOL SYNDROME
The minimal criteria for describing FAS include prenatal and postnatal growth deficiencies, central nervous system impairment, and facial dysmorphology.[8] For individuals with only some of the criteria the designation is either "fetal alcohol effects" (FAE) or "alcohol-related birth defects" (ARBD).

A. Prenatal and Postnatal Growth Retardation
1. Microcephaly
2. Abnormalities in length and weight

B. Central Nervous System (CNS) Involvement
1. Mental retardation; learning disabilities
2. Behavioral dysfunction
3. Poor motor coordination; abnormal gait

4. Hyperactivity; irritability

C. Facial Dysmorphology (Figure 57-1)
1. Eyes: short palpebral fissure (eye openings); epicanthal folds.
2. Thin upper lip, smooth philtrum.
3. Midface: flattened, depressed; underdeveloped maxilla.
4. Nose: Short, upturned, with sunken nasal bridge.
5. Micrognathia.
6. Ears: anomalies of shape and position.

D. Other Characteristics
A variety of other health problems may result from major organ malformations including cardiac, hepatic, muscular, skeletal, and renal. There may be hearing and vision defects. Immune system function may be compromised, leading to susceptibility to infections.

ALCOHOL WITHDRAWAL SYNDROME[1]

Withdrawal consists of the disturbances that occur after abrupt cessation of alcohol intake in the alcohol-dependent person. Withdrawal signs appear within a few hours after drinking has stopped. Even a relative decline in blood concentration can precipitate the syndrome.

I. PREDISPOSING FACTORS
Malnutrition, fatigue, depression, and physical illnesses aggravate withdrawal symptoms.

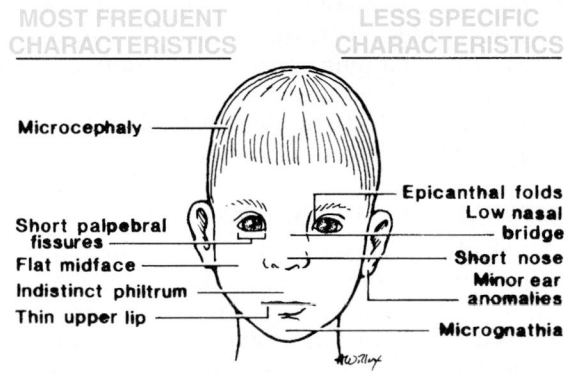

FIGURE 57-1 Fetal Alcohol Syndrome. The characteristic abnormal facial features of a child born to a mother who is alcohol-dependent. Growth deficiency is also a recognized feature, as are many other signs of development and behavioral problems. (Adapted from Little, R.E. and Streissguth, A.P.: *Alcohol, Pregnancy and the Fetal Alcohol Syndrome Unit in Alcohol Use and Its Medical Consequences: A Comprehensive Teaching Program for Biomedical Education. Project Cork of Dartmouth Medical School.* Milner-Fenwick, Inc., 2125 Greenspring Drive, Timonium, MD 21093.

II. FEATURES

   A. Tremor of hands, tongue, eyelids.
   B. Nervousness and irritation; anxiety.
   C. Malaise, weakness, headache.
   D. Dry mouth.
   E. Autonomic hyperactivity; sweating, rapid pulse rate, elevated blood pressure.
   F. Transient visual, tactile, or auditory hallucinations.
   G. Insomnia.
   H. Grand mal seizures.
   I. Nausea or vomiting.

III. COMPLICATIONS

A. Alcohol Withdrawal Delirium (Delirium Tremens, "DTs")
   1. May occur within 1 week of cessation of heavy alcohol intake.
   2. Features
      a. Marked autonomic hyperactivity: rapid heart beat, sweating.
      b. Vivid hallucinations (visual, auditory, tactile).
      c. Delusions and agitated behavior; tremor.
      d. Confusion and disorientation.

B. Alcohol Hallucinosis
   1. Auditory and visual hallucinations develop within 48 hours after abruptly stopping or reducing heavy alcohol intake of long-standing dependency.
   2. Features
      a. May last weeks or months.
      b. Impairment is severe, with schizophrenic symptoms, although schizophrenia is not a predisposing factor.
      c. Delirium is not present.

TREATMENT

The overall objective of treatment is to help the person achieve and maintain total abstinence. An alcohol-dependent person probably can never drink even small amounts of alcohol without eventually resuming dependency.

Treatment includes a combination of medical and psychiatric therapy with self-help. Patients are encouraged not to take other psychoactive drugs, including minor tranquilizers and caffeine.

I. EARLY INTERVENTION

When problem drinkers who are not yet dependent can be identified, counseling may help to reduce and perhaps eliminate the use of alcohol.

II. DETOXIFICATION

The term detoxification applies to the management of acute intoxication and the withdrawal syndrome. A variety of treatments may be involved.

A. Treatment for Immediate Emergencies
An alcoholic may have been in an accident or have a medical emergency other than that of the alcohol withdrawal syndrome. Fractures, head injury, internal bleeding, or other problems may require initial attention. In fact, alcohol dependency may be revealed after a patient is admitted for other reasons and withdrawal symptoms appear within a few hours or days.

B. Removal From Source of Alcohol: Abstinence
One of the advantages of hospitalization is that supervision is available. The patient does not have access to usual sources of alcohol.

C. Rest, Sleep, Exercise, and Proper Diet
One goal of therapy is to restore general physical health by treating nutritional deficiencies and encouraging a normal daily pattern of sleep and meals.

D. Treatment for Medical Complications
Possible medical complications were described with their systemic effects earlier in this chapter. Most alcoholics have additional illnesses.

E. Relief From Acute Withdrawal Signs
Tranquilizers may be prescribed for short-term use. Vitamins, particularly thiamine, are usually administered.

III. PHARMACOTHERAPY[9,10]

A. Medications Used in Alcoholism Treatment
Agents for withdrawal management include:
   1. Alcohol sensitizing agents (cause aversive reactions in combination with alcohol).
   2. Anticraving agents (decrease desire for and consumption of alcohol).
   3. Amethystic agents (reverse the acute intoxicating and depressant effects of alcohol).
   4. Medications for treatment of coexisting psychiatric disorders such as depression and anxiety (Chapter 56, pages 825 to 830).

B. Disulfiram (Antabuse): Alcohol Sensitizing Agent
The drug disulfiram interferes with the metabolism of alcohol by acting on the enzyme that converts acetaldehyde to acetone in the liver. As a result, acetaldehyde accumulates in the tissues. When both alcohol and disulfiram are taken at the same time, nausea and vomiting with hypotension result, and the patient becomes very ill. The drug acts as a deterrent to provide an adjunct to comprehensive therapy in selected patients.

C. Naltrexone (Trexan): Anticraving Agent
The drug naltrexone produces an aversive reaction. It can help decrease craving and consump-

tion by the alcohol-dependent person. Although there are some side effects, it has been shown to be efficacious as an adjunct to psychosocial treatment.

IV. REHABILITATION

A. Counseling and Education

The patient must recognize that alcoholism is a serious disease and must be willing to be helped. Family and work associates may be recruited to cooperate with the program. Behavior therapy and psychotherapy have been used.

B. Group Therapy

Alcoholics Anonymous (AA) is one source of possible help for motivated individuals. Other people prefer special clinics and centers for treatment.

AA is a fellowship of men and women who help themselves and others to recover from alcoholism. Al-Anon is a separate program for parents, adult children, siblings, and spouses, as well as other persons concerned with the recovering alcoholic. Alateen is a program for teenage children.

C. Psychiatry

Treatment is needed for patients with psychiatric disorders. An increased frequency of schizophrenia, psychoneurosis, sociopathy, and manic-depressive diseases is being recognized among alcohol-dependent people.

D. Aftercare Services

Because recovery takes a long time, an extended period of aftercare is needed. Early relapse is more likely when a recovering alcoholic leaves a treatment system too early. A typical follow-up includes weekly aftercare group meetings for 9 to 12 months.

DENTAL HYGIENE CARE

Only a small percentage of individuals with an alcohol-use problem are incapacitated, homeless, shabbily dressed, or socially disoriented. Most alcohol-dependent people continue to maintain home, work, and social relationships, at least initially, and many for a span of years.

In dental and dental hygiene practice, patients who consume alcohol include the occasional social drinker, the light to moderate drinker, the problem drinker, the alcohol abuser, and the alcohol-dependent person. The abstainer or "teetotaler" is particularly important to identify because that patient may be a recovering alcoholic.

Many patients with an alcohol use disorder are polysubstance abusers. They may use other psychoac-tive drugs, such as cocaine, heroin, amphetamines, marijuana, and assorted sedatives or hypnotics.

I. PATIENT ASSESSMENT

The quality of the content and the frequent updating of the medical history are essential to patient care because of the many general health-related problems of alcohol ingestion that can influence oral health and treatment procedures.

A. Obtain Patient Confidence

Information about substance use and abuse must be obtained from patients of all age levels. Adolescents of all socioeconomic groups may be involved. The number of elderly alcohol consumers is ever increasing; some of these are alcoholics.[11]

Unfortunately, people are hesitant to reveal personal information about alcohol use because of the social stigma attached to alcoholism. A patient first needs to understand the reasons for obtaining the information as a health-safety measure. More than that, the patient must know that personal information will remain confidential.

B. Present Questions Carefully

Questions must be asked privately and without sign of disapproval or judgment. A patient's family members may provide an alert to the patient's problem.

The basic questionnaire or interview format must have a few leading questions to provide basic facts. Care must be taken not to place the patient on the defensive.

1. *Suggested Content for Routine Questions*
   a. Pattern of alcohol consumption, frequency, amount on an average day.
   b. Systemic conditions suggestive of alcohol-related diseases.
   c. Hospitalizations suggestive of alcohol-related accidents or detoxification program.
   d. Information about medications; self-prescribed, over-the-counter, and prescribed drugs. A relationship to polydrug abuse or treatment for alcoholism may be evident.
   e. History of drinking problem.
2. *Screening for Alcohol Abuse or Dependency.* Various questionnaires have been used in the attempt to detect alcoholism. One of these, the **CAGE,** has four selected questions. Although these questions may not provide a positive diagnosis, research has shown that they can alert the interviewer and provide a high index of suspicion. One positive reply can lead to further inquiry. The four questions are as follows[12]:
   a. Have you ever felt you ought to **C**ut down on your drinking?

b. Have people **A**nnoyed you by criticizing your drinking?

c. Have you ever felt bad or **G**uilty about your drinking?

d. Have you ever had a drink first thing in the morning to steady your nerves or to get rid of a hangover (**E**ye-opener)?

II. PATIENT EXAMINATION[13]

Except for the increased risk of oral cancer in persons who use alcohol heavily, no specific oral finding can be attributed directly to alcohol as the etiologic agent. The characteristics listed here have been observed frequently. When present, they assist in patient evaluation and dental hygiene care planning.

A. Extraoral Examination

1. *Breath and Body Odor of Alcohol and of Tobacco.* Many alcohol users are also heavy tobacco users.

2. *Tremor of Hands, Tongue, Eyelids.* Signs of withdrawal.

3. *Skin.* Redness of forehead, cheeks, nose; acne rosacea; dilated blood vessels that produce spider petechiae on the nose.

4. *Face Color.* Light yellowish brown may indicate jaundice from liver disease.

5. *Eyes.* Red, baggy eyes or puffy facial features; bloated appearance.

6. *Evidences of Trauma.* Facial injuries related to falls when intoxicated. Alcohol abusers are especially prone to traumatic accidents.

7. *Lips.* Angular cheilitis related to poor nutrition.

8. *Parotid Glands.* Swelling.

B. Intraoral Examination

1. *Mucosa, Lips, Tongue.* Dry; xerostomia.

2. *Tongue.* Coated; glossitis related to nutritional deficiencies.

3. *Periodontal Infection*

   a. Generalized poor oral hygiene; heavy plaque not unusual.

   b. Calculus deposits may be generalized, depending on patient neglect.

   c. Gingiva that bleeds spontaneously or on probing.

4. *Teeth*

   a. Chipped and fractured from falls and injuries; stained from tobacco use.

   b. Attrition secondary to bruxism.

   c. Erosion secondary to frequent vomiting.

   d. Dental caries. Except for neglect of dental care, dental caries incidence may be no different from that for the usual population of the age level. An alcoholic who uses primarily wine or sweetened cocktails and frequently snacks on cariogenic foods is likely to have more carious lesions, particularly if gingival recession and root exposures have

occurred. Lack of bacterial plaque removal also favors increased incidence of dental caries.

5. *Evidence of Minimal Dental Care.* Although subject to great variation, the overall tendency is for the alcoholic patient to put off dental and dental hygiene care, sometimes in the interest of money needed to purchase alcohol or, for the polysubstance abuser, additional drugs.

   The alcohol-dependent person also may tend to use dental care primarily for emergency purposes for pain relief. The evidence may be noted in a patient who has more missing teeth than treated teeth. The indication can be that dental caries was neglected to the point where extraction was requested.

6. *Dentures.* Chipped, missing; may require frequent repairs.

III. CONSULTATION

Information in the patient history may not reveal accurately the extent of a patient's alcohol use, but clinical observations along with the medical history may provide a high degree of suspicion. From that, further inquiry and consultation with the patient's physician may help to confirm precautions needed during clinical procedures.

When a patient does not have a regular physician and has not had a recent medical evaluation, referral to a physician should be made.

IV. VITAL SIGNS

Routine recording of vital signs is indicated. Blood pressure is frequently increased. Fluctuations can be particularly significant.

V. CLINICAL TREATMENT PROCEDURES

The clinical procedures for dental hygiene care are greatly influenced by the many health problems that can result from chronic ingestion of alcohol. Some of the effects were described earlier in this chapter.

A. Nonalcoholic Rinses

Preprocedural rinse, antibacterial agents, or any oral hygiene product that contains alcohol must be avoided for all patients suffering from an alcohol use problem. This is absolutely necessary for the recovering alcoholic because recovery depends on a medication-free lifestyle. The most minute amount of alcohol ingested by a patient being treated with disulfiram can cause an emergency.

B. Scaling and Debridement

The usual oral tissue response expected following periodontal instrumentation may be limited by the changes in the patient's tissues. These can be summarized as follows:

1. Decreased overall reserve that has resulted

from degeneration of multiple organ systems.

2. Impaired healing
   a. Prolonged bleeding time; impaired clotting mechanism from chronic liver disease.
   b. Interference with collagen formation and deposition.
   c. Decreased immune system function.
3. Increased susceptibility to infection.

C. Power-Driven Instruments

The patient with chronic alcohol abuse or dependency, particularly one who also inhales tobacco smoke, most likely has pulmonary complications. Lung infections are common. Lung abscesses can be caused by bacteria taken into the lungs from the oral cavity or by abnormal breathing during intoxication.

Power-driven instruments, particularly ultrasonic scalers and air-powder stain-removal devices, must be used with caution to prevent inhalation of oral microorganisms by the patient. High-powered suction applied by an assistant is essential.

PATIENT INSTRUCTION

I. BACTERIAL PLAQUE CONTROL

Teaching oral health and cleanliness can be especially important. Motivation may be difficult because many patients with alcohol or polysubstance dependency are preoccupied with alcohol or drugs and place less priority on personal hygiene.

A preventive care program for a recovering alcoholic should become part of the total rehabilitation process.

II. DIET AND NUTRITION

A. Relation of Diet to Alcoholism

1. Alcoholic beverages contain calories; a day's allotment of calories may be ingested when alcohol is used in excess.
2. The calories of alcohol are "empty" calories without nutritional elements, and the balance of the diet can be very limited.
3. Alcohol unfavorably affects the absorption and digestion of many nutrients by the changes it produces in the mucosa of the gastrointestinal tract.
4. Liver damage has a major detrimental influence on the metabolism of nutrients.

B. Dietary Deficiencies

Malnutrition is clearly associated with alcohol abuse. The severe malnutrition that has been described applies primarily to the derelict or "skid row" alcoholic who has limited resources for proper food.

Many middle and upper class alcohol dependents do not consume an acceptable "balanced" diet, but they cannot be considered with the severely malnourished group.

C. Instruction

After a dietary assessment is reviewed with the patient, help can be provided by reviewing the basic dietary needs and encouraging the use of foods from the food guide pyramid (Figure 28-2, page 445).

III. CONTINUING CARE

Compliance with self-care measures and keeping scheduled appointments for dental hygiene care are major problems. A special effort must be made to provide the patient with the supervision and periodic treatment needed. The moderate and excess user of alcohol, especially when tobacco is also used, is at risk for oral cancer and periodontal bone and attachment loss. Regular screening is necessary.

FACTORS TO TEACH THE PATIENT

I. Alcohol abuse is a great risk to overall health.
II. Incidence of oral cancer is increased by the use of alcohol and tobacco.
III. Mixing alcohol with other drugs (prescription or over-the-counter) can lead to medical emergencies. Always check each drug and its actions before using it in combination with alcohol.
IV. Alcoholism is a disease with serious implications. Advise young people of the dangers involved and discourage them from drinking alcohol.
V. Commercial antibacterial and fluoride mouthrinses may contain up to 30% alcohol. Labels must be read carefully. Keep mouthrinse bottles out of reach of children.
VI. Use of alcohol during pregnancy must be avoided because of possible devastating effects on the baby. Be alert to the alcohol content of certain foods and drugs.
VII. Alcohol readily enters breast milk and is transmitted to the infant during nursing.

REFERENCES

1. **American Psychiatric Association:** *Diagnostic and Statistical Manual of Mental Disorders* (DSM-IV). Washington, DC, American Psychiatric Association, 1994, pp. 195–199.
2. **United States Department of Health and Human Services,** Secretary of Health and Human Services: *Eighth Special Report to the U.S. Congress on Alcohol and Health.* Rockville, MD, National Institute on Alcohol Abuse and Alcoholism, September, 1993, pp. 61–77.
3. **United States Department of Health and Human Services:** op. cit., pp. 147–149.
4. **United States Department of Health and Human Services:** op. cit., p. 89.
5. **United States Department of Health and Human Services:** op. cit., p. 175.

6. **Lieber**, C.S.: Medical Disorders of Alcoholism, *N. Engl. J. Med., 333*, 1058, October 19, 1995.

7. **United States Department of Health and Human Services:** op. cit., pp. 180–181.

8. **Sokol**, R.J. and Clarren, S.K.: Guidelines for Use of Terminology Describing the Impact of Prenatal Alcohol on the Offspring, *Alcohol. Clin. Exp. Res., 13*, 597, August, 1989.

9. **Kranzler**, H.R.: Alcoholism, in Rakel, R.E., ed.: *Conn's Current Therapy, 1997.* Philadelphia, W.B. Saunders, 1997, p. 1139.

10. **United States Department of Health and Human Services:** op. cit., pp. 332–335.

11. **Friedlander**, A.H. and Solomon, D.H.: Dental Management of the Geriatric Alcoholic Patient, *Gerodontics, 4*, 23, February, 1988.

12. **Ewing**, J.A.: Detecting Alcoholism. The CAGE Questionnaire, *JAMA, 252*, 1905, October 12, 1984.

13. **Friedlander**, A.H., Mills, M.J., and Gorelick, D.A.: Alcoholism and Dental Management, *Oral Surg., Oral Med., Oral Pathol., 63*, 42, January, 1987.

with Alcohol-Related Liver Disease, *J. Am. Dent. Assoc., 128*, 61, January, 1997.

Halsted, C.H.: Alcohol: Medical and Nutritional Effects, in Ziegler, E.E. and Filer, L.J., eds.: *Present Knowledge in Nutrition*, 7th ed. Washington, DC, ILSI Press, 1996, pp. 547–556.

Harris, C.K., Warnakulasuriya, K.A.A.S, Johnson, N.W., Gelbier, S., and Peters, T.J.: Oral Health in Alcohol Misusers, *Community Dent. Health, 13*, 199, December, 1996.

Leonard, R.H.: Alcohol, Alcoholism, and Dental Treatment, *Compend. Cont. Educ. Dent., 12*, 274, April, 1991.

McDiarmid, M.: Dental Treatment and the Alcoholic, *N. Zeal. Dent. J., 92*, 83, September, 1996.

Michels, R. and Marzuk, P.-M.: Progress in Psychiatry (Second of Two Parts), *N. Engl. J. Med., 329*, 628, August 26, 1993.

Robb, N.D. and Smith, B.G.N.: Chronic Alcoholism: An Important Condition in the Dentist-Patient Relationship, *J. Dent., 24*, 17, January/March, 1996.

Talamini, R., Franceschi, S., Barra, S., and La Vecchia, C.: The Role of Alcohol in Oral and Pharyngeal Cancer in Non-smokers, and of Tobacco in Non-drinkers, *Int. J. Cancer, 46*, 391, September 15, 1990.

SUGGESTED READINGS

Biron, C.R.: Help Patients Before They Hit Rock Bottom, *RDH, 15*, 20, August, 1995.

Boffetta, P., Mashberg, A., Winkelmann, R., and Garfinkel, L.: Carcinogenic Effect of Tobacco Smoking and Alcohol Drinking on Anatomic Sites of the Oral Cavity and Oropharynx, *Int. J. Cancer, 52*, 530, October 21, 1992.

Brickley, M.R. and Shepherd, J.P.: Alcohol Abuse in Dental Patients, *Br. Dent. J., 169*, 329, November 24, 1990.

Dobkin, P.L., Tremblay, R.E., Desmarais-Gervais, L., and Depelteau, L.: Is Having an Alcoholic Father Hazardous for Children's Physical Health? *Addiction, 89*, 1619, December, 1994.

Glick, M.: Medical Considerations for Dental Care of Patients

Fetal Alcohol Syndrome

Coles, C.D.: Impact of Prenatal Alcohol Exposure on the Newborn and the Child, *Clin. Obstet. Gynec., 36*, 255, June, 1993.

Haney, K. and Bothwell, E.: Fetal Alcohol Syndrome. Implications for Dental Health Professionals, *DentalHygienistNews, 7*, 8, Summer, 1994.

Lewis, D.D. and Woods, S.E: Fetal Alcohol Syndrome, *Am. Family Physician, 50*, 1025, October, 1994.

Seo, P.: Treating the Patient with Fetal Alcohol Syndrome, *Access, 11*, 60, May–June, 1997.

Spohr, H.-L., Willms, J., and Steinhausen, H.-C.: Prenatal Alcohol Exposure and Long-term Developmental Consequences, *Lancet, 341*, 907, April 10, 1993.

58

The Patient With a Cardiovascular Disease

Cardiovascular, as the names implies, includes diseases of the heart and blood vessels. Diseases of the heart are the leading causes of death in the United States. Key words and terminology describing the cardiovascular diseases are defined in Box 58-1. Prefixes and suffixes to clarify the terminology are listed on pages 919 to 921.

Patients with cardiovascular conditions are encountered frequently in a dental office or clinic and may be from any age group, although the highest incidence is among older people. A heart disease may be present for many years before the symptoms are recognized. The patients seen in the dental office range from those with no obvious symptoms to the nearly disabled.

I. CLASSIFICATION

Classification of the diseases is made on either an anatomic or an etiologic basis. In an anatomic system,

BOX 58-1 KEY WORDS: Cardiovascular Disease

Aneurysm (an'ū-rizm): sac formed by the localized dilatation of the wall of an artery, a vein, or the heart.

Angina (an-jī'nah): a disease marked by spasmodic suffocative attacks.

Angina pectoris: acute pain in the chest from decreased blood supply to the heart muscle.

Anoxia (ah-nok'sē-ah): absence of oxygen in the tissues; may be accompanied by deep respirations, cyanosis, increased pulse rate, and impairment of coordination.

Anticoagulant (an'tī-kō-ag'ū-lant): a substance that suppresses, delays, or nullifies coagulation of the blood.

Apnea (ap'nē-ah): temporary cessation of breathing.

Arrhythmia (ah-rith'mē-ah): variation from the normal rhythm, especially with reference to the heart.

Arterial blood: oxygenated blood carried by an artery away from the heart to nourish the body tissues.

Asphyxia (as-fik'sē-ah): a condition in which there is a deficiency of oxygen in the blood and an increase in carbon dioxide.

Atheroma (ath'er-ō'mah): lipid (cholesterol) deposit on the intima (lining) of an artery; also called atheromatous plaque.

Bradycardia (brād'e-kar'dē-ah): slowness of heartbeat with slowing of pulse rate to less than 60 per minute.

Cyanosis (sī'ah-nō'sis): bluish discoloration of the skin and mucous membranes caused by excess concentration of reduced hemoglobin in the blood.

Dyspnea (disp'ne-ah): labored or difficult breathing.

Echocardiography (ek'ō-kar'dē-og'rah-fē): recording of the position and motion of the heart walls and internal structures of the heart and neighboring tissue by the echo obtained from beams of ultrasonic waves directed through the chest wall; used to show valvular and other structural deformities; the record produced is called an **echocardiogram.**

Edema (ĕ-dē'mah): abnormal accumulation of fluid in the intercellular spaces of the body.

Electrocardiography (ē-lek'trō-kar'dē-og'rah-fē): the graphic recording from the body surface of the potential of electric currents generated by the heart as a means of studying the action of the heart muscle; the record produced is called an **electrocardiogram (EKG).**

Embolism (em'bō-lizm): the sudden blocking of an artery by a clot of foreign material, an **embolus,** that has been brought to its site of lodgment by the blood stream; the embolus may be a blood clot (most frequently), or an air bubble, a clump of bacteria, or a fat globule.

Heparin (hep'ah-rin): anticoagulant; prevents platelet agglutination and thrombus formation.

Hypoxia (hi-pok'sē-ah): diminished availability of oxygen to blood tissues.

Infarct (in'farkt): localized area of ischemic necrosis produced by occlusion of the arterial supply or venous drainage of the part.

Ischemia (is-kē'mē-ah): deficiency of blood to supply oxygen in part resulting from functional constriction or actual obstruction of a blood vessel.

Lumen (loo'men): the cavity or channel within a tube or tubular organ, such as a blood vessel or the intestine.

Murmur (mur'mur): irregularity of heartbeat caused by a turbulent flow of blood through a valve that has failed to close.

Myocardium (mī"ō-kar'dē-um): the middle and thickest layer of the heart wall, composed of cardiac muscle.

Occlusion (o-kloo'zhun): blockage; state of being closed.

Prolapse (pro'laps): downward displacement.

Sclerosis (skle-rō'sis): induration, hardening.

Arteriosclerosis: group of diseases characterized by thickening and loss of elasticity of the arterial wall.

Stenosis (stĕ nō'sis): narrowing or contraction of a body passage or opening.

Tachycardia (tak'kar'dē-ah): abnormally rapid heart rate, usually taken to be over 100 beats per minute.

Tetralogy (tĕ-tral'ō-je): a group or series of four.

Tetralogy of Fallot: congenital, cyanotic malformation of the heart that includes pulmonary stenosis, ventricular septal defect, hypertrophy of the right ventricle, and dextroposition of the aorta.

Thrombus (throm'bus): blood clot attached to the intima of a blood vessel; may occlude the lumen; contrast with embolus, which is detached and carried by the blood stream.

Venous blood: nonoxygenated blood from the tissues; blood pumped from the heart to the lungs for oxygenation.

diseases of the pericardium, myocardium, endocardium, heart valves, and blood vessels are defined. In an etiologic system, the diseases are named by the cause. The principal causes of heart diseases are infectious agents, atherosclerosis, hypertension, immunologic mechanisms, and congenital anomalies.

II. MAJOR CARDIOVASCULAR DISEASES

The five major cardiovascular diseases are congenital heart disease, rheumatic heart disease, infective endocarditis, ischemic heart disease, and hypertensive heart disease. Characteristics and symptoms are complex and overlapping. In this chapter, each of the major diseases is described by its principal symptoms and treatments as well as the applications in dental hygiene care.

CONGENITAL HEART DISEASES[2,3]

Anomalies of the anatomic structure of the heart or major blood vessels result following irregularities of development during the first 9 weeks *in utero*. The fetal heart is completely developed by the ninth week.

Early diagnosis is important because between one fourth and one half of the infants born with cardiovascular anomalies require treatment during the first year. Treatment usually involves surgical correction.

I. TYPES[1]

Many types of heart defects exist. Those that occur most frequently are the ventricular septal defect, patent ductus arteriosus, atrial septal defect, and transposition of the great vessels.

A diagram of the normal heart is shown in Figure 58-1 to provide a comparison with the anatomic changes that may appear in a defective heart. Congenital anomalies either produce abnormal pathways in the blood flow or interfere with the flow itself. The two most common anomalies are described here.

A. Ventricular Septal Defect

In this type of defect, the left and right ventricles are connected through an opening in their dividing wall (septum). The oxygenated blood from the lung, which is normally pumped by the left ventricle to the aorta and then to the entire body, can pass across to the right ventricle as shown in Figure 58-2.

When the opening is very small, only a heart murmur and little disability result. If the opening is large, the heart enlarges to compensate for overwork.

B. Patent Ductus Arteriosus

A patent ductus arteriosus means the passageway (shunt) is open between the two great arteries that arise from the heart, namely the aorta and the pulmonary artery. Normally, the opening is closed during the first few

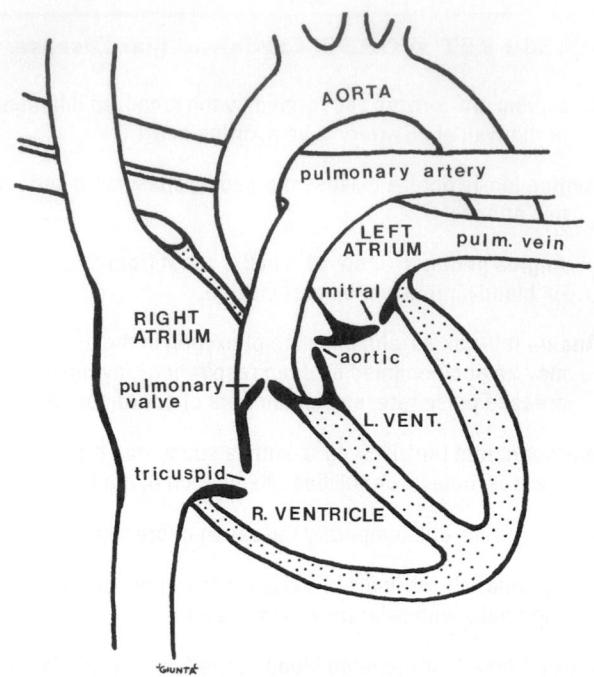

FIGURE 58-1 The Normal Heart. The major vessels and the location of the tricuspid, pulmonary, aortic, and mitral valves are shown.

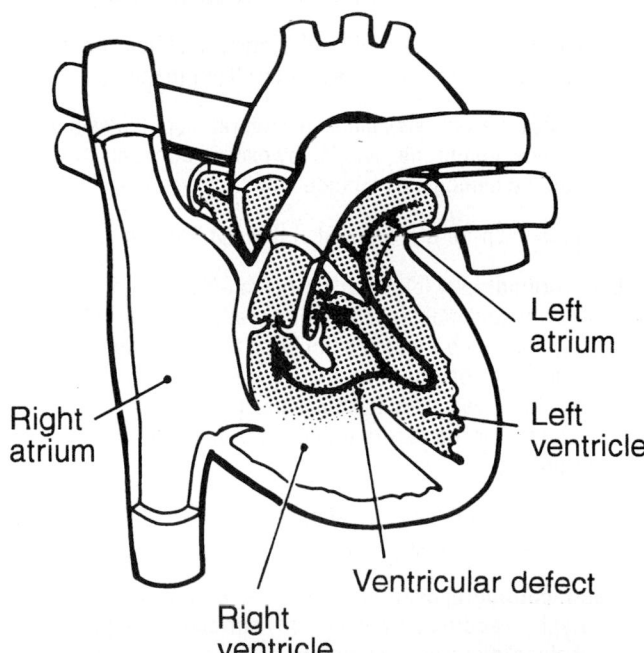

FIGURE 58-2 Ventricular Septal Defect. The right and left ventricles are connected by an opening that permits oxygenated blood from the left ventricle to shunt across to the right ventricle and then recirculate to the lungs. Compare with Figure 58-1 in which the septum separates the ventricles. (Adapted from Bleck, E.E. and Nagel, D.A.: *Physically Handicapped Children. A Medical Atlas for Teachers.* New York, Grune & Stratton, 1975.)

weeks after birth. When the opening does not close, blood from the aorta can pass back to the lungs, as shown in Figure 58-3. The heart compensates in the attempt to provide the body with oxygenated blood and becomes overburdened.

II. ETIOLOGY

Causes are genetic, environmental, or a combination. Many are unknown.

A. Genetic

Heredity is apparent in some types of defects. An example of a chromosomal defect is Down's syndrome, in which congenital heart anomalies occur frequently (page 815).

B. Environmental

Most congenital anomalies originate between the fifth and eighth weeks of fetal life, when the heart is developing.
1. Viral infections (rubella, cytomegalovirus).
2. Drugs.
   a. Chronic maternal alcohol abuse. The fetal alcohol syndrome is described on page 840.
   b. Thalidomide.

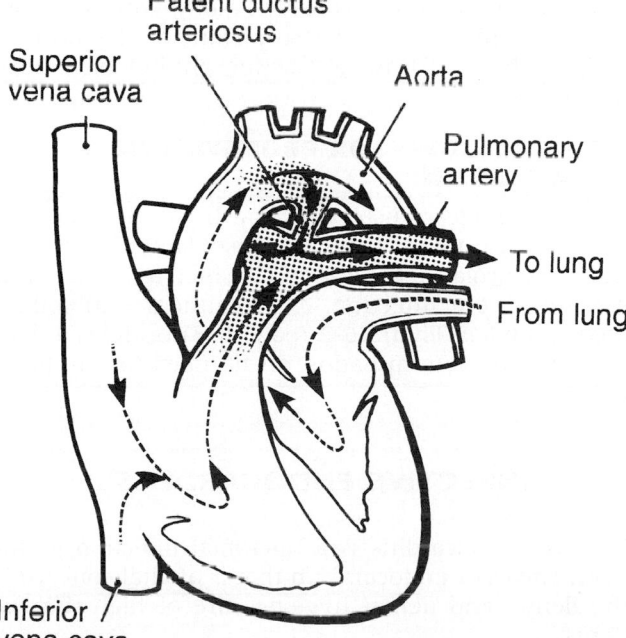

FIGURE 58-3 Patent Ductus Arteriosus. An open passageway between the aorta and the pulmonary artery permits oxygenated blood from the aorta to pass back into the lungs. Arrows show directions of flow through the patent ductus. Compare with normal anatomy in Figure 58-1. (Adapted from Bleck, E.E. and Nagel, D.A.: *Physically Handicapped Children. A Medical Atlas for Teachers.* New York, Grune & Stratton, 1975.)

III. PREVENTION

A. Use of rubella vaccine for childhood immunization. Vaccination confers indefinite immunity. Vaccination for women of childbearing age is highly advised for women not vaccinated in childhood. The vaccine should not be given during pregnancy, and not within 3 months of becoming pregnant, because of potential risks to the fetus.
B. No medications used during pregnancy without prior consultation with the physician.
C. Appropriate use of radiologic equipment. A lead apron should be used when oral radiographs are made.
D. Control of tobacco, drug, and alcohol addictions.
E. Genetic counseling.

IV. CLINICAL CONSIDERATIONS

A. Signs and Symptoms of Congenital Heart Disease

General conditions that may be present and that influence patient management are:
1. Easy fatigue.
2. Exertional dyspnea; fainting.
3. Cyanosis of lips and nailbeds.
4. Poor growth and development.
5. Chest deformity.
6. Heart murmurs.

B. Dental Hygiene Concerns

1. *Prevention of Infective Endocarditis.* Defective heart valves are susceptible to endocarditis from bacteremia produced during oral treatments.
2. *Elimination of Oral Disease.* Maintenance of a high level of oral health.

RHEUMATIC HEART DISEASE[2,3]

Rheumatic heart disease is a complication following rheumatic fever. A rather high percentage of patients with a history of rheumatic fever have permanent heart valve damage. The damaged heart valve, as in congenital heart disease, is susceptible to infective endocarditis.

I. RHEUMATIC FEVER

A. Incidence

Approximately 90% of initial attacks occur between ages 5 and 15. The patient is left susceptible to future attacks, which may cause additional damage to previously damaged heart valves. The tendency to recurrence diminishes with age.

B. Etiology
1. The onset of acute rheumatic fever usually

appears 2 to 3 weeks after a beta-hemolytic group A streptococcal pharyngeal infection.

2. Rheumatic fever and rheumatic heart disease are believed to be immunologic disorders caused by sensitization to antigens of beta-hemolytic group A streptococci.

C. Prevention

The persistence and severity of the pharyngeal infection are significant factors in whether rheumatic fever follows; therefore, early diagnosis and treatment of streptococcal throat and pharyngeal infections are necessary.

D. Symptoms of Rheumatic Fever

Over a period of several months of low-grade fever, the joints, heart muscles, central nervous system, skin, and subcutaneous tissues become involved. All the following symptoms disappear with recovery except the cardiac valve damage.

1. *Arthritis.* Migratory polyarthritis is present, which may affect more than one joint at a time. The temporomandibular joint is rarely involved.

2. *Carditis.* In a severe case, death may result from heart failure during the acute stage of rheumatic fever, or valvular damage may be sustained with disability. Severity varies, and many patients do not have heart symptoms at the time of the acute illness, some never, and others may have rheumatic heart disease diagnosed later in life without having had evidence of rheumatic fever.

   The mitral valve is most commonly affected, followed by the aortic valve (Figure 58-1). Rheumatic carditis is almost always associated with a significant murmur of insufficiency. The damaged valves are susceptible to infection, leading to infective endocarditis.

II. THE COURSE OF RHEUMATIC HEART DISEASE

Many factors influence the outlook after rheumatic fever symptoms subside. Usually, no symptoms persist except the effects of the valvular deformity.

A. Symptoms

1. Stenosis or incompetence of valves; most commonly, the aortic and mitral valves.
2. Heart murmur influenced by the amount of scarring of the valves and myocardium.
3. Cardiac arrhythmias.
4. Late symptoms include shortness of breath, murmur, angina pectoris, epistaxis, elevation of diastolic blood pressure, enlargement of the left ventricle, and increasing signs of congestive cardiac failure.

B. Practice Applications

The significance in dental and dental hygiene practice is the same as that for congenital heart disease.

1. Maintenance of a high level of oral health to prevent a need for treatment of advanced disease.
2. Prevention of infective endocarditis by antibiotic premedication.

MITRAL VALVE PROLAPSE

I. DESCRIPTION

The mitral valve is between the left atrium and the left ventricle (Figure 58-1). Oxygenated blood from the lungs passes from the pulmonary vein into the left atrium and on into the left ventricle, where it is pumped into the aorta for distribution to the body cells.

When the mitral valve leaflets are damaged, the closure is imperfect, and oxygenated blood can backflow or regurgitate. Mitral valve prolapse is the most common disorder of the valve that causes regurgitation.

II. SYMPTOMS

Most patients with mitral valve prolapse are without symptoms. A small number of cases will have symptoms of palpitations, fatigue, atypical chest pain, and a late systolic murmur.

When there is more severe involvement, an increase in frequency of palpitations and progressive mitral regurgitation is apparent along with a systolic click and murmur. Initial suspicion for diagnosis of valvular heart disease is the recognition of a heart murmur.

III. INDICATIONS FOR PROPHYLACTIC ANTIBIOTIC

Infective endocarditis occurs at a higher incidence in patients with mitral valve prolapse. Patients with mitral valve prolapse have been classified as at moderate risk for severe infection.[4] Pretreatment antibiotic is recommended. Figure 6-2 (page 103) outlines a decision tree for determination of the need for antibiotic prophylaxis.

INFECTIVE ENDOCARDITIS[5,6]

Infective endocarditis is a microbial infection of the heart valves or endocardium that is of vital concern in the dental and dental hygiene care of high-risk patients.

A bacteremia, or presence of microorganisms in the blood stream, is necessary for the development of infective endocarditis. A transitory bacteremia usually is created during invasive dental and dental hygiene treatment when bleeding occurs.

Infective endocarditis is a serious disease, the prognosis of which depends on the degree of cardiac damage, the valves involved, the duration of the infection, and the treatment. Patients are prone to develop heart failure leading to death unless the infection is promptly controlled.

Infective endocarditis is characterized by the formation of vegetations composed of masses of bacteria and blood clots on the heart valves. The vegetations may arise on normal valves, but are most likely to occur on previously damaged valves. When bacteremia occurs, the heart valves may become infected, and infective endocarditis can develop.

I. ETIOLOGY

A. Microorganisms

Almost any species of microorganisms may cause infective endocarditis. Streptococci and staphylococci are responsible in most cases, with alpha-hemolytic streptococci being the most prevalent. Because yeast, fungi, and viruses have been implicated, the choice of the name "infective" endocarditis is more inclusive than "bacterial" endocarditis.

B. Risk Factors

1. *Preexisting cardiac abnormalities.* Bacteria lodge on the endocardial (valvular) surface during bacteremia.
2. *Prosthetic heart valves.* There is an increased number of patients who have had valve replacement surgery who are susceptible.
3. *Intravenous drug abuse.* Infected material is injected by contaminated needles directly into the blood stream. Intravenous drug abusers are at high risk for endocarditis, which can initiate on previously normal valves.

C. Precipitating Factors

1. *Self-induced Bacteremia.* In the oral cavity, self-induced bacteremias may result from eating, bruxing, chewing gum, or any activity that can force bacteria through the wall of a diseased sulcus or pocket.
2. *Infection at Portals of Entry.* Infections at sites where microorganisms may enter the circulating blood provide a constant source of potential infectious microorganisms. In the oral cavity, organisms enter the blood by way of periodontal and gingival pockets, where multitudes of many species of microorganisms are harbored. An open area of infection, such as an ulcer caused by an ill-fitting denture, may also provide a site of entry.
3. *Trauma to Tissues by Instrumentation.* Bacteremias are created during general or oral surgery, endodontic procedures, periodontal therapy, scaling, and, particularly, any therapy that causes bleeding.

II. DISEASE PROCESS

A. Bacteremia Initiated

1. Trauma from instrumentation can rupture blood vessels in the gingival sulcus or pocket.

2. Pressure from trauma forces oral microorganisms into the blood. Ease of entry of organisms directly relates to the severity of trauma and the severity of the gingivitis or periodontitis.

B. Bacterial Implantation

1. Circulating microorganisms attach to a damaged heart valve, prosthetic valve, or other susceptible area. The mitral valve is most often affected.
2. Microorganisms proliferate to form vegetative lesions containing masses of plasma cells, fibrin, and bacteria.
3. Heart valve becomes inflamed; function is diminished.
4. Clumps of microorganisms (emboli) may break off and spread by way of the general circulation; complications result.

C. Clinical Course

1. Symptoms may appear within 2 weeks. Severe symptoms of fever, loss of appetite and weight loss, weakness, arthralgia, and heart murmurs require hospitalization.
2. Emboli can lead to paralysis and chest and other body pains.
3. Complications lead to eventual susceptibility to reinfection with infective endocarditis, congestive heart failure, and cerebrovascular disease.

III. PREVENTION

The three basic areas for attention in dental and dental hygiene care that contribute to the prevention of infective endocarditis are shown in Table 58-1.

A. Patient History

1. *Special Content.* Specific questions should be directed to elicit any history of rheumatic fever and its related symptoms, congenital heart defects, cardiac surgery, presence of prosthetic valves or pacemaker, or previous episode of infective endocarditis.
2. *Consultation With Patient's Physician.* Consultation can be assumed necessary for all patients with a history of rheumatic fever, heart defects, and any other condition sug-

---

TABLE 58-1 Prevention of Infective Endocarditis

- Identification of Risk Patients
  - Medical and personal history
  - Consultation with physician
- Prophylactic Antibiotic Coverage During Appointments
- Upgrading and Maintenance of the Patient's Oral Health
  - Personal: daily bacterial plaque removal
  - Professional: supervision, instruction, and motivation through frequent maintenance appointments

gesting the need for prophylactic antibiotic premedication. Instrumentation, including the use of a probe or explorer during assessment of the patient, must be withheld until the medical status is cleared.

B. Prophylactic Antibiotic Premedication
1. *Recommended Regimens.* The recommendations of the American Heart Association are outlined on pages 101 to 104.
2. *Objectives of the Recommended Regimen*
   a. Prevent, or reduce the severity and magnitude of, bacteremia.
   b. Administer antibiotic 1 hour before, so the blood level at the time of the actual procedure is adequate to control infection and prevent infective endocarditis.

C. Dental Hygiene Care
Maintenance of a high degree of oral health is important to each patient susceptible to infective endocarditis.
1. *Instruction.* Instruction in brushing and flossing at initial appointments should be provided while the patient is under antibiotic coverage.
2. *Sequence of Treatment.* Plaque removal instruction should precede instrumentation for scaling to bring the tissues to as healthy a state as possible. The more severe the disease, the higher the incidence of bacteremia during and following instrumentation.
3. *Instrumentation.* Reduce the microbial population about the teeth and on the oral mucosa prior to instrumentation by having the patient brush, floss, and rinse thoroughly with an antiseptic mouthrinse.

HYPERTENSION[7]

Hypertension means an abnormal elevation of blood pressure. It is a symptom, not a disease entity. It is a contributing risk factor in many vascular diseases, or it may be a result or an effect of underlying pathologic changes.

Detection of blood pressure for dental and dental hygiene patients has become an essential step in patient assessment prior to treatment. Early detection, with referral for additional diagnosis and treatment when indicated, can prove to be life saving for certain people. In addition, knowledge of the health problems of patients is needed so treatment can be safe and free from dangers of emergencies that may arise.

I. ETIOLOGY

A. Primary or Essential Hypertension
1. *Incidence.* Approximately 90% of all hypertension is primary or essential.
2. *Predisposing or Risk Factors.* Combinations of

the factors listed are more significant than any one alone.
   a. *Cigarette Smoking.* Risk factors for atherosclerosis are interrelated (page 855).
   b. *Heredity.*
   c. *Overweight.*
   d. *Race.* The incidence is higher among African Americans than among white Americans, the illness is more severe, and the mortality rate is higher at a younger age.
   e. *Climate.* Hypertension is less common in tropical and semitropical countries.
   f. *Salt.* Particularly in excess in the diet.
   g. *Sex.* Men are more affected before age 45; women slightly more than men in later years.
   h. *Age.* General increase from birth to age 20; leveling off until 40 years of age; then a slow increase into the older age group.
   i. *Oral Contraceptives.* Severe hypertension from contraceptives is uncommon. Increased hypertension over years of using contraceptives has been shown, particularly when other risk factors are also involved.
   j. *Environment.* Environmental conditions that increase stress factors.

B. Secondary Hypertension
About 10% of all hypertension is secondary. A specific cause can be identified, in which the pathologic elevation of blood pressure is secondary to a major underlying disease. Examples are disorders of the kidney or of the adrenal or pituitary glands.

II. BLOOD PRESSURE LEVELS
The blood pressure is the pressure exerted by the blood within the arteries. It is determined by the cardiac output, resistance of the capillary bed, and volume and viscosity of the blood. Diseases can alter each of the parts and, thus, alter the blood pressure.

Procedures for blood pressure determination are described with other vital signs in Chapter 7, pages 113 to 114.

Blood pressure fluctuates, so that more than one reading is needed. The blood pressure should be measured two or three times and the average reading entered in the patient's record. When physicians plan treatment for a hypertensive patient, the individual's pattern is usually studied by making at least three determinations on at least two different days.

A. Normal and High Blood Pressure[8]
Table 58-2 shows the normal and high normal readings for blood pressure, and the stages of hypertension for adults 18 years and over.

B. Low Blood Pressure
Many healthy people have a normal diastolic pressure under 90 mmHg or even under 80

TABLE 58-2 Classification of Blood Pressure for Adults Age 18 Years or Older*

Category	Systolic (mmHg)	Diastolic (mmHg)
Optimal[†]	<120	<85
Normal[†]	<130	<85
High normal	130–139	85–89
Hypertension[‡]		
Stage 1	140–159	90–99
Stage 2	160–179	100–109
Stage 3	180–209	110–119

*Not taking antihypertensive drugs and acutely ill. When systolic and diastolic pressures fall into different categories, the higher category should be selected to classify the individual's blood pressure status. For instance, 160/92 mmHg should be classified as Stage 2, and 174/120 mmHg should be classified as Stage 3. Isolated systolic hypertension (ISH) is defined as SBP of 140 mmHg or greater and DBP below 90 mmHg and staged appropriately (for example, 170/82 mmHg is defined as stage 2 ISH).
[†]Optimal blood pressure with respect to cardiovascular risk is SBP <120 mmHg and DBP <80 mmHg. Unusually low readings, however, should be evaluated for clinical significance.
[‡]Based on the average of two or more readings taken at each of two or more visits following an initial screening. (From *The Sixth Report of the Joint National Committee on Prevention, Detection, Evaluation, and Treatment of High Blood Pressure.* National High Blood Pressure Education Program, NIH National Heart, Lung, and Blood Institute, NIH Publication No. 98-4080, November, 1997.)

mmHg, which may be considered "low blood pressure." Such a level is normal for that person and no clinical problems are evident.

A marked sudden drop in blood pressure is usually associated with an emergency, such as severe blood loss, shock, myocardial infarction, or other medical problem. Immediate attention, in the category of a medical emergency, is indicated. Referral to specific procedures can be found in Table 61-6 (pages 911 to 912, 915).

C. Postural Hypotension
Postural or orthostatic hypotension is a condition in which fainting, nausea, or feelings of faintness or dizziness occur when a person sits up quickly from a supine position. One predisposing factor for postural hypotension is the medication used for hypertension.

III. CLINICAL SYMPTOMS OF HYPERTENSION

Hypertension frequently goes unrecognized because of the lack of apparent clinical symptoms.

A. High Blood Pressure
Evidence of the following may be present:
1. Headaches.
2. Dizziness, fainting.
3. Shortness of breath, particularly on effort.
4. Disturbances of concentration or memory impairment.

B. Long-Standing Severe Elevation of Blood Pressure
Hypertensive crisis is a life-threatening disorder. The brain, eyes, heart, or kidney may undergo marked changes in function. In the severe state, if any or all of the following are noted, the patient should be referred immediately.
1. Occipital headaches, more severe in the morning.
2. Mental confusion leading to stupor, coma, convulsions.
3. Blurring of vision; possible loss of sight.
4. Severe dyspnea.
5. Chest pains similar to angina pectoris.

C. Major Sequelae
1. Hypertensive heart disease; enlarged heart with eventual cardiac failure.
2. Cerebral vascular accident (stroke, page 775).
3. Hypertensive renal disease.
4. Ischemic heart disease (pages 854 to 856).

IV. TREATMENT

A. Goals
1. *Primary Hypertension*
   a. Achieve and maintain diastolic pressure level at 90 mmHg or below with minimal adverse effects.
   b. Lower the risk of serious complications and premature death.
2. *Secondary Hypertension.* Surgical or other correction of the cause is needed.

B. Lifestyle Changes (Table 58-3)
1. *Diet.* Salt restriction and weight loss may be all that are needed for the control of mild elevations of blood pressure.
2. *Cigarette Smoking.* All forms of tobacco must be eliminated.
3. *Other Risk Factors.* Factors that contribute to

TABLE 58-3 Lifesetyle Modifications for Hypertension Control and/or Overall Cardiovascular Risk

- Lose weight if overweight.
- Limit alcohol intake to no more than 1 ounce of ethanol per day (24 ounces of beer, 8 ounces of wine, or 2 ounces of 100-proof whiskey).
- Exercise (aerobic) daily.
- Reduce sodium intake to less than 100 mmol per day (2.4 g of sodium or <6 g of sodium chloride).
- Maintain adequate dietary potassium, calcium, and magnesium intake.
- Stop smoking and reduce dietary saturated fat and cholesterol intake for overall cardiovascular health. Reducing fat intake also helps to reduce caloric intake—important for control of weight and type 2 diabetes.

(From *The Sixth Report of the Joint National Committee on Prevention, Detection, Evaluation, and Treatment of High Blood Pressure.* National High Blood Pressure Education Program, NIH National Heart, Lung, and Blood Institute, NIH Publication No. 98-4080, November, 1997.)

stress and tension must be decreased or minimized. Risk factors are listed on page 852.

C. Antihypertensive Drug Therapy

1. *Selection of Therapy.* The decision by the physician to prescribe drug therapy at the various levels depends on the severity of the hypertension, as well as on all factors related to the patient's health.
2. *Categories of Drugs Used in Therapy*
   a. Diuretics to promote renal excretion of water and sodium ions.
   b. Beta-blockers.
   c. Vasodilators to act directly on the blood vessels.
3. *Duration.* Management of hypertension must be considered a lifelong endeavor. Dental personnel can encourage their patients to continue treatment even when a normal reading is maintained. Because many antihypertensive drugs have undesirable side effects, the patient may become discouraged and discontinue treatment.
4. *Side Effects.* The effects of the different drugs prescribed vary, but some of the problems confronted by patients may actually influence the behavior at dental and dental hygiene appointments. Cancellation of an appointment could be anticipated. Side effects may include some or all of the following:
   a. Fatigue.
   b. Gastrointestinal disturbances, including nausea, diarrhea, or cramps.
   c. Xerostomia (potential for dental caries).
   d. Postural hypotension with dizziness and fainting.
   e. Impotence.
   f. Depression.

V. HYPERTENSION IN CHILDREN

Children 3 years of age and older need to have blood pressure determinations made at least annually. A variety of cuff sizes are available, and other procedural suggestions are described on pages 112 to 114.

When a child between ages 3 and 12 has a diastolic pressure greater than 90 mmHg, or if over age 12, greater than 100 mmHg, further investigation is indicated. Because hypertension has a familial tendency, determining the pressure levels for children of parents known to have hypertension may reveal important information about the health of the child.

HYPERTENSIVE HEART DISEASE[9]

Hypertensive heart disease results from the increased load on the heart because of elevated blood pressure. When the peripheral arterial resistance to the flow of blood pumped from the heart is increased, the blood pressure rises. The heart attempts to maintain its normal output. To cope with the increased workload resulting from the peripheral resistance, muscle fibers are stretched and the heart enlarges.

The effect of hypertension on the heart is at first a thickening of the left ventricle. In later stages, the entire heart is enlarged. This may be discerned by radiographic and medical examination.

Cardiac enlargement has no specific symptoms, but the patient may have symptoms of hypertension, such as headaches, weakness, and others listed on page 853. When undiagnosed and untreated, the severity increases and left ventricular congestive failure occurs, resulting from the disturbance of cardiac function.

ISCHEMIC HEART DISEASE

Ischemic heart disease is the cardiac disability, acute and chronic, that arises from reduction or arrest of blood supply to the myocardium.

The heart muscles (myocardium) are supplied through the coronary arteries, which are branches of the descending aorta. Because of the relationship to the coronary arteries, the disease is often referred to as *coronary heart disease* or *coronary artery disease.*

Ischemia means oxygen deprivation in a local area from a reduced passage of fluid into the area. Ischemic heart disease is the result of an imbalance of the oxygen supply and demand of the myocardium, which, in turn, results from a narrowing or blocking of the lumen of the coronary arteries.

I. ETIOLOGY[10]

Other factors may be involved, but the principal cause of the reduction of blood flow to the heart muscle is *atherosclerosis* of the vessel walls, which narrows the lumen, thus obstructing the flow of blood.

A. Definition of Atherosclerosis

Atherosclerosis is a disease of medium and large arteries in which atheromas deposit on and thicken the intimal layer of the involved blood vessel. An atheroma is a fibro-fatty deposit or plaque, containing several lipids, especially cholesterol. With time, the plaques continue to thicken and, eventually, close the vessel (Figure 58-4). Some plaques calcify, whereas others may develop an overlying thrombus.

B. Predisposing Factors for Atherosclerosis

Each of the risk factors listed here is significant alone. When these factors occur in combinations, the risk of atherosclerosis, and therefore of ischemic heart disease, is increased. Prevention depends on educational programs along with early identification of persons at risk.

1. Elevated levels of blood lipids; the result of an increased dietary intake of cholesterol, saturated fat, carbohydrate, especially sucrose, alcohol, and calories.
2. Elevated blood pressure.
3. Cigarette smoking.
4. Diabetes.
5. Obesity.
6. Insufficient physical activity.
7. Increased tensions; emotional stress.
8. Family history. Genetic inheritance can be one factor along with the perpetuation of familial lifestyle habits. Diet, smoking habits, tensions, and tendencies toward lack of exercise are typical examples.

II. MANIFESTATIONS OF ISCHEMIC HEART DISEASE

A. Components
1. Angina pectoris.
2. Myocardial infarction.
3. Congestive heart failure.
4. Sudden death.

B. Treatment
1. *Counseling.* With a brief history of angina pain, the patient is counseled to be reassured that lifestyle changes are necessary but that a productive life can be led.
2. *Lifestyle Changes.* Necessary changes in lifestyle (Table 58-3) are encouraged, notably diet, exercise, and no smoking.
3. *Medications.* A variety of medications may be required depending on individual needs, including
   a. Antianginal (vasodilators). Prevent anginal pain by decreasing systolic blood pressure.
   b. Antihypertensives (diuretics). Blood pressure control.
   c. Antidysrhythmics. Fibrillation; ventricular dysrhythmias.

Normal Vessel

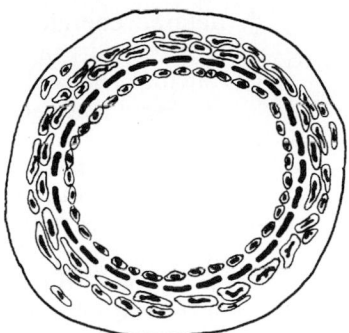

Atherosclerotic Vessel showing Atheroma

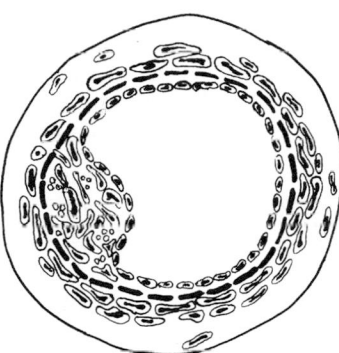

Partially Blocked Vessel

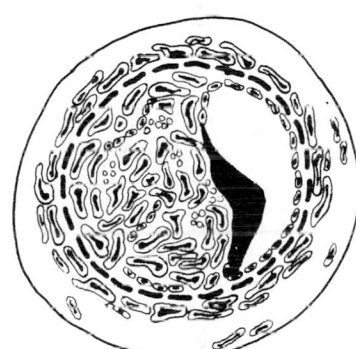

Occluded Vessel

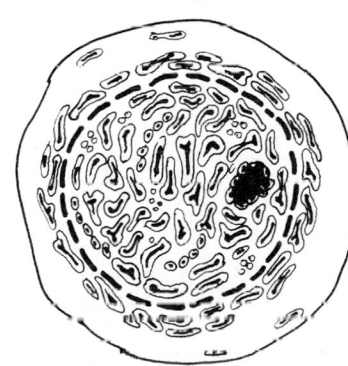

FIGURE 58-4 Atherosclerosis. An atheroma develops within the lining of the normal blood vessel. The atheroma is made of a fatty deposit containing cholesterol. At first, the atheroma is small and no symptoms are apparent, but eventually it enlarges and completely blocks the vessel, thus depriving the area served by the vessel of oxygen. (From *Arteriosclerosis 1981.* Report of the Working Group on Arteriosclerosis of the National Heart, Lung, and Blood Institute, National Institutes of Health, United States Department of Health and Human Services, NIH Publication No. 81–2034, June, 1981.)

d. Beta-adrenergic blocking agents. Decreased heart rate and blood pressure.

e. Calcium channel blockers. Decreased cardiac workload; act as vasodilators.

4. *Surgery*

a. Percutaneous transluminal coronary angioplasty (coronary dilation).

b. Coronary bypass for patients with significant obstruction. The purpose is to "jump-pass" over arteries that have been narrowed with atherosclerosis. The beneficial effects are relief from anginal pains, less workload for the heart, and an increase of oxygen and blood supply to the myocardium. Figure 58-5 shows the use of a vein graft and the internal mammary artery for bypasses.

ANGINA PECTORIS

Angina pectoris is a symptom complex or syndrome of discomfort in the chest and adjacent areas that results from transient and reversible myocardial oxygen deficiency. Although other forms of coronary disease may cause similar pain symptoms, approximately 90% of angina attacks are related to coronary artery atherosclerosis.

I. PREDISPOSING FACTORS

An attack of angina pectoris may be precipitated by exertion or exercise, emotion, or a heavy meal. In the dental office or clinic, a preventive atmosphere of calmness and quiet can do much to alleviate stress.

II. SYMPTOMS

A. Chest Pain

Each person who suffers from angina has a characteristic pattern of pain symptoms. When changes in the usual pain occur, the physician must be notified.

Commonly, the patient has thoracic pain, which is substernal and radiates down the left arm and up to the mandible. It may last for seconds or minutes.

The pain is squeezing or crushing, paroxysmal, or pressing, with a feeling of weight on the chest. The patient stops and tends to stiffen.

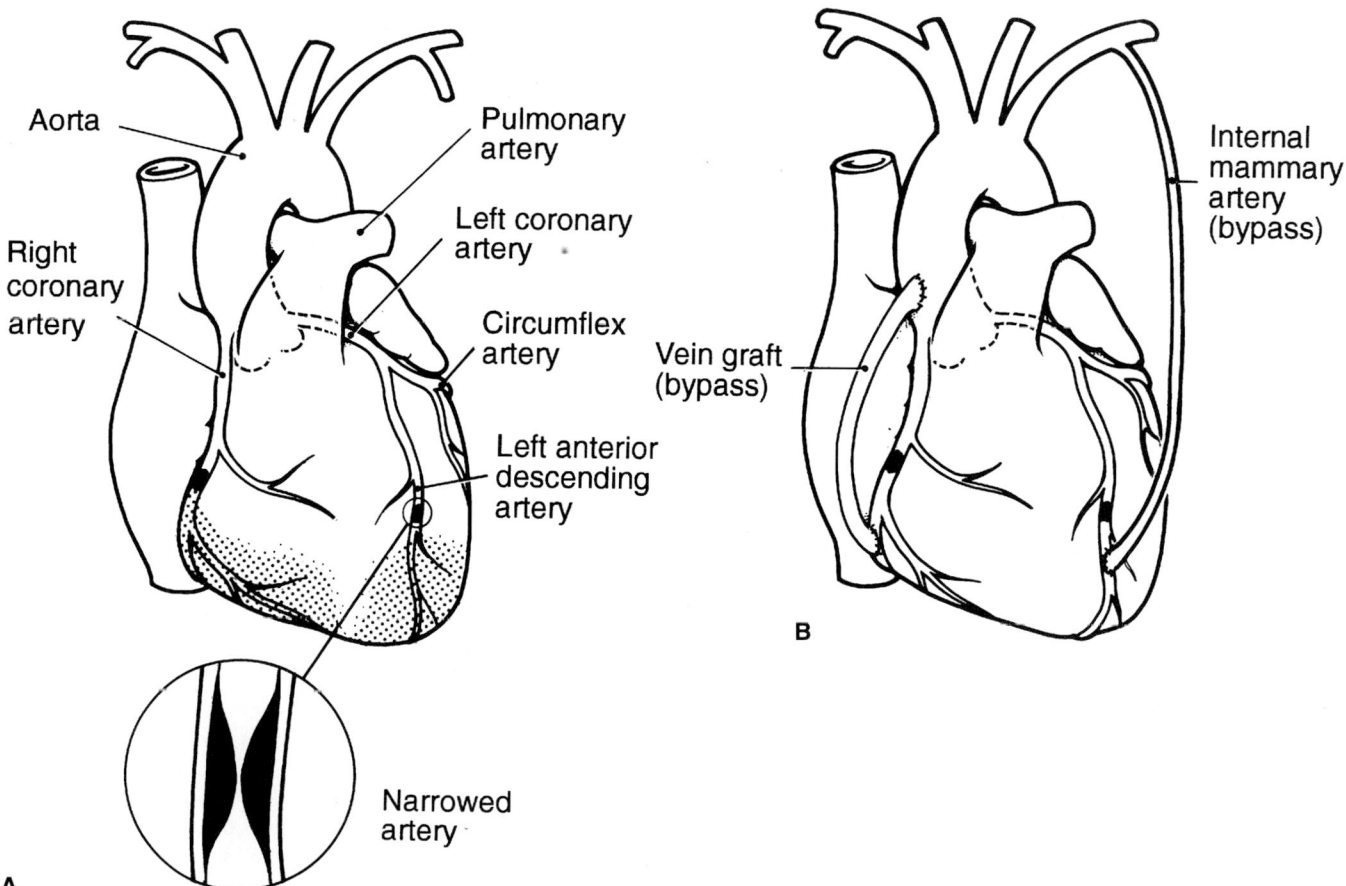

FIGURE 58-5 Coronary Bypass Surgery. (A) Heart showing infarcted (shaded) areas created by coronary arteries narrowed by atherosclerosis. **(B)** Vein graft from saphenous vein connected with aorta to bypass narrowed area of right coronary artery, and internal mammary artery used to bypass narrowed left anterior descending artery.

B. Other Symptoms

The patient may be pale and also experience faintness, sweating, difficulty in breathing, anxiety, or fear.

III. TREATMENT

A vasodilator, usually nitroglycerin, is administered sublingually.

IV. PROCEDURE DURING AN ATTACK IN THE DENTAL OFFICE

A. Terminate Treatment

Stop the dental or dental hygiene procedure. Call for assistance and the emergency kit or cart.

B. Position Patient

Bring seat up to a comfortable position; reassure the patient.

C. Administer Vasodilator

Administer nitroglycerin sublingually. Use of the patient's own supply is preferable. Prior to starting procedures of the appointment, the patient's supply should be placed within reach. The patient can be asked when the nitroglycerin was purchased, because the potency is lost after 6 months out of a sealed storage container.

Patient with xerostomia may not have sufficient saliva to moisten the nitroglycerin. A few drops of water from the unit syringe can be placed on the tablet under the tongue.

D. Check Patient Response

Give additional vasodilator. Usually, the first tablet relieves the condition within minutes. When it is suspected that the patient's supply may not be fresh and the first tablet has been ineffective, use of a second tablet from the dental office emergency kit may be advisable.

E. Call for Medical Assistance

When the patient does not respond to the second dose of vasodilator, assume the attack to be a myocardial infarction. Oxygen administration may be indicated.

F. Record Vital Signs

1. Use *Medical Emergency Report,* Figure 61-1, page 898.
2. Measure blood pressure, take pulse rate, and count respirations.

G. Observe Recovery

For the patient who recovers without additional medical assistance, allow a rest period before dismissal. Record vital signs again.

V. SUBSEQUENT DENTAL AND DENTAL HYGIENE APPOINTMENTS

Keep a copy of the *Medical Emergency Report* in the patient's permanent file for reference when planning future appointments.

MYOCARDIAL INFARCTION

Myocardial infarction is the most extreme manifestation of ischemic heart disease. It is also called *heart attack, coronary occlusion,* or *coronary thrombosis.* It results from a sudden reduction or arrest of coronary blood flow.

The most common artery associated with a myocardial infarction is the anterior descending branch of the left coronary artery. That is also the most common site of advanced atherosclerosis.

I. ETIOLOGY

The immediate cause often is a thrombosis that blocks an artery already narrowed by atherosclerosis. In turn, the blockage creates an area of infarction, which leads to myocardial necrosis of the area. Necrosis of the area can occur within a few hours.

A few patients die immediately or within a few hours. Sudden death may be caused by ventricular fibrillation.

II. SYMPTOMS

A. Pain

1. *Location.* Pain symptoms may start under the sternum, with feelings of indigestion, or in the middle to upper sternum. Pain may last for extended periods, even hours. When the pain is severe, it gives a pressing or crushing heavy sensation and is not relieved by rest or nitroglycerin.
2. *Onset.* The pain may have a sudden onset, sometimes during sleep or following exercise. The pain may be radial, similar to angina pectoris, which extends to the left arm and mandible.

B. Other Symptoms

Cold sweat, weakness and faintness, shortness of breath, nausea, and vomiting may occur. Blood pressure is lowered.

III. MANAGEMENT DURING AN ATTACK

A. Terminate Treatment

Sit the patient up for comfortable breathing, give nitroglycerin, and reassure the patient.

B. Summon Medical Assistance.

1. When nitroglycerin does not reduce the angina-like pain within 3 minutes, call both a physician and an ambulance with paramedical personnel (Table 61-5, page 912).
2. Use *Medical Emergency Report,* Figure 61-1, page 898, and record vital signs.
3. Administer oxygen.
4. Apply cardiopulmonary resuscitation if indicated while waiting for medical assistance.
5. Transport to hospital.

IV. TREATMENT AFTER ACUTE SYMPTOMS

A. Medical Supervision

Current medical care for heart attack calls for a shortened rest period with increased activity, in keeping with the strength and progress of the patient. Most patients experience extreme fatigue during their convalescence.

B. Lifestyle Changes

Limited diet and elimination of smoking and stressful activities are essential. Many patients need considerable education, reassurance, and motivation.

C. Subsequent Appointments

Elective dental and dental hygiene appointments may be postponed 3 months or more until the patient's physician has given consent.

CONGESTIVE HEART FAILURE

Heart failure is a syndrome in which an abnormality of cardiac function is responsible for the inability or failure of the heart to pump blood at a rate necessary to meet the needs of the body tissues. Because of the collection of fluids in various body organs, the term *congestive heart failure* is used.

I. ETIOLOGY

The many causes for heart failure fall into two categories: underlying and precipitating causes.

A. Underlying Causes

Examples of cardiovascular disease that result in heart failure are
1. Heart valve damage (rheumatic heart disease, congenital heart disease).
2. Myocardial failure as a result of an abnormality of heart muscle or secondary to ischemia.

B. Precipitating Causes

Examples that place an additional load on a chronically burdened myocardium are
1. *Acute Hypertensive Crisis.* Severe symptoms of headache, mental confusion, dizziness, shortness of breath, and chest pain may predispose to heart failure.
2. *Massive Pulmonary Embolism.* A thrombus may form in a lower extremity of an inactive person with low cardiac output and circulatory stasis. The thrombus may break loose and, carried by the blood, lodge in the pulmonary artery to cause a pulmonary embolism. Severe dyspnea, cyanosis, congestive failure, and shock result.
3. *Arrhythmia.* After resuscitation of a person with myocardial infarction, ventricular fibrillation, a type of arrhythmia, is the major risk leading to sudden death.

II. CLINICAL MANIFESTATIONS

The clinical manifestations coincide with the parts of the heart involved. Signs and symptoms are different, depending, in general, on whether the left or the right side of the heart or both are affected. The general effects are extreme weakness, fatigue, fear, and anxiety.

A. Left Heart Failure

The left side of the heart receives oxygenated blood from the lungs and pumps the blood into the aorta to the rest of the body. A pathologic condition of the left ventricle or the mitral valve alters output, and causes respiratory difficulty because of the backup of fluid and blood into the lungs.

Clinical symptoms are more prominent at night. The patient rests better in a sitting or semisitting position with more than one pillow.
1. *Subjective Symptoms*
   a. Weakness, fatigue.
   b. Dyspnea, particularly evident on exertion. Shortness of breath on lying supine, relieved when sitting up.
   c. Cough and expectoration.
   d. Nocturia.
2. *Objective Symptoms*
   a. Pallor; sweating, cold skin.
   b. Breathing obviously difficult.
   c. Diastolic blood pressure increased.
   d. Heart rate rapid.
   e. Anxiety, fear.

B. Right Heart Failure

The right heart receives the venous blood from the vena cava and pumps it to the lungs for oxygenation. Right heart failure shows evidence of systemic venous congestion with peripheral edema. When left heart failure precedes right heart failure, the heart is already congested. Resistance to receiving the venous blood is an additional factor.
1. *Subjective Symptoms*
   a. Weakness, fatigue.
   b. Swelling of the feet and/or ankles. The edema progresses to the thighs and abdomen (ascites) in advanced stages of heart failure.
   c. Cold hands and feet.
2. *Objective Symptoms*
   a. Cyanosis of mucous membranes and nailbeds.
   b. Prominent jugular veins.
   c. Congestion with edema in various organs: enlarged spleen and liver; gastrointestinal distress with nausea and vomiting; central nervous system involvement with headache and irritability.
   d. Anxiety, fear.

III. TREATMENT DURING CHRONIC STAGES

A patient with an appointment in a dental office or

clinic may be receiving a variety of medical treatments. These should be revealed by questioning during preparation of histories. Nearly all patients with heart failure complications have the following in their medical treatment plan:

A. Drug Therapy
Physicians may prescribe many different medications for patients with cardiovascular disease. The general types are listed in Table 6-3, page 98.

B. Dietary Control
1. Limited sodium intake to alleviate fluid retention.
2. Weight reduction.

C. Limitation of Activity
Activity should be limited depending on the severity of the health problem and the advice of the physician.

IV. EMERGENCY CARE FOR HEART FAILURE AND ACUTE PULMONARY EDEMA

A medical emergency that demands urgent attention may occur anywhere. The patient with heart failure or acute pulmonary edema is usually conscious.
A. Position the patient upright for comfortable breathing (Table 61-5, page 911).
B. Administer oxygen.
C. Use *Medical Emergency Report*, Figure 61-1, page 898 and monitor vital signs (blood pressure, respiratory rate, and pulse).
D. Reassure the patient.
E. Obtain medical assistance, including both physician and ambulance.

SUDDEN DEATH

Clinical death that occurs within 24 hours after onset of symptoms is known as sudden death, whereas death within 30 seconds is instantaneous death. Biologic death occurs when permanent cellular damage has been done, primarily from lack of adequate oxygen supply. Biologic death takes place when oxygen delivery to the brain is inadequate for 4 to 6 minutes.

I. ETIOLOGY

Nearly all sudden deaths are from a cardiovascular cause, predominantly coronary atherosclerosis. Examples of noncardiac causes are cerebral hemorrhage, drug overdose or toxicity, and pulmonary thromboembolism.

II. MECHANISM OF SUDDEN CARDIOVASCULAR DEATH

A. Definition and Description
Most sudden deaths are caused by *ventricular fibrillation*. Because of many premature beats in which individual muscle bundles fibrillate or contract independently, the ventricle cannot be refilled. Insufficient blood is pumped into the coronary arteries to supply the myocardium. A severe lack of oxygen to the heart muscles causes ventricular standstill, which is one form of cardiac arrest.

B. Clinical Signs of Death
1. Loss of consciousness.
2. No respiration, no pulse, no blood pressure.
3. Dilated pupils.

III. EMERGENCY CARE

A. Immediate Need: Oxygen
Every second counts; only 4 minutes, or 6 at the most, can elapse before enough brain cells die from lack of oxygen to produce biologic death.

B. Basic Life Support
Details of the procedures are described on pages 900 to 906.
1. Provide artificial ventilation.
2. Provide artificial circulation.
3. Provide transportation to a hospital.

CARDIAC PACEMAKER

The natural pacemaker, or center where the normal heartbeat is initiated, is the sino-atrial (S-A) node located in the right atrium or auricle. From that node, impulses are sent along the muscle walls to stimulate and regulate the contractions of the ventricles, which pump the blood throughout the body.

When the natural pacemaker cells are not able to maintain a reliable rhythm, or when the impulses are interrupted because of heart block, cardiac arrest, various arrhythmias, or other disease conditions, treatment by a cardiologist may include the placement of an artificial pacemaker.

I. DESCRIPTION

A. Definition
A cardiac pacemaker is an electronic stimulator used to send a specified electrical current to the myocardium to control or maintain a minimum heart rate. It may be single chambered (to ventricle or atrium) or dual chambered to sense and pace both heart chambers.

B. Parts and Power
A permanently implanted pacemaker has electrodes inserted transvenously to the endocardium. Less commonly, the leads may go to the pericardium of the external heart wall.
The electrodes are connected to the power source, a plastic- or metal-encased, hermetically sealed pulse generator containing a lithium anode battery. The pulse generator is implanted under the skin in the thorax or upper abdomen. The area selected depends on the indi-

vidual condition as determined by the cardiologist (Figure 58-6).

C. Types

Research has provided many advancements in pacemaker technology. Current systems involve rate-responsive or physiologic pacing. Sensors may be alert to muscle or physical activity vibrations, body temperature, or respiration rate. The research will have a significant impact on the future of pacing. The two general types are demand and fixed rate.

1. *Demand.* The demand pacemaker stimulates the heart only when the rate varies from a predetermined norm. By sensing a discrepancy in the electrical signals produced by natural means, the pacemaker sends a signal or stimulus, which regulates the heartbeat.

2. *Fixed Rate.* A preset rate of electrical stimuli is provided independent of the natural heart activity when the natural beat is too slow. Each patient is evaluated for the type of pacemaker that is best for the condition of that individual's heart. The fixed rate is used infrequently.

II. INTERFERENCES AND THEIR EFFECTS

External electromagnetic interferences can stop or alter the function of a pacemaker. Different models of pacemakers and their sensitivities to interference vary. Newer models are made with a special shielding to protect against interference.

Historically, ultrasonic scaling units, electrodesensitizing equipment, pulp testers, electric toothbrushes, electrosurgery machines, certain casting equipment, and the Myomonitor were among the potential sources of interference with a pacemaker in a dental care setting. Dental devices that apply an electric current directly to the patient were considered those most likely to interfere.

The dental environment has been shown to be a source of moderate electromagnetic interference. All dental equipment should be kept in good repair. Electric devices that contact or can contact the patient should be checked for leakage, because leakage can be a source of interference. Electric appliances must be earth-grounded.

The effect of distance has not been sufficiently researched; hence patients in adjacent dental treatment rooms should be checked before equipment is used.

Although the evidence for interferences in the dental setting is not great, concern must be shown because all pacemakers are not the same.

III. PACEMAKER MALFUNCTION

A. Symptoms

A patient may mention feelings of discomfort. At the same time, the clinician must be aware of possible changes and signs in the event of stopping or altering of a pacemaker.

1. Difficulty in breathing.
2. Dizziness, light-headedness, feelings of faintness, or syncope.

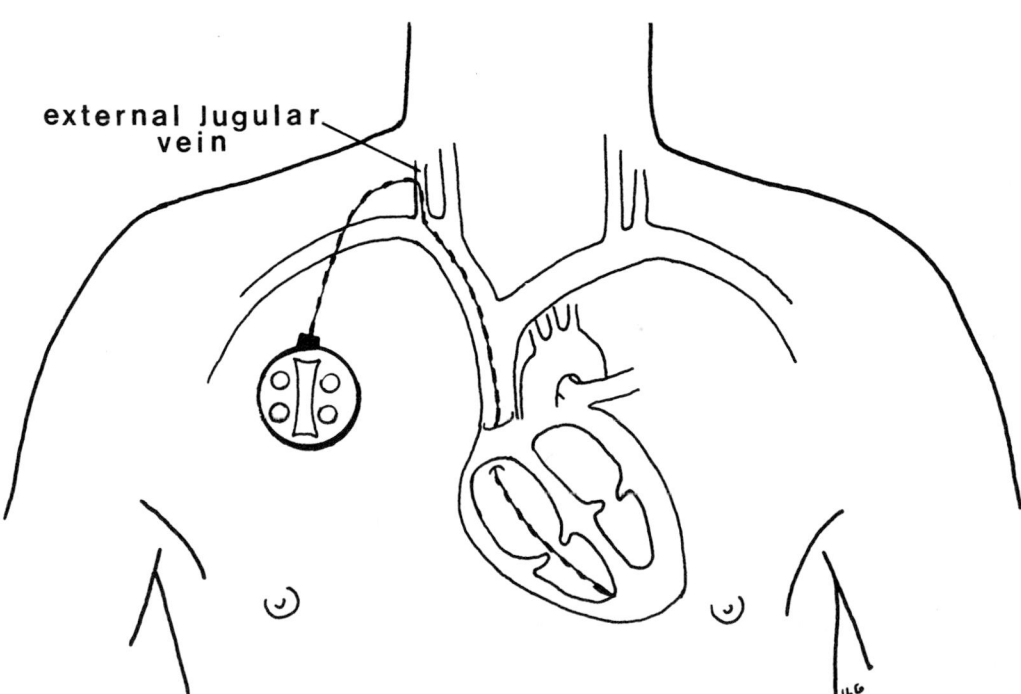

FIGURE 58-6 Cardiac Pacemaker. The pulse generator is implanted under the skin in the thorax or upper abdomen. The lead electrodes may go to the ventricle or to the atrium or both to provide the necessary stimulus for regulation of the heartbeat.

3. Changes in pulse rate.
4. Swelling of legs, ankles, arms, wrists.
5. Chest pain.
6. Prolonged hiccoughing.
7. Muscle twitching.

B. Emergency Procedures

In the event a pacemaker should be turned off, immediate action is needed.

1. Turn off all suspected sources of interference.
2. Call for medical assistance; a defibrillator may be needed.
3. Position the patient for cardiopulmonary resuscitation.
4. Open airway, check for breathing, and begin mouth-to-mouth ventilation. The complete procedure is described on pages 904 to 906.
5. Observe the patient. When the heart is forced to assume its rhythm again as a result of artificial circulation, the pacemaker is set into action to resume the generation and regulation of the pulse.

IV. APPOINTMENT GUIDELINES FOR THE PATIENT WITH A PACEMAKER

General procedures for all patients with cardiovascular involvement apply to the patient wearing a pacemaker. In addition, certain adaptations are recommended.

A. Informed Consent

The signature of the patient or the patient's parent or guardian on a formal statement is a necessary protection against any legal liability in the event of complications or undesirable effects. The patient should receive careful instruction in the anticipated procedures and materials used. Dental and dental hygiene records should be accurate and all-inclusive with a detailed record for each appointment.

B. Patient Histories

The usual health history should be supplemented with information about the type of pacemaker, how long it has been in use, where it is located, the underlying disease condition, and other information pertinent to the patient's safety during dental and dental hygiene appointments. Consultation with the patient's cardiologist is indicated.

C. Prophylactic Antibiotic Premedication

The underlying cardiovascular disease is the basic determinant for the use of antibiotic prophylaxis. Infective endocarditis has occurred in patients with pacemakers.

Antibiotic prophylaxis may be indicated during the first 6 months following placement of a pacemaker. After implantation, the pulse generator and the electrodes are usually covered by endothelium. Although the patient with a pacemaker appears to be at low risk of endocarditis, the dentist and the cardiologist may choose to use antibiotics to cover dental and dental hygiene procedures.

D. Patient Preparation

1. *Chair Position.* Positioning the patient to support breathing and circulation is important. If the patient experiences difficulty in breathing when in the supine position, the chair back should be elevated to reduce stress.

   The patient may experience some discomfort from wire tension or strain at the implant site if the chair is positioned too far back. That depends on the location of the pulse generator. Care must be taken that no pressure is placed over the site of a pacemaker in the patient's chest.

2. *Lead Apron.* Protection of the pulse generator and the lead wires may be indicated. A lead apron can serve to interrupt interferences that may be created by electric devices, including handpieces. A lead apron can be heavy and uncomfortable, however, and therefore may require some consideration.

E. Instrumentation

The use of manual procedures is advisable. Ultrasonic instruments should be avoided.

ANTICOAGULANT THERAPY

Anticoagulants are used in the treatment of many cardiovascular diseases to prevent embolus and thrombus formation. A prescribed drug may be continued indefinitely in the patient's life as a preventive measure.

Drugs most commonly used to prevent or delay blood coagulation are heparin (hospital-administered intravenous) and coumarin derivatives. Although precautions are needed to prevent hemorrhage, discontinuing the drug may be more hazardous for the patient than performing dental and dental hygiene therapy with precautions. When extensive surgical procedures are required, the patient may be hospitalized.

I. CLINICAL PROCEDURES

A. Consultation

Information about the patient's prothrombin time is obtained from the physician during an initial consultation. The prothrombin time is a test of the coagulation phase of blood clotting used to monitor therapy with anticoagulants. A therapeutic range of 1½ to 2½ times the normal level is preferred.

B. Treatment Planning[11]

1. *Pretest for Prothrombin Time*

a. Determine the prothrombin time within 24 hours before an appointment. The patient can have the test made on the day of a dental appointment by preplanning with the physician and the laboratory. Most patients have a routine appointment for monitoring of the blood, and dental appointment dates can be planned to coincide.

b. Safe level for dental and dental hygiene procedures is considered to be 1½ times the normal, provided precautions are taken during instrumentation and postoperative care.

2. *Quadrant Scaling and Root Planing*

a. Treat the most healthy quadrant first. The least bleeding will occur.

b. Teach and emphasize daily bacterial plaque control procedures in a series of appointments to prepare the gingival tissue for instrumentation. Healthy, healed tissue does not bleed as readily or as profusely.

c. Complete treatment, including removal of all calculus and subgingival plaque and other irritants, is necessary to contribute to the goal of healthy tissue that does not bleed.

C. Local Hemostatic Measures

Instrumentation can be performed for most patients without complication, provided precautions are taken to minimize tissue trauma and control bleeding, and not to dismiss the patient until bleeding has stopped.

1. *Pressure.* Pressure with sponges or cotton pellets packed interdentally can aid in control.

2. *Suture.* Sutures may be used to close and adapt the tissue interdentally following deep scaling and root planing.

3. *Periodontal Dressing.* Placement of a dressing is sometimes advisable to provide pressure and protection from trauma that may initiate bleeding. Dressing placement is described on pages 590 to 592.

II. POSTPROCEDURAL INSTRUCTIONS

The practice by oral surgeons of closely observing patients for 6 to 8 hours following a surgical procedure has application following certain dental and dental hygiene procedures for selected patients. At the least, a check that postcare instructions are being followed is advisable.

The patient is advised to avoid vigorous toothbrushing and rinsing for several hours or until the next day. The use of extraoral icepacks may be helpful. General postcare instructions may be found on page 592; for the care of an area with a dressing, see Table 36-1, page 593.

The use of a soft diet, cool rather than hot foods, and general moderation in activity may be advisable.

Long-term instruction must emphasize the maintenance of gingival health to prevent future bleeding problems.

CARDIOVASCULAR SURGERY[12]

Cardiac surgery has become widely used. Patients in dental offices and clinics who have had or will have surgery should be identified and need special procedures. Because the patient with a cardiac prosthesis is at risk for infective endocarditis, all possible dental treatment must be completed before the date of cardiac surgery and preventive measures must be emphasized.

I. PRESURGICAL

Before elective cardiac surgery, the patient should be brought to a state of optimum oral health, with all sources of infection removed. All restorations and other dental procedures must be completed.

Patients requiring cardiac surgery need information and motivation relative to the importance of oral health in eliminating a potential source of infective endocarditis. Vigilance in a preventive program including plaque control and self-applied fluorides is essential.

II. POSTSURGICAL

A. Maintenance Appointments

Frequent appointments are necessary for supervision and maintenance.

B. Prophylactic Antibiotics

1. Antibiotic coverage for all dental and dental hygiene procedures for patients with synthetic prostheses is essential. Because of the high susceptibility to infections, a special regimen for high-risk patients may be indicated.

2. Patients with implanted vascular autographs generally do not need antibiotic premedication before dental and dental hygiene appointments. An example of an implanted vascular autograph is the use of a patient's own blood vessel to provide a coronary bypass (Figure 58-5). The saphenous vein and the internal mammary artery are most commonly used.

C. Immunosuppressive Therapy[13]

Principle drugs used for patients with transplants are cyclosporin, azathioprine, and prednisolone to prevent rejection of the transplant. Among the side effects, particularly of cyclosporin, is gingival enlargement. Many also receive medication with the nifedipine group, also effective in causing gingival enlargement. Special periodontal care will be needed.

TECHNICAL HINTS

I. RECORD PRESCRIPTIONS

Record all prescriptions by date, drug, dose, and directions in the patient's permanent record.

II. DETERMINE STATUS OF PRESCRIPTION

Check that the patient has filled the prescriptions.

III. PREPARE FOR APPOINTMENT

Before each appointment for a patient with a cardiovascular disease:

A. Determine and record blood pressure.
B. Review patient history and notes relative to previous appointments to prepare adequately for the current appointment.
C. Check with the patient to be sure that prescribed medications have been taken and at the proper time.
  1. Antibiotic premedication must be taken 1 hour before the appointment.
  2. Question the patient concerning drugs that may have been taken on the same day as the appointment, such as cocaine, a sedative, alcoholic beverage, or other that may influence the premedication or the effect of an anesthetic to be given.

IV. SOURCE OF MATERIALS

Local Heart Association and American Heart Association
7320 Greenville Avenue
Dallas, TX 75231

FACTORS TO TEACH THE PATIENT

I. HYPERTENSION THERAPY

Encourage patients who have been diagnosed as hypertensive to continue their prescribed therapy.

II. STRESS REDUCTION PROCEDURES[14]

A. Select an appointment time that is optimum with respect to time of day when the patient is feeling best and may be less fatigued. Most anxious patients prefer a morning appointment.
B. Get adequate sleep and rest, and engage in nonfatiguing activities during the 24 hours before the appointment.
C. Use premedication as prescribed for sleeping the night before. A sedative may be prescribed to be taken 60 minutes before an appointment or at the dental office, if possible. When taken at home 1 hour before, the patient should not drive a car.
D. Allow time to get to the dental office or clinic; bring own reading material, knitting or sew-

ing, or other relaxing activity in the event waiting is unavoidable.
E. Eat breakfast, lunch, or other usual between-meal food and take usual medications on schedule.
F. When other family members, especially children, have dental or dental hygiene appointments, do not add to their stress by relaying personal negative feelings.

REFERENCES

1. **Burns**, D.K. and Kumar, V.: The Heart, in Kumar, V., Cotran, R.S., and Robbins, S.L.: *Basic Pathology*, 6th ed. Philadelphia, W.B. Saunders Co., 1997, pp. 333–336.
2. **Burns** and Kumar: op. cit., pp. 321–324.
3. **Little**, J.W., Falace, D.A., Miller C.S., and Rhodus, N.L.: *Dental Management of the Medically Compromised Patient*, 5th ed. St. Louis, Mosby, 1997, pp. 131–143.
4. **Dajani**, A.S., Taubert, K.A., Wilson, W., Bolger, A.F., Bayer, A., Ferrieri, P., Gewitz, M.H., Shulman, S.T., Nouri, S., Newberger, J.W., Hutto, C., Pallasch, T.J., Gage, T.W., Levison, M.E., Peter, G., and Zuccaro, G.: Prevention of Bacterial Endocarditis. Recommendations by the American Heart Association, *Circulation*, 96, 358, July 1, 1997.
5. **Little**, Falace, Miller, and Rhodus: op. cit., pp. 103–117.
6. **Burns** and Kumar: op. cit., pp. 326–328.
7. **Kumar**, V., Cotran, R.S., and Robbins, S.L.: *Basic Pathology*, 6th ed. Philadelphia, W.B. Saunders Co., 1997, pp. 289–292.
8. **United States National Institutes of Health**, National Heart, Lung, and Blood Institute: *The Sixth Report of the Joint National Committee on Prevention, Detection, Evaluation, and Treatment of High Blood Pressure*. Washington, DC, National Heart, Lung, and Blood Institute, NIH Publication No. 98-4080, November, 1997.
9. **Burns** and Kumar: op. cit., pp. 318–319.
10. **Little**, Falace, Miller, and Rhodus: op. cit., pp. 192–196.
11. **Little**, Falace, Miller, and Rhodus: op. cit., pp. 46 47, 485–488.
12. **Little**, Falace, Miller, and Rhodus: op. cit., pp. 66–67, 156–175, 579–581.
13. **Thomason**, J.M., Seymour, R.A., Ellis, J.S., Kelly, P.J., Parry, G., Dark, J., and Idle, J.R.: Iatrogenic Gingival Overgrowth in Cardiac Transplantation, *J. Periodontol.*, 66, 742, August, 1995.
14. **Malamed**, S.F.: *Handbook of Medical Emergencies in the Dental Office*, 4th ed. St. Louis, Mosby, 1993, pp. 44–48.

SUGGESTED READINGS

Boraz, R.A. and Myers, R.: A National Survey of Dental Protocols for the Patient With a Cardiac Transplant, *Spec. Care Dentist.*, 10, 26, January–February, 1990.

Carabello, B.A. and Crawford, F.A.: Valvular Heart Disease, *N. Engl. J. Med.*, 337, 32, July 3, 1997.

Carlson-Mann, L.D.: Case Study: Dental Management of a Heart Transplant Patient, *Canad. Dent. Hyg. (Probe)*, 30, 77, March/April, 1996.

Hays, G.L., McMahon, J.C., Zimmerman, S.J., Lusk, S.S., and DeVoll, R.E.: Screening for Cardiovascular Disease, *Gen. Dent.*, 40, 26, January–February, 1992.

Herman, W.W. and Konzelman, J.L.: Angina: An Update for Dentistry, *J. Am. Dent. Assoc.*, 127, 98, January, 1996.

Hollander, J.E.: The Management of Cocaine-associated Myocardial Ischemia, *N. Engl. J. Med.*, 333, 1267, November 9, 1995.

Mueller-Joseph, L.: Cardiovascular Diseases. Implications for Dental Hygiene Care, *DentalHygienistNews*, 8, 5, Number 3, 1995.

Muzyra, B.C. and Glick, M.: The Hypertensive Dental Patient, *J. Am. Dent. Assoc.*, 128, 1109, August, 1997.

Roelke, M. and Bernstein, A.D.: Cardiac Pacemakers and Cellular Telephones (Editorial), *N. Engl. J. Med., 336*, 1518, May 22, 1997.

Ross, R.: Atherosclerosis—An Inflammatory Disease, *New Engl. J. Med., 340*, 115, January 14, 1999.

Sandor, G.K.B., Vasilakos, S.S., and Vasilakos, J.S.: Mitral Valve Prolapse: A Review of the Syndrome with Emphasis on Current Antibiotic Prophylaxis, *J. Can. Dent. Assoc., 57*, 321, April, 1991.

Souliman, S.K. and Christie, J.: Pacemaker Failure Induced by Radiotherapy, *Pace, 17*, 270, March, 1994.

Vongpatanasin, W., Hillis, L.D., and Lange, R.A.: Prosthetic Heart Valves, *N. Engl. J. Med. 335*, 407, August 8, 1996.

Treatment

Biron, C.R.: Antianginal Therapy, *RDH, 15*, 44, October, 1996.

Biron, C.R.: Drug Therapy for Congestive Heart Failure Poses Several Risks During Dental Treatment, *RDH, 16*, 46, February, 1996.

Bittl, J.A.: Advances in Coronary Angioplasty, *N. Engl. J. Med., 335*, 1290, October 24, 1996.

Bypass Angioplasty Revascularization Investigation (BARI) Investigators: Comparison of Coronary Bypass Surgery with Angioplasty in Patients with Multivessel Disease, *N. Engl. J. Med., 335*, 217, July 25, 1996.

Caplan, L.R.: Diagnosis and Treatment of Ischemic Stroke, *JAMA, 266*, 2413, November 6, 1991.

Cowper, T.R.: Pharmacologic Management of the Patient with Disorders of the Cardiovascular System. Infective Carditis, *Dent. Clin. North Am., 40*, 611, July, 1996.

Ganzberg, S.: Cardiovascular Drugs, in *ADA Guide to Dental Therapeutics*, Chicago, ADA Publishing Co., 1998, pp. 295–318.

Kusumoto, F.M. and Goldschlager, N.: Cardiac Pacing, *N. Engl. J. Med., 334*, 99, January 11, 1996.

Parker, J.D. and Parker, J.O.: Nitrate Therapy for Stable Angina Pectoris, *N. Engl. J. Med., 338*, 520, February 19, 1998.

Periodontal Relationships

American Academy of Periodontology, Committee on Research, Science and Therapy: Periodontal Management of Patients with Cardiovascular Diseases, *J. Periodontol., 67*, 627, June, 1996.

Beck, J., Garcia, R., Heiss, G., Vokonas, P.S., and Offenbacher, S.: Periodontal Disease and Cardiovascular Disease, *J. Periodontol., 67*, 1123, October, 1996, Supplement.

Khocht, A. and Schneider, L.C.: Periodontal Management of Gingival Overgrowth in the Heart Transplant Patient: A Case Report, *J. Periodontol., 68*, 1140, November, 1997.

Loesche, W.J.: Periodontal Disease as a Risk Factor for Heart Disease, *Compend. Cont. Educ. Dent., 15*, 976, August, 1994.

Infective Endocarditis

Biancaniello, T.M. and Romero, J.R.: Bacterial Endocarditis After Adjustment of Orthodontic Appliances, *J. Pediatr., 118*, 248, February, 1991.

Doerffel, W., Fietze, I., Baumann, G., and Witt, C.: Severe Prosthetic Valve-related Endocarditis Following Dental Scaling: A Case Report, *Quintessence Int., 28*, 271, April, 1997.

Duffin, P.R., McGimpsey, J.G., Pallister, M.L., and McGowan, D.A.: Dental Care of Patients Susceptible to Infective Endocarditis, *Br. Dent. J., 173*, 169, September 19, 1992.

Felder, R.S., Nardone, D., and Palac, R.: Prevalence of Predisposing Factors for Endocarditis Among an Elderly Institutionalized Population, *Oral Surg. Oral Med. Oral Pathol., 73*, 30, January, 1992.

Franklin, C.D.: The Aetiology, Epidemiology, Pathogenesis and Changing Pattern of Infective Endocarditis, with a Note on Prophylaxis, *Br. Dent. J., 172*, 369, May 23, 1992.

Knox, K.W. and Hunter, N.: The Role of Oral Bacteria in the Pathogenesis of Infective Endocarditis, *Aust. Dent. J., 36*, 286, August, 1991.

Children

Creighton, J.M.: Dental Care for the Pediatric Cardiac Patient, *J. Can. Dent. Assoc., 58*, 201, March, 1992.

Hallett, K.B., Radford, D.J., and Seow, W.K.: Oral Health of Children with Congenital Cardiac Diseases: A Controlled Study, *Pediatr. Dent., 14*, 224, July/August, 1992.

Liberthson, R.R.: Sudden Death from Cardiac Causes in Children and Young Adults, *N. Engl. J. Med., 334*, 1039, April 18, 1996.

Sinaiko, A.R.: Hypertension in Children, *N. Engl. J. Med., 335*, 1968, December 26, 1996.

Anticoagulant

Carr, M.M. and Mason, R.B.: Dental Management of Anticoagulated Patients, *J. Can. Dent. Assoc., 58*, 838, October, 1992.

Herman, W.W., Konzelman, J.L., and Sutley, S.H.: Current Perspectives on Dental Patients Receiving Coumarin Anticoagulant Therapy, *J. Am. Dent. Assoc., 128*, 327, March, 1997.

Kearon, C. and Hirsh, J.: Management of Anticoagulation Before and After Elective Surgery, *N. Engl. J. Med., 336*, 1506, May 22, 1997.

Martinowitz, U., Mazar, A.L., Taicher, S., Varon, D., Gitel, S.N., Ramot, B., and Rakocz, M.: Dental Extraction for Patients on Oral Anticoagulant Therapy, *Oral Surg. Oral Med. Oral Pathol., 70*, 274, September, 1990.

Meehan, S., Schmidt, M.C., and Mitchell, P.F.: The International Normalized Ratio as a Measure of Anticoagulation: Significance for the Management of the Dental Outpatient, *Spec. Care Dentist., 17*, 94, May/June, 1997.

Pellegrino, S.V. and Berardi, T.R.: Dental Management of Patients on Anticoagulant Therapy, *Gen. Dent., 43*, 351, July–August, 1995.

Steinberg, M.J. and Moores, J.F.: Use of INR to Assess Degree of Anticoagulation in Patients Who Have Dental Procedures, *Oral Surg. Oral Med. Oral Pathol., 80*, 175, August, 1995.

Stern, R., Karlis, V., Kinney, L., and Glickman, R.: Using the International Normalized Ratio to Standardize Prothrombin Time, *J. Am. Dent. Assoc., 128*, 1121, August, 1997.

Terezhalmy, G.T. and Lichtin, A.E.: Antithrombotic, Anticoagulant, and Thrombolytic Agents, *Dent. Clin. North Am., 40*, 649, July, 1996.

The Patient With a Blood Disorder

Oral soft tissue changes, lowered resistance to infection, and bleeding tendencies are major factors to be considered for a patient with a blood disorder. Oral manifestations of blood disorders are generally exaggerated in the presence of bacterial plaque and local predisposing factors.

In this chapter, anemias, leukemias, and hemorrhagic disorders are described. Box 59-1 lists and defines terminology used to describe hematologic conditions. Prefixes, suffixes, and other word derivatives to clarify the terminology are listed on pages 919 to 921.

ORAL FINDINGS SUGGESTIVE OF BLOOD DISORDERS

Early signs of systemic conditions frequently appear in the oral soft tissues. The patient's medical history may not reveal the existence of a blood disorder, but clinical examination may reveal tissue characteristics suggestive of disease. An important referral for medical examination may lead to diagnosis and treatment of a serious disease. In addition, the findings of a laboratory blood examination may provide essential information for safe and effective treatment.

Oral soft tissue changes that may occur in patients with blood diseases are not necessarily exclusive to systemic blood disorders. The important thing is to recognize change in a previously healthy patient, or an apparently exaggerated response in a patient being examined at an initial appointment.

Findings that may suggest a blood disorder include the following:

A. Gingival bleeding, spontaneously or upon gentle probing.
B. History of difficulty in controlling bleeding by usual procedures.

BOX 59-1 KEY WORDS: Blood Disorders

Anaplasia (an' ah-plā'zē-ah): loss of structural differentiation with reversion to a more primitive type of cell.

Aplasia (ah-plā'zē-ah): defective development or congenital absence of an organ or tissue.

Coagulation factor: factor essential to normal blood clotting contained within the blood plasma; designated by Roman numerals I to V and VII to XIII; their absence, diminution, or excess may lead to abnormality of clotting.

Differential cell count: record of number of white blood cells, including the determination of the percent of each type of cell present; the "differential" is used in the diagnosis of various blood disorders, infections, and other abnormal conditions of the body.

Ecchymosis (ek'ĭ-mō'sis): hemorrhagic spot larger than a petechia in the skin or mucous membrane; nonelevated, blue or purplish.

Epistaxis (ep'i-stak'sis): hemorrhage from the nose.

Erythropoiesis (ĕ-rith"rō-poi-ē'sis): formation of red blood cells.

Glossitis (glaw sī'tis): inflammation of the tongue.

Glossodynia (glos'ō-dīn"e-ah): pain in the tongue.

Hemarthrosis (hem'ar-thro'sis): blood in a joint cavity.

Hematocrit (hē-mat'ō-krit): volume percentage of erythrocytes (red blood cells) in whole blood.

Hematopoiesis (hem-ah'-tō-poi-ē'sis): the formation and development of blood cells, usually in bone marrow.

Hemoglobin (he'mo-glo'bin): protein in the erythrocyte that transports molecular oxygen to body cells.

Oxyhemoglobin: oxygenated arterial blood; bright red and about 97% saturated with oxygen; venous blood is a darker color and contains only 20% to 70% oxygen.

Hemolysis (he-mol'ĭ-sis): rupture of erythrocytes with the release of hemoglobin into the plasma.

Leukocytosis (loo"kō-sī-to'sis): increase in the total number of leukocytes.

Leukopenia (loo"kō-pē'nē-ah): reduction in total number of leukocytes in the blood; count under 500 per mL.

Lysis (lī'sis): destruction or decomposition, as of a cell, bacterium, or other substance.

Macrocyte (mak'rō-sīt): abnormally large red blood cell; contrast with **microcyte,** abnormally small erythrocyte.

Myelocyte (mī'ě-lō-sit): young cell of the granulocyte series; occurs normally in bone marrow; found in circulating blood in certain diseases.

Neutropenia (nu"trō-pē'nē-ah): diminished number of neutrophils (polymorphonuclear leukocytes or PMNs).

Petechia (pě-te'kē-ah): minute, pinpoint, round, nonraised, purplish-red spot in the skin or mucous membrane, caused by hemorrhage.

Phagocytosis (fag"ō-sī-tō'sis): engulfing of microorganisms and foreign particles by phagocytes, such as macrophages.

Purpura (pur'pu-rah): hemorrhage into the tissues, under the skin, and through the mucous membranes; produces petechiae and ecchymoses.

Thrombocytic purpura: when circulating platelets are decreased.

C. History of bruising easily, with large ecchymoses.
D. Numerous petechiae.
E. Marked pallor of the mucous membranes.
F. Atrophy of the papillae of the tongue.
G. Persistent sore or painful tongue (glossodynia).
H. Acute or chronic infections, such as candidiasis, that do not respond to usual treatment.
I. Severe ulcerations associated with a lack of response to treatment.
J. Exaggerated gingival response to local irritants, sometimes with characteristics of necrotizing ulcerative gingivitis (ulceration, necrosis, bleeding, pseudomembrane).

NORMAL BLOOD[1]

I. COMPOSITION

The blood is composed of 55% plasma fluid and 45% formed elements. The formed elements are categorized by type into *erythrocytes (red blood cells or corpuscles), leukocytes* (white blood cells), and *thrombocytes* (platelets). The cell forms and nuclei are shown in Figure 59-1.

The red blood cells comprise about 44% and the white blood cells 1% of the 45% total formed elements.

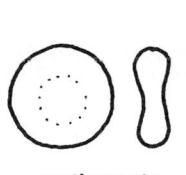 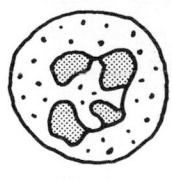 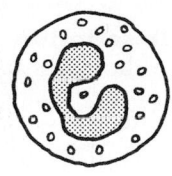 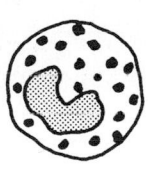 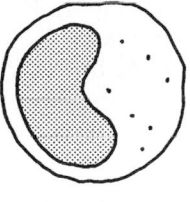 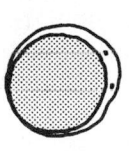 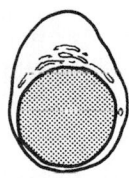

| erythrocyte | neutrophil | eosinophil | basophil | monocyte | lymphocyte | plasma cell |

FIGURE 59-1 Red and White Blood Cells. Diagram shows normal cell forms drawn to scale for comparison of cell size. Note the shape of nuclei in each of the white blood cells. The erythrocyte or red blood cell does not have a nucleus; its biconcave disc shape is shown in the lateral view second from the left.

The *hematocrit* is the percentage of packed volume of blood cells, the normal value for which approximates 45%, as shown in Table 59-1. The test for the hematocrit is commonly used in general health evaluations.

leave the bone marrow in immature forms and go to the lymphoid tissues for later maturing. In certain blood diseases and cancers, the immature cell forms predominate.

II. ORIGIN

In adults, all blood cells originate in the bone marrow. The erythrocytes and granulocytes pass through a series of transformations from the stem cell (cell of origin), the *hemocytoblast,* and leave the bone marrow as mature cells to enter the circulating blood.

The bone marrow also produces the stem cells for the agranulocytes. The lymphocytes and monocytes

III. PLASMA

The constituents of the fluid portion of the blood are similar to the fluid constituents of the connective tissue. The plasma is comprised 90% of water and 10% of the following:

A. Plasma Proteins
1. Albumin (functions to maintain tissue fluid pressure).

TABLE 59-1 Tests Used for Blood Evaluation

Test	Normal Range*	Causes of Deviations
Hemoglobin	Males: 14–18 g/100 mL Females: 12–16 g/100 mL	Increased in: polycythemia, dehydration Decreased in: anemias, hemorrhage, leukemias
Hematocrit (volume of packed red cells)	Males: 40%–54% Females: 37%–47%	Increased in: polycythemia, dehydration Decreased in: anemias, hemorrhage, leukemias
Bleeding time	Duke: 1–3 1/2 minutes Ivy: less than 5 minutes Modified Ivy: 2 ½–10 minutes (Mielke template)	Prolonged in: disorders of platelet function, Thrombocytopenia, von Willebrand's disease, leukemias, with aspirin and certain other drug use
Clotting time	Glass tube: 4–8 minutes	Prolonged in: vitamin K deficiency, severe hemophilia, anticoagulant therapy, liver diseases
Prothrombin time (PT)	11–15 seconds	Prolonged in: polycythemia vera, prothrombin deficiency, anticoagulant therapy, vitamin K deficiency, liver diseases, aspirin use
Partial thromboplastin time (PTT)	68–82 seconds	Prolonged in: hemophilia A and B, von Willebrand's disease, anticoagulant therapy

*The normal range varies with the specificity of the technique used. There is also a range variation, depending on the health facility and the laboratory.

2. Gamma globulins (circulating antibodies essential in the immune system).
3. Beta globulins (transport of hormones, metallic ions, and lipids).
4. Fibrinogen and prothrombin (blood clotting).

B. Inorganic Salts

Sodium, potassium, calcium, bicarbonate, chloride.

C. Gases

Dissolved oxygen, carbon dioxide, and nitrogen.

D. Substances Being Transported

Hormones, nutrients, waste products, enzymes.

IV. RED BLOOD CELLS (ERYTHROCYTES)

A. Description

Although usually called red blood cells, they are more properly termed corpuscles because they have no nuclei (Figure 59-1). They are biconcave discs that contain hemoglobin. The cells are sensitive and flexible and change shape readily as they pass through small capillaries.

Table 59-2 contains reference values for blood cells and the names of conditions in which increases or decreases in the normal values occur.

B. Functions

Hemoglobin carries oxygen to the body cells in

TABLE 59-2 Blood Cells Reference Values

Cell Type	Normal Value	Causes of Increase	Causes of Decrease
Red Blood Cells (Erythrocytes)	Male 4.5–6.0 Female 4.3–5.5 million per mm³	Polycythemia Dehydration	Anemias Leukemias Hemorrhage
Platelets (Thrombocytes)	150,000–400,000 per mm³ Wintrobe method: 140,000– 440,000 per mm³	Polycythemia vera Chronic myelocytic leukemia Sickle cell anemia Rheumatic fever Hemolytic anemias Bone fractures	Acute severe infections Cirrhosis of the liver Thrombocytopenic purpura Acute leukemias Aplastic anemias Pernicious anemia
White Blood Cells (Leukocytes)	5,000–10,000 per mm³	Inflammation Overexertion Polycythemia vera Leukemia	Aplastic anemia Granulocytopenia Drug poisoning Thrombocytopenia Radiation Severe infections (HIV-AIDS)
Differential White Cell Count **Granulocytes** 1. Neutrophils	60%–70%	Acute infections Myelogenous leukemia Poisoning Erythroblastosis	Aplastic anemia Granulocytopenia
2. Eosinophils	1–3%	Allergic diseases Dermatitis Hodgkin's disease Scarlet fever	Aplastic anemia Typhoid fever
3. Basophils	1%	Certain chronic infections	Aplastic anemia
Agranulocytes 1. Lymphocytes	20%–35%	Lymphocytic leukemia Chronic infections Viral diseases	Aplastic anemia Myelogenous leukemia Radiation
2. Monocytes	2%–6%	Monocytic leukemias Tuberculosis Infective endocarditis Hodgkin's disease	Aplastic anemia

the form of oxyhemoglobin. Carbon dioxide is transported from the cells.

The hemoglobin is measured in grams (g) per 100 milliliters (mL). Normal values are shown in Table 59-1 and range from 12 to 18 g per 100 mL. The values reflect the anemic state when the hemoglobin is lowered. They also reflect pathologic conditions in which the hemoglobin is increased to a level higher than normal.

V. WHITE BLOOD CELLS (LEUKOCYTES)

A. Types

White blood cells are divided into two general groups, the granulocytes and the agranulocytes. Granulocytes have granules in their cytoplasm, whereas the agranulocytes do not. They are further subdivided as shown here:

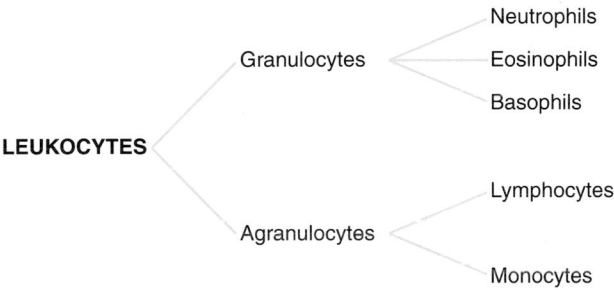

B. Functions

All white cells are amoeboid or motile, thus permitting them to pass through the walls at the terminal ends of capillaries and into the connective tissue. Their work is done within the connective tissue, where they have phagocytic, immunologic, and other functions related to the inflammatory process.

The cells respond to an injury or invasion of microorganisms and migrate into the area in large numbers. Neutrophils arrive first and are active in the phagocytosis of foreign material and microorganisms.

The blood functions as a transport medium for the white cells as they pass to areas in the connective tissue where they are needed. Their numbers and proportions in the blood maintain a constant level in health, as shown in Table 59-2.

A *differential cell count* of the white blood cells is used in the detection and monitoring of diseased states. Increases and decreases of each cell type can be associated with certain conditions.

C. Agranulocytes

1. *Lymphocytes.* A mature lymphocyte is a small round cell with a round nucleus that nearly fills the cell, leaving only a narrow rim of cytoplasm (Figure 59-1). Less mature forms are larger, with more cytoplasm.

    In the connective tissue, certain lymphocytes may differentiate into plasma cells, which produce and secrete antibody. The *plasma cell* is a relatively large oval cell with an eccentric nucleus. Lymphocytes and plasma cells are common in areas of chronic inflammation.

2. *Monocytes.* A monocyte is a large cell with a bean-shaped or indented nucleus. It is actively phagocytic. In the connective tissue, monocytes differentiate into macrophages, which are important in immunologic processes.

D. Granulocytes

1. *Neutrophils.* Neutrophils are the most numerous of all the white blood cells. They are also named polymorphonuclear leukocytes and referred to as "PMNs" or "polys." The nucleus of a neutrophil has three to five lobes connected by thin chromatin threads.

    In circulation, the cells are round, but in the tissues they are more or less amoeboid as they function in phagocytosis. Neutrophils are part of the first line of defense of the body.

2. *Eosinophils.* An eosinophil usually has a two-lobed nucleus and larger, coarser granules than those of a neutrophil. The granules stain a distinct bright pink, so that microscopically the cells can be readily recognized, even though they are few in number. The numbers increase markedly during allergic conditions.

3. *Basophils.* In contrast to the eosinophil or neutrophil, the nucleus of a basophil is usually in "U" or "S" form. The functions of the basophil are related to increasing vascular permeability during inflammation, thus permitting phagocytic cells to pass into the area.

VI. PLATELETS

A platelet is a small round or oval formed element without a nucleus. It is approximately one fourth the size of a red blood cell. Platelets are active in the blood clotting mechanism and essential in the maintenance of the integrity of blood capillaries by closing them at a time of injury. After healing, the platelets participate in clot dissolution.

ANEMIAS

Anemia means a reduction of the hemoglobin concentration, the hematocrit, or the number of red blood cells to a level below that which is normal for the individual. As a result of anemia, oxygen-carrying capacity to the cells is diminished. Oxygen is essential in all body tissues for normal maintenance.

I. CLASSIFICATION BY CAUSE

Anemias are usually classified into three groups by general causes. The categories and an example of each are listed here. Later in the chapter, selected specific anemias with their oral implications are described.

A. Caused by Blood Loss
1. *Acute.* Blood loss from trauma or disease.
2. *Chronic.* An internal lesion with constant slow bleeding, usually of gastrointestinal or gynecologic origin, can lead to a chronic loss of blood. An *iron deficiency anemia* can result.

B. Caused by Increased Hemolysis
Hemolysis means the destruction of red blood cells. These types of anemias are called "hemolytic anemias" because of the cell destruction.
1. *Hereditary Hemolytic Disorders*
      Example: *sickle cell disease,* which belongs to the group of hereditary disorders called the hemoglobinopathies.
2. *Acquired Hemolytic Disorders*
      Examples: drugs, infections, and certain physical and chemical agents that may cause red cell destruction. In the category of antibody-mediated anemia, *erythroblastosis fetalis* occurs when a mother is Rh negative and develops antibodies against a fetus that is Rh positive. It is sometimes called hemolytic disease of the newborn.

C. Caused by Diminished Production of Red Blood Cells
A nutritional deficiency or bone marrow failure may be the reason for diminished production.
1. *Nutritional Deficiency*
   a. Inadequate dietary choices or inadequate intake.
   b. Defective absorption from the gastrointestinal tract.
      Example: *pernicious anemia,* which results from a B_{12} vitamin absorption deficiency.
   c. Increased demand for nutrients.
      Example: *iron deficiency anemia,* which may occur during pregnancy or during a growth spurt.
2. *Bone Marrow Failure*
      Example: *aplastic anemia,* which may result from bone marrow failure because of drug use, irradiation, or chemicals. In aplastic anemia, a combination occurs of anemia, neutropenia, and thrombocytopenia, which means a quantitative decrease in all cells formed in the bone marrow.

II. CLINICAL CHARACTERISTICS OF ANEMIA

When a patient's medical history shows the presence of anemia, certain general characteristics may be anticipated for which clinical adaptations may be needed.
   The general signs and symptoms are
   A. Pale and thin skin.
   B. Weakness, malaise, easy fatigability.
   C. Dyspnea on slight exertion, faintness.
   D. Headache, vertigo, tinnitus.
   E. Dimness of vision, spots before the eyes.
   F. Brittle nails with loss of convexity.

IRON DEFICIENCY ANEMIA

Iron deficiency anemia is a hypochromic microcytic anemia, which means that the hemoglobin is deficient (hypochromic) and the red blood corpuscles are smaller than normal and deficient in hemoglobin (microcytic). In general, it is found more in younger than in older people, and more in females than in males.

I. CAUSES
   A. Malnutrition or malabsorption.
   B. Chronic infection.
   C. Increased body demand for iron over and above the daily intake. Example: during pregnancy.
   D. Chronic blood loss. When iron deficiency anemia occurs in men or in postmenopausal women, it usually indicates internal bleeding, and tests are needed to find the source.
   1. Causes of internal bleeding
      a. Gastrointestinal diseases, such as ulcer, cancer.
      b. Drugs, notably aspirin.
      c. Hemorrhoids.
   2. Excessive menstrual flow.
   3. Frequent blood donations.

II. SIGNS AND SYMPTOMS
A. General
Clinical manifestations of iron deficiency anemia include general weakness, headache, pallor, and fatigue on slight exertion.

B. Oral
1. Pallor of the mucosa and gingiva.
2. Tongue changes
   a. Atrophic glossitis with loss of filiform papillae. In moderate and severe anemia, when the hemoglobin is at 10 or below, the tongue is smooth and shiny. The patient may have burning, painful sensations (glossodynia).
   b. Secondary irritations to the thinned, atrophic mucosa may result from smoking, mechanical trauma, or hot, spicy foods.

III. THERAPY
Iron deficiency anemia is treated with oral ferrous iron tablets. Liquid preparations, which are some-

times used for children, may stain the teeth. Administering the medicine by way of a straw is advised.

MEGALOBLASTIC ANEMIAS[2]

Megaloblastic anemias are characterized by abnormally large (megalo-) red blood cells, many of which are oval shaped. The two principal types of megaloblastic anemias are *pernicious anemia* and *folate deficiency anemia.*

Pernicious anemia is caused by a deficiency of vitamin B_{12}, and folate deficiency anemia is from a deficiency of folate, or folic acid. These two vitamins are essential in red blood cell production in the bone marrow. When one or the other is deficient, the basic precursor cell ("-blast") is altered, thus leading to a derangement in the formation of red blood cells and resultant abnormal, megaloblastic cells. A megaloblastic anemia can result from a deficiency of either vitamin B_{12} or folate, or both.

I. PERNICIOUS ANEMIA

The implication of "fatality" when the word "pernicious" is used can be misleading, because synthetic vitamin B_{12} is now available for treatment and disease control. The traditional name is still in use, however.

A. Etiologic Factors
Vitamin B_{12} deficiency can be caused by decreased intake (inadequate diet or impaired absorption) or increased requirement (pregnancy, hyperparathyroidism, disseminated cancer). Pernicious anemia is caused by *impaired absorption* of B_{12} because of failure of production of *intrinsic factor (IF)* by the gastric mucosa.

Pernicious anemia is primarily a disease of people over 40 years of age. Frequently, the reason for lack of production of *intrinsic factor* is either chronic atrophic gastritis or surgical removal or partial removal of the stomach.

In the childhood form of the disease, other causes are in effect; no gastric abnormality exists. Although more research is needed, the cause may be either that a hereditary inability to produce intrinsic factor exists, or the intrinsic factor produced is ineffective.

B. Clinical Findings
1. *General.* Weakness, tingling or numbness of fingers and toes, and weight loss are usually found. Symptoms of central nervous system involvement may include difficulty in walking, some lack of coordination, loss of position sense, and mental confusion.
2. *Oral*
   a. Tongue (atrophic glossitis, burning tongue). The tongue may be painful and inflamed, flabby, red, smooth, and shiny, with loss of filiform papillae. Secondarily, sensitivity to hot or spicy foods and other irritants and painful swallowing may be expected.
   b. Gingiva and mucosa. Soft tissues may be pale and atrophic and appear similar to those in general vitamin B deficiency.

C. Treatment
Vitamin B_{12} is administered by injection twice weekly until the condition is controlled, and then monthly, indefinitely.

The main sources of vitamin B_{12} are meat and dairy products, that is, all foods containing animal protein. Liver is a rich source and was originally used in therapy before the development of synthetic B_{12}.

II. FOLATE DEFICIENCY ANEMIA

Folate deficiency anemia has the same characteristics as pernicious anemia, except clinically, no neurologic changes are evident.

A. Etiologic Factors[2]
Folate deficiency can be caused by decreased intake (inadequate diet, impaired absorption), increased requirement (pregnancy, disseminated cancer), or blocked activation (certain drugs impair the utilization of folate, for example, cancer chemotherapy drugs).

B. Dietary Factors
Folates are abundant in green vegetables (spinach, lettuce, cabbage, asparagus), yeast, and liver. Only minimal subsistence diets or special diets influenced by such factors as poverty, food fadism, or alcoholism, when the use of alcohol takes precedence over food, are likely to be deficient in folates. Folate deficiency anemia is not uncommon, but it may be more frequently related to malabsorption than to inadequate intake.

C. Fetal Development
A deficiency of folic acid during pregnancy has been implicated in the development of neural tube defects such as spina bifida[3] (page 773).

SICKLE CELL DISEASE[4]

Sickle cell disease is a hereditary form of hemolytic anemia, resulting from a defective hemoglobin molecule. The name is derived from the crescent or "sickle" shape the erythrocytes assume when they become deoxygenated.

The disease occurs primarily in the African American population and in white populations of Mediterranean origin. Tests are available for screening and diagnosis of those with sickle cell trait. Genetic counseling can play an important role in prevention. Detection of the presence of sickle cell disease is possible before birth, so that proper observation and supervision of the infant and young child can be provided.

I. DISEASE PROCESS

Signs and symptoms do not appear until after approximately the sixth month, when hemoglobin has matured. Growth and development may be impaired during the early years. Young children are markedly susceptible to communicable diseases and especially to pneumococcal infections.

The disease abnormality is in the type and solubility of hemoglobin. The defective hemoglobin loses oxygen, and the red blood cells become distorted into sickled shapes (Figure 59-2). Increases in blood fluid viscosity result, and blood stasis occurs, which can lead to thrombosis formation and infarction.

The initial presentation in infancy may include "hand-foot" syndrome due to impaired circulation to the extremities.[5] Aseptic necrosis of long bones is very common. The sickled cells may collect in the vital organs and lead to serious involvement and organ enlargement, particularly of the liver and spleen. In addition to vaso-occlusive crisis, sickle cell disease is also characterized by severe hemolytic anemia, predisposition to bacterial infections, and chronic hyperbilirubinemia.[5]

II. CLINICAL COURSE

A. Severe Hemolytic Anemia

In adults, chronic hemolytic sickle cell disease can be severe. The hematocrit may range between 18% and 30%. The life span of red blood cells normally is from 90 to 120 days, whereas in hemolytic anemia, such as sickle cell anemia, the red blood cell survival rate is about 10 to 15 days.

B. Sickle Cell Crisis

Periodic recurrences of clinical exacerbations of the disease with periods of remission characterize childhood and adolescence. The acute form of the disease is called sickle cell crisis.

1. *Precipitating Factors.* Crises may appear at any time with or without stimuli. Viral or bacterial infections, other systemic diseases, exer-

tion, trauma, and temperature changes (dehydration in summer, reflex vasospasm in cold weather) may be specific precipitating factors, however.

2. *Clinical Signs and Symptoms.* A crisis is characterized by severe pain. Infarctions occur in various tissues and organs. When the central nervous system becomes involved, symptoms of seizure, stroke, or coma may develop.

   The effects of a crisis may be reversible to some degree, severe physical conditions can result, or a crisis can be fatal. The high mortality rate in young children may be the result of the effects of crisis or of severe infections.

C. Systemic Changes That May Occur

Chronic changes may occur in any organ system at any age. The kidney is a major organ affected; changes in the cardiopulmonary system can result in enlargement of the heart, heart murmurs, and coronary insufficiency. Ocular disturbances, even leading to blindness, are not uncommon in adults. Certain patients may be susceptible to cerebrovascular accidents with hemiplegia.

Changes that occur in all bones, including the mandible, result from thrombosis and infarction and from infection.

D. Treatment

1. *Preventive Procedures*
   a. Use folate supplements daily to cope with increased need by the bone marrow.
   b. Avoid and/or promptly treat infections; administer pneumococcal polyvalent vaccine to children.
   c. Obtain genetic counseling for those with sickle cell trait.
   d. Allogeneic stem-cell transplantation may provide a cure for young patients with symptomatic sickle cell disease.[6]
2. *Treatment for Disease State*
   Supportive and palliative treatments include those for specific symptoms during crises, such as pain relief and the use of antibiotics for infectious diseases. Oxygen therapy and blood transfusions have limited selective use.

III. ORAL IMPLICATIONS

A. Radiographic Findings[7,8]

Although radiographic findings of bone changes cannot be considered exclusive to sickle cell disease, the high incidence of characteristics listed here provides a relationship that may, in time, contribute to diagnosis. The bone changes can be observed in patients with sickle cell trait, as well as in those with sickle cell disease.

1. Decreased radiodensity; increased osteoporosis.

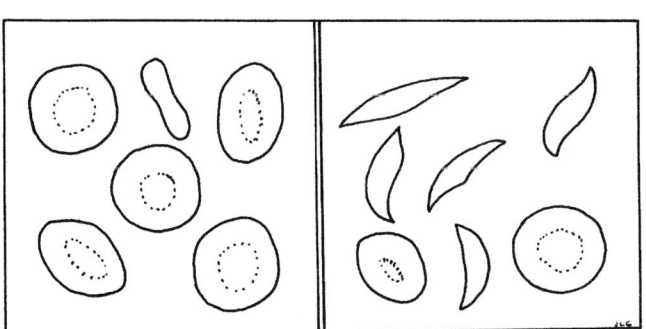

FIGURE 59-2 Sickle Cell Disease. *Left,* diagrammatic drawing of normal red blood cells. ***Right,*** sickle shapes of red blood cells of a patient with sickle cell disease.

2. Coarse trabecular pattern appearing as horizontal rows between teeth ("step-ladder"[7]), with large marrow spaces.
3. Significant bone loss in children, indicating the presence of periodontitis.

B. Oral Soft Tissues

The tissues may show the pallor typical of anemias, and because of the specific destruction of tissues in the liver of the patient with sickle cell disease, the gingiva may have a jaundiced color.

Periodontal evaluation for all ages is likely to reveal pockets, infection, bleeding, and the need for a strict preventive and treatment program.

C. General Suggestions for Appointment Management[9,10]

The objective during therapy is to provide care without precipitating a sickle cell crisis. In general, during a sickle cell crisis, treatment should be limited to emergency relief.

1. Plan routine care in non-crisis periods; short appointments.
2. Prepare or review the comprehensive medical history.
3. Use prophylactic antibiotics. For a patient so highly susceptible to infection, antibiotics should be considered routine, because any form of tissue manipulation can create a bacteremia.
4. Obtain a hematocrit and a hemoglobin determination immediately prior to each treatment appointment. The patient's physician can provide the interpretation and advise whether the patient is able to have a dental or dental hygiene appointment that day.
5. Use local anesthesia without epinephrine.
6. Teach and supervise a comprehensive preventive program to minimize oral infection and control etiologic factors.

POLYCYTHEMIAS

Polycythemia means an increase in the number and concentration of red blood cells above the normal level. Hemoglobin and hematocrit values are raised. The three general categories are described in the following sections.

I. RELATIVE POLYCYTHEMIA

When a loss of plasma occurs without a corresponding loss of red blood cells, the concentration of cells increases and a relative polycythemia results. The causes of fluid loss may be such conditions as dehydration, diarrhea, repeated vomiting, sweating, or loss of fluid from burns.

Other contributing factors may be smoking, hypertension, obesity, and stress, particularly in middle-aged men.

II. POLYCYTHEMIA VERA (PRIMARY POLYCYTHEMIA)[11]

In contrast to "relative" polycythemia, which results from fluid loss, primary, "absolute," or "true" polycythemia results from an actual increase in the number of circulating red blood cells. In addition to an increased red blood cell count and hemoglobin value, the white cell and platelet counts are also elevated. The viscosity of the blood is increased, thereby affecting the oxygen transport to the tissues.

A. Cause

Polycythemia vera is a neoplastic condition resulting from a bone disorder in which the primitive red cells or stem cells proliferate. It occurs more frequently after age 40 and more often in men.

B. Clinical Signs and Symptoms

Clinical manifestations relate to increased blood volume and viscosity and the tendencies to thrombosis and hemorrhage.

1. *General.* Hemorrhagic spots, such as petechiae or ecchymoses, appear on the skin. The patient suffers from headaches, dizziness, nasal and gastric bleeding, and abdominal pain. Elevated blood pressure and enlarged spleen are found along with high blood test values. A few cases transform into leukemia.
2. *Oral*
   a. The tongue, mucous membranes, and gingiva are deep purplish-red.
   b. The gingiva are enlarged, with bleeding on slight provocation.

C. Treatment

1. Chemotherapy or radiation.
2. Phlebotomy, to reduce the total volume, and particularly the red cell volume, of the blood.

D. Dental Hygiene Treatment Considerations

Increased health of the gingival tissues can result from frequent maintenance appointments for the supervision of personal daily plaque removal procedures. When supplemented by professional treatment, especially calculus removal, bleeding tendencies can be lessened.

III. SECONDARY POLYCYTHEMIA

Secondary polycythemia is also called erythrocytosis, which simply means an increase in numbers of red blood cells. The increased red cell production can result from hypoxia, such as occurs in residents of high altitudes.

Another cause for increased numbers of red blood cells is an increase in the body's production of erythropoietin, a hormone essential to stimulate the development of the red blood cells in bone marrow. A variety of diseases and tumors can cause excess erythropoietin production. Treatment of the underlying condition is necessary to correct the secondary polycythemia.

WHITE BLOOD CELLS

Disorders of the white blood cells may occur because of a decrease (leukopenia) or an increase (leukocytosis) in cell numbers. The types of white blood cells are described in Table 59-2 and illustrated in Figure 59-1.

I. LEUKOPENIA

A decrease in the total number of white blood cells results when cell production cannot keep pace with the turnover rate or when an accelerated rate of removal of cells occurs, as in certain disease states.

A. Conditions in Which Leukopenia Occurs
1. *Specific Infections.* HIV/AIDS, typhoid fever, influenza, malaria, measles (rubeola), and German measles (rubella) are examples.
2. *Disease or Intoxification of the Bone Marrow.* Chronic drug poisoning, radiation, and autoimmune or drug-induced immune reactions may be implicated.

B. Agranulocytosis[12]
Agranulocytosis, or malignant neutropenia as it is sometimes called, is a rare, serious disease involving the destruction of bone marrow. Antipsychotic drugs or an autoimmune process are causes.
1. *Clinical Course.* With a sharp drop in white blood cells, bacterial invasion may be rapid, and acute illness may develop. Malaise, chills, and fever are followed by extreme weakness. With complete depression of the bone marrow, blood cells cannot be produced, and death can occur within a few days.
2. *Oral Lesions.* Ulceration in the mouth and pharynx is common in agranulocytosis. Symptoms also include gingival bleeding, increased salivation, and a fetid odor. During the severe illness, only palliative relief is possible by using a soft diet and attempting to clean the mouth with a soft toothbrush, possibly a suction brush (pages 764 to 765).
3. Referral for medical care is indicated.

II. LEUKOCYTOSIS

An increase in the numbers of circulating white blood cells may be caused by inflammatory and infectious states, trauma, exertion, and other conditions listed in Table 59-2. The most extreme abnormal cause of leukocytosis is leukemia.

LEUKEMIAS

Leukemias are malignant neoplasias of immature white blood cells. They are characterized by abnormally large numbers of specific types of leukocytes and their precursors located within the circulating blood and bone marrow and infiltrated into other body tissues and organs.

I. CLASSIFICATION[13]

Leukemias are first named by whether they are acute or chronic and then are subdivided by the maturity and type of white cell predominating, whether lymphocytic, myelocytic, or myelogenous.

A basic classification of leukemias includes the following types:
A. Acute lymphocytic (lymphoblastic) leukemia (ALL).
B. Chronic lymphocytic leukemia (CLL).
C. Acute myelocytic (myeloblastic) leukemia (AML).
D. Chronic myelocytic leukemia (CML).

II. DISEASE PROCESS AND EFFECTS

Leukemias are characterized by (1) generalized replacement of bone marrow with proliferating leukemic cells, (2) large numbers of immature white cells in the circulating blood, and (3) widespread infiltrates of white cells throughout the body. The changes that result may be divided into primary and secondary. Tertiary effects also are associated with the treatment given.

A. Primary Changes
The primary changes are those directly related to the increase in numbers of white blood cells.
1. *Bone Marrow.* All the active red marrow is affected; the marrow is replaced by the neoplastic cells.
2. *Lymph Nodes.* Nodes throughout the body are usually enlarged in all forms of leukemia, because of the accumulation of increased numbers of leukemic cells.
3. *Spleen and Liver.* Both liver and spleen are enlarged, the spleen to the greater degree.
4. *Other Leukemic Infiltrates.* Many organs and tissues become involved, for example, the kidneys, adrenals, thyroid, and myocardium. Infiltrates in the gingiva are described in the section "Oral Manifestations," page 875.

B. Secondary Changes
Secondary changes are the result of complications that arise from the destructive effects of the leukemic infiltrates on the bone marrow. Myelosuppression results from the displacement of hematopoietic tissue in the bone marrow by immature leukocyctes.
1. *Anemia.* Red cells cannot develop because of the infiltrated bone marrow. Severe anemia can result.
2. *Thrombocytopenia.* Abnormal bleeding tendency is a significant characteristic of all forms of leukemia. The platelet count is very low.
3. *Susceptibility to Infection.* Circulating white

cells do not have their usual defense capacities.

4. *Osteoporosis*. Expansion of the marrow spaces and changes in the bone by the leukemic infiltrate lead to osteoporosis and radiographic radiolucency. Osseous changes in the maxilla and mandible are not uncommon.

III. CLINICAL SIGNS AND SYMPTOMS

A. Acute Form
1. Onset: sudden and severe.
2. Fatigue, pallor, weakness (from anemia).
3. Purpura and ecchymoses of the skin, bleeding from the nose and gingiva (from thrombocytopenia).
4. Lymphadenopathy, splenomegaly, hepatomegaly.
5. Fever, indicating an infection (from lowered resistance).
6. Headache, nausea, vomiting, and sometimes seizures and coma (from leukemic infiltration of the meninges).

B. Chronic Form
1. Onset: insidious.
2. Low-grade fever, night sweats.
3. Weight loss, weakness, easy fatigability.
4. Anemia with exertional dyspnea.
5. Lymphadenopathy, splenomegaly, hepatomegaly.

IV. TREATMENT FOR LEUKEMIA[14]

A. Induction of Remission
1. *Objective*. To return the blood and bone marrow at least to minimally normal blood test levels.
2. *Methods*. Chemotherapy and/or radiation.

B. Stabilization Therapy
Treatment for anemia, bleeding, infections, and other complications is needed.

C. Continuation Therapy
During remission, therapy is continued to prevent bone marrow relapse. Therapy may be stopped after 2 to 4 years of remission.

Children in remission go to school and participate in normal activities. Physically, the only difference is alopecia, a side effect of chemotherapy, which is often reversible when chemotherapy is completed. Remission periods are used for routine dental and dental hygiene therapy.

D. Bone Marrow Transplant
When indicated, transplants may be performed during remission, while the patient is stronger and the numbers of cancer cells may be fewer. Chemotherapy and total body radiation precede the marrow transplant to eradicate leukemic cells and suppress immunoreactivity (pages 732 to 733).

V. ORAL MANIFESTATIONS

Patients with acute leukemias have more oral problems than do those with chronic disease. The oral lesions result from the effects of infiltration, treatment, and depression of bone marrow and lymphoid tissue.

A. Leukemic Infiltrate of the Gingiva
1. *Occurrence*. More severe lesions in monocytic leukemia than other types.
2. *Characteristics*. Bluish red, blunted papillae, soft spongy consistency, and grossly enlarged even to cover a large portion of the anatomic crown.

B. Effects of Treatment: Direct Drug Toxicity
1. *Oral Complications*. Painful ulcerations, spontaneous gingival bleeding, tongue desquamation, xerostomia, and secondary infections.
2. *Direct Drug Toxicity*. Effects and management of chemotherapy are described on pages 730 to 732.

DENTAL HYGIENE CARE

Selection of procedures centers around the patient's problem of susceptibility to infection and bleeding. During acute exacerbations, the patient is usually very ill, and may be hospitalized. Consultation with the patient's physician, hematologist, or oncologist is mandatory to explain the precautions which may be indicated prior to oral treatment and to obtain information about the patient's hematologic status.

I. PRIOR TO AND DURING CHEMOTHERAPY INDUCTION

A. Prophylactic Antibiotic Premedication
(pages 101 to 104)
The patient with leukemia is susceptible to infection, and drugs used in therapy are immunosuppressive. In addition, the patient may possess an indwelling catheter.

B. Blood Evaluation
Complete blood evaluation tests, including a minimum of those listed in Table 59-1, are essential shortly before dental and dental hygiene treatment.

C. Oral Examination
Routine, thorough examinations are needed. Dental and periodontal conditions without symptoms may become acute problems during chemotherapy.

D. Meticulous Oral Hygiene and Nutritious Diet
Although all severe tissue reactions during periods of chemotherapy cannot be alleviated, much suffering can be prevented if the oral cavity is in a state of health at the outset.

1. *Gingiva.* Palliative care for enlarged, bleeding, ulcerated gingiva includes frequent warm saline rinses and bacterial plaque removal procedures using a very soft toothbrush.
2. *Suction toothbrush.* In the hospital setting a suction brush may be of value (pages 764 to 765).
3. *Diet.* Instruction is provided for a nutritious liquid diet with dietary supplements.

II. DURING REMISSION

A. Preventive Care

Complete preventive care with supervised plaque removal, daily self-applied fluoride, sealants, and a noncariogenic nutritious diet are basic.

B. Dental Treatment Completed

HEMORRHAGIC DISORDERS

Hemorrhagic disorders have in common tendencies to spontaneous bleeding and moderate to excessive bleeding following trauma or a surgical procedure. Spontaneous bleeding occurs as small hemorrhages into the skin or mucous membranes and other tissues, and appears as petechiae or purpura. Moderate to excessive bleeding or prolonged bleeding may follow dental hygiene therapy, especially nonsurgical instrumentation. A history or suspicion of a bleeding problem should be fully evaluated before treatment is started.

I. DETECTION

A. Patient's Medical and Dental Histories

1. *Basic Health Questionnaire.* Includes items related to bleeding, bruising, blood transfusions (and for what reasons they were needed), blood disorders, familial blood disorders, and previous abnormal bleeding that may have followed past dental or dental hygiene appointments.
2. *Consultation and Follow-up.* Follow-up conversational questioning after "yes-no" answers on a written questionnaire can delve into sufficient detail to determine the need for blood tests before treatment is started. Additional information is also obtained by consultation with the patient's physician. When blood tests have been made in the past but are not recent, new reports can be requested.

B. Laboratory Blood Tests

Selected basic tests are listed in Table 59-1 with their normal values. Additional tests are frequently needed for a thorough evaluation of specific conditions.

Certain tests may be needed on the same day as treatment, because blood values may fluctu-

ate. For example, the patient taking anticoagulants is required to have a prothrombin time determination within 24 hours of appointment time (pages 861 to 862). A patient with leukemia also needs immediate pre-evaluation, as described on page 875.

The types and numbers of tests vary. For example, the information required prior to subgingival instrumentation and periodontal surgery depends on the severity of the patient's condition. For a patient with leukemia, the tests recommended may include a prothrombin time, partial thromboplastin time, thrombin time, fibrinogen level, and platelet count, in addition to routine blood counts and a differential white count.[14]

II. TYPES OF HEMORRHAGIC DISORDERS

A. Abnormalities of the Blood Capillaries

1. *Characteristics.* Vascular fragility is increased; petechial and purpuric hemorrhages in the skin or mucous membranes, including the gingiva.
2. *Conditions Predisposing to Bleeding*
   a. Severe infections (septicemias, severe measles, typhoid fever).
   b. Drug reactions (sulfonamides, phenacetin).
   c. Scurvy or vitamin C deficiency (impaired collagen of vessel wall).

B. Platelet Deficiency or Dysfunction

1. *Thrombocytopenia.* A lowered number of platelets may be caused by decreased production in the bone marrow. The cause of bone marrow depression may be invasive disease, such as leukemia, or deficiencies, such as folate or vitamin B_{12} deficiency anemias.
2. *Platelet Dysfunction.* Interference with the blood clotting mechanism leads to a prolonged bleeding time. Defects occur as a result of certain hereditary states, uremia, von Willebrand's disease, and certain drugs such as salicylates (aspirin).

C. Blood Clotting Defects

A possible irregularity or disorder is associated with each of the many clotting factors.

1. *Acquired Disorders*
   a. Vitamin K deficiency. Vitamin K is essential for prothrombin synthesis and factors VII, IX, X.
   b. Liver disease. Nearly all the clotting factors are produced in the liver. When the liver is not functioning properly, the clotting factors may be altered.
2. *Hereditary Disorders.* At least 30 hereditary coagulation disorders exist, each resulting from a deficiency or abnormality of a plasma protein. Clinically, their signs and symptoms are

similar. The following three are described in detail in the next section:

a. Hemophilia A (factor VIII abnormality).

b. Hemophilia B (factor IX abnormality).

c. von Willebrand's disease (von Willebrand factor, which chemically forms a large part of the factor VIII complex, is either too low or does not function properly).

HEMOPHILIAS[15]

The hemophilias are a group of congenital disorders of the blood clotting mechanism. The three most common types are classic hemophilia A, hemophilia B or Christmas disease, and von Willebrand's disease.

Hemophilias A and B are inherited by males through an X-linked recessive trait carried by females, and von Willebrand's disease is transmitted by an autosomal co-dominant trait. Rarely is a female affected by hemophilias A or B, but von Willebrand's disease occurs in males and females.

I. LEVEL OF CLOTTING FACTOR

The severity of the disease can be related directly to the level of the clotting factor in the circulating blood. Normal concentrations of the clotting factors are between 55% and 150%.

Patients with severe hemophilia have a clotting factor VIII or IX of less than 1%. They have spontaneous bleeding into muscles, joints, and soft tissues, and severe, prolonged bleeding after minor trauma.

When the hemophilia is less severe, the clotting factor is in the 2% to 5% range. Spontaneous bleeding may be only occasional; gross bleeding occurs after light but definite trauma.

II. EFFECTS AND LONG-TERM COMPLICATIONS

A. Effects of Minor Trauma

Bleeding and bruising from minor trauma vary, depending on the severity of the disease.

B. Hemarthroses

Bleeding into the soft tissue of joints (knees, ankles, elbows) begins in the very young with severe hemophilia. Much swelling, pain, and incapacitation are created.

C. Joint Deformity and Crippling

Permanent joint damage can result, and the patient may need splints, braces, or orthopedic surgery.

D. Intramuscular Hemorrhage

Hemorrhage into the muscles is accompanied by pain and limitation of motion.

E. Oral Bleeding

Bleeding from the gingiva is common and more extensive when periodontal infection is more severe. Because of the fear of bleeding, patients may neglect toothbrushing and flossing; doing so can lead to increased plaque accumulation and inflammation. Small children may injure the oral area when they tumble, and severe bleeding can result.

III. HOME INFUSION PROGRAM

Hemophilia care-center teams work with health personnel in the patient's home community to plan and carry out an individual program of instruction for the parents of a young patient. Instruction for a young patient is given as soon as the child is capable of self-care. Some patients have an intravenous port-a-cath surgically placed which simplifies the infusion. The prescribed concentrates of clotting factor can be stored in the home refrigerator and reconstituted as needed for infusion.

The parents and child are taught to recognize the symptoms of the beginning of a bleeding episode or bleeding from injury, and how to administer the treatment. For patients who have bleeding episodes often, such as more than once each week, a prophylactic schedule may be appropriate. Many patients do not require more than one infusion each month, so that routine prophylaxis is not needed.

IV. DENTAL HYGIENE CARE

Although prevention and control of bleeding are the central issues when planning appointments for a patient with hemophilia, other factors also require adaptations and attention. A few of these patients are multihandicapped as a result of internal hemorrhages, which have led to mental and physical problems. Suggestions for appointments from Chapter 50 may prove useful for the patient who has had hemarthroses and orthopedic treatment.

A few patients have suffered brain damage as a result of cerebral hemorrhage and may be limited intellectually. Others have emotional stresses related to the disease, its treatment, and the excessive cost. New channels for adjustment have opened since patients have been able to develop the responsibility for self-care. This is in contrast to previous requirements of long hospitalizations, childhood separations from family and school, and dependency on others.

A. Preparation for Appointments

1. *Preliminary Evaluation.* The patient's medical and dental histories must include the pertinent hemophilic history with information about the type, severity, treatment, medications used for pain and other symptoms, and family history.

   Most patients are now vaccinated for hepatitis B unless they have previously been exposed to the virus. Replacement therapy may be the origin of HIV. Additional information from the hematologist contributes to planning safe and effective appointments.

2. *Factor Replacement.* In preparation for local anesthetic administration, subgingival in-

strumentation, surgical procedures, or any procedure likely to cause bleeding, replacement therapy is given just prior to the appointment in accord with medical consultation.

3. *Premedication.* Prophylactic antibiotic premedication is usually indicated because of the susceptibility to infection, joint prostheses, and/or indwelling catheter. Consultation with the patient's physician and/or orthopedic surgeon is advised.

B. Preventive Program

The prevention and control of gingival and dental diseases constitute essential aspects of care for patients with hemophilia. Not only are dental and periodontal treatments complicated by necessary special precautions, but spontaneous oral bleeding problems can be at least partially controlled by the elimination of oral infections.

1. *Anticipatory Guidance.* To ensure that all possible preventive measures are started while the child is very young, fluorides, sealants, bacterial plaque control, diet for caries control, and early professional supervision are all included.

2. *Bacterial Plaque Removal.* Complete instruction is given as for any patient. A soft brush is indicated.
   a. Flossing. Teach flossing carefully and correctly to prevent cutting the gingiva and inducing proximal bleeding.
   b. Aids for disabilities. Patients with limited range of motion may benefit from the special adaptations described on pages 749 to 751.

C. Instrumentation

All instrumentation is performed carefully but thoroughly to minimize tissue trauma and prevent unnecessary bleeding. Care planning for a series of appointments is appropriate.

1. *Tissue Conditioning.* When oral care has been neglected and the gingiva are soft and spongy, and bacterial plaque is abundant, a tissue conditioning program is advised. Patient instruction in plaque control procedures is given, practiced, and repeated as necessary over a series of appointments.

   Scaling can be accomplished in small segments. As the tissue begins to shrink, heal, and become more firm, subgingival scaling and root debridement can be completed.

2. *Probing and Periodontal Treatment Planning.* Depending on the bleeding tendencies of the gingival tissues, probing and charting for complete periodontal treatment planning may need to be postponed for a few appointments while tissue conditioning is carried out.

   Many patients can be brought to a state of periodontal health through conservative measures. Complete treatment should be accomplished, including periodontal surgery. As with all oral surgery for a patient with hemophilia, coordination with the medical team and hospitalization when indicated can provide the patient with safe and effective treatment.

D. Miscellaneous Treatment Suggestions

Techniques and procedures should be analyzed to make sure that all excess trauma to the patient is prevented. The same procedures should be applied to all patients, but they are more significant with a patient who has a bleeding problem.

1. *Rubber Dam.* A thin rubber dam may be more gentle to the oral tissues than a heavy one. The use of a Young's frame may eliminate pressure, especially at the corners of the mouth. Rubber dam clamps can be checked for sharp corners and placed carefully without damage to the gingival tissues.

2. *Film Placement.* Films can cut and press on the mucous membranes. Care in placement must be exercised.

3. *Impressions.* Beading the rims of the trays protects the mucosa from pressure and damage from a hard, possibly rough surface (page 175).

4. *Evacuation.* High-vacuum suction tips may be sharp. Caution in the use of suction is necessary to prevent pulling the sublingual or other mucosal tissues into the suction tip and causing hematomas.

5. *Periodontal Dressing.* After subgingival scaling and planing, a periodontal dressing can provide pressure and adapt the tissue against the teeth as an aid for the prevention of postappointment bleeding.

6. *Treatment for Hematoma.* Ice pack application may limit the spread of a hematoma as a temporary measure. Prompt replacement therapy may be needed.

7. *Aspirin.* Never suggest the use of aspirin for pain relief for a patient with a bleeding disorder. The bleeding tendency is greatly increased by drug-induced platelet dysfunction.

8. *Frequency of Maintenance Care.* Frequent appointments can aid in keeping the oral tissues in an optimum state of health and help to prevent the need for complex dental treatments.

REFERENCES

1. **Borysenko**, M. and Beringer, T.: *Functional Histology,* 3rd ed. Boston, Little, Brown and Company, 1989, pp. 87–102.
2. **Cotran**, R.S., Kumar, V., and Robbins, S.L.: *Robbins Pathologic Basis of Disease,* 5th ed. Philadelphia, W.B. Saunders Co., 1994, pp. 603–610.

3. **Selhub,** J. and Rosenberg, I.H.: Folic Acid, in Ziegler, E.E. and Filer, L.J., eds.: *Present Knowledge in Nutrition,* 7th ed. Washington, DC, ILSI Press, 1996, pp. 215–216.

4. **Cotran,** Kumar, and Robbins: op. cit., pp. 592–596.

5. **Sansevere,** J.J. and Milles, M.: Management of the Oral and Maxillofacial Surgery Patient with Sickle Cell Disease and Related Hemoglobinopathies, *J. Oral Maxillofac. Surg., 51,* 912, August, 1993.

6. **Walters,** M.C., Patience, M., Leisenring, W., Eckman, J.R., Scott, J.P., Mentzer, W.C., Davies, S.C., Ohene-Frempong, K., Bernaudin, F., Matthews, D.C., Storb, R., and Sullivan, K.M.: Bone Marrow Transplantation for Sickle Cell Disease, *N. Engl. J. Med., 335,* 369, August 8, 1996.

7. **Taylor,** L.B., Nowak, A.J., Giller, R.H., and Casamassimo, P.S.: Sickle Cell Anemia: A Review of the Dental Concerns and a Retrospective Study of Dental and Bony Changes, *Spec. Care Dentist., 15,* 38, January/February, 1995.

8. **Ibsen,** O.A.C., Phelan, J.A., and Vernillo, A.T.: Oral Manifestations of Systemic Diseases, in Ibsen, O.A.C. and Phelan, J.A.: *Oral Pathology for the Dental Hygienist,* 2nd ed. Philadelphia, W.B. Saunders Co., 1996, pp. 404–405.

9. **Little,** J.W., Falace, D.A., Miller, C.S., and Rhodus, N.L.: *Dental Management of the Medically Compromised Patient,* 5th ed. St. Louis, Mosby, 1997, pp. 50, 507.

10. **May,** O.A.: Dental Management of Sickle Cell Anemia Patients, *Gen. Dent., 39,* 182, May–June, 1991.

11. **Cotran,** Kumar, and Robbins: op. cit., p. 616.

12. **Shafer,** W.G., Hine, M.K., and Levy, B.M.: *A Textbook of Oral Pathology,* 4th ed. Philadelphia, W.B. Saunders Co., 1983, pp. 732–734.

13. **Cotran,** Kumar, and Robbins: op. cit., pp. 648–656.

14. **Little,** Falace, Miller, and Rhodus: op. cit., pp. 502–505, 508–511.

15. **Mosher,** D.F.: Disorders of Blood Coagulation, in Bennett, J.C. and Plum, F., eds.: *Cecil Textbook of Medicine,* 20th ed. Philadelphia, W.B. Saunders Co., 1996, pp. 987–1001.

SUGGESTED READINGS

Badner, V.M., Lawrence, C., and Mehler, S.: Polycythemia Vera: Dental Management Considerations, *Spec. Care Dentist., 11,* 227, November/December, 1991.

Bergmann, O.J., Ellegaard, B., Dahl, M., and Ellegaard, J.: Gingival Status During Chemical Plaque Control with or Without Prior Mechanical Plaque Removal in Patients with Acute Myeloid Leukaemia, *J. Clin. Periodontol., 19,* 169, March, 1992.

Dreizen, S.: The Many Faces of Adult Leukemia, *Compend. Cont. Educ. Dent., 12,* 46, January, 1991.

Epstein, J.B., Vickars, L., Spinelli, J., and Reece, D.: Efficacy of Chlorhexidine and Nystatin Rinses in Prevention of Oral Complications in Leukemia and Bone Marrow Transplantation, *Oral Surg. Oral Med. Oral Pathol., 73,* 682, June, 1992.

George, J.N. and Shattil, S.J.: The Clinical Importance of Acquired Abnormalities of Platelet Function, *N. Engl. J. Med., 324,* 27, January 3, 1991.

Imbery, T.A., Camm, J.H., and Anderson, L.D.: Dental Management of a Patient with Aplastic Anemia, *Gen. Dent., 40,* 316, July–August, 1992.

Luker, J., Scully, C., and Oakhill, A.: Gingival Swelling as a Manifestation of Aplastic Anemia, *Oral Surg. Oral Med. Oral Pathol., 71,* 55, January, 1991.

Miyasaki, K.T.: The Neutrophil: Mechanisms of Controlling Periodontal Bacteria, *J. Periodontol., 62,* 761, December, 1991.

Pernu, H.E., Pajari, U.H., and Lanning, M.: The Importance of Regular Dental Treatment in Patients with Cyclic Neutropenia. Follow-up of 2 Cases, *J. Periodontol., 67,* 454, April, 1996.

Pui, C.-H.: Childhood Leukemias, *N. Engl. J. Med., 332,* 1618, June 15, 1995.

Schaedel, R. and Goldberg, M.H.: Chronic Lymphocytic Leukemia of B-cell Origin: Oral Manifestations and Dental Treatment Planning, *J. Am. Dent. Assoc., 128,* 206, February, 1997.

Toh, B.-H., van Driel, I.R., and Gleeson, P.A.: Pernicious Anemia, *N. Engl. J. Med., 337,* 1441, November, 13, 1997.

Sickle Cell Anemia

Arowojolu, M.O. and Savage, K.O.: Alveolar Bone Patterns in Sickle Cell Anemia and Non-sickle Cell Anemia Adolescent Nigerians: A Comparative Study, *J. Periodontol., 68,* 225, March, 1997.

Bunn, H.F.: Pathogenesis and Treatment of Sickle Cell Disease, *N. Engl. J. Med., 337,* 762, September 11, 1997.

Cherry-Peppers, G., Davis, V., and Atkinson, J.C.: Sickle Cell Anemia: A Case Report and Literature Review, *Clin. Prev. Dent., 14,* 5, July/August, 1992.

Kelleher, M., Bishop, K., and Briggs, P.: Oral Complications Associated with Sickle Cell Anemia, *Oral Med. Oral Surg. Oral Pathol., 82,* 225, August, 1996.

Patton, L.L., Brahim, J.S., and Travis, W.D.: Mandibular Osteomyelitis in a Patient with Sickle Cell Anemia: Report of Case, *J. Am. Dent. Assoc., 121,* 602, November, 1990.

Shroyer, J.V., Lew, D., Abreo, F., and Unhold, G.P.: Osteomyelitis of the Mandible as a Result of Sickle Cell Disease. Report and Literature Review, *Oral Surg. Oral Med. Oral Pathol., 72,* 25, July, 1991.

Thornton, J.B. and Sams, D.R.: Preanesthesia Transfusion and Sickle Cell Anemia Patients: Case Report and Controversies, *Spec. Care Dentist., 13,* 254, November/December, 1993.

Hemophilia/Bleeding Disorder

Kelly, M.A.: Common Laboratory Tests—Their Use in the Detection and Management of Patients with Bleeding Disorders, *Gen. Dent., 38,* 282, July–August, 1990.

Luke, K.H.: Comprehensive Care for Children with Bleeding Disorders. A Physician's Perspective. *Can. Dent. Assoc. J., 58,* 115, February, 1992.

Mulherin, J.: Hospital Offers Perfect Setting for RDH to Help Special Patients, *RDH, 13,* 26, August, 1993.

Mulherin, J. and Sanders, B.: Coagulation Disorders. Considerations in Dental Care, *DentalHygienistNews, 9,* 3, Number 1, 1996.

Patton, L.L. and Ship, J.A.: Treatment of Patients with Bleeding Disorders, *Dent. Clin. North Am., 38,* 465, July, 1994.

Ublansky, J.H.: Comprehensive Dental Care for Children with Bleeding Disorders—A Dentist's Perspective, *Can. Dent. Assoc. J., 58,* 111, January, 1992.

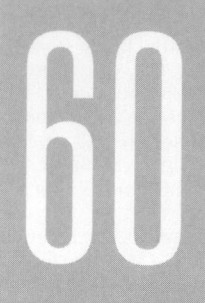

The Patient With Diabetes Mellitus

An effective dental hygiene program is vital for the patient with diabetes mellitus. Signs and symptoms can be identified from a thorough medical history and clinical assessment. Oral changes may be indicative of systemic disease. Dental professionals are able to recognize the warnings and refer the patient for early diagnosis.

A patient with diabetes may have a lowered resistance to infections and delayed healing, and be prone to life threatening emergencies. The presence of infection, including periodontitis, may intensify symptoms and make diabetes more difficult to regulate. The dental team has a significant responsibility to provide instruction and oral care aimed at maintaining health and preventing infections and emergencies, and to be able to recognize and treat acute emergencies.

Modifications in dental and dental hygiene procedures may be indicated. No treatment should be at-

tempted until the state of the diabetes has been confirmed. Key words and abbreviations used in this chapter are found in Box 60-1 and Table 60-1, respectively.

DIABETES MELLITUS

I. DEFINITION[1]

  A. Diabetes mellitus is a group of metabolic diseases characterized by hyperglycemia.
  B. Hyperglycemia results from a defect in insulin secretion, insulin action, or both. There is a relative or absolute lack of insulin or an inadequate function of insulin.

II. IMPACT

  A. About 6% of adults in the United States have

BOX 60-1 KEY WORDS: Diabetes Mellitus

Beta cells: insulin-producing cells of the islets of Langerhans in the pancreas.

Brittle diabetes: term formerly used to describe very unstable juvenile diabetes; characterized by unexplained oscillation between hypoglycemia and diabetic ketoacidosis.

Casual plasma glucose: Glucose level at any time of day with no regard to time of eating.

Exocrine (ex′so-krin): secreting externally via a duct.

Exogenous insulin: insulin from source outside patient.

Gestational diabetes (jes-ta′shun-al): diabetes that occurs during pregnancy.

Gluconeogenesis (gloo′ko-ne-o-jen-e-sis): synthesis of glucose from noncarbohydrate sources, such as amino acids and glycerol; can occur in the liver and kidneys when the carbohydrate intake is insufficient to meet the body's needs.

Glycemia (gli-se′-me-a): presence of glucose in blood.

Hyperpnea (hi′perp-ne′ah): abnormal increase in depth and rate of respiration.

Hypoglycemia (hi′po-gli-se′-me-ah): an abnormally low level of glucose in the blood; opposite of **hyperglycemia**, very high blood glucose.

Insulin (in′su-lin): a powerful hormone secreted by the beta cells in the islets of Langerhans of the pancreas; the major fuel-regulating hormone; enters the blood in response to a rise in concentration of blood glucose and is transported immediately to bind with cell surface receptors throughout the body.

Ketoacidosis (ke′to-ah′si-do′sis): diabetic coma; too little insulin; accumulation of ketone bodies in the blood.

Ketone bodies: normal metabolic products of lipid (fat) within the liver; excess production leads to urinary excretion of these chemicals.

Ketonuria (ke′to-nu′re-ah): excess concentration of ketone bodies in the urine.

Oral glucose tolerance test: a test of the body's ability to utilize carbohydrates; aid to the diagnosis of diabetes mellitus. After ingestion of a specific amount of glucose solution, the fasting blood glucose rises promptly in a nondiabetic person, then falls to normal within an hour. In diabetes mellitus, the blood glucose rise is greater and the return to normal is prolonged.

Ural hypoglycemic agent: synthetic drug that lowers the blood sugar level; stimulates the synthesis and release of insulin from the beta cells of the islets of Langerhans in the pancreas; used to treat patients with non-insulin-dependent diabetes mellitus.

Polydipsia (pol′e-dip′se-ah): excessive thirst.

Polyphagia (pol′e-fa′je-ah): excessive ingestion of food.

Polyuria (pol′e-u′re-ah): excessive excretion of urine.

Postprandial (post-pran′de-al): after a meal.

Pruritus (proo ri′tus): itching.

Retinopathy (ret-i-nop′ah-the): noninflammatory degenerative disease of the retina; called **diabetic retinopathy** when it occurs with diabetes of long standing.

---

been diagnosed with diabetes. About half who have the disease have not yet been diagnosed.

B. As the population ages, diabetes becomes more prevalent.

C. Due to the prevalence, cost of treatment, and lost productivity, diabetes is one of the most costly health problems.

INSULIN

I. DEFINITION

Insulin is a hormone produced by the beta cells in the pancreas. It directly or indirectly affects every organ in the body.

II. DESCRIPTION

A. Insulin is synthesized and released into the blood in proportion to the amount of glucose in the blood.

B. When the blood glucose level rises, as a result of digestion, insulin is released.

C. Insulin allows glucose transport into cells. Cells use glucose for energy.

D. Blood glucose level then decreases.

III. FUNCTIONS

The functions of insulin are listed in Table 60-2. Without insulin, glucose accumulates in the blood, resulting in hyperglycemia. Normal blood glucose levels in healthy individuals usually range from 60–150 mg/dL. In diabetes, levels range much higher.

IV. EFFECTS OF DECREASED INSULIN

A. Less glucose is transmitted through cell walls into the cells.

B. Glucose increases in the circulating blood

TABLE 60-1 Key of Abbreviations: Diabetes Mellitus

EMS	Emergency Medical Service
FPS	Fasting plasma glucose
GDM	Gestational diabetes mellitus
HbA$_{1c}$	Glycosylated hemoglobin
HDL	High-density lipoprotein
IDDM	Insulin-dependent diabetes mellitus
IFG	Impaired fasting glucose
IGT	Impaired glucose tolerance
LDL	Low-density lipoprotein
NIDDM	Non-insulin-dependent diabetes mellitus
OGTT	Oral glucose tolerance test
PP	Postprandial
WHO	World Health Organization

(hyperglycemia) until a threshold is reached when glucose spills over into the urine (glucosuria).

C. Without glucose in the cells to use for energy, the starving cells utilize fat.
1. End products of fat metabolism (ketones) accumulate in the blood.
2. Ketones are acidic. Usually, when they accumulate, they are neutralized in the blood. When the quantity is large, the neutralizing effect is depleted rapidly and an acidic condition (acidosis) results.
3. In severe, untreated, or inadequately controlled diabetes, acidosis leads to diabetic coma (ketoacidosis).

V. INSULIN COMPLICATIONS

Earlier diagnosis, improved treatment, and better informed patient, family, and friends have reduced the occurrence of emergencies. Constant verbal and visual contact must be maintained with a patient to identify early behavioral and physical changes indicative of a developing crisis.

A. Hypoglycemia/Insulin Shock
Too much insulin (hyperinsulinism), with lower levels of blood glucose (hypoglycemia).

TABLE 60-2 Functions of Insulin

1. Facilitates glucose uptake from blood into tissues, which lowers blood glucose level.
2. Speeds the oxidation of glucose within the cells to use for energy.
3. Speeds the conversion of glucose to glycogen to store in the liver and skeletal muscles and to prevent the conversion of glycogen back to glucose.
4. Facilitates conversion of glucose to fat in adipose tissue.

Hypoglycemia is the emergency more likely to occur in the dental setting.

B. Hyperglycemic Reaction/Diabetic Coma (Ketoacidosis)
Too little insulin (hypoinsulinism) with increased levels of blood glucose (hyperglycemia). Table 60-3 shows a comparison of the characteristics of hyperglycemic and hypoglycemic reactions along with the respective treatment procedures.

DIABETES MELLITUS: ETIOLOGIC CLASSIFICATION[1]

In 1997, an international expert committee, organized by the American Diabetes Association, revised the classification of diabetes. The new system is based on the etiology of the disease wherever possible. A comparison of Types 1 and 2 diabetes is found in Table 60-4.

I. TYPE 1 DIABETES

A. Description
1. An absolute insulin deficiency.
2. Due to the destruction of beta cells in the pancreas. The loss of beta cells is due either to (1) a cellular-mediated autoimmune or (2) an idiopathic etiology.
3. Dependent on exogenous insulin to sustain life and prevent ketosis.
4. Prone to ketoacidosis.
5. Usually arises in childhood or puberty, but may occur at any age.

B. Former Names
Type I diabetes, insulin-dependent diabetes mellitus (IDDM), juvenile diabetes, juvenile onset diabetes, ketosis prone diabetes, brittle diabetes.

II. TYPE 2 DIABETES

A. Description
1. Pancreatic insulin secretion may be low, normal, or even higher than normal, but the patient exhibits an insulin resistance that impairs the use of the insulin that is secreted.
2. Insulin resistance is the inability of the peripheral tissues to respond to the insulin that is produced.
3. Most prevalent type of diabetes, more than 90% of all patients with diabetes.
4. Onset typical after 30 years of age, but may occur in younger individuals.

B. Screening[2]
Because of the severe complications, screening should be done for those who are asymptomatic. Basic criteria for testing:
1. Age 45 and above, repeated every 3 years.

TABLE 60-3 Comparison of Insulin Reaction and Diabetic Coma

	Hypoglycemia/Insulin Shock	Diabetic Coma/Ketoacidosis
History/Predisposing Factors	Too much insulin Too little food: omitted or delayed Excessive exercise Stress	Too little insulin: omission of medication or failure to increase dose when requirements increased Too much food Stress Illness of any sort
Cause	Lowered blood glucose with excess insulin in proportion	Decreased glucose utilization when insufficient insulin leads to prolonged hyperglycemia, increasing acidosis
Occurrence	In type I diabetes, particularly the unstable or severe type	Type I diabetes that is poorly controlled, unstable, omits or reduces insulin
Physical Findings	Skin: moist, sweaty, perspiration Hunger Headache Tremor, shakiness, weakness Pallor Dilated pupils Dizziness, staggering gait	Skin: flushed, dry Abdominal pain Nausea, vomiting Lack of appetite, anorexia Dry mouth, thirst Increased urination Soft, sunken eyeballs

Vital Signs:
  Temperature
  Respiration
  Pulse
  Blood Pressure
	Normal or below
	Normal
	Fast, irregular
	Normal or slightly elevated
		Elevated when infection
		Hyperpnea, acetone/fruity breath
		Weak, rapid
		Lowered, person may go into shock

Behavior	Drowsy, restless Anxious, irritable, agitated Incoordination Stupor, confusion Eventual coma, possible convulsions, leading to death	Progressive drowsiness Confusion Tired, lethargic Weak Eventual coma and death
Treatment	GIVE SUGAR to raise blood glucose level (apple juice, cake frosting) Revival is prompt If unconscious/unresponsive; injection of glucagon or intravenous glucose	Immediate professional care Activate EMS, hospitalize Monitor vital signs Keep patient warm Fluids for conscious patient Insulin injection
Prevention	Smooth regulation of blood sugar level	Early diagnosis Well-regulated patient

2. Testing should begin earlier and more frequently if patient has any risk factors listed in Table 60-5.

C. Former Names

Type II diabetes, non-insulin-dependent diabetes mellitus (NIDDM), adult-onset diabetes, maturity-onset diabetes, ketosis-resistant diabetes.

III. GESTATIONAL DIABETES MELLITUS (GDM)

A. Description

1. Defined as any degree of glucose intolerance with onset or first recognition during pregnancy.

2. Related to genetics, obesity, and hormones causing insulin resistance around 24th week of pregnancy.

3. Occurs in about 4% of pregnancies in the United States.

4. Diagnosis is reclassified 6 or more weeks after pregnancy ends.

5. Insulin adjustment, carefully supervised prenatal care, and improved obstetric practices have lessened much of the potential danger for the mother.

6. Infants are larger; premature births more frequent; incidence of congenital malformations and perinatal death high; lower rate with improved prenatal care.

TABLE 60-4 Comparison of Type I and Type 2 Diabetes Mellitus

Characteristic	Type I	Type 2
Age of onset	Young, usually before or during puberty, but may appear later	Adult, usually after 30 years, but may occur at younger age
Body weight	Normal or thin	Obesity is most important risk factor
Ethnicity	More common in Caucasians	More common in African Americans, Asian Americans, Hispanics, and Native Americans
Hereditary	Yes, but less frequent occurrence in families than type 2	Much more frequent occurrence in families
Lifestyle	Restrictions very difficult for young patients.	More frequent in sedentary individuals with high-fat diets
Onset of symptoms	Rapid, abrupt symptoms of hyperglycemia	Slow, insidious progression over years
Symptoms	Weight loss, weakness Polyuria Polydipsia Polyphagia Blurred vision Mimic flu	Any type 1 symptom Frequent/recurrent infections Slow healing Tingling/numb extremities Fatigue Eye/kidney/cardiovascular problems
Severity	Severe, life-threatening	Early mild but progressively serious
Complications	Acute hypo/hyperglycemic emergencies and chronic long-term complications common	Acute complications rare, chronic long-term complications common
Stability	Unstable, difficult and much effort to control	More stable, easier to manage
Exogenous insulin required	All	Some
Chronic manifestations	Uncommon before 20 years, prevalent and severe by 30 years	Develop slowly at later ages

7. Have tendency to develop Type 2 diabetes later in life.

B. Testing
Selective screening between the 24th and 28th week of gestation is recommended for any woman with one or more risk factors:
1. Age over 25 years.
2. Has any risk factor for Type 2 diabetes in Table 60-5.

TABLE 60-5 Risk Factors for Type 2 Diabetes

Obesity, especially around midsection
Immediate blood relative has diabetes
High-risk population: Native/African/Hispanic/Asian American
Had baby weighing 9 pounds or more
Had gestational diabetes mellitus
Hypertensive (>140/90 mmHg)
Age greater or equal to 45 years
HDL cholesterol level greater than or equal to 35 mg/dL
Triglyceride level greater than or equal to 250 mg/dL
Prior test had IGT or IFG

IV. OTHER SPECIFIC TYPES OF DIABETES[1]
Other types of diabetes result from genetic defects, diseases, endocrinopathies, surgery, drugs, malnutrition, infections, and injury.

A. Genetic Defects of
1. Beta cell function.
2. Insulin action.

B. Diseases of the Pancreas
1. Diseases that injure or destroy beta cells.
2. Includes: pancreatitis, trauma, pancreatectomy, neoplasia, cystic fibrosis.

C. Endocrinopathies
1. Several hormones antagonize or inhibit insulin action.
2. Includes: acromegaly, Cushing's syndrome, hyperthyroidism.

D. Drug- or Chemical-Induced Diabetes
1. Chemicals do not cause diabetes but may impair insulin secretion, impair insulin action, destroy beta cells, and precipitate diabetes.
2. Includes: glucocorticoids, thyroid hormone, dilantin, thiazides.

E. Infections
1. Some viruses can destroy beta cells.
2. Includes: congenital rubella, cytomegalovirus.

F. Immune-Mediated Diabetes: Uncommon Forms of Diabetes

G. Other Genetic Syndromes Sometimes Associated With Diabetes
Includes: Down's syndrome, Huntington's chorea, Prader-Willi syndrome.

DIAGNOSIS OF DIABETES

I. PATIENTS WITH SYMPTOMS SUGGESTIVE OF DIABETES

Questions can be directed to obtain the risk factors (Table 60-5) and symptoms (Table 60-4).

II. DIAGNOSTIC TESTS

A. Patients with signs or symptoms suggestive of diabetes should be referred to a physician immediately for evaluation.
B. Routine Tests
1. Symptoms of diabetes plus casual plasma glucose greater than or equal to 200 mg/dL.
2. Fasting plasma glucose: greater than or equal to 126 mg/dL.
C. Routine blood tests must be repeated on another day to confirm diagnosis of diabetes.

EFFECTS OF DIABETES

I. INFECTION

A. Susceptibility
Patients are more susceptible to infections and they exhibit impaired healing, especially when inadequately controlled.

B. Infections
Infections involve the urinary tract, skin, lungs (pneumonia or tuberculosis), and the oral cavity (opportunistic infections such as oral candidiasis and chronic infections such as periodontitis).

C. Effect of Treatment
Failure to treat any infection intensifies the symptoms and increases severity of diabetes; can progress to life threatening infections or precipitate diabetic coma.

D. Increased Insulin
Insulin requirements may increase with any of the following: fever, infection, inflammation, trauma, bleeding, or pain. When the condition is eliminated, it may be possible to decrease the prescribed insulin.

E. Factors Involved
Factors involved are alterations in metabolism of carbohydrate and protein, impaired circulation, altered nutritional state, and abnormal immunologic response.

II. LONG-TERM COMPLICATIONS

Patients with tightly controlled blood glucose levels develop fewer complications and later than those whose diabetes is less well controlled.[3,4]

A. Neuropathy
Diabetes is a major cause of limb amputation (usually foot). Lack of feeling can delay patient identification of the infection. Neuropathy also can cause oral and facial symptoms.

B. Nephropathy
Diabetes is a leading cause of renal disease, which may require dialysis or kidney transplant, also may result in impotence.

C. Retinopathy
Diabetes is a leading cause of blindness.

D. Vascular Disease
Includes cardiovascular disease, atherosclerosis, arteriosclerosis, and leads to myocardial infarction and stroke.

E. Depression
Daily life is significantly affected by diabetes.
1. Treatment regimens may be difficult to cope with and lead to depression.
2. Make an appropriate referral for professional help, which may improve quality of life.

F. Silent Killer
Average life span is reduced; diabetes is a leading cause of death.

MEDICAL TREATMENT FOR DIABETES CONTROL

There is no known cure for diabetes. Treatment methods depend on the severity of the disease and on the age, activity, vocation, and psychologic needs, as well as the health status and nutritional and weight problems of the patient.

I. OBJECTIVES

A. Prevent complications of diabetes through tight glycemic control.
B. Attain the best possible general health: control hypertension; keep reasonable weight; maintain personal, physical, and mental health.

II. GENERAL PROCEDURES

A. Early diagnosis.
B. Preventive physical examinations on routine basis.

C. Immediate treatment to manage acute symptoms.
   1. Aggressive treatment of infections.
   2. Eliminate sources of infection, including oral diseases.
   3. Prevent injuries.
D. Patient education for self-care.

SELF CARE

I. INFLUENCING FACTORS
A. Knowledge, understanding, and attitude of the patient.
B. Physical and genetic factors of patient.
C. Psychologic factors.
   1. Reaction to the initial diagnosis and years of treatments with restrictions may influence behavior.
   2. Periods of emotional distress can lead to alterations in the blood glucose levels.

II. INSTRUCTION
A. Health Team
   1. Initial and ongoing individualized education must be provided by the health team.
   2. Members include the physician, registered nurse, dietitian, mental health professional, dental professionals, and other specialists.

B. Instructional Materials
   1. *Books and Journals.* A number of excellent books and other printed materials have been prepared for the patient and for health professionals. Review of these materials can provide the dental team members with greater insight into the background and knowledge of the patient in preparation for oral health instruction.
   2. *Internet.* An extensive resource for information, support groups, products.

III. EXERCISE
A. An essential part of the treatment program.
B. Contributes to lowering insulin requirements.
C. Lowers the cardiovascular risk factors of obesity, inactivity, and LDL cholesterol level.
D. Many cases of type 2 diabetes can be controlled with weight reduction and exercise alone.

IV. DIET
Diet counseling is basic and is planned by the physician and dietitian. Diet planning is ongoing and based on individual needs and treatment goals. There is no specific diabetic diet. Healthy, well-controlled individuals can have a diet very similar to a healthy person without diabetes. No foods are prohibited but eaten in moderation at strictly observed times.

A. Goals of Nutritional Therapy[5]
   1. Maintain near-normal blood glucose levels by balance of food intake with medications.
   2. Maintain optimal serum lipid levels.
   3. Provide adequate calories for individual needs and reasonable weight.
   4. Prevent and treat acute complications.
   5. Improvement of overall health.

B. Fundamentals of Diet
   1. *Carbohydrates.* Monitor and control amount consumed with less regard to source. Foods containing high proportions of sugars should be used sparingly.
   2. *Total Food Intake.* The daily intake may be identical with normal for the patient's age and stature, with appropriate adjustments for growth and degree of activity in the young patient. The obese patient needs a weight-reduction diet. Food lost as in vomiting may affect glucose balance.
   3. *Diet Selection.* Based on individual quantitative need. Proper nutrition is stressed so adequate calories are provided to attain and maintain ideal body weight and prevent hyperglycemia. High fiber, low fat to normalize serum cholesterol and triglycerides to reduce risk of vascular and heart disease.
   4. *Timing of meals/snacks.* Consistent, specific times for medication and food intake to control blood glucose levels. Usually three on-time meals and three interval feedings are followed.

V. HABITS
   1. *Tobacco.* Patient must avoid all types of tobacco. Smoking is a major health hazard for everyone and especially dangerous for those with diabetes. It increases risk of heart disease, stroke, myocardial infarction, limb amputations, periodontal disease, and numerous other health problems.
   2. *Alcohol.* Avoid excessive alcohol; alcohol can raise blood pressure and contribute to other health problems (page 839).

MEDICATION

I. INSULIN THERAPY
All patients with type 1 diabetes require exogenous insulin for survival. Type 2 patients may need to use insulin for control.

A. Types of Insulin
Insulin is classified as rapid, short, intermediate, or long-acting based on the onset, peak, and duration of action. The types of insulin and range of peak action are found in Table 60-6.

TABLE 60-6 Types and Action of Insulin

Class of Insulin	Type	Peak Action
Rapid acting	Lispro	30–90 minutes
Short acting	Regular	2–3 hours
Intermediate acting	NPH Lente	4–10 hours 4–12 hours
Long acting	Ultralente	12–16 hours

B. Dosage

Depends on the individual.

1. *Objective.* Attain optimum utilization of glucose throughout each 24 hours.
2. *Factors affecting the need for insulin.* Food intake, illness, stress, variations in exercise, or infections.
3. *"Sick Day Rules."* Insulin dose is supplemented if there are any factors that are affecting the need for insulin.

C. Methods for Insulin Administration

1. Subcutaneous injection with syringe.
2. Insulin pump through a battery-operated subcutaneous insulin infusion catheter.

II. ORAL HYPOGLYCEMIC AGENTS

Oral agents are commonly used to treat type 2 diabetes in conjunction with diet, exercise, and possibly the injection of insulin. The agents used are listed in Table 60-7.

PANCREAS TRANSPLANTATION[6,7]

Pancreas and islet cell transplantation are options for treatment for selected patients. Successful transplantation has eliminated the need for exogenous insulin in thousands of type 1 patients.

Life-long immunosuppression therapy is required to prevent rejection and the autoimmune process that may destroy the islet cells again. Suggestions for the care of an immunosuppressed patient are found on pages 730 to 732. A complete medical history must be confirmed along with any additional recommendations for antibiotic premedication for these patients.

Due to the shortage of donors, an artificial implantable device is under research and development. It consists of three components: a continuous blood glucose monitor, an insulin pump to deliver the appropriate amount, and a control system to complete a closed feedback loop.

BLOOD GLUCOSE TESTING

Blood glucose testing is used to diagnose diabetes and to monitor blood glucose levels. Patients with type 1 diabetes typically do self monitoring of blood glucose level three to four times per day. Blood glucose testing can be accomplished in the dental setting to confirm a safe blood glucose level for treatment. Interpretation of the levels of routine tests is in Table 60-8.

I. SELF-ADMINISTERED TESTS

Self administered tests also may be sent to a laboratory for analysis.

A. Fasting Plasma Glucose (FPG)

1. *Timing.* Test blood after fasting at least 8 hours.
2. *Diagnosis.* Repeated results greater or equal to 126 mg/dL are used to diagnose diabetes.

B. Postprandial (PP)

Blood tested after consuming meal.

C. Self-Testing Methods to Obtain and Analyze Blood Samples

1. *Test Strip.* Finger prick blood placed on a test strip. Color change of strip is compared to a chart; used at home or in the dental setting.
2. *Glucose Meter.* Finger prick blood placed in the glucose meter; self-monitoring equipment for accurate measurement of blood glucose level; used at home or in the dental setting.

TABLE 60-7 Oral Agents Used for Treatment of Type 2 Diabetes

Sulfonylureas	First generation: chlorpamide, tolbutamide, tolazamide Second generation: glyburide, glipizide	Act by stimulating insulin release from the beta cells in pancreas May cause hypoglycemia
Diguanides	Metformin	Prevents liver glycogen breakdown to glucose Increases tissue sensitivity to insulin
Thiazolidinediones	Troglitazone	Increases tissue sensitivity to insulin
Alpha-glucosidase inhibitors	Acarbose	Slows digestion and glucose uptake into blood

TABLE 60-8 Blood Glucose Test Values as Related to Control of Diabetes

	FPG	PP	HbA$_{1c}$
Normal, well controlled	<126 mg/dL	<160 mg/dL	<6%
Moderate control	<160 mg/dL	160–200 mg/dL	6%–7%
Uncontrolled	>160 mg/dL	>200 mg/dL	>8%

Key: FPG = Fasting plasma glucose; PP = postprandial; HbA$_{1c}$ = glycosylated hemoglobin.

II. LABORATORY TESTS

A. Oral Glucose Tolerance Test (OGTT)
1. *Procedure.* Fast 10–16 hours, glucose given, blood samples taken at time intervals.
2. *Results.* Normal or indicative of diabetes.
3. *Intermediate Results.* Categorized as **impaired fasting glucose** (IFG) or **impaired glucose tolerance** (IGT), which are considered a risk factor for diabetes and cardiovascular disease.

B. Glycosylated Hemoglobin Assay (HbA$_{1c}$)
1. *Objective.* To measure amount of glucose irreversibly bound to a hemoglobin molecule.
2. *Use.* Value is proportional to blood glucose status over half-life of the red blood cell; complements daily monitoring and helps predict risk for developing complications by indicating glycemic control of a longer period of time.

C. Urine Test
1. *Objective.* To measure ketones; indicates burning of fat instead of glucose.
2. *Use.* Used during illness or stress; indicates glucose level over the past few hours; not as accurate as blood tests.

ORAL RELATIONSHIPS

The oral cavity of a patient with diabetes may show unusual susceptibility and marked reactions to injury, infections, and all local irritants. Responses are related to lowered resistance and the delayed healing that is especially prevalent in undiagnosed, uncontrolled, and poorly controlled diabetes. Oral findings may be indicative of undiagnosed diabetes and should be referred for early detection testing.

I. PERIODONTAL INVOLVEMENT[8,9]

Diabetes is a significant risk factor for periodontal infections. Periodontal infections also affect control of blood glucose levels in diabetes.

A. Diabetes Effect on Periodontal Disease
1. Marked periodontal disease at young age, particularly in patients with type 1 diabetes, and is related to lack of glycemic control.
2. Patients with uncontrolled glucose levels have more severe periodontal disease at younger ages.
3. Diabetes acts as a conditioning, modifying, and accelerating factor for disease.
4. Inadequate bacterial plaque control contributes to more severe tissue response because of decreased resistance.

B. Periodontal Status Effect on Diabetes
1. Poorly controlled periodontal health may alter blood glucose levels. Infection affects insulin requirements and may lead to unstable diabetes.
2. Treatment of periodontal infection and reduction of periodontal inflammation is associated with a reduction in level of glycosylated hemoglobin (HbA$_{1c}$).[10]

II. OTHER ORAL FINDINGS

Diabetes does not cause oral disease but may lower resistance and increase susceptibility to the oral findings listed in Table 60-9.

DENTAL HYGIENE CARE PLAN

The control of oral infections is vital. Infection can alter the course and treatment of diabetes. Frequent, thorough care, with supervision, is needed and requires the patient's utmost cooperation and motivation.

The patient with diabetes is prone to life-threatening emergencies. The dental team must practice to prevent an emergency, identify early indications of a developing emergency, and act swiftly and appropriately.

I. PATIENT HISTORY

A. Refer for Early Diagnosis
Questions regarding signs and symptoms of diabetes are basic on any standard medical history questionnaire. For commonly asked questions refer to Table 60-10. If an unexplained positive

TABLE 60-9 Oral Findings That May Occur With Diabetes

Location	Findings
Gingiva	Increased gingival inflammation
Periodontium	Periodontitis: more frequent, severe, longer duration Attachment loss: more frequent, more extensive Probing depths: more teeth with deep pockets Alveolar bone loss: more Tooth mobility and migration: increased Healing: delayed, increased infection after surgery
Teeth	Poorly controlled diabetes: increased caries related to decreased saliva, diet Well controlled diabetes: decreased caries related to low sugar, regular eating habits, dental maintenance appointments
Lips	Dry, cracking, angular cheilitis
Saliva	Decreased flow Glucose in sulcular fluid Xerostomia associated with medications, contributes to opportunistic infection such as oral candidiasis
Mucosa	Edematous, red Oral candidiasis Burning mouth and/or tongue, altered taste Poor tolerance for removable prostheses Delayed healing

response is present, the patient is referred to a physician. Pertinent questions for undetected diabetes apply to weight loss, excess thirst and urination, hunger, and family history of diabetes.

B. Medical History

1. Supplement the basic medical history with additional questions about diabetes found in Table 60-11.
2. Update at each appointment.
3. Inquire about recent hypoglycemic reactions: patient who recently had a hypoglycemic reaction may be more likely to have another.
4. Identify other health problems, complications of diabetes, that may influence dental treatment. Refer to specialist when indicated.
5. Ask about exercise and tobacco use; review effect on health.

II. CONSULTATION WITH PHYSICIAN

If unable to obtain complete and accurate information from a patient, a consultation between dental professional and physician is necessary before any treatment.

III. APPOINTMENT PLANNING

Stress, including that created during a dental or dental hygiene appointment, increases glycemia and a

TABLE 60-10 Common Medical History Questions to Screen for Diabetes

1. Have you ever been diagnosed with diabetes?	YES	NO
2. Have any members of your family ever been diagnosed with diabetes?	YES	NO
3. Do you urinate (pass water) more than six times per day?	YES	NO
4. Are you thirsty much of the time?	YES	NO
5. Does your mouth frequently become dry?	YES	NO
6. Have you had any unexplained weight loss?	YES	NO

TABLE 60-11 Information to Obtain From Patient With Diabetes

Adherence to treatment prescribed
Medications taken on schedule
Meals and snacks eaten on schedule
Recent history of glycemic control
History of hypo/hyperglycemia and symptoms experienced
Symptoms suggestive of complications
Results of recent blood glucose level testing
Medical changes, other illnesses
Current medications
Exercise, tobacco use
Stress such as life, psychological, and social changes

tendency toward diabetic acidosis and coma. Appointment planning centers around many factors including stress prevention.

A. Antibiotic Premedication

1. *Well-controlled diabetes.* In general, the patient with well-controlled diabetes is treated the same as a patient without diabetes and requires no premedication related to diabetes.
2. *Uncontrolled, unstable diabetes.* Routine dental treatment is deferred until diabetes is stabilized. Only emergency care is given to the uncontrolled patient. Antibiotic premedication may be required due to the reduced ability to resist infection.

B. Time

Treat on full stomach, avoid peak insulin level noted in Table 60-6.
1. *Choice.* Morning after the patient's normal breakfast and medication, during the descending portion of the blood glucose level curve.
2. *Alternative.* After lunch. Always ask if patient has eaten.

C. Precautions: Prevent/Prepare for Emergency

1. Do not keep the patient waiting.
2. Do not interfere with the patient's regular meal and between-meal eating schedule.
3. Avoid long periods of stressful procedures; dental and dental hygiene care should be divided into short appointments appropriate to the individual's needs.
4. Take additional precautions indicated for the patient with long-term diabetes with complications related to atherosclerosis and other cardiovascular diseases (Chapter 58). Needs of the gerodontic patient may be applied (pages 690 to 694).
5. Prepare for diabetic emergency. Keep a tube of cake frosting or a jar of apple juice for the conscious patient as part of the office emergency supplies (pages 896 to 897, and Table

61-5, page 913). These items have long shelf life and are less likely to be consumed in a non-emergency.
6. Prevent and treat all infections.

IV. CLINICAL PROCEDURES

A. Instrumentation

1. *Quadrant or Area Scaling.* Limit number of teeth treated at each visit. Complete scaling and root planing in deep pockets reduces the possibility of periodontal abscess formation. Allow several short appointments if needed for stress management.
2. *Healing.* Undue trauma to tissues must be avoided to encourage healing without complications.

B. Fluoride Application

Home use of fluoride is encouraged. Methods for daily self-fluoride application are described on pages 469 to 472.

V. PATIENT INSTRUCTION

A. Bacterial Plaque Control

Due to the impact of diabetes on periodontal health and the effect of oral infection on diabetes status, daily home care is crucial. A plaque check and individualized self-care measures for plaque control must be reviewed continuously.

B. Diet

1. Most patients limit concentrated sweets which complements caries control measures. Correlate information about dental caries prevention with the elimination of cariogenic foods.
2. Reinforce principles of a nutritious diet as provided by the physician and dietitian.

C. Smoking Cessation

For smokers, discuss importance of cessation. Offer assistance (pages 436 to 438).

VI. MAINTENANCE PHASE

A. Appoint for supervision and examination on regular 3- to 4-month basis as needed. Calculus should not accumulate.
B. Probe carefully to detect early gingival bleeding and evidence of pocket formation.
C. Assess soft tissue with attention to areas of irritation related to fixed and removable prostheses.
D. Identify changes that require referral to patient's physician, dietitian, mental health professional, or other specialist.
E. Check for bacterial plaque control and review with the patient at each appointment. Gingival health is of major importance.

DIABETES INSIPIDUS

Diabetes insipidus should not be confused with diabetes mellitus. Diabetes insipidus is a rare disease characterized by polyuria and polydipsia. It is induced by an antidiuretic hormone deficiency.

REFERENCES

1. **American Diabetes Association**: Report of the Expert Committee on the Diagnosis and Classification of Diabetes Mellitus, *Diabetes Care, 21,* S5, Supplement 1, January, 1998.
2. **American Diabetes Association**: Screening for Type 2 Diabetes, *Diabetes Care, 21,* S20, Supplement 1, January, 1998.
3. **American Diabetes Association, Diabetes Control and Complications Trial Research Group**: The Effect of Intensive Treatment of Diabetes on the Development and Progression of Long-term Complications of Insulin-dependent Diabetes Mellitus, *N. Engl. J. Med., 329,* 977, September 30, 1993.
4. **American Diabetes Association, Diabetes Control and Complications Trial Research Group**: Hypoglycemia in the Diabetes Control and Complications Trial, *Diabetes, 46,* 271, February, 1997.
5. **American Diabetes Association**: Nutrition Recommendations and Principles for People with Diabetes Mellitus, *Diabetes Care, 21,* S32, Supplement 1, January, 1998.
6. **Porte,** D., Baker, L., Bollinger, R.R., Genuth, S., Scharp, D.W., and Sutherland, D.E.R.: Pancreas Transplantation for Patients with Diabetes Mellitus (Technical Review), *Diabetes Care, 15,* 1668, November, 1992.
7. **Jaremko,** J. and Rorstad, O.: Advances Toward the Implantable Artificial Pancreas for Treatment of Diabetes, *Diabetes Care, 21,* 444, March, 1998.
8. **American Academy of Periodontology, Committee on Research, Science and Therapy**: Position Paper. Diabetes and Periodontal Diseases, *J. Periodontol., 67,* 166, February, 1996.
9. **American Academy of Periodontology, Committee on Research, Science and Therapy**: Periodontal Disease as a Potential Risk Factor for Systemic Diseases, *J. Periodontol., 69,* 841, July, 1998.
10. **Grossi,** S.G., Skrepcinski, F.B., DeCaro, T., Robertson, D.C., Ho, A.W., Dunford, R.G., and Genco, R.J.: Treatment of Periodontal Disease in Diabetics Reduces Glycated Hemoglobin, *J. Periodontol., 68,* 713, August, 1997.

SUGGESTED READINGS

American Diabetes Association: Standards of Medical Care for Patients With Diabetes Mellitus, *Diabetes Care, 21,* S23, Supplement 1, January, 1998.

Biron, C.R.: Alert Dentist's Suspicions About Diabetes Reminds Us of Importance of Detecting Disease, *RDH, 18,* 44, February, 1998.

Blanchaert, R.H.: Implants in the Medically Challenged Patient, *Dent. Clin. North Am., 42,* 35, January, 1998.

Fioretto, P., Steffes, M.W., Sutherland, D.E.R., Goetz, F.C., and Mauer, M.: Reversal of Lesions of Diabetic Nephropathy After Pancreas Transplantation, *N. Engl. J. Med., 339,* 69, July 9, 1998.

Harris, M.I., Flegal, K.M., Cowie, C.C., Eberhardt, M.S., Goldstein, D.E., Little, R.R., Wiedmeyer, H.-M., and Byrd-Holt, D.D.: Prevalence of Diabetes, Impaired Fasting Glucose, and Impaired Glucose Tolerance in U.S. Adults, *Diabetes Care, 21,* 518, April, 1998.

Jacobson, A.M.: The Psychological Care of Patients With Insulin-dependent Diabetes Mellitus, *N. Engl. J. Med., 334,* 1249, May 9, 1996.

Mealey, B.L.: Impact of Advances in Diabetes Care on Dental Treatment of the Diabetic Patient, *Compend. Cont. Educ. Dent., 19,* 41, January, 1998.

Parker, R.C., Rapley, J.W., Isley, W., Spencer, P., and Killoy, W.J.: Gingival Crevicular Blood for Assessment of Blood Glucose in Diabetic Patients, *J. Periodontol., 64,* 666, July, 1993.

Pérusse, R., Goulet, J.-P., and Turcotte, J.-Y.: Contraindications to Vasoconstrictors in Dentistry: Part II. Hyperthyroidism, Diabetes, Sulfite Sensitivity, *Oral Surg. Oral Med. Oral Pathol., 74,* 687, November, 1992.

Rees, T.D.: The Diabetic Dental Patient, *Dent. Clin. North Am., 38,* 447, July, 1994.

Slavkin, H.C.: Diabetes, Clinical Dentistry and Changing Paradigms, *J. Am. Dent. Assoc., 128,* 638, May, 1997.

Sreebny, L.M., Yu, A., Green, A., and Valdini, A.: Xerostomia in Diabetes Mellitus, *Diabetes Care, 15,* 900, July, 1992.

Tavares, M., DePaola, P., Soparkar, P., and Joshipura, K.: The Prevalence of Root Caries in a Diabetic Population, *J. Dent. Res., 70,* 979, June, 1991.

Twetman, S., Nederfors, T., Stahl, B., and Aronson, S.: Two-year Longitudinal Observations of Salivary Status and Dental Caries in Children with Insulin-dependent Diabetes Mellitus, *Pediatr. Dent., 14,* 184, May–June, 1992.

Periodontal Infection

Bridges, R.B., Anderson, J.W., Saxe, S.R., Gregory, K., and Bridges, S.R.: Periodontal Status of Diabetic and Non-diabetic Men: Effects of Smoking, Glycemic Control, and Socioeconomic Factors, *J. Periodontol., 67,* 1185, November, 1996.

Christgau, M., Palitzsch, K.-D., Schmalz, G., Kreiner, U., and Frenzel, S.: Healing Response to Non-surgical Periodontal Therapy in Patients With Diabetes Mellitus: Clinical, Microbiological, and Immunologic Results, *J. Clin. Periodontol., 25,* 112, February, 1998.

Grossi, S.G., Skrepcinski, F.B., DeCaro, T., Zambon, J.J., Cummins, D., and Genco, R.J.: Response to Periodontal Therapy in Diabetics and Smokers, *J. Periodontol., 67,* 1094, October, Supplement, 1996.

Löe, H.: Periodontal Disease: The Sixth Complication of Diabetes Mellitus, *Diabetes Care, 16,* 329, Supplement 1, January, 1993.

Mandell, R.L., Dirienzo, J., Kent, R., Joshipura, K., and Haber, J.: Microbiology of Healthy and Diseased Periodontal Sites in Poorly Controlled Insulin Dependent Diabetes, *J. Periodontol., 63,* 274, April, 1992.

Nishimura, F., Takahashi, K., Kurihara, M., Takashiba, S., and Murayama, Y.: Periodontal Disease as a Complication of Diabetes Mellitus, *Ann. Periodontol., 3,* 20, July, 1998.

Soskolne, W.A.: Epidemiological and Clinical Aspects of Periodontal Diseases in Diabetics, *Ann. Periodontol., 3,* 3, July, 1998.

Taylor, G.W., Burt, B.A., Becker, M.P., Genco, R.J., Shlossman, M., Knowler, W.C., and Pettitt, D.J.: Non-insulin Dependent Diabetes Mellitus and Alveolar Bone Loss Progression Over 2 Years, *J. Periodontol., 69,* 76, January, 1998.

Tervonen, T. and Oliver, R.C.: Long-term Control of Diabetes Mellitus and Periodontitis, *J. Clin. Periodontol., 20,* 431, July, 1993.

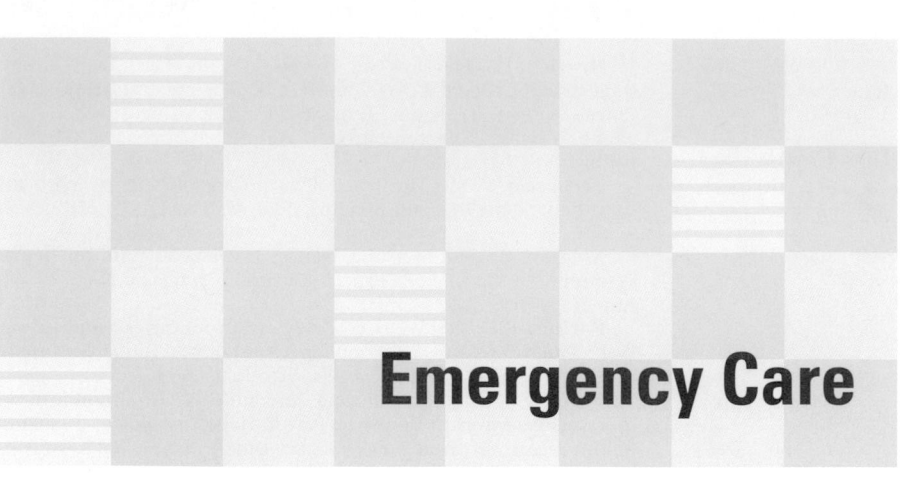

Emergency Care

It is relatively easy to be skillful in techniques that are repeated frequently. Emergency care is performed only occasionally and, in instances that involve life-saving measures, may be performed once in many years. To be prepared for that rare moment is difficult, but the public expects an individual trained in a health profession to be able to act in an emergency. Periodic review of procedures is necessary if application is to be effective.

Emergencies may occur within or in the vicinity of a dental office or clinic. Readiness involves having not only knowledge of proper procedures, but equipment kept in a convenient place. A quick, handy reference of emergency measures, which may be in the form of a posted chart with characteristic symptoms and related treatment, is important.

The information included in this chapter is basic and is presented with no attempt to mention all types of emergencies that may arise, particularly those of complex traumatic injuries. The principal objectives are to list the symptoms and management of the more common emergencies that can occur, and to provide a list of the equipment that should be readily available. Other up-to-date references should be kept in the dental office and all dental personnel should familiarize themselves with such sources of information.

Key words and definitions are provided in Box 61-1.

PREVENTION OF EMERGENCIES

I. ATTENTION TO PREVENTION

The best way to prevent an emergency is to employ proper patient assessment techniques, including thorough medical history questionnaires, documentation of vital signs, and the completion of a physical assessment of the patient. Extraoral and intraoral examinations are an integral part of the patient assessment.

Having gathered the information from the patient assessment, proper risk management and stress reduction protocols can be incorporated into the patient care plan. Prior to each appointment, the record must be reviewed and updated so that preparatory steps can be taken. Table 61-1 suggests a basic five-point plan for emergency prevention.

Prevention of emergencies requires preparedness, alertness, and anticipation. Some of the procedures that contribute to meeting the requirements are described here.

BOX 61-1 KEY WORDS: Emergencies

Angioneurotic edema (an'jē-ō-nu-rot'ik ĕ-dē'mah): sudden and temporary appearance of large areas of painless swelling in the subcutaneous tissue or submucosa; a symptom related to allergy; also called angioedema.

Arrhythmia (ah-rĭth'mē-ah): variation from normal rhythm, especially the heartbeat.

Basic life support: the phase of emergency cardiac care that supports the ventilation of a victim of respiratory arrest with rescue breathing and supports the ventilation and circulation of a victim of cardiac arrest with cardiopulmonary resuscitation.

Cannula (kan'u-lah): a tube for insertion into a duct or cavity.

> **Nasal cannula:** a semicircle of plastic tubing with two plastic tips that fit into the patient's nostrils.

Cardiac arrest (kar'dē-ak): sudden and often unexpected stoppage of heart action; circulation ceases and vital organs are deprived of oxygen.

Crepitation (krep'ĭ-tā'shun): dry crackling sound, such as that produced by the grating of the ends of a fractured bone.

Cricothyrotomy (kri'kō-thi-rot'ō-mē): incision through the skin and the cricothyroid membrane to secure a patent airway for emergency relief of upper airway obstruction.

Defibrillation (dē-fib'rĭ-lā'shun): termination of atrial or ventricular fibrillation usually accomplished by electric shock.

Defibrillator (dē-fib'ri-lā-tor): an apparatus used to produce defibrillation by application of brief electric shock to the heart directly or through electrodes placed on the chest wall.

Dyspnea (disp-knee'ah): labored or difficult breathing; indication of inadequate ventilation, or of insufficient oxygen in the circulating blood.

Fibrillation (fi-brĭ-lā'shun): involuntary muscular contraction caused by spontaneous activation of single muscle cells or fibers.

> **Ventricular fibrillation:** a cardiac arrhythmia marked by fibrillary contractions of the ventricular muscle caused by rapid repetitive excitation of myocardial fibers without coordinated ventricular contraction; a frequent cause of cardiac arrest.

Hypoxemia (hī'pok-se'me-ah): deficient oxygenation of the blood; insufficient oxygenation of the blood eventually leads to **hypoxia**, which is diminished oxygen to body tissues.

Kussmaul breathing (koos' mowl): loud, slow, labored breathing common to patients in diabetic coma.

Parenteral (pah-ren'ter-al): not through the alimentary canal; administered by subcutaneous, intramuscular, or intravenous injection.

Rescue breathing: a rescuer delivers a volume of 800 to 1200 mL with each ventilation; the exhaled air contains 16% to 17% oxygen, sufficient for the needs of the victim.

Syncope (sin'kō-pē): temporary loss of consciousness caused by a sudden fall in blood pressure resulting in generalized cerebral ischemia; can have serious consequences, particularly in patients with a cardiovascular disease; commonly referred to as **fainting.**

Trendelenburg's position (tren-del'en-bergz): the patient is supine with the heart higher than the head on a surface inclined downward about 45°.

Urticaria (ur'tĭ-ka'rē-ah): vascular reaction of the skin with transient appearance of slightly elevated patches (wheals) that are redder or paler than the surrounding skin; may be accompanied by severe itching; also called hives.

TABLE 61-1 Five-Step Plan to Prevent Emergencies

1. Use careful, routine patient assessment procedures.
2. Document and update accurate, comprehensive patient records.
3. Implement stress reduction protocols.
4. Recognize early signs of emergency distress.
5. Organize team management plan for emergency preparedness.

II. FACTORS CONTRIBUTING TO THE RISK OF MEDICAL EMERGENCIES

A. Increased number of older patients in society with natural teeth and dental diseases that require invasive procedures.
B. Older patients and many other patients are taking medications that interact adversely with drugs used in dentistry.
C. More complex dental procedures require longer appointments.
D. Increased use of drugs in dentistry
   1. Anesthesia: local, general, conscious sedation
   2. Tranquilizers
   3. Pain medications (CNS depressants)
   4. Antibiotics

PATIENT ASSESSMENT

I. ASSESSMENT FOR ROUTINE TREATMENT

A. First Contact
1. Start with the first interaction with the patient.
2. Note abnormalities of patient's voice on the telephone during appointment scheduling.
3. Assess overall appearance and gait when patient enters the dental office or clinic.
4. Document findings in the patient's chart.

B. Parts of the Assessment
1. Physical assessment (signs and symptoms)
2. Comprehensive medical history
3. Vital signs
4. Extraoral and intraoral examination
5. Comprehensive documentation of findings

C. Emergency Indicators
Changes in a patient's appearance on the day of an appointment may suggest indicators that encourage preparation for emergencies.

II. THE PATIENT'S MEDICAL HISTORY

A. Update and Document Changes
1. Review at each appointment.
2. Discuss changes with dental team members who are providing treatment for the patient.

3. A comprehensive medical history includes all the items listed in Tables 6-1, 6-2, and 6-3, pages 93 to 100.

B. Use of Medical Alert Box
A "Medical Alert Box" at the top of the inside front page of the patient's record folder should include information that may predispose the patient to medical emergencies. *Confidentiality must be maintained.* Significant items include:
1. Physical conditions that may lead to an emergency.
2. Diseases the patient has or previously had.
3. Medical emergencies the patient experienced previously.
4. Medications the patient has taken within the last 2 years.
5. Allergies and adverse drug reactions.
6. Previous adverse reactions to dental treatments.

III. VITAL SIGNS

Vital signs are essential to assess a patient's overall health status, and to evaluate the severity of a medical emergency. A well-prepared dental team takes vital signs routinely, not only during the earliest sign of emergency distress.

A. The Eight Vital Signs
Pulse, blood pressure, respirations, temperature, height, weight, age, and the information from the Medical Alert Tag (bracelet, necklace, anklet), provide essential information for patient care.

B. Baseline Vital Signs
The vital signs taken at a routine appointment are considered baseline. The ranges of vital signs are described in Table 7-1, page 107.

C. During Emergency
In a medical emergency the vital signs that are taken are compared to the baseline findings.
1. *"Compensating."* In most medical emergencies, patients will experience a "fight or flight" reaction during which time they are said to be compensating. The vital signs are elevated above the baseline findings.
2. *"Decompensating."* The vital signs have fallen below baseline, and the patient could be going into a state of shock.
3. *Shock.* A state of lack of perfusion (saturation) of oxygenated blood to all cells of the brain and body. When brain cells are deprived of oxygenated blood, they cease to provide respiratory and circulatory function.

IV. EXTRAORAL AND INTRAORAL EXAMINATIONS

Extraoral and intraoral examinations can provide significant findings that are clues to underlying disease processes that predispose a patient to a medical emergency. Thorough examinations are an integral part of the prevention of medical emergencies.

A. Extraoral
Blood disorders and endocrine disorders may be discovered from extraoral palpation, skin color changes, abnormalities of the eyes, and asymmetry of the face or neck.

B. Intraoral
Oral manifestations and lesions can be indications of many disease states such as diabetes, anemia, leukemia, lupus, or AIDS.

V. RECOGNITION OF INCREASED RISK FACTORS

The carefully prepared and regularly updated medical and personal history, with adequate follow-up consultation with the patient's physician for integration of dental and medical care, can prevent many emergencies by alerting dental personnel to the individual patient's needs and idiosyncrasies. Special needs may include:

A. Specific physical conditions that may lead to an emergency, for example, genetic predispositions, seizures, diabetes.

B. Diseases for which the patient is (or has been) under the care of a physician and the type of treatment, including medications.

C. Allergies or drug reactions.

VI. COMPREHENSIVE RECORD KEEPING

All details about the patient, the treatments, reactions, healing, and comments by the patient, provide crucial information should a medical emergency or post-treatment complication occur.

A. Document
1. All medical findings and changes.
2. Treatments provided including types and amounts of local anesthesia, general anesthesia, and nitrous oxide.
3. Regimens of medications prescribed for patients are crucial information should a medical emergency or a post-treatment complication occur.

B. Consults
Document in the patient's record telephone and written responses of consultations with physicians.

C. New Entries
1. *Response to Treatment.* Document a patient's reactions and responses to treatments, whether they are unremarkable or remarkable.
2. *Previous Appointment Review.* Complete a comprehensive review of previous appointment documentations before providing additional treatment at sequential appointments.
3. *Current Information.* Update information

about the patient's health status as an integral part of the prevention of medical emergencies.

STRESS MINIMIZATION

Stress and anxiety are the basis for many of the common emergencies that occur in a dental office or clinic. The office atmosphere and the warmth and sincerity of the personnel can help a patient feel accepted and secure. The apprehension and anxiety that can be associated with dental treatment compounds the risk factors for medical emergencies.

I. RECOGNIZE THE PATIENT WITH STRESS PROBLEMS

A. Apprehensive about any dental appointment.

B. Elderly patients are especially prone to medical emergencies, as they may have cardiovascular diseases that have or have not been diagnosed.

C. Essential medications: certain prescriptions must be taken on schedule or the patient is at risk for an emergency.

II. SUGGESTIONS FOR EFFECTIVE COMMUNICATION

Any patient who is apprehensive or medically predisposed to emergencies should be provided with a stress reduction plan. Reduction of stress includes the development of patient rapport through effective communication between the dental team and the patient.

A. Actively Listen to a Patient's Fears.
1. Develop rapport so the patient senses that the listener is empathetic and interested in alleviating the apprehension.
2. Communicate with a patient about fear. A discussion can be very beneficial for emergency prevention.

B. Effects of Fear
Patients who try to repress their fears are more likely to hyperventilate or experience syncopal episodes.

III. REDUCTION OF STRESS
A. Appointment Scheduling[1]
1. *New Patient.* Initial appointment for a new patient used for consultation and assessment will build rapport and provide opportunity to evaluate the level of anxiety. Stress reduction can be built into treatment appointments.
2. *Time of Appointment.* Plan in accord with personal health requirements.
3. *Waiting Time Minimized.* First appointment in the morning prevents building of anxiety by waiting all day for the appointment.
4. *Eating Requirements.* Usual meal time and

previous meal checked to prevent hunger anxiety or hypoglycemia.

5. *Length of Appointment:* limited to the patient's durability.

B. Medication

1. Premedication when indicated and recommended by the physician and dentist.
2. Pain control during treatment.
3. Patient's own prescriptions. Patients who are subject to emergencies are instructed to bring their own prescribed medicines; for example, the patient with asthma or one who is subject to attacks of angina pectoris.

C. Post-treatment Care

1. Postcare instructions for prevention and/or relief of discomfort.
2. Follow-up telephone call for anxious patient.

EMERGENCY MATERIALS AND PREPARATION

Organization is a key concept in being prepared for an emergency. Group planning and individual acceptance of responsibility can provide the team with efficiency, composure, and freedom from fear at the time of crisis.

I. COMMUNICATION: TELEPHONE NUMBERS FOR MEDICAL AID

Telephone numbers should be posted near each extension from which outside calls can be made.

A. Rescue squads with paramedics (fire, police, flying squad, or 911 in many cities in the United States).
B. Ambulance service.
C. Nearest hospital emergency room.
D. Poison information center.
E. Physicians
   1. Patient's physician should be listed in the permanent record in a standard, convenient place.
   2. Physicians available for emergency calls.

II. EQUIPMENT FOR USE IN AN EMERGENCY

Every dental office or clinic should have an emergency kit or cart,[1,2] and everyone in the office must be familiar with its contents. The kit should be in order, its contents replenished, and outdated materials replaced as needed.

The emergency equipment should be portable and kept in a place readily accessible to all treatment rooms. Materials are plainly marked and kept separate from other office supplies. Materials included are selected to accomplish emergency treatment by current methods.

The items included in the kit imply proper training in their use. A team should work out additions to the list in keeping with their training and abilities.

A. Essential Equipment

1. *Pocket Masks.* Each rescuer has personal mask.
2. *Series E Portable Oxygen Tank.*
   a. Low-flow regulator to allow administration at different concentrations.
   b. Delivery systems include nasal cannula, simple face mask, nonrebreather bag, bag-valve mask (Ambu Bag), demand valve.
3. *Airways.* Various sizes for oropharyngeal and nasopharyngeal—child and adults; water-soluble lubricant for insertion of nasopharyngeal airways (petroleum jelly is combustible, hence contraindicated).
4. *Suction Tips.* Wide diameter with smooth edges to prevent damage to mucous membranes.
5. *Blood Pressure Equipment.* Sphygmomanometer; stethoscope; child, regular, and large blood pressure cuffs.
6. *Magill Forceps.* Blunt-ended instrument designed to grasp objects from the mouth or throat.
7. *Cricothyrotomy Equipment.* Included only with advanced training.
8. *Defibrillator.* Included only for use for those with advanced training.

B. Injectable Drugs

1. *Essential (critical)*
   a. Antiallergy. Epinephrine 1:1000 in preloaded syringe.
   b. Antihistamine. Chlorpheniramine; diphenhydramine.
2. *Secondary (noncritical)*
   In a clinical setting where trained individuals are available, an emergency kit may contain a variety of drugs for specific emergencies. Included may be an anticonvulsant, an analgesic, a vasopressor, an antihypoglycemic, a corticosteroid, an antihypertensive, and an anticholinergic.
3. *Equipment*
   a. Syringes. Disposable sterile 2- to 3-mL-capacity syringes (Luer-Lok-Tip) with 18- or 21-gauge disposable needles. Syringes and tourniquet are only included for parenteral drug administration.
   b. Tourniquet. Rubber or Velcro; rubber tubing or the blood pressure cuff can be used.

C. Noninjectable Treatment Items

1. *Essential (critical)*
   a. Oxygen.
   b. Vasodilator. Nitrostat tablets (nitroglycerin); nitrolingual spray.
2. *Secondary (noncritical)*
   a. Respiratory stimulant. Aromatic ammonia in gray vaporoles.

b. Bronchodilator. Albuterol inhaler.

c. Antihypoglycemic (for conscious person). Frosting mix (tube), sugar cubes, apple juice.

d. Antihypertensive. Nifedipine or nitroglycerin capsule form.

e. Sterile irrigating solution for eyes.

f. Brown paper bags (for hyperventilation).

D. Supplementary Equipment

1. Pen flashlight.
2. Stopwatch.
3. Scissors.
4. Emesis basin.
5. Blanket (nonallergenic).
6. Board, 12 × 24 inches, to place under patient in a soft dental chair for CPR when patient cannot be moved to floor.
7. Commercial cold pack (nonrefrigerated quick-forming cold bag).
8. Blank pad of *Medical Emergency Report* (Figure 61-1) forms with pen.
9. Bandages and dressings are purchased in individual packages and maintained in the sealed sterile state.
   a. Adhesive bandages.
   b. Sterile dressings in sealed envelopes: 2 × 2 inches, and 4 × 4 inches.
   c. Rolled bandage: 1-inch (5 yards); 2-inch (5 yards).
   d. Adhesive tape.
   e. Gauze sponges: 4 × 4 inches.
   f. Inflatable splints (assorted sizes).

III. CARE OF DRUGS

All dental personnel must be familiar with the emergency drugs maintained in the particular office or clinic. Only specially trained, experienced persons should administer injectable medications. If no one on the team has the proper background and experience, the drugs should not be kept in the office with the emergency supplies.[3]

A. Identification

The purpose and method of administration of each drug should be clearly identified with the container. A compartmentalized clear plastic cabinet or box can be particularly useful for this purpose, because the labels and instructions can be seen from the outside and efficient selection can be made.

The replacement date must appear clearly on each item with a limited shelf life. When narcotics are included in the list of drugs available for emergencies, storage in a less accessible place than an emergency kit and purchase in small amounts are indicated to prevent them from being stolen easily.

B. Record of Drugs

A complete record of each available drug is kept. Recorded are the name, dosage, date purchased, address of source if different from the usual local pharmacy, with each itemized record signed by the staff member responsible.

As each drug is used, a specific entry is made. Expiration dates can be checked at routine intervals.

IV. RECORD OF EMERGENCY

Figure 61-1 shows an example of a form that can be used to record the essential information during an emergency. Such a form can be printed into pads for the convenience of having a carbon copy to place in the patient's permanent record when the original accompanies the patient to a hospital or other medical facility.

A. Purposes

1. Organize data collected during the emergency.
2. Serve as a time reference during the monitoring of vital signs.
3. Prepare a record from which the medical personnel can interpret the patient's condition at the time of transfer from the dental facility.

B. Uses

1. Evaluation for planning dental and dental hygiene appointments so that future emergencies for the patient can be avoided.
2. Provide a reference in the event legal questions arise. A well-kept record can be vital, and each emergency, however insignificant the incident may seem, should be recorded.[4]

V. PRACTICE AND DRILL

A. Staff Instruction

Each member of the clinic or office staff must be thoroughly familiar with the location, purpose, effect, and application of each item of equipment and its source.

B. Assignments

Specific responsibilities must be assigned to each staff member to prevent confusion. Each must know the order of procedures in all types of emergencies, however, and be able to assume any role when needed. Moments count, and there is no time for fumbling or discussion.

C. Flowchart

Figure 61-2 shows an example of possible distribution of duties when three people are available to attend the patient. Although a chart can be posted for study, it must be memorized by the persons concerned. In a real emergency, no one would have time to consult a flowchart.

1. *Advantages*
   a. Organization efficiently uses personnel.
   b. Sharing responsibility relieves pressure.
   c. Duties can be carried out quietly, without excess discussion.

Medical Emergency Report

Patient's Name: _____ Today's Date: _____

Description of Incident: _____

_____

_____

Time of Onset:

Stopwatch:	Clock TIme:

Time EMS Summoned:

Stopwatch:	Clock TIme:

Time EMS Arrived:

Stopwatch:	Clock TIme:

Time Patient Released:

Stopwatch:	Clock TIme:

Patient Released to:

	Finding:	Stopwatch Time:	Finding:	Stopwatch Time:	Finding:	Stopwatch Time:
Blood Pressure	/		/		/	
Pulse:						
Respirations:						
Oxygen Delivery Method:						

Cessation of Breathing | Stopwatch: |

Cessation of Pulse | Stopwatch: |

CPR Initiated | Stopwatch: |

Drugs Administered	Route	Dosage	Stopwatch Time:

FIGURE 61-1 Medical Emergency Report. The form is prepared in duplicate. One copy accompanies the patient to the emergency clinic, and the second copy is retained in the patient's dental record file. (From Biron, C.R.: *Dental Team Management of Medical Emergencies.* Philadelphia, W.B. Saunders, 2000)

Team Member 2

1. Starts stopwatch
2. Brings cart and oxygen
3. Assists with oxygen
4. Prepares medications
5. Assists Team Leader
6. Assists with CPR

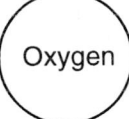

Oxygen

Emergency Kit
or Cart

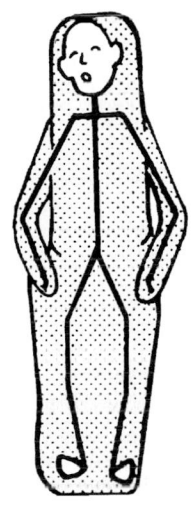

Team Leader 1

1. Provides basic life support
2. Evaluates vital signs
3. Initiates CPR
4. Positions patient
5. Manages airway
6. Directs emergency care
7. Administers oxygen
8. Administers drugs

Team Member 3

1. Calls for medical aid
2. Monitors vital signs
3. Records data
4. Assists Team Leader
5. Suctions
6. Loosens tight clothing
7. Relieves others in CPR

FIGURE 61-2 Emergency Team Flowchart: Three People. Suggested distribution of responsibilities to be memorized and practiced by the dental personnel who form the emergency team.

d. Necessary work gets done without duplication and without omissions.

2. *Preparation.* The preparation of a flowchart and the assignment of all duties related to emergencies should be a result of planning by the whole team.

3. *Substitutions.* Because a staff member may be absent from the scene at the time of an emergency, each person should know the duties for all positions so that substitutions can be made and duties doubled with a minimum of discussion and no confusion.

D. Drills

1. Regular reviews and rehearsals for each type of emergency should be conducted, preferably on a "surprise" basis, at least once a month. A specific code call can be used when an intercom or other message system is available.

2. Practice in the use of all procedures, including oxygen administration, resuscitation, and

airway maneuvers, as well as of specific positioning of a patient for all emergencies, is indicated.

3. Equipment and materials can be checked at the time of the drill to ensure their availability and that each is in working order. Outdated supplies can be replaced. One staff member should be in charge of the emergency supplies.

4. Keep a record of drills by making a diary of dates and names of those present.

E. New Staff Member

1. Assignment of duties and practice for the new member should be a part of the first working day's orientation.

2. New members must be expected to renew CPR certificates by taking necessary refresher courses within a specified time. Such a procedure is not necessary in a state where a renewal certificate is required for annual licensure.

F. Procedures Manual

A loose-leaf manual, reviewed and updated three or four times each year, can provide a valuable study and work reference. It is particularly useful during the orientation of a new member.

The notebook can contain work assignments and check lists for equipment and resources. Direct reference information concerning specific emergencies with their symptoms and initial treatment may be placed in alphabetic order in a specially color-coded section. Members of the team can keep the manual current by bringing references and notes from readings and courses.

BASIC LIFE SUPPORT[5]

Sudden cessation of effective respiration and circulation must be treated immediately. Without breathing and heart action, oxygen cannot be carried to the cells and a deficiency occurs quickly. The flow chart in Figure 61-3 shows the steps to take in every emergency.

Irreversible brain tissue damage may occur within 4 to 6 minutes in the absence of oxygenated blood. After 6 minutes, brain damage nearly always occurs.

The cause of collapse, respiratory arrest, or cardiac arrest cannot always be determined at the outset. Survival rates depend on prompt entry into emergency medical service (EMS) for state-of-the-art medical attention. Preliminary assessment of the state of consciousness (response, breathing, and pulse rate) must be made quickly, and the EMS activated promptly.

Basic patient care in an emergency is defined by the letters A-B-C-D.

It is necessary to keep calm and act promptly, but not hastily. The incorrect procedure may be more harmful than none at all. Each member of the dental team should have participated in courses in emergency procedures and resuscitation techniques while in school and periodically since graduation for refresher, renewal, and updating.

This section is intended to provide an outline for reference and review. Abbreviations pertaining to emergency care are listed in Table 61-2. The steps described are carried out in rapid succession.

I. QUICKLY LOWER DENTAL CHAIR (IN DENTAL SETTING)

A. Adjust patient for supine position.

TABLE 61-2 Emergency Care: Abbreviations	
ACLS	Advanced Cardiac Life Support
AED	Automated External Defibrillator
AHA	American Heart Association
ALS	Advanced Life Support
BLS	Basic Life Support
BCLS	Basic Cardiac Life Support
CAD	Coronary Artery Disease
CPR	Cardiopulmonary Resuscitation
ECC	Emergency Cardiac Care
ECG	Electrocardiogram
EMD	Emergency Medical Dispatcher
EMS	Emergency Medical Service
EMT	Emergency Medical Technician
EMT-D	Emergency Medical Technician-Defibrillation

B. Remove a round or wedge-shaped accessory head or shoulder support to permit the head to lie flat and the chin to be raised without resistance.

II. DETERMINE STATE OF CONSCIOUSNESS (FIGURE 61-4)

A. Tap or gently shake the shoulder and shout "Are you OK?" If fractures are suspected, the shake must be light.

B. Unconscious patient does not respond.

C. Call for help. When available, use an alert (buzzer) system of an office or clinic.

D. Start the stopwatch (Figure 61-5).

III. OPEN AIRWAY

A. Head Tilt with Chin Lift

1. Place palm of hand on the forehead to apply a backward pressure.
2. Place fingertips (not thumb) of other hand under the chin with light pressure on the mandible to bring the chin up (Figure 61-6).

B. Modified Jaw Thrust

1. Indication. When a neck or spinal injury is suspected, the airway can be opened without extending the neck. DO NOT use head tilt/chin lift maneuver when spinal injury is suspected.
2. Procedure
   a. From over the top of the head, place thumbs on zygomas and grasp angles of the mandible with fingertips.
   b. Lift fingers upward to open airway.

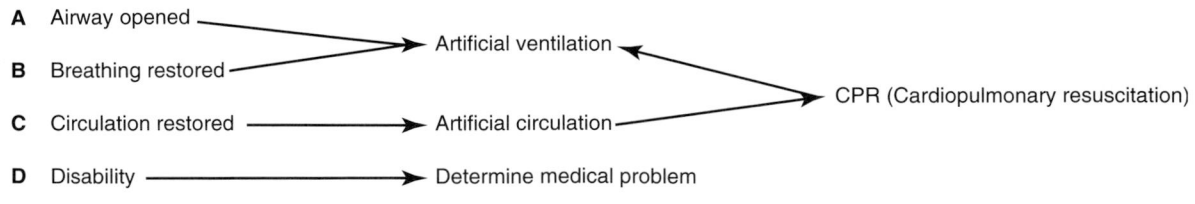

A Airway opened ⟶ Artificial ventilation

B Breathing restored ⟶

C Circulation restored ⟶ Artificial circulation ⟶ CPR (Cardiopulmonary resuscitation)

D Disability ⟶ Determine medical problem

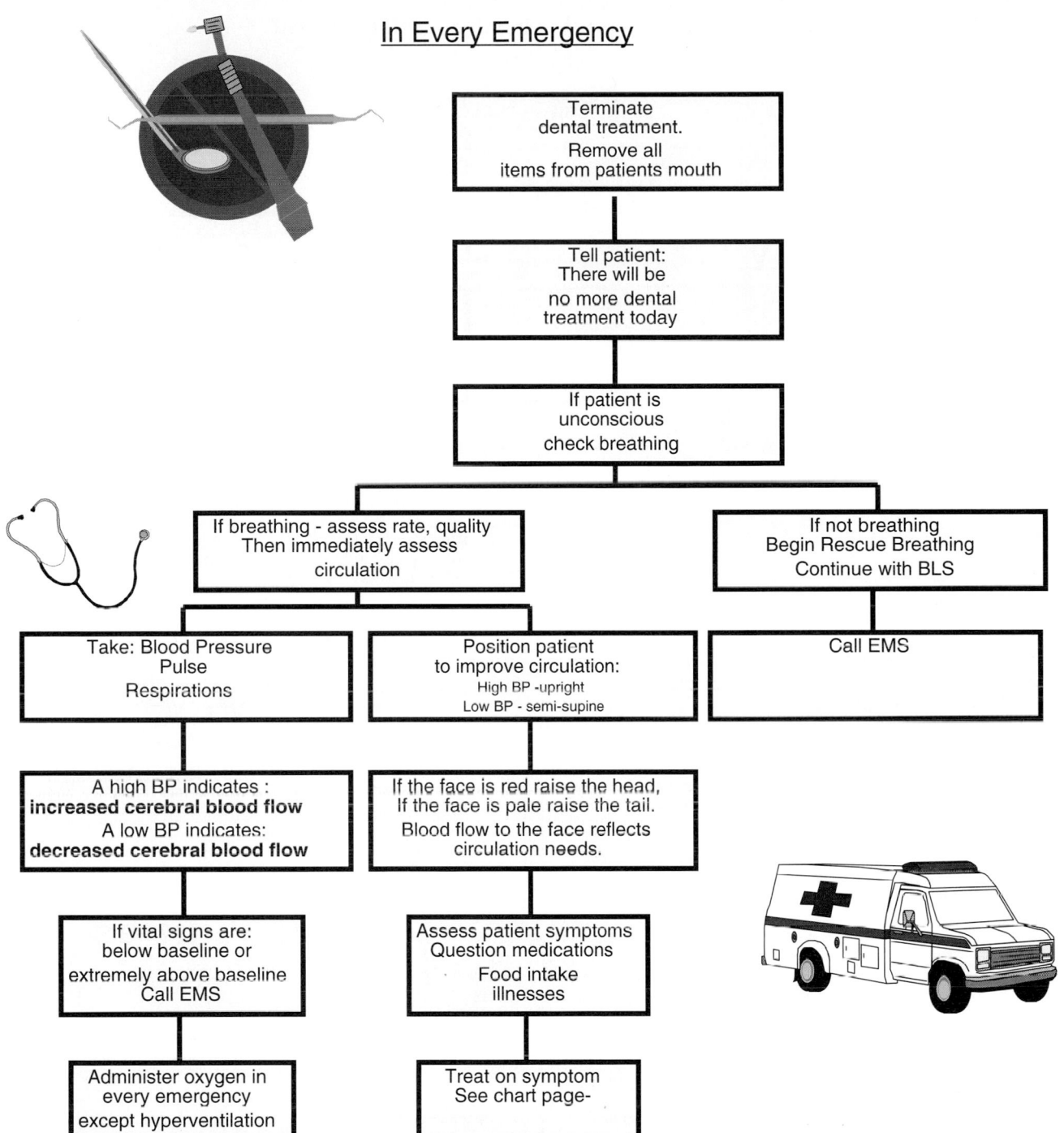

In Every Emergency

Terminate dental treatment. Remove all items from patients mouth

↓

Tell patient: There will be no more dental treatment today

↓

If patient is unconscious check breathing

If breathing - assess rate, quality Then immediately assess circulation

If not breathing Begin Rescue Breathing Continue with BLS

Take: Blood Pressure Pulse Respirations

Position patient to improve circulation: High BP -upright Low BP - semi-supine

Call EMS

A high BP indicates : **increased cerebral blood flow** A low BP indicates: **decreased cerebral blood flow**

If the face is red raise the head, If the face is pale raise the tail. Blood flow to the face reflects circulation needs.

If vital signs are: below baseline or extremely above baseline Call EMS

Assess patient symptoms Question medications Food intake illnesses

Administer oxygen in every emergency except hyperventilation

Treat on symptom See chart page-

FIGURE 61-3 Flowchart: IN EVERY EMERGENCY. (From Biron, C.R.: *Dental Team Management of Medical Emergencies.* Philadelphia, W.B. Saunders, 2000)

c. Never tilt the head when spinal injury is suspected.

IV. CHECK BREATHING (3 TO 5 SECONDS)

A. From beside the patient at the shoulder (kneeling if patient is on the floor), place ear over the patient's mouth and nose while looking at the chest.

B. LOOK for chest movement.

C. LISTEN for and FEEL air from the nose and mouth.
1. If patient is unconscious and breathing, check pulse.
2. If patient is unconscious with no breathing, say "No breathing" when signaling second rescuer.

D. When NO breathing: immediately administer two full breaths.

Assessment of the Unconscious Patient

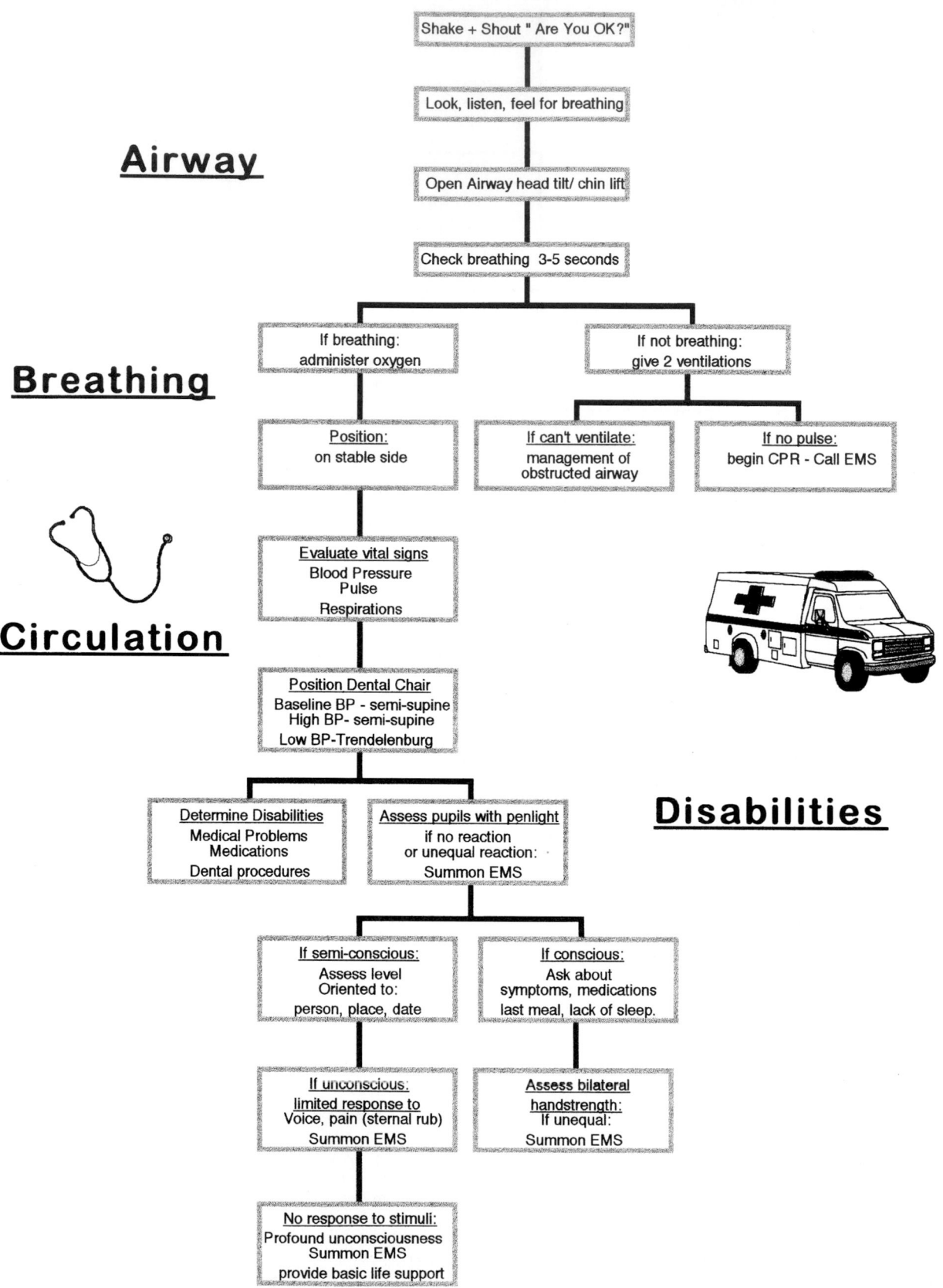

Airway

Breathing

Circulation

Disabilities

Shake + Shout " Are You OK?"

Look, listen, feel for breathing

Open Airway head tilt/ chin lift

Check breathing 3-5 seconds

If breathing:
administer oxygen

If not breathing:
give 2 ventilations

Position:
on stable side

If can't ventilate:
management of
obstructed airway

If no pulse:
begin CPR - Call EMS

Evaluate vital signs
Blood Pressure
Pulse
Respirations

Position Dental Chair
Baseline BP - semi-supine
High BP- semi-supine
Low BP-Trendelenburg

Determine Disabilities
Medical Problems
Medications
Dental procedures

Assess pupils with penlight
if no reaction
or unequal reaction:
Summon EMS

If semi-conscious:
Assess level
Oriented to:
person, place, date

If conscious:
Ask about
symptoms, medications
last meal, lack of sleep.

If unconscious:
limited response to
Voice, pain (sternal rub)
Summon EMS

Assess bilateral
handstrength:
If unequal:
Summon EMS

No response to stimuli:
Profound unconsciousness
Summon EMS
provide basic life support

☐**FIGURE 61-4 Assessment of the Unconscious Patient.** (From Biron, C.R.: *Dental Team Management of Medical Emergencies.* Philadelphia, W.B. Saunders, 2000)

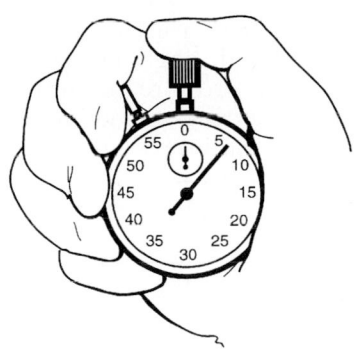

FIGURE 61-5 Stopwatch. An essential part of every emergency kit. It is turned on at the onset of an emergency and turned off when the EMS takes the patient to the hospital, or when the medical emergency is over. Time is recorded on the *Medical Emergency Report.*

1. Position patient on stable side.
2. Place resuscitation mask on patient.
3. Place thumbs on each side of mask (to obtain seal).
4. Place fingers on border of ramus.
5. Utilize a modified jaw thrust to open airway.
6. Holding the tight seal around mask, force air in until the chest is seen to rise, then release.
7. **When patient cannot be ventilated**, obstruction is apparent. Proceed to **Airway Obstruction** management (page 906).

V. CHECK PULSE

A. Location

1. *Adult.* Carotid pulse in neck (Figure 61-7).
2. *Child* (ages 1 to 8 years). Carotid pulse in neck.
3. *Infant* (younger than 1 year). Brachial pulse of the inner upper arm (Figure 7-4, page 110).

B. Determine Need for Cardiopulmonary Resuscitation (CPR)

1. **If pulse present** and patient not breathing, **proceed with rescue breathing.**
2. Position on stable side.
3. **If NO pulse**, but patient breathing, **proceed with CPR.**

VI. ACTIVATE EMERGENCY MEDICAL SERVICES

Telephone 911 or appropriate number for the given community.

RESCUE BREATHING

I. CLEAR THE MOUTH

Turn the patient's head to the side to clear the mouth of mucus, vomitus, and other foreign material. Use suction, gauze, and finger. Dentures should be left in

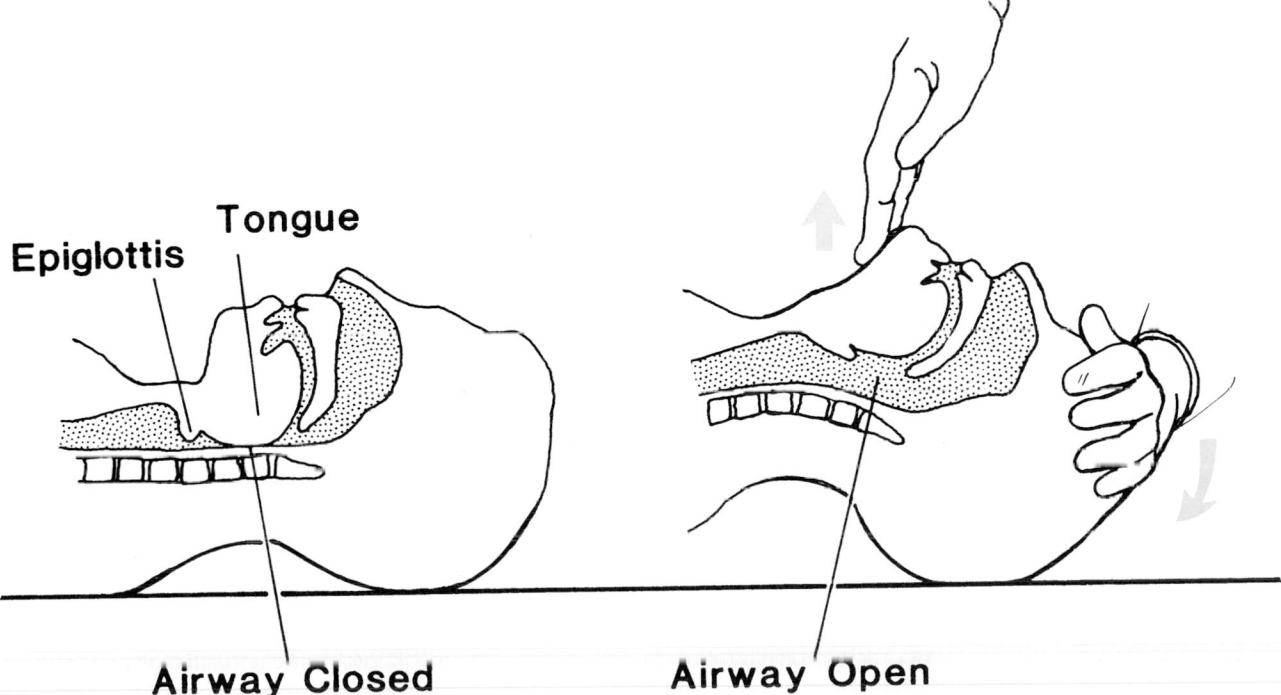

Epiglottis Tongue

Airway Closed   Airway Open

FIGURE 61-6 Chin Lift to Open Airway. *Left,* Unconscious person with tongue falling back against posterior wall of pharynx and obstructing the air passage. ***Right,*** Head is tilted back and chin is lifted by light pressure under the mandible. When neck injury is suspected, a jaw thrust is used. See text for instructions. (After Malamed, S.F.: *Handbook of Medical Emergencies in the Dental Office,* 4th ed. St. Louis, Mosby, 1993, page 106.)

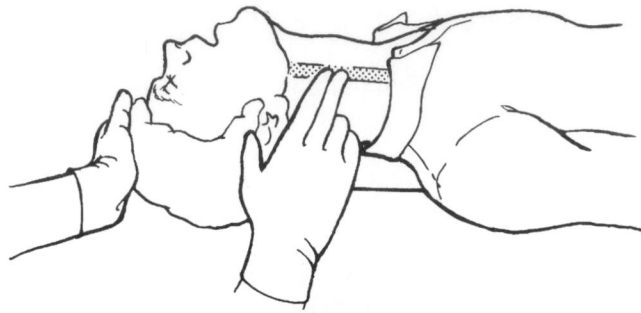

FIGURE 61-7 Carotid Pulse. To locate the pulse, two or three fingers are placed on the patient's pharynx. The fingers are then slid down into the groove between the trachea and the neck muscles. With gentle pressure, the pulse can be detected.

place to provide support unless the dentures are very loose and could cause throat obstruction if displaced.

II. RESCUE BREATHING

A. Place resuscitation mask on patient.
B. Hold with thumbs (on sides of mask) and place fingers on the border of the ramus to obtain a seal.
C. Apply modified jaw thrust to open airway.
D. Deliver two breaths (1½ to 2 seconds each breath).
E. Remove mouth and take in fresh air between each breath. The rescuer must take care not to become hyperventilated by taking too many deep breaths.
F. For child or infant, use only enough breath volume for chest to rise and fall.

III. REPEAT THE VENTILATIONS

A. For adult, repeat one ventilation every 5 seconds (12 per minute).
B. For child, repeat one ventilation every 3 seconds (20 per minute).
C. For infant, repeat one ventilation every 3 seconds (20 per minute).
D. Rescue breathing is considered effective when the patient's chest rises with each ventilation.

IV. MAKE A PULSE CHECK EACH MINUTE

A. **If no pulse**, start CPR.
B. **With pulse present**, continue rescue breathing.

EXTERNAL CHEST COMPRESSION

There are two mechanisms for blood flow during CPR. One is the principle that rhythmic pressure applied over the lower half of the sternum compresses the heart to produce artificial circulation. The procedure is also called *external cardiac compression*.

The second mechanism involves the intrathoracic pressure, which rises during chest compression. The rise in intrathoracic pressure provides a significant mechanism for movement of blood to the brain. Both cardiac and intrathoracic pressures may be in effect during resuscitation efforts.

Chest compressions are always accompanied by rescue breathing.

I. POSITION

The patient is in a supine position. When working in a dental chair, lower the chair to its lowest position and place a cardiac arrest board or other firm flat object under the patient's back to provide a solid surface for compression.

II. ADULT

A. Locate Point for Compression

1. Run the middle finger of hand 1 along the lower edge of the rib cage to the notch in the midline.
2. With the middle finger in the notch and the index finger beside it, place the heel of hand 2 next to the index finger on the midline of the sternum.
3. Place the heel of hand 1 on top of hand 2 with the fingers in the same direction. Link and close the fingers.
4. Hold the fingers up so that only the heel of hand 2 is on the sternum (Figure 61-8).

B. Compression

1. Lean forward over the positioned hands, arms straight, until shoulders are directly over the sternum.
2. Use a firm, steady, vertical pressure (not a blow). The sternum moves down 1½ to 2 inches (Figure 61-8).
3. Release pressure but maintain contact and position of the hands with sternum.
4. Compress at a rate of 80 to 100 times per minute.
5. Make the compressions smooth and uninterrupted, with compression and relaxation of equal duration.
6. Use the natural weight of the upper body to prevent pushing from the shoulders or depending on arm strength.
7. As the heart is compressed between the sternum and the spine, blood is forced out of the heart into the circulation.
8. Release of pressure allows blood to flow into the heart.
9. An interruption in compression results in a return of blood flow to zero.

III. CHILD

A. Locate Point for Compression

1. Follow the lower edge of the rib cage to the notch where sternum and ribs meet.

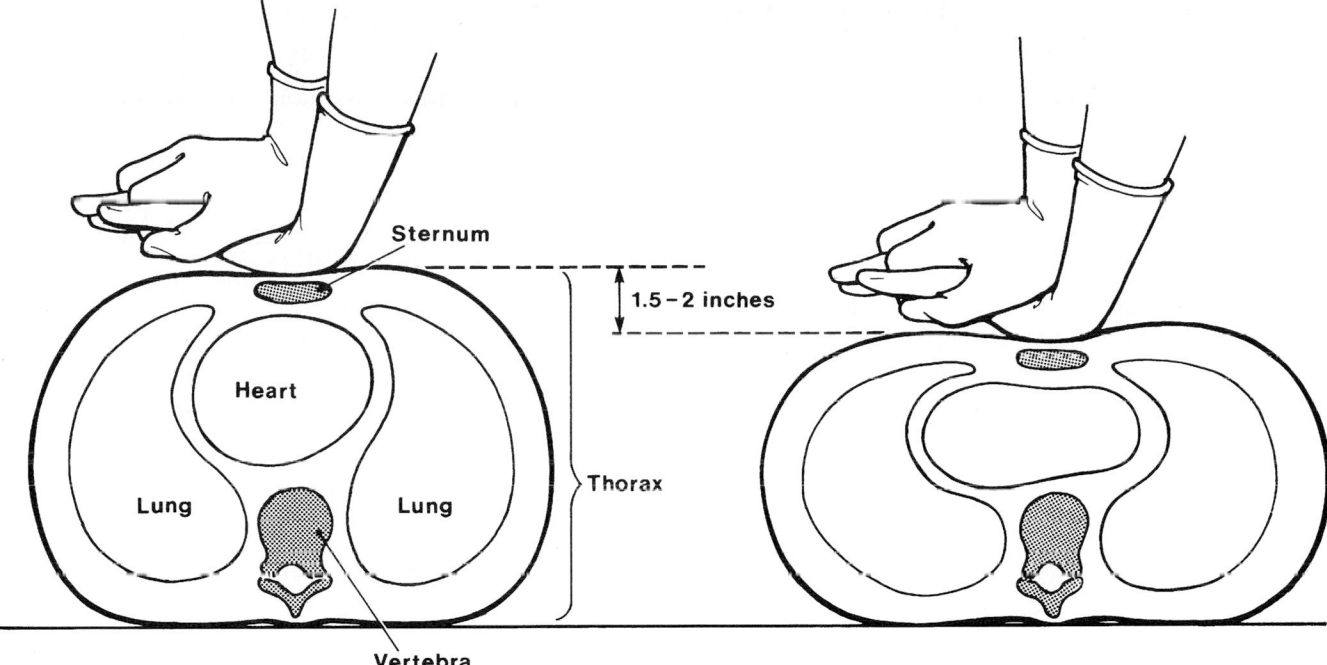

Sternum

1.5 – 2 inches

Heart

Thorax

Lung   Lung

Vertebra

FIGURE 61-8 External Chest Compression. *Left,* Hands in position on the sternum with fingers turned up. ***Right,*** Application of firm vertical pressure compresses the heart. The sternum should be compressed 1 1/2 to 2 inches and then released. Hands are held in position for the next compression. For an adult, compressions are repeated at a rate of 80 to 100 per minute.

2. Place the middle finger in the notch with the index finger beside it.
3. Place the heel of the other hand next to the index finger.

B. Compression
1. Use the heel of one hand only; compress to a depth of 1 to 1½ inches.
2. Release to allow chest to return to normal level.
3. Compress at a rate of 80 to 100 per minute, using a smooth, even rhythm.
4. Keep fingers up, off the chest.

IV. INFANT

A. Locate Point for Compression
1. Place fingers along the sternum, with the index finger just below an imaginary line between the nipples. Lift the index finger. If the fingers are on the xiphoid process, move the fingers closer to the nipples.
2. Use the area under the middle and ring fingers.

B. Compression
1. Compress with two fingers to a depth of ½ to 1 inch; release to allow chest to return to normal after each compression.
2. Compress at a rate of at least 100 per minute, using a smooth rhythm.

V. COORDINATED ACTIVITY FOR CPR

A. Lone Rescuer
1. Provide ventilation and compressions.
2. *Adult Patient*
   a. Use ratio 15 compressions followed by 2 lung inflations.
   b. Compress at the rate of 80 to 100 per minute (count "1 and, 2 and, 3 and . . .").
   c. Check carotid pulse after four cycles of compressions and ventilations; continue if no pulse; check pulse regularly.
3. *Child and Infant*
   a. Use a ratio of five compressions with a slight pause for one ventilation.
   b. Compress at the rate of 80 to 100 per minute for a child; minimum of 100 for an infant.
   c. Reassess pulse after 10 cycles, and every few minutes.

B. Two Rescuers
1. First person begins airway, breathing, and circulation treatment as has been described.
2. Second person calls for medical assistance and ambulance, then promptly takes over compression.
3. Use coordinated rhythm of one lung inflation after five compressions.
4. The rescuer at the patient's head maintains the open airway, monitors the carotid pulse, and provides rescue breathing.

5. The compressor calls the time for a switch of positions between ventilation and compression.
6. Always finish the cycle with a ventilation and after a pulse check.
7. Start the cycle with a ventilation.

VI. LENGTH OF TREATMENT

A. Signs of recovery: normal skin color returns, patient may gasp or show other sign of breathing, and the body may move or wiggle.
B. Do not stop heart compressions while patient is being transported to the hospital.
C. When circulation and breathing appear to have returned do not leave patient; watch for need to continue resuscitation in case of relapse.

VII. SEQUELAE

Cardiopulmonary resuscitation must be continued until medical assistance arrives or the patient begins to recover. While the patient is transported to a hospital, resuscitation must continue.

For emergencies that do not require hospitalization, the patient can be moved to a couch for rest, but must be watched carefully. The cause of the emergency must be determined and additional treatment provided when indicated.

The *Medical Emergency Report* with monitored vital signs should accompany the patient to the medical care facility for reference by the persons assuming responsibility. The carbon copy for the patient's dental files is marked clearly with recommendations for prevention of future emergencies.

AIRWAY OBSTRUCTION[5]

A procedure of subdiaphragmatic abdominal thrusts, the Heimlich maneuver, is recommended for removal of a foreign body obstructing an airway in adults and children.

I. PREVENTION

With thought and planning, care can be exercised to prevent aspiration of objects by a patient during a dental or dental hygiene appointment. A few of the procedures that contribute to safety are as follows:

A. Place the patient in supine position during examination and treatment. The throat is closed (Figure 61-6).
B. Use a rubber dam for all appropriate procedures.
C. Use a length of floss to tie to small objects, such as a rubber dam clamp or a bite block. Floss hangs out from angle of lips.
D. Use low-speed handpiece to prevent splashing or spinning masses of agents into the throat.
E. Have assistant use aspirator for various procedures that involve large pieces of calculus, copious blood clots, excess saliva, excess water for ultrasonic scaling, restorative materials, and other potentially inhalable items.
F. Pay attention to mobile permanent or exfoliating primary teeth that could be inadvertently displaced.

II. RECOGNITION OF AIRWAY OBSTRUCTION

Immediate recognition is essential. Differentiation from other emergencies, such as fainting, heart attack, or stroke, in which a sudden respiratory failure may also occur, may be necessary when no object or material was involved that could have been inhaled.

When no doubt exists that an object has been inhaled, medical aid must be obtained. A radiograph may be needed to confirm the location of a radiopaque object.

A. Signs and Symptoms of Partial Obstruction
1. Air exchange
   a. Poor air exchange with gasping and irregular respirations.
   b. Good air exchange with wheezing and forceful coughing.
2. Patient's face is red or cyanotic.
3. Treat poor air exchange as a complete obstruction.

B. Signs of Complete Obstruction
1. No air exchange with attempts at breathing; no sounds from larynx or pharynx.
2. Patient demonstrates the *universal distress signal* (clutches neck with hand).
3. Cyanosis and unconsciousness follow unless emergency care is provided quickly.

III. OUTLINE OF TREATMENT

An airway must be established within 4 to 6 minutes to prevent possible brain damage from oxygen deficiency. With total obstruction, the patient may become unconscious within a few seconds.

Treatment begins with the A-B-C-D of Basic Life Support, unless inhalation of a specific item was observed. When the inspiration is known, the rescuer can proceed directly to attempt to dislodge the obstructing object.

A. Conscious Adult Patient
1. With good air exchange, let patient cough.
2. Object may become dislodged; follow up with medical examination.
3. **If poor air exchange or complete obstruction, apply Heimlich maneuver.**
4. Patient may become unconscious; proceed for unconscious patient.

B. Unconscious Adult Patient
1. Initiate A-B-C-D of Basic Life Support (page 900).
2. When breathing attempt is not successful, readjust airway and attempt again.

3. **Activate EMS.**
4. Proceed with airway obstruction management.
   a. Heimlich maneuver: 6 to 10 abdominal thrusts.
   b. Examine mouth for object; apply finger sweep.
   c. Place resuscitation mask; open airway; give two breaths.
   d. Repeat steps a and b until object is expelled.

IV. HEIMLICH MANEUVER: ABDOMINAL THRUST

Manual thrusts are made to the upper abdomen or, in selected cases, the chest. The abdominal thrust should not be used during pregnancy.

The thrusts are given to provide pressure against the diaphragm that compresses the lungs. In turn, the pressure in the lungs is increased, thereby forcing air through the trachea and perhaps forcing out the obstructing object.

A. Patient Standing or Sitting: Conscious
1. From behind, wrap the arms around the waist of the patient. Make a fist.
2. Hold thumb side of the fist on the patient's upper abdomen above the navel and below the xiphoid. Grab the fist with the other hand.
3. Press the fist into the abdomen with quick upward thrusts until the object is dislodged, or the patient may become unconscious.

B. Patient in Supine Position: Unconscious
1. Open the airway.
2. Stand beside and facing the head of the chair when the patient is in the dental chair. On the floor, a more direct thrust can be applied from astride the patient.
3. Hold the heel of one hand over the upper abdomen, with the other hand on top.
4. Apply 6 to 10 quick upward thrusts followed by a finger sweep and 2 ventilations.
5. Repeat abdominal thrusts, finger sweeps, and ventilations.

V. CHEST THRUST

The chest thrust is not used routinely, but is recommended only when it is not possible to use the abdominal thrust, such as during pregnancy and for very obese individuals.

A. Patient Standing or Sitting with Clinician Behind
1. From behind, wrap arms around the chest of the patient at level of armpits.
2. Make a fist. Position the thumb side of the fist on the sternum. The thrust definitely should not be made on the ribs or on the xiphoid because fracture is possible.

3. Grasp the fist with the other hand and apply quick backward thrusts.

B. Patient in Supine Position
1. Open the airway.
2. Position hands on the lower sternum in the same position as for external cardiac compression (page 904 and Figure 61-8).
3. Apply quick downward thrusts.

VI. FINGER SWEEP: UNCONSCIOUS

After each series of 6 to 10 abdominal thrusts, an attempt should be made to remove the offending object by examination of the mouth and throat and by using the fingers, gauze, or suction appropriately. Care must be taken not to force the object deeper.

Finger sweeps are not used for children and infants unless the object is visible.

A. Open the Mouth
Lift the tongue and mandible with the thumb and index finger of nondominant hand.

B. Index Finger Sweep
1. Slide the index finger of other hand along the buccal mucosa and deep into the throat to the base of the tongue.
2. Anticipate contact with an object, move slowly, with care not to push the object farther into the throat.
3. Hook the end of the finger under and around to remove the object.

C. Repeat
1. Repeat abdominal thrusts, mouth examination, and finger sweep until object is expelled.
2. Place resuscitation mask, open airway, give two ventilations.

VII. INFANT

A. Conscious
1. If good air exchange, encourage coughing.
2. If poor air exchange or complete obstruction, proceed with airway obstruction management.
3. Hold the infant face down over the forearm, with the head supported in the hand. Head is lower than the body.
4. Apply four back blows with the heel of the hand, between the infant's shoulder blades.
5. Turn the infant over by placing the free arm over the back and supporting the infant's head with the hand. Place the infant across the thigh with the infant's head lower than its body.
6. Apply four chest thrusts. The point of pressure is the same as for external cardiac compression in the infant (page 905).
7. Repeat back blows and chest thrusts until object is dislodged or infant becomes unconscious.

B. Unconscious
1. Initiate A-B-C-D of Basic Life Support (page 900).
2. When breathing attempt is not successful, reposition airway and attempt again.
3. **Activate EMS.**
4. Proceed with airway obstruction management as for conscious infant, with four back blows and four chest thrusts.
5. Examine mouth for object; if visible, use a finger sweep to remove it.
6. Give two ventilations.
7. Repeat steps 3 to 5 until object is expelled.
8. Check airway, breathing, and pulse.

OXYGEN ADMINISTRATION

Oxygen is an important agent, useful in most emergencies. High concentration of oxygen is contraindicated for chronic obstructive lung diseases, especially emphysema. Oxygen is also not indicated in the presence of hyperventilation because the patient is receiving increased amounts of air and is in need of carbon dioxide.

The use of oxygen is beneficial in all other emergencies. When the patient is not breathing, *positive pressure oxygen* (also known as demand valve resuscitator) delivery is needed.

I. EQUIPMENT

Oxygen delivery systems with indications, flow rate, and percent oxygen delivered are shown in Table 61-3.

A. Parts

Oxygen resuscitation equipment consists of an oxygen tank, a reducing valve, a flow meter, tubing, mask, and a positive pressure bag. The *E* cylinder, which can provide oxygen for 30 minutes, is the minimum size recommended. Smaller tanks provide too little oxygen for a real emergency, and larger tanks are less portable.

B. Directions

Table 61-4 outlines the steps for operation of an oxygen tank. Clear, readable directions should be permanently attached to the tank. Practice is a definite part of team drills.

TABLE 61-3 Oxygen Delivery Systems   LAMINATE AND AFFIX TO THE OXYGEN TANK

Device	Indications	Flow Rate	Oxygen Delivery
Cannula	For patient who is breathing and needs low levels of oxygen.	2–6 liters per minute	25%–40%
Face Mask	For patient who is breathing and needs moderate levels of oxygen: • when cannula is not tolerated • when more oxygen is desired • patient is in shock	8–12 liters per minute	60%
Non-Rebreather Mask	For patient who is breathing and needs high level of oxygen • patient is in shock • when more oxygen is desired	10–12 liters per minute	60%–90%
Bag-Valve Mask	When patient has stopped breathing or needs respiratory assistance due to respiratory depression. Bag-valve mask is used instead of mouth-to-mouth resuscitation.	10–12 liters per minute	90%–100%
Demand Valve Resuscitator	Positive-pressure delivery of oxygen on demand.	Used by EMTs or others professionally trained	100%

(From Biron, C.R.: *Dental Team Management of Medical Emergencies.* Philadelphia, W. B. Saunders, 2000.)

TABLE 61-4 Operation of Oxygen Tank

TO TURN ON:

1. Attach oxygen delivery system to tank.
2. Turn **key** on top of tank in *counter-clockwise direction* to open flow of oxygen.
3. Read **Low Flow Regulator Knob:**
   To increase O₂ flow: turn the knob in the direction the arrow indicates. (Many regulators are the opposite of sink faucets and open clockwise instead of counter-clockwise.)
4. Attach oxygen delivery system to patient.

TO TURN OFF:

1. Remove oxygen delivery system from patient.
2. Turn **key** on top of tank in *clockwise direction* to shut off flow of oxygen.
3. Turn the **Low Flow Regulator Knob** to open position to bleed oxygen from the system.
4. After bleeding, gently close the **Low Flow Regulator Knob.**

LAMINATE AND AFFIX TO OXYGEN TANK

II. PATIENT BREATHING: USE SUPPLEMENTAL OXYGEN

A. Apply a full-face clear mask or a nasal cannula.
B. Supplemental oxygen is started at 4 to 6 L per minute.
C. Monitor breathing; if breathing stops, proceed with positive pressure oxygen.

III. PATIENT NOT BREATHING: USE POSITIVE PRESSURE

For persons not trained in the use of the bag-valve-mask or positive pressure delivery, a mouth-to-mask procedure should be used.

A. Apply full-face clear mask; must fit with a tight seal. One dental team member may need to apply pressure to the face mask to maintain a complete seal.
B. Adjust oxygen flow so that the positive pressure bag remains filled.
C. Compress the bag manually at 5-second intervals to provide 12 respirations per minute for an adult. For a child, use 4-second intervals.
D. Watch chest rise and fall. When the chest does not rise and fall, recheck airway for obstruction. Proceed with airway obstruction management.
E. Obtain medical assistance.

IV. DEFIBRILLATION

A defibrillator may be used only by dental professionals who are trained in a special program on how to use the defibrillation equipment.

SPECIFIC EMERGENCIES

Certain systemic disease conditions and physical injuries require specific treatment during an emergency. In Tables 61-5 and 61-6, the *Emergency Reference Charts*, several conditions are listed with their symptoms and treatment procedures. Some of the same conditions have been described in detail in Section VI of this book.

TECHNICAL HINTS

I. PRECAUTIONS DURING MOUTH-TO-MOUTH VENTILATION

Infection may be transmitted or acquired. Dental personnel may gain proficiency in the use of a face mask with one-way delivery to prevent unnecessary contact with ill, debilitated patients or those known or suspected to be carriers of a disease.

II. CARE OF DRUGS

A. Label each with information about shelf life and due date for replacement. Nitroglycerin, for example, must be changed at 6 months.

(text continues on page 916)

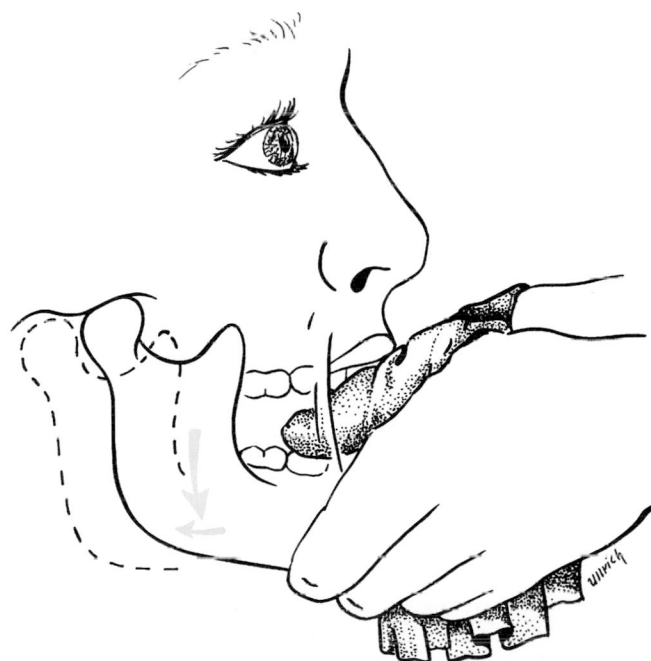

■ **FIGURE 61-9 Treatment for a Dislocated Mandible.** With thumbs wrapped in toweling and placed on the buccal cusps of the mandibular teeth, the fingers are curved under the body of the mandible. The jaw is pressed down and back with the thumbs while pulling up and forward with the fingers to permit the condyle to pass over the articular eminence into its normal position in the glenoid fossa. As the jaw slips into place, the thumbs must be moved quickly aside.

TABLE 61-5 Emergency Reference Chart: Medical Emergencies

Emergency	Signs/Symptoms	Procedure

All Cases		1. Determine consciousness (shake and shout); yell for help
		2. Place on stable side (unconscious)
		3. Identify major problem—Primary Assessment
		   A. Airway: open with head tilt/chin lift maneuver
		   B. Breathing
		   C. Circulation: pulse + blood pressure
		   D. Disability: chief complaint, medical problems, drugs
		4. Act in accord with findings
		     Positioning: "If face is red, raise the head, if face is pale, raise the tail."
		5. Activate EMS

Respiratory Failure	Labored or weak respirations or cessation of breathing
	Cyanosis or ashen-white with blood loss
	Pupils dilated
	Loss of consciousness
		Position: stable side (not breathing)
		     upright (breathing)
		Check for and remove foreign material from mouth
		Establish airway
		Rescue Breathing
		   Adult: 1 breath every 5 seconds
		   Child (1–8): 1 breath every 3 seconds
		   Infant (younger than 1 year): 1 breath every 3 seconds
		Monitor vital signs: blood pressure, pulse, respirations
		Administer oxygen by nonrebreather bag

Airway Obstruction	Good air exchange, coughing, wheezing (patient can speak)	Sit patient up Loosen tight collar, belt No treatment; let patient cough
Partial	Poor air exchange; noisy breathing; weak, ineffective cough; difficult respirations; gasping (usually patient cannot talk, but makes crowing sounds on taking in air.) Patient is panicky	Reassure patient Treat for complete obstruction (page 906)

Complete	Gasping with great effort; no noises
	Patient clutches throat
	Unable to speak, breathe, cough
	Cyanosis
	Dilated pupils
		Conscious patient
		   Perform Heimlich maneuver
		   Patient becomes unconscious: proceed for unconscious<hr>**Unconscious patient**
		   Initiate A-B-C-D of Basic Life Support
		   Unsuccessful breathing attempts: proceed with airway obstruction management
		   Perform Heimlich maneuver: 6 to 10 thrusts
		   Examine mouth: apply finger sweep
		   Open airway: give 2 ventilations
		   Repeat manual thrusts and finger sweep until object is expelled
		   Try rescue breathing again
		Obtain medical assistance

Hyperventilation Syndrome	Light-headedness, giddiness Anxiety, confusion Dizziness Overbreathing (25 to 30 respirations per minute) Feelings of suffocation Deep respirations Palpitations (heart pounds) Tingling or numbness in the extremities	Terminate oral procedure Remove rubber dam and objects from mouth Position upright Immediately tell patient: "There will be no more dental treatment today." Loosen tight collar Reassure patient. Explain overbreathing; request that each breath be held to a count of 10

(continued)

TABLE 61-5 Emergency Reference Chart: Medical Emergencies (Continued)

Emergency	Signs/Symptoms	Procedure
Hyperventilation Syndrome (continued)		Ask patient to breath deeply (7 to 10 per minute) into a paper bag adapted closely over nose and mouth. Never use a bag for a patient with diabetes or patients exhibiting signs of diabetic coma, e.g. fruity breath odor, Kussmaul breathing, lethargy, dry skin. **Carbon dioxide is indicated, NOT oxygen**
Heart Failure (page 858)	Difficult or labored breathing Pulmonary congestion with cough and difficulty breathing May cough up blood Rapid, weak pulse Dilated pupils May have chest pain	Urgent medical assistance needed Place patient in upright position Make patient comfortable: cover with blanket Administer oxygen by nonrebreather bag Reassure patient
Cardiac Arrest	Skin: ashen gray, cold, clammy No pulse No heart sounds No respirations Eyes fixed, with dilated pupils; no constriction with light Unconscious	Position: supine Basic life support Check oral cavity for debris or vomitus; leave dentures in place for a seal **Begin cardiopulmonary resuscitation: minutes count**
Asthma Attack	Difficulty breathing, wheezing, (extreme cases—silence, indicating little to no air exchange) Cyanosis Dilated pupils Confusion due to lack of oxygen Chest pressure Sweating	Position patient upright with arms up and supported forward Assist with patient's own bronchodilator Administer supplemental oxygen by nasal cannula Epinephrine if patient decompensates Supplemental cortisone to patients who are or have been on corticosteroid therapy Basic life support—may need demand valve resuscitator if patient experiences respiratory depression **Activate EMS**
Syncope (Fainting)	Pale gray face, anxiety Dilated pupils Weakness, giddiness, dizziness, faintness, nausea Profuse cold perspiration Rapid pulse at first, followed by slow pulse Shallow breathing Drop in blood pressure Loss of consciousness	Position: Trendelenburg Loosen tight collar, belt Place cold, damp towel on forehead Crush ammonia vaporole under patient's nose Keep warm (blanket) Monitor vital signs: blood pressure, pulse, respirations Keep airway open Administer oxygen by nasal cannula Keep in supine position 10 minutes after recovery to prevent nausea and dizziness Reassure patient, especially during recovery
Shock	Skin: pale, moist, clammy Rapid, shallow breathing Low blood pressure Weakness and/or restlessness Nausea, vomiting Thirst, if shock is from bleeding Eventual unconsciousness if untreated	Position: Trendelenburg Keep quiet and warm Monitor vital signs: blood pressure, respirations, pulse Keep airway open Administer oxygen by nonrebreather bag **Summon medical assistance**

(Continued)

TABLE 61-5 Emergency Reference Chart: Medical Emergencies (Continued)

Emergency	Signs/Symptoms	Procedure
Stroke (Cerebrovascular Accident) (page 775)	*Premonitory* 　Dizziness, vertigo 　Transient paresthesia or weakness on 　　one side 　Transient speech defects *Serious* 　Headache (with cerebral hemorrhage) 　Breathing labored, deep, slow 　Chills 　Paralysis one side of body 　Nausea, vomiting 　Convulsions 　Loss of consciousness (slow or sudden 　　onset)	**Conscious patient** 　Turn patient on paralyzed side; semiupright 　Loosen clothing about the throat 　Reassure patient; keep calm, quiet 　Monitor vital signs: blood pressure, pulse, 　　respirations 　Administer oxygen by nasal cannula 　Clear airway; suction vomitus because the throat muscles may 　　be paralyzed **Seek medical assistance promptly** **Unconscious patient** 　Position: supine 　Basic life support 　Cardiopulmonary resuscitation if indicated
Cardiovascular Diseases	Symptoms vary depending on cause	**For all patients** Be calm and reassure patient Keep patient warm and quiet; restrict effort Always administer oxygen when there is chest pain. **Call for medical assistance**
Angina Pectoris (page 856)	Sudden crushing, paroxysmal pain in 　substernal area Pain may radiate to shoulder, neck, arms Pallor, faintness Shallow breathing Anxiety, fear	Position: upright, as patient requests, for comfortable breathing Place nitroglycerin sublingually only when the blood pressure is 　at or above baseline Administer oxygen by nasal cannula Reassure patient Without prompt relief after a second nitroglycerin, treat as a 　myocardial infarction
Myocardial Infarction (Heart Attack) (page 857)	Sudden pain similar to angina pectoris, 　which also may radiate, but of longer 　duration Pallor; cold, clammy skin Cyanosis Nausea Breathing difficulty Marked weakness Anxiety, fear Possible loss of consciousness	Position: with head up for comfortable breathing Symptoms are not relieved with nitroglycerin Monitor vital signs: blood pressure, pulse, respirations Administer oxygen by nonrebreather bag Alleviate anxiety; reassure **Call for medical assistance for transfer to hospital**
Adrenal Crisis (Cortisol Deficiency)	Anxious, stressed Mental confusion Pain in abdomen, back, legs Muscle weakness Extreme fatigue Nausea, vomiting Lowered blood pressure Elevated pulse Loss of consciousness Coma	**Conscious patient** 　Terminate oral procedure 　Call for help and emergency kit 　Place patient in supine position with legs slightly raised 　Request telephone call for medical assistance 　Administer oxygen by nonrebreather bag 　Monitor blood pressure and pulse **Unconscious patient** 　Place patient on stable side with legs slightly raised 　Basic life support 　Try ammonia vaporole when cause is undecided 　Administer oxygen **Summon medical assistance;** **Transport to hospital**

(continued)

TABLE 61-5 Emergency Reference Chart: Medical Emergencies (Continued)

Emergency	Signs/Symptoms	Procedure

Insulin Reaction (Hyperinsulinism, hypoglycemia)	Sudden onset
	Skin: moist, cold, pale
	Confused, nervous, anxious
	Bounding pulse
	Salivation
	Normal to shallow respirations
	Convulsions (late)
		Conscious patient
		    Administer oral sugar (cubes, apple juice, candy or frosting)
		    Observe patient for 1 hour before dismissal
		    Determine time since previous meal, and arrange next appointment following food intake
		Unconscious patient
		    Basic life support
		    Position: supine
		    Maintain airway
		    Administer oxygen by nonrebreather bag
		    Monitor vital signs
		Summon medical assistance
		Administer intravenous glucose

Diabetic Coma (Ketoacidosis) (Hyperglycemia)	Slow onset
	Skin: flushed and dry
	Breath: fruity odor
	Dry mouth, thirst
	Low blood pressure
	Weak, rapid pulse
	Exaggerated respirations (Kussmaul breathing)
	Coma
		Conscious patient
		    Terminate oral procedure
		    Obtain medical care; hospitalization indicated
		    Keep patient warm
		    Administer oxygen by nasal cannula
		Unconscious patient
		    Basic life support
		Urgent medical assistance needed

Epileptic Seizure 1. Generalized tonic-clonic (page 804)	Anxiety or depression Pale, may become cyanotic Muscular contractions Loss of consciousness	Position: supine. Do not attempt to move from dental chair Make safe by placing movable equipment out of reach Do not force anything between the teeth; a soft towel or large sponges may be placed while mouth is open Open airway; monitor vital signs Administer oxygen by nasal cannula Allow patient to sleep during post-convulsive stage Do not dismiss the patient if unaccompanied
2. Generalized absence (page 804)	Brief loss of consciousness Fixed posture Rhythmic twitching of eyelids, eyebrows, or head May be pale	Take objects from patient's hands to prevent their being dropped

Allergic Reaction
1. Delayed
	Skin
	    Erythema (rash)
	    Urticaria (wheals, itching)
	    Angioedema (localized swelling of mucous membranes, lips, larynx, pharynx)
	Respiration
	    Distress, dyspnea
	    Wheezing
	    Extension of angioedema to larynx: may have obstruction from swelling of vocal apparatus
		Skin
		    Administer antihistamine
		Respiration
		    Position: upright
		    Administer oxygen by nasal cannula
		    Epinephrine
		Airway obstruction
		    Position: supine
		    Airway maintenance
		    Epinephrine
		Summon medical assistance

2. Immediate Anaphylaxis (Anaphylactic shock)	Skin
	    Urticaria (wheals, itching)
	    Flushing
	Nausea, abdominal cramps, vomiting, diarrhea
		Rapid treatment needed (epinephrine)
		Position: supine (except when dyspnea predominates)
		Administer oxygen by nonrebreather bag
		Basic life support
		Monitor vital signs

(continued)

TABLE 61-5 Emergency Reference Chart: Medical Emergencies (Continued)

Emergency	Signs/Symptoms	Procedure
Allergic Reaction (continued)	Angioedema 　Swelling of lips, membranes, eyelids 　Laryngeal edema with difficult swallowing Respiration distress 　Cough, wheezing 　Dyspnea 　Airway obstruction 　Cyanosis Cardiovascular collapse 　Profound drop in blood pressure 　Rapid, weak pulse 　Palpitations Dilation of pupils Loss of consciousness (sudden) 　Cardiac arrest	Cardiopulmonary resuscitation **Summon medical assistance; transfer to hospital**
Local Anesthesia Reactions 1. Psychogenic	Reaction to injection, not the anesthetic Syncope Hyperventilation syndrome	Page 911 (syncope) Page 910 (hyperventilation)
2. Allergic 　(very rare)	Anaphylactic shock Allergic skin and mucous membrane 　reactions Allergic bronchial asthma attack	See earlier in this table (page 913)
3. Toxic 　Overdose	Effects of intravascular injection rather than 　increased quantity of drug are more 　common Stimulation phase 　Anxious, restless, apprehensive, 　　confused 　Rapid pulse and respirations 　Elevated blood pressure 　Tremors 　Convulsions Depressive phase 　Follows stimulation phase 　Drowsiness, lethargy 　Shock-like symptoms: pallor, 　　sweating 　Rapid, weak pulse and respirations 　Drop in blood pressure 　Respiratory depression or respiratory 　　arrest 　Unconsciousness	Mild reaction 　Stop injection 　Position: supine 　Loosen tight clothing 　Reassure patient 　Monitor blood pressure, heart rate, respirations 　Administer oxygen by nasal cannula **Summon medical assistance** Severe reaction 　Basic life support: maintain airway 　Administer oxygen by nonrebreather bag 　Continue to monitor vital signs 　Cardiopulmonary resuscitation 　Administration of anticonvulsant

TABLE 61-6 Emergency Reference Chart: Traumatic Injuries

Emergency	Signs/Symptoms	Procedure

Hemorrhage	Prolonged bleeding
	   Spurting blood: artery
	   Oozing blood: vein
		Compression over bleeding area
		a. Apply gauze pack with direct pressure
		b. Bandage pack into place firmly where possible
		c. Elevate injury above the heart if possible
		Severe bleeding: digital pressure on pressure point of supplying vessel
		Watch for shock symptoms

	Bleeding from tooth socket	Pack wtih folded gauze; do not dab Have patient bite down firmly. If bleeding does not stop instruct patient to gently bite down on a damp tea bag and hold in place for 10 minutes. Do not rinse
	Bleeding of an extremity	Elevate the part: support with pillows or substitute Apply tourniquet only when limb is amputated, mangled, or crushed
	Nosebleed	Tell patient to breathe through mouth Apply cold application to nose Press nostril on bleeding side for a few minutes Advise patient not to blow the nose for an hour or more If bleeding does not stop, wet cotton rolls with water and lubricate with water soluble lubricant. Pack nostril. Instruct patient to breathe through the mouth. Leave packing in place until medical assistance is available to the patient.
Burns 1. First degree 2. Second degree (partial thickness)	Skin reddened Swelling Pain Skin reddened, blisters Swelling Wet surface Pain (more than third degree) Heightened sensitivity to touch	*First- and Second-degree Burns* Do not give food or liquids; anticipate nausea Be alert for signs of shock Do not apply ointment, grease, or bicarbonate of soda Immerse in cool water to relieve pain; do not apply ice Gently clean with a mild antiseptic Dress lightly with a dry sterile bandage Elevate burned part **Obtain medical assistance**
3. Third degree (full thickness)	Leathery look Insensitive to touch	Request medical assistance and transport system Treat for shock Basic life support: maintain airway Check for other injuries Wrap in clean sheet; transport
4. Chemical burn	Reddened, discolored	Immediate, copious irrigation with water for ½ hour Check directions on container from which the chemical came for antidote or other advice Burn caused by an acid may be rinsed with bicarbonate of soda, burn caused by alkali may be rinsed in weak acid such as acetic (vinegar) **Medical assistance needed**
Internal Poisoning	Signs of corrosive burn around or in oral cavity Evidence of empty container or information from patient Nausea, vomiting, cramps	Be calm and supportive Basic life support: airway maintenance Artificial ventilation (inhaled poison) Record vital signs **Call Poison Control Center**

(continued)

TABLE 61-6 Emergency Reference Chart: Traumatic Injuries (Continued)

Emergency	Signs/Symptoms	Procedure
Poisoning (continued)		**Conscious patient** 　Dilute poison in the stomach with 1 or 2 glasses of water or milk. 　Induce vomiting by giving 1 tablespoon of syrup of ipecac followed by 1 to 2 glasses of water. 　Do not induce vomiting if caustic, corrosive, or petroleum products have been ingested Avoid nonspecific and questionably effective antidotes, stimulants, sedatives, or other agents, which may do more harm **Obtain medical assistance**
Foreign Body in Eye	Tears Blinking	Wash hands Ask patient to look down Bring upper lid down over lower lid for a moment; move it upward Turn down lower lid and examine: if particle is visible, remove with moistened cotton applicator Use eye cup: wash out eye with plain water When unsuccessful, seek medical attention: prevent patient from rubbing eye by placing gauze pack over eye and stabilizing with adhesive tape
Chemical Solution in Eye	Tears Stinging	Irrigate promptly with copious amounts of water. Turn head so water flows away from inner aspect of the eye. Continue for 15 to 20 minutes
Dislocated Jaw	Mouth is open: patient is unable to close	Stand in front of seated patient Wrap thumbs in towels and place on occlusal surfaces of mandibular posterior teeth Curve fingers and place under body of the mandible Press down and back with thumbs, and at same time pull up and forward with fingers (Figure 61–9, page 909) As joint slips into place, quickly move thumbs outward Place bandage around head to support jaw
Facial Fracture	Pain, swelling Ecchymoses Deformity, limitation of movement Crepitation on manipulation Zygoma fracture: depression of cheek Mandibular fracture: abnormal occlusion	Place patient on side Basic life support Support with bandage around face, under chin, and tied on the top of the head (Barton) **Seek prompt transport to emergency care facility**
Tooth Forcibly Displaced (avulsed tooth)	Swelling, bruises, or other signs of trauma, depending on the type of accident	Instruct patient or parent to rinse tooth gently in cool water and place in water or wrap in wet cloth. Bring to dental office or clinic *immediately*. The longer the time lapse between avulsion and replantation, the poorer the prognosis.

B. Check weekly to maintain emergency kit in workable order.

C. Dispose of an outdated narcotic drug in the presence of a witness to prevent question that the drug may have been stolen.

III. MEDIC ALERT IDENTIFICATION

Identification for patients with medical problem. A metal emblem is worn as a bracelet or a pendant to provide specific information pertinent to an emergency that may arise. Information about the emblems is available by writing the Medic Alert Foundation International, Turlock, CA 95380. Note patients who wear the identification and record in the patient history.

REFERENCES

1. **Malamed,** S.F.: *Handbook of Medical Emergencies in the Dental Office,* 4th ed. St. Louis, Mosby, 1993, pp. 44–45.
2. **Malamed:** op. cit., pp. 50–89.
3. **Biron,** C.R.: Emergency Drugs, *RDH, 13,* 48, July, 1993.

4. **Robbins**, K.S.: Medicolegal Considerations, in Malamed, S.F.: *Handbook of Medical Emergencies in the Dental Office*, 4th ed. St. Louis, Mosby, 1993, pp. 91–101.

5. **American Heart Association:** Guidelines for Cardiopulmonary Resuscitation and Emergency Cardiac Care. Recommendations of the 1992 National Conference, *JAMA, 268,* 2171–2302, October 28, 1992.

SUGGESTED READINGS

Assael, L.A.: Acute Cardiac Care in Dental Practice, *Dent. Clin. North Am., 39,* 555, July, 1995.

Bavitz, J.B.: Emergency Management of Hypoglycemia and Hyperglycemia, *Dent. Clin. North Am., 39,* 587, July, 1995.

Becker, D.E.: Management of Immediate Allergic Reactions, *Dent. Clin. North Am., 39,* 577, July, 1995.

Biron, C.R.: Allergic Reactions to Dental Materials, Drugs Require an Alert Response from Practitioner, *RDH, 17,* 42, February, 1997.

Biron, C.R.: Quick Retrieval of Swallowed Objects Prevents Further Complications Such as Peritonitis, *RDH, 17,* 38, May, 1997.

Camp, J.: Emergency Dealing With Sports-related Dental Trauma, *J. Am. Dent. Assoc., 127,* 812, June, 1996.

Diem, S.J., Lantos, J.D., and Tulsky, J.A.: Cardiopulmonary Resuscitation on Television, *N. Engl. J. Med., 334,* 1578, June 13, 1996.

Gutman, M.E., Prater, S.L., Naugher, A.M., and Gutman, J.L.: Practical Considerations in the Management of an Avulsed Tooth, *J. Pract. Hyg., 7,* 25, January/February, 1998.

Hodges, E.D., Durham, T.M., and Stanley, R.T.: Management of Aspiration and Swallowing Incidents: A Review of the Literature and Report of Case, *ASDC J. Dent. Child., 59,* 413, November–December, 1992.

Hyman, F.N., Klontz, K.C., and Tollefson, L.: Eating as a Hazard to Health: Preventing, Treating Dental Injuries Caused by Foreign Objects in Food, *J. Am. Dent. Assoc., 124,* 65, November, 1993.

Kerr, I.L., Bigsby, G.A., Haeseler, G.A., Kerr, D.R., and Kerr, L.P.: Prevention and Emergency First-aid Treatment for Sports-related Dentofacial Injuries, *Compend. Cont. Educ. Dent., 14,* 1142, September, 1993.

Malamed, S.F.: Emergency Medicine: Beyond the Basics, *J. Am. Dent. Assoc., 128,* 843, July, 1997.

Monafo, W.W.: Initial Management of Burns, *N. Engl. J. Med., 335,* 1581, November 21, 1996.

Norris, L.H. and Papageorge, M.B.: The Poisoned Patient. Toxicologic Emergencies, *Dent. Clin. North Am., 39,* 595, July, 1995.

Rivera, F.P., Grossman, D.C., and Cummings, P.: Injury Prevention (First of Two Parts), *N. Engl. J. Med., 337,* 543, August 21, 1997.

Rivera, F.P., Grossman, D.C., and Cummings, P.: Injury Prevention (Second of Two Parts), *N. Engl. J. Med., 337,* 613, August 28, 1997.

Rogers, S.N. and Vale, J.A.: Oral Manifestations of Poisoning, *Br. Dent. J., 174,* 141, February 20, 1993.

Talan, D.A.: Infectious Disease Issues in the Emergency Department, *Clin. Infect. Dis., 23,* 1, July, 1996.

Preparation

Alexander, R.E.: Office Medical Emergencies. A Prevention-Oriented, Team Approach, *DentalHygienistNews, 7,* 10, Spring, 1994.

Biron, C.R.: Are You Prepared? *RDH, 12,* 10, January, 1992.

Chapman, P.J.: Medical Emergencies in Dental Practice and Choice of Emergency Drugs and Equipment: A Survey of Australian Dentists, *Aust. Dent. J., 42,* 103, April, 1997.

McCarthy, F.M.: A Minimum Medical Emergency Kit, *Compend. Cont. Educ. Dent., 15,* 214, February, 1994.

Scaramucci, M.K. and Cook, S.: Medical Emergencies in the Dental Office, *J. Pract. Hyg., 6,* 41, November/December, 1997.

Wakeen, L.M.: Dental Office Emergencies: Do You Know Your Legal Obligations? *J. Am. Dent. Assoc., 124,* 54, August, 1993.

Children

Harding, A.M. and Camp, J.H.: Traumatic Injuries in the Preschool Child, *Dent. Clin. North Am., 39,* 817, October, 1995.

Kawashima, Z. and Pineda, F.R.: Replanting Avulsed Primary Teeth, *J. Am. Dent. Assoc., 123,* 90, October, 1992.

Schindler, M.B., Bohn, D., Cox, P.N., McCrindle, B.W., Jarvis, A., Edmonds, J., and Barker, G.: Outcome of Out-of-hospital Cardiac or Respiratory Arrest in Children, *N. Engl. J. Med., 335,* 1473, November, 14, 1996.

Wilson, S., Smith, G.A., Preisch, J., and Casamassimo, P.S.: Nontraumatic Dental Emergencies in a Pediatric Emergency Department, *Clin. Pediatr., 36,* 333, June, 1997.

Prefixes, Suffixes, and Combining Forms

A

a-, an- absence, lack, without, e.g. *a*morphous
ab- from, away, e.g. *ab*normal
ad- (change d to c, f, g, p, s, or t before words beginning with those consonants) to, toward, e.g. *ad*hesion, *ac*cretion
adeno- gland, e.g. *adeno*fibroma
-algia pain, e.g. neur*algia*
ambi- all (both) sides, round, e.g. *ambi*dexterity
amelo- enamel, e.g. *amelo*genesis
amphi-, ampho- on both sides, double, e.g. *ampho*diplopia
ana- up, excessive, again, e.g. *ana*bolism
andro- masculine, male, e.g. *andro*gen
angio- vessel, e.g. *angio*ma
ante- before, e.g. *ante*febrile
anti- against, e.g. *anti*dote
aqu-, aqua- water, e.g. *aqu*eous
arthro-, arth- joints, e.g. *arthr*itis
-ase denotes an enzyme, e.g. dextrin*ase*
-asthenia weakness, e.g. my*asthenia* gravis
auto-, aut- self, e.g. *auto*transplant

B

bi- two, twice, double, e.g. *bi*furcation
bio-, bi- life, living, e.g. *bio*psy
-blast formative cell, e.g. osteo*blast*
-brachy- short, e.g. *brachy*dactylic
brady- slow, e.g. *brady*cardia
bucc- cheek, e.g. *bucc*inator

C

calc- stone, calcium, lime, e.g. *calc*ification
cardio-, cardi- heart, e.g. *cardio*vascular
cata- down, against, e.g. *cata*bolism
-cele swelling, protrusion, hernia, e.g. meningo*cele*
cephalo-, cephal- head, e.g. *cephalo*metry
cerebro-, cerebr- brain, e.g. *cerebr*al palsy
cheilo-, cheil- lip, e.g. *cheil*itis
chloro-, chlor- pale green, e.g. *chloro*phyll
chromo-, chromat- color, pigmentation, e.g. *chromo*genic
-cidal killing, e.g. bacteri*cidal*
-clast break up, divide into parts, e.g. osteo*clast*

-clus- shut, e.g. oc*clus*ion
co-, com-, con-, cor- with, together, e.g. *con*genital
coll- glue, e.g. *coll*oid
contra- opposite, e.g. *contra*lateral
cryo, cry- cold, freezing, e.g. *cryo*therapy
cuti- skin, e.g. *cuti*cle
cyan- blue, e.g. *cyan*otic
-cyto-, -cyt- cell, e.g., leuko*cyt*e

D

-dactyl, dactylo- fingers, e.g. *dactyl*edema
de- down, away from, separation, e.g. *de*calcification
denti-, dent- tooth, e.g. *dent*ition
-derm-, derma- skin, e.g. hypo*derm*ic
dextr-, dextro- right, toward right, e.g. *dextro*cardia
di- twice, two, e.g. *di*plopia
dia- (drop *a* before words beginning with a vowel) through, apart, e.g. *dia*phragm
dis- separation, opposite, taking apart, e.g. *dis*infect
disto-, dist- posterior, distant from center, e.g. *disto*buccal
-drome course, e.g. syn*drome*
dur- hard, e.g. in*dur*ation
dys- bad, ill, difficult, e.g. *dys*trophy

E

ecto-, ect- without, outer side, e.g. *ecto*derm
-ectomy surgical removal, e.g. gingiv*ectomy*
-emia (-aemia) blood condition, e.g. bacter*emia*
en- in, on, into, e.g. *en*demic
encephal-, encephalo- brain, e.g. *encephalo*meningitis
endo- inside, e.g. *endo*dontics
entero-, enter- intestine, e.g. *entero*toxin
epi- upon, after, in addition, e.g. *epi*dermis
erythro-, eryth- red, e.g. *eryth*ema
esthesio-, esthesia (-aesthesia) sensation, perception, e.g. an*esthesia*
ex- beyond, from, out of, e.g. *ex*udate
extra- outside of, beyond the scope of, e.g. *extra*cellular

F

faci- face, e.g. *faci*al

-facient causes or brings about, e.g. rube*facient*
-ferent carry, bear, e.g. af*ferent*
fibro-, fibr- fibers, fibrous tissue, e.g. *fibro*blast
fract- break, e.g. *fract*ional

G

galacto-, galact- milk, e.g. *galact*ose
gastro-, gastr- stomach, e.g. *gastr*itis
-gen- produced, e.g. glyco*gen*
genio- chin, lower jaw, e.g. *genio*plasty
germ- bud, early growth, e.g. *germ*inal
gero- old age, e.g. *gero*dontics
glosso-, gloss- tongue, e.g. *gloss*itis
gluco-, gluc- glucose e.g. *gluco*neogenesis
glyco-, glyc- sweet, e.g. *glyc*erin
gnatho-, gnath- jaw, e.g. *gnath*odynamometer
-gnosis knowledge, e.g. pro*gnosis*
-gram, -graph write, draw, e.g. radio*graphic*
gran- grain, particle, e.g. *gran*uloma
gyn-, gyne-, gynec- woman, e.g. *gyne*cology

H

hemi- half, e.g. *hemi*section
hemo- (haemo-) blood, e.g. *hemo*rrhage
hepato-, hepat- liver, e.g. *hepat*itis
hetero-, heter- other, different, e.g. *hetero*geneous
histo-, hist- tissue, e.g. *histo*logy
homo-, homeo- like, similar, e.g. *homeo*stasis
hydro-, hydr- water, e.g. *hydro*cephalic
hygro-, hygr- moisture, e.g. *hygro*phobia
hyper- abnormal, excessive, e.g. *hyper*trophy
hypno-, hypn- sleep, e.g. *hypno*tic
hypo-, hyp- deficiency, lack, below, e.g. *hypo*tonic
hystero-, hyster- uterus or hysteria, e.g. *hyster*ectomy

I

-ia state or condition, e.g. glycosur*ia*
iatro- relation to medicine, a physician, dentist, or other health professional, e.g. *iatro*genic
-ic of, pertaining to, e.g. gastr*ic*
idio- one's own, separate, distinct, e.g. *idio*pathic
in- not, without, e.g. *in*activate
infra- beneath, below, e.g. *infra*orbital
inter- between, among, e.g. *inter*cellular
intra- within, into, e.g. *intra*oral
ischo-, isch- suppression, stoppage, e.g. *isch*emia
iso- equality, similarity, e.g. *iso*tonic
-ist one who practices, holds certain principles, e.g. hygien*ist*
-itis inflammation, e.g. dermat*itis*

J

-ject- throw, e.g. in*ject*ion
juxta- next to, near, e.g. *juxta*position

K

karyo-, kary- nucleus of a cell, e.g. *karyo*lysis
kerato-, kerat- horny, keratinized tissue, e.g. *kera*tinization
kin- move, e.g. *kin*etic

L

labio- lip, e.g. *labio*version
lacto-, lact- milk, e.g. *lact*ation
laryngo-, laryn- larynx, e.g. *laryn*gitis
later- side, e.g. *later*oversion
leuko-, leuk- white, e.g. *leuko*plakia
linguo, lingu- tongue, e.g. *lingu*al
lipo-, lip- fat, fatty, e.g. *lip*oma
-logy doctrine, science, e.g. periodonto*logy*
lympho-, lymph- lymph, e.g. *lymph*angioma
-lysin, -lysis, -lytic dissolving, destructive, e.g. hemo*lysis*

M

macro-, macr- enlargement, elongated part, e.g. *macro*dontia
mal- bad, ill, e.g. *mal*nutrition
mast-, mastro- breast, e.g. *mast*ectomy
-megalo-, -megal- large, great, e.g. *megalo*blast
melano- dark-colored, relating to melanin, e.g. *melano*genesis
meningo-, mening- meninges, e.g. *mening*itis
meno- month, e.g. *meno*pause
mes-, medi, mesio- middle, intermediate, e.g. *meso*derm
meta-, met- over, beyond, transformation, e.g. *meta*bolism
metro-, metra- uterus, e.g. *metro*fibroma
-metry measure, e.g. cephalo*metry*
micro-, micr- small, e.g. *micro*organism
mono- one, single, e.g. *mono*saccharide
morpho-, morph- form, shape, e.g. *morph*ology
muco-, muc- relating to mucous membrane, e.g. *muco*gingival
myel-, myelo- bone marrow, spinal cord, e.g. *myelo*blast
mylo- molar teeth or posterior portion of mandible, e.g. *mylo*hyoid
myo-, my- muscle, e.g. *myo*cardium

N

naso- nose, e.g. *naso*palatine
necr- death, e.g. *necr*otic
neo-, ne- new, recent, e.g. *neo*plasm
nephro-, nephr- kidneys, e.g. *nephr*itis
neuro-, neuri-, neur- pertaining to nerves, e.g. *neur*asthenia
nucleo-, nucle- pertaining to nucleus, e.g. *nucleo*protein

O

ob- (change b to c before words beginning with c) against, toward, e.g. *oc*clusion
odonto-, odont- tooth, e.g. *odont*algia
-oid like, resembling, e.g. ameb*oid*
-olig-, oligo- a few, a little, e.g. *oligo*dontia
oma swelling, tumor, e.g. lip*oma*
-opia, -opy sight, eye defect, e.g. my*opia*
oro- mouth, oral, e.g. *oro*nasal
ortho-, orth- straight, normal, e.g. *orth*odontics
-osis condition, state, e.g. cyan*osis*
osteo-, oste- bone, e.g. *osteo*porosis
oto-, ot- ear, e.g. *oto*plasty
-ous full of, having, e.g. aque*ous*
ovi-, ovo-, ovu- egg, e.g. *ovu*lation

P

pan- all, every, general, e.g. *pan*acea
para- beyond, beside, near, e.g. *para*site
patho-, path- disease, e.g. *patho*gnomonic
pedia-, pedo- (paedo-) child, e.g. *pedo*dontics
-penia deficiency, e.g. leuko*penia*
per- throughout, completely, e.g. *per*cussion
peri- around, near, e.g. *peri*apical
phago- to eat, e.g. *phago*cytic
-phile, -phil- loving, e.g. hemo*phil*ia
phlebo-, phleb- vein, e.g. *phleb*itis
-phobe, -phobia fear, dread, e.g. photo*phobia*
pilo- hair, e.g. *pilo*erection
-plas- mold, shape, e.g. gingivo*plas*ty
plasmo-, plasm form, e.g. cyto*plasm*
-plegia, -plexy paralysis, stroke, e.g. hemi*plegia*
pleo- more, e.g. *pleo*morphism
-pnea (-pnoea) breathing, e.g. dys*pnea*
pneumo- air, lung, e.g. *pneumo*thorax
-poiesis, -poietic production, e.g. erythro*poietic*
poly- many, much, e.g. *poly*saccharide
pont- bridge, e.g. *pont*ic
poro-, -por- opening, pore, duct, e.g. *poro*us
post- behind, after, e.g. *post*natal
pre- before, in front of, e.g. *pre*maxilla
pro- before, in front of, e.g. *pro*gnathic
proprio- one's own, e.g. *proprio*ceptive
proto- first, e.g. *proto*plasm
pseudo- false, deceptive, e.g. *pseudo*membrane
psycho-, psych- mind, mental processes, e.g. *psycho*somatic
pulmo- lung, e.g. *pulmo*nary
pur- pus, e.g. *pur*ulent
pyo- pus, e.g. *pyo*rrhea
pyro- fever, heat, e.g. *pyro*genic

R

re- back, again, e.g. *re*gurgitate
-renal kidney, e.g. ad*renal*
retro- back, backward, behind, e.g. *retro*molar
-rhage breaking, bursting forth, profuse flow, e.g. hemor*rhage*
-rhea (-rhoea) flow, discharge, e.g. pyor*rhea*
rhino-, rhin- nose, e.g. *rhin*itis
rube- red, e.g. *rube*facient

S

sarco- flesh, muscle, e.g. *sarco*ma
sclero hard, e.g. *sclero*derma
-scopy examination, inspection, e.g. micro*scopy*
semi- half, partly, e.g. *semi*permeable
sero- serum, serous, e.g. *sero*purulent
sial-, sialo- saliva, e.g. *sialo*graphy
somat-, somato-, -some body, e.g. chromo*some*
-squam- scale, e.g. de*squam*ative
stomat- mouth, e.g. *stomat*itis
sub- beneath, under, deficient, e.g. *sub*acute
super- above, upon, excessive, e.g. *super*numerary tooth
syn- with, together, e.g. *syn*drome

T

tachy- swift, e.g. *tachy*cardia
tact- touch, e.g. *tact*ile
tera-, terato- monster, malformed fetus, e.g. *terato*genic
thermo- heat, e.g. *thermo*phile
thrombo-, thromb- clot, coagulation, e.g. *thromb*in
-thym-, thymo- mind, soul, emotions, e.g. dys*thym*ia
trans- beyond, through, across, e.g. *trans*plantation
tropho-, trophic nutrition, nourishment, e.g., hyper*trophic*
-tropic turning toward, changing, e.g. hydro*tropic*

U

-ule diminutive, small, e.g. tub*ule*
-uria urine, e.g. glucos*uria*

V

vaso- blood vessels, e.g. *vaso*dilation
vita- life, e.g. *vita*min

X

xero- dry, e.g. *xero*stomia

Glossary

Introduction

Each chapter has included a table of "Key Words and Abbreviations" with their definitions. By having the definitions readily available at the lead of a chapter, it is expected that study and learning can be facilitated.

This *Glossary* includes additional words of a general nature. All words that have been defined in this book can be located through the *Index* starting on page 940.

The meaning of words from the basic medical and dental sciences frequently can be determined from the list of word prefixes, suffixes, and combining forms on the previous pages. A medical dictionary is an important adjunct to guide professional reading.

A

Absorption (ab-sorp'shun). taking up of fluids or other substances by the skin or mucous surfaces; passage of substances to the blood, lymph, and cells from the alimentary canal after digestion.

Accessory (ak-ses'e-rē). subordinate, attached, or added for convenience.

Acid (as'id). a chemical substance that undergoes dissociation with the formation of hydrogen ions in aqueous solution; pH less than 7.0.

Acne vulgaris (ak'ne vul-ga'ris). a chronic inflammatory disease of the sebaceous glands that appears on the face, back, and chest in the form of eruptions.

Acquired characteristics. those obtained after birth, as a result of environment.

Acuity (a-ku'i-tē). sharpness or clearness, especially of the special senses.

Acute (a-kut'). having rapid onset, short, severe course, and pronounced symptoms; opposite of chronic.

Adenopathy (ad-e-nop'ah-the). swelling or enlargement of lymph nodes.

Adsorption (ad-sorp'shun). the attachment of one substance to the surface of another substance.

Agar (ah'gar). gelatin extracted from seaweed, used as a nutrient solidifying agent in bacteriologic culture media; constituent of a reversible hydrocolloid impression material.

Agglutination (a-glu'ti-na'shun). state of being united; adhesion of parts; clumping, as of bacteria or other cells.

Alkali (al'kah-lī). a strong water-soluble base; see **Base.**

Allergen (al'er-jen). an antigenic substance that produces hypersensitivity; may be inhaled, ingested, or injected or may produce a reaction upon contact with the skin.

Allergy (al'er-je). a hypersensitive state gained from exposure to a specific substance or allergen, re-exposure to which causes a heightened capacity to react.

Alloplast (al'lo-plast). a graft of an inert metal or plastic material.

Alloy (al'loi). a substance composed of a mixture of two or more metals.

Alopecia (al'ō-pe'shi-ah). loss of hair.

Amelia (ah-mel'e-ah). congenital absence of a limb or limbs.

Ameloblast (ah-mel'-ō-blast). epithelial cell of the enamel organ; functions in the formation of enamel.

Amylase (am'i-laze). an enzyme that converts starch into sugar.

Anaphylaxis (an-ah-fi-lak'sis). an acute, severe, allergic reaction characterized by sudden collapse, shock, or respiratory and circulatory failure following the injection of an allergen; increased susceptibility to an allergen resulting from previous exposure to it.

Anhydrous (an-hī'drus). containing no water.

Anlage (ahn'lah-gheh). earliest primary stage in the development of an organ.

Anodyne (an'ō-dīne). any agent that neutralizes or relieves pain.

Anomaly (a-nom'a-le). deviation from the normal.

Anorexia (an-o-rek'se-ah). lack or loss of appetite for food.

Anoxia (an-ok'si-ah). oxygen deficiency; a condition in which the cells of the body do not have or cannot utilize sufficient oxygen to perform normal functions.

Antidote (an-ti-dōte). a medicine or other remedy for counteracting the effects of a poison.

Antimicrobial therapy. treatment using agents for the control or destruction of microorganisms that cause the disease or condition.

Aphthous ulcer (af'thus ul'ser). aphthous stomatitis; canker sore, vesicle that ruptures after 1 or 2 days and forms a depressed, spherical, painful ulcer with elevated rim.

Aqueous (a'kwe-us). water; prepared with water.

Armamentarium (ar'mah-men-ta're-um). the equipment, such as books, materials, and instruments essential to professional practice.

    Dental hygiene armamentarium: all the instruments and equipment used during a dental hygiene procedure.

    Dental hygiene instrumentarium: set of instruments used for a particular clinical procedure by the dental hygienist.

Arthroplasty (ar'thrō-plas"te). plastic repair of a joint.

    Total hip arthroplasty: replacement of the femoral head and acetabulum with a prosthesis that is cemented to the bone.

    Acetabulum (as"e-tab'u-lum): the cup-shaped cavity on the lateral surface of the hip bone that receives the head of the femur.

Articulation (ar-tik"u-la'shun). the place where two or more bones of the skeleton join or unite; bony joint that may or may not be movable.

Artifact (ar'ti-fact). caused by the technique used, not a natural occurrence; in radiography, a structure, blemish, or unintended radiographic image that may result from the faulty manufacture, manipulation, exposure, or processing of an x-ray film.

ASA Classification. physical status classification of the American Society of Anesthesiologists (Table 21-2, page 324).

Ascites (a-si'tez). accumulation of fluid in the abdominal cavity.

Aspirator (as"pi-ra'tor). an apparatus employing suction.

Atom (at'om). the small particle of an element that is composed of protons, neutrons, and electrons.

Attrition (a-trish'un). gradual wearing away of tooth structure, resulting from mastication.

Autogenous (au-toj'en-us). originating from within; self generated; an autogenous graft (autograft) uses tissue transferred from one position to another within the same individual.

Autograft (aw'tō-graft). a graft in which the tissue is obtained from the same individual.

Autoimmune disease (aw'tō-im-mun'). disease caused by immunologic action of an individual's own cells or antibodies on components of the body.

Autonomic (aw tō-nom'ik). a division of the nervous system that supplies the sensory innervation for the smooth muscles, heart, and glands. It is divided into the parasympathetic (craniosacral) and the sympathetic (thoracolumbar) systems.

Auxiliary (awk-sil'e-ar-e). giving support; helping; aiding; assisting.

Avulsion (a-vul'zhun). traumatic or forcible separation; an avulsed tooth has been traumatically removed from its socket.

B

Bacterial spore. a resistant form of bacteria encapsulated by a thick cell wall that enables the cell to survive in environments unfavorable to immediate growth and division; not a reproductive mechanism.

Bactericide (bak'ter-i-sīd). capable of destroying bacteria.

Bacteriostatic (bak-ter"i-o-stat'ik). capable of inhibiting the growth and multiplication of bacteria.

Barodontalgia (aerodontalgia) (barō-don-tal'ji-ah). the sudden acute pain response in a tooth under reduced atmospheric pressure, notably during high-altitude flying.

Base (bās). a chemical substance that in solution yields hydroxyl ions and reacts with an acid to form a salt and water. A base turns red litmus paper blue and has a pH higher than 7.0.

Bevel (bev'el). the inclination a line or surface makes with another when they are not at right angles.

Bifid (bi'fid). cleft into two parts or branches.

Biocidal (bi"o-si'dal). ability of a physical or chemical agent to kill microorganisms.

Biocompatible (bi"ō-kom-pat'i-bel). harmonious with life; no toxic or injurious effects on biologic function.

Bruxism (bruk'sizm). a neurogenically related habit of grinding, clenching, or clamping the teeth. Damage to the teeth and attachment apparatus can result.

Buffer (büf'er). any substance in a fluid that tends to lessen the change in hydrogen ion concentration (reaction) that otherwise would be produced by adding acids or alkalis.

C

Cachexia (ka-kek'si-ah). lack of nutrition; wasting; may occur in the course of chronic disease.

Calcification (kal"si-fi-ka'shun). the process by which organic tissue becomes hardened by a deposit of calcium and other inorganic salts within its substance.

Cancer (kan'ser). malignant and invasive neoplasm; see **Neoplasm, Precancerous lesion.**

Canker sore: see **Aphthous ulcer.**

Capnophilic (kap-nō-fil'ik). growing best in the presence of carbon dioxide; usually used in reference to bacteria.

Carbohydrate (kar"bō-hi'drate). organic compound of carbon, hydrogen, and oxygen: includes starches, sugars, cellulose; formed by plants and used for growth and source of energy.

Caries: see **Dental caries.**

Caries activity test. Test to determine the presence or absence of specific microorganisms in saliva and bacterial plaque, salivary secretion rate, salivary components and buffering effect, or sugar clearance time, in order to predict occurrence of new carious lesions.

Carious (ka're-us). affected with caries or decay; in dentistry, a carious lesion is a cavity in a tooth that is the result of dental caries.

Cartilage (kar'ti-lij). firm, elastic, flexible connective tissue that is attached to articular bone surfaces and that forms certain parts of the skeleton.

Caustic (kaws'tik). an agent that burns or corrodes; destroys living tissue; having a burning taste.

Cauterize (kaw'ter-īze). to burn, corrode, or destroy living tissue by means of a caustic substance, a heated metal, or an electric current.

Cementicle (ce-men'ti-kel). small globular mass of cementum (diameter 0.2 to 0.3 mm); may lie free within the periodontal ligament or be attached to the cementum of the root surface.

Cephalometry (sef"ah-lom'e-tre). measurement of the bony structure of the head using reproducible lateral and anteroposterior radiographs.

Cheilosis (ke-lō'sis). a condition marked by fissuring and dry scaling of the surface of the lips and angles of the mouth; characteristic of riboflavin deficiency.

Chemotaxis (ke"mō-tak'sis). attraction of living protoplasm to chemical stimuli; for example, movement of neutrophils to an area of inflammation; a host defense mechanism.

Chorea (kō-re'ah). a nervous disorder characterized by irregular and involuntary action of the muscles of the extremities and the face.

Chronic (kron'ik). characterized by a long, slow course; opposite of acute.

Cicatrix (sik'ah-triks). a scar; fibrous tissue left after the healing of a wound.

Clean (klēn). freedom from or removal of all matter in which microorganisms may find favorable conditions for continued life and growth.

Cleidocranial dysostosis (klī"dō-kra'ni-al di-os-tō'sis). developmental defect characterized by absence of development of clavicles and abnormal shape of skull.

Coagulation (kō-ag-u-la'shun). changing of a soluble into an insoluble protein; process of changing into a clot.

Coaptation (kō-ap-ta'shun). proper adaptation or union of parts to each other, such as the ends of a fractured bone or the edges of a wound without overlap.

Commissure (kom'i-shur). angle or corner of eye or lips.

Communicable (ko-mu'ni-kah-bel). capable of being transmitted from one person to another.

Contagious (kon-ta'jus). communicable; transmissible by contact with an infected or sick person.

Contracture (kon-trak'chur). shortening or distortion; permanent, as from shrinkage of muscles, or temporary, from sudden stimulus.

Corticosteroid (kor"ti-kō-ste'roid). hormone produced by the adrenal cortex and synthetic equivalent; various steroids have different physiologic effects.

Glucocorticoid: used in treatment of a variety of conditions, including inflammations, allergies, collagen diseases, and certain neoplasms.

Cryosurgery (krī"ō-ser'jer-ē). surgery performed with the use of extremely low temperature.

Cryotherapy (krī"ō-ther'ah-pē). therapeutic application of cold.

Cryptogenic (krip"tō-jen'ik). of obscure, doubtful, or undeterminable origin.

Current (kur'rent). the number of electrons per second passing a given point on a conductor. Electrons are negatively charged and move toward the positive.

Cuticle, primary (ku'ti-kel). a delicate membrane covering the crown of a newly erupted tooth; produced by the ameloblasts after they produce the enamel rods. Also called Nasmyth's membrane.

Cyst (sist). a sac, normal or pathologic, containing fluid or other material.

> **Dentigerous cyst**: formed by a dental follicle, containing one or more well-formed teeth.

> **Radicular cyst**: an epithelial-lined sac, formed at the apex of a pulpless tooth, containing cystic fluid.

Cystic fibrosis (sis'tik fī-brō'sis). a generalized hereditary disorder of young children primarily; characterized by signs of chronic pulmonary disease (as a result of excess mucus production in the respiratory tract) and pancreatic deficiency.

D

Defense mechanism. in psychiatry, an unconscious mental process or coping mechanism that lessens the anxiety associated with a situation or internal conflict and protects the person from mental discomfort.

Deglutition (deg"loo-tish'un). the act of swallowing.

Dehiscence (dē-his'ens). isolated area in which a root is denuded of bone when the denuded area extends to the margin of the bone. Compare with **Fenestration.**

Dehydration (dē-hī-dra'shun). removal of water; the condition that results from undue loss of water.

Dental caries (den'tal kar'ēz). a disease of the calcified structures of the teeth, characterized by decalcification of the mineral components and dissolution of the organic matrix.

Dental prosthetic laboratory procedures. the steps in the fabrication of a dental prosthesis that do not require the presence of a patient for their accomplishment.

Dental public health: see under **Public health.**

Denticle (den'ti-kel). a pulp stone; relatively large body of calcified substance in the pulp chamber of a tooth.

Denturist (den'tur-ist). any non-dentist who makes, fits, and repairs dentures directly for the public; a non-dentist licensed to provide complete dentures directly to the public.

Denudation (den"u-da'shun). laying bare; surgical or pathologic removal of epithelial covering.

Desensitization (de-sen"si-ti-za'shun). process of removing reactivity or sensitivity.

Detritus (de-tri'tus). debris that adheres to tooth, gingival, and mucosal surfaces.

Diagnosis (di"ag-nō'sis). a scientific evaluation of existing conditions; the process of determining by examination the nature and circumstances of a diseased condition; the decision reached as to the nature of a disease.

> **Differential diagnosis**: the art of distinguishing one disease from another.

Digital (dij'i-tal). of, pertaining to, or performed with a finger.

Dilaceration (di-las"er-a'shun). abnormal angulation or curve in the root or crown of a tooth.

Dislocation: see **Luxation.**

Distilled water. water that has been subjected to a process of vaporization and subsequent condensation for purification.

DNA (deoxyribonucleic acid) (de-ok"se-rī"-bō-nu-kle'ik as'id). occurs in nuclei (chromosomes) of all animal and vegetable cells; repository of hereditary characteristics.

Donor site (dō'nor sīt). area from which tissue is obtained during surgical procedures such as for a graft.

Dorsum (dor'sum). the back surface or a part similar to the back in position; opposite of ventral surface.

Duct (dukt). a passage with well defined walls; especially a tube for the passage of excretions or secretions.

Dysarthria (dis-ar'thre-ah). disturbances of articulation as a result of emotional stress or paralysis, incoordination, or spasticity of the muscles used for speaking.

Dyslexia (dis-lek'se-ah). inability or difficulty in reading, including word blindness and a tendency to reverse letters and words in reading and writing.

Dysmorphism (dis-mor'fizm). abnormality of shape.

Dysplasia (dis-pla'zi-ah). abnormal development or growth; an alteration in adult cells characterized by variations in their size, shape, and organization.

Dystrophy (dis'trō-fe). degeneration associated with atrophy and dysfunction.

E

Ecology (e-kol'ō-je). the science that deals with the study of the environment and the life history of organisms.

Echocardiography (ek"o-kar"de-og'rah-fe). use of ultrasound in the diagnosis of cardiovascular lesions, especially mitral valve disease; recorded in an **echocardiogram**.

Ectopic (ek-top'ik). out of place. An **ectopic pregnancy** is one that occurs elsewhere than in the cavity of the uterus.

Edema (e-de'mah). collection of abnormally large amounts of fluid in the intercellular spaces, causing swelling.

> **Pitting edema**: pressure on edematous area

causes pits, which remain for prolonged period after pressure is released.

Edentulous (e-den'tu-lus). without teeth.

Emaciation (e-ma"se-a'shun). condition of excessive leanness or wasted body tissues.

Emesis basin (em'e-sis). a basin, usually kidney shaped, used for receiving material expectorated or vomited.

Emollient (e-mōl'ē-ent). softening or soothing; an agent used to soften the skin or other body surface.

Emphysema (em"fi-se'mah). pathologic accumulation of air in tissues or organs; commonly used to designate the chronic pulmonary disorder in which the terminal bronchioles become plugged with mucus and breathing becomes difficult.

Endemic (en-dem'ik). present in a community or among a group of people; the continuing prevalence of a disease as distinguished from an epidemic.

Endodontics (en"dō-don'tiks). that branch of dentistry concerned with the etiology, diagnosis, and treatment of diseases of the dental pulp and their sequelae.

Endometrium (en"dō-me'tri-um). the mucous membrane lining the uterus.

Enzyme (en'zīm). an organic compound, frequently protein in nature, that can accelerate or produce by catalytic action some change in a specific substance.

Ephebodontics (e-fe"bō-don'tiks). dentistry for the individual undergoing the transition from childhood to adulthood; that is, the period of life known as adolescence.

Epidemic (ep'i-dem'ik). the occurrence in a community or region of a group of illnesses of similar nature, clearly in excess of normal expectancy and derived from a common source.

Epithelialization (ep"i-the"le-al-i-za'shun). growth of epithelium over a denuded surface.

Eruption (e-rup'shun). the act of breaking out, appearing, or becoming visible; a visible pathologic lesion of the skin, marked by redness, swelling, or both.

> **Tooth eruption**: the combination of movements of a tooth both before and after the emergence of its crown into the oral cavity, which serves to bring the tooth and maintain it in occlusion with the tooth or teeth of the opposing arch.

Erythrocyte (e-rith'rō-sīte). red blood cell; specialized cell for the transport of oxygen.

Erythroplakia (e-rith"rō-pla'ke-ah). lesions of the oral mucosa that appear as bright red patches or plaques that cannot be characterized clinically or pathologically as any other disease.

Erythropoiesis (e-rith"rō-pō-e'sis). formation of red blood cells.

Escharotic (es"ka-rot'ik). corrosive; capable of producing sloughing.

Ethics (eth'iks). rules or principles that govern right conduct. Each practitioner upon entering a profession is invested with the responsibility to adhere to the standards of ethical practice and conduct set by the profession (Appendix 1, page 934).

Etiology (e"ti-ol'o-je). the science or study of the cause of disease; that which is known about the causes of a disease.

Exfoliate (eks-fŏ'le-āt). to fall off in scales or layers; in dentistry, to shed primary teeth.

Exostosis (ek"sos-to'sis). benign new growth projecting from a bone surface; examples: torus mandibularis or torus palatinus.

Extirpation (ek"stir-pa'shun). complete removal or eradication of a part; in dentistry, the removal of the dental pulp from the pulp chamber and root canal.

F

Febrile (fe'bril). pertaining to fever; feverish.

Fenestration (fen"es-tra'shun). isolated area in which a root is denuded of bone when the marginal bone is intact. Compare with **Dehiscence.**

Fermentable (fer-men'ta-bel). term applied to a substance that is capable of undergoing chemical change as a result of the influence of an enzyme; usually applied to substances that break down to an acid or an alcohol; applied to carbohydrate breakdown to form acid in bacterial plaque.

Fetus (fe'tus). the unborn offspring in the uterus, after the second month.

Fistula (fis'tu-lah). commonly used term for a narrow passage or duct leading from one cavity to another, as from a periapical abscess to the oral cavity; see **Sinus tract.**

Flora (flŏ'rah). the entire plant life of a geographic area; used to indicate the microorganisms that live together in a specific location.

    Oral flora: the microorganisms that inhabit the oral cavity of an individual, that are usually saprophytic, and that live together in a symbiotic relationship.

Focal infection. infection caused by bacteria or toxins carried in the blood from a distant lesion or focus.

Follicle (dental) (fol'i-kel). the sac that encloses the developing tooth before its eruption.

Forensic dentistry (fo-ren'sik). the aspect of dental science that relates and applies dental facts to legal problems; encompasses dental identification, malpractice litigation, legislation, peer review, and dental licensure.

Frenectomy (fre-nek'tŏ-me). complete removal of a frenum.

Frenotomy (fre-not'o-me). partial removal of a frenum.

Frenum, pl. frena (fre'num) (fre'na). a narrow fold of mucous membrane passing from a more fixed to a movable part, as from the gingiva to the lip, cheek, or undersurface of the tongue, serving in a measure to check undue movement of the part.

Friable (fri'a-bel). easily broken or crumbled.

G

Germicide (jer'mi-sīd). anything that destroys bacteria; applied especially to chemical agents that kill disease germs but not necessarily bacterial spores; applied to both living tissue and inanimate objects.

Gerodontics (jer"ō-don'tiks). that branch of dentistry that treats all problems peculiar to the oral cavity in old age and the aging population. Also called geriatric dentistry.

Gestation (jes-ta'shun). pregnancy.

Gingivectomy (jin"ji-vek'tō-me). The surgical removal of diseased gingiva to eliminate periodontal pockets.

Gingivoplasty (jin'ji-vō-plas"te). the surgical contouring of the gingival tissue to produce the physiologic architectural form necessary for the maintenance of tissue health and integrity.

Gnathodynamometer (nath"ō-dī"nah-mom'e-ter). an instrument for measuring the force exerted in closing the jaws.

Graft (graft). tissues transferred from one site to replace damaged structures in another site.

    Free graft: tissue for grafting is completely removed from its donor site.

    Pedicle graft: the graft remains attached to its donor site. See also **Autograft; Heterograft; Homograft.**

H

Habilitation (ha-bil"i-ta'shun). application of measures that will assist a person in obtaining a state of health, efficiency, and independent action.

Halitosis (hal"i-tō'sis). offensive or bad breath, may be related to systemic disease or uncleanliness of the oral cavity.

Health (helth). state of complete physical, mental, and social well-being, not merely the absence of disease.

Hemangioma (he-man'ji-ō"mah). a benign tumor composed of newly formed capillaries filled with blood.

Hemorrhage (hem'o-rij). bleeding; an escape of blood from the blood vessels.

Hemostat (he'mo-stat). an instrument or other agent used to arrest the escape or flow of blood.

Heterograft (het'er-ō-graft). a heterologous graft in which the tissue is obtained from another species.

Holistic (ho lis'tik). pertaining to totality, the whole; in holistic health care emotional, social, and physical needs are dealt with together.

Homograft (hŏ'mō-graft). a homologous graft in which the tissue is obtained from a different individual of the same species.

Hydrophilic (hī"drō-fil'ik). having a strong affinity for water; as opposed to hydrophobic, repelling water.

Hygiene (hī'jen). the science that deals with the preservation of health.

Hygroscopic (hi"gro-sco'pik). capable of readily absorbing and retaining moisture.

Hyperkeratosis (hi"per-ker"ü-to'sis). abnormal increase in the thickness of the keratin layer (stratum corneum) of the epithelium. **Benign hyperkeratosis** is one of the most common white lesions of the oral mucous membrane.

Hyperkinesis (hi"per-ki-ne'sis). excessive motility; excessive muscular activity.

Hyperthermia (hi"per-ther'me-a). therapeutically induced hyperpyrexia (high fever).

   Malignant hyperthermia: rapid onset of extremely high fever with muscle rigidity.

Hypertonic (hi"per-ton'ik). having excessive tone, tonicity, or activity.

   Hypertonic solution: one that has a higher molecular concentration than another with which it is compared; of greater concentration than isotonic.

Hyperventilation (hi"per-ven"til-a'shun). increased alveolar ventilation with carbon dioxide pressure below normal.

Hypnotic (hip-not'ik). inducing sleep.

Hypocalcification (hi"po-kal"si-fi-ka'shun). deficiency in the mineral content of a calcified tissue, for example in the enamel that results from disturbance in the maturation phase during development; may be caused by systemic, local, or hereditary factors.

Hypodontia (hi"po-don'she-ah). condition of congenitally missing teeth; partial anodontia.

Hypoplasia (hi"po-pla'ze-ah). defective or incomplete development; enamel hypoplasia results when the enamel matrix formation is disturbed.

Hypotonic (hi"po-ton'ik). having diminished tone; tonicity, or activity.

   Hypotonic solution: one that has a lesser molecular concentration than another to which it is compared; of less concentration than isotonic.

I

Iatrogenic (i-at"ro-jen"ik). caused by inadvertent or erroneous diagnosis and/or treatment by a professional.

Idiopathic (id"e-o-path'ik). self-originated; of unknown cause.

Idiosyncrasy (id"e-o-sin'krah-se). any tendency, characteristic, or the like, peculiar to an individual.

Immunity (i-mu'ni-te). an inherited, congenital, or naturally or artificially acquired ability to resist the occurrence and effects of a specific disease.

   Acquired immunity: that possessed as a result of having recovered from a disease or from building up resistance against vaccines, toxins, or toxoids.

   Natural immunity: that inherited by the child from the mother or from the race.

   Passive immunity: that possessed as a result of injection of antibodies or antitoxins of serum from an immune individual or from an animal.

Implant (im'plant). a material or body part that is grafted or inserted within body tissues.

Implantation (im"plan-ta'shun). the placement within body tissues of a foreign substance, for example metal or plastic, for restoration by mechanical means. In dentistry, a foreign material placed into or onto the jawbone to support a crown, partial or complete denture.

Incipient (in-sip'e-ent). beginning to exist; coming into existence.

Incubation (in"ku-ba'shun). the keeping of a microbial or tissue culture in an incubator to facilitate growth and development.

Inert (in-ert'). without intrinsic active properties; no inherent power of action, motion, or resistance.

Infection (in-fek'shun). invasion of the body by pathogenic microorganisms and the body's response to the microorganisms and their toxic products; transfer of disease from one part to another or one person to another.

Infectious (in-fek'shus). capable of being transmitted; producing an infection.

Inflammation (in"flah-ma'shun). reaction of living tissue to injury; a defense reaction of the body characterized by heat, redness, swelling, pain, and loss of function.

Informed consent (kon-sent'). voluntary agreement of a patient with the professional that an action can take place; person giving consent must be of sufficient mental capacity and in possession of all essential information to give valid consent.

Inhibitor (in-hib'i-tor). a substance that arrests or restrains physiologic, chemical, or enzymatic action or the growth of microorganisms.

Inoculation (i-nok"u-la'shun). introduction of microorganisms or some substance into living tissues or culture media: introduction of a disease agent into a healthy individual to induce immunity.

Inorganic (in-or-gan'ik). not characterized by organization of living bodies or vital processes; also, pertaining to compounds not containing carbon, except cyanides and carbonates.

Insidious (in-sid'e-us). coming on gradually or almost imperceptibly; as in a disease, the onset of which is gradual, with a more serious effect than is apparent.

Intermaxillary (in"ter-mak'si-lar-e). between the maxilla and the mandible.

Intervention (in"ter-ven'shun). action selected to meet a treatment need of a patient; item in the care plan.

In vitro (in ve'tro). outside the living body: in a test tube or other artificial environment.

In vivo (in ve'vo). in the living body of a plant or animal.

Ion (i'on). an electrically charged atom or group of atoms.

   Anion (an'i-on): negatively charged ion, which passes to the positive pole in electrolysis.

   Cation (kat'i-on): positively charged ion, which passes to the negative pole in electrolysis.

I.Q.: Intelligence Quotient. the relationship between intelligence and chronologic age.

Isoniazid (ī″sō-nī′ah-zid). antibacterial compound used in the treatment of tuberculosis.

Isotonic (ī″sō-ton′ik). having a uniform tonicity or tension. See also **Hypertonic, Hypotonic.**

    Isotonic solution: one which has the same molecular concentration as another with which it is compared.

Isotope (ī′sō-tōp). any of two or more forms of a chemical element that have different mass numbers because their nuclei contain different numbers of neutrons. Radioactive isotopes are widely used as tracers in research.

J

Jaundice (jawn′dis). condition in which there are bile pigments in the blood and deposition of bile pigments in the skin and mucous membranes, with resulting yellowish appearance.

Jurisprudence (joor″is-proo′dens). the science of law, its interpretation and application.

K

Kaolin (ka′ō-lin). a fine white clay; used in pharmacy in ointments and for coating pills.

Keratin (ker′ah-tin). a protein material formed as a transformation product of the cellular proteins of the flat cells on the surface of the epithelium; form of protective adaptation to function.

Keratinization (ker″ah-tin-i-za′shun). process of formation of a horny protective layer on the surface of stratified squamous epithelium of certain body surfaces, including the epidermis and masticatory oral mucosa.

L

Laceration (las″er-a′shun). a wound produced by tearing or irregular cutting.

Latent (la′tent). concealed, not apparent, potential.

Learning disorders. academic skills disorders; developmental arithmetic disorder (dyscalculia); writing disorder (dysgraphia); and reading disorder (dyslexia).

Lethargy (leth′ar-je). condition of drowsiness or sleepiness.

Leukoplakia (lu″kō-pla′ke-ah). a white patch or plaque that cannot be characterized clinically or pathologically as any other disease and is not associated with any physical or chemical causative agent except the use of tobacco.

Local (lō′kel). restricted to one spot or area; not generalized.

Luxation (luk-sa′shun). a dislocation. For example, dislocation of the temporomandibular joint occurs when the head of the condyle moves anteriorly over the articular eminence and cannot be returned voluntarily.

Lymphadenopathy (lim″fad-e-nop′ah-the). disease process affecting a lymph node or lymph nodes.

M

Maintenance phase. series of appointments after initial therapy for periodic reexamination and additional therapy as needed to keep the teeth and periodontal tissues in health without recurrence of disease.

Malaise (mal-az′). any vague feeling of illness, uneasiness, or discomfort.

Mandrel (man′drel). a spindle, axle, or shaft designed to fit a dental handpiece for the purpose of supporting a revolving instrument.

Manifestation (man″i-fe-sta′shun). that which is made evident, especially to the sight and understanding.

    Oral manifestation: a symptom or sign of a disease in the oral cavity.

Manikin (man′i-kin). model of the human body or a part; used for teaching purposes.

Massage (mah-sahzh′). manipulation of tissues for remedial or hygienic purposes with the hand or other instrument; the systematic application of frictional rubbing and stroking to the gingival tissues for increasing the circulation of blood through the tissues and for increasing the keratinization of the surface epithelium.

Mastication (mas″ti-ka′shun). a series of highly coordinated functions that involve the teeth, tongue, muscles of mastication, lips, cheeks, and saliva in the preparation of food for swallowing and digestion.

Matrix (ma′triks). the form or substance within which something originates, takes form, or develops; intercellular substance of a tissue.

    Amalgam matrix: a thin metal form, usually stainless steel, adapted to a prepared cavity to supply the missing wall so the amalgam will be confined when condensed into the cavity preparation.

Medication (med″i-ka′shun). use of medicine or medicaments for treatment of a disease.

Metabolism (me-tab′ō-liz″m). the sum total of the chemical changes occurring in the body; chemical process of transforming foods into complex tissue elements and of transforming complex body substances into simple ones, along with the production of heat and energy.

    Anabolism (ah-nab′ō-liz″m): the building up of tissue; maintenance and repair of the body.

    Catabolism (kah-tab′ō-liz″m): the breaking down of tissue into simpler constituents for energy production and excretion.

Micron (mī′kron). unit of linear measurement; one-thousandth of a millimeter.

Milliliter (mil′i-le″ter). one-thousandth part of a liter, usually abbreviated **mL.** It is approximately equal to 1 cubic centimeter.

Miscible (mis′i-bel). capable of being mixed.

Monitoring (mon'i-tor-ing). the overall surveillance of a patient by methods employing the senses of touch, sight, hearing, or smell or by means of devices that operate chemically, physically, or electronically to measure the adequacy of the various physiologic functions.

Morbidity (mor-bid'i-te). the morbidity rate is the ratio to the total population of individuals who are ill or disabled.

Mortality (mor-tal'i-te). the mortality rate is the death rate; the ratio of the number of deaths to the total population.

Morphology (mor-fol'ō-je). the science that deals with form and structure without reference to function.

Motivation. internal knowledge, incentive, and will of an individual to act.

    Internal motivation: from within; the individual's willingness or personal wish to change behavior.

    External motivation: from outside sources; dependency or reliance on other people to guide.

Mucin (mu'sin). secretion of the mucous or goblet cell; a polysaccharide protein that, combined with water, forms a lubricating solution called mucous; contained in saliva.

Myotonia (mī"ō-tō'ne-ah). disorder involving the tonic (continuous tension) spasm of a muscle cell.

N

Nasmyth's membrane: see Cuticle, primary.

Necrosis (ne-kro'sis). cell or tissue death within the living body.

Neoplasm (ne'ō-plaz"m). a new growth comprised of an abnormal collection of cells, the growth of which exceeds and is uncoordinated with that of the normal tissues; see **Cancer; Precancerous lesion.**

Nidus (ni'dus). the point of origin or focus of a process.

Nosocomial (nōs"ō-kō'mi-al). denotes a disorder associated with being treated in a hospital, which is unrelated to the primary reason for being in the hospital.

Nostrum (nos'trum). a quack, patent, or secret remedy.

O

Obstetrician (ob'ste-trish'un). a physician who specializes in the management of pregnancy, labor, and the period of confinement after delivery.

Obtundent (ob-tun'dent). having the power to dull sensibility or soothe pain; a soothing or partially anesthetic medicine.

Occupational hazard. potential exposure to injury or disease within the workplace.

Odontalgia (ō"-don-tal'je-ah). toothache; pain in a tooth.

Odontoblast (ō-don'tō-blast). connective tissue cell that functions in the formation of dentin.

Odontolysis (ō"don-tol'i-sis). dissolution or resorption of tooth structure.

Olfactory (ol-fak'tō-re). pertaining to the sense of smell.

Oncology (ong-kol'ō-je). study or science of neoplastic growth.

Oral and maxillofacial surgery. that part of dental practice that deals with the diagnosis and surgical and adjunctive treatment of the diseases, injuries, and defects of the oral and maxillofacial region.

Orthopnea (or"thop-ne'ah). ability to breathe easily only in the upright position.

Orthostatic hypotension. fall in blood pressure associated with dizziness, syncope, and blurred vision occurring upon standing. Also called **postural hypotension**.

Osmosis (oz-mo'sis). the passage of a solvent through a semipermeable membrane into a solution of higher molecular concentration, thus equalizing the concentrations on either side of the membrane.

Osteoblast (os'te-ō-blast"). cell whose activity initiates the formation of new bone.

Osteoclast (os'te-ō-klast"). large multinucleated cell that brings about the resorption of bone; found only during the process of active bone or root resorption.

Osteoectomy, ostectomy (os"-te-ō-ek'tō-me; os-tek'tō-me). removal of tooth-supporting bone for correction of pockets and nonphysiologic bony contours.

Osteomyelitis (os"te-ō-mī"e-lī'tis). acute or chronic inflammation of the bone marrow or of the bone and marrow.

Osteoplasty (os'te-ō-plas"te). reshaping of bone.

    Alveoloplasty: plastic contouring of the alveolar process to achieve physiologic contours in the bone and gingival tissues.

Otolaryngologist (o"tō-lar"in-gol'ō-jist). medical specialist who treats the ears, throat, pharynx, larynx, nasopharynx, and tracheobronchial tree.

P

Palliative (pal'e-a-tiv). affording relief but not cure.

Pallor (pal'or). paleness.

Palpitation (pal-pi-ta'shun). rapid beating of the heart with or without irregularity in rhythm.

Parasympathetic (par"ah-sim"pah-thet'ik). craniosacral division of the autonomic nervous system.

Pathogenesis (path"ō-jen'e-sis). the course of development of disease, including the sequence of processes or events from inception to the characteristic lesion or disease.

Pathogenic (path"-ō-jen'ik). causing disease: disease-producing.

Pathognomonic (path"og-nō-mon'ik). a sign or

symptom significantly unique to a disease to distinguish the disease from other diseases.

Pathosis (path-ō'sis). a disease entity.

Pediatric dentistry (pe"de-at'rik). the practice, teaching of, and research in comprehensive preventive and therapeutic oral health care of children from birth through adolescence; includes care for special patients beyond the age of adolescence who demonstrate mental, physical, and/or emotional problems.

Pedodontics: see **Pediatric dentistry.**

Periapical (per"e-ap'i-kal). around the apex of a tooth.

    Periapical tissues: the tissues surrounding the apex of a tooth, including the periodontal ligament and the alveolar bone.

Pericoronitis (per"i-kor"ō-ni'tis). inflammation of the soft tissues surrounding the crown of an erupting tooth; frequently seen in association with erupting mandibular third molars and usually accompanied by infection.

Periodontics (per"e-ō-don'tiks). the branch of dentistry that deals with the diagnosis and treatment of diseases and conditions of the supporting and surrounding tissues of the teeth or their implanted substitutes.

Periodontology (per"e-ō-don-tol'ō-je). the scientific study of the periodontium in health and disease.

Periodontopathic (per"e-ō-don"tō-path'ik). refers to an agent able to induce and/or initiate periodontal pathosis.

Periradicular (per"i-rah-dik'u-lar). around or surrounding the root of a tooth.

Petri plate (pe'tre). a small, shallow dish of thin glass with a loosely fitting, overlapping cover, used for plate cultures in microbiology.

pH: symbol commonly used to express hydrogen ion concentration, the measure of alkalinity and acidity. Normal (neutral) pH is 7.0. Above 7.0 the solution is alkaline; below, acidic.

Phosphorescence (fos"fo-res'ens). emission of radiation by a substance as a result of previous absorption of radiation of shorter wave length; contrasts with fluorescence in that the emission may continue for a time after cessation of the ionizing radiation.

Physiologic saline solution. a 0.9% sodium chloride solution, which exerts an osmotic pressure equal to that exerted by the blood, and thus is compatible with blood.

Pipette (pī-pet'). a slender, graduated tube for measuring and transferring liquids from one vessel to another.

Placebo effect (plah-se'bō). a positive response to a pain-relieving technique that is enhanced through the power of suggestion.

Potentiation (pō-ten"she-a'shun). enhancement of one agent by another so that the combined effect is greater than the sum of the effects of each agent alone.

Precancerous lesion. a morphologically altered tissue in which cancer is more likely to occur than in its apparently normal counterpart. A **precancerous condition** is a generalized state associated with a significantly increased risk of cancer.

Precipitate (pre-sip'i-tate). to cause a substance in solution to separate out in solid particles (verb); that which is separated out is called the **precipitate** (noun).

Predisposition (pre"dis-pō-zish'un). a concealed but present susceptibility to disease, which may be activated under certain conditions.

Premaxilla (pre"mak-sil'ah). the intermaxillary bone situated in front of the maxilla proper; carries the incisor teeth.

Premedication (pre"med-i-ka'shun). preliminary treatment, usually with a drug, to prevent untoward results that may be effected by the treatment to be performed.

Prescribe (pre-skrīb'). to designate or recommend a remedy for administration; to direct in writing the dosage, preparation, and dispensing of a remedy or drug.

Prodrome (prō'drōm). early or premonitory symptom of a disease.

Prognosis (prog-nō'sis). a forecasting of the probable course and termination of a disease and the response to treatment; the prospect of recovery from a disease as indicated by the nature and symptoms of the case.

Proliferation (prō-lif"e-ra'shun). reproduction or multiplication of similar forms.

Prone (prōn). flat, prostrate; **prone position,** lying flat.

Prosthodontics (pros"thō-don'tiks). the branch of dentistry pertaining to the restoration and maintenance of oral function, comfort, appearance, and health of the patient by the restoration of natural teeth and/or the replacement of missing teeth and contiguous oral and maxillofacial tissues with artificial substitutes.

Protein (prō'ten). any one of a group of complex organic nitrogenous compounds widely distributed in plants and animals that form the principal constituents of cell protoplasm. They are essentially combinations of alpha amino acids and their derivatives.

Proteolytic (prō"te-ō-lit'ik). effecting the digestion of proteins.

Protoplasm (prō'tō-plaz"m). the only known form of matter in which life is apparent; it composes the essential material of all plant and animal cells.

Psychiatry (sī-kī'ah-tre). that branch of medicine which deals with the diagnosis and treatment of mental diseases.

Psychosomatic (sī"kō-sō-mat'ik). pertaining to the mind-body relationship; having body symptoms of a psychic, emotional, or mental origin.

Ptosis (tō'sis). falling or sinking down; drooping of the upper eyelid.

Ptyalin (tī'ah-lin). an enzyme occurring in the saliva that converts starch into maltose and dextrose.

Public health. the science and art of preventing disease, prolonging life, and promoting physical health and efficiency through organized community efforts.

> **Dental public health:** art of preventing and controlling dental diseases and promoting oral health through organized community efforts.

Pulp stone: see **Denticle.**

Pulpectomy (pul-pek'tō-me). removal of the pulp chamber and root canals of a tooth.

Pulpotomy (pul-pot'o-me). the removal of a portion of the pulp of a tooth, usually meaning the coronal portion.

Purulent (pu'roo-lent). containing or forming a pus.

Pyorrhea (pī"-ō-re'ah). a purulent discharge; discharge of pus. Formerly a name for advanced, severe periodontal disease.

Pyramidal (pi-ram'i-dal). shaped like a pyramid.

> **Pyramidal tracts:** collection of motor nerve fibers arising in the brain and passing down through the spinal cord to motor cells in the anterior horns.

Q

Quadrant (kwod'rant). any one of the four parts or quarters of the dentition, with the dividing line of the maxillary or mandibular teeth at the midline between the central incisors.

R

Raphe (ra'fe). a ridge, furrow, or seam-like union between two parts or halves of an organ or structure.

Rarefaction (rar"e-fak'shun). being or becoming less dense.

Recurrent (re-kur'ent). returning after intermissions.

Reflux (re'fluks). backward or return flow.

> **Gastroesophageal reflux:** reflux of stomach contents into the esophagus.

Refractory (re-frak'to-re). not readily yielding to treatment.

Rehabilitation (re"ha-bil-i-ta'shun). restoration to former state of health, efficiency, and independent action; regeneration.

Remission (re-mish'un). a decrease or arrest of the symptoms of a disease; also the period during which such decrease occurs.

Replantation (re"plan-ta'shun). replacement into its own alveolar socket of a traumatically or otherwise removed tooth.

Resection (re-sek'shun). operation in which a part of a tissue or an organ is removed.

> **Root resection:** removal of a root from a multi-rooted tooth.

> **Hemisection:** removal of half of a tooth.

Resorption (re-sorp'shun). removal of bone or tooth structure by pressure; gradual destruction of dentin and cementum of the root, as the primary teeth prior to shedding; in orthodontic tooth movement, bone formation on one side compensates for resorption of bone on the other side.

Resuscitation (re-sus"i-ta'shun). restoration of life or consciousness; restoration of heartbeat and respiration.

Rh factor. agglutinogens of red blood cells responsible for isoimmune reactions such as occur in erythroblastosis fetalis and incompatible blood transfusions; erythroblastosis fetalis results when a mother is Rh negative and develops antibodies against the fetus, which is Rh positive.

Rheostat (re'ō-stat). an appliance for regulating the resistance and thus controlling the amount of current entering an electric circuit; the dental unit control usually is located in a device operated by the foot.

Rheumatic (roo-mat'ik). pertaining to or affected with **rheumatism,** which is a general term pertaining to conditions characterized by inflammation or pain in muscles or joints.

Risk factor. an attribute or exposure that increases the probability of occurrence of disease.

RNA (ribonucleic acid) (rī"bō-noo-kla'ik as'id). occurs in nuclei and cytoplasm of all cells; stores and transfers genetic information.

Ruga (roo'gah). ridge, wrinkle, fold.

> **Palatal rugae** (roo'ge). the irregular ridges in the mucous membrane covering the anterior part of the hard palate.

S

Scoliosis (skō"le-ō'sis). curvature of the spine.

Sedation (se-da'shun). allaying stress, irritability, or excitement; act of calming, especially by the administration of a sedative drug by inhalation, oral administration, or parenteral injection (intramuscular or intravenous).

> **Conscious sedation:** a minimally depressed level of consciousness that retains the patient's ability to maintain an airway independently and continuously and to respond to verbal command or physical stimulation; may be produced by pharmacologic or nonpharmacologic methods or a combination of the two.

> **Deep sedation:** a controlled state of depressed consciousness accompanied by partial loss of reflexes, including inability to respond purposefully to verbal command; produced by a pharmacologic or nonpharmacologic method, or combination of the two.

Senescence (se-nes'ens). process or condition of growing old; physiologic aging not necessarily related to chronologic age.

Senility (se-nil'i-te). old age; feebleness of body and mind occurring with old age.

Septum (sep'tum). a dividing wall, partition, or membrane.

Sequestrum (se-kwes'trum). a piece of necrosed bone that has become separated from the surrounding bone; usually the necrosed bone is being expelled from the body.

Serrated (ser'at-ed). having a sawlike edge.

Serum (se'rüm). the clear, liquid part of blood separated from its more solid elements after clotting; the blood plasma from which fibrinogen has been removed in the process of clotting.

Shunt. to divert, to bypass; a passage between two natural channels, especially between blood vessels (e.g., cardiovascular shunt); to relieve hydrocephalus, a shunt between a cerebral ventricle and a cardiac atrium or the peritoneum.

Sinus tract (si'nus trakt). a pathologic sinus or passage leading from an abscess cavity or hollow organ to the surface, or from one cavity to another; formerly known as a fistula.

Slough (sluf). a mass of dead tissue in, or cast out of, living tissue.

Spondylitis (spon'di-lī'tis). inflammation of the vertebrae.

Spore: see **Bacterial spore.**

Stabile (sta'bīl). not moving, stationary, resistant; opposite of labile.

   Heat stabile (thermostabile): resistant to moderate degrees of heat.

Standards of care. levels of professional performance expected of dental hygiene practitioners; provision of same level of care as provided by other practitioners under similar conditions.

Stomatitis (stō"ma-tītis). inflammation of the oral mucosa, because of local or systemic factors.

Subclinical (süb-klin'i-kel). without clinical manifestations; said of early stages of a disease.

Subluxation (süb-lük-sa'shun). partial or incomplete dislocation; see **Luxation.**

Submerged tooth (süb-merjd'). one which is below the line of occlusion and may be ankylosed; intrusion; infraocclusion.

Substantivity. ability of an antimicrobial agent to be retained in the oral cavity for continued activity at effective levels over an extended time period.

Supernumerary tooth (su"per-nu'mer-ar-e). extra tooth; one which is in excess of the normal number.

Suppuration (süp"ü-ra'shun). formation of pus.

Sympathetic nervous system: that part of the autonomic (involuntary) nervous system that arises in the thoracic and the first three lumbar segments of the spinal cord.

Syndrome (sin'drom). a group of symptoms and signs that, when considered together, characterize a disease or lesion.

Synergistic (sin"er-jis'tik). acting jointly; enhancing the effect of another drug, force, or agent.

Systemic (sis-tem'ik). pertaining to or affecting the whole body.

T

Tactile (tak'til). pertaining to the touch; perceptible to the touch.

Technician, dental laboratory. a technician who performs any type of dental laboratory procedure not requiring the presence of a patient; see also **Dental prosthetic laboratory procedures.**

Teratoma (ter"a-tō'mah). A neoplasm composed of multiple tissues, including tissues not normally found in the organ in which it arises.

Therapeutic (ther"ah-pu'tik). pertaining to the treating or curing of disease; curative.

Therapy (ther'ah-pe). the treatment of disease.

Threshold (thresh'old). that amount of stimulus that just produces a perceptible sensation.

   Pain threshold: that amount of stimulus which just produces a sensation of pain.

Tic. an involuntary purposeless movement of muscle, which usually occurs under emotional stress; a twitching, especially of facial muscles.

Tincture (tingk'chur). an alcoholic solution of a drug or other chemical substance.

Tone (tōn). the normal degree of vigor and tension; a healthy state of a part.

Tonguetie (tung'tī). abnormal shortness of the frenum of the tongue, resulting in limitation of the motion of that organ.

Topical (top'i-kel). on the surface; pertaining to a particular spot; local.

Topography (tō-pog'rah-fe). the detailed description and analysis of the features of an anatomic region or of a special part.

Toxic (tok'sik). poisonous.

Toxicity (toks-is'i-te). the state or quality of being poisonous; degree of virulence of a toxic microbe or of a poison; the capacity of a drug to damage body tissue or seriously impair body functions.

Toxin (tok'sin). any poisonous substance of microbial, vegetable, or animal origin that causes symptoms after a period of incubation; can induce the elaboration of specific antitoxins in suitable animals.

Tracheotomy (tra"ke-ot'ō-me). surgical operation to provide an artificial opening into the trachea.

Transdermal medication. drug delivered by patch on skin; a mode for slow release over extended time.

Transmissible (trans-mis'si-bel). capable of being carried across from one person to another.

Transplant (trans'plant). tissue removed from one part of the body and placed at a different site.

Transplantation (trans-plan-ta'shun). implanting a tissue or organ that has been taken from another part of the same body or from another person.

   Autotransplant: transfer of a tissue or organ to another place in the same person.

Trauma (traw'mah). an injury; damage; impairment; external violence, producing body injury or degeneration.

Treatment (tret'ment). the management and care of a patient for the purpose of curing a disease or disorder.

Tremor (trem'or). involuntary trembling or quivering.

U

Urticaria (ur"ti-ka're-ah). hives; nettle rash; an eruption of itching wheals usually of systemic origin. It may be caused by a state of hypersensitivity to foods or drugs, foci of infection, physical agents (heat, cold, light, friction), or psychic stimuli.

V

Vehicle (ve'i-kel). a substance possessing little or no medicinal action, used as a medium to confer a suitable consistency or form to a drug.

Ventral (ven'tral). anterior, front surface: opposite of dorsal surface.

Virulent (vir'u-lent). capable of causing infection or disease.

Viscosity (vis-kos'i-te). stickiness; ability of a fluid to resist change in shape or arrangement during flow.

Volatile (vol'ah-til). tending to evaporate readily.

Vulcanite (vul'kan-īt). a hard rubber prepared by vulcanizing India rubber with sulfur; formerly used for making removable dentures.

W

Wheal (hwēl, wēl). an acute circumscribed transitory area of edema of the skin; an urticarial lesion; see **Urticaria.**

Whitlow (hwit'lo). a purulent infection or abscess involving the end of a finger; also called a felon.

X

Xerostomia (ze"ro-stŏ'me-ah). dryness of the mouth caused by functional or organic disturbances of the salivary glands.

American Dental Hygienists' Association Code of Ethics for Dental Hygienists

1. Preamble

As dental hygienists, we are a community of professionals devoted to the prevention of disease and the promotion and improvement of the public's health. We are preventive oral health professionals who provide educational, clinical, and therapeutic services to the public. We strive to live meaningful, productive, satisfying lives that simultaneously serve us, our profession, our society, and the world. Our actions, behaviors, and attitudes are consistent with our commitment to public service. We endorse and incorporate the Code into our daily lives.

2. Purpose

The purpose of a professional code of ethics is to achieve high levels of ethical consciousness, decision making, and practice by the members of the profession. Specific objectives of the Dental Hygiene Code of Ethics are:

- to increase our professional and ethical consciousness and sense of ethical responsibility.
- to lead us to recognize ethical issues and choices and to guide us in making more informed ethical decisions.
- to establish a standard for professional judgement and conduct.
- to provide a statement of the ethical behavior the public can expect from us.

The Dental Hygiene Code of Ethics is meant to influence us throughout our careers. It stimulates our continuing study of ethical issues and challenges us to explore our ethical responsibilities. The Code establishes concise standards of behavior to guide the public's expectations of our profession and supports existing dental hygiene practice, laws and regulations. By holding ourselves accountable to meeting the standards stated in the Code, we enhance the public's trust on which our professional privilege and status are founded.

3. Key Concepts

Our beliefs, principles, values and ethics are concepts reflected in the Code. They are the essential elements of our comprehensive and definitive code of ethics, and are interrelated and mutually dependent.

4. Basic Beliefs

We recognize the importance of the following beliefs that guide our practice and provide context for our ethics:

- The services we provide contribute to the health and well being of society.
- Our education and licensure qualify us to serve the public by preventing and treating oral disease and helping individuals achieve and maintain optimal health.
- Individuals have intrinsic worth, are responsible for their own health, and are entitled to make choices regarding their health.
- Dental hygiene care is an essential component of overall healthcare and we function interdependently with other healthcare providers.
- All people should have access to healthcare, including oral healthcare.
- We are individually responsible for our actions and the quality of care we provide.

5. Fundamental Principles

These fundamental principles, universal concepts and general laws of conduct provide the foundation for our ethics.

UNIVERSALITY

The principle of universality assumes that, if one individual judges an action to be right or wrong in a given situation, other people considering the same action in the same situation would make the same judgement.

COMPLEMENTARITY

The principle of complementarity assumes the existence of an obligation to justice and basic human rights. It requires us to act toward others in the same way they would act toward us if roles were reversed. In all relationships, it means considering the values and perspectives of others before making decisions or taking actions affecting them.

ETHICS

Ethics are the general standards of right and wrong that guide behavior within society. As generally accepted actions, they can be judged by determining the extent to which they promote good and minimize harm. Ethics compel us to engage in health promotion/disease prevention activities.

COMMUNITY

This principle expresses our concern for the bond between individuals, the community, and society in general. It leads us to preserve natural resources and inspires us to show concern for the global environment.

RESPONSIBILITY

Responsibility is central to our ethics. We recognize that there are guidelines for making ethical choices and accept responsibility for knowing and applying them. We accept the consequences of our actions or the failure to act and are willing to make ethical choices and publicly affirm them.

6. Core Values

We acknowledge these values as general for our choices and actions.

INDIVIDUAL AUTONOMY AND RESPECT FOR HUMAN BEINGS

People have the right to be treated with respect. They have the right to informed consent prior to treatment, and they have the right to full disclosure of all relevant information so that they can make informed choices about their care.

CONFIDENTIALITY

We respect the confidentiality of client information and relationships as a demonstration of the value we place on individual autonomy. We acknowledge our obligation to justify any violation of a confidence.

SOCIETAL TRUST

We value client trust and understand that public trust in our profession is based on our actions and behavior.

NONMALEFICENCE

We accept our fundamental obligation to provide services in a manner that protects all clients and minimizes harm to them and others involved in their treatment.

BENEFICENCE

We have a primary role in promoting the well being of individuals and the public by engaging in health promotion/disease prevention activities.

JUSTICE AND FAIRNESS

We value justice and support the fair and equitable distribution of healthcare resources. We believe all people should have access to high-quality, affordable oral healthcare.

VERACITY

We accept the obligation to tell the truth and assume that others will do the same. We value self-knowledge and seek truth and honesty in all relationships.

7. Standards of Professional Responsibility

We are obligated to practice our profession in a manner that supports our purpose, beliefs, and values in accordance with the fundamental principles that support our ethics. We acknowledge the following responsibilities:

TO OURSELVES AS INDIVIDUALS . . .

- Avoid self-deception, and continually strive for knowledge and personal growth.
- Establish and maintain a lifestyle that supports optimal health.
- Create a safe work environment.
- Assert our own interests in ways that are fair and equitable.
- Seek the advice and counsel of others when challenged with ethical dilemmas.
- Have realistic expectations of ourselves and recognize our limitations.

TO OURSELVES AS PROFESSIONALS . . .

- Enhance professional competencies through continuous learning in order to practice according to high standards of care.
- Support dental hygiene peer-review systems and quality-assurance measures.
- Develop collaborative professional relationships and exchange knowledge to enhance our own lifelong professional development.

TO FAMILY AND FRIENDS . . .

- Support the efforts of others to establish and maintain healthy lifestyles and respect the rights of friends and family.

TO CLIENTS . . .

- Provide oral healthcare utilizing high levels of professional knowledge, judgement, and skill.
- Maintain a work environment that minimizes the risk of harm.
- Serve all clients without discrimination and avoid action toward any individual or group that may be interpreted as discriminatory.

- Hold professional client relationships confidential.
- Communicate with clients in a respectful manner.
- Promote ethical behavior and high standards of care by all dental hygienists.
- Serve as an advocate for the welfare of clients.
- Provide clients with the information necessary to make informed decisions about their oral health and encourage their full participation in treatment decisions and goals.
- Refer clients to other healthcare providers when their needs are beyond our ability or scope of practice.
- Educate clients about high-quality oral health care.

TO COLLEAGUES . . .

- Conduct professional activities and programs, and develop relationships in ways that are honest, responsible, and appropriately open and candid.
- Encourage a work environment that promotes individual professional growth and development.
- Collaborate with others to create a work environment that minimizes risk to the personal health and safety of our colleagues.
- Manage conflicts constructively.
- Support the efforts of other dental hygienists to communicate the dental hygiene philosophy and preventive oral care.
- Inform other healthcare professionals about the relationship between general and oral health.
- Promote human relationships that are mutually beneficial, including those with other healthcare professionals.

TO EMPLOYEES AND EMPLOYERS . . .

- Conduct professional activities and programs, and develop relationships in ways that are honest, responsible, open, and candid.
- Manage conflicts constructively.
- Support the right of our employees and employers to work in an environment that promotes wellness.
- Respect the employment rights of our employers and employees.

TO THE DENTAL HYGIENE PROFESSION . . .

- Participate in the development and advancement of our profession.
- Avoid conflicts of interest and declare them when they occur.
- Seek opportunities to increase public awareness and understanding of oral health practices.
- Act in ways that bring credit to our profession while demonstrating appropriate respect for colleagues in other professions.
- Contribute time, talent, and financial resources to support and promote our profession.

- Promote a positive image for our profession.
- Promote a framework for professional education that develops dental hygiene competencies to meet the oral and overall health needs of the public.

TO THE COMMUNITY AND SOCIETY . . .

- Recognize and uphold the laws and regulations governing our profession.
- Document and report inappropriate, inadequate, or substandard care and/or illegal activities by a healthcare provider, to the responsible authorities.
- Use peer reviews as a mechanism for identifying inappropriate, inadequate, or substandard care provided by dental hygienists.
- Comply with local, state, and federal statutes that promote public health and safety.
- Develop support systems and quality-assurance programs in the workplace to assist dental hygienists in providing the appropriate standard of care.
- Promote access to dental hygiene services—for all, supporting justice and fairness in the distribution of healthcare resources.
- Act consistently with the ethics of the global scientific community of which our profession is a part.
- Create a healthful workplace ecosystem to support a healthy environment.
- Recognize and uphold our obligation to provide pro bono service.

TO SCIENTIFIC INVESTIGATION . . .

We accept responsibility for conducting research according to the fundamental principles underlying our ethical beliefs in compliance with universal codes, governmental standards, and professional guidelines for the care and management of experimental subjects. We acknowledge our ethical obligations to the scientific community:

- Conduct research that contributes knowledge that is valid and useful to our clients and society.
- Use research methods that meet accepted scientific standards.
- Use research resources appropriately.
- Systematically review and justify research in progress to ensure the most favorable benefit-to-risk ratio to research subjects.
- Submit all proposals involving human subjects to an appropriate human subject review committee.
- Secure appropriate institutional committee approval for the conduct of research involving animals.
- Obtain informed consent from human subjects participating in research that is based on specification published in Title 21 Code of Federal Regulations Part 46.
- Respect the confidentiality and privacy of data.

- Seek opportunities to advance dental hygiene knowledge through research by providing financial, human, and technical resources whenever possible. Report research results in a timely manner.
- Report research findings completely and honestly, drawing only those conclusions that are supported by the data presented.
- Report names of investigators fairly and accurately.
- Interpret the research and the research of others accurately and objectively, drawing conclusions that are supported by the data presented and seeking clarity when uncertain.
- Critically evaluate research methods and results before applying new theory and technology in practice.
- Be knowledgeable concerning currently accepted preventive and therapeutic methods, products, and technology and their application to our practice.

APPENDIX 2

Average Measurements
of Human Teeth

TABLE A-1 Average Measurements of the Primary Teeth (in Millimeters)					
		Overall Length	Length of Crown	Length of Root	Width of Crown (mesial-distal at widest point)
Maxillary	Central Incisor	16.0	6.0	10.0	6.5
	Lateral Incisor	15.8	5.6	11.4	5.1
	Canine	19.0	6.5	13.5	7.0
	First Molar	15.2	5.1	10.0	7.3
	Second Molar	17.5	5.7	11.7	8.2
Mandibular	Central Incisor	14.0	5.0	9.0	4.2
	Lateral Incisor	15.0	5.2	10.0	4.1
	Canine	17.5	6.0	11.5	5.0
	First Molar	15.8	6.0	9.8	7.7
	Second Molar	18.8	5.5	11.3	9.9

(From Black, G.V.: *Descriptive Anatomy of the Human Teeth,* 4th ed. Philadelphia, The S.S. White Dental Manufacturing Company, 1897, according to Ash, M.M.: *Wheeler's Dental Anatomy, Physiology, and Occlusion,* 7th ed. Philadelphia, W.B. Saunders, Co., 1993, p. 58.)

TABLE A-2 Average Measurements of the Permanent Teeth (in Millimeters)

		Overall Length	Length of Crown	Length of Root	Width of Crown (mesial-distal at widest point)
Maxillary	Central Incisor	23.5	10.5	13.0	8.5
	Lateral Incisor	22.0	9.9	13.0	6.5
	Canine	27.0	10.0	17.0	7.5
	First Premolar	22.5	8.5	14.0	7.0
	Second Premolar	22.5	8.5	14.0	7.0
	First Molar	B* L 19.5 20.5	7.5	B L 12 13	10.0
	Second Molar	B L 17.0 19.0	7.0	B L 11 12	9.0
	Third Molar	17.5	6.5	11.0	8.5
Mandibular	Central Incisor	21.5	9.0	12.5	5.0
	Lateral Incisor	23.5	9.5	14.0	5.5
	Canine	27.0	11.0	16.0	7.0
	First Premolar	22.5	8.5	14.0	7.0
	Second Premolar	22.5	8.0	14.5	7.0
	First Molar	21.5	7.5	14.0	11.0
	Second Molar	20.0	7.0	13.0	10.5
	Third Molar	18.0	7.0	11.0	10.0

*B = Buccal measurement; L – Lingual measurement
(From Ash, M.M.. *Wheeler's Dental Anatomy, Physiology, and Occlusion,* 7th ed. Philadelphia, W.B. Saunders Co., 1993, p. 15.)

INDEX

NOTE: A *t* following a page number indicates tabular material, an *f* following a page number indicates a figure, and a *b* following a page number indicates boxed material. Drugs are listed under their generic names. When a drug trade name is listed, the reader is referred to the generic name.

Clinical crown, 187, 188f
Clinical root, 187
Clinical trial, 294
Clinician. *See also* Dental hygienist; Dental personnel
  preparation for radiographs and, 148
  radiation exposure limits for, 145, 145t
  radiation protection for, 146–147, 147f
Clinician positioning, 75, 77, 77f, 521
  for four-handed dental hygiene, 79, 79f
  neutral positions for instrumentation and, 521–522, 522f
  for radiation protection while making exposures, 147, 147f
Clinician's stool, 75, 76f
  infection control and, 58, 58f
CLL. *See* Chronic leukemia, lymphocytic
Clock system, for toothbrushing, 356
Clomid. *See* Clomiphene
Clomiphene, adverse effects of on fetus and infant, 655t
Clonic, definition of, 803b
Clonic phase, of seizure, definition of, 803b
Closed reduction, for jaw fracture, 713
Clostridium tetani, 17
Clotting defects, 876–877
  hereditary, 876–877. *See also* Hemophilia
Clotting (coagulation) factors
  definition of, 866b
  levels of, hemophilia severity and, 877
  replacement of
    home program for, 877
    pretreatment, 877–878
Clotting time, 867t
CML. *See* Chronic leukemia, myelocytic
CMV. *See* Cytomegalovirus
CO₃. *See* Carbonate
Coagulation, definition of, 924
Coagulation defects, 876–877
  hereditary, 876. *See also* Hemophilia
Coagulation factors
  definition of, 866b
  level of, hemophilia severity and, 877
  replacement of
    home program for, 877
    pretreatment, 877–878
Coapt, definition of, 586b
Coaptation, definition of, 924
Cocaine, abuse of, 130t
  adverse effects of on fetus and infant, 655t
Cocci,
  in plaque, 268t, 269, 269f
Coccobacilli
  morphologic form of, 265f
Code of Ethics for Dental Hygienists, 7–8, 934–937
Coe-Pak dressing, 591
Cognitive, definition of, 822b
Cognitive-behavioral therapy, for anxiety disorders, 829
Cognitive domain, definition of, 334b
Cognitive impairment disorders, 821t
Coherent (Thompson/unmodified) scattering, definition of, 139b
Coitus, definition of, 675b
Coke (cocaine), abuse of, 130t
Col, 191–192, 192f, 372
  definition of, 371b
  epithelium of, 372
  flossing precautions and, 373
Cold sore (herpes labialis), 19t, 30, 31
Cold test, of pulpal vitality, 250
Collagen, definition of, 226b
Collagenase, definition of, 226b
Collagen dressings, 591
Collimating film holder, 153, 157f
Collimation
  protection from radiation and, 146–147
  radiograph quality affected by, 140–141, 142f
Collimator, 137, 137f, 141
Collis method (simultaneous sulcular), 357–358, 358f
Color blindness, definition of, 791b

Coloring agents
  in dentifrices, 388
  in mouthrinses, 385
Coma. *See also* Unconscious patient
  definition of, 762b
  diabetic, 882, 883t
    emergency treatment of, 913t
  postconvulsive, 804
Comatose, definition of, 762b
Combined push and pull stroke, 525
Come, sign for, 797f
Comminuted fracture, 712, 712f
Commissure, definition of, 924
Communicable, definition of, 924
Communicable disease. *See* Infection
Communicable period
  definition of, 14b
  for hepatitis A, 23
  for hepatitis B, 26
Communication
  autistic patient and, 816, 816t
  definition of, 334b
  disabled patient and, 742
  disorders of, 811t
  hearing impaired patient and, 794–795, 796f, 797–799f
Community periodontal index of treatment needs, 308–309
Community water fluoridation. *See* Fluoridation
Compensating patient, vital signs indicating, 894
Competency, definition of, 4b
Complete denture prosthodontics, definition of, 698b
Complete dentures, 403–404, 403f. *See also* Dentures
  base of, 403
  care of, 699, 700t
    for helpless/unconscious patient, 764
  cleaning, 404–405, 405–407, 406f, 700t, 702
    by clinician, 615–616, 703
    by disabled patient, 752, 753f
    purposes of, 404
  components of, 403–404, 403f
  definition of, 395b, 698b
  deposits on, 404
    prevention of, 407
  ill-fitting
    lesions caused by, 701
    in terminally ill patient, 766
  immediate, 698–699
    care of, 699
    definition of, 395b, 698b
  implant-supported, 698
  maintenance care and, 700t
  marking, 703–705
  mucosa underlying
    care of, 407–408, 702
    daily removal providing rest for, 700t, 701, 702–703
  oral changes associated with, 699–701
  oral lesions caused by, 701–702
  overdenture, 408, 408f, 698
    care of, 408–409
    definition of, 698b
    dental caries control and, 703
  patient teaching and, 699, 700t, 705
  postinsertion care and, 699, 700t
  prevention and maintenance and, 702–703
  provisional (interim) prosthesis, 698
  in rehabilitated mouth, 413
  removal of
    by clinician, 615
    during sleep, mucosal rest provided by, 700t, 701, 702–703
    as splint for fractured jaw, 715
  storage of, 700t
  surfaces of, 403–404, 403f
  teeth of, 404
  tissue-supported, 698
  types of, 698–699
Complete examination, 83. *See also* Examination procedures; Extraoral and intraoral examination

Complete history, 89. *See also* History
Complete overdenture, 408, 408f, 698
  care of, 408–409
  definition of, 698b
  dental caries control and, 703
Complete rehabilitation. *See* Oral rehabilitation
Complex cavity, 238
Complex partial seizure, 803–804
Compliance, definition of, 334b, 643b
Composites, 627–628
  definition of, 625b
Compound cavity, 238
Compound fracture, 712, 712f
Compressed air, supragingival calculus identification and, 280
Compressed air syringe, 203–204
Compressed gas cylinders, for nitrous oxide-oxygen sedation, 494
Compromise periodontal maintenance therapy, 644
Compton scatter radiation, definition of, 139b
Compulsions, 829
Computer-controlled anesthesia deliver system (WAND), 503
Computerized charting, 315
Computerized digital radiography, 139–140
Computers, in administering maintenance plans, 646
Conditioner, definition of, 481b
  enamel
    for brackets, 638
    for sealant, 480, 485
Conditioning, tissue, 324
  for hemophilia patient, 878
  nonsurgical periodontal instrumentation and, 546, 547
Conductive hearing loss, 794
Cone-cut, 141
  definition of, 136b
Cone, sharpening, 537–538, 538f
Cone socket handles, 515
Congenital, definition of, 666b
Congenital cytomegalovirus infection, 30
Congenital heart disease, 848–849
  dental hygiene concerns related to, 849. *See also* Endocarditis
  in Down's syndrome patients, 815
  history of, 98t
Congenital hypothyroidism, mental retardation and, 813
Congenital malformations, oral, 746
Congenital rubella syndrome, 20t, 812
Congenital syphilis, 20t, 812–813
  hypoplasia associated with, 243, 244f
Congenital toxoplasmosis, 813
Congestive heart failure, 858–859
  emergency treatment of, 859, 911t
  local anesthesia and, 502
Connective tissue, in advanced gingivitis, 226
Connector, of fixed partial denture, 399, 400f
Conscious, definition of, 493b
Consciousness
  assessing, in medical emergency, 900, 902f, 903f
  definition of, 803b
  loss of. *See also* Unconscious patient
    in absence seizure, 804
    in tonic-clonic seizure, 804
Conscious sedation
  advantages and disadvantages of, 498
  definition of, 493b, 931
  nitrous oxide-oxygen, 492–498. *See also* Nitrous oxide-oxygen sedation
Consent
  definition of, 322b
  for disabled patient, 739
  informed, 328, 328t
    definition of, 88b, 322b, 927
    for mentally retarded patient, 818
    pacemaker patient and, 861
    for oral and maxillofacial surgery, 719
Consultation, 101
  alcohol-dependent patient and, 843